Textbook of Assisted Reproduction

Gautam Nand Allahbadia • Baris Ata
Steven R. Lindheim • Bryan J. Woodward
Bala Bhagavath
Editors

Textbook of Assisted Reproduction

Springer

Editors
Gautam Nand Allahbadia
Consultant Reproductive Endocrinology & IVF
Millennium Medical Center MMC IVF
Dubai Health Care City
Dubai
UAE

Bourn Hall Fertility Clinic
Jumeira
Dubai
UAE

Steven R. Lindheim
Department of Obstetrics and Gynecology
Wright State University
Boonshoft School of Medicine
Dayton, OH
USA

Baris Ata
Division of Reproductive Endocrinology
and Infertility
Department of Obstetrics and Gynecology
Koç University School of Medicine
Istanbul
Turkey

Bryan J. Woodward
X&Y Fertility
Leicester
UK

Bala Bhagavath
School of Medicine and Dentistry
University of Rochester Medical Center
Newyork
USA

ISBN 978-981-15-2379-3 ISBN 978-981-15-2377-9 (eBook)
https://doi.org/10.1007/978-981-15-2377-9

This Springer imprint is published by the registered company Springer Nature Singapore Pte Ltd.
The registered company address is: 152 Beach Road, #21-01/04 Gateway East, Singapore 189721, Singapore

Thank you to all of the healthcare workers who selflessly give themselves to others. Your work is truly incredible and does not go unnoticed. You are true heroes of the COVID-19 crisis that stopped our world, and this book is dedicated to your hard work and sacrifices in the front line helping people.

Foreword

It is more than 60 years since we learned how to stimulate the ovary and the testis and more than 40 years that IVF was introduced.

These two events together with the development of the clinical use of gonadotropins, GnRH agonists, and antagonists allowed us to help more than 11 million couples to have children. However, there is still much to learn to improve patient pathways to overcome infertility. According to the WHO, 48.5 million couples worldwide were still unable to have a child after 5 years of trying. This necessitates the creation of many more treatment centers and to educate many more clinicians to treat infertility.

More than 90% of infertile couples may today have their genetic offspring if we educate them to seek treatment before the age of 35 and make optimal use of methods and products available today. This book will help students, practicing physicians, and scientists working in the field of reproductive medicine and endocrinology to achieve this goal.

This textbook *Assisted Reproduction* written by highly experienced and well-recognized specialists from all over the world will help the readers to better understand the physiology of reproduction and therapeutic agents they use and in managing patients with sub-fertility and infertility to obtain the best possible and most cost-effective results.

The book has over 900 pages, divided into 93 chapters with strong content ranging from basic diagnostic aspects of female and male infertility to different etiologies, relevant endocrine aspects such as polycystic ovaries, and premature ovarian insufficiency. It explores medically assisted reproduction from low to high complexity, types of treatment, fertility preservation, related genetics, ethical aspects, and laboratory techniques.

I am truly delighted to pen the foreword for a textbook on ART being brought out from a collaboration of editors from three continents.

I sincerely hope that postgraduates and practicing physicians, teachers, and scientists working in the field of reproductive medicine and endocrinology will find this book stimulating and helpful.

Moreover, I sincerely hope that this compendium will stimulate new work and a continuous dialogue between basic scientists and clinicians and between gynecologists and reproductive endocrinologists.

I wish the book many editions to come in the future and look forward to holding this impressive work of medical literature in my hands.

Bruno Lunenfeld
Prof Emeritus of the Faculty of Life Sciences
Bar-Ilan University
Ramat Gan, Israel

Preface

Setting goals is the first step in turning the invisible into the visible.—Tony Robbins

The idea for this book came about from a spark ignited by one of the neurons in the mind of my colleague and co-editor, Dr Gautam Nand Allahbadia. For those of you who do not know Gautam, he is a gynaecologist and entrepreneur extraordinaire from Mumbai, India. Gautam has a lot of sparks that go off in his head on a regular basis, no doubt as a result of all of the neurons! It is a bit like a firework party in there, but the world is a better place for it.

Gautam's spark lit a fuse, which led him to contact Prof Baris Ata (Istanbul, Turkey), Prof Bala Bhagavath (Rochester, New York, USA) and myself (Leicester, UK). We were invited to attend a conference organised by Gautam: the 3rd World Congress on Ovulation Induction & Ovarian Stimulation Protocols (WOOSP) held in September 2015 in the Seychelles. It was here that we met with Springer and planned the contents and structure of this book. With 90 chapters proposed, we knew it would be a massive undertaking and there was understandable trepidation at the size of our challenge. However, we were no doubt influenced by our location, after all the Seychelles is a sun-kissed paradise in the Indian Ocean. We were also encouraged by the quality of the conference presentations we all enjoyed and our mutual enthusiasm for this once-in-a-lifetime project, so we agreed to commit to the task. With the high number of chapters though, we agreed we needed one more co-editor to make our team complete. Our colleague Prof Steven Lindheim (Dayton, Ohio, USA) was the obvious choice, and fortuitously, he agreed to join us.

An advantage of having five international co-editors is that, between us, we have been privileged to meet many of the top experts in the field of assisted reproductive technology (ART). Thus, when we came up with the chapter titles, we were able to ask these experts to contribute chapters. We were very lucky to receive positive responses from them all and are deeply indebted to our authors, not only for providing brilliant chapters but also for their patience over the length of time it has taken to bring all of their work together.

The purpose of the book is to provide the latest knowledge from across the whole scope of ART. The book is aimed at all disciplines of ART practitioners, including clinicians, embryologists, reproductive biologists, fertility nurses and all other staff who contribute to helping people conceive via ART. Our goal is to present, in a straightforward manner, the best practice approaches for overcoming the challenge of infertility. The book can be read in its entirety or be used to dip into as a source of reference.

The book covers all aspects of ART from the diagnostic stage to the delivery of a healthy baby. We split the chapters into specific sections to help the reader navigate topics of interest. We begin with the initial assessment of the male and female, before addressing the topic of ovarian stimulation and egg retrieval. The latest superovulation protocols are discussed alongside natural cycle IVF programmes. The next section looks at various facets of ART, covering diverse topics ranging from the effect of obesity and autoimmunity to treating people identifying as transgender. We then look at the current options available for improving ART outcomes. Success rates have significantly improved since Steptoe, Edwards and Purdy helped to conceive the world's first IVF baby, but there is still much to learn to improve patient pathways to overcome infertility. We also look at how ART involving a third party is now helping people to realise their dream of parenthood, not only via gamete donation but also by uterine transplantation.

With improvements to gamete and embryo cryopreservation protocols, we have dedicated a section to fertility preservation (FP). This provides updates in FP for prepubertal children and of gonadal tissue. This is followed by sections on counselling and genetic testing, the importance of which is becoming increasingly recognised. The final section looks at the IVF laboratory, with nineteen chapters dedicated to all aspects of setting up and managing a successful IVF lab.

Bringing these chapters together has been an epic adventure. In line with the quote by Tony Robbins, once we had managed to take those first goal-setting steps, we were able to turn the invisible into the visible. In a way, we adopt a similar approach when we help our patients, by taking the first steps to turn their gametes, invisible to the naked eye, into a blastocyst, then a foetal heartbeat visible via ultrasound scan, culminating in the shared joy and wonder when their baby is born. We are always humbled by our role in assisting nature with conception, and we are both humbled and honoured to present the insights from our authors' chapters for you in this book.

I hope you enjoy reading and learning from the book, as much as my co-editors and I enjoyed liaising with the contributors and ourselves. We are also very grateful to Margaret Burns who provided considerable editorial expertise to keep us on track. Finally, we are indebted to our family and friends for their support and patience. It has been four long years in the conception and gestation, and we hope you like what we have delivered.

Leicester, UK
2019

Bryan J. Woodward

The original version of this book was revised. Copyright page text has been updated. A correction to this chapter can be found at https://doi.org/10.1007/978-981-15-2377-9_93

Contents

Part VI Fertility Preservation

Part VIII Genetic Testing

Editors and Contributors

About the Editors

Gautam Nand Allahbadia is Consultant Reproductive Endocrinology & IVF at the Millennium Medical Center MMC IVF, DHCC; Canadian Specialist Hospital, Dubai; and Bourn Hall Fertility Clinic, Jumeira, Dubai, UAE. He is the founder and academic mentor of Rotunda—The Center for Human Reproduction, the world-renowned fertility clinic in Mumbai. He is a noted world authority on ultrasound-guided embryo transfers and one of the pioneers in third-party reproduction in Southeast Asia. Dr. Allahbadia was responsible for India's first trans-ethnic surrogate pregnancy involving a Chinese couple's baby delivered by an unrelated Indian surrogate mother. Gautam N Allahbadia is the Emeritus Editor of the *Journal of Obstetrics and Gynecology* of India as well as the *IVF Lite* (Journal of Minimal Stimulation IVF).He cherishes over 150 peer-reviewed publications, 142 book chapters and 31 textbooks, the latest being a comprehensive two-book set published by Springer International, entitled *Textbook of Assisted Reproduction*, and is on the Editorial Board of several international journals. Dr Allahbadia was elected as the Vice President of the World Association of Reproductive Medicine (WARM), headquartered in Rome, and "Mumbai's Top Doc" for 2012 by a peer nomination process.

Baris Ata, MD, MSc, is Professor of Obstetrics and Gynecology, Chair of the Department of Obstetrics and Gynecology, Koç University School of Medicine, and the Director of the Assisted Reproduction Unit, Koç University Hospital, Istanbul. He authored over 100 peer-reviewed publications and numerous book chapters on infertilty, assisted reproduction and endometriosis. He sits on the editorial boards of several renowned journals in the field. He is the recipient of multiple awards of excellence in clinical practice and research. He is the vice president of the Turkish Society of Reproductive Medicine and an executive committee member of the European Society of Human Reproduction and Embryology.

Steven R. Lindheim is Professor of Obstetrics and Gynecology, Division Chief of Reproductive Endocrine and Infertility at Wright State University, Boonshoft School of Medicine in Dayton, Ohio. He currently is President of the Society of Reproductive Surgeons and Associate Editor for *Fertility and Sterility*. Dr Lindheim has published more than 200 peer-reviewed articles and book chapters and has been voted "Top Doctor" on multiple occasions throughout his career.

Bryan J. Woodward, BSc, MMedSci, PhD, FRCPath has been a reproductive scientist since 1990, when he began his career at Sheffield Fertility Centre, South Yorkshire, UK. He was then invited to direct the IVF laboratory at the BUPA Hospital in Leicester, UK, in 1995. He has since helped to establish numerous IVF clinics in Africa, Asia and the Caribbean. In the UK, Bryan has served on the Executive Committees of the Association of Clinical Embryologists (ACE) and the Association of Biomedical Andrologists (ABA). He is passionate about training reproductive scientists and is presently the Coordinator of the ESHRE Embryology Certification Committee.

Bala Bhagavath, MD, is Professor of Obstetrics and Gynecology (CHS) at the University of Wisconsin, Madison. In the past, he has been faculty at Brown University and the University of Rochester. In addition to his expertise in management of infertility, he is an accomplished reproductive surgeon and has been President of the Society of Reproductive Surgeons. He has practised medicine in India, Singapore, the UK and the USA.

Contributors

Suleyman Akarsu, MD In Vitro Fertilization Unit, Izmir Medicalpark Hospital, Karsiyaka, Izmir, Turkey

Akanksha Allahbadia Gupta, MS Consultant Gynecologist & IVF Specialist, Indira IVF, New Delhi, India

Gautam Nand Allahbadia Millennium Medical Center MMC IVF, Dubai Health Care City, Dubai, UAE

Bourn Hall Fertility Clinic, Jumeira, Dubai, UAE

Charlene A. Alouf, PhD, TS/HCLD (AAB) Invitae, San Francisco, CA, USA

Chelsea Fertility, New York, NY, USA

Reproductive Science Center of NJ, Eatontown, NJ, USA

South Jersey Fertility Center, Marlton, NJ, USA

Alessandra Alteri, PhD Obstetrics and Gynaecology Department, IRCCS San Raffaele Scientific Institute, Milan, Italy

Leslie Coker Appiah, MD Department of Obstetrics and Gynecology, Nationwide Children's Hospital, Pediatric and Adolescent Gynecology, The Ohio State University College of Medicine, Columbus, OH, USA

The Fertility Preservation and Reproductive Health Program, OSU Comprehensive Cancer Center, James Cancer Hospital and Solove Research Institute, Columbus, OH, USA

Baris Ata, MD Division of Reproductive Endocrinology and Infertility, Department of Obstetrics and Gynecology, Koç University School of Medicine, Istanbul, Turkey

Pooja Awasthi, MSc Origin IVF & Fertility Centre, Kaushambi, Ghaziabad, Uttar Pradesh, India

Pinar Caglar Aytac, MD Department of Obstetrics and Gynecology, Division of Reproductive Endocrinology and IVF Unit, Baskent University Faculty of Medicine, Adana, Turkey

Gulam Bahadur, MD Reproductive Medicine Unit, North Middlesex University Hospital, London, UK

Homerton Fertility Unit, Homerton University Hospital, London, UK

Mustafa Bahceci, MD Department of Obstetrics and Gynecology, Bahçeci Fulya IVF Centre, Istanbul, Turkey

Amy Barrie, PhD Countess of Chester Hospital, CARE Fertility Chester, Chester, UK

Mohamed Bedaiwy, MD, PhD, FACOG, FRCSC Division of Reproductive Endocrinology and Infertility, Department of Obstetrics and Gynaecology, The University of British Columbia, Vancouver, BC, Canada

Neerja Bhatla, MD, FICOG, FAMS Department of Obstetrics and Gynaecology, All India Institute of Medical Sciences, New Delhi, India

Christophe Blockeel, PhD, MD Centre for Reproductive Medicine, Universitair Ziekenhuis Brussel, Vrije Universiteit Brussel, Brussels, Belgium

Department of Obstetrics & Gynaecology, School of Medicine of the University of Zagreb, Zagreb, Croatia

Zeev Blumenfeld, MD Reproductive Endocrinology, Obsterics/Gynecology, Rappaport Faculty of Medicine, Technion – Israel Institute of Technology, Haifa, Israel

Ernesto Bosch, PhD, MD Instituto Valenciano de Infertilidad, València, Spain

Gurkan Bozdag, MD Department of Obstetrics and Gynecology, Hacettepe University School of Medicine, Ankara, Turkey

Normand Brais, PEng, MASc, PhD Sanuvox Technologies, Inc., Quebec, Canada

Mats Brännström, MD Department of Obstetrics and Gynecology, Sahlgrenska Academy, University of Gothenburg and Stockholm IVF, Stockholm, Sweden

Jonathan Briggs, MD Royal Victoria Infirmary, Adult Cystic Fibrosis Centre, Newcastle upon Tyne, Newcastle upon Tyne, UK

Stephen Brown, MD Department of Obstetrics, Gynecology and Reproductive Sciences, University of Vermont, Lerner College of Medicine, Burlington, VT, USA

Orhan Bukulmez, MD Division of Reproductive Endocrinology and Infertility, Department of Obstetrics and Gynecology, UT Southwestern Medical Center, Dallas, TX, USA

Corey Burke Cryos International USA, Orlando, FL, USA

Jorge F. Carrillo, MD, FACOG Department of Obstetrics and Gynecology, University of Central Florida, Orlando, FL, USA

Paula Celada, MD Instituto Valenciano de Infertitidad, València, Spain

Gerard F. Celia Jr, PhD, TS/HCLD (AAB) The Jones Institute for Reproductive Medicine, Norfolk, VA, USA

Ciler Celik-Ozenci, DDS, PhD Department of Histology & Embryology, Akdeniz University Faculty of Medicine, Akdeniz University, Antalya, Turkey

Grace Centola, PhD, HCLD/CC/ALD (AAB) (CC) Reproductive Laboratory and Tissue Bank Consultant, Manhattan Cryobank, New York, NY, USA

Daphne Chong, MB, ChB, MRCOG The Hewitt Fertility Centre, Liverpool Women's NHS Foundation Trust Hospital, Liverpool, UK

Meenakshi Choudhary Newcastle Fertility Centre for Life, Newcastle upon Tyne Hospitals NHS Foundation Trust, Biomedicine West Wing, Newcastle upon Tyne, UK

Mindy S. Christianson, MD Division of Reproductive Endocrinology and Infertility, Department of Gynecology and Obstetrics, Johns Hopkins University School of Medicine, Baltimore, MD, USA

Jin-Tae Chung, MSc MUHC Reproductive Centre, Department of Obstetrics and Gynecology, McGill University Health Center (MUHC), McGill University, Quebec, Canada

D. Cimadomo, MSc GENERA, Center for Reproductive Medicine, Valle Giulia Clinic, Rome, Italy

La Tasha B. Craig, MD Department of Obstetrics and Gynecology, University of Oklahoma Health Sciences Center, Oklahoma City, OK, USA

Ivor Cullen, MD University Hospital Waterford, Waterford, Ireland

Blackrock Clinic, Dublin, Ireland

Rachel Cutting, MBE Human Fertilization and Embryology Authority, Spring Gardens, London, UK

Michael H. Dahan, MD, FACOG, FRCSC Division of Reproductive Endocrinology and Infertility, Department of Obstetrics and Gynecology, McGill University, Quebec, Canada

Chloë De Roo, MD Department of Reproductive Medicine, Ghent University Hospital, Ghent, Belgium

Petra De Sutter Department of Reproductive Medicine, Ghent University Hospital, Ghent, Belgium

Jane Denton, CBE, FRCN The Multiple Births Foundation/Co-lead Elizabeth Bryan Multiple Births Centre, Queen Charlotte's & Chelsea Hospital, Imperial College Health Care NHS Trust, London, UK

Tim Dineen, PhD Waterstone Clinic, Lotamore House, Cork, Ireland

Panagiotis Drakopoulos, MD, PhD Centre for Reproductive Medicine, Universitair Ziekenhuis Brussel, Vrije Universiteit Brussel, Brussels, Belgium

School of Medicine of the University of Zagreb, Department of Obstetrics & Gynaecology, Zagreb, Croatia

Jamie P. Dubaut, MD Department of Obstetrics and Gynecology, University of Oklahoma Health Sciences Center, Oklahoma City, OK, USA

Jennifer Dundee, MD Department of Obstetrics, Gynecology and Reproductive Sciences. University of Vermont, Burlington, VT, USA

Caitlin Dunne, MD, FRCSC Pacific Centre for Reproductive Medicine (PCRM), University of British Columbia, Vancouver, BC, Canada

Stephanie J. Estes, MD, FACOG Division of Reproductive Endocrinology and Infertility, Department of Obstetrics and Gynecology, Penn State Health, Hershey, PA, USA

Necati Findikli, PhD Bahçeci Fulya IVF Centre, Istanbul, Turkey

Austin D. Findley, MD, MSCR Department of Obstetrics and Gynecology, Wright-Patterson Medical Center, Wright-Patterson Air Force Base, OH, USA

Benjamin Fisch, MD, PhD IVF and Infertility Unit, Beilinson Hospital, Petach Tikva, Israel

Kellie Flood-Shaffer, MD, FACOG Department of Obstetrics & Gynecology, JPS Health, Fort Worth, TX, USA

Gary N. Frishman, MD Division of Reproductive Endocrinology and Infertility, Department of Obstetrics and Gynecology, Women & Infants Hospital, Alpert Medical School of Brown University, Providence, RI, USA

Barry Fuller, PhD Division of Surgery & Interventional Science, UCL Medical School, Royal Free Hospital, London, UK

Pascal Gagneux, PhD Department of Pathology and Anthropology, University of California San Diego, La Jolla, CA, USA

Goral Gandhi, MSc Indo Nippon IVF, Mumbai, Maharashtra, India

Rebecca A. Garbose, MD Division of Reproductive Endocrinology and Infertility, Department of Gynecology and Obstetrics, Johns Hopkins University School of Medicine, Baltimore, MD, USA

Laura C. Gemmell, MD Case Western Reserve University School of Medicine, Cleveland, OH, USA

Adrienne Gentry, DO Carilion Clinic, Reproductive Medicine and Fertility, Roanoke, VA, USA

Natalie Getreu, PhD Institute of Reproductive Health, Division of UCL, London, UK

Luwam Ghidei, MD Department of Obstetrics and Gynecology, Women & Infants Hospital, Alpert Medical School of Brown University, Providence, RI, USA

E. Giacomini, PhD Division of Genetics and Cell Biology, Reproductive Sciences Laboratory, IRCCS San Raffaele Hospital Institute, Milan, Italy

Tanya L. Glenn, MD Department of Obstetrics & Gynecology, Wright State University, Dayton, OH, USA

Marjorie Gloff, MD Department of Anesthesiology and Perioperative Medicine, University of Rochester, Rochester, NY, USA

Funda Gode, MD, PhD In Vitro Fertilization Unit, Izmir Medicalpark Hospital, Karsiyaka, Izmir, Turkey

Jeffrey M. Goldberg, MD Reproductive Endocrinology and Infertility, Department of Obstetrics and Gynecology, Cleveland Clinic, Cleveland, OH, USA

Valentina Grisendi, MD Mother-Infant Department, University of Modena and Reggio Emilia, and Clinica Eugin Modena, Modena, Italy

Jon Havelock, MD Division of Reproductive Endocrinology & Infertility, Department of Obstetrics & Gynecology, University of British Columbia, Vancouver, BC, Canada

Logan Havemann, MD Wright State University School of Medicine, Dayton, OH, USA

Bulent Haydardedeoglu, MD Department of Obstetrics and Gynecology, Division of Reproductive and Endocrinology Unit, Baskent University Faculty of Medicine, Adana, Turkey

Sara Henderson MUHC Reproductive Centre, Department of Obstetrics and Gynecology, McGill University Health Center (MUHC), McGill University, Quebec, Canada

Sheryl Homa, PhD Andrology Solutions, London, UK

Roy Homburg, FRCOG Homerton Fertility Unit, Homerton University Hospital, London, UK

Ciara Hughes, BMedSc, PG Dip (Biomed), MSc Embroyology Department, Beacon Care Fertility, Dublin, Ireland

Helen Hunter, BSc, MSc Department of Reproductive Medicine, Old St Mary's Hospital, Manchester, UK

Kanna Jayaprakasan, MBBS, MD, DNB, MRCOG, PhD Derby Fertility Unit, Royal Derby Hospital, Derby, UK

Karen Jessup, DO Wright-Patterson Medical Center, Department of Obstetrics and Gynecology, Wright-Patterson, OH, USA

Esra Bulgan Kılıçdağ, MD Department of Obstetrics and Gynecology, Division of Reproductive Endocrinology and IVF Unit, Baskent University Faculty of Medicine, Adana, Turkey

Martina Kollmann, MD, PhD Division of Obstetrics and Maternal Fetal Medicine, Department of Obstetrics and Gynecology, Medical University of Graz, Graz, Austria

George Koustas, PhD, M Med Sc The Agora Clinic, Hove, UK

Peter Kovacs, MD, PhD IVF Center, Kaali Institute, Budapest, Hungary

Melissa Kreso, MD Departments of Anesthesiology and Perioperative Medicine, University of Rochester Medical Center, School of Medicine and Dentistry, Rochester, NY, USA

Antonio La Marca, MD, PhD Department of Obstetrics and Gynecology, University Hospital of Modena, Modena, Italy

Elena Labarta, PhD, MD Instututo Valenciano de Infertiidad, València, Spain

Stephanie C. Laniewski, MS, CGC Division of Maternal-Fetal Medicine, Department of Obstetrics and Gynecology, University of Rochester Medical Center, Rochester, NY, USA

Peter Larsen Cryos International, Aarhus, Denmark

Angela K. Lawson, PhD Departments of Clinical Obstetrics and Gynecology and Psychiatry, Northwestern University Feinberg School of Medicine, Chicago, IL, USA

Lawrence C. Layman, MD Section of Reproductive Endocrinology, Infertility, & Genetics, Department of Obstetrics & Gynecology, Department of Neuroscience & Regenerative Medicine, Department of Physiology, Medical College of Georgia, Augusta University, Augusta, GA, USA

Veronika Levin, MD Department of Obstetrics and Gynecology, Reading Medical Center, West Reading, PA, USA

Sylvie Lierman, BSc Department of Reproductive Medicine, Ghent University Hospital, Ghent, Belgium

Steven R. Lindheim, MD, MMM Department of Obstetrics and Gynecology, Wright State University, Boonshoft School of Medicine, Dayton, OH, USA

Federica Lopes, PhD Centre for Discovery Brain Sciences, University of Edinburgh, Hugh Robson Building, Edinburgh, UK

Yolianne Lozada-Capriles, MD Department of Obstetrics and Gynecology, University of Puerto Rico, Medical Sicences Campus, San Juan, PR, USA

Mariusz Łukaszuk, MD Invicta Fertility Clinic Gdansk, Gdansk, Poland

Stewart Lustik, MD, MBA Department of Anesthesiology, University of Rochester, Rochester, NY, USA

Jody Lyneé Madeira, JD, PhD Center for Law, Society and Culture, Indiana University Bloomington, Bloomington, IN, USA

Lone Bruhn Madsen, MSc, PhD Cryos International, Aarhus, Denmark

A. H. Maham Millennium Medical Center MMC IVF, Dubai, UAE

Jacqueline Y. Maher, MD Division of Reproductive Endocrinology and Infertility, Department of Gynecology and Obstetrics, Johns Hopkins University School of Medicine, Baltimore, MD, USA

Reeva Makhijani, MD Women & Infants' Fertility Center, Providence, RI, USA

Henry E. Malter, PhD, HCLD (ABB) Department of Obstetrics and Gynecology, University of South Carolina School of Medicine, Greenville, SC, USA

Fertility Center of the Carolinas, University of South Carolina School of Medicine, Greenville, SC, USA

Monique Marguerie, MSc Department of Obstetrics and Gynaecology, BC Women's Hospital, Vancouver, BC, Canada

Hayley Marshall, DO Department of Obstetrics and Gynecology, John Peter Smith Hospital, Ft. Worth, TX, USA

Erin M. Masaba, MD Department of Obstetrics/Gynecology, University of Rochester, Rochester, NY, USA

Nadine Massiah, MBBS Newcastle Fertility Centre for Life, Newcastle upon Tyne Hospitals NHS Foundation Trust, Newcastle upon Tyne, UK

Virginia Mensah, MD Reproductive Science Center of New Jersey, Eatontown, NJ, USA

Cornelia G. A. Meyer, Dipl-Biol, MSc Cryos International, Aarhus, Denmark

David Miller, PhD Discovery and Translational Science Department, University of Leeds, Leeds Institute of Cardiovascular and Metabolic Medicine (LICAMM), Leeds, UK

Shahab Minassian, MD Department of Obstetrics and Gynecology, Reading Hospital, West Reading, PA, USA

Rod T. Mitchell, MBChB, PhD MRC Centre for Reproductive Health, University of Edinburgh, The Queen's Medical Research Institute, Edinburgh, UK

Carmen Morales, PhD The PGD Laboratory, Kuwait City, Jabriya Medical Center, Jabriya, Kuwait

Sezcan Mumusoglu, MD Department of Obstetrics and Gynecology, Hacettepe University School of Medicine, Ankara, Turkey

Asıf Muneer, MD, FRCS(Urol) Department of Urology and NIHR Biomedical Research Centre, University College London Hospitals NHS Foundation Trust, London, UK

Division of Surgery and Interventional Science, University College London, London, UK

Maximilian Murtinger IVF Centers Prof. Zech, Bregenz, Austria

Jeanne O'Brien, MD Department of Urology, University of Rochester Medical Center, Rochester, NY, USA

Kathleen O'Leary, MD Institute for Reproductive Health, Cincinnati, OH, USA

Galia Oron, MD IVF and Infertility Unite, Beilinson Hospital, Petah Tikva, Israel

Ajibike Oyewumi Lagoon Hospital, Apapa, Logos, Nigeria

Kelly Pagidas, MD Department of Obstetrics and Gynecology, University of Louisville, Louisville, KY, USA

J. Preston Parry, MD, MPH Department of Obstetrics & Gyncology, University of Mississippi Medical Center, Jackson, MS, USA

Valerie L. Peddie Department of Obstetrics and Gynaecology, School of Medicine and Dentistry, Division of Applied Health Sciences, University of Aberdeen, Aberdeen Maternity Hospital, Aberdeen, Scotland

Jana E. C. Pittman Western Sydney University School of Medicine, Campbelltown, NSW, Australia

Shayne Plosker, MD Department of Obstetrics and Gynecology, University of South Florida Morsani College of Medicine, Tampa, FL, USA

Kimball O. Pomeroy, PhD The World Egg Bank, Phoenix, AZ, USA

Csaba Pribenszky, PhD University of Veterinary Medicine, Budapest, Hungary

David Prokai, MD Division of Reproductive Endocrinology and Infertility, Department of Obstetrics and Gynecology, University of Texas Southwestern Medical Center, Dallas, TX, USA

Osbourne Quaye, PhD Virology Laboratory, West African Centre for Cell Biology of Infectious Pathogens, Department of Biochemistry, Cell & Molecular Biology, University of Ghana, Accra, Ghana

Michael L. Reed, PhD The Fertility Center of New Mexico, Albuquerque, NM, USA

Ilana B. Ressler, MD Department of Reproductive Endocrinology, Reproductive Medicine Associates of Connecticut, Norwalk, CT, USA

L. Rienzi, MSc GENERA, Center for Reproductive Medicine, Valle Giulia Clinic, Rome, Italy

John S. Rushing, MD Department of Obstetrics and Gynecology, University of Mississippi Medical Center, Jackson, MS, USA

Richard Thomas Russell, MD The Hewitt Fertility Centre, Liverpool Women's NHS Foundation Trust Hospital, Liverpool, UK

Francisco Javier Ruiz Flores, MD IVI Abu Dhabi, Abu Dhabi, UAE

Sana M. Salih, MD, MS RMA of Central Pennsylvania at PinnacleHealth, Mechanicsburg, PA, USA

V. Sarais, MD Obstetrics and Gynaecology Department, IRCCS San Raffaele Scientific Institute, Milan, Italy

Megan Schneiderman Department of Obstetrics and Gynecology, McGill University, Quebec, Canada

Neil Seligman, MD, MS Division of Maternal-Fetal Medicine, Department of Obstetrics and Gynecology, University of Rochester Medical Center, Rochester, NY, USA

Munevver Serdarogullari, PhD British Cyprus IVF Hospital, Nicosia, Cyprus

Shrenik Shah, MSc Department of Obstetrics and Gynecology, University of Rochester School of Medicine & Dentistry, Rochester, NY, USA

K. Aparna Sharma, MD, DNB, MNAMS Department of Obstetrics and Gynaecology, All India Institute of Medical Sciences, New Delhi, India

Erhan Şimşek, MD Baskent University Faculty of Medicine, Adana, Turkey

Mehmet Sipahi, MD Department of Obstetrics and Gynecology, Giresun University School of Medicine, Merkez/Giresun, Turkey

Heather Skanes-DeVold, MD Department of Obstetrics and Gynecology, Morehouse School of Medicine, Atlanta, GA, USA

Megan C. Smith, BA Department of Obstetrics and Gynecology, Wright State University Boonshoft School of Medicine, Dayton, OH, USA

Weon-Young Son, MD MUHC Reproductive Centre, Department of Obstetrics and Gynecology, McGill University Health Center (MUHC), McGill University, Quebec, Canada

Rajesh K. Srivastava, PhD Department of Obstetrics and Gynecology, Director IVF and Andrology Laboratories, Strong Fertility Center, Rochester, NY, USA

University of Rochester Medical Center, Rochester, NY, USA

Jason E. Swain, PhD, HCLD CCRM IVF Network, Lone Tree, CO, USA

Pankaj Talwar, MBBS, MD HOD, ART Centre, Army Hospital (Research and Referral), New Delhi, India

Justin Tan, MD, MPH Department of Obstetrics and Gynecoogy, BC Women's Hospital, Vancouver, BC, Canada

Seang Lin Tan Department of Obstetrics and Gynecology, James Edmund Dodds Chair in ObGyn, McGill University, Quebec, Canada

OriginElle Fertility Clinic and Women's Health Centre, Quebec, Canada

McGill Reproductive Centre, Quebec, Canada

Eleanor Taylor, PhD The Hewitt Fertility Centre, Liverpool Women's NHS Foundation Trust, Liverpool, UK

Kelly Tilleman, PhD Department of Reproductive Medicine, Ghent University Hospital, Ghent, Belgium

Pinar Tokdemir Calis, MD Department of Obstetrics and Gynecology, Gazi University School of Medicine, Yenimahalle/Ankara, Turkey

Keshia Torres-Shafer, MD Department of Obstetrics & Gynecology, Wright State University Boonshoft School of Medicine, Dayton, OH, USA

Stephen Troup, PhD Reproductive Science Consultancy Ltd, Wilmslow, UK

Engin Turkgeldi, MD Department of Obstetrics and Gynecology, Koc University Hospital, Istanbul, Turkey

Karla Turner, BSc (Hons) Bristol Centre for Reproductive Medicine, Southmead Hospital, Bristol, UK

F. M. Ubaldi, MD GENERA Center for Reproductive Medicine, Rome, Italy

Bulent Urman, MD Department of Obstetrics and Gynecology, Koc University Faculty of Medicine, Istanbul, Turkey

A. Vaiarelli, MD GENERA, Center for Reproductive Medicine, Rome, Italy

Juan Antonio García Velasco, MD, PhD Department of Obstetrics and Gynecology, Universidad Rey Juan Carlos, Madrid, Spain

IVI Madrid, Madrid, Spain

Esther Velilla, PhD PGDlabs Kuwait, Jabriya Medical Center, Jabriya, Kuwait

P. Viganò, PhD Division of Genetics and Cell Biology, Reproductive Sciences Laboratory, IRCCS San Raffaele Hospital Institute, Milan, Italy

Wendy Vitek, MD Department of Obstetrics and Gynecology, University of Rochester School of Medicine & Dentistry, Rochester, NY, USA

UR Medicine – Strong Fertility Center, Rochester, NY, USA

Ian Waldman, MD Department of Obstetrics and Gynecology, Penn State Milton S. Hershey Medical Center, Hershey, PA, USA

Stephanie Welsh, MPH Wright State University Boonshoft School of Medicine, Dayton, OH, USA

Carol Wheeler, MD Women & Infants' Fertility Center, Providence, RI, USA

Leah D. Whigham, PhD Center for Community Health Impact, Department of Health Promotion and Behavioral Sciences, UTHealth School of Public Health El Paso, El Paso, TX, USA

Linsey White Assisted Conception Service, NHS Greater Glasgow and Clyde, Glasgow, UK

Paul Wilson Bristol Centre for Reproductive Medicine, Southmead Hospital, Bristol, UK

Ashley Wiltshire, MD Department of Obstetrics and Gynecology, Morehouse School of Medicine, Atlanta, GA, USA

Michael W. Witthaus, MD Department of Urology, University of Rochester Medical Center, Rochester, NY, USA

Maureen Wood, PhD Department of Obstetrics and Gynaecology, University of Aberdeen, Aberdeen, UK

Bryan J. Woodward, PhD X&Y Fertility, Leicester, UK

John Wu, MD Division of Reproductive Endocrinology and Infertility, Department of Obstetrics and Gynecology, University of Texas Southwestern Medical Center, Dallas, TX, USA

Michael Bright Yakass, MPhil Virology Laboratory, West African Centre for Cell Biology of Infectious Pathogens, Department of Biochemistry, Cell & Molecular Biology, University of Ghana, Accra, Ghana

Assisted Conception Unit, Lister Hospital & Fertility Centre, Accra, Ghana

Kayhan Yakin, MD Department of Obstetrics and Gynecology, Koc University Faculty of Medicine, Istanbul, Turkey

Sule Yildiz, MD Department of Obstetrics and Gynecology, Koc University Hospital, Istanbul, Turkey

Herbert Zech, MD IVF Centers, Bregenz, Austria

Ahmet Zeki Isik, MD Izmir Medicalpark Hospital, In Vitro Fertilization Unit, Karsiyaka, Izmir, Turkey

Julianne E. Zweifel, PhD Department of Obstetrics and Gynecology, University of Wisconsin School of Medicine & Public Health, Madison, WI, USA

Part I

Assessment

1 Assessment of Tubal Patency

Erin M. Masaba

1.1 Tubal Factor Infertility

The fallopian tube serves as the main conduit between the ovary and the uterus. It provides mechanical transport and physiological support of gametes and cleavage stage embryos. Tubal damage can either be due to external or internal injury which leads to dysfunctional transport of gametes. Assessment of tubal disease plays a major role in determining a woman's fertility potential.

The World Health Organization defines infertility as "a disease of the reproductive system defined by the failure to achieve a clinical pregnancy after 12 months or more of regular unprotected sexual intercourse" [1]. The American Society of Reproductive medicine recommends evaluation after 6 months in women 35 and older [2]. Tubal disease accounts for 25–30% of all cases of infertility. This includes proximal obstruction and distal obstruction as well as narrowing and dilation of the fallopian tube. This ranges from conditions that change tubal function due to changes to the internal structure of the tube as well as external pathology that results in compromise of normal tubal architecture. Causes of tubal disease include infection, prior abdominal/pelvic surgery, and endometriosis. Tubal disease as a result of infection is typically due to salpingitis from pelvic inflammatory disease. Other infectious/inflammatory processes that may cause tubal damage include tuberculosis and gastrointestinal disease (i.e., appendicitis, Crohn's disease). Proximal tubal blockage which is present in 10–25% of women with tubal disease can be caused by obstruction as a result of tubal spasm, tubal debris, or blockage by intrauterine pathology (endometrial polyps, submucosal myomas, and intrauterine adhesions) or by occlusion as a result of fibrosis due to infection or endometriosis [3].

E. M. Masaba (✉)
Department of Obstetrics and Gynecology, University of Rochester, Rochester, NY, USA
e-mail: erin_masaba@urmc.rochester.edu

A diagnostic test should be cost-effective and minimally invasive while maintaining a relatively high sensitivity and specificity [4]. The current "gold standard" in tubal assessment is laparoscopy with chromopertubation with or without concomitant hysteroscopy. However, the hysterosalpingogram (HSG) has become the first-line diagnostic tool for the assessment of tubal patency [2]. This chapter aims to review the different diagnostic tools available to assess tubal patency. The technical aspects of the procedures as well as the risks, advantages, and utility of each will be discussed.

1.2 Chlamydia Antibody Testing

Salpingitis is thought to account for greater than 50% of cases of tubal factor infertility. Ascending infection from the lower genital tract causes destruction of the tubal epithelial cells. Tubal occlusion due to infection is most commonly seen at the cornual and fimbrial ends. *Chlamydia trachomatis* is the leading bacterial cause of sexually transmitted disease in the world.

Chlamydia antibody tests (CAT) present a low-cost, noninvasive way of assessing for tubal disease. There are four different serologic methods to detect chlamydia antibodies: microimmunofluorescence (MIF), immunofluorescence (IF), immunoperoxidase (IP) assay, and ELISA. The only method that specifically detects *Chlamydia trachomatis* is MIF. The other methods are not genus specific resulting in a high false positive rate. A meta-analysis comparing CAT with hysterosalpingogram while using laparoscopy with chromopertubation as the standard showed that MIF had a sensitivity of less than 75% and a specificity of greater than 75% [5]. In a more recent study looking at the diagnostic accuracy of a more specific ELISA test for chlamydia antibody compared to HSG and laparoscopy, the authors found that the ELISA test had a sensitivity of 45% and a specificity of 83% in predicting tubal pathology. Comparable diagnostic accuracy of the hysterosalpingogram was found in this study [6].

G. N. Allahbadia et al. (eds.), *Textbook of Assisted Reproduction*, https://doi.org/10.1007/978-981-15-2377-9_1

Limitations of testing for chlamydia antibodies include false positive results due to cross reactivity to other bacteria and the inability to assess the contour of the uterus and cervix. Some have suggested that it is most suitable for classifying women as low or high risk for tubal disease. Women in the high-risk group would go on to have further diagnostic testing, and the women in the low-risk group could avoid invasive procedures. No well-defined role of CAT testing has been established [7]. CAT testing will not be able to diagnose tubal pathology secondary to causes other than chlamydial infection.

1.3 Hysterosalpingogram

In 1910, Rindfleisch injected bismuth into the uterine cavity in an attempt to diagnose pregnancy in a young woman. An x-ray was obtained which showed the uterine cavity and the left fallopian tube. In 1913, Rubin and Cary injected a silver salt (Collargal) into the uterine cavity and were able to demonstrate bilateral tubal patency by delayed (x-ray) imaging. In 1925, the first iodine preparation, Lipiodol®, was introduced. The oil-based contrast agent remained popular throughout the 1960s because of its ability to produce good-quality delayed images. Once fluoroscopy became more widely available, allowing for high-quality real-time imaging, a switch to water-based contrast medium was made.

There has been debate in the literature as to whether hysterosalpingography enhances fertility and if oil contrast media has a greater therapeutic role. A recent Cochrane review identified five studies that compared oil-based contrast media to water-based contrast media. Only two of these studies had live birth as their primary outcome [8]. Rasmussen et al. reported a higher live birth rate when oil-based contrast media was utilized, whereas Spring et al. found no difference between the groups [9, 10]. A meta-analysis by Watson et al. concluded that there was a consistently higher pregnancy rate with oil-based contrast in all four randomized controlled trials (RCT) that were evaluated. However, only one RCT reached statistical significance. This benefit was greatest in patients with unexplained infertility [11].

Oil contrast media fell out of favor due to reports of an increased risk of oil embolism and anaphylaxis. Another disadvantage of oil-based medium is its slow absorption rate which was found to cause granuloma and adhesion formation in rabbits [12]. Water-based medium is considered to be safer and less expensive. It has the advantage of enhancing tubal mucosal folds and ampullary rugae [13]. However, it has also been associated with increased procedural pain when compared to oil contrast media [13]. Oil-based and water-based contrast media contain iodine. Patients should be questioned about potential iodine allergy. If allergy is not severe, the patient can be pre-medicated with steroids and/or anti-histamines prior to intracavitary instillation.

A hysterosalpingogram (HSG) is performed by placing either a cannula (Cohen or Jarcho) or a balloon catheter (typically 5–7 French) into the cervical canal. An oil- or water-based radio-opaque contrast agent is then administered transcervically into the uterine cavity. The cannula or catheter should be flushed prior to placement in order to avoid the introduction of air bubbles into the uterine cavity. Intermittent fluoroscopy is used to visualize the endometrial cavity as well as the fallopian tubes. If the uterus is noted to be retroverted, a tenaculum can be placed on the anterior lip of the cervix to ensure thorough evaluation of the uterine cavity. The speculum should be removed in order to obtain imaging of the cervical canal and lower uterine segment. If a balloon is utilized, it should be deflated at the end of the study in order to evaluate the entire uterine cavity. This study should be performed during the follicular phase in order to prevent disruption of an early pregnancy.

There are many studies on the accuracy of HSG. These studies are limited by the fact that the gold standard, laparoscopy with chromopertubation, is itself not a perfect test and not an ideal standard for assessing tubal patency. A meta-analysis reported that compared to laparoscopy with chromopertubation, the HSG has a sensitivity of 65% and specificity of 85%. In this study, they also concluded that HSG is unreliable in the diagnosis of peritubal adhesions. Also, a finding of proximal tubal occlusion should be interpreted with caution as this may be secondary to tubal spasm in up to 20% of cases or plugging of tubes by debris in 40% of cases [14].

When proximal occlusion is encountered, selective salpingography and tubal recanalization are useful tools to determine if this is a true obstruction. This diagnostic test is typically performed in an interventional radiology suite with intravenous sedation. A catheter is passed through the cervix and into the proximal tubal ostium. Contrast medium is then injected under fluoroscopic guidance. This procedure can also be performed during hysteroscopy with concomitant laparoscopy [15]. Recanalization is successful 85% of the time with re-occlusion occurring in approximately 30% of patients. Histologic exam of tubes that were unsuccessfully recanalized revealed tubal disease in 93% of the specimens [16]. Therefore, if recanalization is attempted and not successful, then there is likely intrinsic tubal disease and occlusion.

The major complication of HSG is infection which occurs in 1–3% of patients. Empiric antibiotic prophylaxis with doxycycline is not currently recommended unless the patient has a history of pelvic infection. If a hydrosalpinx is noted at the time of HSG, doxycycline should be prescribed post procedure. The typical dose is 100 mg twice daily for 5 days. Other complications include allergic reaction to contrast media (as previously described) and pain. Pain can be reduced by administering a nonsteroidal anti-inflammatory agent 30 min to 1 h prior to the procedure.

1.4 Saline Instillation Sonography/Saline Sonohysterography

Uterine cavity images were found to be superior when hematometra was present. This led to the idea that instillation of saline into the uterine cavity may better depict the endometrial lining. Saline instillation sonography (SIS) or saline sonohysterography (SSH) was described by Nannini in 1981 [17]. The procedure requires instillation of saline via a catheter placed transcervically. This infusion is performed under continuous visualization via transvaginal ultrasonography in order to better detect intrauterine cavity defects. The endometrium should appear symmetric and surround an anechoic, distended uterine cavity. This diagnostic test aids in determining if intracavitary pathology is arising from the endometrium or submucosal.

While transvaginal ultrasonography and SIS/SSH are a good diagnostic tool for assessment of the uterine cavity as well as ovarian architecture, it has little utility in tubal assessment. Tubal pathology such as hydrosalpinx may be visualized via transvaginal ultrasonography with great accuracy [18]. However, the normal fallopian tube does not provide the defined interfaces necessary to visualize it via ultrasonography. In order to better visualize the tube, a hyperechoic contrast can be used to distend the uterine cavity. This contrast can then be visualized flowing through the fallopian tubes. This procedure was coined HyCoSy or hysterosalpingosonography (sono-HSG) and was first described in 1986. Another method of imaging the fallopian tubes with ultrasonography is with instillation of saline with air bubbles into the uterine cavity. The FemVue® Sono Tubal Evaluation System is an FDA-approved device that simultaneously delivers saline and air in order to visualize the fallopian tubes.

Hysterosalpingosonography is a short, well-tolerated outpatient procedure. It has the advantage over traditional HSG of having a greater sensitivity and specificity in detecting intrauterine pathology as well as the ability to assess the adnexa simultaneously. There is no risk of iodine allergy or exposure to ionizing radiation with this procedure. A meta-analysis concluded that there was no statistically significant difference between sono-HSG and HSG as compared to laparoscopy with chromopertubation in regard to the detection of tubal occlusion [19]. Despite this, sono-HSG has not gained widespread acceptance in clinical practice, and HSG continues to be the most utilized test for evaluation of uterine cavity and tubal patency.

1.5 Laparoscopy with Chromopertubation

The most widely accepted method to evaluate tubal patency is laparoscopy with chromopertubation. It is currently considered the "gold standard" diagnostic procedure for tubal assessment. Laparoscopy usually requires general anesthesia. The patient is placed in dorsal lithotomy position and is prepped and draped using aseptic technique. The peritoneal cavity is insufflated using CO_2. Trocars are then placed typically in the umbilicus as well as the right and left lower quadrants or the midline suprapubic location. Abdominal and pelvic survey is then taken with the use of a 0^0 or 30^0 laparoscopic telescope. Chromopertubation is often performed simultaneously by instillation of a methylene blue dye via a transcervical catheter. The dye passes through the uterine cavity and through the fallopian tubes into the peritoneal cavity which is visualized via the laparoscope. Laparoscopy allows for assessment of the entire abdominal and pelvic cavity. This allows for the simultaneous diagnosis and treatment of various tubal and pelvic pathologies. Concomitant hysteroscopy can be performed to assess intrauterine pathology and to assist in tubal cannulation if proximal tubal blockage is discovered.

Laparoscopy is the most commonly performed gynecologic surgical procedure and is thought to be relatively safe. In a prospective trial in the Netherlands, a complication rate of approximately 0.6% was observed in gynecologic laparoscopic procedures. The most commonly observed complications were vascular and intestinal injuries. There was a difference in the complication rate of diagnostic laparoscopies and operative laparoscopies (0.3 vs. 1.8%, respectively) [20]. A similar retrospective study looking at gynecologic laparoscopies worldwide showed an overall complication rate ranging from 0.2 to 10.3%, with only 20–25% of these recognized at the time of surgery [21]. Even though laparoscopy has a low complication rate, its role in the infertility evaluation has been extensively debated. Historically, laparoscopy was thought to be a first-line diagnostic tool for infertility. However, with the introduction of less invasive and less expensive office procedures as well as the advancement in artificial reproductive technology, it is not an ideal first-line screening test. Laparoscopy is no longer considered to be indicated in cases of a normal HSG or unilateral obstruction on HSG due to the fact that very few patients will have a change in treatment plans based on the results of a surgical procedure. Laparoscopy should be recommended for patients who are found to have bilateral tubal occlusion on HSG. Approximately one third of these patients are likely to have patent tubes at the time of laparoscopy [22].

1.6 Conclusion

Assessment of tubal patency plays a major role in determining a woman's fertility potential. Tubal disease account for 25–30% of all cases of infertility. A diagnostic test should be accurate, cost-effective, and reliable as well as minimally invasive with a low-risk profile. In this chapter we have reviewed the different imaging and laboratory modalities currently utilized to assess for tubal disease. While hysterosalpingosonography appears to provide the most comprehensive study with the ability to assess the endometrial cavity, fallopian tubes, as well as the adnexa, it is not currently widely used. The first-line test should be either sono-HSG or HSG unless otherwise indicated. When these office procedures indicate tubal disease, a laparoscopy should be performed for a definitive diagnosis and possible treatment.

References

1. Zegers-Hochschild F, Adamson GD, de Mouzon J, Ishihara O, Mansour R, Nygren K, et al. International Committee for Monitoring Assisted Reproductive Technology (ICMART) and the World Health Organization (WHO) revised glossary of ART terminology, 2009. Fertil Steril. 2009;92(5):1520–4.
2. Practice Committee of the American Society for Reproductive Medicine. Diagnostic evaluation of the infertile female: a committee opinion. Fertil Steril. 2015;103(6):e44–50.
3. Practice Committee of the American Society for Reproductive Medicine. Committee opinion: role of tubal surgery in the era of assisted reproductive technology. Fertil Steril. 2012;97(3):539–45.
4. Panchal S, Nagori C. Imaging techniques for assessment of tubal status. J Hum Reprod Sci. 2014;7(1):2–12.
5. Mol BW, Dijkman B, Wertheim P, Lijmer J, van der Veen F, Bossuyt PM. The accuracy of serum chlamydial antibodies in the diagnosis of tubal pathology: a meta-analysis. Fertil Steril. 1997;67(6):1031–7.
6. Perquin DA, Beersma MF, de Craen AJ, Helmerhorst FM. The value of Chlamydia trachomatis-specific IgG antibody testing and hysterosalpingography for predicting tubal pathology and occurrence of pregnancy. Fertil Steril. 2007;88(1):224–6.
7. Dun EC, Nezhat CH. Tubal factor infertility: diagnosis and management in the era of assisted reproductive technology. Obstet Gynecol Clin N Am. 2012;39(4):551–66.
8. Mohiyiddeen L, Hardiman A, Fitzgerald C, Hughes E, Mol BW, Johnson N, et al. Tubal flushing for subfertility. Cochrane Database Syst Rev. 2015;5:CD003718.
9. Rasmussen F, Lindequist S, Larsen C, Justesen P. Therapeutic effect of hysterosalpingography: oil- versus water-soluble contrast media—a randomized prospective study. Radiology. 1991;179(1):75–8.
10. Spring DB, Barkan HE, Pruyn SC. Potential therapeutic effects of contrast materials in hysterosalpingography: a prospective randomized clinical trial. Kaiser Permanente Infertility Work Group. Radiology. 2000;214(1):53–7.
11. Watson A, Vandekerckhove P, Lilford R, Vail A, Brosens I, Hughes E. A meta-analysis of the therapeutic role of oil soluble contrast media at hysterosalpingography: a surprising result? Fertil Steril. 1994;61(3):470–7.
12. Miyamoto Y, Tsujimoto T, Iwai K, Ishida K, Uchimoto R, Miyazawa T, et al. Safety and pharmacokinetics of iotrolan in hysterosalpingography. Retention and irritability compared with Lipiodol. Investig Radiol. 1995;30(9):538–43.
13. Soules MR, Spadoni LR. Oil versus aqueous media for hysterosalpingography: a continuing debate based on many opinions and few facts. Fertil Steril. 1982;38(1):1–11.
14. Swart P, Mol BW, van der Veen F, van Beurden M, Redekop WK, Bossuyt PM. The accuracy of hysterosalpingography in the diagnosis of tubal pathology: a meta-analysis. Fertil Steril. 1995;64(3):486–91.
15. Novy MJ, Thurmond AS, Patton P, Uchida BT, Rosch J. Diagnosis of cornual obstruction by transcervical fallopian tube cannulation. Fertil Steril. 1988;50(3):434–40.
16. Letterie GS, Sakas EL. Histology of proximal tubal obstruction in cases of unsuccessful tubal canalization. Fertil Steril. 1991;56(5):831–5.
17. Nannini R, Chelo E, Branconi F, Tantini C, Scarselli GF. Dynamic echohysteroscopy: a new diagnostic technique in the study of female infertility. Acta Eur Fertil. 1981;12(2):165–71.
18. Sokalska A, Timmerman D, Testa AC, Van Holsbeke C, Lissoni AA, Leone FP, et al. Diagnostic accuracy of transvaginal ultrasound examination for assigning a specific diagnosis to adnexal masses. Ultrasound Obstet Gynecol. 2009;34(4):462–70.
19. Maheux-Lacroix S, Boutin A, Moore L, Bergeron ME, Bujold E, Laberge P, et al. Hysterosalpingosonography for diagnosing tubal occlusion in subfertile women: a systematic review with meta-analysis. Hum Reprod. 2014;29(5):953–63.
20. Jansen FW, Kapiteyn K, Trimbos-Kemper T, Hermans J, Trimbos JB. Complications of laparoscopy: a prospective multicentre observational study. Br J Obstet Gynaecol. 1997;104(5):595–600.
21. Magrina JF. Complications of laparoscopic surgery. Clin Obstet Gynecol. 2002;45(2):469–80.
22. Lavy Y, Lev-Sagie A, Holtzer H, Revel A, Hurwitz A. Should laparoscopy be a mandatory component of the infertility evaluation in infertile women with normal hysterosalpingogram or suspected unilateral distal tubal pathology? Eur J Obstet Gynecol Reprod Biol. 2004;114(1):64–8.

Assessment of Uterine Anatomy and Implications of Müllerian Disorders and Acquired Uterine Lesions on Fertility

2

Adrienne Gentry and Kelly Pagidas

2.1 Anatomy and Physiology

Uterine factor infertility is a relatively uncommon cause of female infertility occurring in <5% of women. Many uterine causes for infertility, both acquired and congenital, have been described. Although uterine factors may be diagnosed during investigation of infertility, a thorough investigation and management of all other causes of infertility should be undertaken at the same time.

Knowledge of the anatomy, physiology, and function of the uterus is paramount to the understanding of the development of congenital müllerian disorders and acquired uterine lesions and their potential impact on fertility. In brief, the uterus is a thick-walled muscular structure, with its sole function being to allow implantation of the developed embryo, and subsequently serving as the incubation chamber for the growing fetus during gestation. Hence, the development of a normal uterus is a key element in optimizing one's reproductive potential. The uterus is comprised of three main parts: the uterine corpus, isthmus, and cervix (Fig. 2.1). The uterine corpus, or body of the uterus, consists of three main layers [1]. The first layer and most internal layer, the endometrium, forms the inner layer of the triangle-shaped uterine cavity. This layer consists of mucus secreting columnar epithelium. The endometrium is under hormonal control in the reproductively active female and is divided into two phases of menses. During the proliferative phase, estrogen produced by the ovary promotes growth in the columnar epithelium, angiogenesis, and glandular development. The secretory phase, under the control of progesterone produced by the corpus luteum of the ovary post ovulation, is characterized by secretion of substances from the endometrial glands, to allow for an optimal implantation site for an embryo. If an embryo is not implanted, progesterone levels decrease and ultimately result in the breakdown of endometrium, resulting in menses. The second layer of the uterine corpus is the myometrium. The myometrium contains smooth muscle that is responsible for the contractile activity of the uterus during labor and delivery. The third layer, and most outer layer of the uterine corpus, is the serosa and is equivalent to the peritoneum. The isthmus is the most inferior part of the uterine corpus and is adjacent to the cervix, directly above the internal cervical os. The cervix is the lowest part of the uterus, is approximately 4 cm long, and connects the uterus to the vagina. The cervix allows transport of sperm into the uterus, passage of menstrual blood out of the uterus, and dilates and thins during labor to allow passage of the fetus. The uterus is highly vascularized to support the implanted embryo and growing fetus, and its main blood supply is the uterine artery.

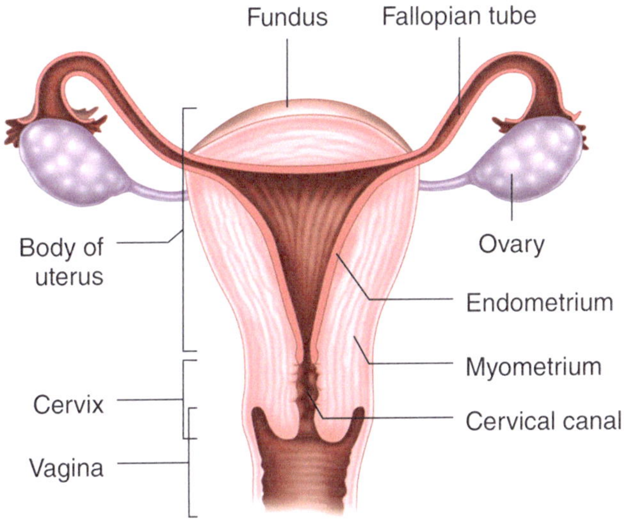

Fig. 2.1 Normal uterine anatomy

A. Gentry
Carilion Clinic, Reproductive Medicine and Fertility, Roanoke, VA, USA

K. Pagidas (✉)
Department of Obstetrics and Gynecology, University of Louisville, Louisville, KY, USA
e-mail: kelly.pagidas@louisville.edu

G. N. Allahbadia et al. (eds.), *Textbook of Assisted Reproduction*, https://doi.org/10.1007/978-981-15-2377-9_2

The uterine artery arises from the anterior division of the interior iliac artery.

A sequence of purposeful events occurs during the embryological development of the uterus, cervix, and vagina, both structurally and ultra-structurally, resulting in a normal-sized uterus, cervix, and vagina that is able to support implantation of the embryo and serve as the carrying vessel for the remainder of gestation until term. Any disruption prenatally along this programmed sequence of events can lead to an alteration in the structure and/or ultrastructure of the uterus, resulting in an array of congenital müllerian disorders that may impact the ability to conceive and/or ability to carry a pregnancy to term. Post-natally, the uterus is also susceptible to a variety of acquired uterine lesions that may impair fertility and/or reproductive outcomes.

2.2 Congenital Müllerian Disorders

In order to fully appreciate the anatomy of müllerian disorders, also known as congenital uterine anomalies, it is important to understand the embryological development of the uterus. There are a number of classification systems to describe the array of simple and complex müllerian anomalies in existence; the most commonly used and widely accepted classification is the American Fertility Society (AFS, now American Society for Reproductive Medicine) classification scheme [2]. The AFS scheme characterizes its classifications of uterine anomalies based on the embryological development of the uterus [2]. Other classification systems that have been recently proposed but have not yet found wide acceptance include European Society for Human Reproduction and Embryology/European Society for Gynecologic Endoscopy (ESHRE/ESGE) classification and Congenital Uterine Malformation by Experts (CUME) classification.

The female reproductive tract is completely developed by approximately the 22nd week of pregnancy. It arises from the urogenital ridge and begins to develop at 6 weeks of gestation, giving rise to the paired paramesonephric (müllerian) ducts that eventually give rise to the fallopian tubes, uterus, cervix, and upper vagina. The development occurs in a particular scheduled series of events that include müllerian duct elongation, fusion, canalization, and septal resorption. Any disruption in these events leads to what is known as a congenital müllerian (uterine) anomaly. The AFS classification describes seven classes of congenital müllerian anomalies, Class I to Class VII, based on the stage at which the arrest of the embryological development of the müllerian system occurred (Fig. 2.2). These classes can be further grouped into three major categories: anomalies with underdevelopment of the müllerian ducts, Classes I and II; non-fusion anomalies of the müllerian ducts, Classes III and IV; and non-resorption anomalies of the müllerian ducts, Classes V and VI.

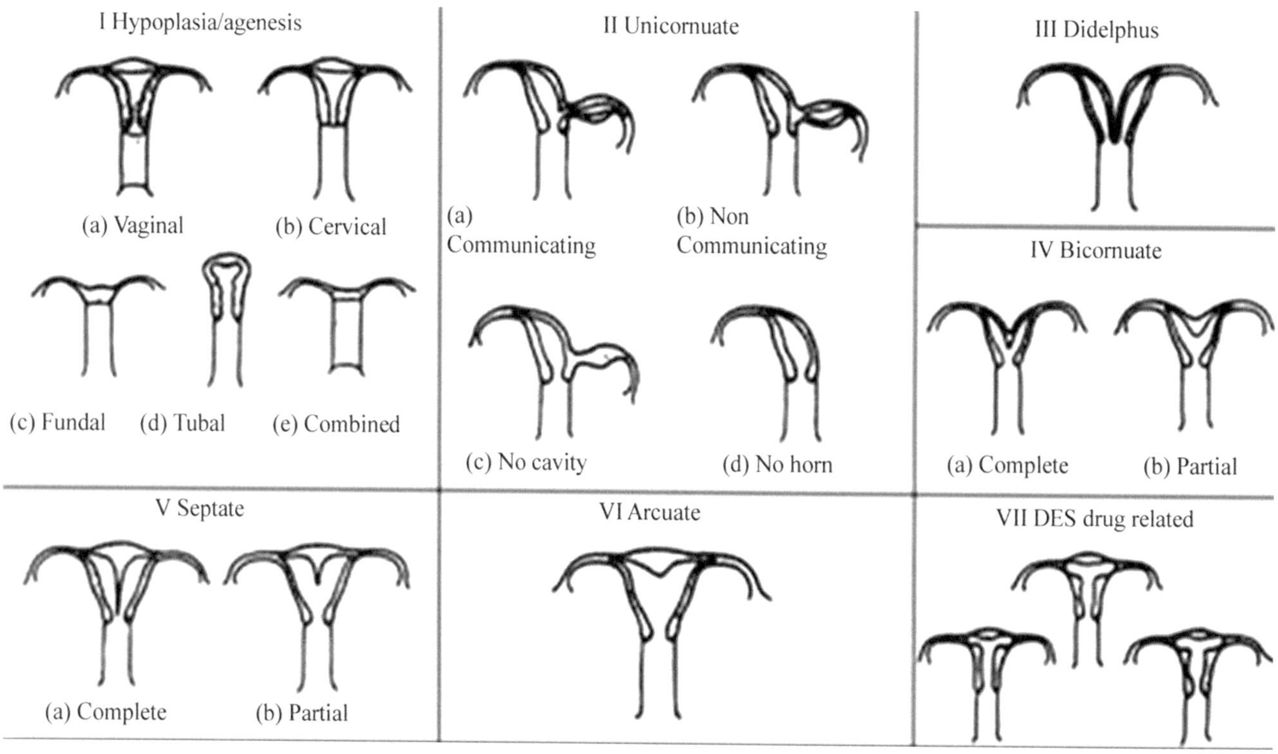

Fig. 2.2 The classification system of müllerian duct anomalies used by the American Fertility Society. (From the American Fertility Society classifications of adnexal adhesions, distal tubal occlusion, tubal occlusion secondary to tubal ligation, tubal pregnancies, mullerian anomalies and intrauterine adhesions. Fertil Steril 1988;49(6):944–955, with permission)

2.3 Diagnosis, Treatment, and Fertility Implications of Congenital Müllerian Disorders

The prevalence of müllerian duct anomalies has historically been estimated to be approximately 1%; however, advances in diagnostic imaging modalities now estimate the prevalence to be closer to 5.5% in the general population [3, 4]. Further, if we look at women with recurrent pregnancy loss, the prevalence has been reported to be as high as 13% [3, 4]. Müllerian anomalies can often go unrecognized because many of the women with these uterine anomalies have minimal to no symptoms and are often only detected during pregnancy or as part of an infertility workup.

What remains a conundrum is whether or not uterine anomalies have a negative impact on the reproductive potential of women and which, if any, treatment may be of benefit. Despite recent systematic reviews and meta-analysis, there remains a lack of sufficiently powered well-designed randomized controlled trials exploring surgical versus expectant management of congenital uterine anomalies with regard to optimizing reproductive potential.

The type of uterine anomaly dictates whether or not it is associated with a women's inability to conceive and/or carry a pregnancy to term. Hence, an assessment of the uterine cavity is paramount in women presenting with infertility or recurrent pregnancy loss. Historically, the gold standard for making a diagnosis of any congenital uterine anomaly is a diagnostic hysteroscopy and laparoscopy as it provides direct visualization of both the exterior and interior contour of the uterus. At present, radiological imaging has taken the lead in the diagnosis of müllerian anomalies. The most commonly used imaging modalities include ultrasonography, sonohysterography or saline infusion sonography (SIS), hysterosalpingography (HSG), and magnetic resonance imaging (MRI). One imaging modality may be more appropriate than another for a given congenital uterine anomaly with the goal in mind being to identify surgically correctable from inoperable uterine anomalies. Overall, ultrasound is routinely used as the initial modality for the diagnosis of congenital uterine anomalies with an accuracy approximating 90% [5, 6]. Transvaginal sonography (TVUS) is superior to transabdominal, as it provides higher-resolution images, as the female reproductive organs lay low in the pelvis, and thus the vaginal transducer is closer to the structures to be imaged. Further, three-dimensional (3D) ultrasound yields a greater degree of accuracy than two-dimensional (2D) ultrasound. However, MRI is overall considered clinically the gold standard imaging modality for the delineation of uterine anomalies as it can differentiate between surgically correctable from inoperable forms of uterine anomalies [6, 7]. The accuracy of MRI in the diagnosis of congenital uterine anomalies approaches 100% [6]. MRI also has the added advantage of identifying renal anomalies commonly associated with certain classes of uterine anomalies that are overall seen in approximately 11–30% of müllerian disorders. With MRI, T2-weighted sequences depict the classic inherent contrast for delineating the anatomy of the müllerian system, and a single-shot, fast spin echo image with a larger field of view can also be obtained and enable visualization of the kidneys [6]. Recent reports note that 3D sonography with saline infusion has a 100% accuracy when compared with laparoscopy and hysteroscopy for the diagnosis of septate, bicornuate, and arcuate uterus [8]. In addition, saline infusion sonogram with 3D ultrasonography has been shown to diagnose müllerian anomalies with the same sensitivity and specificity and accuracy as a diagnostic hysteroscopy [9, 10]. The 3D technology allows for visualization of the coronal view of the uterus, which assists in accurate assessment of the uterine contour and degree of myometrial/septal indentation, if it is present [11–13]. Swift advances in 3D/4D sonographic technology will soon be the new clinical imaging gold standard, if it is not already, for the diagnosis of congenital müllerian disorders.

With any imaging modality, there are three key anatomical elements that need to be ascertained in order to assist in the accurate diagnosis of the class of uterine anomaly present [6]:

1. Is the uterus present or absent, and if present, is it normal or smaller in size?
2. If the uterus is present, is the outer contour of the uterine fundus normal in configuration (convex)?
3. If the uterus displays an abnormal fundal contour, is the degree of myometrial/septal indentation into the uterine cavity less than or greater than 1 cm?

2.3.1 Müllerian Disorders

2.3.1.1 Class I

Hypoplasia/agenesis occurs when the paired müllerian ducts fail to or incompletely develop, resulting in the absence or rudimentary development of the uterus, cervix, and upper vagina [1, 6]. This is a result of failure of the first stage of development. Müllerian agenesis is characterized by variable degrees of uterine and vaginal non-development. Approximately 90–95% of patients are reported to have complete absence of vagina and uterus with presence normal fallopian tubes and ovaries due to the separate embryological origin of these structures. Class I disorders are the rarest form of müllerian disorders, representing >4% of the uterine anomalies. Mayer-Rokitansky-Kuster-Hauser syndrome is the most common Class I disorder.

The patient with uterine hypoplasia or agenesis will typically present with primary amenorrhea and possibly dyspareunia. It is the second most common cause of primary

Table 2.1 Congenital uterine anomalies

Class of müllerian disorder	Diagnostic imaging	Fertility impact	At risk for early pregnancy loss	At risk for adverse pregnancy outcome	Surgical repair of uterus
Class I	US, MRI	+	NA	NA	–
Class II	HSG, US, MRI	–	–	+	–
Class III	US, MRI	–	–	+	–
Class IV	US, SIS, MRI	–	–	+	–
Class V	US, SIS, MRI	–	+	+	+
Class VI	US, SIS, MRI	–	–	–	–
Class VII	HSG	+	–	–	–

US refers to 2D/3D ultrasound imaging

amenorrhea after gonadal dysgenesis. The initial imaging modality commonly used is the ultrasound. Typically an absent or hypoplastic uterus with no normal zonal anatomy which is characteristic for the diagnosis is noted [6]. The upper two-thirds of the vagina is absent or atretic, as well. The MRI is not necessary to make this diagnosis; however if the ultrasound is diagnostic, then it is recommended to proceed with an MRI for complete detailed evaluation of the female abdomen and pelvis, as over 50% of women with Class I disorders also have other congenital or renal anomalies [14].

Class I uterine disorders are associated with total reproductive failure (Table 2.1). At the present time, there are no surgical treatment options for Class I uterine anomalies. Recent surgical advances in uterine transplantation hold promise. Even without uterine transplantation, women with uterine hypoplasia or agenesis have the ability to have their own biological offspring as their ovaries are unaffected, with the use of a gestational carrier through assisted reproductive technology.

2.3.1.2 Class II

A unicornuate uterus is the result of incomplete and/or failed development of one of the müllerian ducts, leaving a functional uterine cavity with a single horn referred to as a single-horned uterus [1, 6]. There can be a contralateral rudimentary horn that is communicating or non-communicating with the single horn. This is as a result of failure of the first stage of development, as a result of a lateral fusion defect. A unicornuate uterus represents approximately 4.4% of the uterine anomalies [15].

Patients with a unicornuate uterus may be asymptomatic, and diagnosis is often made at time of an infertility workup. However, if there is a non-communicating functional horn, i.e., presence of an endometrial cavity, the patient may experience painful periods, endometriosis, hematometra, and hematosalpinx. Ectopic pregnancy may occur in a communicating horn. Counterintuitively, ectopic pregnancy can occur in a non-communicating uterine horn as well [16].

Initial imaging usually consists of an HSG as it is part of the standard infertility workup. Imaging by HSG, as well as ultrasound and MRI, is notable for a fusiform "banana-shaped" endometrial cavity, which is laterally displaced [1]. When diagnosed, it is recommended to perform an MRI to evaluate the presence of a rudimentary horn, as well as the presence of renal anomalies, which are often seen with this anomaly. In particular, contralateral renal agenesis to the dominant uterine horn is most commonly seen.

In a recent meta-analysis, no significant difference was noted in the probability of spontaneous pregnancy or pregnancy after assisted reproductive techniques in women with Class II müllerian disorders [17]. The unicornuate uterus is associated with pregnancy complications and poor obstetrical outcomes, including malpresentation and preterm delivery, but the impact on fertility, i.e., implantation and ability to achieve a pregnancy, remains unaffected. However, there is no surgical option to improve the uterine size/volume in a unicornuate uterus. The management is conservative with vigilant prenatal care at time of pregnancy. In cases where the unicornuate uterus is associated with a functional rudimentary horn, surgery may be prudent to alleviate the symptoms associated with an obstructed horn and minimize the risk of an ectopic pregnancy. A pregnancy in the partially developed horn requires emergency removal via laparotomy or laparoscopy. If there is an asymptomatic, non-functioning, non-communicating horn, it can be left untreated.

2.3.1.3 Class III

A didelphys uterus occurs when there is failure of the müllerian ducts to fuse, resulting in two uteri and two cervices (Fig. 2.3) [1, 6]. Failure of fusion of the vaginal portion of the müllerian duct is common resulting in the presence of a longitudinal vaginal septum seen in 75% of didelphys uteri. A didelphys uterus represents approximately 11% of the uterine anomalies [15]. A horizontal uterine septum may also be present which can lead to unilateral hematocolpos (OHVIRA syndrome—obstructed hemivagina, ipsilateral renal agenesis).

Imaging modalities to make the diagnosis include transvaginal sonography and MRI. An HSG can also be performed, but failure to identify the presence of two cervices and hence cannulate both cervices can lead to the erroneous diagnosis of a unicornuate uterus. Class III uterine anomaly is most commonly associated with renal agenesis. Hence, once the diagnosis is made, MRI is recommended to rule out any coexisting renal anomalies.

Uterine didelphys often goes undetected as pregnancy is not precluded and rare reports exist of simultaneous pregnancies in both uteri. In a recent meta-analysis, no significant

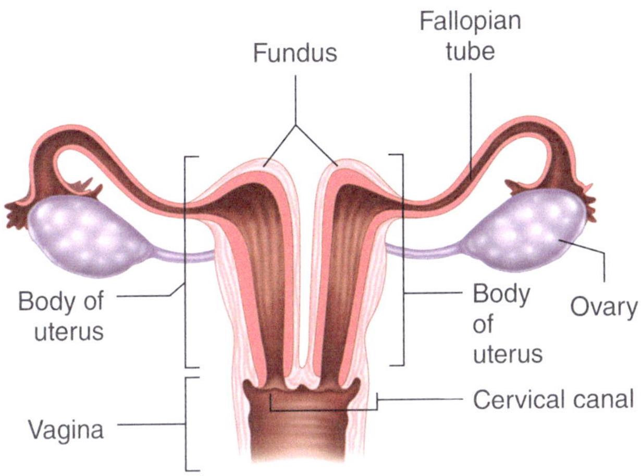

Fig. 2.3 A Class III congenital uterine anomaly; the didelphys uterus occurs when there is failure of the müllerian ducts to fuse, resulting in two uteri and two cervices

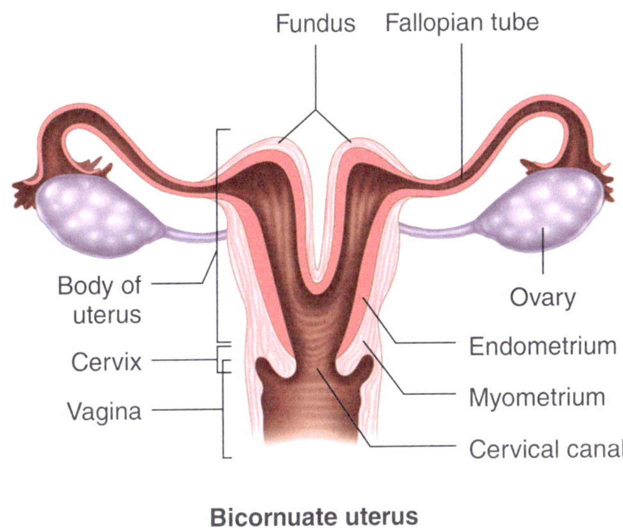

Fig. 2.4 Class IV congenital uterine anomaly, the bicornuate uterus

difference was noted in the probability of spontaneous pregnancy or pregnancy after assisted reproductive techniques in women with Class III müllerian disorders [17]. A uterine didelphys has a good prognosis for achieving a pregnancy, as well as maintaining a pregnancy. Hence, there is no indication for surgical unification of the two uteri. There is no data to support any proven benefit in surgically correcting the non-fused component of a uterine didelphys [18]. Hence, expectant management is prudent with adequate surveillance in pregnancy.

2.3.1.4 Class IV

A bicornuate uterus occurs when the inferior portion of the müllerian ducts fuse correctly; however, the superior (upper-mid) portion of the paired ducts fail to fuse (Fig. 2.4). Lack of fusion of the upper-mid uterine horns results in a significant fundal cleft (>1 cm) [1, 6]. It is characterized by a heart-shaped uterus with an external groove in the uterine dome where a muscular, intrauterine septum divides the uterus. The bicornuate uterus accounts for approximately 46% of the diagnosed müllerian disorders and is typically undetected until caesarean section [15].

The imaging modalities of choice are a transvaginal ultrasound or MRI. Both sonography and MRI will detect the presence of a fundal uterine cleft >1 cm with divergent uterine horns. Although an HSG may be the initial imaging performed as part of the infertility workup and findings suggestive of a bicornuate uterus based on a widened angle, >105°, between the uterine horns and widened intercornual distance of >4 cm, it cannot rule out a septate uterus as the external fundal uterine contour cannot be evaluated with an HSG [1].

The patient with a bicornuate uterus is also typically asymptomatic. The bicornuate uterus is associated with pregnancy complications and poor outcomes, including malpresentation, preterm delivery, and early pregnancy loss if associated with uterine septum, but overall the obstetrical outcomes are much better than those seen with a unicornuate uterus. Fertility rates also do not appear to be significantly reduced with Class IV anomalies from the general population [3, 15]. In a recent meta-analysis, no significant difference was noted in the probability of spontaneous pregnancy or pregnancy after assisted reproductive techniques in women with Class IV müllerian disorders [17].

In the early 1900s, Dr. Strassmann developed a surgical technique, termed the Strassmann metroplasty, to correct a bicornuate uterus. The Strassmann metroplasty begins with a laparotomy, with wedge resection of the medial aspects of the uterine horns, and then reapproximation to produce a single uterine cavity. This surgical procedure is no longer recommended due to the minimal change in obstetrical outcomes post repair and because of the improved management and outcomes of premature neonates [19]. Other metroplasty technique described by Bret-Palmer is also typically performed via laparotomy. The only time a bicornuate uterus may be surgically managed is if it is associated with a uterine septum and the patient has experienced early recurrent pregnancy loss with no other cause noted. There is no indication for surgical correction of bicornuate uterus for the diagnosis for infertility alone. There is no data to support any proven benefit in surgically correcting the non-fused component of a bicornuate uterus [18]. Hence, expectant management is prudent with adequate surveillance in pregnancy.

2.3.1.5 Class V

A septate uterus arises from failure of resorption of the poorly vascularized fibromuscular septum once the müllerian tract fuses earlier in development [1, 6]. The septate

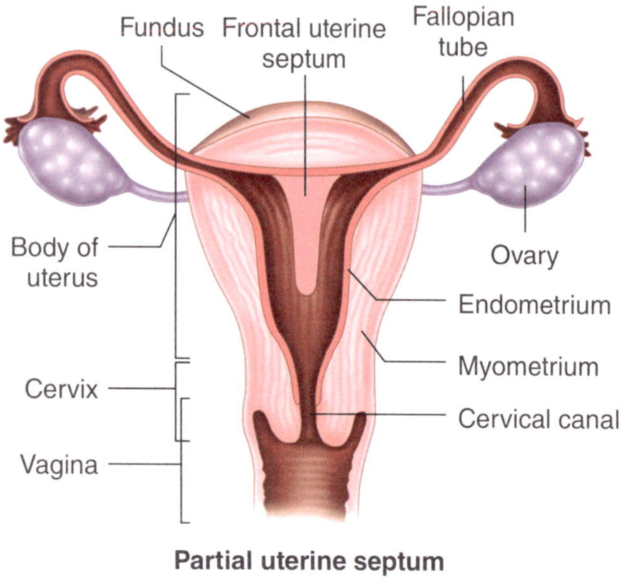

Fig. 2.5 Class Va congenital uterine anomaly, the partial uterine septum

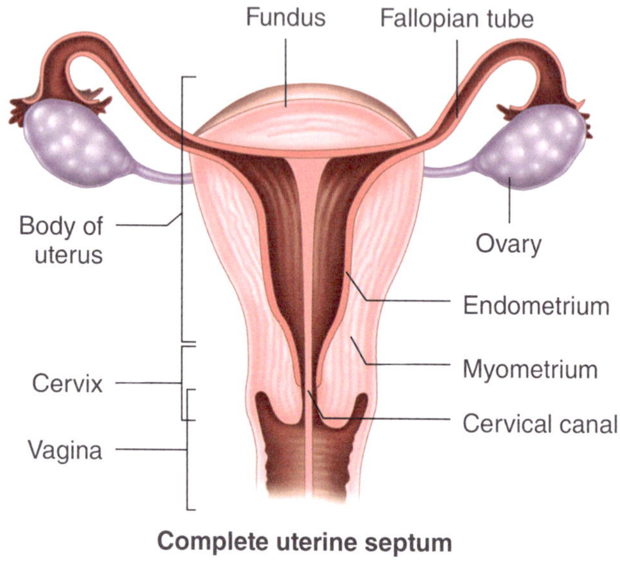

Fig. 2.6 Class Vb congenital uterine anomaly, complete uterine, cervical and vaginal septum

uterus can be partial, due to only partial resorption of the septum, or complete, when none of the septum resorbed. It is the most common congenital uterine anomaly associated with early pregnancy loss and accounts for approximately 22% of the diagnosed müllerian disorders [15]. The diagnostic hallmark for the septate uterus is that the uterine fundal contour is normal (convex) or minimally indented (<1 cm); however, the myometrial/septal indentation or invagination into the uterine cavity is >1.5 cm [20, 21]. A partial septum is when the septum does not reach the cervix, and a complete septum is when the septum reaches the external os of the cervix (Fig. 2.5). The septum can vary in both length and width. A longitudinal vaginal septum may also be present.

The deciding factor to assist in differentiating between a septate, arcuate, and bicornuate uterus is the degree of myometrial/septal indentation into the uterine cavity, which can be accomplished with either 3D ultrasound or MR imaging modality. The determination is made by drawing a line connecting the cornua of the uterus, then a perpendicular line along the visualized indentation of the myometrium or fibrous septum is drawn, and the distance between this line and the indentation is measured [20]. If the indentation measures <1 cm, it is an arcuate uterus, and if it measures >1.5 cm, it is a septate uterus (Figs. 2.6 and 2.7) [20].

Historically, the gold standard for making a diagnosis of a septate uterus and in particular to differentiate a bicornuate uterus is diagnostic hysteroscopy and laparoscopy. Although a hysterosalpingogram is most often the initial infertility test, it is associated with a low diagnostic accuracy for distinguishing a septate, bicornuate, or arcuate uterus. At present, given the remarkable advancement in ultrasound, many of these can be diagnosed with a less invasive approach, and sonography has taken the lead in the diagnosis of a uterine septum. The use of 3D transvaginal ultrasonography has been able to distinguish the bicornuate uterus and uterine septum, with the same accuracy and reproducibility as the MRI with a sensitivity as high as 100% [11–13]. In addition, the saline infusion sonogram with 3D ultrasonography has been shown to diagnose müllerian anomalies with the same sensitivity and specificity as a diagnostic hysteroscopy [9]. The 3D technology allows for visualization of the coronal view of the uterus, which assists in accurate measurements of a uterine septum if it is present and determines the fundal contour [11–13]. Another report notes that 3D sonography with saline infusion had a 100% accuracy when compared with laparoscopy and hysteroscopy for the diagnosis of septate, bicornuate, and arcuate uterus [8]. Overall, MRI is an accurate method to diagnose uterine anomalies but is only about 70% accurate for the diagnosis of uterine septum [20]. An added advantage to using the MRI is information gained with regard to the composition of the septum, and a low T2 signal is seen with a thin fibrous septum and an intermediate signal with a thick myometrial septum [1]. In summary, 3D ultrasound, sonohysterography, and MRI are good diagnostic tests to differentiate between a bicornuate and septate uterus, and the use of laparoscopy/hysteroscopy should not be first line. Further, if hysteroscopy is used for the diagnosis of a septate uterus, a concurrent laparoscopy is no longer recommended, but consideration can be given for concomitant transabdominal ultrasound guidance.

Data is conflicting with regard to uterine septum and its association with female infertility [12, 22–24]. Though evidence is clearer that recurrent pregnancy loss is indeed associated with a uterine septum, the exact pathophysiol-

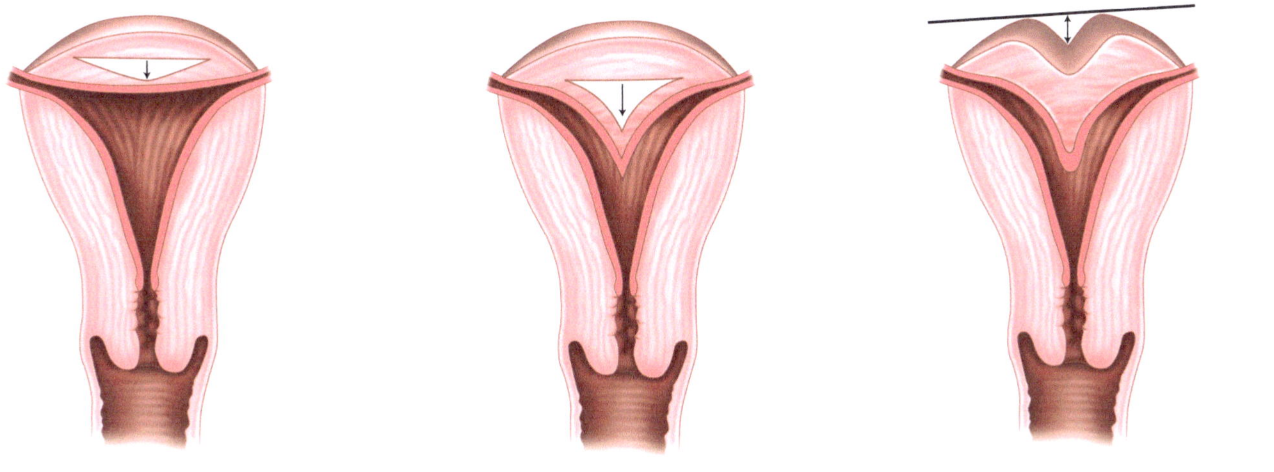

Fig. 2.7 ASRM definition of Class IV (bicornuate), V (septate), and VI (arcuate) congenital uterine anomalies

ogy that causes the loss is truly unknown and still up for debate. However, the most common mechanism postulated for the increase loss rate observed with a septate uterus is likely secondary to the poor blood supply of the septum providing suboptimal support for the implanted embryo and growing fetus.

Infertility is not seen more frequently in women with a septate uterus [25]. Primary infertility has also been noted to be less common in women with a septate uterus than controls. Review of the existing data has shown no difference in the cumulative pregnancy rates or monthly fecundity in women with septate uteri compared to women with normal uterine cavities [17]. At present, the evidence to date does not support an association between uterine septum and infertility.

Although many women with a uterine septum have an uncomplicated reproductive history, the uterine septum has been associated with pregnancy loss and poor obstetrical outcomes. No randomized controlled trials (RCT) exist, but small observation studies suggest that a septate uterus is associated with a higher rate of pregnancy loss and preterm delivery compared to controls. The incidence of first-trimester miscarriage in patients with a septate uterus has been reported to be as high as 42% compared to 12% ($p < 0.01$) in women with a normal cavity, yet no difference was seen in the rate of second-trimester loss or preterm delivery [21]. A meta-analysis noted that a septate uterus had a higher rate of miscarriage compared to controls with a RR 2.65 (95% CI 1.39–5.06) [17]. Additional adverse outcomes noted were preterm delivery, malpresentation, IUGR, and placental abruption [17]. The evidence to date supports the possibility that a septate uterus contributes to miscarriage and preterm birth and it may increase the risk of adverse obstetrical outcomes. Data is also lacking with regard to differing obstetrical outcomes based on the size (length or width) of a uterine septum [20].

Additionally, there is ongoing controversy in regard to the indication for surgical management of a uterine septum, mostly due to a lack of randomized controlled trials. The primary indication for surgical treatment is when a patient has a uterine septum and history of recurrent pregnancy loss. Regardless, many providers will surgically correct a uterine septum if the patient has experienced only one loss or has a diagnosis of primary infertility, termed a "prophylactic metroplasty." There are no RCT evaluating hysteroscopic metroplasty for women with septate uterus and ≥2 prior miscarriages. However, case series report improvement in the miscarriage rate pre- and post-surgery, 100 versus 13%, respectively, and improvement in obstetrical outcomes such as ability to carry to term, pre- and post-surgery, of 14 and 55%, respectively. Combined data for a total of 466 patients with hysteroscopic septum division reported an overall term and preterm delivery, miscarriage, and live birth rate of 76.2, 6.8, 16.4, and 83.2%, respectively, approaching rates for women without uterine anomalies [26]. In a meta-analysis with a mixed population of women with infertility, miscarriage, and/or recurrent pregnancy loss, the overall pregnancy rate and the live birth rate after septum division were 63.5 and 50.2%, respectively [24]. Another meta-analysis that looked at the effect of uterine septum division on pregnancy outcome noted that women who had a septum division had a significantly decreased probability of spontaneous abortion compared to those that did not, RR 0.37, 95% CI 0.25–0.55 [17], while other studies do not support an improvement in reproductive outcome post-uterine septum division [20, 27].

Several small observational studies suggest that hysteroscopic septum division is associated with improved clinical pregnancy rates in women with infertility including women undergoing IVF-ET. A retrospective matched controlled study of three groups of women undergoing embryo transfer reported significantly lower pregnancy and live birth rates in women with an intact uterine septum compared with controls, 12.4 versus 29.2% and 2.7 versus 21.7%, respectively [28]. Also, pregnancy rates were higher in the groups that had undergone a septum division compared to those that did not, OR 2.507, 95% CI 1.539–4.111, and miscarriage rate was significantly higher in the septate uterus group than controls, 77.1 versus 16.7%, respectively [28]. After surgery the live birth rate was comparable to that of women with a normal uterus. More controversy exists about whether a complete uterine septum that is noted incidentally even requires division unless it is associated with pregnancy loss or poor obstetrical outcome [29]. The controversy extends further to whether or not the cervical part of the septum should be divided due to potential risk of cervical incompetence during pregnancy post resection, and the decision is often left to the discretion of the operating surgeon.

The surgical management of a uterine septum, termed metroplasty, was first performed through an abdominal approach (Tompkins metroplasty and Jones metroplasty) and has evolved to a minimally invasive approach via the transcervical route with the use of a hysteroscopy. The two main hysteroscopic techniques are the use of a resectoscope or with an operative hysteroscope [30]. Recently, the use of a hysteroscopic morcellator for metroplasty has been suggested; however, the cost-effectiveness and outcomes have not been evaluated. There is no one specific technique that is best for hysteroscopic septum division. Regardless of the instrument used for the septum division, the purpose of the surgical management is to restore a normal uterine cavity, by dividing the septum starting at the apex inferiorly and progressing superiorly until both tubal ostia are visualized in the same plane, without compromising the integrity of the uterine fundus.

In summary, there is no consensus regarding management of a uterine septum. What we conclude here is based on limited data: A decrease in miscarriage rates with associated improvement in live birth rates in women with recurrent pregnancy loss may be achieved with hysteroscopic division of septum. Women with infertility may benefit from septum division as well. Hence, it is reasonable to consider septum division in women with infertility, prior pregnancy loss, or poor obstetrical outcome after appropriate counseling regarding potential risks and benefits of the procedure.

2.3.1.6 Class VI

The arcuate uterus, though still considered normal, is due to incomplete resorption of the superior aspect of the septum, leaving a focal bulge at the uterine fundus [1, 6] (Fig. 2.8). An arcuate uterus is a less severe form of a septate uterus. The uterus has a normal fundal contour with minimal indentation of the myometrium at the uterine fundus. The depth of the indentation into the endometrial cavity is <1–1.5 cm. The

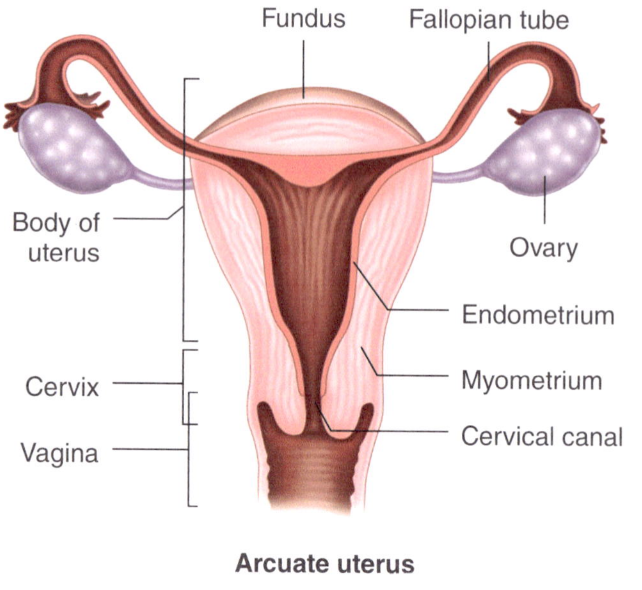

Fig. 2.8 Class VI congenital uterine anomaly, arcuate uterus

arcuate uterus accounts for approximately 15% of the diagnosed müllerian disorders. An ultrasound or MRI would be notable for a single uterine cavity with a smooth, broad indentation of the myometrium (<1 cm) at the level of the fundus and normal external fundal uterine contour. Its exact incidence is not known, nor is it associated with an adverse impact on fertility or clinical outcomes such as pregnancy loss, although some controversy exists regarding this as well. An arcuate uterus is a normal variant, and women with an arcuate uterus do not benefit from surgical correction.

2.3.1.7 Class VII

Hypoplastic, T-shaped, diethylstilbestrol (DES, a non-steroidal estrogen)-related uterine anomaly is seen in women whose mothers ingested DES during pregnancy. HSG is the imaging modality of choice as the classic T-shaped uterus and shortened irregular contour of the fallopian tubes are well appreciated. Women who received in utero exposure to DES had a higher chance of a Class VII müllerian disorder. Also, DES-exposed children presented with infertility. There are no medical or surgical modalities to correct this disorder. Given its use predominantly in the 1940s–1970s, this class of müllerian disorders is becoming extinct in women of reproductive age but must be kept in mind in women undergoing ART in their late fourth or early fifth decade of life with the use of autologous preexisting gametes/embryos or donor gametes/embryos.

In summary, each class of müllerian anomaly as defined by the AFS classification scheme can be traced back to the stage at which the müllerian system arrested. The three major categories within this classification system can be grouped into underdevelopment disorders, Classes I and II; nonfusion disorders, Classes III and IV; and non-degeneration anomalies, Classes V and VI. Although the type of müllerian disorder often dictates the imaging modality of choice, overall, MRI and 3D ultrasound are the clinical modalities of choice for the diagnosis of a given class of müllerian disorder. At present there is lack of evidence to support an adverse impact on fertility for any of the müllerian disorders, Classes II–VI with the exception of Class I disorders; hence, the only class of müllerian disorder that may benefit from surgical intervention in improving clinical outcomes is Class V, a septate uterus (Table 2.1).

2.4 Diagnosis, Treatment, and Fertility Implications of Acquired Uterine Lesions

Acquired uterine lesions differ from congenital uterine anomalies, in that acquired uterine lesions are not present at birth and develop most commonly after the second decade of life. The etiology of acquired uterine lesions is diverse in origin and in clinical presentation. Some acquired lesions are completely asymptomatic, and others may be associated with pelvic discomfort, abnormal uterine bleeding, and possibly infertility and pregnancy loss (Table 2.2).

Table 2.2 Acquired uterine lesions

Acquired uterine lesion	Diagnostic imaging	Fertility impact	Surgical removal
Endometrial polyp	HSG±, US, SIS	±	+
Uterine synechiae	HSG, US, SIS	+	+
Uterine myoma			
Intramural no cavitary distortion	US, MRI	–	–
Intramural with cavitary distortion	HSG±, US, SIS, MRI	+	+
Submucosal	HSG, US, SIS, MRI	+	+
Serosal	US, MRI	–	–

2.4.1 Uterine Myomas

One of the most common acquired uterine lesions is a uterine myoma or leiomyoma, also known as uterine fibroid. A myoma is a benign, estrogen-dependent smooth muscle lesion that originates from the myometrium of the uterus. Myomas can vary in size, locations, and number. Approximately 20–40% of reproductive age women have uterine myomas [31, 32]. Myomas can arise from any part of the uterus, and the most commonly used subclassification system is by the International Federation of Gynecology and Obstetrics (FIGO) [33]. There are four main myoma groups:

1. Submucosal (Types 0–2) subdivided based on complete intracavitary (O), <50% intramural [1], and ≥50% intramural component.
2. Intramural (Types 3–4) contacts the endometrium but 100% intramural [3] and intramural [4].
3. Subserosal (Types 5–7), ≥50% intramural [5], <50% intramural [6] component and pedunculated [7].
4. Other (Type 8) such as cervical (Fig. 2.9) [33].

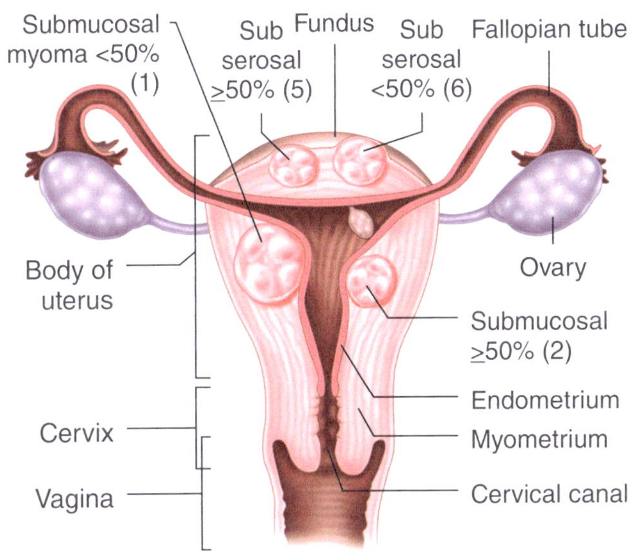

Fig. 2.9 Subclassification of uterine myomas

The best initial imaging modality for location of the uterine myoma is the transvaginal ultrasound. On ultrasound, myoma appears as a focal heterogeneous appearing mass and can have both hypo- and hyperechoic areas within. A TVUS can identify myomas with uterine cavity disruption; however, 3D technology and SIS can determine the location of myoma and the degree of uterine cavity distortion with 100% sensitivity and specificity [34]. An HSG can identify myoma early in the filling phase; however, it is not specific, and it is difficult to determine exact location and its impact on the endometrial cavity. An MRI can also be helpful though certainly not necessary, unless further delineation of myoma location, number, and extent is needed for pre-surgical mapping [32, 35].

Surgical treatment of myomas is considered for symptomatic relief of myoma-related symptoms such as abnormal uterine bleeding and/or pelvic pressure, pain, or discomfort when all other options have failed. However, treatment recommendations for the removal of myomas in women with infertility and/or recurrent pregnancy loss in the absence of other symptoms are less clear given the limited quality of existing data. The surgical removal of a myoma (myomectomy) can be accomplished hysteroscopically for Class 0–1-type myomas; otherwise, a laparoscopic or open approach is best.

The majority of the data to assess the impact of myomectomy on reproductive or fertility outcomes in women with infertility or pregnancy loss come from observational studies that are inherently associated with selection bias and confounding variables that, most importantly, lack appropriate control groups [35]. A systematic review based on the only RCT found no significant effect of myomectomy on clinical pregnancy rate based on the location of the myoma removed [35, 36].

Systematic reviews of the current literature conclude that there is insufficient evidence that the removal of intramural or serosal myomas improves fertility and reproductive outcomes in infertile women (including women undergoing ART) [34, 35, 37]. Further, in the only RCT, no improvement in clinical pregnancy rate was seen in women with intramural or subserosal myomas that underwent myomectomy compared to no intervention (56.5 and 63.6%, respectively) [38]. Also, observational cohort studies that assess the impact of myomectomy for intramural or subserosal myomas on ART pregnancy rates report no improvement in clinical pregnancy rate compared to the nonsurgical groups regardless of route of procedure [39, 40]. However, if a myomectomy is performed, it does not appear to impair the clinical or live birth rate following ART [41].

In addition, in the only RCT, there was no difference in miscarriage rates in women with intramural or submucosal myomas randomized to surgery or no surgery [38]. Further, a systematic review showed no difference in the miscarriage rate after myomectomy versus nonintervention [34, 36]. Also, no difference in miscarriage rate was seen after laparoscopy versus open myomectomy. In summary, there is insufficient evidence that myomectomy reduces miscarriage rates [34–37].

With regard to the benefit of myomectomy for submucosal myomas, the data is more favorable for removal. In a single small RCT, an improvement in the clinical pregnancy rate in women who had undergone surgery compared to those who had not (43.3 and 27.2%, $p < 0.05$, respectively) was demonstrated [38]. Further, a systematic review of women who had a hysteroscopic myomectomy of a submucosal myoma had higher rates of clinical pregnancy when compared to women with the myoma left in situ, RR 2.03 (CI 1.08–3.82), $p = 0.028$ [34]. However, in the same review, an improvement in the miscarriage rate could not be demonstrated [34].

In summary, the effect of myomas on achieving and maintaining pregnancy is not clear. Based on reasonable evidence, it appears likely that hysteroscopic myomectomy improves clinical pregnancy rate when cavity-distorting myomas are present; it is still unclear in these cases if myomectomy improves the likelihood of early pregnancy loss or live birth. In the absence of cavity-distorting myomas, myomectomy is not recommended in otherwise asymptomatic women with infertility. In unique cases it may be reasonable to consider myomectomy, if the myoma causes severe distortion of the pelvic anatomy compromising safe ovarian access during oocyte retrieval [35].

2.4.2 Endometrial Polyp

An endometrial polyp is a common, usually benign, acquired uterine lesion of unknown etiology. It is characterized by a focal, intrauterine, endometrial overgrowth of endometrial glands and stroma around a vascular pedicle originating from a spiral artery (Fig. 2.10). There are three types of endometrial polyps, hypertrophic polyps that are similar to endometrial hyperplasia and at risk for endometrial cancer, atrophic polyps noted in post-menopausal patients, and functional polyps that are associated with the menstrual cycle [32]. The true incidence of endometrial polyps is unknown as they typically are asymptomatic and are often identified incidentally during imaging. If symptomatic, the most common presentation is abnormal uterine bleeding. It remains controversial where or not endometrial polyps are associated with subfertility.

The imaging modality of choice for an endometrial polyp is a transvaginal ultrasound. The endometrial polyp usually appears as a focal, hyperechoic lesion with regular contours within the uterine cavity. The use of a 3D ultrasound or color flow Doppler can further increase the ability of TVUS to diagnose a polyp. With color flow Doppler, a single feeding vessel seen within the endometrial layers is quite typical for the presence of an endometrial polyp. Depending on polyp size and location, the saline infusion sonogram with or without 3D imaging will have a better detection rate than TVUS alone and further improves the diagnostic accuracy for pol-

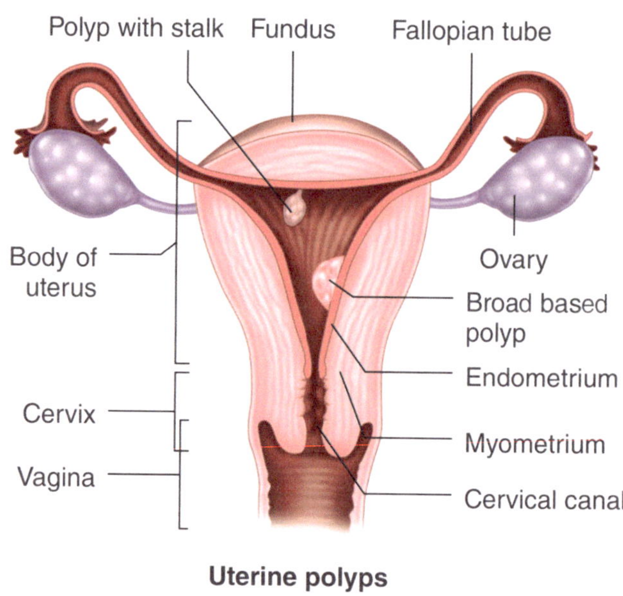

Fig. 2.10 Uterine polyps

yps [42]. On SIS imaging, a polyp appears as a smooth, echogenic, intracavitary lesion with a stalk or broad base surrounded by fluid. HSG is not the best modality to distinguish between a polyp and myoma, and an MRI is reserved for cases where there is concern about the type of mass seen within the uterus.

Hysteroscopic polypectomy is the gold standard for treatment, and it can be performed as an office procedure, or in the operating room, and is associated with a minimal recovery time. However, conservative management is acceptable, especially for small, asymptomatic polyps as they may regress spontaneously.

Endometrial polyps are often seen in women with subfertility and pregnancy loss, but it is uncertain if they have a causal role in their etiology as the pathophysiology is not clearly understood. There are few observational studies and only one RCT assessing the effects of polypectomy on infertility. In the RCT, the cumulative pregnancy rate in the group that underwent hysteroscopic polypectomy prior to IUI cycles was 63.4% compared to 28.2% in the control group ($P < 0.001$), but live birth rates were not reported [43]. Of note, 65% of the pregnancies in the polypectomy group occurred before the first IUI. In addition, two controlled studies found no effect of small endometrial polyps on IVF outcomes. If a hysteroscopic polypectomy is performed just prior to an IVF-ET cycle, patients can undergo ovarian stimulation with their next menses without affecting IVF-ET outcomes [44].

Due to possible adverse effect of endometrial polyps on fertility, their removal prior to any fertility treatment to include IVF-ET cycle is widely practiced despite the lack of further clinical evidence and benefit in improving reproductive outcome and live birth rate [45, 46]. Additional well-designed RCT are lacking, and no good-quality data exists supporting the routine removal of endometrial polyps identified in women undergoing ART such as IVF at the present time. On the other hand, the procedure is minimally invasive with low risks with additional benefit of providing an opportunity for histological diagnosis.

2.4.3 Uterine Synechiae

Uterine synechiae, also known as intrauterine adhesions (IUA), are permanent adhesions of the endometrial cavity (Fig. 2.11). It is postulated that any cause that is destructive to the endometrium including local uterine infection can lead to uterine synechiae. Common causes include uterine infections, missed abortion, prior pregnancy, and curettage. Asherman was the first to describe the frequency of uterine synechiae and the etiological symptoms associated with the condition, and this condition is therefore referred to as Asherman syndrome. The exact incidence of IUA is not known, but the estimated prevalence is 1.5%. The most common presentation is menstrual disturbance, and severe cases present with amenorrhea. IUA may be associated with infertility and recurrent pregnancy loss. If conception occurs, it is often complicated by abnormal placentation.

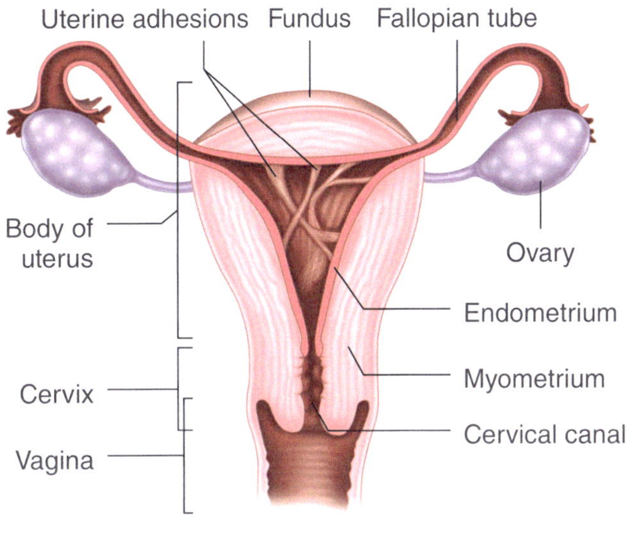

Fig. 2.11 Uterine synechiae or intrauterine adhesions

Table 2.3 AFS classification system for uterine synechiae

Extent of cavity involved Score	<1/3 1	1/3–2/3 2	>2/3 4
Type of adhesions Score	Filmy 1	Filmy and dense 2	Dense 4
Menstrual pattern Score	Normal 0	Hypomenorrhea 2	Amenorrhea 4
Prognostic classification		*HSG score*[a]	*Hysteroscopy score*
Stage I (Mild) Stage II (Moderate) Stage III (Severe)	1–4 5–8 9–12	______ ______ ______	______ ______ ______

[a]All adhesions should be considered dense

Multiple classification systems have been described for IUA based on location of pathology, extent of uterine adhesions, and even menstrual pattern (AFS classification) [2]. The presence of viable endometrium available for regeneration after adhesiolysis may be indicated by menstruation and could be of prognostic significance. According in to AFS classification scheme, synechiae are classified into three stages, Stages I–III. Stage III indicates complete obliteration of the uterine cavity (Table 2.3).

The imaging modality of choice for the diagnosis of synechiae is an HSG. The classic finding on HSG is irregular, well-defined, angular, and/or linear filing defects within the cavity. If the synechiae are extensive, they can lead to partial or complete obliteration of the endometrial cavity. However, saline infusion sonography is equally effective in making the diagnosis of intrauterine adhesions as is an HSG and is beginning to replace HSG as the imaging modality of choice [47]. However, a transvaginal ultrasound alone is not adequate to make the diagnosis. Mild adhesions are often asymptomatic and only noted at the time of imaging, yet moderate to severe adhesions may be associated with menstrual abnormalities (hypo- or amenorrhea), recurrent pregnancy loss, or infertility.

Early detection for IUA is a key preventive feature as early adhesions that are filmy, thin, and avascular are easily managed with adhesiolysis. Surgical management of uterine synechiae by hysteroscopic removal of adhesions and scars in an attempt to restore a normal uterine cavity is recommended. Studies have shown that pregnancy rate after surgical management is based on the extent of adhesions preoperatively [48]. Furthermore, it sometimes requires two or more operations to restore normal uterine cavity and achieve normal menstruation and improved pregnancy rates [49]. Despite such interventions, reformation rate of IUA in moderate to severe cases remains high.

A number of studies have been published reporting outcomes of hysteroscopic adhesiolysis of IUA, but no RCT exist. Overall, there appears to be an improvement in the reproductive outcomes especially in women with recurrent pregnancy loss with increase in delivery rate compared to women with infertility. Further, the delivery rate is highest in women with Stage I and Stage II IUA compared to III. Stage III IUA has a grave prognosis, and the use of a gestational carrier should be considered an option. In a large series of 332 women desiring fertility, the reproductive outcomes were followed for an average duration of 27 months, and the overall conception rate after hysteroscopic adhesiolysis was 48.2%. The conception rate decreases with increasing IUA severity (mild, 60.7%; moderate, 53.4%; severe, 25%) [50]. In a smaller series of women with IUA and infertility, the overall conception rate after hysteroscopic adhesiolysis was 40.4%, with the highest rate seen in mild cases, compared to moderate and severe, 58, 30, and 33%, respectively [51]. No pregnancies occurred in women who needed repeat adhesiolysis.

The key to managing IUA is early detection and surgical treatment. Moderate to severe adhesions in addition to any adhesion blocking tubal ostia should be promptly managed with hysteroscopic lysis. When mild adhesions are encountered, surgical treatment should be reserved for cases where no other cause for infertility or recurrent pregnancy loss can be found. The minimum endometrium needed to attain and sustain a normal pregnancy remains unknown.

2.4.4 Adenomyosis

One final acquired lesion that is worth mentioning is adenomyosis. Adenomyosis is typically noted in women in their third and fourth decades of life. It is a benign process characterized by endometrial glands and stroma invading the myometrium, and it can be diffuse or focal (adenomyoma).

The initial imaging modality of choice is the transvaginal ultrasound [52]. Ultrasound images demonstrate the loss of the endometrial-myometrial junctional zone and an enlarged, globular uterus [52]. MRI is also equally effective in the diagnosis demonstrating diffusely enlarged junctional zone with poorly defined margins and small, bright T2-weighted signal intensity projecting into the myometrium consistent with endometrial glands. Further, the MRI has added value in distinguishing between a myoma and an adenomyoma [52].

Typically, patients experience abnormal uterine bleeding and dysmenorrhea, and there may be a role for hormonal therapy to alleviate such symptoms prior to adenomyomectomy or hysterectomy. There is a lack of good-quality evidence to suggest that adenomyosis is associated with infertility, and although some advocate surgery to remove the adenomyosis, surgical management is not widely recommended for treatment of infertility.

In summary, overall, the imaging modality of choice for acquired uterine lesions is transvaginal sonography, preferably with 3D imaging and/or SIS, and reserving MRI only if further characterization and/or presurgical mapping is needed. The type of acquired uterine lesion dictates the potential adverse impact on fertility. At present surgical intervention may be of benefit for cavitary-distorting myomas, uterine synechiae, and possibly endometrial polyps in improving clinical pregnancy rate, but improvement in live birth rate remains to be elucidated.

References

1. Kaproth-Joslin K, Dogra V. Imaging of female infertility. A pictorial guide to the hysterosalpingography, ultrasonography, and magnetic resonance imaging findings of the congenital and acquired causes of female fertility. Radiol Clin N Am. 2013;51(6):967–81.
2. American Fertility Society Classification of adnexal adhesions, distal tubal occlusion, tubal occlusion secondary to tubal ligation, tubal pregnancies, mullerian anomalies and intrauterine adhesions. Fertil Steril. 1988;49:944–55.
3. Chan YY, Jayaprakasan R, Zamora J, Thornton JG, Raine-Fenning N, Coomarasamy A. The prevalence of congenital uterine anomalies in unselected and high-risk populations: a systematic review. Hum Reprod Update. 2011;17:761–71.
4. Saravelos SH, Cocksedge KA, Li TC. Prevalence and diagnosis of congenital uterine anomalies in women with reproductive failure: a critical appraisal. Hum Reprod Update. 2008;14:415–29.

5. Moini A, Mohammadi S, Hosseini R, Eslami B, Ahmadi F. Accuracy of 3dimsneional sonography for diagnosis and classification of congenital uterine anomalies. J Ultrasound Med. 2013;32:923–7.
6. Robbins JB, Broadwell C, Chow LC, Parry JP, Sadowski EA. Mullerian duct anomalies: embryological development, classification, and MRI assessment. Magn Reson Imaging. 2014;41:1–12.
7. Li Y, Phelps A, Zapala MA, et al. Magnetic resonance imaging of mullerian duct anomalies. Pediatr Radiol. 2016;46:796–805.
8. Ludwin A, Pityriski K, Ludwin I, Banas T, Knafel A. Two- and three-dimensional ultrasonography and sonohysterography versus hysteroscopy with laparoscopy in the differential diagnosis of septate, bicornuate, and arcuate uteri. J Minim Invasive Gynecol. 2013;20:90–9.
9. Makris N, Kalmantis K, Skartados N, et al. Three-dimensional hysterosonography versus hysteroscopy for the detection of intracavitary uterine abnormalities. Int J Gynecol Obstet. 2007;97:6–9.
10. Ludwin A, Ludwin I, Kudla M, Pitynski K, Banas T, Jach R, Knafel A. Diagnostic accuracy of three-dimensional sonohysterography compared with office hysteroscopy and its interrater/intrarater agreement in uterine cavity assessment after hysteroscopic metroplasty. Fertil Steril. 2014;101:1392–9.
11. Groszmann Y, Benacerraf B. Complete evaluation of anatomy and morphology of the infertile patient in a single visit; the modern infertility pelvic ultrasound examination. Fertil Steril. 2016;105:1381–93.
12. Detti L. Ultrasound assessment of uterine cavity remodeling after surgical correction of subseptations. Am J Obstet Gynecol. 2014;210:262.e1–6.
13. Graupera B, Pascual MA, Hereter L, Browne L, Ubeda B, Rodriguez I, Pedrero C. Accuracy of three-dimensional ultrasound compared with magnetic resonance imaging in diagnosis of mullerian duct anomalies using ESHRE-ESGE consensus on the classification of congenital anomalies of the female genital tract. Ultrasound Obstet Gynecol. 2015;46:616–22.
14. Fedele L, Dorta M, Brioschi D, Giudici MN, Candiani GB. Magnetic resonance imaging in Mayer-Rokitansky-Kuster-Hauser syndrome. Obstet Gynecol. 1990;76:593–6.
15. Acien P. Incidence of mullerian defects in fertile and infertile women. Hum Reprod. 1997;12:1372–6.
16. Reichman D, Laufer MR, Robinson BK. Pregnancy outcomes in unicornuate uteri: a review. Fertil Steril. 2009;91:1886–94.
17. Venetis CA, Papadopoulos SP, Campo R, Gordts S, Tartlatzis BC, Grimbizis GF. Clinical implications of congenital uterine anomalies: a meta-analysis of comparative studies. Reprod Biomed Online. 2014;29:665–83.
18. Vallerie AM, Breech LL. Update in Mullerian anomalies: diagnosis, management, and outcomes. Curr Opin Obstet Gynecol. 2010;22:381–7.
19. Rysavy MA, Li L, Bell EF, et al. Between hospital variation in treatment and outcomes in extremely preterm infants. N Engl J Med. 2015;372:1801–11.
20. Practice Committee of the American Society for Reproductive Medicine. Uterine septum: a guideline. Fertil Steril. 2016;106:530–40.
21. Woelfer B, Salim R, Banerjee S, Elson J, Regan L, Jurkovic D. Reproductive outcomes in women with congenital uterine anomalies detected by three dimensional ultrasound screening. Obstet Gynecol. 2001;98:1099–103.
22. Paradisi R, Barzanti R, Natali F, et al. Hysteroscopic metroplasty: reproductive outcome in relation to septum size. Arch Gynecol Obstet. 2014;289:671–6.
23. Heinonen PK, Pustynen PP. Primary infertility and uterine anomalies. Fertil Steril. 1983;40:311–6.
24. Valle RF, Ekpo GE. Hysteroscopic metroplasty for the septate uterus: review and meta-analysis. J Minim Invasive Gynecol. 2013;20:22–42.
25. Acien P. Reproductive performance of women with uterine malformations. Hum Reprod. 1993;8:122–6.
26. Grimbizis GF, Camus M, Tarlatzis BC, et al. Clinical implications of uterine malformations and hysteroscopic treatment results. Hum Reprod Update. 2001;7:161–74.
27. Grynberg M, Gervaise A, Faivre E, Deffieux X, Frydman R, Fernandez H. Treatment of twenty-two patient with complete uterine and vaginal septum. J Minim Invasive Gynecol. 2012;19:34–9.
28. Tomazevic T, Ban-Frangez H, Virant-Klun I, Verdenik I, Poziep B, Vrtacnik-Bokai E. Septate, subseptate and arcuate uterus decrease pregnancy and live birth rates in IVF/ICSI. Reprod Biol Online. 2010;21:700–5.
29. Heinonen PK. Complete septate uterus with longitudinal vaginal septum. Fertil Steril. 2006;85:700–5.
30. Nappi C, Di Spiezio Sardo A. State of the art. Hysteroscopic approach to the pathologies of the genital tract. Tuttlingen: Endopress; 2014.
31. Ciarmela P, Islam S, Reis FM, et al. Growth factors and myometrium: biologic effects in uterine fibroid and possible clinical implications. Hum Reprod Update. 2011;17:772–90.
32. Griffin Y, Sudigali V, Jacques A. Radiology of benign disorders of menstruation. Semin Ultrasound CT MR. 2010;116:747–58.
33. Munro MG, Critchley HO, Broder MS, Fraser IS, FIGO Working Group on Menstrual Disorders. FIGO classification system (PALM-COEIN) for causes of abnormal uterine bleeding in nongravid women of reproductive age. Int J Gynecol Obstet. 2011;113:3–13.
34. Pritts EA, Parher WH, Olive DL. Fibroids and infertility; an updated systematic review of the evidence. Fertil Steril. 2009;91:1215–23.
35. Practice Committee of the American Society for Reproductive Medicine. Removal of myomas in asymptomatic patients to improve fertility and/or reduce miscarriage rate: a guideline. Fertil Steril. 2017;108:416–25.
36. Metawally M, Cheong YC, Horne AW. Surgical treatment of fibroids for subfertility. Cochrane Database Syst Rev. 2012;11:CD003857.
37. Galliano D, Bellver J, Diaz-Garcia C, Simon C, Pellicer A. ART and uterine pathology: how relevant is the maternal side for implantation? Hume Reprod Update. 2015;21:13–38.
38. Casini MI, Rossi F, Agostini R, Unifer V. Effects of the position of fibroids on fertility. Gynecol Endocrinol. 2006;22:106–9.
39. Aboulghar MM, Al-Inany HG, Aboulghar MA, Serour GI, Mansour RT. The effect of intramural fibroids on the outcome of IVF. Middle East Fertil Soc J. 2004;9:263–7.
40. Seoud M, Patterson R, Musher S, Coddington C. Effects of myoma or prior myomectomy on in vitro fertilization (IVF) performance. J Assist Reprod Genet. 1992;9:217–21.
41. Surrey E, Minjarez D, Stevens J, Schoolcraft W. Effect of myomectomy on the outcome of assisted reproductive technologies. Fertil Steril. 2005;83:1473–9.
42. Bittencourt CA, Dos Santos Simoes R, Bernardo WM, Fuchs LFP, Soares Junior JM, Pastore AR, Bracat EC. Accuracy of saline contrast sonohysterography in detection of endometrial polyps and submucosal leiomyomas in women of reproductive age with abnormal uterine bleeding: systematic review and meta-analysis. Ultrasound Obstet Gynecol. 2017;50:32–9.
43. Perez-Medina T, Baj-Arenas J, Salazar F, Redondo T, Sanfrutos L, Alvarez P, Engels V. Endometrial polyps and their implication in the pregnancy rates of patient undergoing intrauterine insemination. Hum Reprod. 2005;20:1632–5.
44. Pereira N, Amrane S, Estes JL, Lekovich JP, Elias RT, Chung PH, Rosenwaks Z. Does the time interval between hysteroscopic polypectomy and start of in vitro fertilization affect outcomes? Fertil Steril. 2016;105:539–44.
45. Jayaprakasan K, Polanski L, Sahu B, Thornton JG, Raine-Fenning N. Surgical intervention versus expectant management for endometrial polyps in subfertility women. Cochrane Database Syst Rev. 2014;8:CD009592.

46. Kodaman PH. Hysteroscopic polypectomy for women undergoing IVF treatment: when is it necessary? Curr Opin Obstet Gynecol. 2016;28:184–90.
47. Deans R, Abborr J. Review of Intrauterine adhesions. J Minim Invasive Gynecol. 2010;17:555–69.
48. Valle RF, Sciarra JJ. Intrauterine adhesions: hysteroscopic diagnosis, classification, treatment, and reproductive outcome. Am J Obstet Gynecol. 1988;158:1459–70.
49. Hanstede MM, van der Meij E, Goedemans L, Emanuel MH. Results of centralized Asherman 1 surgery, 2003–2013. Fertil Steril. 2015;104:1561–8.
50. Chen L, Zhang H, Wang Q, Xie F, Gao S, Song Y, Dong J, Feng H, Xie K, Sui L. Reproductive outcomes in patients with intrauterine adhesions following hysteroscopic adhesiolysis: experience from the largest women's hospital in China. Arch Gynecol Obstet. 2010;281:355–61.
51. Roy KK, Baruah J, Sharma JB, Kumar S, Kachawa G, Singh N. Reproductive outcome following hysteroscopic adhesiolysis in patients with infertility due to Asherman's syndrome. Arch Gynecol Obstet. 2010;281:355–61.
52. Valentini AL, Gul SS, Sogali BG, et al. Adenomyosis: from the sign to the diagnosis, imaging, diagnostic pitfall and differential diagnosis: a pictorial review. Radiol Med. 2011;116:1267–87.

3 Assessment of Ovarian Reserve and Its Implications on Fertility

Caitlin Dunne and Jon Havelock

The goal of the patient who is experiencing infertility is to achieve a healthy live birth at term. Prior to embarking on treatment directed towards that outcome, it is invaluable to be able to provide the patient(s) with prognostic information on their proposed treatments. Towards that aim, ovarian reserve tests (ORT) have been developed, with the goal of being able to predict the probability of fertility treatment success. However, in spite of the limited value of many of these tests in predicting the gold standard of fertility treatment success (live birth), they are routinely performed without a clear understanding by the physician or patient as to the clinical utility of the result. Furthermore, some of these ovarian reserve tests have now been advocated for mass screening as a predictor of fertility potential in women not currently trying to conceive. Such widespread testing of fertility potential by ORT without meeting the requisite principles of a valid screening test can lead to unnecessary interventions for individuals who may be advised to consider fertility treatments when scant evidence demonstrates they are needed [1].

3.1 Ovarian Reserve Testing: What Are We Measuring and Why Are We Measuring It?

While the literature has described a multitude of ORTs, there are a select number that are most commonly utilized. Currently, the most common ORTs consist of female age, day 3/basal FSH, antral follicle count (AFC), and anti-Müllerian hormone (AMH). To further understand their utility in the context of fertility, it is important to understand their predictive value for spontaneous conception in the fertile population, predictive value of live birth in the context of fertility treatment, and the value of ORT in predicting ovarian response in IVF. When ordering and interpreting an ORT, it is important that the test is interpreted in the context of one of these specific scenarios.

3.2 Age as an Ovarian Reserve Test

In the literal and figurative sense, female age is the oldest and most widely accepted ORT. Spontaneous and treatment-related reproductive senescence has no greater influence than chronologic age (Fig. 3.1). At age 20, the inability for a live birth is approximately 2.4%, with significant reduction in fertility in the fourth and fifth decades, with 35% of women unable to achieve a live birth at age 40, 50% of women

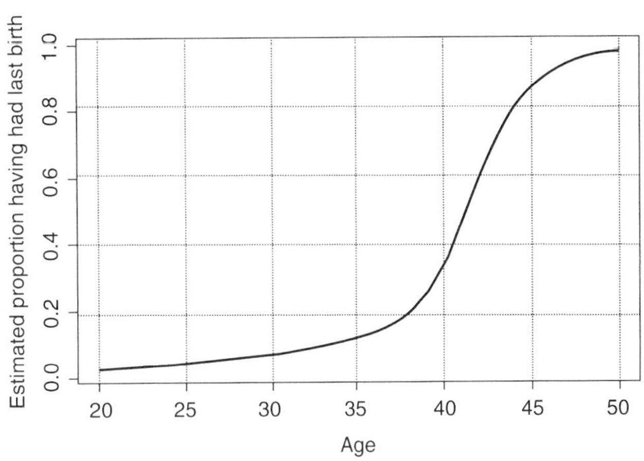

Fig. 3.1 Age at live birth curve for six natural fertility populations. (From Eijkemans MJC, van Poppel F, Habbema DF, Smith KR, Leridon H, Velde te ER. Too old to have children? Lessons from natural fertility populations. Human Reproduction. 2014 Jun;29(6):1304–12, with permission)

C. Dunne (✉)
Pacific Centre for Reproductive Medicine (PCRM), University of British Columbia, Vancouver, BC, Canada
e-mail: cdunne@pacificfertility.ca

J. Havelock
Division of Reproductive Endocrinology and Infertility, Department of Obstetrics and Gynecology, University of British Columbia, Vancouver, BC, Canada

G. N. Allahbadia et al. (eds.), *Textbook of Assisted Reproduction*, https://doi.org/10.1007/978-981-15-2377-9_3

unable to achieve a live birth at age 41, and 90% at age 45 [2]. Nothing has greater impact in reducing the risk of unwanted childlessness or the inability to achieve the desired number of children than attempting conception at a younger female age. However, the effect of primary interventions to achieve the aim of decreasing the age at attempted conception (i.e., through the implementation of fertility assessment clinics) remains unknown [3].

Advancing female reproductive age is immutable and is associated with increasing disease prevalence. As a result, a larger cohort of older patients will subsequently experience infertility and pursue assisted reproductive technologies (ART) or medically assisted reproduction (MAR) in an effort to compensate for the loss in natural fertility. The probability of achieving the desired family size can be improved through the use of MAR. If a female patient is willing to accept a 90% probability of having either a one-, two-, or three-child family, she can delay childbearing by 3–5 years, if she is willing to undergo IVF treatment to achieve the desired family size (Table 3.1) [4]. However, this prediction model assumes that the patient is willing to undergo up to three full IVF cycles. However, on a per IVF cycle using non-donor eggs, the chance of a live birth per fresh IVF cycle which started in the USA in 2014 was 37% for female age under 35 years, 30% for age 35–37, 19% for age 38–40, 10% for age 41–42, 4% for age 43–44, and 1% for age 45 and greater [5]. While the reduction in pregnancy rates is partially explained due to an increase in cycle cancellations and embryo transfer cancellations due to an increasing prevalence of poor ovarian response with advancing female age, the predominant factor for failure to achieve live birth is due to failed ongoing embryo implantation. Comprehensive chromosomal screening data has demonstrated that while the blastocyst development yield is attenuated with age, the greatest factor is the high prevalence of embryonic aneuploidy with advancing female age (Fig. 3.2) [6].

While live birth remains the most important IVF outcome, poor ovarian response (POR) is an important surrogate outcome, as POR is related to low probability of live birth with IVF. Using conventional ovarian stimulation protocols, cycle cancellation, or retrieval of three or fewer oocytes occurs in approximately 15% of females under age 30 undergoing IVF and increases to 50% after age 40 [7]. Such prognostic information, in the absence of the addition of other ORTs, provides an initial crude estimate of the probability of cycle cancellation or suboptimal oocyte yield, leading to decreased likelihood of IVF treatment success.

Table 3.1 Maximum female age (years) at which couples should start building a one-, two-, or three-child family, for a 50, 75, and 90% chance of realizing the desired family size, with and without IVF

Chance of realization	One-child family	Two-child family	Three-child family
Without IVF			
50%	41	38	35
75%	37	34	31
90%	32	27	23
With IVF			
50%	42	39	36
75%	39	35	33
90%	35	31	28

From Habbema JDF, Eijkemans MJC, Leridon H, Velde te ER. Realizing a desired family size: when should couples start? Human Reproduction. 2015 Sep;30(9):2215–21, with permission

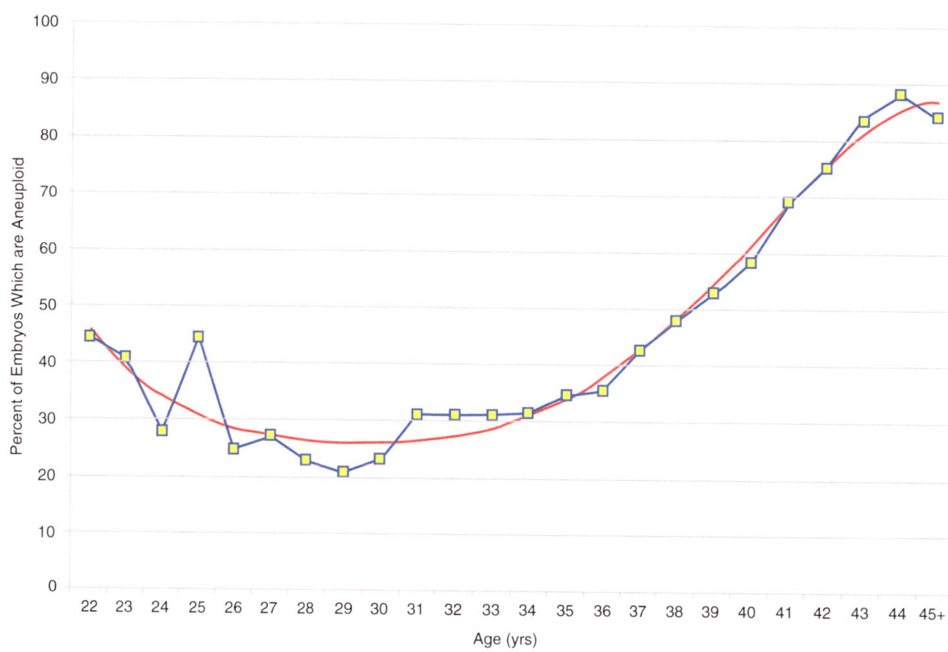

Fig. 3.2 The prevalence of aneuploidy from trophectoderm biopsies of embryos obtained at IVF, relative to the female age. (From Franasiak JM, Forman EJ, Hong KH, Werner MD, Upham KM, Treff NR, et al. The nature of aneuploidy with increasing age of the female partner: a review of 15,169 consecutive trophectoderm biopsies evaluated with comprehensive chromosomal screening. Fertility and Sterility. 2014 Mar;101(3):656–663.e1, with permission)

3.3 Follicle-Stimulating Hormone

Follicle-stimulating hormone (FSH) is the dimeric glycoprotein produced by the anterior pituitary, responsible for testicular spermatogenesis and ovarian folliculogenesis, acting on its cognate receptor on the Sertoli cell and granulosa cell, respectively. Documentation of early follicular phase (basal/cycle day 2–4) FSH elevations with reproductive aging was first established more than 40 years ago [8]. Through observation of the endocrine characteristics in IVF cycles of poor responders, it was determined that early follicular FSH levels were frequently elevated [9]. FSH has been the most ubiquitous and accepted initial endocrine ovarian reserve test. However, it is an ORT with significant limitation, and in most circumstances should be used as a prognostic aid, rather than an exclusionary test.

The regulation of FSH production and secretion is under the control of gonadal sex steroids, as well as inhibin B (another ORT of limited value and now infrequently used). Loss of gonadal function at menopause results in significant elevations of FSH through the interruption of the classic endocrine negative feedback loop of the hypothalamic-pituitary-ovarian axis. This FSH elevation at menopause is the sine qua non laboratory result, such that measurement of FSH at menopause has no clinical value in making the diagnosis. It has been the goal of many clinician scientists to determine the threshold value of FSH to predict either successful or unsuccessful outcomes of fertility treatments and, to a limited extent, predict spontaneous conception.

There has been limited research on the value of basal FSH testing in the prediction of spontaneous conception, as earlier fertility research and testing have largely been targeted towards treatment rather than prevention of disease. The largest study to date on basal FSH levels in spontaneous pregnancy examined 3519 subfertile women and found that FSH levels of 8 IU/L were associated with reduction in the probability of spontaneous pregnancy within the subsequent 12 months of attempted conception (Hazard Ratio 0.93 IU/L) [10]. However, this study was conducted in an unexplained, subfertile population, where the ongoing pregnancy rate over the subsequent 12 months was only 16%, indicating that past subfertility was the greatest predictor of future subfertility.

There is high-quality evidence from two large randomized controlled trials to suggest that moderate elevations in basal FSH levels (10–15 IU/L) in conjunction with mildly elevated day 3 estradiol levels (40–100 pg/ml) in women aged 21–42 undergoing controlled ovarian stimulation and intrauterine insemination (COH/IUI) are associated with futile outcomes [11]. This subset of 19 patients (58 COH/IUI cycles) in a study of 603 patients had a 0% live birth rate, with a 33% live birth rate when undergoing IVF. Women with FSH levels of 10–15 IU/L and day 3 estradiol levels under 40 pg/ml had similar live birth rates when undergoing COH/IUI, when compared to women with FSH levels <10 IU/L. The value of the day 3 estradiol in conjunction with the FSH result serves to confirm the proper timing of the FSH level in the early follicular phase, as well as to effectively rule out artificially low basal FSH due to a functional ovarian cyst. However, this study suggests that even moderately elevated follicular phase estradiol levels, in conjunction with a moderately elevated FSH, may be further suppressing an otherwise higher FSH level through negative inhibition and that the combination of these two ORT findings should provide consideration to counsel the patient/couple into more intensive but successful treatment (IVF). A recent analysis of 2019 IUI cycles with the husband's sperm revealed that FSH levels ≤7 IU/L were associated with an odds ratio of 1.4 for pregnancy [12].

The use of basal FSH testing seems to have its greatest utility in conjunction with prediction of IVF outcomes. Unfortunately, it is a very insensitive test (normal results are poor in determining whether IVF will be successful) but does have good positive predictive value (PPV—elevated FSH levels are good in determining that IVF will be unsuccessful). A 2004 meta-analysis, using basal FSH cut-offs ranging from 11 to 25 IU/L for patients undergoing fertility treatments (predominantly IVF), found a test sensitivity of 6.6%, with a PPV of 92% when disease prevalence was 40% [13]. There is demonstrable inter-cycle variability with basal FSH testing, leading to the rationale to attempting IVF and ovarian stimulation during a cycle with a lower basal FSH. The largest study to date looking at repetitive basal FSH levels in women undergoing multiple IVF cycles found that overall maximum FSH levels predicted IVF cycle cancellation rates better than current cycle FSH level [14]. When comparing cycles where the prior maximum FSH level was >13 IU/L, subsequent IVF cycles with a current normalized FSH level resulted in an increase of 0.5 metaphase II oocytes when compared to IVF cycles where the FSH level was persistently elevated, without a corresponding increase in pregnancy rates. It appears then that using an improved, current basal FSH level as an indicator for treatment initiation has very little supportive evidence. Rather, it appears ovarian reserve screening by repetitive basal FSH measurements to determine maximal basal FSH levels is a way to modestly improve the sensitivity of basal FSH testing. However, such a screening strategy may result in treatment delay and at FSH threshold levels of above 13 IU/L will result in the loss of the ability for adequate treatment intervention in a latent stage of the disease.

The best use for basal FSH seems to be to use threshold levels for predicting IVF success (live birth rates). Basal FSH level of <7 IU/L seems to correlate with highest live birth rates when stratified by age, and basal FSH levels of >18 IU/L correlate with live birth rates of <2% (Fig. 3.3) [15]. FSH levels are not reassuring at any age, and any

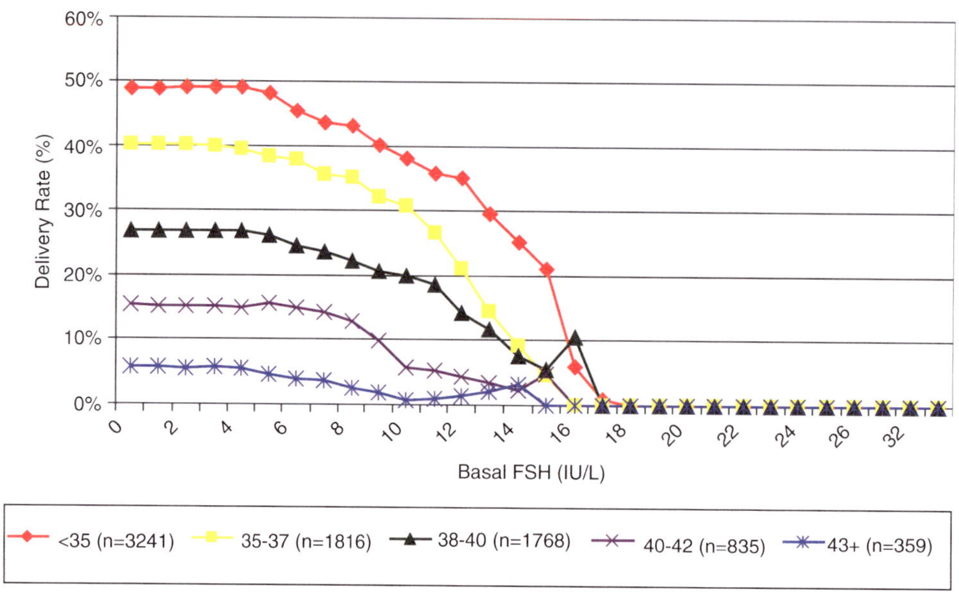

Fig. 3.3 Greater-than-efficiency curve calculations for basal FSH levels, calculated in 1-IU/L increments. Efficiency curves involve sequential calculation of the delivery rate at every possible threshold, starting at 1 IU/L and moving upward to the highest level in the population. (From Scott RT, Elkind-Hirsch KE, Styne-Gross A, Miller KA, Frattarelli JL. The predictive value for in vitro fertility delivery rates is greatly impacted by the method used to select the threshold between normal and elevated basal follicle-stimulating hormone. Fertility and Sterility. Elsevier; 2008 Apr;89(4):868–78, with permission)

elevation above 7 IU/L should cause concern. Moreover, progressive rise in the FSH levels above 7 IU/L should cause increasing concern.

3.4 Antral Follicle Count (AFC)

The decline in natural fertility parallels the primordial follicle depletion with ovarian aging. The transition of select primordial follicles into the growing follicular pool allows for direct visualization by endovaginal ultrasound when these growing follicles develop a fluid-filled antrum reaching a diameter of 2 mm. Although direct measurement of the primordial follicle pool is not possible, histologic studies from ovaries removed at surgery have shown a good correlation between the primordial follicle number and the ovarian antral follicle count measured on endovaginal ultrasound [16]. It is this correlation that serves as the rationale for antral follicle count (AFC) measurements as an ORT.

Certain limitations exist in the use of AFC measurements as an ORT. The test requires adequate visualization of both ovaries by ≥7 MHz frequency, 2D-endovaginal ultrasound, in order to determine the total AFC. The AFC result could be imprecise in the presence of ovarian pathology (i.e., ovarian endometrioma or other ovarian mass). The AFC should optimally be performed in the early follicular phase (preferably not during oral contraceptive use (OCP), as there may be a modest reduction in AFC in OCP users) [17]. All follicles between 2 and 10 mm should be counted in each ovary, and a total AFC should be determined by combining each individual ovarian AFC [18]. Even with the attempt to standardize the AFC measurement process, the test has significant intra- and inter-observer variability, with limits of agreement of AFC between +8 and −7 follicles when two measurements are performed by the same operator and similar results when performed by two different operators [19]. Additionally, improvements in ultrasound resolution have resulted in raising the AFC cut-offs predicting poor ovarian response. Such variance can hamper the performance characteristics of AFC as an ORT. In spite of these limitations, when measuring the AFC across consecutive menstrual cycles, there seems to be minimal inter-cycle variability, with inter-class coefficient of 0.71 [20]. The AFC still remains an attractive ORT as it is a simple, point of care test that additionally yields useful anatomic information in the female fertility work-up.

There is a demonstrable decline in the ovarian AFC with age in women with proven natural fertility, with a decline of AFC of 4.8% per year before age 37, and an 11.7% annual decline thereafter [21]. Additionally, this decline has shown to occur at a similar rate in the infertile population as well. However, there does not seem to be measurable differences in AFC measurements in fertile and infertile women under age 40, suggesting that a single AFC measurement in the fertile population should not be used in an attempt to predict future infertility [22]. Additionally, the observation of infertile women with poor ovarian response may simply represent the expected, age-related decline that would be seen in equivalent proportion if fertile women underwent controlled ovarian stimulation. AFC, when controlling for age, does not predict oocyte quality, with similar clinical pregnancy rates and miscarriage rates in women undergoing therapeutic donor insemination [23]. Together, these findings would suggest that a low AFC discovered incidentally, or in the course of fertility investigations, should not be a reason for expedited IVF treatment.

The value of AFC as an ORT is in its predictive value for ovarian response. In an individual patient data (IPD) meta-analysis of 5705 women undergoing IVF, while age was the best predictor of poor ovarian response (area under receiver-operating characteristic curve (AUC) 0.61), AFC improved the prediction model (AUC 0.76). The addition of AMH to AFC and age did not improve prediction of poor response, and AMH and age had an equivalent AUC to AFC and age [24]. The best AFC threshold for predicting poor ovarian response is not accurately defined, with AFC cut-offs ranging between <3 and <12 [25]. In addition to predicting poor ovarian response, numerous retrospective and prospective observational studies have shown that high AFC is predictive of ovarian hyper-response (>15–20 oocytes). The most commonly used AFC threshold for predicting ovarian hyper-response is 14 [25], with a positive predictive value (PPV) of 58% for retrieval of more than 20 oocytes [26]. Increasing the AFC cut-off to 18 will improve the PPV to 71%. AFC does not appear to have any incremental value in predicting IVF outcome, with age being the best predictor [24].

3.5 Anti-Müllerian Hormone

3.5.1 The History of AMH

Long before it was touted as the possible "holy grail" of ovarian reserve testing, anti-Müllerian hormone (AMH) was described by Professor Albert Jost for its role in sexual differentiation [27, 28]. His series of experiments in the 1940s demonstrated that Sertoli cell-derived AMH (also called Müllerian-inhibiting substance (MIS)) was required in combination with testicular testosterone to virilize the Wolffian ducts, urogenital sinus, and external genitalia while simultaneously inducing regression of the Müllerian ducts to form a male fetus [27]. Several decades later, AMH production by adult ovarian granulosa cells in hens suggested that the hormone was important for normal reproductive physiology even after the Müllerian ducts were gone [29].

AMH is a dimeric glycoprotein with a molecular weight of 140 kD, encoded by a gene on the short arm of chromosome 19 [30]. It is a member of the transforming growth factor-beta (TGF-β) superfamily [31]. The expression of AMH is markedly different in males and females, both in concentration and temporality. In males, Sertoli cells maintain a high concentration of AMH in utero which peaks shortly after birth and then drops precipitously at puberty [32]. In females, granulosa cells produce very low levels of AMH in utero followed by a transient spike in the neonatal period. Concentrations of the hormone then rise steadily through adolescence to a peak in the mid-twenties and subsequently decline until becoming undetectable in menopause [33]. Nomograms of serum AMH concentration have been validated throughout the life span (Fig. 3.4) [33, 34].

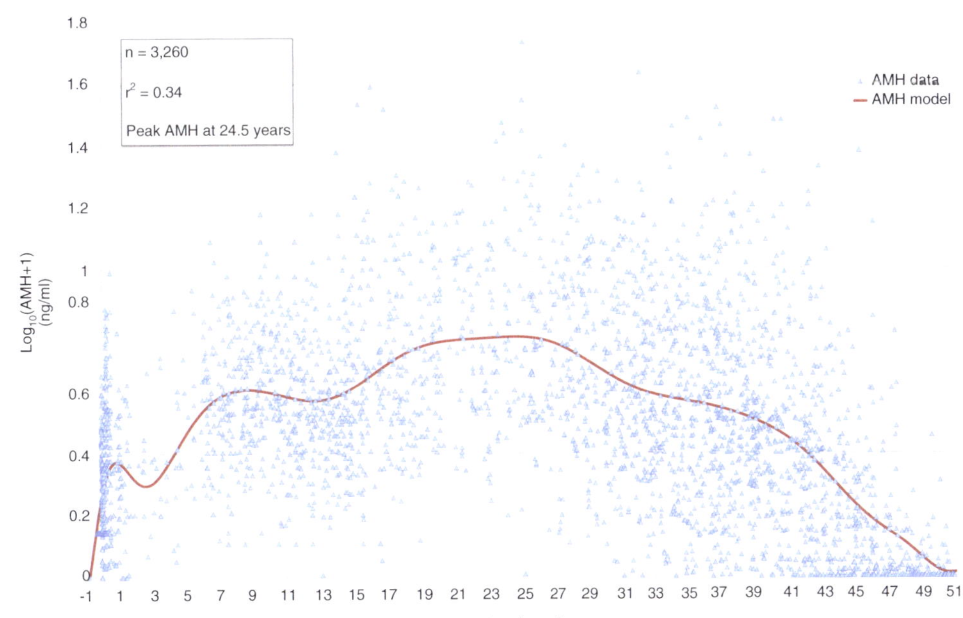

Fig. 3.4 Serum top right corner: AMH data. The red line is the model that best fits the 3260 datapoints shown as triangles. The coefficient of determination, r^2, is 0.34, indicating that 34% of variation in serum AMH concentrations is due to age alone. Peak serum AMH is at 24.5 years. (From Kelsey TW, Wright P, Nelson SM, Anderson RA, Wallace WHB. A validated model of serum anti-müllerian hormone from conception to menopause. Vitzthum VJ, editor. PLoS ONE. Public Library of Science; 2011;6(7):e22024, with permission)

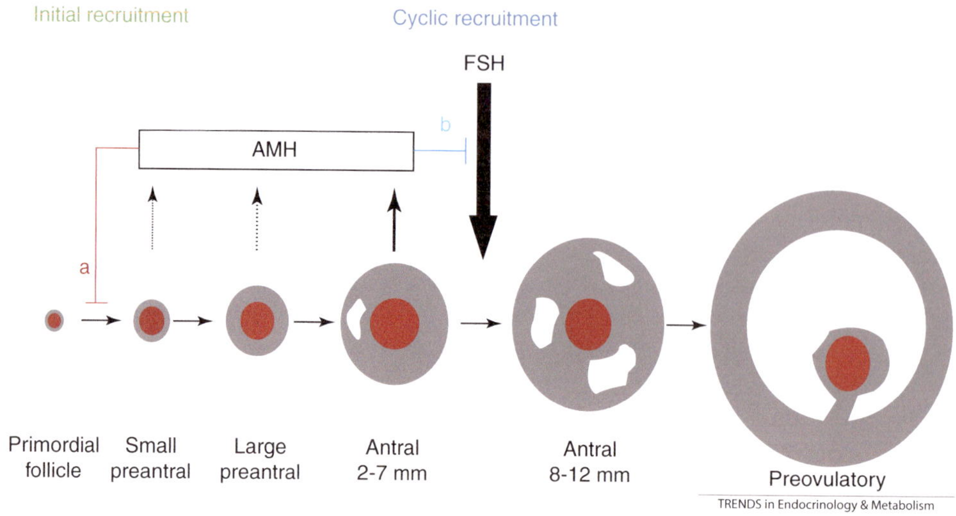

Fig. 3.5 AMH is only produced by pre-antral and small antral follicles which have ascended from the much larger primordial follicle pool. (From Broekmans FJ, Visser JA, Laven JSE, Broer SL, Themmen APN, Fauser BC. Anti-Müllerian hormone and ovarian dysfunction. Trends Endocrinol Metab. 2008 Nov;19(9):340–7, with permission)

Early clinical applications of AMH included the diagnostic workup of intersex disorders, differentiating between cryptorchidism and anorchia and clinical monitoring of sex cord-stromal tumors [32, 35]. In recent years AMH has been increasingly utilized to assess a woman's ovarian reserve. It can be used to assess the effect of chemotherapy, pelvic irradiation, and ovarian surgery, all of which are known to be detrimental to ovarian reserve. More commonly, AMH is used to plan controlled ovarian stimulation in an in vitro fertilization (IVF) cycle.

3.5.2 AMH as an Ovarian Reserve Test

A woman's true "ovarian reserve" comprises her pool of oogonia formed during fetal life and then arrested in primordial follicles. Anti-Müllerian hormone has been described as the "follicular gatekeeper" that limits the size of the cohort available to respond to pituitary gonadotropins each month [36, 37]. AMH is only produced by pre-antral and small antral follicles which have ascended from the much larger primordial follicle pool and is therefore perhaps more appropriately termed a "functional" ovarian reserve test (Fig. 3.5) [38]. However, because both true and functional ovarian reserves decline in parallel as a woman ages, AMH represents an accurate, indirect hormonal assessment of a woman's remaining egg number [39].

The dominant follicle and corpus luteum do not secrete AMH and accordingly, AMH levels have been demonstrated to remain relatively stable throughout the menstrual cycle [36, 40]. A small amount of intra-individual variability exists across menstrual cycles, although it is likely not substantial enough to warrant repeated measurement [41]. Younger women appear to have more pronounced variation in AMH between cycles and this fluctuation decreases with age [42].

Patient characteristics and lifestyle factors that can influence AMH have been identified. In a linear regression analysis of 887 women seeking fertility assessment, AMH was found to be 19% lower (95% CI 9.1–29.3%) in users of the oral contraceptive pill compared with non-users, irrespective of age, BMI, smoking status, and maternal age at menopause [17]. AMH levels also decline during pregnancy and the peripartum period [43]. Ethnicity may influence AMH, with one study finding lower levels in African-American (25%) and Hispanic (24%) women compared to women of Caucasian descent [44]. Obesity and increasing body mass index (BMI) have been associated with lower AMH in some studies, while others have not demonstrated a difference [36, 45]. Smoking has been associated with an earlier age of menopause [46] but not consistently with lower AMH values [47]. Although ovarian reserve is of obvious importance to reproductive potential, a history of infertility per se does not appear to influence AMH. A prospective study of women under 40 years old compared AMH levels in 382 women with infertility to 350 controls and reported a similar prevalence of very low AMH levels (<0.7 ng/ml) in both groups [22]. Vitamin D deficiency, physical exercise, alcohol use, age at menarche, and socioeconomic status all do not appear to have an effect on AMH [48, 49].

3.5.3 AMH as a Clinical Tool

AMH has been investigated as a tool to help predict age of natural menopause with only modest success. This is arguably because of the complex interaction of genetic, familial, and lifestyle factors that contribute to age of menopause [36]. A recently published long-term observational study followed women recruited in three different settings between 1983 and 2001. They included interval measurements of AMH along with a questionnaire that assessed menstrual status. Regression analysis demonstrated that AMH alone was an independent predictor of time to menopause (Hazard Ratio 0.70, 95% CI 0.56–0.86, $p < 0.001$); however, its predictive effect declined substantially as subjects aged through their late 40s and early 50s [50]. These results are consistent with previous reports that showed menopause is predictable using AMH, only with wide confidence intervals and marked variation between women [36, 51]. AMH appears to add accuracy to menopause forecasting models beyond mother's age at menopause alone, but further refinements are required to make it clinically useful [52]. Variations in the AMH and AMH receptor II (AMHR2) genes are believed to influence the onset of natural menopause via the signaling pathway controlling follicular recruitment [53]. Paradoxically, a study on AMH and AMHR2 polymorphisms failed to find a link between premature ovarian failure and the AMH signal transduction pathway [54]. AMH and AMHR2 polymorphisms are also not associated with ovarian response or outcomes in controlled ovarian stimulation cycles [55].

Natural fecundability is not reduced in young women with low AMH (<1.96 ng/ml) compared to those with normal AMH levels [56]. High AMH (5.6–25.6 ng/ml) has been associated with a reduced probability of conceiving, even when controlling for irregular cycles [56]. In women with a history of recurrent miscarriage, neither low AMH (<1 ng/ml) nor high AMH (>3.5 ng/ml) levels were associated with fecundability in unassisted conceptions [57]. Clinical and biochemical pregnancy loss have also been investigated and found to have no relationship to AMH [58].

3.5.4 AMH in Assisted Reproductive Technology

In 2002 Seifer et al. published a report demonstrating an association between serum AMH levels and the number of retrieved oocytes [59]. Since that publication, the clinical uses for AMH in assisted reproductive technology have been intensely studied and refined.

AMH can reliably be used to predict hyper-response to gonadotropins in a controlled ovarian stimulation cycle. Women known to have a high AMH prior to ovarian stimulation can be expected to produce a similarly high number of oocytes [60, 61]. One publication seeking a consensus among reproductive medicine physicians concluded that hyper-response is a risk when AMH is above 3 ng/ml or antral follicle count (AFC) is higher than 14 [62]. In a retrospective study of patients who experienced ovarian hyperstimulation syndrome compared to matched controls, AMH was noted to be significantly higher in the over-responders compared to the normo-responders (AMH = 3.62 ng/ml vs. 0.63 ng/ml, $p = 0.0036$) [63]. AMH can be helpful to individualize treatment protocols for controlled ovarian stimulation. A prospective cohort study of 538 subjects found that AMH could be used as a tool to assign patients at high risk of over-response (AMH > 2.1 ng/ml) to an antagonist protocol, whereas those with a normal AMH (0.7–2.1 ng/ml) could be treated with a long-agonist protocol. The authors concluded that this approach helped to minimize clinical risk and treatment burden while maintaining pregnancy rates [60].

Women with a very low AMH can be predicted to produce a low number of oocytes with controlled ovarian stimulation. This information can be useful to guide IVF protocol selection and gonadotropin dosing as well as provide an objective measure from which to set expectations. For example, AMH levels below 0.7 ng/ml have a 63% probability of an antral follicle count less than eight [64]. The Bologna criteria requires two of three of the following features to define poor ovarian response (POR): advanced maternal age (≥40 years) or any other risk factor for POR; and a previous POR (≤3 oocytes with a conventional stimulation protocol); an abnormal ovarian reserve test (i.e., AFC < 5–7 or AMH < 0.5–1.1 ng/ml) [7]. A woman over 40 years old with a low AMH could therefore be counseled to expect a low egg number, even with no prior history of stimulation. A finding of low AMH (<0.5–1.1 ng/ml) is considered to perform better than AFC (<5–7) and basal follicle-stimulating hormone (FSH > 10–15 IU/L) for the prediction of poor response to controlled ovarian stimulation (≤3 oocytes) [7]. Some fertility clinics may use low or undetectable AMH levels as a reason not to offer autologous-oocyte IVF. However, because IVF is not universally futile in these cases, it has been argued that preemptive denial of treatment is unjustified [36].

AMH has advantages over day 3 FSH measurement. FSH is highly cycle day-dependent and must be interpreted in the context of estradiol. It is also prone to inter-cycle fluctuations and is not considered valid in some clinical situations, such as women currently taking hormonal contraceptives [65]. As a woman approaches perimenopause and her smaller follicular pool secretes decreasing amounts of inhibin B, the anterior pituitary is permitted to release increasing amounts of FSH. This makes FSH a relatively late marker for ovarian depletion. Even the original publication in 2002 that introduced the association between AMH and mature oocyte yield for IVF showed that high day 3 FSH had a substantially weaker correlation ($r = -0.26$, $p < 0.005$) than low AMH ($r = 0.48$, $p < 0.0005$).

Several studies have compared antral follicle count (AFC) to AMH for ovarian reserve testing and predictive value. The visible (2–9 mm) ovarian follicles on ultrasound that comprise AFC are derived from the pre-antral and small antral pool (1–2 mm follicles) producing the majority of AMH. It logically follows that the correlation between these two biomarkers should be strong. Two reasons have been proposed for why studies favoring one or the other exist in the litera-

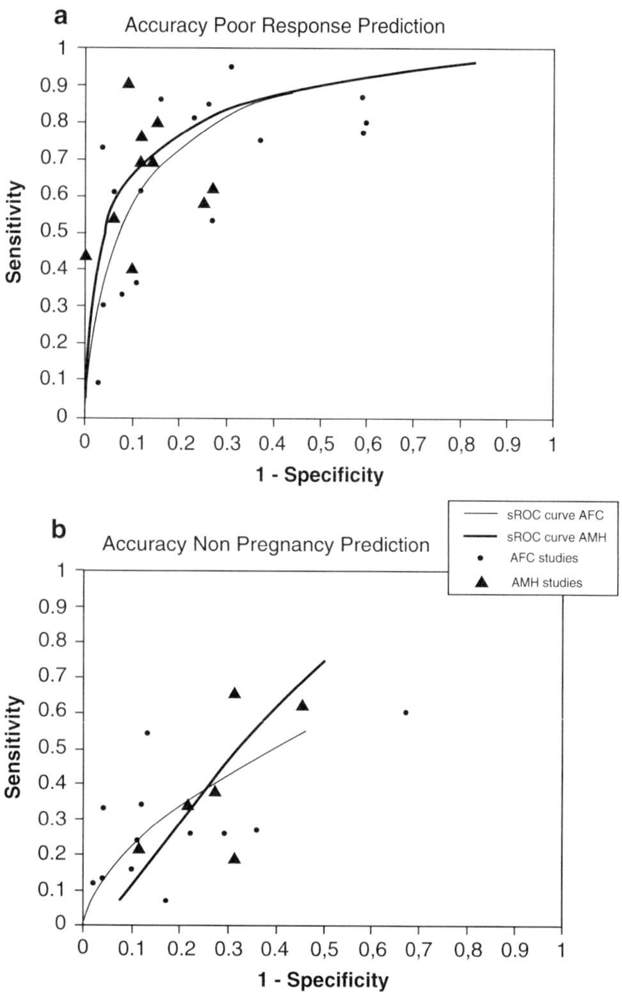

Fig. 3.6 AMH has similar predictive abilities for oocyte yield and poor response with the potential added outcomes of embryo quality, clinical pregnancy, and live birth. (From Broer SL, Mol BWJ, Hendriks D, Broekmans FJM. The role of antimullerian hormone in prediction of outcome after IVF: comparison with the antral follicle count. Fertility and Sterility. Elsevier; 2009 Mar;91(3):705–14, with permission)

ture. First, AFC cannot take into account the health of follicles, and therefore, atretic follicles can contribute to AFC when they would unlikely be producing a normal quantity of AMH [36]. Second, AFC is ultrasound operator-dependent, and it incorporates a wide range of follicle sizes (2–9 mm) compared to AMH [36]. A recent publication compared AMH to AFC separately and in combination with clinical characteristics, to create a model to predict live birth at IVF. They reported that its predictive power was highest when incorporating clinical characteristics and AMH. Receiver operating characteristic (ROC) analysis showed an area under the curve of 0.716 for AMH while adding AFC provided no additional value [66]. A 2015 review paper, which was published as a follow-up to the live debate held at the 2013 American Reproductive Society Annual Meeting, summarized the predictive abilities of AMH and AFC for use in assisted reproduction [49]. AFC has predictive value for number of retrieved oocytes, response to gonadotropins, poor response, and cycle cancellation [49]. AMH has similar predictive abilities for oocyte yield and poor response with the potential added outcomes of embryo quality, clinical pregnancy, and live birth [49, 61] (Fig. 3.6). Those authors concluded that both tests had merit, but that the "objectivity, convenience of untimed sampling, and potential standardization of AMH level make this a preferred method for the evaluation of ovarian reserve in most women" [49].

AMH has recently been validated as a biomarker to optimize and individualize ovarian responsiveness in women undergoing IVF. In a randomized controlled trial (RCT) comparing follitropin delta (with fixed daily dosing based on body weight and serum AMH levels determined using Elecsys AMH immunoassay (Roche Diagnostics International)) to follitropin alpha at 150 IU/day (with subsequent, clinician-determined dose adjustments based on ovarian responsiveness) revealed similar ongoing pregnancy rates (30.7 vs. 31.6%) [67]. However, the AMH determined follitropin-delta dose resulted in fewer poor responses (fewer than 4 oocytes in women with AMH < 15 pM) (11.8 vs. 17.9%), and fewer excessive responses (≥20 oocytes in women with AMH ≥ 15 pM) (10.1 vs. 15.6%), and fewer measures taken to prevent ovarian hyperstimulation. It appears that using AMH-dependent, standardized, and fixed gonadotropin dosing protocols validated through this RCT will result in improvement in MAR outcomes and optimization of ovarian stimulation.

3.6 Conclusions

In spite of the numerous ovarian biomarkers in predicting ovarian reserve, female age remains the best predictor of fecundity. Significantly elevated basal FSH levels (using efficiency curve methodology for threshold determination) can provide high predictive value of probability of absence of live birth approaching 100%. While AFC and AMH provide similar predictive value in predicting ovarian responsiveness in retrospective and observational trials, recent RCT trials suggest that AMH is the best ORT for predicting and individualizing gonadotropin dosing for appropriate ovarian responsiveness and minimizing both poor ovarian response and ovarian hyper-response.

References

1. Wilson JMG, Jungner G. Principles and practice of screening for diseases. Geneva: World Health Organization; 1968. p. 1.
2. Eijkemans MJC, van Poppel F, Habbema DF, Smith KR, Leridon H, te Velde ER. Too old to have children? Lessons from natural fertility populations. Hum Reprod. 2014;29(6):1304–12.

3. Hvidman HW, Petersen KB, Larsen EC, Macklon KT, Pinborg A, Nyboe Andersen A. Individual fertility assessment and pro-fertility counselling; should this be offered to women and men of reproductive age? Hum Reprod. 2015;30(1):9–15.
4. Habbema JDF, Eijkemans MJC, Leridon H, te Velde ER. Realizing a desired family size: when should couples start? Hum Reprod. 2015;30(9):2215–21.
5. art-2014-national-summary-report.pdf.
6. Franasiak JM, Forman EJ, Hong KH, Werner MD, Upham KM, Treff NR, et al. The nature of aneuploidy with increasing age of the female partner: a review of 15,169 consecutive trophectoderm biopsies evaluated with comprehensive chromosomal screening. Fertil Steril. 2014;101(3):656–63.e1.
7. Ferraretti AP, La Marca A, Fauser BCJM, Tarlatzis B, Nargund G, Gianaroli L, et al. ESHRE consensus on the definition of "poor response" to ovarian stimulation for in vitro fertilization: the Bologna criteria. Hum Reprod. 2011;26(7):1616–24.
8. Sherman BM, Korenman SG. Hormonal characteristics of the human menstrual cycle throughout reproductive life. J Clin Invest. 1975;55(4):699–706.
9. Muasher SJ, Oehninger S, Simonetti S, Matta J, Ellis LM, Liu HC, et al. The value of basal and/or stimulated serum gonadotropin levels in prediction of stimulation response and in vitro fertilization outcome. Fertil Steril. 1988;50(2):298–307.
10. van der Steeg JW, Steures P, Eijkemans MJC, Habbema JDF, Hompes PGA, Broekmans FJ, et al. Predictive value and clinical impact of Basal follicle-stimulating hormone in subfertile, ovulatory women. J Clin Endocrinol Metab. 2007;92(6):2163–8.
11. Kaser DJ, Goldman MB, Fung JL, Alper MM, Reindollar RH. When is clomiphene or gonadotropin intrauterine insemination futile? Results of the fast track and standard treatment trial and the forty and over treatment trial, two prospective randomized controlled trials. Fertil Steril. 2014;102(5):1331–1.
12. Dinelli L, Courbière B, Achard V, Jouve E, Deveze C, Gnisci A, et al. Prognosis factors of pregnancy after intrauterine insemination with the husband's sperm: conclusions of an analysis of 2,019 cycles. Fertil Steril. 2014;101(4):994–1000.
13. Jain T, Soules MR, Collins JA. Comparison of basal follicle-stimulating hormone versus the clomiphene citrate challenge test for ovarian reserve screening. Fertil Steril. 2004;82(1):180–5.
14. Gingold JA, Lee JA, Whitehouse MC, Rodriguez-Purata J, Sandler B, Grunfeld L, et al. Maximum basal FSH predicts reproductive outcome better than cycle-specific basal FSH levels: waiting for a "better" month conveys limited retrieval benefits. Reprod Biol Endocrinol. 2015;13(1):91.
15. Scott RT, Elkind-Hirsch KE, Styne-Gross A, Miller KA, Frattarelli JL. The predictive value for in vitro fertility delivery rates is greatly impacted by the method used to select the threshold between normal and elevated basal follicle-stimulating hormone. Fertil Steril. 2008;89(4):868–78.
16. Hansen KR, Hodnett GM, Knowlton N, Craig LB. Correlation of ovarian reserve tests with histologically determined primordial follicle number. Fertil Steril. 2011;95(1):170–5.
17. Birch Petersen K, Hvidman HW, Forman JL, Pinborg A, Larsen EC, Macklon KT, et al. Ovarian reserve assessment in users of oral contraception seeking fertility advice on their reproductive lifespan. Hum Reprod. 2015;30(10):2364–75.
18. Broekmans FJM, de Ziegler D, Howles CM, Gougeon A, Trew G, Olivennes F. The antral follicle count: practical recommendations for better standardization. Fertil Steril. 2010;94(3):1044–51.
19. Deb S, Jayaprakasan K, Campbell BK, Clewes JS, Johnson IR, Raine-Fenning NJ. Intraobserver and interobserver reliability of automated antral follicle counts made using three-dimensional ultrasound and SonoAVC. Ultrasound Obstet Gynecol. 2009;33(4):477–83.
20. van Disseldorp J, Lambalk CB, Kwee J, Looman CWN, Eijkemans MJC, Fauser BC, et al. Comparison of inter- and intra-cycle variability of anti-Mullerian hormone and antral follicle counts. Hum Reprod. 2010;25(1):221–7.
21. Scheffer GJ, Broekmans FJ, Dorland M, Habbema JD, Looman CW, te Velde ER. Antral follicle counts by transvaginal ultrasonography are related to age in women with proven natural fertility. Fertil Steril. 1999;72(5):845–51.
22. Hvidman HW, Bentzen JG, Thuesen LL, Lauritsen MP, Forman JL, Loft A, et al. Infertile women below the age of 40 have similar anti-müllerian hormone levels and antral follicle count compared with women of the same age with no history of infertility. Hum Reprod. 2016;31(5):1034–45.
23. Ripley M, Lanes A, Léveillé M-C, Shmorgun D. Does ovarian reserve predict egg quality in unstimulated therapeutic donor insemination cycles? Fertil Steril. 2015;103(5):1170–2.
24. Broer SL, van Disseldorp J, Broeze KA, Dólleman M, Opmeer BC, Bossuyt P, et al. Added value of ovarian reserve testing on patient characteristics in the prediction of ovarian response and ongoing pregnancy: an individual patient data approach. Hum Reprod Update. 2013;19(1):26–36.
25. La Marca A, Sunkara SK. Individualization of controlled ovarian stimulation in IVF using ovarian reserve markers: from theory to practice. Hum Reprod Update. 2014;20(1):124–40.
26. Kwee J, Elting ME, Schats R, McDonnell J, Lambalk CB. Ovarian volume and antral follicle count for the prediction of low and hyper responders with in vitro fertilization. Reprod Biol Endocrinol. 2007;5(1):9.
27. Josso N. Professor Alfred Jost: the builder of modern sex differentiation. Sex Dev. 2008;2(2):9.
28. Lambalk CB. Anti-müllerian hormone, the holy grail for fertility counselling in the general population? Hum Reprod. 2015;30(10):2257–8.
29. Hutson J, Ikawa H, Donahoe PK. The ontogeny of Mullerian inhibiting substance in the gonads of the chicken. J Pediatr Surg. 1981;16(6):822–7.
30. Cohen-Haguenauer O, Picard JY, Mattéi MG, Serero S, Nguyen VC, de Tand MF, et al. Mapping of the gene for anti-müllerian hormone to the short arm of human chromosome 19. Cytogenet Cell Genet. 1987;44(1):2–6.
31. Cate RL, Mattaliano RJ, Hession C, Tizard R, Farber NM, Cheung A, et al. Isolation of the bovine and human genes for müllerian inhibiting substance and expression of the human gene in animal cells. Cell. 1986;45(5):685–98.
32. Guibourdenche J, Lucidarme N, Chevenne D, Rigal O, Nicolas M, Luton D, et al. Anti-müllerian hormone levels in serum from human foetuses and children: pattern and clinical interest. Mol Cell Endocrinol. 2003;211(1–2):55–63.
33. Kelsey TW, Wright P, Nelson SM, Anderson RA, Wallace WHB. A validated model of serum anti-müllerian hormone from conception to menopause. PLoS One. 2011;6(7):e22024.
34. Nelson SM, Messow MC, McConnachie A, Wallace H, Kelsey T, Fleming R, et al. External validation of nomogram for the decline in serum anti-müllerian hormone in women: a population study of 15,834 infertility patients. Reprod Biomed Online. 2011;23(2):204–6.
35. Chang HL, Pahlavan N, Halpern EF, MacLaughlin DT. Serum müllerian inhibiting substance/anti-müllerian hormone levels in patients with adult granulosa cell tumors directly correlate with aggregate tumor mass as determined by pathology or radiology. Gynecol Oncol. 2009;114(1):57–60.
36. Dewailly D, Andersen CY, Balen A, Broekmans F, Dilaver N, Fanchin R, et al. The physiology and clinical utility of anti-Mullerian hormone in women. Hum Reprod Update. 2014;20(3):370–85.
37. Durlinger AL, Kramer P, Karels B, de Jong FH, Uilenbroek JT, Grootegoed JA, et al. Control of primordial follicle recruitment

by anti-müllerian hormone in the mouse ovary. Endocrinology. 1999;140(12):5789–96.

38. Broekmans FJ, Visser JA, Laven JSE, Broer SL, Themmen APN, Fauser BC. Anti-müllerian hormone and ovarian dysfunction. Trends Endocrinol Metab. 2008;19(9):340–7.
39. Anderson RA, Nelson SM, Wallace WHB. Measuring anti-müllerian hormone for the assessment of ovarian reserve: when and for whom is it indicated? Maturitas. 2012;71(1):28–33.
40. La Marca A, Stabile G, Artenisio AC, Volpe A. Serum anti-Mullerian hormone throughout the human menstrual cycle. Hum Reprod. 2006;21(12):3103–7.
41. Fanchin R, Taieb J, Lozano DHM, Ducot B, Frydman R, Bouyer J. High reproducibility of serum anti-Mullerian hormone measurements suggests a multi-staged follicular secretion and strengthens its role in the assessment of ovarian follicular status. Hum Reprod. 2005;20(4):923–7.
42. Overbeek A, Broekmans FJ, Hehenkamp WJ, Wijdeveld ME, van Disseldorp J, van Dulmen-den Broeder E, et al. Intra-cycle fluctuations of anti-müllerian hormone in normal women with a regular cycle: a re-analysis. Reprod Biomed Online. 2012;24(6):664–9.
43. Köninger A, Schmidt B, Mach P, Damaske D, Nießen S, Kimmig R, et al. Anti-Mullerian-hormone during pregnancy and peripartum using the new Beckman Coulter AMH Gen II Assay. Reprod Biol Endocrinol. 2015;13(1):86.
44. Seifer DB, Golub ET, Lambert-Messerlian G, Benning L, Anastos K, Watts DH, et al. Variations in serum müllerian inhibiting substance between white, black, and Hispanic women. Fertil Steril. 2009;92(5):1674–8.
45. Steiner AZ, Stanczyk FZ, Patel S, Edelman A. Antimullerian hormone and obesity: insights in oral contraceptive users. Contraception. 2010;81(3):245–8.
46. Ertunc D, Tok EC, Aytan H, Gozukara YM. Passive smoking is associated with lower age at menopause. Climacteric. 2015;18(1):47–52.
47. La Marca A, Spada E, Grisendi V, Argento C, Papaleo E, Milani S, et al. Normal serum anti-müllerian hormone levels in the general female population and the relationship with reproductive history. Eur J Obstet Gynecol Reprod Biol. 2012;163(2):180–4.
48. Drakopoulos P, van de Vijver A, Schutyser V, Milatovic S, Anckaert E, Schiettecatte J, et al. The effect of serum vitamin D levels on ovarian reserve markers: a prospective cross-sectional study. Hum Reprod. 2017;32(1):208–14.
49. Fleming R, Seifer DB, Frattarelli JL, Ruman J. Assessing ovarian response: antral follicle count versus anti-müllerian hormone. Reprod Biomed Online. 2015;31(4):486–96.
50. Depmann M, Eijkemans MJC, Broer SL, Scheffer GJ, van Rooij IAJ, Laven JSE, et al. Does anti-müllerian hormone predict menopause in the general population? Results of a prospective ongoing cohort study. Hum Reprod. 2016;31(7):1579–87.
51. Tehrani FR, Solaymani-Dodaran M, Tohidi M, Gohari MR, Azizi F. Modeling age at menopause using serum concentration of anti-mullerian hormone. J Clin Endocrinol Metabol. 2013;98(2):729–35.
52. Dólleman M, Verschuren WMM, Eijkemans MJC, Broekmans FJM, van der Schouw YT. Added value of anti-müllerian hormone in prediction of menopause: results from a large prospective cohort study. Hum Reprod. 2015;30(8):1974–81.
53. Braem MGM, Voorhuis M, van der Schouw YT, Peeters PHM, Schouten LJ, Eijkemans MJC, et al. Interactions between genetic variants in AMH and AMHR2 may modify age at natural menopause. PLoS One. 2013;8(3):e59819.
54. Yoon SH, Choi YM, Hong MA, Kim JJ, Lee GH, Hwang KR, et al. Association study of anti-Mullerian hormone and anti-Mullerian hormone type II receptor polymorphisms with idiopathic primary ovarian insufficiency. Hum Reprod. 2013;28(12):3301–5.
55. Cerra C, Newman WG, Tohlob D, Byers H, Horne G, Roberts SA, et al. AMH type II receptor and AMH gene polymorphisms are not associated with ovarian reserve, response, or outcomes in ovarian stimulation. J Assist Reprod Genet. 2016;33(8):1085–91.
56. Hagen CP, Vestergaard S, Juul A, Skakkebæk NE, Andersson A-M, Main KM, et al. Low concentration of circulating anti-müllerian hormone is not predictive of reduced fecundability in young healthy women: a prospective cohort study. Fertil Steril. 2012;98(6):1602–2.
57. Zarek SM, Mitchell EM, Sjaarda LA, Mumford SL, Silver RM, Stanford JB, et al. Is anti-müllerian hormone associated with fecundability? Findings from the EAGeR trial. J Clin Endocrinol Metabol. 2015;100(11):4215–21.
58. Zarek SM, Mitchell EM, Sjaarda LA, Mumford SL, Silver RM, Stanford JB, et al. Antimüllerian hormone and pregnancy loss from the effects of aspirin in gestation and reproduction trial. Fertil Steril. 2016;105(4):946–52.e2.
59. Seifer DB, MacLaughlin DT, Christian BP, Feng B, Shelden RM. Early follicular serum müllerian-inhibiting substance levels are associated with ovarian response during assisted reproductive technology cycles. Fertil Steril. 2002;77(3):468–71.
60. Nelson SM, Yates RW, Lyall H, Jamieson M, Traynor I, Gaudoin M, et al. Anti-müllerian hormone-based approach to controlled ovarian stimulation for assisted conception. Hum Reprod. 2009;24(4):867–75.
61. Broer SL, Mol BWJ, Hendriks D, Broekmans FJM. The role of antimullerian hormone in prediction of outcome after IVF: comparison with the antral follicle count. Fertil Steril. 2009;91(3):705–14.
62. La Marca A, Ferraretti AP, Palermo R, Ubaldi FM. The use of ovarian reserve markers in IVF clinical practice: a national consensus. Gynecol Endocrinol. 2016;32(1):1–5.
63. Nakhuda GS, Chu MC, Wang JG, Sauer MV, Lobo RA. Elevated serum müllerian-inhibiting substance may be a marker for ovarian hyperstimulation syndrome in normal women undergoing in vitro fertilization. Fertil Steril. 2006;85(5):1541–3.
64. Anderson RA, Anckaert E, Bosch E, Dewailly D, Dunlop CE, Fehr D, et al. Prospective study into the value of the automated Elecsys antimüllerian hormone assay for the assessment of the ovarian growing follicle pool. Fertil Steril. 2015;103(4):1074–4.
65. Practice Committee of the American Society for Reproductive Medicine. Testing and interpreting measures of ovarian reserve: a committee opinion. Fertil Steril. 2012;98(6):1407–15.
66. Nelson SM, Fleming R, Gaudoin M, Choi B, Santo-Domingo K, Yao M. Antimüllerian hormone levels and antral follicle count as prognostic indicators in a personalized prediction model of live birth. Fertil Steril. 2015;104(2):325–32.
67. Nyboe Andersen A, Nelson SM, Fauser BCJM, García-Velasco JA, Klein BM, Arce J-C, et al. Individualized versus conventional ovarian stimulation for in vitro fertilization: a multicenter, randomized, controlled, assessor-blinded, phase 3 noninferiority trial. Fertil Steril. 2017;107(2):387–96.e4.

4 AMH and Medically Assisted Reproduction

Valentina Grisendi and Antonio La Marca

4.1 Individualization of Controlled Ovarian Stimulation

In assisted reproduction technologies (ART) or medically assisted reproduction (MAR), the controlled ovarian stimulation (COS) therapy is the starting point from which a good oocyte retrieval depends. In recent years, several treatment protocols have been studied and tested on various kinds of patients, searching for the therapy that ensures the best outcome for the single patients, in terms of pregnancy and live birth, minimizing iatrogenic risks and the rate of cycle cancellation due to absent or excessive response. For this reason, there has been the evolution from the concept of "one size fits all" to the concept of "individualization." This should guarantee also more advantages, including a reduction in costs and in the dropout rate of patients of ART programs, often caused by failure and by physical and psychological burden [1]. If we look to the possible risks for patients [2, 3], the prescription of a standard COS may even be considered not ethical.

Ovarian response prediction is the first step for the individualization of therapy. Ovarian response to COS depends first of all on a woman's ovarian reserve, secondly on the monthly variability of ovarian functional activity, and lastly on the stimulation regimen itself. An accurate analysis of the individual ovarian reserve through ovarian reserve markers is therefore essential. In particular, serum AMH and ultrasound antral follicle count (AFC) have shown to be the most reliable markers. A therapeutic strategy based on the outcome of a previous IVF cycle is also recommended, while in the absence of a previous cycle, a treatment grossly based on age, BMI, anamnestic data such as previous ovarian surgery, or cycle characteristics is to be considered careless.

Using the Italian scenario as an example, a large consensus exists among the Italian clinicians about the use of ovarian reserve markers, namely, AMH and AFC, to identify the ovarian reserve of a single woman and to predict her possible response to ovarian stimulation with the aim to individualize ovarian stimulation itself [4].

Surely the choice of the COS protocol may not be a simple clinical decision, because of the variety of drugs now available. Moreover, the selection of the FSH starting dose is very important for the outcome of the cycle [2, 5–9].

In this chapter, we will discuss about these issues.

4.2 Literature Search

We scanned literature (Medline, Cochrane Library, and Web of Science databases) in search for papers about ovarian reserve markers, in particular AMH, and their role in MAR. Key words used were ovarian reserve markers, AMH, anti-Müllerian hormone, poor/high response, and IVF.

Additional journal articles were identified from the bibliographies of included studies. Literature available up to February 2017 was included.

4.3 Predictive Value of Ovarian Reserve Markers

4.3.1 FSH

Serum FSH was one of the first ovarian reserve markers proposed for use in clinical practice. But FSH has several limitations. First of all, in order for FSH to be interpretable, it needs to be dosed on 3–5 of the menstrual cycle together with estradiol. Secondly, it begins to rise in serum only when ovarian reserve is severely compromised. Thirdly, it can't be

V. Grisendi
Mother-Infant Department, University of Modena and Reggio Emilia and Clinica Eugin Modena, Modena, Italy

A. La Marca (✉)
Department of Obstetrics and Gynecology, University Hospital of Modena, Modena, Italy

G. N. Allahbadia et al. (eds.), *Textbook of Assisted Reproduction*, https://doi.org/10.1007/978-981-15-2377-9_4

used for ovarian response prediction and therapy individualization in IVF, because of its low sensitivity and specificity. This knowledge limits the usefulness of the marker.

4.3.2 AMH and AFC

Serum AMH and AFC performed by ultrasound are the most recent and direct markers of ovarian reserve as they can accurately measure the pool of small antral follicles present in both ovaries. As antral follicles are related to the full amount of primordial follicles, AMH and AFC are considered capable of reflecting oocyte quantity and are, for this reason, highly correlated [10].

Regarding MAR, both AMH and AFC have an optimal predictive ability on ovarian response to controlled ovarian stimulation and on the number of oocytes retrieved [11–20]. In literature, a few studies are in favor of AMH as the strongest predictor of ovarian response, having failed to show an independent association between AFC and oocyte yield, while other studies demonstrated a stronger predictive value for AFC [21–26].

Undoubtedly the data regarding AMH result from much larger cohorts compared with any other marker, contributing further to the robustness of AMH as a predictive tool. Serum AMH has the advantage of very little intra- and inter-cycle variability, and the introduction of new automated essays for AMH dosage has overcome previous problems of low reliability and repeatability of dosages among laboratories. On the other hand, AFC is known for its intra-cycle variability, and it is hampered by an important intra- and inter-observer variability, which derives from technical limitations and differences in methodology for counting antral follicles. Experts are still discussing about what class of antral follicles may better correlate with the number of retrieved oocytes (2–5 mm, 4–6 mm, or 5–10 mm); however, counting all identifiable antral follicles of 2–10 mm in diameter seems the most simple and accurate way in clinical practice [27–29]. The recent application of three-dimensional (3D) ultrasound technology to the antral follicle count showed to reduce both intra- and inter-observer variability [30], so we hope that this technology will be most largely available in the next future.

In the end, both markers can be applied to tailor stimulation protocol and FSH starting dose in IVF patients [10, 23, 31, 32]. In case of a fixed FSH starting dose, serum AMH seems able to efficiently predict the need to modify the dose on stimulation day 6 [33].

Regarding the outcome live birth, the predictive value of AFC is instead less clear, while several studies report a positive correlation between AMH and live birth rates [23, 34, 35], so that a few authors suggest AMH level may even predict embryo quality. It seems that AMH could be used in the counselling with the couple regarding chances of live birth, not AFC.

4.4 The Choice of the FSH Starting Dose Based on Markers

In the attempt to tailor controlled ovarian stimulation on the single patient, female age alone can't be considered a sufficient criterion to predict ovarian response, because women of similar age may have a large variability in the ovarian reserve and therefore in the ovarian response itself [36].

Field markers of ovarian reserve have a major role in this. Although the use of markers is an agreed-upon approach by most experts, literature is still lacking of practical algorithms which may help clinician to formulate the correct therapy.

Few studies proposed to base individualization on a single marker, AFC, or AMH.

Regarding AFC, a large RCT is now studying the live birth rate and the cost-effectiveness resulting from the individualization of the gonadotrophin starting dose versus a standard dose [37].

Two studies have been published reporting predictive models for gonadotrophin dose selection based only on AMH [2, 38]. In the prospective non-randomized study by Nelson, choosing the therapeutic protocol (standard long agonist or antagonist protocol) and the FSH starting dose on the basis of serum AMH brought to a reduction of both excessive responses and cancelled cycles [2].

A retrospective study by Yates comparing COS based on serum AMH versus one based on FSH levels confirmed that AMH-based treatment reduced the incidence of ovarian hyperstimulation syndrome (OHSS) and reduced costs; moreover, it resulted in a significant increase in both pregnancy and live birth rates [38].

Finally, a recent pilot study compared the efficacy and safety of two strategies, one based on AMH and the other on AFC, to determine the starting dose of recombinant FSH (rFSH) for ovarian stimulation in 348 women. No differences emerged regarding clinical pregnancy, multiple pregnancy, and miscarriage rate between the two groups, but in the AFC group, a major proportion of hyper-responses was noticed [39].

4.4.1 Complex Algorithms to Establish FSH Starting Dose

The fact that ovarian response may be due to different variables acting together induced a few experts to elaborate predictive algorithms based on more than one variable [40–43].

A first algorithm included age, AFC, ovarian volume, Doppler ovarian score, and smoking status [40], but some of these variables were too complex, and the model couldn't have a wide clinical application. Subsequently, it was proposed a model based on age, BMI, day 3 serum FSH, and AFC [44] that was later tested in the CONSORT study [45] and in another more recent prospective study on 197 women [46]. These studies showed that the predicted gonadotrophin starting doses were often lower than those dictated by clinical practice and led to iatrogenic poor responses. Moreover, this model cannot be used by clinicians because the coefficients for computing the algorithm were never published [46].

Another retrospective study created a simple model based on age, AFC, and day 3 serum FS and showed that AFC was the most significant predictor of ovarian response [47]. For example, in a woman aged 30 years with a day 3 FSH of 4 IU/L and an AFC of 16, the most appropriate FSH starting dose would be 150 IU daily. This model seems to be useful but needs to be validated in an independent cohort.

Regarding AMH, a simple algorithm was developed including AMH, age, and day 3 serum FSH [48]. This model would prescribe a gonadotrophin dose of 150 IU/daily for a woman aged 30 years with a day 3 FSH of 4 IU/L and a serum AMH of 4 ng/ml. The efficacy of the model was later retrospectively tested in the patients' population of two IVF centers in Italy, and it was confirmed that the use of the nomogram would have generated more appropriate FSH starting doses compared to those actually given, in order to obtain optimal ovarian responses [49].

The reliability of the AMH-based approach for COS individualization is such that a new recombinant gonadotrophin (follitropin delta) with dosing based on patient's AMH and body weight has been created. The new drug promises similar live births rates with fewer poor responses and fewer hyper-responses compared to the traditional rFSH [50].

4.5 Ovarian Response Prediction and Management

Individualizing FSH starting dose on ovarian reserve markers seems definitely the correct way to go. Moreover, markers may be useful for the choice of the stimulation protocol. Aim of COS is an optimal oocyte retrieval, defined as the retrieval of 5–15 oocytes, which should guarantee the highest chances of pregnancy with the minimal risks for the patient. In fact, an egg retrieval of less than 5 oocytes would probably end in few and poor-quality embryos. A retrieval of more than 15 oocytes puts the patient at risk of OHSS, a condition potentially life-threatening.

The clinician should therefore use a maximizing approach in predicted normal responders, while in high responders, ovarian stimulation must be cautious and safe. For predicted poor responders, an optimizing therapeutic protocol does not exists, and the clinician should choose the treatment less stressful for the patient.

4.5.1 Predicted Poor Response

Poor ovarian response is defined as the retrieval of <4 oocytes following a standard IVF protocol [51]. The incidence of poor ovarian response in IVF ranges from 10 to 20%, and the prevalence increases with advancing woman's age.

Poor ovarian response has a multifactorial origin, and its causes are only in minimal part reversible. An iatrogenic poor response caused by a suboptimal FSH starting dose can be easily recovered increasing FSH dose in the next cycle. A poor response caused by a functional ovarian cyst won't probably repeat in the following cycle. But in most cases this condition is due to a critical depletion of oocytes in the ovaries, which is the effect of advancing age, previous ovarian surgery, and genetic defects. As a consequence, there is no stimulation therapy that could allow a good follicular recruitment and an optimal oocyte retrieval. It was shown that increasing FSH dose is not useful to improve egg collection in these patients [20]. The subsequent difficulty in obtaining good embryos to transfer has the effect to reduce pregnancy rates, so that MAR is often ineffective in poor responder patients.

Criteria to identify poor responder patients are based on anamnestic evaluation (age, shortening of the menstrual cycle, previous ovarian surgery, outcome of a previous cycle) and on ovarian reserve assessment. Although in literature markers cut-off values for poor response prediction are quite variable, due to the variability in the measuring methods of markers and the different definitions of poor ovarian response, reference ranges can be identified. Regarding AMH, a cut-off value ranging between 0.7 and 1.3 ng/ml showed a good sensitivity and specificity [17, 42]. On the other hand, the most frequently reported AFC cut-off values for prediction of poor response range between AFC <5 and <7 [28, 52].

The assessment of ovarian reserve in these patients is useful first of all to help during pre-treatment counselling. Being conscious beforehand of the possible cycle cancellation and of the low success rates is useful for these couples on one hand to limit the psychological impact due to the possible negative outcome and on the other hand to reduce treatment drop out. By the way, experts recommend to not exclude women predicted as poor responders from IVF programs, because the predictive accuracy of markers of ovarian reserve is not 100%, especially in the prediction of pregnancy [6, 7], and the possibility to achieve pregnancy exists in young women [53]. Only in very poor prognosis patients, the clinician may decide to recommend a heterologous IVF cycle with eggs donation.

As previously reported, there isn't nowadays a COS protocol better than another that could guarantee a positive reproductive outcome in these patients. Several studies compared the old GnRH agonist long protocol, very suppressive in the phase of follicular recruitment, with the short GnRH antagonist one, but results show that both protocols are comparable in terms of oocyte retrieval and pregnancy rate [54, 55]. It can be concluded that, at the same reproductive outcome, GnRH antagonist protocol could be preferred because it is more patient friendly and allows a reduction in costs through a lower gonadotrophin consumption.

In this context, a mild ovarian stimulation strategy with GnRH antagonist has been proposed and compared with a standard long protocol. Ongoing pregnancy rate was not different between the two protocols (95% CI: 0.57–1.57), while the duration of ovarian stimulation and the amount of gonadotrophins used were significantly lower in the mild stimulation strategy [56].

In conclusion, prediction of poor response can have positive results in terms of patient compliance and reduction of costs, but it does not seem to produce a significant improvement of IVF outcome [53, 57, 58].

4.5.2 Predicted Normal/High Response

The term "hyper-response" refers to the retrieval of more than 15 oocytes following a standard COS protocol [6, 7, 17]. It involves until 7% of MAR cycles and decreases with advancing woman's age.

Clues of a possible high response come from clinical criteria and anamnestic characteristics, such as young age, long menstrual cycles, symptoms of PCOS, and hyper-response in a previous cycle [59, 60]. But the study of ovarian reserve through reliable markers appears fundamental for an accurate prediction. An AMH serum level >3.5 ng/ml [23, 31] or an AFC >16 seems able to identify the most of hyper-responder patients [15].

The prediction of a high response has a relevant value. First of all, it allows to inform couples accurately on the possibility to achieve pregnancy through MAR and on the potential risks connected to treatment, OHSS in the first place. Secondly, it permits to consistently modify the treatment according to predicted response: in these patients COS individualization is crucial, because it really permits to improve IVF outcome and to avoid the main complication that is OHSS.

The first step of COS individualization is the choice of FSH starting dose. In high responder patients, a FSH too low starting dose could cause an iatrogenic poor response, whereas a dose which is too high could lead to OHSS. As previously described, the right FSH starting dose can be efficiently calculated using algorithms based on ovarian reserve markers [47, 48].

Among COS protocols, the GnRH antagonist protocol seems to be the best for women predicted as high responders, since the latter showed to significantly reduce the incidence of OHSS and the following risks of cycle cancellation and patient's hospitalization, as well as to reduce costs [2, 38, 61, 62]. A large RCT including 1050 first IVF cycles has recently demonstrated that the incidence of severe OHSS (5.1 vs. 8.9%; $P = 0.02$) and moderate OHSS (10.2 vs. 15.6%; $P = 0.01$) was significantly lower in the GnRH antagonist group compared with the agonist group, respectively, while pregnancy rates were similar in the two groups [61].

The GnRH antagonist protocol gives another advantage, that is, the possibility to induce final oocyte maturation with a single bolus of a GnRH analogue instead of the traditional human chorionic gonadotrophin (hCG). This regimen has a great efficacy on OHSS prevention, but it is associated in fresh IVF cycles with lower pregnancy rates, because of an adverse effect on endometrium receptivity and the induction of early luteolysis [59, 63]. On the other hand, it was demonstrated that implantation rate, clinical pregnancy rate, ongoing pregnancy rate, and survival rate of frozen-thawed embryos are similar independent of the stimulation protocol used, to indicate that the GnRH antagonist protocol plus GnRH agonist triggering doesn't impact on oocyte quality [64].

The strategies proposed to solve the detrimental effect of GnRH agonist triggering are the following. First it was suggested to add a low-dose (1500 IU) HCG bolus 35 h or 5 days after triggering, but there are doubts on the ability of this approach to eliminate severe OHSS [65]. Another possible option derives from improvement in vitrification technologies: it is IVF cycle segmentation. It consists in freezing all embryos produced in the fresh cycle in order to perform transfer of frozen-thawed embryos in subsequent cycles. This seems to be the winning strategy to cut down the risk of OHSS maintaining elevated pregnancy rates [66, 67].

4.6 Conclusions

At any age of the woman, individual ovarian reserve conditions the prognosis and oocyte retrieval impacts on the chance of live birth. An optimal oocyte retrieval must be the aim of the clinician, who has the task to evaluate globally all anamnestic factors of the patients and to interpret ovarian reserve markers, in order to formulate the most appropriate COS protocol for the single patient. From literature we already have several indications to guide correct management of patients, from predicted poor to predicted hyper-responders, but a lot must still be done to reduce iatrogenic risks and improve IVF outcomes.

References

1. Verberg MF, Eijkemans MJ, Heijnen EM, Broekmans FJ, de Klerk C, Fauser BC, et al. Why do couples drop-out from IVF treatment? A prospective cohort study. Hum Reprod. 2008;23:2050–5.
2. Nelson SM, Yates RW, Lyall H, Jamieson M, Traynor I, Gaudoin M, et al. Anti-Müllerian hormone-based approach to controlled ovarian stimulation for assisted conception. Hum Reprod. 2009;24:867–75.
3. Nardo LG, Fleming R, Howles CM, Bosch E, Hamamah S, Ubaldi FM, et al. Conventional ovarian stimulation no longer exists: welcome to the age of individualized ovarian stimulation. Reprod Biomed Online. 2011;23:141–8.

4. La Marca A, Ferraretti AP, Palermo R, Ubaldi FM. The use of ovarian reserve markers in IVF clinical practice: a national consensus. Gynecol Endocrinol. 2016;32:1–5.
5. Broekmans FJ, Kwee J, Hendriks DJ, Mol BW, Lambalk CB. A systematic review of tests predicting ovarian reserve and IVF outcome. Hum Reprod Update. 2006;12:685–718.
6. La Marca A, Sighinolfi G, Radi D, Argento C, Baraldi E, Artenisio AC, et al. Anti-mullerian hormone (AMH) as a predictive marker in assisted reproductive technology (ART). Hum Reprod Update. 2010;16:113–30.
7. Broer SL, Do'lleman M, Opmeer BC, Fauser BC, Mol BW, Broekmans FJ. AMH and AFC as predictors of excessive response in controlled ovarian hyperstimulation: a meta-analysis. Hum Reprod Update. 2011;17:46–54.
8. Devroey P, Polyzos NP, Blockeel C. An OHSS-free clinic by segmentation of IVF treatment. Hum Reprod. 2011;26:2593–7.
9. Nelson SM. Biomarkers of ovarian response: current and future applications. Fertil Steril. 2013;99:963–9.
10. Fleming R, Seifer DB, Frattarelli JL, Ruman J. Assessing ovarian response: antral follicle count versus anti-Müllerian hormone. Reprod Biomed Online. 2015;31:486–96.
11. Seifer DB, MacLaughlin DT, Christian BP, Feng B, Shelden RM. Early follicular serum Müllerian-inhibiting substance levels are associated with ovarian response during assisted reproductive technology cycles. Fertil Steril. 2002;77:468–71.
12. Fanchin R, Schonäuer LM, Righini C, Frydman N, Frydman R, Taieb J. Serum anti-Müllerian hormone dynamics during controlled ovarian hyperstimulation. Hum Reprod. 2003;18:328–32.
13. Hazout A, Bouchard P, Seifer DB, Aussage P, Junca AM, Cohen-Bacrie P. Serum anti Müllerian hormone/Müllerian-inhibiting substance appears to be a more discriminatory marker of assisted reproductive technology outcome than follicle-stimulating hormone, inhibin B, or estradiol. Fertil Steril. 2004;82:1323–9.
14. Muttukrishna S, Suharjono H, McGarrigle H, Sathanandan M. Inhibin B and anti-mullerian hormone: markers of ovarian response in IVF/ICSI patients? BJOG. 2004;111:1248–53.
15. Kwee J, Elting ME, Schats R, McDonnell J, Lambalk CB. Ovarian volume and antral follicle count for the prediction of low and hyper responders with in vitro fertilization. Reprod Biol Endocrinol. 2007;5:9.
16. La Marca A, Giulini S, Tirelli A, Bertucci E, Marsella T, Xella S, et al. Anti-Müllerian hormone measurement on any day of the menstrual cycle strongly predicts ovarian response in assisted reproductive technology. Hum Reprod. 2007;22:766–71.
17. Nelson SM, Yates RW, Fleming R. Serum anti-Müllerian hormone and FSH: prediction of live birth and extremes of response in stimulated cycles—implications for individualization of therapy. Hum Reprod. 2007;22:2414–21.
18. Elgindy EA, El-Haieg DO, El-Sebaey A. Anti-Müllerian hormone: correlation of early follicular, ovulatory and midluteal levels with ovarian response and cycle outcome in intracytoplasmic sperm injection patients. Fertil Steril. 2008;89:1670–6.
19. Jayaprakasan K, Campbell BK, Hopkisson JF, Clewes JS, Johnson IR, Raine-Fenning NJ. Effect of pituitary desensitization on the early growing follicular cohort estimated using anti-mullerian hormone. Hum Reprod. 2008;23:2577–83.
20. Lekamge DN, Lane M, Gilchrist RB, Tremellen KP. Increased gonadotrophin stimulation does not improve IVF outcomes in patients with predicted poor ovarian reserve. J Assist Reprod Genet. 2008;25:515–21.
21. Nelson SM, Klein BM, Arce JC. Comparison of antimüllerian hormone levels and antral follicle count as predictor of ovarian response to controlled ovarian stimulation in good-prognosis patients at individual fertility clinics in two multicenter trials. Fertil Steril. 2015;103:923–30.e1.
22. Andersen AN, Witjes H, Gordon K, Mannaerts B, Xpect Investigators. Predictive factors of ovarian response and clinical outcome after IVF/ICSI following a rFSH/GnRH antagonist protocol with or without oral contraceptive pre-treatment. Hum Reprod. 2011;26:3413–23.
23. Arce JC, La Marca A, Mirner Klein B, Nyboe Andersen A, Fleming R. Antimüllerian hormone in gonadotropin releasing-hormone antagonist cycles: prediction of ovarian response and cumulative treatment outcome in good-prognosis patients. Fertil Steril. 2013;99:1644–53.
24. Himabindu Y, Sriharibabu M, Gopinathan K, Satish U, Louis TF, Gopinath P. Anti-mullerian hormone and antral follicle count as predictors of ovarian response in assisted reproduction. J Hum Reprod Sci. 2013;6:27–31.
25. Tsakos E, Tolikas A, Daniilidis A, Asimakopoulos B. Predictive value of anti-müllerian hormone, follicle-stimulating hormone and antral follicle count on the outcome of ovarian stimulation in women following GnRH-antagonist protocol for IVF/ET. Arch Gynecol Obstet. 2014;290:1249–53.
26. Hsu A, Arny M, Knee AB, Bell C, Cook E, Novak AL, et al. Antral follicle count in clinical practice: analyzing clinical relevance. Fertil Steril. 2011;95:474–9.
27. Jeppesen JV, Anderson RA, Kelsey TW, Christiansen SL, Kristensen SG, Jayaprakasan K, et al. Which follicles make the most anti-mullerian hormone in humans? Evidence for an abrupt decline in AMH production at the time of follicle selection. Mol Hum Reprod. 2013;19:519–27.
28. Jayaprakasan K, Deb S, Batcha M, Hopkisson J, Johnson I, Campbell B, et al. The cohort of antral follicles measuring 2–6 mm reflects the quantitative status of ovarian reserve as assessed by serum levels of anti-Müllerian hormone and response to controlled ovarian stimulation. Fertil Steril. 2010;94:1775–81.
29. Broekmans FJ, de Ziegler D, Howles CM, Gougeon A, Trew G, Olivennes F. The antral follicle count: practical recommendations for better standardization. Fertil Steril. 2010;94:1044–51.
30. Deb S, Campbell BK, Clewes JS, Pincott-Allen C, Raine-Fenning NJ. Intracycle variation in number of antral follicles stratified by size and in endocrine markers of ovarian reserve in women with normal ovulatory menstrual cycles. Ultrasound Obstet Gynecol. 2013;41:216–22.
31. La Marca A, Sunkara SK. Individualization of controlled ovarian stimulation in IVF using ovarian reserve markers: from theory to practice. Hum Reprod Update. 2014;20:124–40.
32. Iliodromiti S, Nelson SM. Ovarian response biomarkers: physiology and performance. Curr Opin Obstet Gynecol. 2015;27:182–6.
33. Anckaert E, Smitz J, Schiettecatte J, Klein BM, Arce JC. The value of anti-mullerian hormone measurement in the long GnRH agonist protocol: association with ovarian response and gonadotrophin-dose adjustments. Hum Reprod. 2012;27:1829–39.
34. Khader A, Lloyd SM, McConnachie A, Fleming R, Grisendi V, La Marca A, et al. External validation of anti-Müllerian hormone based prediction of live birth in assisted conception. J Ovarian Res. 2013;6:3.
35. Brodin T, Hadziosmanovic N, Berglund L, Olovsson M, Holte J. Antimüllerian hormone levels are strongly associated with live-birth rates after assisted reproduction. J Clin Endocrinol Metab. 2013;98:1107–14.
36. La Marca A, Spada E, Sighinolfi G, Argento C, Tirelli A, Giulini S, et al. Age-specific nomogram for the decline in antral follicle count throughout the reproductive period. Fertil Steril. 2011;95:684–8.
37. van Tilborg TC, Eijkemans MJ, Laven JS, Koks CA, de Bruin JP, Scheffer GJ, et al. The OPTIMIST study: optimisation of cost effectiveness through individualised FSH stimulation dosages for IVF treatment. A randomised controlled trial. BMC Womens Health. 2012;12:29.
38. Yates AP, Rustamov O, Roberts SA, Lim HY, Pemberton PW, Smith A, et al. Anti-mullerian hormone-tailored stimulation protocols improve outcomes whilst reducing adverse effects and costs of IVF. Hum Reprod. 2011;26:2353–62.

39. Lan VT, Linh NK, Tuong HM, Wong PC, Howles CM. Anti-Müllerian hormone versus antral follicle count for defining the starting dose of FSH. Reprod Biomed Online. 2013;27:390–9.
40. Popovic-Todorovic B, Loft A, Lindhard A, Bangsbøll S, Andersson AM, Andersen AN. A prospective study of predictive factors of ovarian response in 'standard' IVF/ICSI patients treated with recombinant FSH. A suggestion for a recombinant FSH dosage normogram. Hum Reprod. 2003;18:781–7.
41. Fauser BC, Diedrich K, Devroey P, Evian Annual Reproduction Workshop Group 2007. Predictors of ovarian response: progress towards individualized treatment in ovulation induction and ovarian stimulation. Hum Reprod Update. 2008;14:1–14.
42. Al-Azemi M, Killick SR, Duffy S, Pye C, Refaat B, Hill N, et al. Multi-marker assessment of ovarian reserve predicts oocyte yield after ovulation induction. Hum Reprod. 2011;26:414–22.
43. Broer SL, van Disseldorp J, Broeze KA, Dolleman M, Opmeer BC, Bossuyt P, et al. Added value of ovarian reserve testing on patient characteristics in the prediction of ovarian response and ongoing pregnancy: an individual patient data approach. Hum Reprod Update. 2013;19:26–36.
44. Howles CM, Saunders H, Alam V, Engrand P, FSH Treatment Guidelines Clinical Panel. Predictive factors and a corresponding treatment algorithm for controlled ovarian stimulation in patients treated with recombinant human follicle stimulating hormone (follitropin alfa) during assisted reproduction technology (ART) procedures. An analysis of 1378 patients. Curr Med Res Opin. 2006;22:907–18.
45. Olivennes F, Howles CM, Borini A, Germond M, Trew G, Wikland M, et al. Individualizing FSH dose for assisted reproduction using a novel algorithm: the CONSORT study. Reprod Biomed Online. 2009;18:195–204.
46. Pouly JL, Olivennes F, Massin N, Celle M, Caizergues N, Contard F, French CONSORT Study Group. Usability and utility of the CONSORT calculator for FSH starting doses: a prospective observational study. Reprod Biomed Online. 2015;31:347–55.
47. La Marca A, Grisendi V, Giulini S, Argento C, Tirelli A, Dondi G, et al. Individualization of the FSH starting dose in IVF/ICSI cycles using the antral follicle count. J Ovarian Res. 2013;6:11.
48. La Marca A, Papaleo E, Grisendi V, Argento C, Giulini S, Volpe A. Development of a nomogram based on markers of ovarian reserve for the individualisation of the follicle-stimulating hormone starting dose in in vitro fertilisation cycles. BJOG. 2012;119:1171–9.
49. Papaleo E, Zaffagnini S, Munaretto M, Vanni VS, Rebonato G, Grisendi V, et al. Clinical application of a nomogram based on age, serum FSH and AMH to select the FSH starting dose in IVF/ICSI cycles: a retrospective two-centres study. Eur J Obstet Gynecol Reprod Biol. 2016;207:94–9.
50. Nyboe Andersen A, Nelson SM, Fauser BC, García-Velasco JA, Klein BM, Arce JC, ESTHER-1 Study Group. Individualized versus conventional ovarian stimulation for in vitro fertilization: a multicenter, randomized, controlled, assessor-blinded, phase 3 noninferiority trial. Fertil Steril. 2017;107:387–96.e4.
51. Ferraretti AP, La Marca A, Fauser BC, Tarlatzis B, Nargund G, Gianaroli L, ESHRE Working Group on Poor Ovarian Response Definition. ESHRE consensus on the definition of 'poor response' to ovarian stimulation for in vitro fertilization: the Bologna criteria. Hum Reprod. 2011;26:1616–24.
52. Frattarelli JL, Levi AJ, Miller BT, Segars JH. A prospective assessment of the predictive value of basal antral follicles in in vitro fertilization cycles. Fertil Steril. 2003;80:350–5.
53. Oudendijk JF, Yarde F, Eijkemans MJ, Broekmans FJ, Broer SL. The poor responder in IVF: is the prognosis always poor? A systematic review. Hum Reprod Update. 2012;18:1–11.
54. Pu D, Wu J, Liu J. Comparisons of GnRH antagonist versus GnRH agonist protocol in poor ovarian responders undergoing IVF. Hum Reprod. 2011;26:2742–9.
55. Sunkara SK, Coomarasamy A, Faris R, Braude P, Khalaf Y. Long gonadotropin-releasing hormone agonist versus short agonist versus antagonist regimens in poor responders undergoing in vitro fertilization: a randomized controlled trial. Fertil Steril. 2014;101:147–53.
56. Youssef MA, van Wely M, Al-Inany H, Madani T, Jahangiri N, Khodabakhshi S, et al. A mild ovarian stimulation strategy in women with poor ovarian reserve undergoing IVF: a multicenter randomized non-inferiority trial. Hum Reprod. 2017;32:112–8.
57. Klinkert ER, Broekmans FJ, Looman CW, Habbema JD, te Velde ER. Expected poor responders on the basis of an antral follicle count do not benefit from a higher starting dose of gonadotrophins in IVF treatment: a randomized controlled trial. Hum Reprod. 2005;20:611–5.
58. Pandian Z, McTavish AR, Aucott L, Hamilton MP, Bhattacharya S. Interventions for 'poor responders' to controlled ovarian hyper stimulation (COH) in in-vitro fertilisation (IVF). Cochrane Database Syst Rev. 2010;1:CD004379.
59. Humaidan P, Quartarolo J, Papanikolaou EG. Preventing ovarian hyperstimulation syndrome: guidance for the clinician. Fertil Steril. 2010;94:389–400.
60. Papanikolaou EG, Humaidan P, Polyzos N, Kalantaridou S, Kol S, Benadiva C, et al. New algorithm for OHSS prevention. Reprod Biol Endocrinol. 2011;9:147.
61. Toftager M, Bogstad J, Bryndorf T, Løssl K, Roskær J, Holland T, et al. Risk of severe ovarian hyperstimulation syndrome in GnRH antagonist versus GnRH agonist protocol: RCT including 1050 first IVF/ICSI cycles. Hum Reprod. 2016;31:1253–64.
62. Lainas TG, Sfontouris IA, Zorzovilis IZ, Petsas GK, Lainas GT, Alexopoulou E, et al. Flexible GnRH antagonist protocol versus GnRH agonist long protocol in patients with polycystic ovary syndrome treated for IVF: a prospective randomised controlled trial (RCT). Hum Reprod. 2010;25:683–9.
63. Griesinger G, Diedrich K, Devroey P, Kolibianakis EM. GnRH agonist for triggering final oocyte maturation in the GnRH antagonist ovarian hyperstimulation protocol: a systematic review and meta-analysis. Hum Reprod Update. 2006;12:159–68.
64. Eldar-Geva T, Zylber-Haran E, Babayof R, Halevy-Shalem T, Ben-Chetrit A, Tsafrir A, et al. Similar outcome for cryopreserved embryo transfer following GnRH-antagonist/GnRH-agonist, GnRH-antagonist/HCG or long protocol ovarian stimulation. Reprod Biomed Online. 2007;14:148–54.
65. Orvieto R. Triggering final follicular maturation—hCG, GnRH-agonist or both, when and to whom? J Ovarian Res. 2015; 8:60.
66. Casper RF. Introduction: gonadotropin-releasing hormone agonist triggering of final follicular maturation for in vitro fertilization. Fertil Steril. 2015;103:865–6.
67. Griesinger G, Schultz L, Bauer T, Broessner A, Frambach T, Kissler S. Ovarian hyperstimulation syndrome prevention by gonadotropin-releasing hormone agonist triggering of final oocyte maturation in a gonadotropin-releasing hormone antagonist protocol in combination with a "freeze-all" strategy: a prospective multicentric study. Fertil Steril. 2011;95:2029–33.e1.

5 Assessment of the Male Partner

Michael W. Witthaus and Jeanne O'Brien

Infertility in a couple can be attributed exclusively to male factor in 20% of couples, and male factor may contribute in some form in an additional 30% of couples [1]. The accepted definition of infertility is the inability to conceive after 12 months of regular sexual intercourse. Couples who present for evaluation earlier than this recommended time could still begin a basic evaluation. Underlying life-threatening conditions in men presenting with infertility have been observed, adding additional importance to evaluation [2].

Gynecologists and primary care physicians are the principal sources of referral to urologists specializing in infertility (ideally a male infertility fellowship-trained urologist). Most academic medical centers have such an urologist available for diagnostic and therapeutic services and collaborate with reproductive endocrinologists and gynecologic physicians to provide coordinated and specialized care. Advancement of assisted reproductive technologies (ART) or medically assisted reproduction (MAR), and microsurgical techniques, have enabled men who were previously considered sterile to father children.

Male factor infertility can be caused by pre-testicular, testicular, and post-testicular abnormalities. History, physical exam, endocrine analysis, and radiologic studies will guide diagnosis and treatment.

M. W. Witthaus · J. O'Brien (✉)
Department of Urology, University of Rochester Medical Center, Rochester, NY, USA
e-mail: jeanne_obrien@urmc.rochester.edu

5.1 Evaluation

5.1.1 History and Physical

Male fertility requires certain factors including good erectile function; spermatogenesis; normal endocrine factors; and normal ejaculation. Intercourse must occur around the ovulatory period. Sperm can live for approximately 5 days in the cervical mucus [3]. However, to ensure adequate sperm in the female genital tract, patients should be advised to have sexual intercourse every 48 h around the time of ovulation [4].

Anxiety and stress are often associated with infertility, and male patients will often describe some degree of erectile dysfunction. Further, the stress of inability to conceive compounds the issue [5]. Understandably, if sexual intercourse is not occurring, then conception is impossible! Erectile dysfunction may also be secondary to various disease states or exposures including diabetes, atherosclerosis, smoking tobacco or cannabis, steroid use, or a history of chemotherapy and radiation. Past history of genitourinary cancers or pelvic surgeries may also cause impaired erectile function.

Spermatogenesis takes between 2 and 74 days [6]. Results of any illness/injury or treatment will take at least 52–72 days to show response in semen parameters.

Follicle-stimulating hormone (FSH) acts on Leydig cells in the testes which in turn secrete testosterone which acts on spermatogonia to stimulate normal spermatogenesis. An elevated FSH is an indication that the testes are not functioning normally. Testicular failure, genetic abnormalities, and toxic exposures (including radiation, chemotherapy, and heat) are some causes for elevated FSH levels. Previously, it was maintained that if FSH was elevated by two times normal, then the probability of finding sperm on testicular biopsy was very low [7]. This has changed, though, with the onset of new microsurgical techniques (including micro TESE—microscopic testicular sperm extraction) [8]. FSH continues to be used as a prognostic indicator of the potential outcomes after treatment. Testosterone is important for libido, erectile

G. N. Allahbadia et al. (eds.), *Textbook of Assisted Reproduction*, https://doi.org/10.1007/978-981-15-2377-9_5

function, and sperm production and is also used to guide treatment evaluation and outcomes of therapy.

A comprehensive history should include all past and current medical problems related to reproductive function, including any previous pregnancies. Men who have not contributed to pregnancy in any female partner have *primary infertility*, and those who have done so have *secondary infertility*. The *ideal frequency of intercourse* is every other day [9]. History of use of artificial lubricants, even water-soluble or natural sources, may indicate a cause for impaired sperm motility [10].

Exposures to pesticides, chemicals, organic solvents, or heat (tanning booths, cooks, and foundry workers) can be significant cause for male infertility. Smoking (tobacco or marijuana) can lead to decreased sperm concentrations (*oligospermia*) and affect motility [11]. Testicular function can be impaired secondary to use of illicit drugs and alcohol abuse by disrupting the hypothalamic-pituitary axis. Anabolic steroid abuse can suppress the hypothalamo-pituitary-gonadal axis and result in testicular atrophy as well as oligo- or azoospermia [12]. Several medications have been documented to have an adverse effect on sperm concentrations and function. A list of potential prescription and over-the-counter medications is given (Table 5.1). All men should be asked about their use of supplements and herbal remedies.

The *surgical history* should include cryptorchidism (undescended testis), hypospadias, inguinal hernia repair, and malignancy. Oligospermia and even azoospermia can result from cryptorchidism. Surgical correction of hypospadias, chordee, hernia, as well as any surgery on the bladder neck, urethra, rectum, or pelvis can be significant causes for abnormal semen parameters and may cause ejaculatory difficulty by injuring sympathetic nerves. Urethral and ductal obstruction can result from urethral strictures and sexually transmitted diseases which in turn reduce sperm count. Certain malignancies including Hodgkin's lymphoma and testicular cancer are often associated with infertility and a low sperm count [13, 14] which may be related to the disease per se or to treatments such as chemotherapy, radiation, and retroperitoneal lymph node dissections.

The *ROS* (Review of Systems) can reveal less common causes for male infertility. Diabetes could be associated with partial or retrograde ejaculation, multiple sclerosis with impaired ejaculation, and spinal cord injuries with erectile dysfunction. Recurrent respiratory infections can indicate primary ciliary dyskinesia (*Kartagener's syndrome*) which is also associated with immotile sperm. Anosmia (inability to smell) could indicate hypogonadotropic hypogonadism (*Kallmann's syndrome*).

A thorough male genitourinary exam cannot be overemphasized. The patient should be examined in a warm room, in an upright position. Extent of virilization should be documented. Presence or absence of gynecomastia should alert the examiner to marijuana use and may be a prompt to rule out a prolactin-producing pituitary tumor. Normal testicular size can vary between 15 and 20 ml, and the normal testicular consistency should be firm but not hard similar to the thenar eminence of the thumb [15]. A *Seager orchidometer* can be used to more accurately assess testicular size [16]. Any thickening of the epididymis and vas deferens noted on palpation should raise the possibility of obstructive causes of infertility. Varicocele—dilation of the spermatic pampiniform plexus—should be ruled out by examining the spermatic cords in the upright position. It has been theorized that varicoceles may impair semen parameters by increasing testicular temperature or by allowing reflux of adrenal metabolites via incompetent veins [17]. Varicoceles as a cause for infertility are controversial as 15% of men with normal fertility have a varicocele and up to 70% of men with secondary infertility have varicocele [18, 19]. Most commonly the varicocele is identified on the left side in 78–93% [20]. Grading of varicoceles is primarily by physical exam although occasionally, ultrasound may be used if body precludes diagnosis by palpation. Similarly, absence of the vas deferens can be discerned by physical exam [21]. The absence can be unilateral or bilateral and may be associated with other genitourinary abnormalities such as absence of the ipsilateral kidney or incomplete epididymis formation [22]. The basis of the association is due to common congenital origin of the ureteric bud and vas from Wolffian structures (*mesonephric duct*). Cystic fibrosis (CF) is the most common (80%) cause of CBAVD and is not associated with congenital absence of kidney or epididymis [21, 23]. Men with CBAVD and their partners should undergo genetic testing and counseling regarding CF mutations.

Table 5.1 Pharmacological and environmental causes of infertility

Diethylstilbestrol (DES)	Calcium channel blockers
Radiation	Lead
Testosterone	Cigarettes
Chemotherapy	Alcohol
Ketoconazole	Cocaine
Heat	Marijuana
Nitrofurantoin	Sulfa drugs
Pesticides	Solvents

5.1.2 Laboratory Studies

All men should have their semen analyzed as part of infertility evaluation. The WHO recommends analysis of two samples, obtained 2 weeks apart with 2 or 3 days of abstinence [24]. Use of lubricant should be avoided during masturbation for collection of specimen when possible. The fifth edition of World Health Organization criteria for normal semen param-

Table 5.2 Semen analysis (based on WHO criteria)

Oligospermia	<20 million sperm/ml
Azoospermia	Absence of sperm in the ejaculate
Teratospermia	<4% normal morphology
Asthenospermia	<40% sperm motile
Leukocyto(pyo)spermia	>1 million/ml WBCs

eters are universally used as reference values (Table 5.2) [19]. It is common to observe more than one abnormal parameter. Low ejaculatory volume should prompt examination of urine sample obtained within minutes of ejaculation to observe any sperm in the urine. Sperm in the urine is highly suspicious of *retrograde ejaculation* if the history is not consistent with obstruction. Low ejaculatory volume coupled with absence of sperm in the post ejaculatory urine could indicate *ejaculatory duct obstruction or ejaculatory duct absence*. Transrectal ultrasound is useful in these cases to recognize enlarged seminal vesicle.

Oligospermia is defined as <10 million sperm per ejaculate, and *azoospermia* is defined as the absence of sperm in the ejaculate [19]. Men with either *oligo-* or *azoospermia* should undergo hormonal analysis to determine the etiology of low sperm volume by categorizing the presentation into one of the following: *pre-testicular*, the hypothalamic-pituitary axis; *testicular*, primary testicular failure; or *post-testicular*, obstruction or absence of the vasa. As one would expect, treatment ultimately depends on the identification of the abnormality in one or a combination of the three categories. There are instances where the patient cannot be categorized and are described as idiopathic male infertility (IMI), which accounts for a remarkable percentage of patients evaluated—around 30% [15]. It is common practice to empirically treat patients with IMI with hormonal, antioxidant, or both regimens with or without assisted reproductive techniques [25].

Asthenospermia denotes poor motility and is often accompanied by other semen abnormalities [19]. Movement of the tails without progression may indicate sperm antibodies attached to sperm or agglutination (clumping) of the sperm. To successfully have pregnancies, couples with antibodies in their semen analysis undergo either sperm washing or either intrauterine insemination (IUI) or in vitro fertilization/intracytoplasmic sperm injection (IVF/ICSI) [26].

Teratospermia is the morphological abnormality of sperm with the expectation of at least 4% of the sperm being classified as structurally normal [19]. These sperm are not likely to fertilize the egg. *Pyospermia*—WBC in the ejaculate—should be treated with antibiotics only in the presence of a documented source of infection. There are various tests to analyze sperm function if the semen analysis appears normal, for example, utilization of electron microscopy for 0% motility. However, these analyses are not usually performed as couples will typically proceed to IVF/ICSI if a functional problem is suspected.

Thorough evaluation for male infertility should comprise a complete medical and reproductive history, a physical exam by a urologist (preferably a male reproductive specialist), and at least two semen analyses.

A patient may require hormone analysis based on history and findings on physical examination. In recent years, hormonal evaluation has become a frequent part of the standard evaluation. Measurements include FSH, LH, and testosterone levels. This helps in differentiating pre-testicular and testicular causes of infertility. It should be noted however that endocrine causes of male infertility are unusual.

The evaluation of the male infertility patient is summarized in Fig. 5.1.

5.1.3 Radiologic Studies

If a testicular mass is detected it should alert the clinician to possibility of cancer and an ultrasound should be performed expeditiously. Infertility may be presenting symptom of testicular cancer [27]. As mentioned earlier, transrectal ultrasound is indicated in the presence of low semen volume and normal vas deferens on palpation. Dilated seminal vesicles >1.5 cm in AP diameter suggest partial or complete obstruction [28]. Non-palpable varicoceles are of little clinical significance and do not require scrotal ultrasound [29].

Abnormal testicular exam should prompt an immediate scrotal ultrasound to eliminate testicular masses which may indicate cancer.

5.2 Management

The physical examination, laboratory evaluation, and semen analyses will guide treatment. Some diagnoses such as CBAVD are made by physical examination. Retrograde ejaculation, for example, may be implied from the patient's history and is diagnosed by semen analysis and post ejaculatory urine analysis. It is further supported by ultrasound, but that is neither necessary nor sufficient for diagnosis. Although a varicocele may be diagnosed by physical exam, 15% of the fertile male population has a varicocele, and clinically significant varicoceles require diagnosis by semen analysis. Differential diagnoses for male infertility are given in Table 5.3.

Azoospermia, the absence of sperm in the ejaculate, can be seen in all three categories of infertility—pre-testicular, testicular, and post-testicular. Pre-testicular etiologies are

Fig. 5.1 Male infertility evaluation

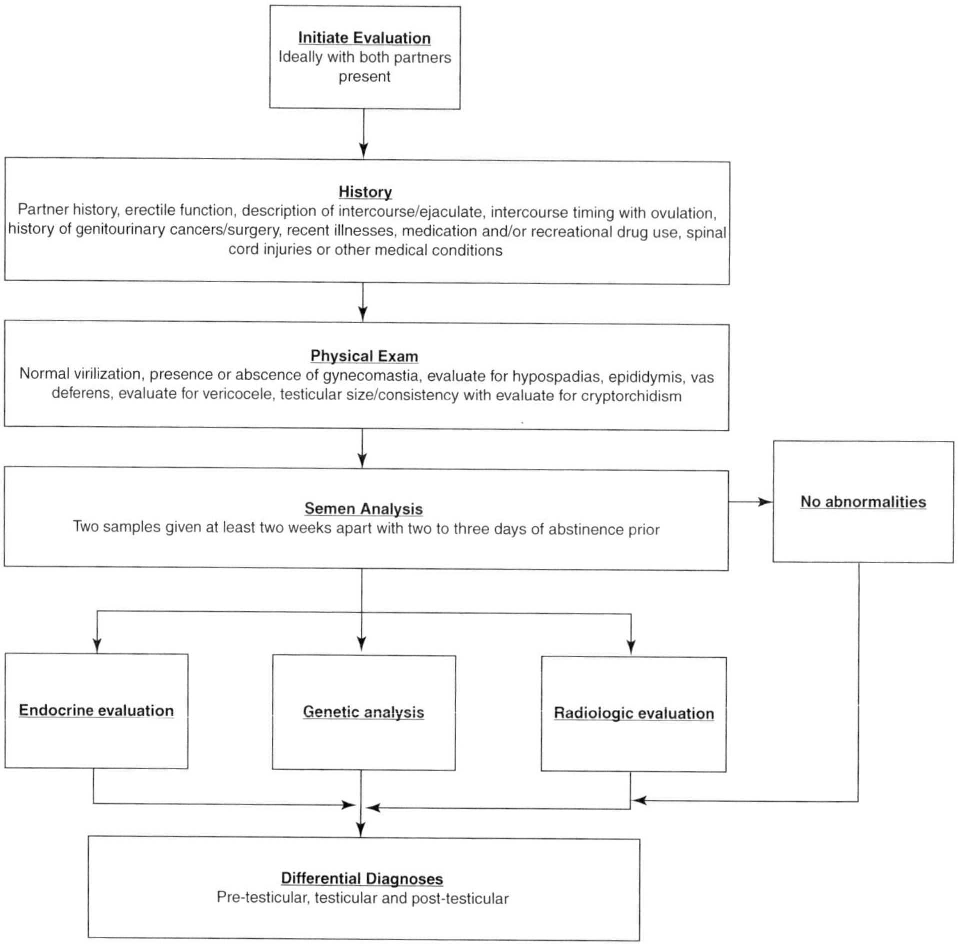

Table 5.3 Differential diagnoses for male infertility

Pre-testicular		
Hypogonadotropic hypogonadism	Anabolic steroids	
Kallmann's syndrome	Excess prolactin	
Isolated FSH deficiency	Other pharmacologic/environmental	
Testicular		
Klinefelter's syndrome	Gonadotoxins	
Noonan's syndrome	Kartagener's syndrome	
Cystic fibrosis trait/disease	Viral orchitis	
Sertoli cell only syndrome	Antisperm antibodies	
Myotonic dystrophy	Testicular cancer	
Y microdeletion	Idiopathic (25% of infertile men)	
Post–testicular		
Ductal obstruction	**Retrograde ejaculation**	**Anejaculation**
CBAVD Ejaculatory duct obstruction Previous vasectomy	Previous surgery (RPLND) Multiple sclerosis Diabetes mellitus	Spinal cord injury RPLND Myotonic dystrophy Diabetes mellitus

differentiated by endocrine analysis [19]. High testosterone and low FSH and LH may be indicative of steroid use [30]. Low FSH, LH, and T and high prolactin may be suggestive of a prolactin pituitary tumor and warrants MRI evaluation. Testicular causes of *azoospermia* may be cryptorchidism, viral orchitis, trauma, infections, and toxins. The physical exam and history of these patients will guide diagnosis. Treatment plan relies on diagnosis with the exception of testicular causes. With the exception of varicoceles, testicular causes can rarely be reversed with treatment. Testicular biopsy may be a last resort when diagnosis cannot be made by physical exam, semen analysis, and endocrine profile.

Many couples will require advanced reproductive techniques (MAR) for successful pregnancy. Repair of varicoceles may reverse azoospermia in 55% of cases [31]. Postoperative pregnancy rates can be as high as 40% for all grades of varicocele after surgical repair with supporting data found on meta-analysis showing highest success rates with palpable varicocele and at least one abnormal semen parameter [32, 33]. *Azoospermic* men with ductal obstruction will have normal hormone parameters and a normal testicular exam. Semen analysis, endocrine profile, and physical examination will aid diagnosis. Although transrectal ultrasound (TRUS) can diagnose ductal obstruction, not all cases of ductal obstruction will be diagnosed by TRUS [34]. Such men can undergo surgical repair of obstruction: vasovasostomy, MAR with sperm taken from a testicular extraction (micro TESE), biopsy, or sperm aspiration from the epididymis.

5.3 Post-treatment Evaluation

A repeat semen analysis should be performed 3 months after any medical or surgical treatment. A lack of improvement, usually 1 year from surgery, and 1–2 spermatogenesis cycles after medical therapy, should prompt the clinician to counsel the couple regarding ART, donor sperm, fostering and adoption.

5.4 Other Surgical and Medical Treatments for Infertility

Retrograde ejaculation is generally treated with a trial of sympathomimetic medications (ephedrine, pseudoephedrine). Another approach can be performed by alkalinizing the urine with oral sodium bicarbonate with subsequent sperm extraction from a urine sample and then used for MAR.

Anejaculation in the spinal cord injury patient can be treated with electrostimulation to the penile glans or prostate/seminal vesicle. Urethral strictures effecting fertility are to be treated with stricture ablation or reconstructive repair.

References

1. Thonneau P, Marchand S, Tallec A. Incidence and main causes of infertility in a resident population (1,850,000) of three French regions (1988–1989). Hum Reprod. 1991;6:811.
2. Honig SC, Lipshultz LI, Jarow J. Significant medical pathology uncovered by a comprehensive male infertility evaluation. Fertil Steril. 1994;62:1028.
3. Wilcox AJ, Weinberg CR, Baird DD. Timing of sexual intercourse in relation to ovulation. Effects on the probability of conception, survival of the pregnancy, and sex of the baby. N Engl J Med. 1995;333(23):1517–21.
4. Scarpa B, Dunson DB, Giacchi E. Bayesian selection of optimal rules for timing intercourse to conceive by using calendar and mucus. Fertil Steril. 2007;88:915–24.
5. Ramezanzadeh F, Aghssa MM, Jafarabadi M, et al. Alterations of sexual desire and satisfaction in male partners of infertile couples. Fertil Steril. 2006;85:139–43.
6. Sigman M, Jarow J. Male infertility. In: Walsh PC, et al., editors. Campbell's urology. Philadelphia: WB Saunders; 2002.
7. Zitzmann M, Nordhoff V, von Schonfeld V, Nordsiek-Mengede A, Kliesch S, Schuring AN, Luetjens CM, Kamischke A, Cooper T, Simoni M, Nieschlag E. Elevated follicle-stimulating hormone levels and the chances for azoospermic men to become fathers after retrieval of elongated spermatids from cryopreserved testicular tissue. Fertil Steril. 2006;86(2):339–47. https://doi.org/10.1016/j.fertnstert.2005.12.058.
8. Tsujimura A. Microdissection testicular sperm extraction: prediction, outcome, and complications. Int J Urol. 2007;14(10):883–9.
9. Levitas E, Lunenfeld E, Weiss N, et al. Relationship between the duration of sexual abstinence and semen quality: analysis of 9,489 semen samples. Fertil Steril. 2005;83:1680–6.
10. Anderson L, Lewis S, McClure N. The effects of coital lubricants on sperm motility in vitro. Hum Reprod. 1998;13:3351–6.
11. Gorzalka BB, Hill MN, Chang SCH. Male-female differences in the effects of cannabinoids on sexual behavior and gonadal hormone function. Horm Behav. 2010;58:91–9.
12. de Souza GL, Hallak J. Anabolic steroids and male infertility: a comprehensive review. BJU Int. 2011;108:1860–5.
13. de Bruin D, de Jong IJ, Arts EG, et al. Semen quality in men with disseminated testicular cancer: relation with human chorionic gonadotropin beta-subunit and pituitary gonadal hormones. Fertil Steril. 2009;91:2481–6.
14. Raman JD, Nobert CF, Goldstein M. Increased incidence of testicular cancer in men presenting with infertility and abnormal semen analysis. J Urol. 2005;174:1819–22.
15. Sigman M, Lipshultz LI, Howards SS. Office evaluation of the subfertile male. In: Lipshultz LI, Howards SS, Niederberger CS, editors. Infertility in the male. 4th ed. New York: Cambridge University Press; 2009. p. 153–76.
16. Niederberger CS. Clinical evaluation of the male. In: Niederberger CS, editor. An introduction to male reproductive medicine. New York: Cambridge University Press; 2011. p. 29–57.
17. Gorelick JI, Goldstein M. Loss of fertility in men with varicocele. Fertil Steril. 1993;59(3):613–6.
18. Khera M, Lipshultz LI. Evolving approach to the varicocele. Urol Clin North Am. 2008;35(2):183–9, viii.
19. Dubin L, Amelar RD. Etiologic factors in 1294 consecutive cases of male infertility. Fertil Steril. 1971;22:469–74.
20. Saypol DC, Lipschultz LI, Howards SS. Varicocele. In: Lipschultz LI, Howards SS, editors. Infertility in the male. New York: Churchill Livingstone; 1983. p. 299–313.
21. Hall S, Oates RD. Unilateral absence of the scrotal vas deferens associated with contralateral mesonephric duct anomalies resulting in infertility: laboratory, physical and radiographic findings, and therapeutic alternatives. J Urol. 1993;150:1161.
22. Schlegel PN, Shin D, Goldstein M. Urogenital anomalies in men with congenital absence of the vas deferens. J Urol. 1996;155:1644–8.
23. Anguiano A, Oates RD, Amos JA, et al. Congenital bilateral absence of the vas deferens. A primarily genital form of cystic fibrosis. JAMA. 1992;267:1794.
24. WHO. Laboratory manual for the examination of human semen and sperm-cervical mucus interaction. 3rd ed. Cambridge: Cambridge University Press; 1992.
25. Gudeloglu A, Brahmbhatt JV, Parekattil SJ. Medical management of male infertility in the absence of a specific etiology. Semin Reprod Med. 2014;32(4):313–8. https://doi.org/10.1055/s-0034-1375184.
26. Van Peperstraten A, Proctor ML, Johnson NP, Philipson G. Techniques for surgical retrieval of sperm prior to ICSI for azoospermia. Cochrane Database Syst Rev. 2006;3:CD002807.
27. Mancini M, Carmignani L, Gazzano G, et al. High prevalence of testicular cancer in azoospermic men without spermatogenesis. Hum Reprod. 2007;22:1042–6.
28. Baker K, Sabanegh E Jr. Obstructive azoospermia: reconstructive techniques and results. Clinics (Sao Paulo). 2013;68(Suppl 1):61–73.
29. Jarow JP, Ogle SR, Eskew LA. Seminal improvement following repair of ultrasound detected subclinical varicoceles. J Urol. 1996;155:1287–90.

30. Carnegie C. Diagnosis of hypogonadism: clinical assessments and laboratory tests. Rev Urol. 2004;6(Suppl 6):S3–8.
31. Matthews GJ, Matthews ED, Goldstein M. Induction of spermatogenesis and achievement of pregnancy after microsurgical varicocelectomy in men with azoospermia and severe oligoasthenospermia. Fertil Steril. 1998;70(1):71–5.
32. Madgar I, Weissenberg R, Lunenfeld B, et al. Controlled trial of high spermatic vein ligation for varicocele in infertile men. Fertil Steril. 1995;63:120–4.
33. Marmar JL, Agarwal A, Prabakaran S, Agarwal R, Short RA, et al. Reassessing the value of varicocelectomy as a treatment for male subfertility with a new meta-analysis. Fertil Steril. 2007;88:639–48.
34. Schroeder-Printzen I, Ludwig M, Köhn F, et al. Surgical therapy in infertile men with ejaculatory duct obstruction: technique and outcome of a standardized surgical approach. Hum Reprod. 2000;15:1364–8.

Part II

Ovarian Stimulation and Egg Retrieval

Analyses and Approaches to Improve IUI Outcome

6

Gulam Bahadur, Roy Homburg, Mariusz Łukaszuk, and Kanna Jayaprakasan

Fertility treatment via intrauterine insemination (IUI) was first practiced in 1962 [1]. The costs for IUI treatment are less expensive than in vitro fertilization (IVF), and the treatment is less invasive whilst providing an acceptable success rate per cycle. Whilst IUI has recently been neglected by some IVF practitioners because of potentially lower success rate per cycle of treatment on a head-to-head comparison, and possibly for commercial reasons, persuasive economic data emphatically backs the use of the IUI procedure as an initial cost-effective treatment choice [2, 3].

When the expenses to provide fertility treatments are considered, IUI works out to be cheaper compared to IVF treatment. The average expense per live birth rate has been calculated at €7187 for IVF treatment versus €5070 for IUI treatment, with an incremental ratio of cost-effectiveness per live birth of €43,375 for IVF [3]. In the UK, typical costs in 2016–2017 to the patient and UK Care Commissioning Groups (CCG) were around £3800–£6500 per IVF cycle versus £800–£1300 per IUI cycle.

If guideline recommendations about sperm quality are adhered to, the costs for provision of all IUI cycles and trigger dose show an incremental net financial gain between €645 and over €7500 per couple [4]. The wider implication of this is that IUI brings substantial economic benefits. Although the threshold for sperm was described as having 'more than 1 million motile spermatozoa should be available for IUI after sperm preparation' [5], it seems cost-effective to have a minimum of 3 million motile sperm for IUI. The financial benefit of IUI over IVF is confirmed when the man provides an ejaculate containing a total motile sperm count (TMSC) of >3 million [6], whilst good outcomes are associated with >5 million TMSC [7].

More than 144,000 IUI cycles are initiated annually in Europe, aiming to help approximately 32,000 couples with infertility (as calculated over the period 2000–2002). As such, this could result in a potential financial saving of over €20 million annually [4]. Thus, there is a need to improve the development and implementation of the current guideline [4].

A misconception exists regarding the finance of gonadotropin use versus clomiphene citrate (CC). Accepting that CC is a cheaper drug, calculations for provision of a live birth need to also take into account the wider running costs (consultations, baseline examinations, numerous visits for ultrasound scans and ovulation monitoring). As well as the emotional toil, additional considerations include the costs linked to multiple births, possible abnormalities in the foetus and failure of the cycle.

An evidenced-based report performed independently by non-fertility expert researchers at the Centre for Evidence-Based Medicine, Oxford University, UK, showed the effect of IUI in a natural cycle on the live birth rate: odds ratio (95% CI) 1.95 (1.10–3.44) in a trial with 396 couples, compared with natural intercourse or expectant management in a cycle using ovarian stimulation [8]. This contrasts with the effect on live birth rate: odds ratio (95% CI), for example, of endometrial scratching having a relative risk of 1.42 (1.08–1.85) compared with no injury to days 2–3 [8]. Compared to endometrial scratching, IUI was superior in practice, but, despite this evidence, there appears a skewed tendency to practice poorly supported IVF add-on techniques.

G. Bahadur (✉)
Reproductive Medicine Unit, North Middlesex University Hospital, London, UK

Homerton Fertility Unit, Homerton University Hospital, London, UK

R. Homburg
Homerton Fertility Unit, Homerton University Hospital, London, UK

M. Łukaszuk
Invicta Fertility Clinic Gdansk, Gdansk, Pomeranian, Poland

K. Jayaprakasan
Derby Fertility Unit, Royal Derby Hospital, Derby, UK

G. N. Allahbadia et al. (eds.), *Textbook of Assisted Reproduction*, https://doi.org/10.1007/978-981-15-2377-9_6

6.1 Indications for IUI Treatment

When considering medically assisted reproduction (MAR), there is need to proportion a high pregnancy rate whilst giving an acceptably low multiple pregnancy rate, avoiding an OHSS risk. Individual risk assessments need to be performed to avoid harm to the patient or foetus.

Protocols are variable, and identifying what is optimal remains a major task. One problem with assessing success is the fact that there may not be optimal provision and practice of the IUI procedure. Patients need to be properly informed of their choices, risks and options to ensure their safety before any treatment.

It is clear that it is preferable to aim for stimulation of two follicles for an IUI cycle. By doing this, the likelihood of obtaining an IUI pregnancy potentially rises by 3.4-fold compared with mono-follicular cycles [9]. Precise follicle monitoring can bring down the absolute rate of multiple pregnancies to 0.3 and 2.8% for mono-follicular growth and multifollicular growth, respectively [10]. Furthermore, depending on whether 2, 3 or 4 follicles are stimulated, the chance of a multiple gestation has been proposed to rise by 6, 14 and 10%, respectively [10].

IUI treatment aims to improve the likelihood that an optimal concentration of healthy sperm reaches the ampulla, for fertilization to take place. For female patients where a cervical mucus problem is suspected, IUI can circumvent a possible cervical factor. Whilst IUI is conventionally performed for subfertility due to unexplained causes, mild male factor and mild endometriosis, IUI is routinely considered as an initial treatment in all patients with the female having a minimum of one patent fallopian tube and the male having a TMSC of >3 million/ml in the ejaculate. Contraindication includes bilateral tubal obstruction, moderate to severe oligo-asthenozoospermia, cervicitis or endometritis.

6.2 IUI Procedures and Insemination Methods

6.2.1 Mode of Insemination

The primary goal of artificial insemination is to deliver a concentrate of highly motile sperm as near to the site of ovulation as possible. Intra-cervical insemination (ICI) is rarely used for patients with a history of subfertility but may occasionally be resorted to. There is no reason why ICI, used to emulate timed intercourse, cannot be used in single or lesbian women with no history of subfertility.

However, IUI with a processed sperm sample is the widely accepted standard approach. Furthermore. it should be noted that using a soft-tip over a hard-tip catheter does not result in any improvement in the IUI live birth rate [11].

6.2.2 Ovulation Induction Methods

Regarding the ovarian stimulation protocols for IUI treatment, several are in use. However, it remains unclear which protocol or dose is most financially viable. Whilst robust evidence is lacking, IUI using gonadotropins could be most effective, according to a Cochrane review [12]. Although low-dose protocols are advised to overcome OHSS and multiple pregnancy risks, there is insufficient information on how this may work in individualised care with a robust cancellation policy [12].

A frequently used ovulation-inducing agent is CC. However, when compared to CC, both the conception and live birth rates have been shown to be higher using hMG with IUI [13, 14]. The relative term pregnancy rate was 2.10 (95% CI 0.77–5.73) for hMG versus CC [13]. Ovarian stimulation with either letrozole or CC, to reduce the dose of gonadotropins prior to IUI, appeared justified with possible reduction in stimulation protocol cost [15].

A significantly higher pregnancy rate following IUI with hMG (OR 0.44 95% CI 0.19–0.99) compared to CC has been reported [16]. However, the mean pregnancy rates per cycle were 8% for CC and 25% for gonadotropins [17]. Pregnancy rates per cycle with use of 75–150 IU hMG or CC led to pregnancy rates per cycle of 13–20 and 4–7%, respectively [16, 18, 19].

Another prospective study [20] indicated that the use of GnRH antagonists had a positive effect on the live birth rate, especially if the multifollicular stimulation was induced [20]. This group reported an overall live birth rate of 11.4% per cycle (ranging between clinics from 8.4 to 17.6% per cycle). Practice difference included use of GnRH antagonists (15.2% with vs. 9.4% without) and the number of mature recruited follicles (9.4% for one vs. 15.2% for two), both having a statistically significant impact on the delivery rate [20].

6.2.3 Gonadotropin Superovulation

A low-dose gonadotropin (50–75 IU/day) to induce controlled ovarian hyperstimulation with preferably bifollicular response has been suggested to achieve a high conception rate with low risk of multiple pregnancy. Bifollicular IUI cycles potentially increase the chance of achieving an IUI pregnancy, where the pregnancy rate against the number of mature recruited follicles is significant (9.4% for one vs. 15.2% for two) [20].

Some fertility clinics use gonadotropins at a higher dose than the standard for controlled ovarian stimulation. A recent review of 170 cycles at one of our clinics showed that use of 150 IU hMG (alternate day) + 50 mg CC (daily) provided cycles with a single follicle (31.5%), two follicles (46%) and three follicles (22.5%), with respective pregnancy rates per cycle of 18%, 18% (three sets of twins) and 26% (no multiple births). The number of follicles that develop is variable and depends on several factors, including BMI and age. However, there can be a benefit for IUI from a multifollicular environment.

In a review of 27 studies, it was shown that pregnancy rate per cycle started improved from 8 to 18% with IUI and gonadotropin stimulation [21]. In another trial, IUI improved fertility in cycles in which CC was combined with gonadotropins [22]. Combination stimulation may have merit in overcoming some elements of unexplained infertility. In our recent cohort of 67 cycles in women aged 35–40 years receiving 150–225 IU hMG plus 50 mg CC, the pregnancy rate per cycle started was 27%, although a larger RCT dataset is needed to validate this approach.

6.2.4 Aromatase Inhibitors

In a large randomised controlled trial (RCT) comparing treatment with gonadotropins, CC or letrozole, clinical pregnancies occurred in 35.5, 28.3 and 22.4% of cycles and live birth in 32.2, 23.3 and 18.7%, respectively. Pregnancy rates with letrozole were lower than with gonadotropin or CC ($P = 0.003$) or gonadotropin alone ($P < 0.001$), but not with CC alone ($P = 0.10$) [23].

It appears that inhibition of oestrogen synthesis by aromatase inhibition induces estrogenic negative feedback, resulting in an increase in endogenous FSH secretion. Moreover, by inhibiting conversion of androgens into oestrogens, accumulating androgens may increase follicular sensitivity to FSH. Such a protocol has the potential to lower FSH treatment cost and may improve response for low responders who require high FSH doses during ovarian stimulation [24].

6.3 What Is Effective?

In a dedicated IUI setting, an ongoing pregnancy rate of 32.6% (43/132) can be achieved per cycle [25]. The pregnancy rate following treatment with hMG-IUI approached that for IVF for most conventionally treated infertility subgroups. The authors suggest that most infertility patients should therefore be offered hMG-IUI therapy prior to IVF referral [25].

A patient-tailored approach is needed, as demonstrated by a multicentre RCT using recombinant follicle-stimulating hormone (rFSH) [26]. In this study, patients were given either an 'individual' ($n = 113$) or a 'standard' dose ($n = 115$) (at 50–100 and 75 IU rFSH/day, respectively). For the 'individual' dose, patient dose was based on a nomogram, taking into account patient BMI and the antral follicle count, resulting in 70% patients developing two to three follicles. This is compared to the 'standard' dose group where 56% of patients develop two to three follicles [95% confidence interval (CI) 2–26, $P = 0.03$]. Where multiple follicles developed, two follicles were observed in 58% 'individual' group patients versus 53% 'standard' group patients ($P = 0.54$). The ongoing pregnancy rates were 20 and 18% for the 'individual' and 'standard' groups, respectively, with multiple gestation rates of 1 versus 4% ($P = 0.21$). Thus, compared to standard dosing, individual dosing according to a nomogram was shown to be beneficial [26].

6.3.1 Luteal Phase Support

Controlled ovarian stimulation combined with IUI is a convenient treatment of infertility with a success rate of 11%/cycle. Luteal phase support appears in common usage, although support for practice appears limited. The supplementation of luteal phase with vaginal progesterone significantly increases live birth among women undergoing IUI when receiving gonadotropins for ovulation induction, although women receiving CC to induce ovulation do not seem to benefit [27].

However, in a recent systematic review of 2842 patients undergoing 4065 cycles, progesterone luteal phase support was beneficial to patients undergoing ovulation induction (OI) with gonadotropins in IUI cycles. Progesterone support did not benefit patients undergoing ovulation induction with CC or CC plus gonadotropins. In patients receiving gonadotropins, clinical pregnancy (relative risk [RR] 1.56, 95% confidence interval [CI] 1.21–2.02) and live birth (RR 1.77, 95% CI 1.30–2.42) were more likely in progesterone-supplemented patients. These findings persisted in analysis of live birth rates per IUI cycle (RR 1.59, 95% CI 1.24–2.04). There was no benefit on clinical pregnancy with progesterone support for patients who underwent OI with CC (RR 0.85, 95% CI 0.52–1.41) or CC plus gonadotropins (RR 1.26, 95% CI 0.90–1.76) [28].

The use of a GnRH agonist to trigger final follicle maturation in stimulated cycles of hyper-responders has been shown to be associated with a favourable reproductive outcome and no incidence of OHSS. However, such treatments resulted in higher multiple pregnancies. This highlights the fact that critical risk assessment needs to be performed before IUI [29].

Use of leuprolide acetate (LA) to trigger a gonadotropin surge as a means of inducing ovulation in FSH-stimulated women could be an alternative to improve the IUI results. One study looked at administration of two s.c. doses of LA or 7500 IU of i.m. hCG when at least one 18-mm-diameter follicle was seen and estradiol levels reached 120 pg/ml per follicle if a ≥16 mm diameter follicle was seen. The pregnancy rates per cycle started were 17.3% (hCG) and 27.3%

(LA), respectively ($P = 0.0007$), and abortion rates 22.2% (hCG) and 24.5% (LA), respectively [30].

6.3.2 Heterogeneity of IUI Practices

It seems the concurrent use of low-dose r-FSH and CC might be cost-effective whilst preventing high-order multiple pregnancies [31]. In protocols with recombinant rFSH (75 vs. 150 UI/day), there was a clear trend to achieve a better pregnancy rate with 150 UI/day without a significant rise in multiple pregnancy rates nor OHSS. The multifollicular development was associated with the 150 UI/day group [32]. AMH in IUI has attracted little application so far, but this can be used as basis for adjusting the drug stimulation dosage [33].

Data for the European Society for Human Reproduction and Embryology (ESHRE) on IUI provides an overall negative picture of IUI with CC where pregnancy rates average 7% per cycle [5]. FSH ovarian stimulation and IUI treatment is only modestly better, with a pregnancy rate of 12% per cycle but multiple birth rates averaging 13%. This study concluded that IUI yields modest results with high multiple pregnancy rates, meaning that it is no more than a poor substitute for IVF treatment. However, a problem with this study was the collection of heterogeneous practices with IUI treatment cycles encompassing >3 follicles which were already at high risk of a multiple pregnancy. Furthermore, most data was generated from IVF centres with little incentive to improve on their IUI procedures [5].

6.3.3 Cycle Numbers

The question as to how many consecutive IUI treatment cycles to perform, before either stopping or moving on to IVF treatment, remains unanswered. Many clinics suggest six cycles [11, 34], whilst one report showed that most of their pregnancies were in the fifth treatment cycle (10.8% (95% CI 6.6–17). There is a need to achieve a bi- or trifollicular environment by increasing the dosages of gonadotropins [34]. An offer of six cycles of IUI is therefore justified practice.

6.3.4 Timing of Insemination

Potentially the most important determinants of success with IUI are the timings of both the ovulation trigger and the actual IUI treatment.

Despite the optimal IUI time being 30 h post-trigger, the majority of IUIs take place 32–36 h post-trigger [7]. Trigger time can differ in CC cycles and hMG cycles according to leading follicle diameter. For example, the optimal time for hCG trigger in CC cycles has been shown to be when the leading follicle reaches 20 mm in diameter, compared to 18 mm in diameter in hMG cycles [35].

A premature LH surge can take place in 25–30% of stimulated IUI cycles, which may interfere with IUI timing [36]. The LH surge is required for luteinization, final maturation of the oocyte and follicle rupture. Whilst GnRH antagonist could be used to prevent premature luteinisation, in certain situations where IUI should intentionally be delayed over the weekend when follicle reaches 17 mm, routine use of GnRH antagonist in IUI cycles does not increase the pregnancy rates [37].

6.3.5 Timing and Stimulation

Without any drug stimulation, the LH level should be monitored daily to achieve a higher pregnancy rate per IUI cycle [38]. Once the LH rise is detected, the IUI should take place the following day, rather than 2 days later, with a respective risk ratio of achieving a clinical pregnancy of 1.78 [95% confidence interval (CI), 1.11–2.88] and a pregnancy rate of 20.5 versus 12.2%, although this difference was not significant [38]. Using this data, one extra clinical pregnancy could be obtained for every 12 IUI cycles, by performing IUI takes on the day following the LH rise, rather than 2 days.

One prospective RCT of 1257 COH-IUI cycles [39] randomised patients into a 'single' IUI group (receiving single insemination 34 h post hCG administration) and a 'double' IUI group (receiving two inseminations 18–24 and 36–48 h post hCG injection). The double IUI group had a significantly better male factor infertility pregnancy rate than the single IUI group (19.9 vs. 11.1%, $p < 0.05$) [39].

This benefit of 'double IUI' is backed up by another study comparing gonadotropin-containing ovarian stimulation protocols or within the ovulatory dysfunction and male factor diagnostic categories [40]. In this report, 110 clinical pregnancies occurred for 508 couples in 999 single IUI cycles (fecundity, 11.0%), whilst 45 clinical pregnancies for 174 couples occurred in 277 double IUI cycles (16.2%, $p < 0.004$). Differences for fecundity were noted regarding diagnostic categories between single and double IUI groups (ovulation dysfunction, 12.9 vs. 19.5%, $p < 0.048$, and male factor, 7.9 vs. 17.5%, $p < 0.030$) and ovulation protocols (CC-Gn-hCG, 13.0 vs. 21.3%, $p < 0.031$, and L-Gn-hCG, 4.2 vs. 25.0%, $p < 0.002$) [40].

6.3.6 Use of Consecutive Ejaculations in IUI

We introduced a unique way to overcome the male factor problem by utilising a 'consecutive ejaculate' which must not be confused with 'consecutive day IUIs'. Men were profiled beforehand for their suitability for IUI. This required the laboratory processing the sperm sample to provide information to the treating clinician about the feasibility of delivering >5 million motile progressive sperm for IUI.

Based on previous recovery rates of motile sperm from processing procedures, it is possible to predict whether the unprocessed ejaculate could deliver the minimum threshold of sperm for IUI. Where a shortfall was expected, the man was asked to provide another ejaculate immediately after the next [7]. The easiest way was to determine if there were ≤10 million total progressive sperm in the whole ejaculate. In such cases, a consecutive ejaculate was requested.

By doing this, patients who would otherwise had been considered as suitable for IVF/ICSI procedures were actually found to be suited for IUI procedures. This phenomenon had never been publicly addressed and has since turned out to be a very powerful and unique tool to overcome male factor infertility.

In these cases, the only hindrance to pregnancy for female partners had been the availability of suitable numbers of motile sperm, and therefore these women should be suitable for pregnancy if this rate-limiting step could be overcome. The initial report suggests that oligozoospermic males can be made to emulate normozoospermia males with consecutive ejaculate application.

From our study, the pregnancy rate in the single ejaculate group was 23%, whilst the pregnancy rate in the consecutive ejaculate group was 19%, giving an overall pregnancy rate of 20.5%. Tables 6.1 and 6.2 highlights the differences in semen

Table 6.1 Semen quality and pregnancy rates for couples having IUI with subfertile males producing initial and consecutive ejaculations

	Mean		Pair-wise differences
Parameter	Sample 1	Sample 2	Mean ± SEM
Abstinence (Days)	4.4	–	–
Abstinence (Hours)	–	0.65	–
Volume (ml)	2.7	1.1	1.6 ± 0.14
Concentration (mill/ml)	17.8	19.7	1.9 ± 1.7
Viscosity (% High)	25%	39%	14 ± 5.6%
Normal morphology	6.1%	7.3%	1.1% ± 0.8
Rapid motility	8.8%	26.5%	17.8 ± 1.6*

*$P < 0.001$

Table 6.2 Pregnancy rates in consecutive and single ejaculates

	No pregnancy		Pregnancy	
Single	37	77%	11	23%
Consecutive	56	81%	13	19%
Overall	93	79.50%	24	20.50%

Initial ejaculate; Sample 2 = consecutive ejaculate
Pearson chi^2 = 0.2884; $P = 0.591$
The pregnancy rate in the single ejaculate group was 23%, whilst the pregnancy rate in the consecutive ejaculate group was 19%, giving an overall pregnancy rate of 20.5%

parameters of a consecutive ejaculate which can often be surprising to clinical practitioners, given the findings are opposite to classical teachings.

To recognise the value of the consecutive ejaculate represents a major leap in our understanding and management of male infertility. It is recommended that consecutive ejaculates should be analysed routinely, especially for the percentage of rapidly progressive sperm, which is one of the positive indicators for sperm fertilization.

6.3.7 Managing Weekend IUI

Weekend management of IUI will impact on the overall outcome. Therefore, timing raises question on managing weekend IUIs and ways to avoid weekend IUIs for clinics that do not operate a 7-day service.

For stimulated IUI programmes, when one or more follicles of 15–16 mm diameter are observed on ultrasound scan on a Friday, and it is not possible for logistic reasons (weekend) to perform the insemination 72 h later, GnRH antagonist can be administered until hCG administration. The IUI can then be performed on Monday.

This approach has been investigated, by reviewing success rates of standard IUI against an IUI 'weekend-free' group [41]. The pregnancy rates per cycle were similar for the weekend-free group (15.7%) and the standard group (16.5%), with no difference in the multiple pregnancy or hyperstimulation rates. The only difference with the weekend-free group was higher estradiol levels, due to the prolonged ovarian stimulation.

Thus, GnRH antagonists can be used to control folliculogenesis to avoid weekend IUIs, without apparently reducing the PR [41]. In one study, IUI was performed at either (1) 26–28 h after hCG injection or (2) 36–38 h after hCG injection. Both groups were advised to have timed intercourse within a 12–18-h period [42]. Pregnancy rates were comparable, and the number of follicles >17 mm diameter per patient was not significantly different between the two groups (23.6 vs. 23.4%).

The different timing but similar efficacy of these two IUI protocols provides a practical choice to clinicians. The availability of both protocols may avoid unnecessary scheduling of clinical and laboratory work on weekends and holidays in women participating in controlled ovarian hyperstimulation and IUI programmes for treatment of non-male infertility [42].

6.3.8 Unilateral Tubal Blockage

Where there is unilateral tube blockage, conception is possible if the egg is released from the ipsilateral ovary and patent fallopian tube [43]. For such patients, a cumulative pregnancy rate (CPR) of 26.3% (10/38) after three IUI cycles has been shown, compared to 44.7% (55/123) in patients with patent fallopian tubes ($p = 0.043$).

Another study showed that for stimulated IU, there were no significant differences in pregnancy rate per cycle between a unilateral tubal occlusion group (17.3%) and a control group (18.9%). There pregnancy rates were not statistically significant if patients had a proximal tubal occlusion (21.7%), a mid-distal tubal occlusion (12.5%) or unexplained infertility (18.9%) [44].

6.3.9 Volume for IUI

What volume to place in the uterus remains an underexplored issue, and yet it is one of the most important factors, since this defines what initial loss of prepared sperm can be expected against what the uterus can hold for IUI in a meaningful way. In fallopian tube sperm perfusion (FSP), 4 ml is possible, whereas in IUI typically 0.2–0.5 ml is injected.

One study of FSP included women who were randomly allocated to group 1 (FSP via Foley catheter with 4 ml of inseminate) or group 2 (standard IUI with 0.5 ml of inseminate) ($n = 60$ for both) [45]. The main outcome measure was CPR. The CPR was significantly higher in group 1 than in group 2 (16 [26.7%] vs. 7 [11.7%]; $P < 0.04$). Whilst FSP appeared to be an effective technique in the management of mild-moderate male factor infertility, it is clear there is scope to increase the IUI volume. We have regularly utilised 1 ml with very slow and careful insemination procedure to minimise spillage, back flow. Initial failed cycles may provide clue on the level of retention and backflow. Bed rest of 15 min is suggested [45].

6.4 Summary

It may also be that the CC-induced IUI cycles were never analysed for the optimal trigger time and only recently have the differences in follicle sizes been noted for hMG and CC cycles.

Clinics need a database to allow a real-time view of their progress. It appears the biggest determinant in the success of IUI is the clinical management of the patient followed by a detailed view of every aspect of the treatment cycle. We should reflect on how progress for IVF had started, but in this case, it relied on a huge number of IUI cases being fast-tracked for IVF, which is unfair to and unethical towards patients.

A number of studies exist with good CPRs and the methods need to be emulated. 150 IU hMG and 10,000 IU hCG appear to provide CPRs at the upper levels of 13–20% per cycle, and CC cycles appear to lag considerably in CPRs, probably because of lack of optimisation. In the future, AMH profiles need to be applied to IUI patients in order to tailor the dose of the gonadotropin.

Low-dose aspirin therapy in IUI appears to support women with a thin endometrium (<8 mm) with significantly better CPRs rates (18.4 vs. 9.0%) [46]. Ultrasound-guided IUI seems not to confer additional benefit [47]. Laboratory detail to sperm preparation is crucial as this will define what motile sperm is available for IUI, with a net effect of converting normozoospermia patients into oligozoospermia status and vice versa [7].

However, we still need to establish the most effective semen handling techniques. This includes optimal abstinence [7], the time interval between ejaculation and sperm processing, the preparation methods, the optimal time between sperm preparation and insemination, temperature during centrifugation, centrifugation speeds, loading volumes in centrifuge tubes and the temperature of storage of processed sperm whilst awaiting insemination.

The impact of the time interval between semen collection and insemination, between semen collection and processing and between processing and insemination needs further evaluation [48, 49]. Higher CPRs were shown where IUI took place within 90 min after semen collection compared to longer time intervals (i.e. 91–120 and >120 min) [48], although another study reported no differences [49]. In our higher performing IUI clinic, sperm preparation occurs immediately after liquefaction, and IUI performed mostly within half an hour of processing, although no longer than 1-h post preparation. The sample is kept in an incubator at 37 °C for any waiting periods.

6.5 Conclusion

The future of IUI is promising if every IUI cycle is optimised, especially if most cycles are performed with two follicles using hMG, whilst having a strict cancellation policy if greater than or equal to three mature follicles are present to minimise multiple births. There is no evidence-based support that IUI is responsible for multiple births given live birth reports rarely exist and excessive multiple births are an IVF phenomenon.

The use of 'consecutive ejaculate' is a new concept. This has shown how male factor definitions can be altered by simply profiling the males beforehand to alter the management of the couple's subfertility in the patient's favour. Although there is little evidence to support the use of luteal phase support, it is in common use and not deemed harmful.

The language of presenting outcomes is becoming clearer, and presenting IUI success rates and renewed focus on optimising IUI outcomes has a major societal contribution. This involves having a strict IUI rejection policy where patients could be better served with IVF.

The use of combination drugs hMG/CC seems promising for the 35–40-year-old group, with a CPR of 27% per cycle. For patients, the largest benefit is the least intrusive and least psychologically demanding procedure and one which can benefit a much bigger subfertile global population.

References

1. Cohen MR. Intra-uterine insemination. Int J Fertil. 1962;7:235–40.
2. Bahadur G, Homburg R, Muneer A, Racich P, Alangaden T, Al-Habib A, Okolo S. First line fertility treatment strategies regarding IUI and IVF require clinical evidence. Hum Reprod. 2016;31(6):1141–6. https://doi.org/10.1093/humrep/dew075.
3. Tjon-Kon-Fat RI, Bensdorp AJ, Bossuyt PM, Koks C, Oosterhuis GJ, Hoek A, Hompes P, Broekmans FJ, Verhoeve HR, de Bruin JP, et al. Is IVF-served two different ways-more cost-effective than IUI with controlled ovarian hyperstimulation? Hum Reprod. 2015;30:2331–9.
4. Haagen EC, Nelen WL, Adang EM, Grol RP, Hermens RP, Kremer JA. Guideline adherence is worth the effort: a cost-effectiveness analysis in intrauterine insemination care. Hum Reprod. 2013;28(2):357–66. https://doi.org/10.1093/humrep/des408.
5. ESHRE Capri Workshop Group. Intrauterine insemination. Hum Reprod Update. 2009;15(3):265–77. https://doi.org/10.1093/humupd/dmp003.
6. Moolenaar LM, Cissen M, de Bruin JP, Hompes P, Repping S, van der Veen F, Mol BWJ. Cost-effectiveness of assisted conception for male subfertility. Reprod Biomed Online. 2015;30:659–66.
7. Bahadur G, Almossawi O, Illahibuccus A, Al-Habib A, Okolo S. Factors leading to pregnancies in stimulated intrauterine insemination cycles and the use of consecutive ejaculations within a small clinic environment. J Obstet Gynaecol India. 2016;66(Suppl 1):513–20. https://doi.org/10.1007/s13224-016-0876-0.
8. Spencer E, Mahtani K, Goldacre B, et al. Claims for fertility interventions: a systematic assessment of statements on UK fertility centre websites. BMJ Open. 2016;6:e013940. https://doi.org/10.1136/bmjopen-2016-013940.
9. Tomlinson MJ, Amissah-Arthur JB, Thompson KA, Kasraie JL, Bentick B. Prognostic indicators for IUI (IUI): statistical model for IUI success. Hum Reprod. 1996;11:1892–6.
10. van Rumste MME, Custers IM, van der Veen F, van Wely M, Evers JLH, Mol BWJ. The influence of the number of follicles on pregnancy rates in IUI with ovarian stimulation: a meta-analysis. Hum Reprod Update. 2008;14:563–70.
11. Vermeylen AM, D'Hooghe T, Debrock S, Meeuwis L, Meuleman C, Spiessens C. The type of catheter has no impact on the pregnancy rate after intrauterine insemination: a randomized study. Hum Reprod. 2006;21(9):2364–7.
12. Cantineau AE, Cohlen BJ, Heineman MJ. Ovarian stimulation protocols (anti-oestrogens, gonadotrophins with and without GnRH agonists/antagonists) for intrauterine insemination (IUI) in women with subfertility. Cochrane Database Syst Rev. 2007;2:CD005356.. Review
13. Manganiello PD, Stern JE, Stukel TA, Crow H, Brinck-Johnsen T, Weiss JE. A comparison of clomiphene citrate and human menopausal gonadotropin for use in conjunction with intrauterine insemination. Fertil Steril. 1997;68(3):405–12.
14. Peeraer K, Debrock S, De Loecker P, Tomassetti C, Laenen A, Welkenhuysen M, Meeuwis L, Pelckmans S, Mol BW, Spiessens C, De Neubourg D, D'Hooghe TM. Low-dose human menopausal gonadotrophin versus clomiphene citrate in subfertile couples treated with intrauterine insemination: a randomized controlled trial. Hum Reprod. 2015;30(5):1079–88.
15. Badawy A, Elnashar A, Totongy M. Clomiphene citrate or aromatase inhibitors combined with gonadotropins for superovulation in women undergoing intrauterine insemination: a prospective randomised trial. J Obstet Gynaecol. 2010;30(6):617–21. https://doi.org/10.3109/01443615.2010.497873.
16. Karlstorm PO, Bergh T, Lundkvist O. A prospective randomized trial of artificial insemination versus intercourse in cycles stimulated with human menopausal gonadotropin or clomiphene citrate. Fertil Steril. 1993;59(3):554–9.
17. Balasch J, Ballesca JL, Pimentel C, Creus M, Fabregues F, Vanrell JA. Late low-dose pure follicle stimulating hormone for ovarian stimulation in intra-uterine insemination cycles. Hum Reprod. 1994;9:1863–6.
18. Karande VC, Rao R, Pratt DE, Balin M, Levrant S, Morris R, Dudkeiwicz A, Gleicher N. A randomized prospective comparison between IUI and fallopian sperm perfusion for the treatment of infertility. Fertil Steril. 1995;64:638–40.
19. Manganiello PD, Stern JE, Stukel TA, Crow H, Brinck-Johnsen T, Weiss JE. A comparison of clomiphene citrate and human menopausal gonadotropin for use in conjunction with IUI. Fertil Steril. 1997;68:405–12.
20. Monraisin O, Chansel-Debordeaux L, Chiron A, Floret S, Cens S, Bourrinet S, Paulhac S, Jimenez C, Parinaud J, Leandri R. Evaluation of intrauterine insemination practices: a 1-year prospective study in seven French assisted reproduction technology centers. Fertil Steril. 2016;105(6):1589–93. https://doi.org/10.1016/j.fertnstert.2016.01.039.
21. Guzick DS, Sullivan MW, Adamson GD, Cedars MI, Falk RJ, Peterson EP. Efficacy of treatment for unexplained infertility. Fertil Steril. 1998;70:207–13.
22. Arcaini L, Bianchi S, Baglioni A, Marchini M, Tozzi L, Fedele L. Superovulation and IUI vs. super ovulation alone in the treatment of unexplained infertility. A randomized study. J Reprod Med. 1996;41:614–8.
23. Diamond MP, Legro RS, Coutifaris C, Alvero R, Robinson RD, Casson P, Christman GM, Ager J, Huang H, Hansen KR, Baker V, Usadi R, Seungdamrong A, Bates GW, Rosen RM, Haisenleder D, Krawetz SA, Barnhart K, Trussell JC, Ohl D, Jin Y, Santoro N, Eisenberg E, Zhang H. Letrozole, gonadotropin, or clomiphene for unexplained infertility. N Engl J Med. 2015;373(13):1230–40. https://doi.org/10.1056/NEJMoa1414827.
24. Mitwally MF, Casper RF. Aromatase inhibition reduces the dose of gonadotropin required for controlled ovarian hyperstimulation. J Soc Gynecol Investig. 2004;11(6):406–15.
25. Hurst FS, Bollmann A, Ciangiola C. Treatment of infertility patients with hMG-IUI in a private practice. Int J Fertil Menopausal Stud. 1993;38(1):28–33.
26. la Cour Freiesleben N, Lossl K, Bogstad J, Bredkjaer HE, Toft B, Rosendahl M, Loft A, Bangsboll S, Pinborg A, Nyboe Andersen A. Individual versus standard dose of rFSH in a mild stimulation protocol for intrauterine insemination: a randomized study. Hum Reprod. 2009;24(10):2523–30. https://doi.org/10.1093/humrep/dep239.
27. Miralpeix E, González-Comadran M, Solà I, Manau D, Carreras R, Checa MA. Efficacy of luteal phase support with vaginal progesterone in intrauterine insemination: a systematic review and meta-analysis. J Assist Reprod Genet. 2014;31(1):89–100.
28. Green KA, Zolton JR, Schermerhorn SM, Lewis TD, Healy MW, Terry N, DeCherney AH, Hill MJ. Progesterone luteal support after ovulation induction and intrauterine insemination: an updated systematic review and meta-analysis. Fertil Steril. 2017;107(4):924–33.e5
29. Awwad JT, Hannoun AB, Khalil A, Younes ZM, Ghazeeri GS. Induction of final follicle maturation with a gonadotropin-releasing hormone agonist in women at risk of ovarian hyperstimulation syndrome undergoing gonadotropin stimulation and

intrauterine insemination: proof-of-concept study. Clin Exp Obstet Gynecol. 2012;39(4):436–9.
30. Romeu A, Monzó A, Peiró T, Diez E, Peinado JA, Quintero LA. Endogenous LH surge versus hCG as ovulation trigger after low-dose highly purified FSH in IUI: a comparison of 761 cycles. J Assist Reprod Genet. 1997;14(9):518–24.
31. Chung MT, Chan TF, Loo TC, Tang HH, Lin LY, Tsai YC. Comparison of the effect of two different doses of recombinant gonadotropin for ovarian stimulationon the outcome of intrauterine insemination. Taiwan J Obstet Gynecol. 2011;50(1):58–61. https://doi.org/10.1016/j.tjog.2010.01.001.
32. Barros Delgadillo JC, Fiszman Amora R, Santibañez Morales A, Sánchez Solis V, Gaviño FG. Preliminary results of effectiveness of two schemes of controlled ovarian hyperstimulation protocols with recombinant foliculle stimulating hormone in intrauterine insemination cycles. Ginecol Obstet Mex. 2012;80(2):61–72.
33. Safdarian L, Khayatzadeh Z, Djavadi E, Mahdavi A, Aghahosseini M, Aleyasin A, Fallahi P, Khayatzadeh S, Ahmadzadeh A, Larijani MB. Prediction of assisted reproductive technique outcome in elevated early follicular phase follicle stimulating hormone with mullerian inhibiting substance level. Iran J Reprod Med. 2012;10(3):201–8.
34. Groeneveld E, Kouijzer IJ, Timmermans AJ, Schats R, Hompes PG. Effectiveness of highly purified human menopausal gonadotropin in intra-uterine insemination. Eur J Obstet Gynecol Reprod Biol. 2011;154(2):182–6. https://doi.org/10.1016/j.ejogrb.2010.10.010.
35. Shalom-Paz E, Marzal A, Wiser A, Hyman J, Tulandi T. Does optimal follicular size in IUI cycles vary between clomiphene citrate and gonadotrophins treatments? Gynecol Endocrinol. 2014;30(2):107–10. https://doi.org/10.3109/09513590.2013.860126.
36. Cantineau AE, Cohlen BJ, Dutch IUI Study Group. The prevalence and influence of luteinizing hormone surges in stimulated cycles combined with IUI during a prospective cohort study. Fertil Steril. 2007;88:107–12.
37. Crosignani PG, Somigliana E, Intrauterine Insemination Study Group. Effect of GnRH antagonists in FSH mildly stimulated intrauterine insemination cycles: a multicentre randomized trial. Hum Reprod. 2007;22(2):500–5.
38. Blockeel C, Knez J, Polyzos NP, De Vos M, Camus M, Tournaye H. Should an intrauterine insemination with donor semen be performed 1 or 2 days after the spontaneous LH rise? A prospective RCT. Hum Reprod. 2014;29(4):697–703. https://doi.org/10.1093/humrep/deu022.
39. Liu W, Gong F, Luo K, Lu G. Comparing the pregnancy rates of one versus two intrauterine inseminations (IUIs) in male factor and idiopathic infertility. J Assist Reprod Genet. 2006;23(2):75–9.
40. Randall GW, Gantt PA. Double vs. single intrauterine insemination per cycle: use in gonadotropin cycles and in diagnostic categories of ovulatory dysfunction and male factor infertility. J Reprod Med. 2008;53(3):196–202.
41. Matorras R, Ramón O, Expósito A, Corcóstegui B, Ocerin I, Gonzalez-Lopera S, Rodríguez-Escudero FJ. Gn-RH antagonists in intrauterine insemination: the weekend-free protocol. J Assist Reprod Genet. 2006;23(2):51–4.
42. Huang FJ, Chang SY, Lu YJ, Kung FT, Tsai MY, Wu JF. Two different timings of intrauterine insemination for non-male infertility. J Assist Reprod Genet. 2000;17(4):213–7.
43. Berker B, Şükür YE, Kahraman K, Atabekoğlu CS, Sönmezer M, Özmen B, Ateş C. Impact of unilateral tubal blockage diagnosed by hysterosalpingography on the success rate of treatment with controlled ovarian stimulation and intrauterine insemination. J Obstet Gynaecol. 2014;34(2):127–30. https://doi.org/10.3109/01443615.2013.853030.
44. Lin MH, Hwu YM, Lin SY, Lee RK. Treatment of infertile women with unilateral tubal occlusion by intrauterine insemination and ovarian stimulation. Taiwan J Obstet Gynecol. 2013;52(3):360–4. https://doi.org/10.1016/j.tjog.2012.01.037.
45. El-Khayat W, El-Mazny A, Abou-Salem N, Moafy A. The value of fallopian tube sperm perfusion in the management of mild-moderate male factor infertility. Int J Gynaecol Obstet. 2012;117(2):178–81. https://doi.org/10.1016/j.ijgo.2011.11.023.
46. Hsieh YY, Tsai HD, Chang CC, Lo HY, Chen CL. Low-dose aspirin for infertile women with thin endometrium receiving IUI: a prospective, randomized study. J Assist Reprod Genet. 2000;17(3):174–7.
47. Oruc AS, Yilmaz N, Gorkem U, Inal HA, Seckin B, Gulerman C. Influence of ultrasound-guided artificial insemination on pregnancy rates: a randomized study. Arch Gynecol Obstet. 2014;289:207–12.
48. Yavas Y, Selub MR. Intrauterine insemination (IUI) pregnancy outcome is enhanced by shorter intervals from semen collection to sperm wash, from sperm wash to IUI time, and from semen collection to IUI time. Fertil Steril. 2004;82:1638–47.
49. Song GJ, Herko R, Lewis V. Location of semen collection and time interval from collection to use for intrauterine insemination. Fertil Steril. 2007;88:1689–91.

7 Letrozole in Fertility Therapy

Monique Marguerie and Mohamed Bedaiwy

Anovulation is a major cause of infertility worldwide. There have been significant efforts to develop a method to medically induce ovulation with the ultimate goal of a viable pregnancy. The gold standard for ovulation induction for over 40 years was the anti-estrogenic drug clomiphene citrate (CC) [1]. Clomiphene citrate has been shown to induce ovulation in approximately 60–80% of treated women [2]; however, successful pregnancies have only been observed to occur in approximately 20–30% of women, cumulatively [3, 4]. The failure of clomiphene citrate was thought to be due to the anti-estrogenic effects it has on the endometrium and cervical mucus as well as the luteal phase abnormalities it causes [5]. This led to the search for new alternatives.

Letrozole, a third-generation aromatase inhibitor (AI), is a newer, safe oral drug, with significant evidence to support its superior efficacy in ovulation induction (OI) and achievement of pregnancy than clomiphene citrate. Third-generation AIs were initially used in the treatment of post menopausal breast cancer and are now approved by the U.S. Food and Drug Administration (FDA) as first-line adjuvant therapy for the treatment of estrogen receptor-positive breast cancer [6]. Letrozole is more commonly used and has been studied more for ovulation induction than other third-generation AIs although anastrozole has also been studied in similar contexts [7, 8].

Letrozole was first proposed by Mitwally and Casper as a viable ovulation induction agent in 2001 in response to the finding that their patients who had previously received substantial CC treatments had significant thinning of their endometrial lining [9]. They were also the first group to demonstrate efficacy of letrozole in patients naïve to therapy and CC-resistant patients [5, 10].

Despite significant evidence supporting the efficacy and safety of letrozole for use in OI, the uptake of letrozole in clinical practice was initially quite slow. This was in part due to premature and unsubstantiated warnings regarding the safety of letrozole in OI [11]. Letrozole has since been demonstrated to have a strong safety profile, and these trends are slowly starting to change. Furthermore, letrozole has been named a safe and efficacious alternative to clomiphene citrate by the Canadian Fertility and Andrology Society (CFAS) and the Society of Obstetricians and Gynaecologists of Canada (SOGC) in March 2017 in their joint-position statement earlier this year [12] (Table 7.1). This statement came in lieu of an announcement earlier this year that the only manufacturer of clomiphene citrate has discontinued its production of the drug and it is likely that their supplies will be exhausted by the end of the 2017. With these pressures on clinical practice, letrozole will become more incorporated into clinical practice in the next several years.

There are many different options available to couples when they are struggling with infertility. In general the first therapy option is ovulation induction, and if this fails, they may be offered intrauterine insemination (IUI), followed by in vitro fertilization (IVF) or intracytoplasmic sperm injection (ICSI). Infertility may be the result of many causes including anovulatory infertility such as polycystic ovarian syndrome (PCOS), endometriosis, or unexplained infertility. Letrozole has been studied in all of these contexts either as a monotherapy or as a combined therapy with another agent (Fig. 7.1). The purpose of this chapter is to review the potential applications for letrozole in ovulation induction and fertility therapy.

7.1 Pharmacology

Aromatase is a member of the cytochrome P450 hemopoietin containing enzyme complex superfamily and is responsible for the conversion of androstenedione to estrone and testosterone to estradiol. Aromatase inhibitors, like their

M. Marguerie
Department of Obstetrics and Gynaecology, BC Women's Hospital, Vancouver, BC, Canada

M. Bedaiwy (✉)
Division of Reproductive Endocrinology and Infertility, Department of Obstetrics and Gynaecology, The University of British Columbia, Vancouver, BC, Canada
e-mail: mohamed.bedaiwy@cw.bc.ca

G. N. Allahbadia et al. (eds.), *Textbook of Assisted Reproduction*, https://doi.org/10.1007/978-981-15-2377-9_7

Table 7.1 Statements and guidelines pertaining to letrozole use in assisted reproduction

Agency	Year	Title	Statement summary/pertinent points
Health Canada [11]	2005	Important Safety Information on the Contraindication of Femara (letrozole) in premenopausal women	• Letrozole is contraindicated in premenopausal, pregnant, and lactating women due to the risk of fetal and maternal toxicity and fetal malformations
The Amsterdam ESHRE/ ASRM-Sponsored PCOS Consensus Workshop Group [13]	2008	Consensus on infertility treatment related to polycystic ovary syndrome	• First-line treatment in patients with PCOS is clomiphene citrate • Metformin should only be used in PCOS patients with glucose intolerance • There is not enough evidence to recommend the use of aromatase inhibitors for ovulation induction in patients with PCOS although preliminary research suggests that letrozole may be as effective as CC • Letrozole can be considered for use "off-label" if all risks and benefits are explained
SOGC [14]	2010	SOGC Clinical Practice Guideline No. 242: Ovulation Induction in Polycystic Ovary Syndrome	• Weight loss and lifestyle modifications should be considered first line for PCOS • CC should be considered first-line therapy and gonadotropins second-line therapy for ovulation induction • Evidence for AIs appears promising; however, caution should be used until they are approved by Health Canada
NICE [15]	2013	Fertility problems: assessment and treatment Clinical guideline 156	• Do not offer ovarian stimulation agents such as CC and letrozole to women with unexplained infertility • Medical management of endometriosis does not enhance fertility and should not be offered • CC, metformin, or a combination of the two are first line for WHO group II ovulation disorders • Letrozole does not result in greater singleton births compared to CC • Letrozole resulted in significantly more clinical pregnancies than CC • No sig diff between number of multiple pregnancies and miscarriages in patients treated with letrozole versus CC
ESHRE [16]	2014	ESHRE guideline: management of women with endometriosis	• Aromatase inhibitors can be considered in patients with endometriosis-associated pain refractory to other medical and surgical treatments in combination with other hormone therapies • Hormonal therapies should not be used for suppression of ovarian function to improve fertility in endometriosis as there is no evidence of any benefit • Hormonal therapy is not recommended as an adjuvant to endometriosis surgery either before or after surgery as there is insufficient evidence that this has a positive benefit on increasing spontaneous pregnancy rates
ACOG [17]	2016	Committee Opinion No 663: Aromatase Inhibitors in Gynecologic Practice	• Letrozole should be used in first-line therapy for women with PCOS and BMI >30 • Letrozole may help manage pain associated with endometriosis in combination with progestins • As compared to treatment with tamoxifen, AIs are associated with lower rates of endometrial cancer, thrombosis, and vaginal bleeding • Data suggests that gonadotropins result in higher birth rates and higher multiple gestation rates than letrozole in unexplained infertility • More research is required to assess whether letrozole or CC is more effective in the treatment of unexplained fertility
CFAS-SOGC joint statement [12]	2017	CFAS-SOGC Joint Position Statement on the Use of Letrozole for the Management of Infertility	• Letrozole is a more effective ovulation induction agent than clomiphene citrate in patients with ovulatory disorders • Letrozole is comparable to clomiphene citrate for ovulation induction in unexplained infertility but is less effective than gonadotropins • Significant research supports the safety of letrozole use for ovulation induction without evidence for increased congenital malformation

name suggests, inhibit this enzyme by competitively binding to the active site of the membrane complex resulting in low levels of circulating estrogen. This hypoestrogenic state releases the negative feedback that circulating estrogen has on central gonadotropin release leading to enhanced growth of ovarian follicles [9, 18].

Letrozole has a relatively short half-life of ~45 h [19, 20]. It is able to reduce serum estrogen by 97–99% [21] while leading to minimal negative effects on estrogen-sensitive tissues and improved endometrial thickness relative to CC [22, 23]. Since AIs do not affect central estrogen receptors, central feedback mechanisms remain intact with letrozole treatment [9]. Thus as a dominant follicle grows, negative feedback on FSH release results in atresia of smaller follicles [9, 24]. This results in the lower rates of multiple ovulation and multiple pregnancy

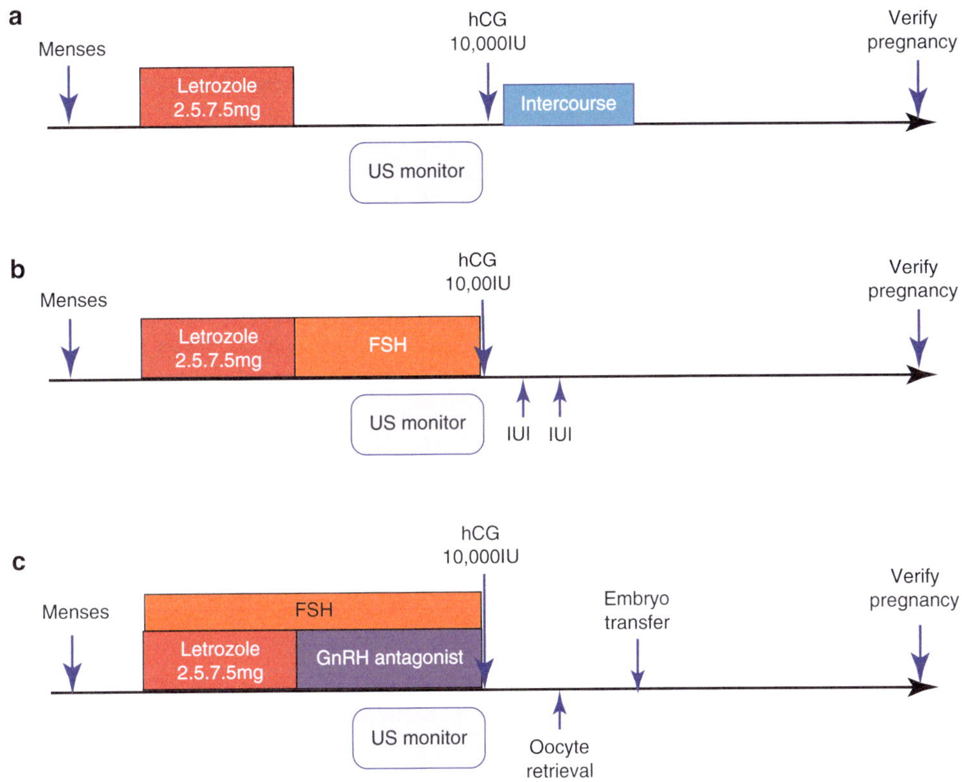

Fig. 7.1 Sample treatment schedules with letrozole. These schedules represent treatment protocols involving letrozole used in ovulation induction and assisted reproductive technology but are not representative of all protocols in use. Doses and schedules vary between studies. (**a**) Representative of an ovulation induction cycle followed by timed intercourse. (**b**) Representative of controlled ovulatory stimulation followed by intrauterine insemination (IUI). (**c**) Representative of in vitro fertilization involving letrozole and FSH combination therapy

rates in letrozole fertility treatments compared to other agents used for OI.

Letrozole has been demonstrated to result in changes in hormonal and follicular dynamics compared to natural cycles without negative effects on pregnancy rates. Bedaiwy et al. demonstrated that letrozole treatment results in lower estradiol levels on day 7 but significantly increased estradiol levels on the day of hCG administration. However estradiol levels per preovulatory follicle were similar between letrozole and natural cycle groups. LH is significantly lower on the day of hCG administration in letrozole-treated patients relative to natural cycle patients [25]. A study by Garcia-Velasco et al. demonstrated that letrozole increases intraovarian androgens which seems to enhance early follicular growth and result in improved IVF outcome [26]. This elevation in intraovarian androgens is thought to increase follicular sensitivity to FSH through amplification of the FSH gene expression or by stimulating insulin growth factor 1 (IGF-1) [27–29].

Compared to natural cycles, letrozole induces development of significantly greater numbers of follicles [25]. Relative to FSH-only cycles however, letrozole +FSH combination therapy results in approximately 33% reduction of follicles without significantly reducing pregnancy rates overall. This is reflective of the lower multiple pregnancy rates in the letrozole combination group relative to FSH treatment on its own [30].

Letrozole is an easy to use medication that is orally administered with complete and rapid absorption [31]. Letrozole is primarily metabolized through CYP 3A4 and CYP 2A6 enzymes, and doses may need to be adjusted in patients with hepatic impairment due to prolongation of letrozole's half-life [31]. Significant drug interactions have not been reported, and age does not affect the drug's pharmacokinetic profile [31].

7.2 Side Effects and Teratogenicity

Side effects associated with letrozole administration are uncommon but include hot flashes (11%), nausea (7%), fatigue (5%), alopecia, headaches, leg cramps, and vaginal bleeding [32–34]. Side effects in women receiving letrozole for OI will be much less common than that experienced in breast cancer patients due to the shorter duration of treatment. Women who receive chronic letrozole treatment should be monitored for bone mineral density due to the increased risk of fractures, osteopenia, and osteoporosis associated with long-term aromatase inhibitor use [35].

The question of the risk of congenital anomalies from letrozole exposure is an important one. In 2005 Novartis Pharmaceuticals issued a warning, endorsed by Health Canada, that letrozole should not be used for ovulation induction due to potential for fetal toxicity and malformation [11]. This warning came following an abstract published at the ASRM in 2005 suggesting an increase in cardiac and locomotor anomalies following letrozole use for ovulation induction [36]. This study was found to be of flawed methodology and was never published, but Health Canada has yet to remove their warning from the product.

Some laboratory studies have demonstrated that exposure of animals to letrozole during pregnancy can lead to intrauterine mortality and teratogenic effects [37]. However in order to have teratogenic effects, an exposure must occur during sensitive phases of development. Given letrozole's short half-life of ~45 h, clearance from the body should be complete prior to implantation, and the embryo is unlikely to be exposed to the drug during the critical developmental period [38]. Care should be taken to avoid administering this drug to individuals who are already pregnant.

There is significant evidence supporting the safety of use of letrozole for ovulation induction in humans. In fact a retrospective study published shortly after the warnings made by Novartis Pharmaceuticals found that there was no difference in the rates of congenital anomalies in babies born to mothers treated with letrozole (2.4%) and CC (4.8%) [38]. In fact, the rates of cardiac anomalies were significantly lower in the letrozole-treated group than the CC-treated group [38]. This is in the context of many previous studies the have demonstrated the safety of CC's use in OI [39–41]. The authors concluded that the concern that letrozole is teratogenic is unfounded based on this study's data.

In 2014, another retrospective analysis [42] as well as a double-blind multicenter trial composed of 750 women by Legro et al. [4] found there was no significant difference in the congenital anomalies between patients receiving OI with CC and with letrozole therapy. In 2017, in a retrospective cohort study investigating patients receiving assisted reproductive therapy (ART), Tatsumi et al. demonstrated that there was no difference in the rate of congenital malformations in women receiving their embryo transfers after a natural cycle or after a letrozole-induced cycle ($p = 0.52$) [43].

Overall data is highly supportive of letrozole's safety for use in clinical practice. The CFAS, SOGC, and ACOG have given their support for the use of letrozole in clinical practice and acknowledge the literature supporting its safety for use in infertility management [12, 17]. Evidence statements published in the NICE 2013 Fertility Guidelines state that there are no significant differences in the number of congenital abnormalities between letrozole and clomiphene citrate [15]. It is important however to note that letrozole is not yet approved either by the FDA or by Health Canada for ovulation induction. In fact, it is labeled as a pregnancy Category X medication by the FDA, and use is not recommended in premenopausal women. Given the significant amounts of data supporting letrozole's safety, it is likely that the guidelines will change with time; however in the interim, patients should be counseled on these warnings prior to use.

7.3 Letrozole Ovulation Induction in PCOS

Normogonadotropic anovulation, referred to as type II anovulation by the World Health Organization, is a main cause of infertility worldwide. Polycystic ovary syndrome (PCOS) affects approximately 5–10% of women worldwide and is the cause for up to 90% of infertility in women with type II infertility [44]. The use of aromatase inhibitors for ovulation induction was first proposed for patients with PCOS in 2001 [10]. Since this time there has been mounting evidence in support of the use of letrozole in anovulatory and infertile PCOS patients [45–48]. For years, studies suggested that relatively higher pregnancy (Fig. 7.2) and birth (Fig. 7.3) rates were attained in letrozole-treated patients compared

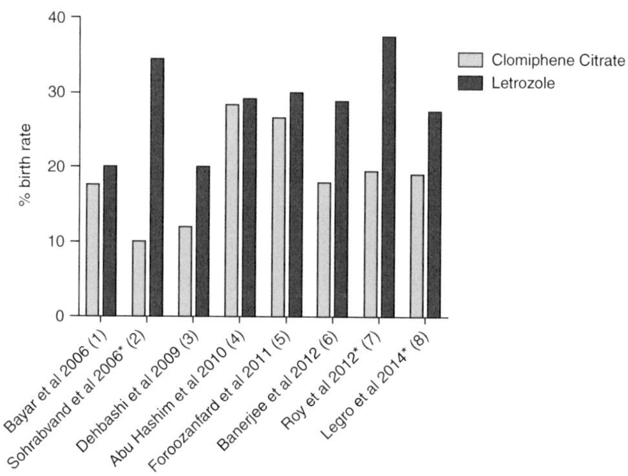

Fig. 7.2 Birth rates (%) in patients with PCOS treated with letrozole versus clomiphene citrate for ovulation induction. Data extracted from Cochrane review by Franik et al. [49]. *Significant difference between birth rates in letrozole- and clomiphene-treated groups. (1) Ovulation induction-naïve women: CC 100 mg/day versus letrozole 5 mg/day [46]. (2) Clomiphene-resistant women: metformin 150 mg/day + CC 100 mg/day versus metformin 150 mg/day + letrozole 2.5 mg/day [50]. (3) Ovulation induction-naïve women: CC 100 mg/day versus letrozole 5 mg/day [51]. (4) Clomiphene-resistant and OI-naïve women: CC 150 mg/day + metformin 1500 mg/day versus letrozole 2.5 mg/day [52]. (5) Clomiphene-resistant women: CC 100 mg/day + hMG 150UI versus letrozole 5 mg/day + hMG 150UI [53]. (6) Unspecified infertile patients: CC 100 mg/day versus letrozole 2.5 mg/day [45]. (7) Unspecified infertile patients: CC 50–100 mg/day versus letrozole 2.5–5 mg/day [48]. (8) Unspecified infertile patients: CC 50–150 mg/day versus letrozole 2.5–7.5 mg/day [4]

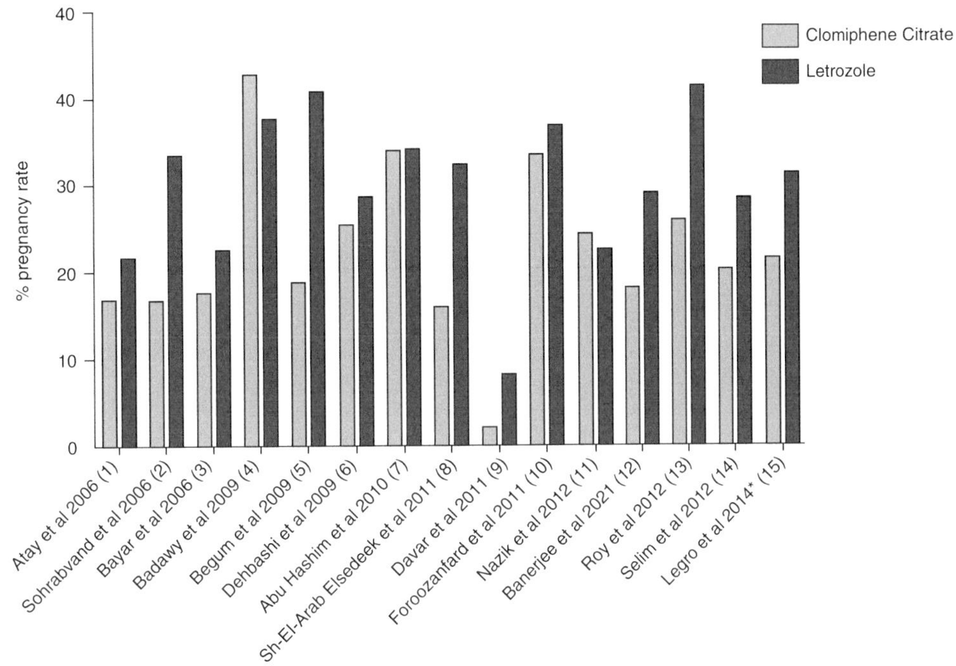

Fig. 7.3 Pregnancy rates (%) in patients with PCOS treated with letrozole versus clomiphene citrate for ovulation induction. Data extracted from Cochrane review by Franik et al. [49]. *Significant difference between birth rates in letrozole- and clomiphene-treated groups. (1) Unspecified infertile patients: CC 100 mg/day versus letrozole 2.5 mg/day [54]. (2) CC-resistant women: metformin 150 mg/day + CC 100 mg/day versus metformin 150 mg/day + letrozole 2.5 mg/day [50]. (3) Ovulation induction-naïve women: CC 100 mg/day versus letrozole 5 mg/day [46]. (4) Ovulation induction-naïve women: CC 100 mg/day versus letrozole 5 mg/day [55]. (5) CC-resistant women: CC 150 mg/day versus letrozole 7.5 mg [47]. (6) Ovulation induction-naïve women: CC 100 mg/day versus letrozole 5 mg/day [51]. (7) CC-resistant and OI-naïve women: CC 150 mg/day + metformin 1500 mg/day versus letrozole 2.5 mg/day [52]. (8) Ovulation induction-naïve women: CC 100 mg/day versus letrozole 5 mg/day [56]. (9) CC-resistant women: metformin 1500 mg/day + CC 100 mg/day versus metformin 150 mg/day + letrozole 5 mg/day [57]. (10) CC-resistant women: CC 100 mg/day + hMG 150UI versus letrozole 5 mg/day + hMG 150UI [53]. (11) Ovulation induction-naïve women: CC 100 mg/day versus letrozole 2.5 mg/day [58]. (12) Unspecified infertile patients: CC 100 mg/day versus letrozole 2.5 mg/day [45]. (13) Unspecified infertile patients: CC 50–100 mg/day versus letrozole 2.5–5 mg/day [48]. (14) Unspecified infertile patients: CC 100 mg/day versus letrozole 5 mg/day [59]. (15) Unspecified infertile patients: CC 50–150 mg/day versus letrozole 2.5–7.5 mg/day [4]

with clomiphene citrate treatment but these studies did not attain statistical significance [45, 47, 48, 51, 53] (Table 7.2). The 2013 NICE guidelines state that the clinical pregnancy rate in patients with PCOS was found to be higher with the use of letrozole for ovulation induction relative to clomiphene citrate, but no significant increase in singleton birth rates was observed [15]. In 2014 a Cochrane review analyzed the data of nine randomized controlled trials (RCT) and found that in patients with PCOS ovulation induction with letrozole and subsequent timed intercourse results in a significantly higher birth rates than CC [49]. It is important to note that the quality of these conclusions was rated as low due to poor reporting of study methods and possible publication bias.

Within the same year, an RCT investigating a similar question was published. Legro et al. studied 750 women with PCOS in a double-blind, multicenter trial [4]. Patients were treated in a 1:1 ratio with either letrozole or clomiphene citrate. Results found that treatment with letrozole resulted in more live births than treatment with clomiphene citrate (27.5 vs. 19.1%, $p = 0.007$). No differences were observed in the rates of congenital anomalies or pregnancy loss. The author concluded that letrozole was superior to clomiphene citrate as treatment for women with PCOS and anovulatory infertility [4]. Despite there being many previous trials addressing a similar question [4, 45, 47, 48, 51, 54, 55], this was the first RCT to have sufficient power to detect such differences.

Patients with PCOS have many factors contributing to their anovulatory state. In part, relative over-suppression of FSH is due to high levels of estrogen secondary to aromatization of circulating androgens [9]. Insulin insensitivity likely also plays an important role [65]. Many lifestyle modifications have been proposed as initial steps to improve fertility including weight loss, exercise, smoking cessation, and reduced alcohol consumption [66, 67]. In their June 2016 Practice Update, the American Committee of Obstetricians and Gynecologists (ACOG) supports that these lifestyle modification strategies should be strongly encouraged as a component of infertility treatment for

Table 7.2 Ovulation induction in letrozole versus clomiphene citrate in polycystic ovary syndrome

Author	Year	Journal	Type of trial	Treatment arms	# patients (# cycles)	Ovulation N (%/cycle)	Pregnancy N (%/pt)	Births N (%/pt)
Atay et al. [54]	2006	J Int Med Res	RCT	Letrozole 2.5 mg Clomiphene 100 mg	51 (55) 55 (55)	42 (76.4) 35 (63.6)	11 (21.6) 5 (9.1)	– –
Conclusion: Letrozole is associated with higher pregnancy rates in patients with PCOS than CC								
Bayar et al. [46]	2006	Fertil Seril	RCT	Letrozole 2.5 mg Clomiphene 100 mg	38 (99) 36 (95)	65 (65.7) 71 (74.7)	9 (23.7) 7 (19.4)	8 (21.1) 7 (19.4)
Conclusion: Letrozole and clomiphene have comparable efficacy in ovulation induction in patients with PCOS								
Sohrabvand et al. [50]	2006	Hum Reprod	RCT	Letrozole 2.5 mg + metformin 1500 mg Clomiphene 100 mg + metformin 1500 mg	29 (53) 30 (67)	48 (90.6) 54 (80.6)	10 (34.5) 5 (16.7)	10 (34.5) 3 (10.0)
Conclusion: Combination of letrozole + metformin leads to more full-term pregnancies than clomiphene +metformin								
Begum et al. [47]	2009	Fertil Steril	RCT	Letrozole 7.5 mg Clomiphene 100 mg	32 (–) 32 (–)	20	13 (40.6) 6 (18.75)	12 (37.5) 6 (18.75)
Conclusion: Letrozole induces superior ovulation and pregnancy rates compared to clomiphene								
Baruah et al. [60]	2009	Arch Gynecol Obstet	Quasi random	Letrozole 2.5–5 mg Clomiphene 100 mg	25 (58) 25 (56)	– –	11 (44.0) 7 (21.9)	– –
Conclusion: Letrozole induces a better endometrial response than clomiphene								
Ganesh et al. [61]	2009	J Assist Reprod Genet	RCT	Letrozole 5 mg Clomiphene 100 mg + rFSH 75–100 IU rFSH FSH 75–100 IU	372 (372) 669 (669) 346 (346)	295 (79.3) 381 (57.0) 311 (90.0)	87 (23.39)* 96 (14.35)* 62 (17.92)	75 (20.2) 80 (12.0) 53 (15.3)
Conclusion: Letrozole is suitable for ovulation induction in PCOS								
Badawy et al. [55]	2009	Fertil Steril	RCT	Letrozole 5 mg Clomiphene 100 mg	218 (540) 220 (523)	365 (68.0) 371 (70.9)	82 (37.6) 94 (42.7)	– –
Conclusion: There is no advantage in using letrozole as first line for ovulation induction over clomiphene								
Dehbashi et al. [51]	2009	Iran J Med Sci	Prospective	Letrozole 5 mg Clomiphene 100 mg	50 50	30 (60)* 16 (32)*	13 (26.0) 7 (14.0)	10 (20.0) 6 (12.0)
Conclusion: OI was sig higher and PR was non-sig higher in letrozole group								
Abu Hashim et al. [52]	2010	Fertil Steril	RCT	Letrozole 2.5 mg Clomiphene 150 mg + metformin 500 mg	123 (285) 127 (297)	185 (64.9) 207 (69.6)	42 (34.1) (14.7)[b] 43 (33.9) (14.4)[b]	38 (30.9) 39 (30.7)
Conclusion: Clomiphene and letrozole are equally effective in ovulation induction in patients with PCOS								
Davar et al. [57]	2011	Iran J Reprod Med	RCT	Letrozole 5 mg + metformin 1500 mg Clomiphene 100 mg + metformin 1500 mg	50 (70) 50 (78)	– –	1(8.3) (1)[b] 4(2) (5)[b]	– –
Conclusion: There is no significant difference in pregnancy rates achieved with OI of clomiphene and letrozole								

Foroozanfard et al. [53]	2011	Pakistani J Med Sci	RCT	Letrozole 5 mg + HMG 150 IU Clomiphene 100 mg + 150 IU	60 60	– –	22 (36.7) 20 (33.3)	18 (30) 16 (26.7)
Conclusion: In combination with gonadotropins letrozole can be an effective ovulation induction agent								
Sheikh-El-Arab Elsedeek et al. [56]	2011	Mid East Fertil Soc J	RCT	Letrozole 5 mg Clomiphene 100 mg	59 57	41 (69.5)[a] 35 (61.4)[a]	20 (33.9) 16 (28)	– –
Conclusion: Letrozole is at least as good as clomiphene in achieving pregnancy by ovulation induction								
Nazik et al. [58]	2011	Health MED		Letrozole Clomiphene				
Selim et al. [59]	2012	J Gynae Surg	Prospective	Letrozole Clomiphene	102 99	72(70.6)[a] 64(64.6)[a]	29 (28.4)* 20 (20.2)*	– –
Conclusion: Letrozole may increase fertility in ovulation induction compared to clomiphene								
Ray et al. [45]	2012	Arch Gynecol Obstet	RCT	Letrozole 2.5 mg Clomiphene 100 mg	69 (132) 78 (156)	60 (86.9)[a] 48 (61.5)[a]	20(28.9)* 14(17.9)*	20 13
Conclusion: Letrozole has beneficial effect on the endometrium which may increase pregnancy rates after OI versus CC								
Roy et al. [48]	2012	J Hum Reprod Sci	RCT	Letrozole 2.5–5 mg Clomiphene 50–100 mg	98 (294) 106 (318)	196 (66.6) 216 (67.9)	43 (43.8) 28 (26.4)	39(39.7)* 21(19.8)*
Conclusion: OI with letrozole resulted in superior endometrial response and pregnancy rates than clomiphene								
Legro et al. [4]	2014	NEJM	RCT	Letrozole 2.5 mg Clomiphene 50 mg	374 (1352) 376 (1425)	834 (61.7)* 668 (48.3)*	117 (31.3)* 81 (21.5)*	103(27.5)* 72(19.1)*
Conclusion: Letrozole is associated with higher live birth rates and ovulation rates than clomiphene								
Elkhateeb and Mahran [62]	2016	Gynecol Obstet Res	RCT	Letrozole 2.5–10 mg Clomiphene 100 mg	100 (242) 100 (249)	165 (68.2) 169 (67.9)	36 (14.8)[b]* 26 (10.4)[b]*	– –
Conclusion: Using letrozole in increasing doses achieves higher pregnancy rates than standard doses of clomiphene								
Ghahiri et al. [63]	2016	Adv Biomed Res	RCT	Letrozole 5 mg Clomiphene 100 mg	50 51	– –	29 (58)[c] 24 (47)[c]	24 (48.0) 18 (35.3)
Conclusion: Letrozole and clomiphene are equally effective in ovulation induction in patients with PCOS								
Al Shaikh et al. [64]	2017	Mid East Fertil Soc J	Prospective	Letrozole 5 mg Clomiphene 100 mg	40 (47) 45 (80)	33 (70.21%) 33 (41.25%)	3 (9.09)[d] 4 (12.12)[d]	1 (2.5) 2 (4.4)
Conclusion: Letrozole induced higher ovulation rates but clomiphene induced higher pregnancy rates in PCOS								

*Significant difference in values
[a]Values represent number of patients that achieved ovulation, while others represent total number of ovulations
[b]Percent pregnancies per cycle
[c]Percent pregnancies per patient
[d]Percent pregnancies per ovulation

PCOS. Furthermore, ACOG suggests that letrozole should be used for OI in patients with PCOS who have a BMI greater than 30 [17].

7.4 Letrozole Ovulation Induction in Unexplained Infertility

Unexplained infertility is a relatively common diagnosis and is estimated to apply to 10–30% of infertile couples [68, 69]. Clomiphene citrate has been used as the drug of choice for decades for superovulation for patients with unexplained infertility prior to IUI; however, as previously outlined, CC is associated with many anti-estrogenic effects which may have deleterious effects on subsequent pregnancy rates. Given that letrozole has shown significant success in ovulation induction in patients with PCOS, it has also been investigated in unexplained infertility.

Studies have shown that there is no significant difference between the pregnancy rates and live birth rates associated with superovulation by letrozole and clomiphene citrate [70, 71]. A large multicenter randomized trial published in 2015 by Diamond et al. examined the efficacy of letrozole compared to clomiphene citrate or gonadotropins followed by IUI. They found that the use of letrozole resulted in similar pregnancy rates and live births as clomiphene citrate. Gonadotropins were associated with significantly greater pregnancy rates (35.5 vs. 22.4%, $P < 0.001$) and live birth rates (32.2 vs. 18.7%, $P < 0.001$) than letrozole; however, they were also associated with significantly higher rates of multiple gestations (32 vs. 13%, $P = 0.006$). The risks associated with gonadotropin use need to be weighed against the risks associated with this treatment. An RCT by Fouda and Sayed demonstrated that treatment with an extended regimen of letrozole of 2.5 mg/day from days 1 to 9 can result in significantly greater pregnancy rates per cycle and cumulative pregnancy rate than clomiphene citrate (18.96 vs. 11.43% and 37.73 vs. 22.86%, respectively) [72]. This is in contrast to the 5-day letrozole that is more often used in letrozole induction. ACOG endorses the need for more research to determine the optimal treatment for unexplained infertility [17]. The recent joint CFAS-SOGC position statement stated that letrozole seems to be at least as effective as clomiphene citrate, while less effective than gonadotropins, and can be used for unexplained infertility management with appropriate workup [12].

7.5 Letrozole in Endometriosis

Endometriosis is defined as the presence of endometrial glands and stroma outside of the uterine cavity and is characterized by chronic pelvic pain, dyspareunia, dysmenorrhea, painful bowel movements, and infertility [73, 74]. Two to ten percent of all women and 50% of infertile women are affected by this disease [75, 76]. While the standard of care is currently surgery and hormonal therapy, there are other new emerging alternatives. Aromatase inhibitors have demonstrated encouraging results in the treatment of both pain and infertility in women with endometriosis resistant to current methods of treatment.

Aromatase expression is elevated in implants and eutopic endometrium of women with endometriosis, while expression is absent in normal endometrium [77]. Molecular differences result in an overproduction of estradiol (E2) and diminished conversion to a less biologically active estrogen [35]. Estrogen stimulates the production of prostaglandin E2 (PGE2) levels, while PGE2 reciprocally stimulates aromatase activity [73]. Prostaglandins mediate the pain, inflammation, and infertility of endometriosis, while estradiol induces inflammation and growth of endometriotic lesions.

Traditional therapies for endometriosis target the E2 produced by ovarian tissues, while AIs target the E2 produced peripherally such as by the endometrial deposits. AIs are commonly combined with oral contraceptives, progestins, or GnRH agonists [78, 79] for the treatment of endometriosis-associated pain to avoid follicular development and cyst formation [80]. These combination therapies have demonstrated significant improvement of pain and disease severity in patients with medical and surgical resistant endometriosis in multiple studies [81–85]. ESHRE supports the use of letrozole combination therapy in otherwise refractory patients [16].

An important concern in endometriosis is the high prevalence of infertility in affected individuals. There is a need for more studies to look at the role of letrozole in endometriosis in the context of fertility preservation, but preliminary studies have shown that AIs do not compromise fertility or pregnancy rates relative to other treatment modalities [80, 86]. A prospective RCT by Alborzi et al. looked at whether using letrozole post-operatively can improve endometriosis-associated infertility [80]. They found no difference in the pregnancy rates between patients treated with letrozole, a GnRH agonist, and no medication (23.4, 27.5, and 28.1%, respectively). Thus, hormone therapy is not recommended post-operatively in women with endometriosis-associated infertility [16].

A recent study by Abu Hashim et al. demonstrated that superovulation with letrozole in patients who have minimal to mild endometriosis followed by IUI is as effective in terms of resulting pregnancy and birth rates as clomiphene citrate [87]. ESHRE supports that superovulation with IUI is more effective than expectant management in patients with mild to moderate endometriosis [16]. With the cessation of clomiphene production by its manufacturer and its inevitable lack of supply unless production resumes, it is important to acknowledge that based on this data letrozole can be used as an alternative to CC for superovulation prior to IUI with the expectation of comparable results. Another preliminary study by Miller et al. suggested that letrozole may be able to improve the poor IVF success rates [88] that are known to occur in patients with reduced integrin expression in endometriosis [89]. More studies are needed to further assess the efficacy of letrozole for superovulation prior to IUI as well as in IVF technology in patients with aberrant integrin expression.

7.6 Letrozole and Gonadotropin Combination Therapy in IUI

One of the major benefits of letrozole for OI is mono-ovulation and thus avoidance of multiple gestations. However in fertility treatments involving intrauterine insemination (IUI), it is often preferable for multiple follicles to develop to increase the rates of a resulting pregnancy. Controlled ovarian stimulation with gonadotropins prior to IUI has been shown to result in much higher pregnancy rates than IUI in patients who did not receive stimulation [90]. However there are risks involved in using gonadotropins for ovarian stimulation such as ovarian hyperstimulation syndrome (OHSS) and multiple gestations. It is also associated with very high costs: each treatment can cost thousands of dollars. Previous studies have investigated the combination of clomiphene citrate with gonadotropin but have not demonstrated encouraging results [1]. While letrozole on its own may not result in sufficient ovarian stimulation for IUI or IVF therapy, it can be combined with low doses of FSH to ensure multiple ovulation [24].

A small observational cohort study by Mitwally and Casper in 2002 demonstrated that poor responders to FSH produced a significantly greater number of follicles in response to combination therapy with FSH + letrozole [91]. A prospective non-randomized study by the same group looking at women undergoing COS and IUI demonstrated that the combination of letrozole + FSH is superior to CC + FSH with respect to pregnancy rates (19.1 vs. 10.5%) and endometrial thickness and equally as effective as higher doses of FSH alone (19.1 vs. 18.7%) [92]. Healy et al. reported that a combined regimen resulted in greater follicular development, a thinner endometrium, but still equivalent pregnancy rates as patients treated with gonadotropin alone [93]. In a retrospective case-control study, Bedaiwy et al. demonstrated that in infertile women over 40 years of age, controlled ovarian stimulation with co-treatment of letrozole + FSH results in lower estradiol levels and fewer follicles, fewer cycle cancellations, and comparable pregnancy rates with those women who received FSH only [94]. Patients receiving FSH-only treatment experience greater cycle cancellations due to over-stimulation, whereas this is far less common in letrozole and gonadotropin co-treatment [94].

These studies and others have demonstrated that the amount of gonadotropin required for equivalent outcomes was much reduced when combined with letrozole [91–93, 95–98]. Thus, the cost per cycle of controlled ovarian stimulation is significantly reduced when letrozole is co-administered without any difference in subsequent pregnancy rates [95, 99]. If the combination of letrozole + FSH makes fertility treatments more affordable, this may increase access to these treatments for those who may have otherwise had a financial barrier to treatment.

7.7 Letrozole and Metformin Combination Therapy

Many studies have shown that treatment with metformin has benefits in patients with PCOS, as supported by fewer complications of pregnancy, decreased metabolic effects, reduced circulating androgens, and improved pregnancy rates [100–102]. Some of the ovulation challenges in patients with PCOS are likely due to insulin resistance [65], and metformin effectively sensitizes tissues to insulin, corrects hyperinsulinemia, and decreases ovarian androgens [103, 104]. In 2007 an RCT published in the *New England Journal of Medicine* demonstrated a significant improvement in birth rate with clomiphene (22.5%) and clomiphene + metformin (26.8%) relative to metformin (7.2%) on its own ($p < 0.001$) [3]. No significant difference was observed between those treated with clomiphene alone and clomiphene + metformin ($p = 0.31$) [3]. While conflicting evidence exists [101], another randomized controlled trial and a meta-analysis also support that that there is no benefit to combination therapy with metformin and CC in terms of live birth rates relative to clomiphene citrate on its own [105, 106]. In fact a Cochrane review published in 2012 found that there was no significant improvement in live birth rates with metformin alone relative to no treatment, despite there being a significant improvement in clinical pregnancy rates [106]. This was contrary to a study by Morin-Papunen published in the same year which demonstrated significantly improved pregnancy rates and live birth rates in women with PCOS who received 3 months of metformin pretreatment [107]. This implies that the benefit of metformin may extend beyond patients with glucose intolerance.

Evidence to date is supportive of superior ovulation induction and pregnancy outcomes with letrozole compared to clomiphene citrate as discussed earlier in this chapter [4, 49, 108, 109]. In 2006 Sohrabvand, Ansari, and Bagheri compared combined metformin-letrozole therapy with metformin-CC therapy in CC-resistant infertile women with PCOS. While not statistically significant, the conceived pregnancy rates in the metformin + letrozole treatment group (34.50%) were double than that of the metformin + CC treatment group (16.67%) [50]. Furthermore, a statistically greater number of full-term pregnancies were observed in patients who received metformin + letrozole than metformin + CC (34.50 vs. 10%) [50]. A study in 2011 demonstrated conflicting results, with no improvement in pregnancy rates in the letrozole + metformin treatment group compared to the clomiphene + metformin treatment group [57]. To our knowledge no studies have compared letrozole on its own to treatment with letrozole + metformin. A study in 2013 demonstrated that the combination of letrozole + metformin has comparable efficacy to bilateral ovarian drilling in terms of ovulation, pregnancy, and abortion rate [110].

Due to insufficient data suggesting benefit in all PCOS patients, the international consensus in 2008 was that metformin use should be restricted to women with glucose intolerance [13]. It is logical that patients with severe insulin resistance should have their insulin resistance corrected before undergoing costly fertility treatments. However, in light of the improvement of live birth rates observed with 3 months of pretreatment with metformin, and the finding that the combination of letrozole + metformin may result in significantly improved live birth rates, there may be bigger role of metformin and letrozole in fertility treatments than we previously thought. More studies are needed to properly elucidate this role.

7.8 Letrozole in Assisted Reproductive Technology

Letrozole has also been studied for superovulation and controlled ovarian stimulation (COS) in the context of ART. While 2–3 follicles may be appropriate for IUI fertility treatments, in IVF/ICSI it is preferable to develop many more follicles to ensure sufficient number of viable oocytes and subsequent embryos for implantation.

A randomized trial in 2006 by Verproest et al. looked at the addition of letrozole to IVF/intracytoplasmic sperm injection (ICSI) in women with normal ovarian response. This study found that both implantation (31.25 vs. 12.5%) and clinical pregnancy rates (50 vs. 12%) were higher in patients receiving combination therapy of letrozole + FSH than in those receiving FSH on its own [111]. This was a pilot study and thus did not have enough power to find a statistically significant difference between groups; however, other studies have observed similar trends [26, 112]. Endometrial thickness was observed to be statistically increased in the group with letrozole co-treatment ($p < 0.05$), but the exact impact of this has yet to be fully elucidated [111]. A randomized single-blind controlled trial by Goswami et al. in 2004 looked at women who had poor responses to gonadotropin (Gn) stimulation for IVF therapy [113]. Thirteen women were stimulated with Gn + letrozole, and 25 underwent a GnRH-agonist protocol followed by stimulation with FSH. Pregnancy rates were found to be statistically comparable, while doses of required FSH in the letrozole combination groups were significantly less [113].

Two studies looking at patients who had poor responses to gonadotropins alone were treated with a GnRH antagonist protocol to induce pituitary downregulation ± letrozole. Garcia-Velasco et al. treated patients with previously cancelled IVF cycles with an antagonist FSH/hMG protocol ± letrozole treatment in the first 5 days of ovarian stimulation. They demonstrated that the IVF implantation rate in the letrozole group was significantly higher than the control group (25 vs. 9.4%, $p = 0.009$) and there was also a higher pregnancy rate per transfer (41.6 vs. 28.9%) but this difference was not statistically significant [26]. While Ozmen et al. did not observe any significant improvement in pregnancy rates in the letrozole-treated group, there was a significant reduction in IVF cycle cancellation due to poor ovarian response [112]. Furthermore they found that the cost associated with each IVF treatment was much less due to reduced gonadotropin requirement [112].

In 2017, a retrospective cohort study looked at women who had received single embryo transfers after either a natural cycle or a letrozole-induced cycle. Letrozole was found not to be associated with increased congenital malformations ($p = 0.52$) and was actually associated with significantly decreased risk of miscarriage ($p < 0.001$) [43].

Together, all of these studies point toward the possible beneficial use of letrozole in ART. With higher implantation rates, lower cycle cancellation rates, lower costs per cycle, and potentially higher pregnancy rates, it seems clear that there could be a benefit in incorporating letrozole into ART for patients who are low responders to Gn stimulation or even into standard ART care. More RCTs are needed to confirm the benefits of letrozole and its safety in ART.

7.9 Letrozole in Fertility Preservation for Patients with Cancer

In recent decades, there have been increasing trends toward childbearing later in life [114], while at the same time, there have been major advances in cancer screening and therapeutics strategies as well as increasing survival rates in patients with cancer. As a result, many women must deal with not only a new cancer diagnosis but also the implications it may have on their childbearing potential [115]. Therapeutic agents, radiation, and curative surgery are all associated with different risks of ovarian dysfunction and infertility. One study quoted amenorrhea rates to be as high as 61% in women under 40 with breast cancer after receiving the classic cyclophosphamide, methotrexate, and 5-FU therapy regimen [116].

While many fertility preservation strategies have been developed, the only fertility preservation technique endorsed by the American Society of Clinical Oncology is oocyte/embryo cryopreservation—all others are still considered experimental [117]. Most commonly this involves COS followed by the cryopreservation of the oocyte or embryo [115] for future reimplantation or transfer to a gestational carrier.

The method of COS selected must take into account how much time the patient can afford to delay therapy [118] as well as whether their cancer is estrogen sensitive. The majority of fertility research in estrogen-sensitive cancers has been in breast cancer, with breast cancer being the second leading cause of cancer-related death in women [119]. While breast cancer increases with age, up to 30% of new breast cancer diagnoses are in pre- or perimenopausal women [120], and up to 29% of these women have said that fertility concerns influenced their choices regarding treatment [121].

Conventional ovarian stimulation protocols involve stimulation with GnRH antagonists and provide the shortest interval to initiation of cancer therapy [115]. Until recently, having an estrogen receptor-positive cancer precluded patients from COS due to the resulting supraphysiologic estrogen levels. Thus, the only fertility preservation option available was natural cycle IVF which only results in an embryo in about 60% of cycles [122]. However, there are now newer COS therapeutic options available such as tamoxifen and letrozole which are not associated with high estrogen levels. A combination therapy of letrozole + FSH is currently the method of choice over tamoxifen since it stimulates development of greater numbers of follicles, mature oocytes, and subsequent embryos [123]. This combination therapy results in significantly reduced circulating estradiol and reduced FSH requirements than conventional therapies [124–126]. Azim et al. demonstrated that letrozole therapy is not associated with any increased breast cancer recurrence or increase mortality compared to individuals who did not receive fertility therapy [127]. While initial evidence suggested comparable oocyte retrieval and fertility rates between individuals receiving letrozole + FSH COS and conventional COS [124, 128], a recent study suggested that the FSH and letrozole therapy results in fewer oocytes [125]. More studies are required to clearly elucidate relative efficacy in cancer patients. Ultimately we may need to consider whether the compromise of efficacy in favor of safety is preferable in the long run.

A recent study by Turan et al. demonstrated that two consecutive ovarian stimulation cycles are safe, with no increased rate of breast cancer recurrence in their study population [129]. Furthermore, a significantly increased oocyte and embryo yield was achieved with two compared to just one COS cycle, with no significant delay in treatment [129]. If a compromise in yield is discovered with letrozole compared with traditional therapy, two consecutive ovarian stimulations may be a way to ameliorate this. Furthermore, case reports have suggested that it may also be possible to use letrozole stimulation in a random-start ovarian hyperstimulation for those patients who require emergent cancer therapy without compromising fertilization rates [130]. This has the potential for significantly reducing the time until cancer therapy.

The advantage of reduced estrogen exposure in the context of fertility treatments seems to be specific to letrozole and is not consistent with all aromatase inhibitors. Breast cancer patients who underwent COS with anastrozole were exposed to significantly higher levels of estradiol than those treated with letrozole [131]. Thus, letrozole is currently the preferred method of ovarian stimulation for women with estrogen-sensitive cancer.

Endometrial cancer is another estrogen-sensitive cancer for which the standard of care in cancer greater than stage 1 grade 2 is a hysterectomy and bilateral salpingectomy. Most cases of endometrial cancer occur in post-menopausal women; however, it can occur in pre- or perimenopausal women as well. If a woman would like to preserve her fertility, she would need to consider oocyte retrieval and a gestational carrier; however, controlled stimulation has traditionally been avoided due to the resulting supraphysiologic estrogen levels. In 2007 Azim and Oktay demonstrated that combined letrozole and gonadotropin therapy could be used in women with endometrial for successful retrieval of oocytes (7 ± 2.85) while avoiding high circulating estradiol levels associated with standard fertility preservation methods [126]. This report was only based on evidence from four women and warrants further investigation, but the results were very encouraging and could have significant implications for young women wanting to preserve their fertility.

7.10 Letrozole in the Prevention of Ovarian Hyperstimulation Syndrome

The Royal College of Obstetricians and Gynecologists describes OHSS as a complication of fertility treatment [132]. Mild OHSS has been generally accepted to affect one third of IVF cycles and moderate to severe to affect 3–8% of patients [133], although a recent US study quoted the incidence to be closer to 1.1% [134]. While the pathophysiology of OHSS is not fully elucidated, it results in increased vascular permeability, third spacing of fluid, and intravascular depletion. Mild OHSS is usually self-limited, but severe cases require hospitalization and can lead to hemodynamic instability, renal failure, adult respiratory distress syndrome, ovarian rupture and hemorrhage, thromboembolism, and even death [135].

OHSS usually occurs as a result of gonadotropin stimulation; however, it has very occasionally been shown to occur in response to other stimulating agents including clomiphene citrate. A recent Cochrane review examined 16 studies comparing letrozole to other ovulation induction agents in patients with PCOS and found that there was not a single case of OHSS in all 882 patients studied who received letrozole [49]. In fact there was no difference in the rates of OHSS between letrozole-treated groups and groups treated with placebo, clomiphene citrate, laparoscopic ovarian drilling, or anastrozole [49]. Low rates of OHSS in OI with letrozole are thought to be due to an intact estrogen feedback loop and resulting in monofollicular ovulation [9].

In ART, while letrozole on its own is insufficient for ovarian stimulation, combining it with low-dose gonadotropin can induce appropriate follicular development while maintaining low estradiol levels. One study reported two events of moderate to severe OHSS in patients stimulated with gonadotropin only and no events in the patients receiving gonadotropins + letrozole [136]. More research is needed to elucidate whether combined gonadotropin + letrozole stimulation for ART results in lower rates of OHSS. If OHSS rates are found to be lower, this would be a safer alternative for COS in high-risk patients than traditional gonadotropin ovarian stimulation.

Preventing the occurrence of OHSS is superior to managing it reactively. Risk factors for developing OHSS include young age, low body weight, PCOS, high doses of exogenous gonadotropins, high or rapidly increasing serum estradiol levels, previous episodes of OHSS, and high numbers of developing ovarian follicles [135]. In 2008 Fatemi et al. performed a pilot study of letrozole administration during the luteal phase of the ovulation cycle. They found that letrozole administration at this time significantly lowers circulating estradiol levels [137]. In 2009 Garcia-Velasco et al. proposed that letrozole could be administered during the luteal phase to high-risk patients to reduce ovarian hyperstimulation [138]. This was supported by a study by He et al. in 2014 that examined 88 patients at high risk for OHSS who were undergoing frozen embryo transfer. They found that administration of 7.5 mg of letrozole starting on the day of oocyte retrieval significantly reduced the incidence of moderate and severe OHSS (9/24 patients vs. 1/20 patients, $p = 0.013$) [139] and that this effect may be dose dependent, although lower doses have been effective in other studies [137, 138, 140].

Low-dose aspirin has been recommended to prevent or reduce the severity of OHSS symptoms [141, 142]. A 238 participant prospective randomized controlled trial published in 2017 by Mai et al. investigated the ability of letrozole relative to aspirin to control OHSS in high-risk patients undergoing embryo cryopreservation [140]. They found that letrozole was more effective than aspirin at decreasing moderate and severe OHSS ($p = 0.044$). This is in contrast to a smaller non-randomized study in 2015 which claimed that letrozole cannot prevent severe OHSS in high-risk patients [143]. This difference may be due to smaller sample size of the earlier study or its non-randomized nature.

More information is needed before we are able to definitively say what is the best method of reducing OHSS in IVF and cryopreservation; both combined FSH + letrozole for COS or stimulation by gonadotropins followed by administration of letrozole in the luteal phase seem like promising viable options.

7.11 Conclusions and Future Directions

Letrozole has significant research supporting its use as an agent for ovulation induction. Multiple societies including ACOG, SOGC, and CFAS have given their support to the use of letrozole in anovulatory infertility based on its superior efficacy as an OI agent than clomiphene citrate and on its safety data (Table 7.3). Endometriosis pain is significantly improved with letrozole, and preliminary data suggests letrozole is at least as effective as CC in treating endometriosis-related infertility. For women with estrogen-sensitive cancers, letrozole has provided fertility preservation options that were not previously available.

The role for letrozole in assisted reproductive therapy is still not clear. It cannot be used as a COS agent on its own, but in combination with gonadotropins, it has demonstrated reduced requirements of FSH, fewer incidents of OHSS, and thicker endometrium, but more studies are needed to fully elucidate if letrozole combination treatment can lead to increased live birth rates.

Letrozole is a promising therapeutic with many potential applications that we are just starting to understand. With a changing climate of available ovulation induction agents that are available, we will undoubtedly see greater uptake of use of letrozole therapy in clinical practice. With more data,

Table 7.3 Important points about letrozole use in fertility therapy

- Letrozole leads to increased pregnancy and birth rates with in patients with PCOS relative to clomiphene citrate
- Letrozole is superior to other ovulation induction agents in its ability to induce mono-ovulation
- Unlike clomiphene citrate, letrozole requires minimal/no ultrasound monitoring of endometrial thickness
- Letrozole is as good as clomiphene citrate for OI in unexplained fertility
- Reduced costs associated with letrozole + gonadotropin controlled ovarian stimulation in ART
- Letrozole has provided fertility preservation options to patients with estrogen sensitive cancers which were not previously available
- Letrozole has an improved safety profile relative to clomiphene citrate and gonadotropin therapy
- We are beginning to understand the potential uses for letrozole in the reduction of OHSS risk in ART

national drug regulation agencies may revisit their warnings about letrozole, further reducing anxiety around its use. As letrozole use becomes more ubiquitous, we will gain a better understanding of its full therapeutic potential in fertility therapy.

References

1. Holzer H, Casper R, Tulandi T. A new era in ovulation induction. Fertil Steril. 2006;85(2):277–84.
2. Brown J, Farquhar C, Beck J, Boothroyd C, Hughes E. Clomiphene and anti-oestrogens for ovulation induction in PCOS. Cochrane Database Syst Rev. 2009;4:CD002249.
3. Legro RS, Barnhart HX, Schlaff WD, Carr BR, Diamond MP, Carson SA, et al. Clomiphene, metformin, or both for infertility in the polycystic ovary syndrome. N Engl J Med. 2007;356(6):551–66.
4. Legro RS, Brzyski RG, Diamond MP, Coutifaris C, Schlaff WD, Casson P, et al. Letrozole versus clomiphene for infertility in the polycystic ovary syndrome. N Engl J Med. 2014;371(2):119–29.
5. Mitwally MF, Casper RF. Use of an aromatase inhibitor for induction of ovulation in patients with an inadequate response to clomiphene citrate. Fertil Steril. 2001;75(2):305–9.
6. Dowsett M, Cuzick J, Ingle J, Coates A, Forbes J, Bliss J, et al. Meta-analysis of breast cancer outcomes in adjuvant trials of aromatase inhibitors versus tamoxifen. J Clin Oncol. 2010;28(3):509–18.
7. Tredway DR, Schertz JC. Anastrozole versus clomiphene citrate: which is better for ovulation induction? Fertil Steril. 2011;95(5):1549–51.
8. Badawy A, Abdel Aal I, Abulatta M. Clomiphene citrate or anastrozole for ovulation induction in women with polycystic ovary syndrome? A prospective controlled trial. Fertil Steril. 2009;92(3):860–3.
9. Casper RF, Mitwally MF. Review: aromatase inhibitors for ovulation induction. J Clin Endocrinol Metab. 2006;91(3):760–71.
10. Mitwally MF, Casper RF. Aromatase inhibition: a novel method of ovulation induction in women with polycystic ovary syndrome. Reprod Technol. 2001;2000(10):244–7.
11. Health Canada. Important safety information on the contraindication of Femara (letrozole) in premenopausal women—for health professionals. In Canada H, editor. healthycanadians.gc.ca: Government of Canada; 2005.
12. SOGC C. CFAS-SOGC joint position statement on the use of letrozole for the management of infertility; 2017.
13. Thessaloniki ESHRE/ASRM-Sponsored PCOS Consensus Workshop Group. Consensus on infertility treatment related to polycystic ovary syndrome. Hum Reprod. 2008;23(3):462–77.
14. Vause TD, Cheung AP, Sierra S, Claman P, Graham J, Guillemin JA, et al. Ovulation induction in polycystic ovary syndrome: no. 242, May 2010. Int J Gynaecol Obstet. 2010;111(1):95–100.
15. Royal College of Obstetricians and Gynaecologists. Fertility: assessment and treatment for people with fertility problems. National Institute for Health and Clinical Excellence: Guidance. London: RCOG Press; 2013.
16. Dunselman GA, Vermeulen N, Becker C, Calhaz-Jorge C, D'Hooghe T, De Bie B, et al. ESHRE guideline: management of women with endometriosis. Hum Reprod. 2014;29(3):400–12.
17. American College of Obstetrics and Gynecology. Committee opinion no. 663: aromatase inhibitors in gynecologic practice. Obstet Gynecol. 2016;127(6):e170–4.
18. Mitwally MF, Casper RF, Diamond MP. The role of aromatase inhibitors in ameliorating deleterious effects of ovarian stimulation on outcome of infertility treatment. Reprod Biol Endocrinol. 2005;3:54.
19. Sioufi A, Gauducheau N, Pineau V, Marfil F, Jaouen A, Cardot JM, et al. Absolute bioavailability of letrozole in healthy postmenopausal women. Biopharm Drug Dispos. 1997;18(9):779–89.
20. Sioufi A, Sandrenan N, Godbillon J, Trunet P, Czendlik C, Howald H, et al. Comparative bioavailability of letrozole under fed and fasting conditions in 12 healthy subjects after a 2.5 mg single oral administration. Biopharm Drug Dispos. 1997;18(6):489–97.
21. Lee VC, Ledger W. Aromatase inhibitors for ovulation induction and ovarian stimulation. Clin Endocrinol. 2011;74(5):537–46.
22. Casper RF, Mitwally MF. A historical perspective of aromatase inhibitors for ovulation induction. Fertil Steril. 2012;98(6):1352–5.
23. Bao SH, Sheng SL, Peng YF, Lin QD. Effects of letrozole and clomiphene citrate on the expression of HOXA10 and integrin alpha v beta 3 in uterine epithelium of rats. Fertil Steril. 2009;91(1):244–8.
24. Casper RF. Letrozole: ovulation or superovulation? Fertil Steril. 2003;80(6):1335–7; discussion 9.
25. Bedaiwy MA, Abdelaleem MA, Hussein M, Mousa N, Brunengraber LN, Casper RF. Hormonal, follicular and endometrial dynamics in letrozole-treated versus natural cycles in patients undergoing controlled ovarian stimulation. Reprod Biol Endocrinol. 2011;9:83.
26. Garcia-Velasco JAML, Pacheco A, Guillen A, Duque L, Requena A, Pellicer A. The AI letrozole increases the concentration of intraovarian androgens and improves *in vitro* fertilization outcome in women with poor ovarian response: a preliminary report. Hum Reprod. 2005;19:2031–5.
27. Palomba S. Aromatase inhibitors for ovulation induction. J Clin Endocrinol Metab. 2015;100(5):1742–7.
28. Vendola KA, Zhou J, Adesanya OO, Weil SJ, Bondy CA. Androgens stimulate early stages of follicular growth in the primate ovary. J Clin Invest. 1998;101(12):2622–9.
29. Weil S, Vendola K, Zhou J, Bondy CA. Androgen and follicle-stimulating hormone interactions in primate ovarian follicle development. J Clin Endocrinol Metab. 1999;84(8):2951–6.
30. Bedaiwy MA, Mousa NA, Esfandiari N, Forman R, Casper RF. Follicular phase dynamics with combined aromatase inhibitor and follicle stimulating hormone treatment. J Clin Endocrinol Metab. 2007;92(3):825–33.
31. Bhatnagar AS. The discovery and mechanism of action of letrozole. Breast Cancer Res Treat. 2007;105(Suppl 1):7–17.
32. Requena A, Herrero J, Landeras J, Navarro E, Neyro JL, Salvador C, et al. Use of letrozole in assisted reproduction: a systematic review and meta-analysis. Hum Reprod Update. 2008;14(6):571–82.
33. Goss PE. Risks versus benefits in the clinical application of aromatase inhibitors. Endocr Relat Cancer. 1999;6(2):325–32.
34. Hamilton A, Piccart M. The third-generation non-steroidal aromatase inhibitors: a review of their clinical benefits in the second-line hormonal treatment of advanced breast cancer. Ann Oncol. 1999;10(4):377–84.
35. Pavone ME, Bulun SE. Aromatase inhibitors for the treatment of endometriosis. Fertil Steril. 2012;98(6):1370–9.
36. Biljan MM, Hemmings R, Brassard N. The outcome of 150 babies following the treatment with letrozole or letrozole and gonadotropins. Fertil Steril. 2005;84:S95.
37. Tiboni GM. AIs and teratogenesis. Fertil Steril. 2004;81:1158–9.
38. Tulandi T, Martin J, Al-Fadhli R, Kabli N, Forman R, Hitkari J, et al. Congenital malformations among 911 newborns conceived after infertility treatment with letrozole or clomiphene citrate. Fertil Steril. 2006;85(6):1761–5.
39. Correy JF, Marsden DE, Schokman FC. The outcome of pregnancy resulting from clomiphene-induced ovulation. Aust N Z J Obstet Gynaecol. 1982;22(1):18–21.
40. Schenker JG, Yarkoni S, Granat M. Multiple pregnancies following induction of ovulation. Fertil Steril. 1981;35(2):105–23.
41. Whiteman D, Murphy M, Hey K, O'Donnell M, Goldacre M. Reproductive factors, subfertility, and risk of neural tube

defects: a case-control study based on the Oxford Record Linkage Study Register. Am J Epidemiol. 2000;152(9):823–8.
42. Sharma S, Ghosh S, Singh S, Chakravarty A, Ganesh A, Rajani S, et al. Congenital malformations among babies born following letrozole or clomiphene for infertility treatment. PLoS One. 2014;9(10):e108219.
43. Tatsumi T, Jwa SC, Kuwahara A, Irahara M, Kubota T, Saito H. No increased risk of major congenital anomalies or adverse pregnancy or neonatal outcomes following letrozole use in assisted reproductive technology. Hum Reprod. 2017;32(1):125–32.
44. ESHRE Capri Workshop Group. Health and fertility in World Health Organization group 2 anovulatory women. Hum Reprod Update. 2012;18(5):586–99.
45. Banerjee Ray P, Ray A, Chakraborti PS. Comparison of efficacy of letrozole and clomiphene citrate in ovulation induction in Indian women with polycystic ovarian syndrome. Arch Gynecol Obstet. 2012;285(3):873–7.
46. Bayar U, Basaran M, Kiran S, Coskun A, Gezer S. Use of an aromatase inhibitor in patients with polycystic ovary syndrome: a prospective randomized trial. Fertil Steril. 2006;86(5):1447–51.
47. Begum MR, Ferdous J, Begum A, Quadir E. Comparison of efficacy of aromatase inhibitor and clomiphene citrate in induction of ovulation in polycystic ovarian syndrome. Fertil Steril. 2009;92(3):853–7.
48. Roy KK, Baruah J, Singla S, Sharma JB, Singh N, Jain SK, et al. A prospective randomized trial comparing the efficacy of Letrozole and Clomiphene citrate in induction of ovulation in polycystic ovarian syndrome. J Hum Reprod Sci. 2012;5(1):20–5.
49. Franik S, Kremer JA, Nelen WL, Farquhar C. Aromatase inhibitors for subfertile women with polycystic ovary syndrome. Cochrane Database Syst Rev. 2014;2:CD010287.
50. Sohrabvand F, Ansari S, Bagheri M. Efficacy of combined metformin-letrozole in comparison with metformin-clomiphene citrate in clomiphene-resistant infertile women with polycystic ovarian disease. Hum Reprod. 2006;21(6):1432–5.
51. Dehbashi SKT, Robati M, Alborzi S, Parsanezhad ME, Shadman A. Comparison of the effects of letrozole and clomiphene citrate on ovulation and pregnancy rate in patients with polycystic ovary syndrome. Iran J Med Sci. 2009;34:23–8.
52. Abu Hashim H, Shokeir T, Badawy A. Letrozole versus combined metformin and clomiphene citrate for ovulation induction in clomiphene-resistant women with polycystic ovary syndrome: a randomized controlled trial. Fertil Steril. 2010;94(4):1405–9.
53. Foroozanfard F, Mahdian M, Mousavi G, Pejmanmanesh M, Soleimani A. Use of letrozole versus clomiphene citrate combined with gonadotropins in patients with clomiphene resistant polycystic ovarian syndrome: a comparative study. Pak J Med Sci. 2011;27(5):967–70.
54. Atay V, Cam C, Muhcu M, Cam M, Karateke A. Comparison of letrozole and clomiphene citrate in women with polycystic ovaries undergoing ovarian stimulation. J Int Med Res. 2006;34(1):73–6.
55. Badawy A, Abdel Aal I, Abulatta M. Clomiphene citrate or letrozole for ovulation induction in women with polycystic ovarian syndrome: a prospective randomized trial. Fertil Steril. 2009;92(3):849–52.
56. Elsedeek MSEA, Elmaghraby HAH. Predictors and characteristics of letrozole induced ovulation in comparison with clomiphene induced ovulation in anovulatory PCOS women. Middle East Fertil Soc J. 2011;16:125–30.
57. Davar R, Javedani M, Fallahzadeh MH. Metformin-letrozole in comparison with Metformin-clomiphene citrate in clomiphene-resistance PCOS patients undergoing IUI. Iran J Reprod Med. 2011;9(1):31–6.
58. Nazik H, Kumtepe Y. Comparison of efficacy of letrozole and clomiphene citrate in ovulation induction for women with polycystic ovarian syndrome. HealthMED. 2011;6:879–83.
59. Selim MF, Borg TF. Letrozole and clomiphene citrate effect on endometrial and subendometrial vascularity in treating infertility in women with polycystic ovary syndrome. J Gynaecol Surg. 2012;28(6):405–10.
60. Baruah J, Roy KK, Rahman SM, Kumar S, Sharma JB, Karmakar D. Endometrial effects of letrozole and clomiphene citrate in women with polycystic ovary syndrome using spiral artery Doppler. Arch Gynecol Obstet. 2009;279(3):311–4.
61. Ganesh A, Goswami SK, Chattopadhyay R, Chaudhury K, Chakravarty B. Comparison of letrozole with continuous gonadotropins and clomiphene-gonadotropin combination for ovulation induction in 1387 PCOS women after clomiphene citrate failure: a randomized prospective clinical trial. J Assist Reprod Genet. 2009;26(1):19–24.
62. Elkhateeb RR, Mahran A. Optimized letrozole dose versus traditional use of clomiphene citrate for ovulation induction in patients with PCOS: a prospective randomized controlled trial. Gynecol Obstet Res Open J. 2016;3(1):7–12.
63. Ghahiri A, Mogharehabed N, Mamourian M. Letrozole as the first-line treatment of infertile women with poly cystic ovarian syndrome (PCOS) compared with clomiphene citrate: a clinical trial. Adv Biomed Res. 2016;5:6.
64. Al-Shaikh SF, Al-Mukhatar EJ, Al-Zubaidy AA, Al-Rubaie BJ, Al-Khuzaee L. Use of clomiphene or letrozole for treating women with polycystic ovary syndrome related subfertility in Hilla city. Middle East Fertil Soc J. 2017;22:105–10.
65. Fleming R, Hopkinson ZE, Wallace AM, Greer IA, Sattar N. Ovarian function and metabolic factors in women with oligomenorrhea treated with metformin in a randomized double blind placebo-controlled trial. J Clin Endocrinol Metab. 2002;87(2):569–74.
66. Huber-Buchholz MM, Carey DG, Norman RJ. Restoration of reproductive potential by lifestyle modification in obese polycystic ovary syndrome: role of insulin sensitivity and luteinizing hormone. J Clin Endocrinol Metab. 1999;84(4):1470–4.
67. Kiddy DS, Hamilton-Fairley D, Bush A, Short F, Anyaoku V, Reed MJ, et al. Improvement in endocrine and ovarian function during dietary treatment of obese women with polycystic ovary syndrome. Clin Endocrinol. 1992;36(1):105–11.
68. Collins JA, Crosignani PG. Unexplained infertility: a review of diagnosis, prognosis, treatment efficacy and management. Int J Gynaecol Obstet. 1992;39(4):267–75.
69. Evers JL. Female subfertility. Lancet. 2002;360(9327):151–9.
70. Badawy A, Elnashar A, Totongy M. Clomiphene citrate or aromatase inhibitors for superovulation in women with unexplained infertility undergoing intrauterine insemination: a prospective randomized trial. Fertil Steril. 2009;92(4):1355–9.
71. Polyzos NP, Tzioras S, Mauri D, Tsappi M, Cortinovis I, Tsali L, et al. Treatment of unexplained infertility with aromatase inhibitors or clomiphene citrate: a systematic review and meta-analysis. Obstet Gynecol Surv. 2008;63(7):472–9.
72. Fouda UM, Sayed AM. Extended letrozole regimen versus clomiphene citrate for superovulation in patients with unexplained infertility undergoing intrauterine insemination: a randomized controlled trial. Reprod Biol Endocrinol. 2011;9:84.
73. Bulun SE. Endometriosis. N Engl J Med. 2009;360(3):268–79.
74. Giudice LC. Clinical practice. Endometriosis. N Engl J Med. 2010;362(25):2389–98.
75. Giudice LC, Kao LC. Endometriosis. Lancet. 2004;364(9447):1789–99.
76. Ilangavan K, Kalu E. High prevalence of endometriosis in infertile women with normal ovulation and normospermic partners. Fertil Steril. 2010;93(3):e10; author reply e2.
77. Bulun SE, Fang Z, Imir G, Gurates B, Tamura M, Yilmaz B, et al. Aromatase and endometriosis. Semin Reprod Med. 2004;22(1):45–50.

78. Ferrero S, Venturini PL, Ragni N, Camerini G, Remorgida V. Pharmacological treatment of endometriosis: experience with aromatase inhibitors. Drugs. 2009;69(8):943–52.
79. Remorgida V, Abbamonte LH, Ragni N, Fulcheri E, Ferrero S. Letrozole and desogestrel-only contraceptive pill for the treatment of stage IV endometriosis. Aust N Z J Obstet Gynaecol. 2007;47(3):222–5.
80. Alborzi S, Hamedi B, Omidvar A, Dehbashi S, Alborzi S, Alborzi M. A comparison of the effect of short-term aromatase inhibitor (letrozole) and GnRH agonist (triptorelin) versus case control on pregnancy rate and symptom and sign recurrence after laparoscopic treatment of endometriosis. Arch Gynecol Obstet. 2011;284(1):105–10.
81. Ailawadi RK, Jobanputra S, Kataria M, Gurates B, Bulun SE. Treatment of endometriosis and chronic pelvic pain with letrozole and norethindrone acetate: a pilot study. Fertil Steril. 2004;81(2):290–6.
82. Agarwal SK, Foster WG. Reduction in endometrioma size with three months of aromatase inhibition and progestin add-Back. Biomed Res Int. 2015;2015:878517.
83. Lall Seal S, Kamilya G, Mukherji J, De A, Ghosh D, Majhi AK. Aromatase inhibitors in recurrent ovarian endometriomas: report of five cases with literature review. Fertil Steril. 2011;95(1):291.e15–8.
84. Ferrero S, Gillott DJ, Venturini PL, Remorgida V. Use of aromatase inhibitors to treat endometriosis-related pain symptoms: a systematic review. Reprod Biol Endocrinol. 2011;9:89.
85. Nawathe A, Patwardhan S, Yates D, Harrison GR, Khan KS. Systematic review of the effects of aromatase inhibitors on pain associated with endometriosis. BJOG. 2008;115(7):818–22.
86. Verma A, Konje JC. Successful treatment of refractory endometriosis-related chronic pelvic pain with aromatase inhibitors in premenopausal patients. Eur J Obstet Gynecol Reprod Biol. 2009;143(2):112–5.
87. Abu Hashim H, El Rakhawy M, Abd Elaal I. Randomized comparison of superovulation with letrozole vs. clomiphene citrate in an IUI program for women with recently surgically treated minimal to mild endometriosis. Acta Obstet Gynecol Scand. 2012;91(3):338–45.
88. Miller PB, Parnell BA, Bushnell G, Tallman N, Forstein DA, Higdon HL 3rd, et al. Endometrial receptivity defects during IVF cycles with and without letrozole. Hum Reprod. 2012;27(3):881–8.
89. Thomas K, Thomson A, Wood S, Kingsland C, Vince G, Lewis-Jones I. Endometrial integrin expression in women undergoing in vitro fertilization and the association with subsequent treatment outcome. Fertil Steril. 2003;80(3):502–7.
90. Hughes EG. The effectiveness of ovulation induction and intrauterine insemination in the treatment of persistent infertility: a meta-analysis. Hum Reprod. 1997;12(9):1865–72.
91. Mitwally MF, Casper RF. Aromatase inhibition improves ovarian response to follicle-stimulating hormone in poor responders. Fertil Steril. 2002;77(4):776–80.
92. Mitwally MF, Casper RF. Aromatase inhibition reduces gonadotrophin dose required for controlled ovarian stimulation in women with unexplained infertility. Hum Reprod. 2003;18(8):1588–97.
93. Healey S, Tan SL, Tulandi T, Biljan MM. Effects of letrozole on superovulation with gonadotropins in women undergoing intrauterine insemination. Fertil Steril. 2003;80(6):1325–9.
94. Bedaiwy MA, Shokry M, Mousa N, Claessens A, Esfandiari N, Gotleib L, et al. Letrozole co-treatment in infertile women 40 years old and older receiving controlled ovarian stimulation and intrauterine insemination. Fertil Steril. 2009;91(6):2501–7.
95. Bedaiwy MA, Forman R, Mousa NA, Al Inany HG, Casper RF. Cost-effectiveness of aromatase inhibitor co-treatment for controlled ovarian stimulation. Hum Reprod. 2006;21(11):2838–44.
96. Mitwally MF, Casper RF. Aromatase inhibition reduces the dose of gonadotropin required for controlled ovarian hyperstimulation. J Soc Gynecol Investig. 2004;11(6):406–15.
97. Yasa C, Bastu E, Dural O, Celik E, Ergun B. Evaluation of low-dose letrozole addition to ovulation induction in IVF. Clin Exp Obstet Gynecol. 2013;40(1):98–100.
98. Papanikolaou EG, Polyzos NP, Humaidan P, Pados G, Bosch E, Tournaye H, et al. Aromatase inhibitors in stimulated IVF cycles. Reprod Biol Endocrinol. 2011;9:85.
99. Hassan A, Shehata N, Wahba A. Cost effectiveness of letrozole and purified urinary FSH in treating women with clomiphene citrate-resistant polycystic ovarian syndrome: a randomized controlled trial. Hum Fertil. 2017;20(1):37–42.
100. Batukan C, Baysal B. Metformin improves ovulation and pregnancy rates in patients with polycystic ovary syndrome. Arch Gynecol Obstet. 2001;265(3):124–7.
101. Vandermolen DT, Ratts VS, Evans WS, Stovall DW, Kauma SW, Nestler JE. Metformin increases the ovulatory rate and pregnancy rate from clomiphene citrate in patients with polycystic ovary syndrome who are resistant to clomiphene citrate alone. Fertil Steril. 2001;75(2):310–5.
102. Nestler JE, Jakubowicz DJ, Evans WS, Pasquali R. Effects of metformin on spontaneous and clomiphene-induced ovulation in the polycystic ovary syndrome. N Engl J Med. 1998;338(26):1876–80.
103. Heard MJ, Pierce A, Carson SA, Buster JE. Pregnancies following use of metformin for ovulation induction in patients with polycystic ovary syndrome. Fertil Steril. 2002;77(4):669–73.
104. Nestler JE, Jakubowicz DJ. Decreases in ovarian cytochrome P450c17 alpha activity and serum free testosterone after reduction of insulin secretion in polycystic ovary syndrome. N Engl J Med. 1996;335(9):617–23.
105. Moll E, Bossuyt PM, Korevaar JC, Lambalk CB, van der Veen F. Effect of clomifene citrate plus metformin and clomifene citrate plus placebo on induction of ovulation in women with newly diagnosed polycystic ovary syndrome: randomised double blind clinical trial. BMJ. 2006;332(7556):1485.
106. Tang T, Lord JM, Norman RJ, Yasmin E, Balen AH. Insulin-sensitising drugs (metformin, rosiglitazone, pioglitazone, D-chiro-inositol) for women with polycystic ovary syndrome, oligo amenorrhoea and subfertility. Cochrane Database Syst Rev. 2012;5:CD003053.
107. Morin-Papunen L, Rantala AS, Unkila-Kallio L, Tiitinen A, Hippelainen M, Perheentupa A, et al. Metformin improves pregnancy and live-birth rates in women with polycystic ovary syndrome (PCOS): a multicenter, double-blind, placebo-controlled randomized trial. J Clin Endocrinol Metab. 2012;97(5):1492–500.
108. Klement AH, Casper RF. The use of aromatase inhibitors for ovulation induction. Curr Opin Obstet Gynecol. 2015;27(3):206–9.
109. Legro RS. Ovulation induction in polycystic ovary syndrome: current options. Best Pract Res Clin Obstet Gynaecol. 2016;37:152–9.
110. Elgafor IA. Efficacy of combined metformin-letrozole in comparison with bilateral ovarian drilling in clomiphene-resistant infertile women with polycystic ovarian syndrome. Arch Gynecol Obstet. 2013;288(1):119–23.
111. Verpoest WM, Kolibianakis E, Papanikolaou E, Smitz J, Van Steirteghem A, Devroey P. Aromatase inhibitors in ovarian stimulation for IVF/ICSI: a pilot study. Reprod Biomed Online. 2006;13(2):166–72.
112. Ozmen B, Sonmezer M, Atabekoglu CS, Olmus H. Use of aromatase inhibitors in poor-responder patients receiving GnRH antagonist protocols. Reprod Biomed Online. 2009;19(4):478–85.
113. Goswami SK, Das T, Chattopadhyay R, Sawhney V, Kumar J, Chaudhury K, et al. A randomized single-blind controlled trial of letrozole as a low-cost IVF protocol in women with poor ovarian response: a preliminary report. Hum Reprod. 2004;19(9):2031–5.

114. Hamilton BE, Martin JA, Ventura SJ. Births: preliminary data for 2011. Natl Vital Stat Rep. 2012;61(5):1–18.
115. Kasum M, Simunic V, Oreskovic S, Beketic-Oreskovic L. Fertility preservation with ovarian stimulation protocols prior to cancer treatment. Gynecol Endocrinol. 2014;30(3):182–6.
116. Goldhirsch A, Gelber RD, Castiglione M. The magnitude of endocrine effects of adjuvant chemotherapy for premenopausal breast cancer patients. The International Breast Cancer Study Group. Ann Oncol. 1990;1(3):183–8.
117. Loren AW, Mangu PB, Beck LN, Brennan L, Magdalinski AJ, Partridge AH, et al. Fertility preservation for patients with cancer: American Society of Clinical Oncology clinical practice guideline update. J Clin Oncol. 2013;31(19):2500–10.
118. Cakmak H, Rosen MP. Ovarian stimulation in cancer patients. Fertil Steril. 2013;99(6):1476–84.
119. Society AC. Cancer facts & figures 2017; 2017.
120. Institute NC. Cancer stat facts: female breast cancer surveillance, epidemiology and end results program; 2017.
121. Partridge AH, Gelber S, Peppercorn J, Sampson E, Knudsen K, Laufer M, et al. Web-based survey of fertility issues in young women with breast cancer. J Clin Oncol. 2004;22(20):4174–83.
122. Oktay K, Buyuk E, Davis O, Yermakova I, Veeck L, Rosenwaks Z. Fertility preservation in breast cancer patients: IVF and embryo cryopreservation after ovarian stimulation with tamoxifen. Hum Reprod. 2003;18(1):90–5.
123. Oktay K, Buyuk E, Libertella N, Akar M, Rosenwaks Z. Fertility preservation in breast cancer patients: a prospective controlled comparison of ovarian stimulation with tamoxifen and letrozole for embryo cryopreservation. J Clin Oncol. 2005;23(19):4347–53.
124. Oktay K, Hourvitz A, Sahin G, Oktem O, Safro B, Cil A, et al. Letrozole reduces estrogen and gonadotropin exposure in women with breast cancer undergoing ovarian stimulation before chemotherapy. J Clin Endocrinol Metab. 2006;91(10):3885–90.
125. Revelli A, Porcu E, Levi Setti PE, Delle Piane L, Merlo DF, Anserini P. Is letrozole needed for controlled ovarian stimulation in patients with estrogen receptor-positive breast cancer? Gynecol Endocrinol. 2013;29(11):993–6.
126. Azim A, Oktay K. Letrozole for ovulation induction and fertility preservation by embryo cryopreservation in young women with endometrial carcinoma. Fertil Steril. 2007;88(3):657–64.
127. Azim AA, Costantini-Ferrando M, Oktay K. Safety of fertility preservation by ovarian stimulation with letrozole and gonadotropins in patients with breast cancer: a prospective controlled study. J Clin Oncol. 2008;26(16):2630–5.
128. Checa Vizcaino MA, Corchado AR, Cuadri ME, Comadran MG, Brassesco M, Carreras R. The effects of letrozole on ovarian stimulation for fertility preservation in cancer-affected women. Reprod Biomed Online. 2012;24(6):606–10.
129. Turan V, Bedoschi G, Moy F, Oktay K. Safety and feasibility of performing two consecutive ovarian stimulation cycles with the use of letrozole-gonadotropin protocol for fertility preservation in breast cancer patients. Fertil Steril. 2013;100(6):1681–5.e1.
130. Sonmezer M, Turkcuoglu I, Coskun U, Oktay K. Random-start controlled ovarian hyperstimulation for emergency fertility preservation in letrozole cycles. Fertil Steril. 2011;95(6):2125.e9–11.
131. Azim AA, Costantini-Ferrando M, Lostritto K, Oktay K. Relative potencies of anastrozole and letrozole to suppress estradiol in breast cancer patients undergoing ovarian stimulation before in vitro fertilization. J Clin Endocrinol Metab. 2007;92(6):2197–200.
132. Royal College of Obstetricians and Gynaecologists. The management of ovarian hyperstimulation syndrome. RCOG Green-top Guideline No 5; 2016.
133. Delvigne A, Rozenberg S. Epidemiology and prevention of ovarian hyperstimulation syndrome (OHSS): a review. Hum Reprod Update. 2002;8(6):559–77.
134. Kawwass JF, Kissin DM, Kulkarni AD, Creanga AA, Session DR, Callaghan WM, et al. Safety of assisted reproductive technology in the United States, 2000–2011. JAMA. 2015;313(1):88–90.
135. Practice Committee of the American Society for Reproductive Medicine. Ovarian hyperstimulation syndrome. Fertil Steril. 2008;90(5 Suppl):S188–93.
136. Ashraf M, Balan A, Sathya B, Sayed S. Letrozole in IVF/ICSI cycles to optimize the number of mature follicles and to maintain estradiol levels within the "safe" range. Int Congr Ser. 2004;1271:97–100.
137. Fatemi HM, Popovic-Todorovic B, Donoso P, Papanikolaou E, Smitz J, Devroey P. Luteal phase oestradiol suppression by letrozole: a pilot study in oocyte donors. Reprod Biomed Online. 2008;17(3):307–11.
138. Garcia-Velasco JA, Quea G, Piro M, Mayoral M, Ruiz M, Toribio M, et al. Letrozole administration during the luteal phase after ovarian stimulation impacts corpus luteum function: a randomized, placebo-controlled trial. Fertil Steril. 2009;92(1):222–5.
139. He Q, Liang L, Zhang C, Li H, Ge Z, Wang L, et al. Effects of different doses of letrozole on the incidence of early-onset ovarian hyperstimulation syndrome after oocyte retrieval. Syst Biol Reprod Med. 2014;60(6):355–60.
140. Mai Q, Hu X, Yang G, Luo Y, Huang K, Yuan Y, et al. Effect of letrozole on moderate and severe early-onset ovarian hyperstimulation syndrome in high-risk women: a prospective randomized trial. Am J Obstet Gynecol. 2017;216(1):42.e1–10.
141. Varnagy A, Bodis J, Manfai Z, Wilhelm F, Busznyak C, Koppan M. Low-dose aspirin therapy to prevent ovarian hyperstimulation syndrome. Fertil Steril. 2010;93(7):2281–4.
142. Varnagy A, Koppan M, Manfai Z, Busznyak C, Bodis J. Low-dose aspirin for prophylaxis of ovarian hyperstimulation syndrome. Fertil Steril. 2008;89(4):1035–6.
143. Wang YQ, Luo J, Xu WM, Xie QZ, Yan WJ, Wu GX, et al. Can steroidal ovarian suppression during the luteal phase after oocyte retrieval reduce the risk of severe OHSS? J Ovarian Res. 2015;8:63.

Gonadotropin-Releasing Hormone and Its Analogues

8

Peter Kovacs

Reproductive functions are regulated by rather complex endocrine mechanisms. There are three levels involved in this function: the hypothalamus, the pituitary, and the ovaries. The hypothalamus serves as the main generator of normal activity by releasing gonadotropin-releasing hormone (GnRH) at regular intervals. GnRH reaches the anterior pituitary via the portal vessels where it induces the synthesis and release of follicle-stimulating hormone (FSH) and luteinizing hormone (LH). These hormones reach the ovaries through the systemic circulation, and they exert their effects on the theca and granulosa cells within the follicles and induce folliculogenesis. There are multiple regulatory mechanisms that control and modify the actions of this axis. There are short-, medium-, and long-loop feedback mechanisms that influence the pulse frequency and amplitude with which GnRH is released. Through the modifications of GnRH release, the synthesis and release of FSH and LH are modified too, and eventually this has an impact on ovarian function.

There are conditions when the malfunction of the hypothalamic-pituitary-ovarian axis results in endocrine and therefore reproductive abnormalities (e.g., Kallmann's syndrome, polycystic ovary syndrome, Sheehan's syndrome, etc.). In addition there are conditions when an interference with the normal hypothalamic-pituitary function is needed to manage a clinical problem (precocious puberty, endometriosis, leiomyomas, etc.). Finally, one has to interrupt the normal GnRH release during fertility treatment when the premature activation of the pituitary-ovarian axis has to be prevented to allow the treatment to proceed successfully.

This chapter will review the physiologic regulatory mechanisms of the hypothalamic-pituitary-ovarian axis and will discuss those clinical scenarios where synthetic GnRH analogues (agonist, antagonist) can be successfully used.

P. Kovacs (✉)
Kaali Institute IVF Center, Budapest, Hungary

8.1 GnRH Release

GnRH is a decapeptide with a short half-life. It is synthesized and released by hypothalamic GnRH neurons. These neurons can be found in the preoptic areas and adjacent sites in the hypothalamus. There are about 1500 GnRH neurons that form a network, and their coordinated activity is required for normal function [1]. GnRH release is episodic and this pulsatile function is an inherent characteristic of the GnRH neurons [2].

The pulsatile function of these neurons is under the control of multilevel feedback mechanisms (Fig. 8.1). GnRH exerts an autocrine effect on the GnRH neurons themselves through transmembrane receptors (very short-loop feedback). GnRH release is Ca dependent. GnRH agonists upon binding to GnRH receptors are coupled to stimulatory G proteins and stimulate cyclic AMP production and Ca signaling. GnRH antagonists upon binding to the receptor are coupled to inhibitory G proteins and interfere with GnRH release [1]. Coupling and uncoupling to stimulatory or inhibitory G proteins is one mechanism through which the pulse frequency and amplitude at which GnRH is released can be adjusted [1].

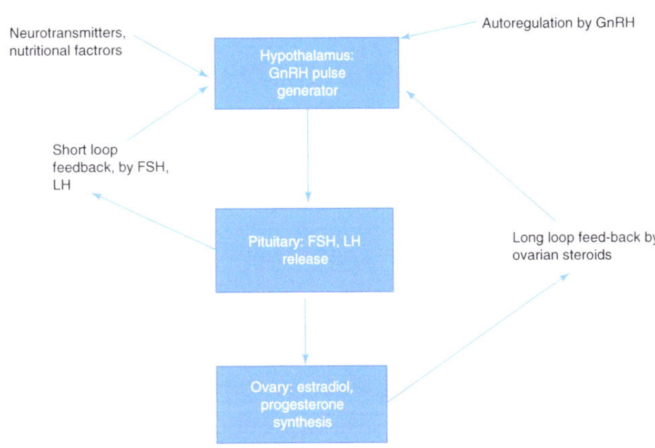

Fig. 8.1 Regulation of the hypothalamic-pituitary-ovarian axis

G. N. Allahbadia et al. (eds.), *Textbook of Assisted Reproduction*, https://doi.org/10.1007/978-981-15-2377-9_8

The activity of the GnRH neurons is also under the control of multiple neurotransmitters (noradrenalin, opioids, GABA, neuropeptide Y, etc.) secreted by neurons that project on GnRH cells [3, 4]. Metabolic factors also play a role in the regulation of hypothalamic GnRH neuron activity. It is well known that the incidence of reproductive dysfunction increases as one deviates from the normal body mass index. The hypothalamus is the site where the connection between energy metabolism and reproduction can be found. Insulin and leptin are believed to be the most important peripheral signals that influence GnRH activity. Leptin receptors cannot be found on GnRH neurons; therefore, they act through interneurons, most probably neuropeptide Y (NPY) releasing interneurons. NPY has a negative effect on GnRH neuron activity, and leptin may suppress this inhibitory effect. Insulin on the other hand seems to have a direct and stimulatory effect on GnRH neurons through its own receptors [5].

GnRH reaches the pituitary through the portal system where it binds to the surface receptors and induces FSH and LH release. Through a short-loop feedback mechanism, hormones secreted by the pituitary (e.g., midcycle LH surge) exert an effect on the hypothalamus and influence the pulsatile release of GnRH (hypothalamic-pituitary loop).

FSH and LH, secreted by the pituitary in response to hypothalamic-pituitary activation, induce follicle development, and the follicles start to secrete increasing amounts of estradiol. Estradiol in return affects GnRH neuronal activity through the long-loop feedback mechanism. For a long time estradiol was thought to influence GnRH neurons indirectly as its receptors (estrogen receptor [ER]) could not be found in the neurons [3]. Subsequently both the ERα and ERβ subtypes were shown to be expressed in GnRH neurons. Estrogen is known to have a negative as well as a positive effect on GnRH activity, the latter required for the midcycle LH surge. This dual activity can be explained by the differential expression of the receptor subtypes. Estradiol upon binding to ERα mediates an inhibitory effect on cyclic AMP production and pulsatile GnRH secretion through the inhibitory effect of G-inhibitory protein (negative feedback). While upon binding to ERβ, estradiol increases cAMP production, and GnRH secretion is achieved consistent with the midcycle positive feedback effect [1, 3, 6]. In addition to estradiol's direct effect through its receptors on GnRH neuronal activity, there is evidence for indirect effects primarily through GABA neurons. Furthermore, estradiol was shown to activate progestin receptors, and this action is required for the LH surge. Antiprogestin successfully blocked the midcycle estradiol-induced LH surge in an animal model, whereas in the absence of antiprogestin, a normal LH surge could be elicited [7].

Table 8.1 Clinical use of GnRH analogues

Female	Male	Both
Benign diseases: uterine fibroids, adenomyosis, endometriosis	Benign disease: benign prostate hypertrophy	Central precocious puberty
Malignant disease: adjuvant therapy in hormone-sensitive cancers (breast, ovarian cancer)	Malignant disease: adjuvant therapy for prostate cancer	Potential for contraception
Gonad protection during chemotherapy		Infertility treatment

8.2 Neuroendocrine Control of Folliculogenesis

GnRH release into the portal vessels is pulsatile (every 60–90 min in the follicular phase and 120–240 min in the luteal phase; besides the frequency, the amplitude changes as well) [3, 4]. Upon reaching the anterior lobe of the pituitary, it binds to its surface receptors and initiates the release of stored FSH and LH. The receptor-ligand complex is then internalized, and upon dissociation the GnRH receptors can be recycled to the cell surface.

There are clinical scenarios when the disruption of intact hypothalamic-pituitary-ovarian/testicular function is desired (Table 8.1). This can be achieved by chronic administration of GnRH agonists or GnRH antagonists. GnRH agonists and antagonists are chemically modified versions of the original decapeptide which was identified in 1971 [8] (Fig. 8.2). By modifying the chemical structure of the original molecule, the half-life of GnRH can be extended, and a chronic effect can be achieved. GnRH agonists are resistant to enzymatic degradation and remain bound to the receptor once internalized. GnRH agonists uncouple GnRH from the second messenger systems (desensitization) and decrease the calcium response, inactivate calcium channels, and reduce inositol phosphate production. Following internalization GnRH analogues remain bound to the receptors, and there is a reduction in receptor recycling to the cell surface resulting in receptor loss preventing GnRH action. Following an initial release of stored FSH/LH, GnRH agonists lead to a decreased gonadotropin output [9].

GnRH antagonists also bind to the GnRH receptors. Unlike GnRH agonists their action is competitive receptor blockage, and they inhibit signal transduction. GnRH antagonists can be replaced from the receptors; their inhibitory effect is competitive and quickly reversible by an appropriate dose of GnRH agonist [9].

Natural GnRH is rapidly metabolized; its degradation is started at the position six amino acid (glycin). The replacement of this amino acid has resulted in increased resistance to degradation (triptorelin, Gly → D-Trp; leuprolide,

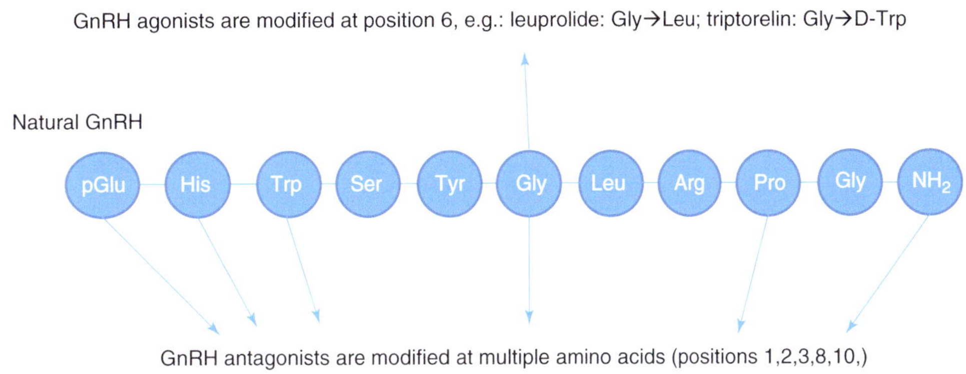

Fig. 8.2 Natural GnRH and sites of chemical modification to obtain agonists/ antagonists

Gly → D-Leu; buserelin, Gly → D-Ser(tBu); goserelin, Gly → D-Ser(tBu)). Furthermore, in some of these compounds, Gly is deleted in position 10 (leuprolide, buserelin). GnRH antagonists are synthesized by chemically modifying the amino acid sequence at multiple sites [9].

8.3 Clinical Use

There are clinical scenarios when the intact function of the hypothalamic-pituitary-ovarian axis is not desired (Table 8.1).

8.3.1 Precocious Puberty

Precocious puberty affects 1:5000–10,000 children and is more common in females. Most cases are idiopathic and are of central origin. Central precocious puberty is associated with the early activation of the hypothalamic-pituitary axis. It leads to premature puberty, accelerated occurrence of secondary sex characteristics, and accelerated bone maturation with eventual short final height and may affect psychosocial development. In untreated cases the growth velocity of long bones is accelerated but is associated with early fusion of the epiphyseal growth plates resulting in short stature [10, 11].

GnRH agonists block the activated hypothalamic-pituitary axis, slow down bone growth, and therefore could improve the final height. The combination of growth hormone with GnRH agonist has been suggested to further improve the clinical findings. Best results can be expected when the treatment is started early on, preferably before the age of 6.

A French study, using decapeptyl in children with precocious puberty, found the final height to be 8.3 cm higher in girls and 13.7 cm higher in boys when compared to historical controls [12]. The Dutch-German study group reported an increase of 6 cm in final height in girls and 10 cm in boys with triptorelin administration when compared to the pretreatment predicted height [13]. A 2014 meta-analysis based on eight studies found a significant increase in the final height with GnRH agonist treatment when compared to pretreatment predicted height. According to the same report, the results are superior when GnRH agonist is combined with growth hormone [10].

Besides the monthly administered GnRH agonist 3-month depot preparations have been successfully used [14]. No significant adverse effect on later ovarian function, bone density, or reproductive function has been documented so far [10]. Best results can be expected with treatment start before the age of 6; later start is of questionable benefit.

8.3.2 Prostate Cancer

Prostate cancer is the third most common cancer when both sexes are considered. 161,360 new cases are estimated in the USA for the year 2017. It is the sixth most common cause of cancer-related death [15]. The estimated incidence is 123/100,000 population. Testosterone has been implicated as both a trigger and a factor to promote prostate cancer [16]. Androgen deprivation therapy (ADT) is considered the first-line treatment of advanced-stage/metastatic prostate cancer. It is used as neoadjuvant or adjuvant therapy as well [17]. ADT may be combined with other antiandrogens that either block the hepatic androgen synthesis or prevent the testosterone-dihydrotestosterone conversion [18]. ADT may involve surgical removal of both testicles or pharmacological suppression of androgen synthesis with GnRH agonists or antagonists.

GnRH agonists were shown to be similarly effective to bilateral orchiectomy [17]. The goal of medical therapy is to suppress testosterone levels to below 1.7 nmol/l. GnRH agonists induce an initial flare effect resulting in transient elevation of serum testosterone levels. Furthermore, microsurges of testosterone can be seen with each additional injection. The clinical significance of the initial flare or subsequent microsurges is questionable though [19].

GnRH antagonists are associated with immediate suppression of testosterone levels, and no microsurges accompany their use. Studies have shown that both GnRH agonists and antagonists are effective in suppressing testosterone levels. GnRH antagonist degarelix was less likely to be associated with prostate-specific antigen elevation or death during therapy when compared to the GnRH agonist leuprolide [20, 21]. Furthermore, levels of serum alkaline phosphatase as an indicator of bone metastasis were lower with degarelix when compared to a GnRH analogue.

ADT is not without side effects. Increased risks for bone loss, fractures, as well as adverse metabolic effects were reported. Lifestyle changes and pharmacologic interventions can be considered if such complications accompany therapy. Intermittent pharmacologic ADT is an alternative for those with significant side effects. In these cases 6–9 months of ADT can be followed by a medication-free period in which PSA levels are monitored. Medical therapy is resumed when PSA starts to rise [17, 18].

8.3.3 Breast Cancer

Breast cancer is the most common cancer (male-female combined) with an estimated 255,000 new cases annually in the USA. It is also estimated that each year, 41,000 of those diagnosed with breast cancer will die as a result of the disease [22].

In up to ¾ of breast cancers, estrogen plays a role in tumor proliferation acting through its receptors [23]. Interfering with estrogen action or the ER pathway has been an integral part of breast cancer treatment. Selective ER modulators (tamoxifen), aromatase inhibitors, GnRH analogues, and ovarian ablation through radiation therapy or surgery are options to reduce circulating estrogen levels [23].

GnRH agonist as an adjuvant therapy was shown to be as effective as oophorectomy in premenopausal women with advanced-stage breast cancer. Disease-free survival was found to be similar to that achieved with chemotherapy [24]. In a randomized trial, 589 premenopausal women with ER+ early breast cancer were assigned either to 2 years of GnRH agonist use or to six cycles of chemotherapy (cyclophosphamide, methotrexate, fluorouracil). At 2 years of follow-up, no difference in disease-free or overall survival was seen [25]. Another randomized trial assigned premenopausal women with hormone-sensitive breast cancer to adjuvant chemotherapy (three cycles of cyclophosphamide, methotrexate, 5-fluorouracil) or GnRH agonist, goserelin for 2 years. Local and distant recurrence, survival, and death rates were similar in the two groups [26]. A 2009 Cochrane review concluded that adjuvant GnRH agonist therapy or adjuvant chemotherapy resulted in similar overall and disease-free survival for the treatment of early-stage breast cancer in premenopausal women. GnRH agonist combined with tamoxifen may provide superior results when compared to agonist alone [27].

Ovarian ablation using GnRH agonist alone or in combination with tamoxifen is an effective adjuvant therapy for early-stage ER+ breast cancer. The optimal duration of use has not been established; studies have investigated use for 2–5 years. For advanced-stage, metastatic breast cancer, the use of tamoxifen combined with GnRH agonist proved to be superior to GnRH agonist alone [28].

8.3.4 Gonad Protection

The number of follicles peaks at 6–7 million at mid-gestation. By birth the number is down to 1–2 million and by puberty to 400–500,000. The loss rate is genetically determined and differs individually [29]. The rate of follicle loss is accelerated by various iatrogenic effects such as gonadotoxic therapy.

Follicle loss related to chemotherapy depends on baseline ovarian reserve, patient age, the chemotherapeutic agent used, and duration of treatment. Chemotherapy may result in premature ovarian failure or transient amenorrhea. It is estimated that each year, about 100,000 women under the age of 45 are diagnosed with cancer [30]. Some of these women are nulliparous or have not completed their family yet and would desire fertility upon completion of successful therapy. Oncologic therapies have significantly improved over the years, and with the increase in the number of patients surviving such treatments, their long-term consequences (fertility, hormonal balance, overall quality of life) have to be considered [30, 31].

Germ cells, especially actively developing cells, are sensitive to chemotherapy-induced damage and undergo apoptosis. These cells are replaced by the recruitment of primordial, dormant cells leading to faster decline in the overall follicle pool. In addition chemotherapy may cause stromal fibrosis and vascular damage reducing ovarian blood supply further augmenting follicle loss [31].

GnRH agonist was proposed to reduce the toxic ovarian effects by inducing a hypogonadotropic state. Inactive follicles are more resistant to damage. GnRH agonist reduces ovarian blood flow and lowers the amount of drug reaching the follicles [31].

There are multiple cohort and randomized studies that assessed the impact of GnRH agonist on ovarian activity during chemotherapy. Patients with different types of cancer, with different baseline characteristics, undergoing heterogeneous chemotherapeutic treatments were evaluated, and not surprisingly the studies reported conflicting outcomes. Lambertini et al. randomly assigned premenopausal women undergoing chemotherapy for breast cancer to triptorelin or no triptorelin during oncotherapy. Over the 5 years of follow-up, menstruation was resumed in 72.6% of women receiving triptorelin, while in 64% of controls (age-adjusted hazard ratio, 1.48; 95% CI, 1.12–1.95) [32]. Moore et al. randomly assigned women undergoing chemotherapy for breast cancer to goserelin versus no goserelin during chemotherapy. Significantly fewer women in the goserelin group developed ovarian failure after chemotherapy, and significantly more of those receiving goserelin became pregnant [33]. Elgindy et al. randomly assigned women with receptor-negative breast cancer undergoing chemotherapy to GnRH agonist or antagonist downregulation or no downregulation. They found no difference in the proportion of women who resumed regular menstruation 12 months after chemotherapy [34]. There are several other randomized or nonrandomized studies that failed to find a benefit with GnRH analogues for gonadal protection [35, 36].

Several meta-analyses were published on the topic of ovarian protection with GnRH agonist. Del Mastro et al. found a significant reduction in premature ovarian failure rates with GnRH agonist use based on the analysis of nine studies [37]. Blumenfeld et al. analyzed the results of 20 retrospective or randomized studies and found significantly lower ovarian failure rates with GnRH administration. According to their analysis, 91% of GnRH agonist-treated patients maintained cycle regularity versus only 41% of those of controls [38]. Vitek et al., on the other hand, found no benefit with GnRH agonist use for the preservation of ovarian function based on the results of four studies in breast cancer patients undergoing chemotherapy [39]. A recent review by Hickman et al. analyzed the results of the various meta-analyses on GnRH agonist use for ovarian protection during chemotherapy. 12 of 14 analyses found a beneficial effect of GnRH on ovarian failure rates. However, only three of the nine studies assessing pregnancy rates reported a favorable outcome with GnRH agonist use [31].

The issue whether GnRH agonist use is beneficial for ovarian protection among premenopausal women undergoing chemotherapy has not been settled yet. Most reports suggest a positive impact on maintenance of ovarian function and chance for pregnancy. Furthermore, the reduction of menstrual flow for those with suppressed hematologic parameters may be an added benefit. Upon proper counseling GnRH agonist could be considered for those who cannot benefit from the proven assisted reproductive technologies (embryo, oocyte cryopreservation) for fertility preservation.

8.3.5 Endometriosis

Endometriosis is diagnosed when endometrial glands and stroma can be found in extrauterine locations. It can be found in 5–10% of the general population and in up to 50% of infertile women. Pain and infertility are the two most common symptoms. Pain can be associated with menstruation (dysmenorrhea) or can manifest as chronic pelvic pain [40]. Symptomatic endometriosis often calls for treatment. This could involve surgery, excision or ablation of endometriotic lesions, or medical therapy [40].

Endometriosis is an estrogen-dependent disease; therefore, any medical therapy that suppresses estrogen levels or creates an androgen- or progesterone-dominant environment could prove to be beneficial. Medical therapy that inhibits folliculogenesis and results in hypoestrogenism typically improves endometriosis-related symptoms.

Prolonged GnRH agonist administration leads to hypogonadism with suppressed steroid hormone levels. The benefit of depot GnRH agonist alone or in combination with other drugs for the treatment of symptomatic endometriosis has been evaluated in several prospective or retrospective trials. A prospective randomized study found GnRH agonist or dienogest + estradiol valerate to be equally effective in improving quality of life postoperatively among women undergoing laparoscopy for chronic pelvic pain [41]. A retrospective study by Morelli et al. found significant improvement in chronic pelvic pain, reduced need for pain medication, and a reduction in loss of productivity among women with endometriosis or adenomyosis using GnRH agonist [42]. Another randomized controlled trial found similar efficacy of pain control with norethisterone acetate and GnRH agonist (both combined with aromatase inhibitor), but norethisterone acetate was better tolerated due to fewer side effects. Reduction in the size of endometriotic lesions was however greater with depot triptorelin [43]. Levonorgestrel intrauterine system was shown to similarly improve the overall endometriosis severity profile at 1, 3, and 6 months when compared to GnRH agonist. However, by the end of the first year of follow-up, compared to pretreatment baseline values, symptom improvement was only shown with GnRH agonist [44]. Several other studies have shown postoperative pain score improvement with GnRH agonist among women undergoing surgery for endometriosis [45, 46]. A 2014 Cochrane review reported GnRH agonist to be effective for the management of endometriosis-related pain [47].

Long-term GnRH agonist use is limited by the side effects related to hypoestrogenism (vasomotor and genitourinary symptoms) and by the adverse lipid and bone effects. Add-back therapy (norethindrone acetate, conjugated equine estrogen, norethindrone) has been recommended to reduce the impact of these side effects. Add-back therapy was not shown to compromise the benefits of GnRH [48].

Endometriosis is common among infertile women, and many of them will eventually require some form of assisted reproduction to achieve success. Pregnancy rates following IVF are lower in women with endometriosis according to the analysis by Barnhart et al. (OR, 0.56; 95% CI, 0.44–0.7) [49]. Medical therapy alone (GnRH, combined contraceptive pill, androgen, progestin) is not effective to manage infertility associated with endometriosis as all these therapies prevent ovulation and therefore the chance to conceive [50]. In addition there is no evidence that the use of GnRH agonist postoperatively to suppress lesions not removed during surgery is of benefit for infertile women [51]. A 2006 Cochrane review based on three trials however found that 3–6-month use of GnRH agonist prior to IVF improved clinical pregnancy rate (OR, 4.28; 95% CI, 2.00–9.15) and live birth rate (OR, 9.19; 95% CI, 1.08–78.22) [52].

8.3.6 Fibroids

Uterine fibroids are common benign, monoclonal tumors of the myometrium. They can be found in up to 70% of women and are associated with symptoms in about 25% of reproductive age women [53]. Symptoms are either associated with menstruation (menometrorrhagia, dysmenorrhea) or are related to size (pressure, fullness). Besides genetic factors, steroid hormones and growth factors (cytokines, chemokines, growth factors) have been implicated in their growth [54, 55]. The definitive therapy is surgery; myomectomy offers short- or long-term benefits, while hysterectomy offers definitive long-term treatment. There are cases when the patient desires to maintain her uterus, and there are cases when the patient is at such high surgical risk that alternative treatment options to surgery are needed. Radiologic interventions or hormonal treatments can be considered for such patients.

GnRH agonist use is associated with suppressed sex steroid levels, interferes with growth factor synthesis, and has direct apoptotic effects on leiomyoma cells and therefore could prove to be beneficial for the management of symptomatic fibroids [55]. Its use was shown to result in significant reduction in myoma size. Friedman et al. randomly assigned premenopausal women to depot leuprolide versus placebo for 6 months. While those in the placebo group experienced no change in the fibroid volume, in the GnRH agonist group, 40% decrease in fibroid volume was achieved. Three months after cessation of leuprolide, the myomas grew back to almost their pretreatment size [56]. Seracchioli et al. also reported a significant 26.5% reduction in myoma volume after 3 months of depot triptorelin in a placebo-controlled randomized trial [57]. GnRH agonist results in an about 30–50% reduction in fibroid and uterine volume, but the effect is temporary and upon discontinuation of therapy the fibroids regain their pretreatment size [58]. The long-term administration of GnRH agonists is limited by its side effects. To avoid adverse bone and metabolic effects, various add-back therapies were explored in combination with GnRH agonist. Raloxifene, progestins, estrogen, and estrogen-progestin combinations have been successfully used to block some of the adverse effects of long-term GnRH agonist use, but they also limit the benefits with GnRH agonist [55].

Due to the significant hypoestrogenic side effects and associated expenses, GnRH agonist does not offer a long-term solution in the management of symptomatic uterine fibroids. The short-term size reduction and the amenorrhea induced by GnRH agonist can be of clinical benefit though. Larger fibroids may require an abdominal surgical approach rather than the vaginal route and may require a vertical abdominal incision rather than a low transverse. Significant reduction in myoma size enables the surgeon to use an approach that is associated with faster postoperative recovery and improved long-term quality of life. Furthermore, a size reduction could be associated with shorter operating time and reduced blood loss and therefore less perioperative morbidity. Significant improvement in preoperative hemoglobin and hematocrit values and reduction in operative blood loss were shown both after laparoscopy and laparotomy following preoperative GnRH agonist treatment [59–61].

Uterine fibroids are common hormone-sensitive tumors that respond favorably to GnRH agonist therapy. The main benefit of such therapy is a reduction in fibroid related menometrorrhagia and therefore an improvement in hematologic parameters. Furthermore, the myoma size reduction enables the surgeon to use the vaginal route instead of the abdominal approach, reduces operating time and blood loss during surgery, and therefore is associated with reduced short-term and long-term morbidity.

8.3.7 ART

The introduction of GnRH agonists in the mid-1980s and subsequently GnRH antagonists into in vitro fertilization (IVF) leads to a revolutionary change in how IVF was practiced [62]. Up until their introduction, premature LH surge/ovulation was a major problem often leading to cycle cancellation. GnRH agonist can be administered as a daily injection or as a depot injection. Initially it induces a flare effect upon binding to the pituitary receptors and induces a transient FSH and LH surge. A continuous exposure to GnRH agonist results in receptor downregulation and desensitization after 5–7 days, and the inhibition of further LH release blocks the preovulatory LH rise. GnRH agonist, when started in the mid-luteal phase of the cycle preceding the stimulation for IVF, results in suppressed gonadotropin levels by the time the cycle ends and the stimulation is initiated. It is then continued throughout the stimulation at a reduced dose (luteal long stimulation). Alternatively it can be stopped as exogenous gonadotropin stimulation is about to get started (luteal stop protocol). For those patients who have irregular cycles, GnRH agonist can be started at the onset of the cycle.

In these cases one has to wait for the suppression to occur after the initial flare effect (follicular long). Alternatively, it can be started overlapping with contraceptive pills to prevent the initial flare effect.

For poor responders the initial gonadotropin flare is desired. Various flare protocols (short, ultrashort, microdose) are in use.

The introduction of GnRH antagonists into stimulation opened up further options for the management of the follicular phase of an IVF cycle. GnRH antagonists immediately inhibit the GnRH receptors, and therefore they can be started once the follicles reach a size when they are at risk for premature ovulation. According to the fixed protocol, it is started on day 6 of the stimulation regardless of follicle size. When the flexible protocol is followed, GnRH antagonist is started once the lead follicle reaches 13–14 mm in size and the estradiol level exceeds 300–500 pmol/l. Once started GnRH antagonist is administered daily up until the final trigger injection prior to oocyte collection. Alternatively a larger, "depot" dose of GnRH antagonist can be used that only has to be supplemented by smaller daily doses if the stimulation lasts for more than 4–5 days beyond the initial depot dose. GnRH antagonist use is considered patient friendly, as antagonist cycles are associated with 1–2 days shorter stimulation, fewer overall injections, and better cycle scheduling when combined with contraceptive pills prior to stimulation start. Unlike GnRH agonist its use is not associated with the hypoestrogenic side effects. Furthermore, the use of GnRH antagonist allows the use of GnRH agonist trigger prior to oocyte collection and can significantly reduce the risk of ovarian hyperstimulation syndrome (OHSS).

A recent Cochrane review compared the efficacy of the different GnRH agonist protocols. It found no difference in the ongoing pregnancy rates and live birth rates when the GnRH agonist long vs. agonist ultrashort, the luteal GnRH agonist long vs. follicular agonist long, or the agonist long vs. agonist stop protocols were compared [63]. GnRH agonist can be administered daily or as a depot injection. Both approaches are equally likely to result in live births. However, the depot injection seems to result in a deeper suppression as patients require more gonadotropins and the stimulation lasts significantly longer [64].

Premature LH rise can successfully be prevented by the administration of GnRH antagonists. Live birth rates in antagonist cycles are similar to live birth rates in GnRH agonist cycles (OR, 1.02; 95% CI, 0.85–1.23). The risk of OHSS is however significantly lower in GnRH antagonist cycles [65]. Using the GnRH antagonist protocol, the stimulations last for fewer days, less gonadotropin is required, peak estradiol level is lower, and the number of oocytes retrieved is fewer [66]. GnRH antagonist results in a quick and deep suppression of LH levels. The available data does not support the addition of LH or the increase of gonadotropin dose upon the start of antagonist [67].

The use of GnRH antagonist allows the use of either human chorionic gonadotropin or GnRH agonist as a trigger injection. GnRH agonist is effective for the induction oocyte maturation and retrieval of mature oocytes and is highly effective in preventing OHSS. It however results in inadequate luteal phase and if not supplemented properly leads to lower live birth rates [68]. With proper luteal support (either intensive luteal phase support with transdermal estradiol and IM progesterone, dual trigger with GnRH agonist and 1000 IU hCG or low dose, 1500 IU hCG on the day of retrieval), high, unaffected pregnancy rates can be maintained [69].

In hCG-induced cycles, luteal administration of GnRH agonist based on low overall quality of evidence was shown to improve live birth rates. This benefit however needs to be further studied [70].

Summary GnRH secreted by the hypothalamus plays a key role in the regulation of the reproductive axis. Its normal pulsatile secretion is required for the pituitary release of FSH and LH hormones that regulate ovarian follicular activity. An intact multilevel feedback mechanism is required for normal function. Any disruption of this finely tuned endocrine axis results in abnormal ovarian function.

GnRH analogues, agonists and antagonists, are now available and can be used to manage various clinical problems. GnRH analogues can be successfully used for the treatment of central precocious puberty, hormone-sensitive cancers, and various benign gynecologic conditions and play an important role in assisted reproduction. Their long-term use is not without side effects however; therefore future research has to focus on developing longer-acting formulas with proper add-back options that do not limit clinical efficacy but improve safety and allow long-term administration.

References

1. Krsmanovic LZ, Hu L, Leung PK, Feng H, Catt KJ. The hypothalamic GnRH pulse generator: multiple regulatory mechanisms. Trends Endocrinol Metab. 2009 Oct;20(8):402–8.
2. Knobil E. The neuroendocrine control of ovulation. Hum Reprod. 1988 May;3(4):469–72.
3. Petersen SL, Ottem EN, Carpenter CD. Direct and indirect regulation of gonadotropin-releasing hormone neurons by estradiol. Biol Reprod. 2003;69:1771–8.
4. Bakker J, Baum MJ. Neuroendocrine regulation of GnRH release in induced ovulators. Front Neuroendocrinol. 2000;21:220–62.
5. Gamba M, Pralong FP. Control of GnRH neuronal activity by metabolic factors: the role of leptin and insulin. Mol Cell Endocrinol. 2006 Jul 25;254-255:133–9.
6. Hu L, Gustofson RL, Feng H, Leung PK, Mores N, Krsmanovic LZ, et al. Converse regulatory functions of estrogen receptor-alpha and -beta subtypes expressed in hypothalamic gonadotropin-releasing hormone neurons. Mol Endocrinol. 2008 Oct;22(10):2250–9.
7. Chappell PE, Levine JE. Stimulation of gonadotropin-releasing hormone surges by estrogen. I. Role of hypothalamic progesterone receptors. Endocrinology. 2000 Apr;141(4):1477–85.
8. Schally AV, Kastin AJ. Stimulation and inhibition of fertility through hypothalamic agents. Drug Ther. 1971;1:29–32.

9. Ortmann O, Weiss JM, Diedrich K. Gonadotrophin-releasing hormone (GnRH) and GnRH agonists: mechanisms of action. Reprod Biomed Online. 2002;5(Suppl 1):1–7.
10. Li P, Li Y, Yang CL. Gonadotropin releasing hormone agonist treatment to increase final stature in children with precocious puberty. A meta-analysis. Medicine. 2014;93:1–8.
11. Heger S, Sippel WG, Partsch CJ. Gonadotropin-releasing hormone analogue treatmnt for precocious puberty. Twenty years of experience. Endocr Rev. 2005;8:94–125.
12. Carel JC, Roger M, Ispas S, Tondu F, Lahlou N, Blumberg J, et al. Final height after long-term treatment with triptorelin slow release for central precocious puberty: importance of statural growth after interruption of treatment. French study group of Decapeptyl in precocious puberty. J Clin Endocrinol Metab. 1999 Jun;84(6):1973–8.
13. Oostdijk W, Drop SL, Odink RJ, Hümmelink R, Partsch CJ, Sippell WG. Long-term results with a slow-release gonadotrophin-releasing hormone agonist in central precocious puberty. Dutch-German precocious puberty study group. Acta Paediatr Scand Suppl. 1991;372:39–45.
14. Lee PA, Klein K, Mauras N, Neely EK, Bloch CA, Larsen L, et al. Efficacy and safety of leuprolide acetate 3-month depot 11.25 milligrams or 30 milligrams for the treatment of central precocious puberty. J Clin Endocrinol Metab. 2012 May;97(5):1572–80.
15. https://cancerstatisticscenter.cancer.org/#/
16. Xu X, Chen X, Hu H, Dailey AB, Taylor BD. Current opinion on the role of testosterone in the development of prostate cancer: a dynamic model. BMC Cancer. 2015 Oct 26;15:806.
17. Shore ND, Abrahamsson PA, Anderson J, Crawford ED, Lange P. New considerations for ADT in advanced prostate cancer and the emerging role of GnRH antagonists. Prostate Cancer Prostatic Dis. 2013 Mar;16(1):7–15.
18. Sharifi N, Gulley JL, Dahut WL. An update on androgen deprivation therapy for prostate cancer. Endocr Relat Cancer. 2010 Oct 29;17(4):R305–15.
19. Vis AN, van der Sluis TM, Al-Itejawi HH, van Moorselaar RJ, Meuleman EJ. Risk of disease flare with LHRH agonist therapy in men with prostate cancer: myth or fact? Urol Oncol. 2015 Jan;33(1):7–15.
20. Tombal B, Miller K, Boccon-Gibod L, Schröder F, Shore N, Crawford ED, et al. Additional analysis of the secondary end point of biochemical recurrence rate in a phase 3 trial (CS21) comparing degarelix 80 mg versus leuprolide in prostate cancer patients segmented by baseline characteristics. Eur Urol. 2010 May;57(5):836–42.
21. Klotz L, Boccon-Gibod L, Shore ND, Andreou C, Persson BE, Cantor P, et al. The efficacy and safety of degarelix: a 12-month, comparative, randomized, open-label, parallel-group phase III study in patients with prostate cancer. BJU Int. 2008 Dec;102(11):1531–8.
22. https://www.cancer.org/research/cancer-facts-statistics/all-cancer-facts-figures/cancer-facts-figures-2017.html
23. Cleator SJ, Ahamed E, Coombes RC, Palmieri C. A 2009 update on the treatment of patients with hormone receptor-positive breast cancer. Clin Breast Cancer. 2009 Jun;9(Suppl 1):S6–S17.
24. Tan SH, Wolff AC. The role of ovarian ablation in the adjuvant therapy of breast cancer. Curr Oncol Rep. 2008 Jan;10(1):27–37.
25. Schmid P, Untch M, Wallwiener D, Kossé V, Bondar G, Vassiljev L, et al. TABLE-study (Takeda adjuvant breast cancer study with Leuprorelin acetate). Cyclophosphamide, methotrexate and fluorouracil (CMF) versus hormonal ablation with leuprorelin acetate as adjuvant treatment of node-positive, premenopausal breast cancer patients: preliminary results of the TABLE-study. Anticancer Res. 2002 Jul-Aug;22(4):2325–32.
26. von Minckwitz G, Graf E, Geberth M, Eiermann W, Jonat W, Conrad B, et al. CMF versus goserelin as adjuvant therapy for node-negative, hormone-receptor-positive breast cancer in premenopausal patients: a randomised trial (GABG trial IV-A-93). Eur J Cancer. 2006 Aug;42(12):1780–8.
27. Goel S, Sharma R, Hamilton A, Beith J. LHRH agonists for adjuvant therapy of early breast cancer in premenopausal women. Cochrane Database Syst Rev. 2009 Oct 7;4:CD004562.
28. Castiglione-Gertsch M. Adjuvant treatment of breast cancer: sequence and duration of hormonal therapy. Ann Oncol. 2006 Sep;17(Suppl 10):x51–3.
29. Gougeon A. Regulation of follicular ovarian development in primates: facts and hypothesis. Endocr Rev. 1996;17:121–55.
30. The Practice Committee of the American Society for Reproductive Medicine. Fertility preservation in patients undergoing gonadotoxic therapy or gonadectomy: a committee opinion. Fertil Steril. 2013;100:1214–23.
31. Hickman LC, Valentine LN, Falcone T. Preservation of gonadal function in women undergoing chemotherapy: a review of the potential role for gonadotropin-releasing hormone agonists. Am J Obstet Gynecol. 2016 Oct;215(4):415–22.
32. Lambertini M, Boni L, Michelotti A, Gamucci T, Scotto T, Gori S, et al. GIM study group. Ovarian suppression with Triptorelin during adjuvant breast cancer chemotherapy and long-term ovarian function, pregnancies, and disease-free survival: a randomized clinical trial. JAMA. 2015 Dec 22-29;314(24):2632–40.
33. Moore HC, Unger JM, Phillips KA, Boyle F, Hitre E, Porter D. Et al; POEMS/S0230 investigators. Goserelin for ovarian protection during breast-cancer adjuvant chemotherapy. N Engl J Med. 2015 Mar 5;372(10):923–32.
34. Elgindy EA, El-Haieg DO, Khorshid OM, Ismail EI, Abdelgawad M, Sallam HN, et al. Gonadatrophin suppression to prevent chemotherapy-induced ovarian damage: a randomized controlled trial. Obstet Gynecol. 2013 Jan;121(1):78–86.
35. Munster PN, Moore AP, Ismail-Khan R, Cox CE, Lacevic M, Gross-King M, et al. Randomized trial using gonadotropin-releasing hormone agonist triptorelin for the preservation of ovarian function during (neo)adjuvant chemotherapy for breast cancer. J Clin Oncol. 2012 Feb 10;30(5):533–8.
36. Gerber B, von Minckwitz G, Stehle H, Reimer T, Felberbaum R, Maass N, et al. German breast group investigators. Effect of luteinizing hormone-releasing hormone agonist on ovarian function after modern adjuvant breast cancer chemotherapy: the GBG 37 ZORO study. J Clin Oncol. 2011 Jun 10;29(17):2334–41.
37. Del Mastro L, Ceppi M, Poggio F, Bighin C, Peccatori F, Demeestere I, et al. Gonadotropin-releasing hormone analogues for the prevention of chemotherapy-induced premature ovarian failure in cancer women: systematic review and meta-analysis of randomized trials. Cancer Treat Rev. 2014 Jun;40(5):675–83.
38. Blumenfeld Z, Evron A. Preserving fertility when choosing chemotherapy regimens - the role of gonadotropin-releasing hormone agonists. Expert Opin Pharmacother. 2015 May;16(7):1009–20.
39. Vitek WS, Shayne M, Hoeger K, Han Y, Messing S, Fung C. Gonadotropin-releasing hormone agonists for the preservation of ovarian function among women with breast cancer who did not use tamoxifen after chemotherapy: a systematic review and meta-analysis. Fertil Steril. 2014 Sep;102(3):808–15.
40. Vercellini P, Viganò P, Somigliana E, Fedele L. Endometriosis: pathogenesis and treatment. Nat Rev Endocrinol. 2014 May;10(5):261–75.
41. Granese R, Perino A, Calagna G, Saitta S, De Franciscis P, Colacurci N, et al. Gonadotrophin-releasing hormone analogue or dienogest plus estradiol valerate to prevent pain recurrence after laparoscopic surgery for endometriosis: a multi-center randomized trial. Acta Obstet Gynecol Scand. 2015 Jun;94(6):637–45.
42. Morelli M, Rocca ML, Venturella R, Mocciaro R, Zullo F. Improvement in chronic pelvic pain after gonadotropin releasing

hormone analogue (GnRH-a) administration in premenopausal women suffering from adenomyosis or endometriosis: a retrospective study. Gynecol Endocrinol. 2013 Apr;29(4):305–8.
43. Ferrero S, Venturini PL, Gillott DJ, Remorgida V. Letrozole and norethisterone acetate versus letrozole and triptorelin in the treatment of endometriosis related pain symptoms: a randomized controlled trial. Reprod Biol Endocrinol. 2011 Jun 21;9:88.
44. Bayoglu Tekin Y, Dilbaz B, Altinbas SK, Dilbaz S. Postoperative medical treatment of chronic pelvic pain related to severe endometriosis: levonorgestrel-releasing intrauterine system versus gonadotropin-releasing hormone analogue. Fertil Steril. 2011 Feb;95(2):492–6.
45. Sesti F, Capozzolo T, Pietropolli A, Marziali M, Bollea MR, Piccione E. Recurrence rate of endometrioma after laparoscopic cystectomy: a comparative randomized trial between post-operative hormonal suppression treatment or dietary therapy vs. placebo. Eur J Obstet Gynecol Reprod Biol. 2009 Nov;147(1):72–7.
46. Bergqvist A, Bergh T, Hogström L, Mattsson S, Nordenskjöld F, Rasmussen C. Effects of triptorelin versus placebo on the symptoms of endometriosis. Fertil Steril. 1998 Apr;69(4):702–8.
47. Brown J, Farquhar C. Endometriosis: an overview of Cochrane reviews. Cochrane Database Syst Rev. 2014 Mar 10;3:CD009590.
48. Zupi E, Marconi D, Sbracia M, Zullo F, De Vivo B, Exacustos C, et al. Add-back therapy in the treatment of endometriosis-associated pain. Fertil Steril. 2004 Nov;82(5):1303–8.
49. Barnhart K, Dunsmoor-Su R, Coutifaris C. Effect of endometriosis on in vitro fertilization. Fertil Steril. 2002 Jun;77(6):1148–55.
50. Hughes E, Brown J, Collins JJ, Farquhar C, Fedorkow DM, Vandekerckhove P. Ovulation suppression for endometriosis. Cochrane Database Syst Rev. 2007 Jul 18;3:CD000155.
51. The Practice Committee of the American Society for Reproductive Medicine. Endometriosis and infertility: a committee opinion. Fertil Fteril. 2012;98:591–8.
52. Sallam HN, Garcia-Velasco JA, Dias S, Arici A. Long-term pituitary down-regulation before in vitro fertilization (IVF) for women with endometriosis. Cochrane Database Syst Rev. 2006 Jan 25;1:CD004635.
53. Bulun SE. Uterine fibroids. N Engl J Med. 2013 Oct 3;369(14):1344–55.
54. Islam MS, Protic O, Giannubilo SR, Toti P, Tranquilli AL, Petraglia F, et al. Uterine leiomyoma: available medical treatments and new possible therapeutic options. J Clin Endocrinol Metab. 2013 Mar;98(3):921–34.
55. Chabbert-Buffet N, Esber N, Bouchard P. Fibroid growth and medical options for treatment. Fertil Steril. 2014 Sep;102(3):630–9.
56. Friedman AJ, Harrison-Atlas D, Barbieri RL, Benacerraf B, Gleason R, Schiff I. A randomized, placebo-controlled, double-blind study evaluating the efficacy of leuprolide acetate depot in the treatment of uterine leiomyomata. Fertil Steril. 1989 Feb;51(2):251–6.
57. Seracchioli R, Venturoli S, Colombo FM, Bagnoli A, Vianello F, Govoni F, et al. GnRH agonist treatment before total laparoscopic hysterectomy for large uteri. J Am Assoc Gynecol Laparosc. 2003 Aug;10(3):316–9.
58. Crosignani PG, Vercellini P, Meschìa M, Oldani S, Bramante T. GnRH agonists before surgery for uterine leiomyomas. A review. J Reprod Med. 1996 Jun;41(6):415–21.
59. Stovall TG, Muneyyirci-Delale O, Summitt RL Jr, Scialli AR. GnRH agonist and iron versus placebo and iron in the anemic patient before surgery for leiomyomas: a randomized controlled trial. Leuprolide acetate study group. Obstet Gynecol. 1995 Jul;86(1):65–71.
60. Vercellini P, Trespìdi L, Zaina B, Vicentini S, Stellato G, Crosignani PG. Gonadotropin-releasing hormone agonist treatment before abdominal myomectomy: a controlled trial. Fertil Steril. 2003 Jun;79(6):1390–5.
61. Chen I, Motan T, Kiddoo D. Gonadotropin-releasing hormone agonist in laparoscopic myomectomy: systematic review and meta-analysis of randomized controlled trials. J Minim Invasive Gynecol. 2011 May-Jun;18(3):303–9.
62. de Ziegler D, Cedars MI, Randle D, Lu JK, Judd HL, Meldrum DR. Suppression of the ovary using a gonadotropin releasing-hormone agonist prior to stimulation for oocyte retrieval. Fertil Steril. 1987 Nov;48(5):807–10.
63. Siristatidis CS, Gibreel A, Basios G, Maheshwari A, Bhattacharya S. Gonadotrophin-releasing hormone agonist protocols for pituitary suppression in assisted reproduction. Cochrane Database Syst Rev. 2015 Nov 9;11:CD006919.
64. Albuquerque LE, Tso LO, Saconato H, Albuquerque MC, Macedo CR. Depot versus daily administration of gonadotrophin-releasing hormone agonist protocols for pituitary down regulation in assisted reproduction cycles. Cochrane Database Syst Rev. 2013 Jan 31;1:CD002808.
65. Al-Inany HG, Youssef MA, Ayeleke RO, Brown J, Lam WS, Broekmans FJ. Gonadotrophin-releasing hormone antagonists for assisted reproductive technology. Cochrane Database Syst Rev. 2016 Apr 29;4:CD001750.
66. Xiao JS, Su CM, Zeng XT. Comparisons of GnRH antagonist versus GnRH agonist protocol in supposed normal ovarian responders undergoing IVF: a systematic review and meta-analysis. PLoS One. 2014 Sep 12;9(9):e106854.
67. Tarlatzis BC, Fauser BC, Kolibianakis EM, Diedrich K, Rombauts L, Devroey P. GnRH antagonists in ovarian stimulation for IVF. Hum Reprod Update. 2006 Jul-Aug;12(4):333–40.
68. Youssef MA, Van der Veen F, Al-Inany HG, Mochtar MH, Griesinger G, Nagi Mohesen M, et al. Gonadotropin-releasing hormone agonist versus HCG for oocyte triggering in antagonist-assisted reproductive technology. Cochrane Database Syst Rev. 2014 Oct 31;10:CD008046.
69. Engmann L, Benadiva C, Humaidan P. GnRH agonist trigger for the induction of oocyte maturation in GnRH antagonist IVF cycles: a SWOT analysis. Reprod Biomed Online. 2016 Mar;32(3): 274–85.
70. Martins WP, Ferriani RA, Navarro PA, Nastri CO. GnRH agonist during luteal phase in women undergoing assisted reproductive techniques: systematic review and meta-analysis of randomized controlled trials. Ultrasound Obstet Gynecol. 2016 Feb;47(2):144–51.

GnRH Agonist Protocols

9

Megan Schneiderman and Michael H. Dahan

In vitro fertilization, commonly referred to as IVF, is a procedure in which infertility of varied etiologies is overcome. The current standard of care requires ovaries to be sufficiently stimulated to allow the collection of many oocytes, which are then fertilized in the laboratory and eventually transferred to a receptive uterine cavity. One difficulty to be overcome with both natural cycle IVF or stimulated cycles is ovulation prior to oocyte collection. There are several protocols to prevent this complication. These protocols achieve pituitary downregulation using gonadotropin-releasing hormone (GnRH) agonists or GnRH antagonists to prevent an undesired spontaneous luteinizing hormone (LH) surge. The three most commonly used protocols are GnRH agonist protocols (long protocol), GnRH agonist flare protocols (microdose or standard-dose flare), and the GnRH antagonist protocols (short protocol). In this chapter, we will address the GnRH agonist protocols for IVF.

9.1 GnRH Agonists

GnRH is a decapeptide produced in the hypothalamus. Transported via the portal circulation, GnRH stimulates gonadotrophs in the anterior pituitary gland to release two gonadotropins: luteinizing hormone (LH) and follicle-stimulating hormone (FSH). LH and FSH then act at the level of the ovaries to regulate both the production of sex steroids and folliculogenesis. LH stimulates the theca cells to produce androgens. FSH stimulates the granulosa cells to support follicular growth, resulting in the production of estrogens. The androgens "feed" the granulosa cells and act as substrate to be aromatized to estrogens, particularly estradiol. FSH initially upregulates its own receptor and by so doing increases granulosa cell stimulation. As estradiol levels increase and the follicle enlarges, the FSH receptor is then downregulated, while LH receptor expression increases. Eventually, the LH surge will be induced by high estradiol levels, which positively feed back on the hypothalamic pituitary axis, prompting follicular ovulation.

Physiologically, GnRH is secreted in a pulsatile manner, which stimulates the timed release of gonadotropins and coordination of follicle development and ovulation. Furthermore, it is known that stimulation of the gonadotrophs by exogenous GnRH agonists in a continuous or nonpulsatile manner eventually results in desensitization of the pituitary gonadotrophs to GnRH. This is achieved by internalization of the FSH receptors in response to a prolonged non-pulsatile GnRH activity [1]. This effect of continuous GnRH stimulation inducing pituitary suppression is the hallmark of ovarian stimulation protocols using GnRH agonists. These were the first nonnatural IVF cycles performed preventing spontaneous ovulation.

GnRH agonist analogues are modifications of the natural decapeptide GnRH, with agonistic effects on the GnRH receptor and subsequent downregulation of the receptors. Commercially available GnRH agonists include triptorelin acetate, nafarelin acetate, buserelin acetate, leuprolide acetate, and goserelin acetate (Table 9.1). The pituitary response to exogenous GnRH agonist administration is biphasic.

Table 9.1 Available synthetic GnRH agonists

Generic name	Brand name	Route
Triptorelin acetate	Decapeptil	Sc IM
Nafarelin acetate	Synarel	Inhalation (nasal)
Buserelin acetate	Suprefact	Sc, inhalation (nasal)
Leuprolide acetate	Lupron Lupron depot	Sc IM depot
Goserelin acetate	Zoladex	Sc implant
Histrelin	Supprelin	Sc implant

Sc subcutaneous, *IM* intramuscular

M. Schneiderman
Department of Obstetrics and Gynecology, McGill University, Quebec, Canada

M. H. Dahan (✉)
Division of Reproductive Endocrinology and Infertility, Department of Obstetrics and Gynecology, McGill University, Quebec, Canada

G. N. Allahbadia et al. (eds.), *Textbook of Assisted Reproduction*, https://doi.org/10.1007/978-981-15-2377-9_9

Firstly, there is an initial flare effect within the first 48 hours of administration, whereby the agonist effect leads to an upregulation of GnRH receptors and an increase in LH and FSH secretion from the gonadotrophs. This flare effect can last for 5 to 14 days. After this time, with continued agonist administration, there is both downregulation and desensitization of GnRH receptors in the anterior pituitary. Ultimately, this leads to reduced gonadotropin production and secretion by the pituitary, as well as decreased responsiveness of the pituitary to GnRH [2, 3].

GnRH agonists were introduced in the 1980s, after the GnRH decapeptide was first isolated in 1971 [4]. Since this time, the approach to ovarian stimulation for IVF has changed significantly as there existed a means to prevent premature ovulation during IVF cycles [5]. Without downregulation of endogenous LH secretion, up to 15–30% of cycles used to be cancelled due to premature ovulation [6]. Using GnRH agonists, the rate of cycle cancellation due to premature ovulation has been reduced to fewer than 2% of treatment cycles [7]. The use of GnRH agonists is based on the known responses of gonadotrophs to continuous GnRH exposure as described above. Through receptor downregulation and desensitization, GnRH agonist treatment biochemically suppresses endogenous gonadotropin secretion and thereby prevents surges in LH from disrupting exogenous ovarian stimulation and causing premature ovulation [8]. This downregulation likely continues for at least 7 days after stopping the GnRH analogue in a typical IVF cycle.

The advantages of GnRH agonist cycles go beyond the prevention of premature ovulation and subsequent cycle cancellation. By preventing the LH surge, patients can be stimulated for longer times to produce a greater number of mature follicles, particularly if a breakaway large follicle is present which would have otherwise caused a spontaneous ovulation prior to the maturation of a lagging follicular cohort. An example of this scenario would be a follicle of 18 mm diameter and ten 12 mm follicles. The 18 mm follicle can be pushed into postmaturity (greater than 21 mm diameter) to allow the 12 mm follicles to grow. Such stimulation ultimately allows the recruitment of a larger number of mature oocytes. Mature oocytes most often occur in follicles of 14–15 mm mean diameters.

Additionally, suppressing endogenous gonadotropin secretion provides an important advantage of scheduling flexibility. By changing the duration of GnRH agonist suppression, prior to the commencement of gonadotropin stimulation, cycles can easily be coordinated for oocyte donation or collections on days the patient is available. Once the gonadotropins have been started, data suggests that retrieving oocytes 1 day earlier or 1 day later than ideal does not change the live birth outcomes, allowing further timing of collections as needed [9].

Often combined oral contraceptives (COCs) are prescribed in GnRH agonist cycles (details described below). The COCs traditionally used contain 30 or 35 micrograms of ethinyl estradiol. It is possible that pills with lower ethinyl estradiol doses can be used without affecting outcomes; however, data related to lower doses of ethinyl estradiol COCs are lacking in IVF cycles. The role of different progestins prior to IVF in COCs is poorly understood. Pre-treatment with COCs firstly provides flexibility in the start time of the cycle and increased convenience for both the patient and fertility center. Secondly, after pre-treatment with COCs, when the protocol is begun, a more uniform cohort of follicles is synchronized at the same developmental stage. Therefore, with gonadotropin stimulation more follicles may reach the same level of maturity close to the same time. Additionally, patients are less likely to develop functional ovarian cysts at the start of GnRH agonist treatment [10]. Taken together, these benefits overall lead to a reduction in cycle cancellation rates and increased convenience in cycle planning. COCs are usually started on a spontaneous or induced menstrual cycle days 1 to 5. They are taken for at least 15 days prior to commencement of the GnRH agonist to prevent cyst development via the GnRH agonist initial flare effect. The GnRH agonist is then overlapped with the COCs for a further 5 days, after which the COCs should be discontinued. Beyond these minimums for scheduling convenience, the COCs duration can be extended. However, use of more than 30 days of COCs can suppress the ovarian response to stimulation, increasing the required dose of gonadotropins and overall reducing the number of follicles ultimately recruited. At least one study evaluated the use of longer duration COC use in women at risk of ovarian hyperstimulation syndrome (OHSS) due to polycystic ovary syndrome. The risk of OHSS was found to be decreased in these patients with 25 to 45 days of COCs [3, 4].

The principal disadvantage to GnRH agonist cycles is the occasionally observed blunted response to exogenous gonadotropins and resulting increase in cost and duration of gonadotropin treatment required to achieve adequate ovarian stimulation (compared to no medications to block GnRH effects). Although at an increased cost, numerous studies have shown that pregnancy and live birth rates were significantly higher when both GnRH agonists and gonadotropins were used, compared to gonadotropins alone [11, 12]. The initial flare-up effect observed after initiating treatment may be another undesired side effect of treatment, which alternatively is taken advantage of in the "flare" protocol as will be explained subsequently.

It has been long established that some patients will form functional ovarian cysts during GnRH agonist treatment. The exact mechanism of cyst formation remains unknown; however, the initial flare effect of GnRH agonists may be contributory [13, 14]. Functional cysts may negatively affect follicular induction in different ways. They may prolong the duration of pituitary suppression required prior to beginning gonadotropin stimulation. The steroids (mainly estradiol and less likely progesterone) produced by functional cysts may negatively impact developing follicles and endometrial receptivity. Finally, by a pressure effect, they may prevent surrounding ovarian tissue and follicles from reaching their growth potential during stimulation. This occurs particularly if the cyst is greater than 1.5 cm in mean diameter or if the serum estradiol level is above 260 pmol/L [15]. Of note, the literature does not support cyst aspiration prior to beginning stimulation, as it has not been found to improve outcomes [14, 16].

Other disadvantages stem from the ovarian suppression induced by the GnRH agonists. Associated with the prolonged suppression, there may be undesired menopausal side effects due to the induced hypoestrogenic state. Furthermore, after agonist cycle completion, pituitary gonadotropin secretion has been found to remain impaired for some time, and luteal phase support with progesterone supplementation is required to maintain a pregnancy after embryo transfer [17]. It should be acknowledged that follicle aspiration also compromises progesterone production by the follicle by disrupting the cells in the follicle, which convert into the corpus luteum. Although many centers also supplement estradiol in the luteal phase, in randomized placebo-controlled studies, this supplementation has failed to improve outcomes [18]. While the benefits of estradiol supplementation remain controversial, progesterone supplementation, either vaginal or intramuscular, does improve results [19]. Lastly a subset of patients complain of headaches while taking the GnRH agonist. This can be alleviated to switching the patient to a GnRH antagonist cycle.

Lastly, the use of GnRH agonist for ovarian suppression increases the risk of developing ovarian hyperstimulation syndrome (OHSS), compared to GnRH antagonist cycles. Since the introduction of GnRH agonists to prevent the spontaneous LH surge in IVF cycles, the incidence of severe OHSS was reported to have increased sixfold [20]. While a GnRH agonist protocol results in the stimulation of more follicles, higher E2 levels, and the subsequent development of more corpus lutea that occurs in a natural cycle, understandably these factors increase the risk of OHSS [21–23]. Although most studies were not designed specifically to assess the risk of OHSS using different protocols, one more recent study demonstrated a higher risk of OHSS among already high-risk patients with the GnRH agonist, compared to antagonist protocol [24].

Considering the numerous advantages, the benefits of suppression of endogenous gonadotropin secretion, prevention of premature ovulation, recruitment of greater number of mature oocytes, fewer cancelled cycles, and most importantly higher pregnancy rates, when compared to unstimulated IVF cycles, GnRH agonist protocols are an excellent choice in an appropriately selected patient population. A recent randomized study comparing the long GnRH agonist cycle, the GnRH agonist microdose flare, and the antagonist cycle in poor responders found poorer pregnancy outcomes with the microdose flare [25]. The study was powered to detect differences in the number of oocytes collected and found that the long protocol collected on average two more oocytes than did the antagonist cycle. Therefore, ideal subjects for use of the GnRH agonist cycles include average-to-low responders and patients with decreased reserve or advanced maternal age. High responders should be treated with GnRH antagonist cycles to decrease the risk of ovarian hyperstimulation syndrome.

9.2 GnRH Agonist Protocols

There are presently two widely used IVF stimulation regimens with GnRH agonists, which differ in the duration of the GnRH agonist treatment:

(i) GnRH agonist gonadotropin stimulation, the "long" protocol.
(ii) GnRH agonist "flare" also known with modification as the "microdose flare" gonadotropin stimulation protocol.

Conceptually, the protocols are similar in that they take advantage of the suppression of endogenous gonadotropin secretion provided by the GnRH agonist to prevent a spontaneous LH surge (Table 9.1). Once suppressed, exogenous gonadotropins (Table 9.2) are provided until adequate fol-

Table 9.2 Gonadotropin preparations for ovarian stimulation

Generic name	Brand name	LH activity	FSH activity	HCG activity	Dosing	Route
Follitropin beta (recombinant FSH)	Follistim (USA) Puregon (CANADA)	–	+	–	75–300 IU (maximum 300 IU daily)	Sc
Follitropin alpha (recombinant FSH)	Gonal-F	–	+	–	75–300 IU (maximum 300 IU daily)	Sc
Urinary products (hMG) (uses hCG mimic LH activity)	Menopur	Minimal	+	+	75–300 IU (maximum 300 IU daily)	Sc
	Repronex	+	+	+		
	Pergonal	+	+	+		
	Humegon	+	+	+		
Lutropin alpha (recombinant LH)	Luveris	+	–	–	75 U–150 daily or FSH:LH ratio 2:1 to 3:1	Sc

[a]hCG: human chorionic gonadotropin
[a]hMG: human menopausal gonadotropins

licular stimulation is achieved. Finally, ovulation is triggered (Table 9.3), and oocytes are retrieved [26]. Collected oocytes can then be fertilized or frozen and ultimately transferred during the same cycle or at a later time.

Ideal dosing regimens for the available GnRH agonists in the different protocols have not been established, and many dose-finding studies examine different regimens. Dosing options are quite broad. We provide a sample-dosing regimen for different GnRH agonists (Table 9.4).

Similarly, there is no ideal gonadotropin dose that applies uniformly to all patients. Rather, the ideal dose is the lowest dose which achieves adequate stimulation, defined as optimal number of follicles developing, oocytes collected, highest live birth rates, and lowest risk of hyperstimulation and subsequent cycle cancellation. Maximum dosage used is controversial with some centers using 450 IU or even 600 IU per day. However, randomized studies suggest no benefit to doses above 300 IU daily [27–29], and the 2013 National Institute for Health and Care Excellence (NICE) guidelines specifically recommend not exceeding 450 IU. In most cases lowest dose used is 100–150 IU daily. In patients weighing more than 170lbs or 77Kg, an additional 75 IU daily should be considered. The ratio of FSH to LH activity should be 2:1 to 3:1 to prevent premature increases in progesterone levels [27] and is independent of patient diagnosis (Table 9.2).

Table 9.4 provides dosing of different GnRH agonists for the long and flair protocols. This is but a partial guide for the uninformed reader. Many other doses have been used in other publications which make an exhaustive list impossible to generate.

Table 9.3 Triggers for ovulation

Generic name	Brand name	Dosing	Route
Recombinant hCG	Ovidrel	250mcg	Sc
Urinary hCG	–	5000–10,000 units	Sc

Table 9.4 Typical dosing of most commonly used GnRH agonists in GnRHa protocols

	Long protocol	Flare protocol	Microdose flare protocol
Nafarelin (Synarel)	100 μg q8h *or* 200–400 μg bid	400 μg twice a day	200 μg twice a day
Buserelin (Suprefact)	*Standard regimen* 0.5 mg sc qd * Reduced dose when GN begun: 0.2 mg sc qd *Low-dose alternative* 0.5 mg sc qd * Reduced dose when GN begun: 0.05 mg sc bid Alterative dosing 0.25 mg qd–1.2 mg qd	0.5 mg sc qd * Reduced dose when GN begun: 0.2 mg sc qd	0.05 mg sc bid
Leuprolide (Lupron)	0.5 mg qd 1.0 (or 0.5) mg qd decrease to 0.5 mg (or 0.25) qd after desensitization 0.04 mg qd	0.0005 mg	40 ug daily
Triptorelin (Decapeptyl)	0.1 mg qd–1 mg qd 3.75 mg qd	0.04–0.05 mg qd 1 mg qd	100 ug daily

N.B. Similar to gonadotropin therapy, studies have yet to identify an "ideal" dose, and different centers/studies use different dosages. Common dosage ranges are included (and not limited to those) in this table.
From Kolibianakis EM, Collins J, Tarlatzis BC, Devroey P, Diedrich K, and Griesinger G. Among patients treated for IVF with gonadotrophins and GnRH analogues, is the probability of live birth dependent on the type of analogue used? A systematic review and meta-analysis. *Hum Reprod Update.* 2006;12 [6]:651–671., with permission.

9.2.1 GnRH Agonist Downregulation Gonadotropin Stimulation: The "Long" Protocol

The general principle of the long protocol is that GnRH agonists are used for varied durations to achieve full suppression of ovarian activity, after which exogenous gonadotropin therapy is initiated to stimulate follicular development. GnRH agonists are continued during gonadotropin stimulation. Response to gonadotropins is monitored, and dosage can be tailored to the patient in a step-up or step-down fashion. Once sufficiently stimulated (with enough follicles of large enough size), oocyte maturation and ovulation is triggered, and oocyte retrieval is scheduled shortly thereafter (Fig. 9.1). If a fresh cycle was planned, fertilization and subsequent transfer with luteal phase support are performed. Otherwise, oocytes or embryos can be frozen and transferred at a later date. In most cases the GnRH agonist is discontinued on the day of hCG triggering for collection. This protocol may be preferred in women with endometriosis due to the degree of endometriosis implants suppression obtained.

Leuprolide acetate, buserelin acetate, and triptorelin acetate are the most commonly used GnRH agonists in IVF cycles. Studies to date have shown no significant difference in pregnancy rates with one of the agonists or dosage regimens compared to others [28, 30]. In the USA, Leuprolide acetate is most commonly used (e.g., 0.5–1.0 mg sc daily), whereas in Europe and elsewhere, buserelin (e.g., 0.1 mg sc or intranasal spray daily) and triptorelin (e.g., 0.1 mg sc daily) are more popular. Depot leuprolide, the long-acting GnRH agonist given in the form of monthly (or longer) injections, can also be used. There is no evidence of inferiority of long-acting formulations compared to daily dosing. However when using long-acting agonists, higher doses of gonadotropins have found to be required over longer dura-

CD1: Day 1 Menstruation. **Begin COC**	**COC**	**COC**	**COC**	**COC**	**COC**	**COC**
COC	**COC**	**COC**	**COC**	**COC**	**COC**	**COC**
COC Begin GnRHa	**COC GnRHa**	**COC GnRHa**	**COC GnRHa**	**COC GnRHa**	**GnRHa**	**GnRHa**
GnRHa ** bleeding?*	**GnRHa** ** bleeding?*	**GnRHa**	**GnRHa**	**GnRHa**	**GnRHa**	**GnRHa**
*Baseline US **GnRHa (reduced dose) GN**	**GnRHa (reduced dose) GN**	**GnRHa (reduced dose) GN**	**GnRHa (reduced dose) GN**	**GnRHa (reduced dose) GN**	**GnRHa (reduced dose) GN**	**GnRHa (reduced dose) GN**
GnRHa (reduced dose) GN	*Monitoring US & estradiol **GnRHa (reduced dose) ?? GN** * Adequate stim: NO GN *incomplete stim: continue GN +/-dose adjustment	* Adequate stim: **hCG** *Incomplete stim: **GnRHa (reduced dose) GN** *repeat US & estradiol q1-3days	* Adequate stim: ---- *Incomplete stim: **GnRHa (reduced dose) GN** *repeat US & estradiol q1-3days	* Adequate stim: Collection ***Luteal phase support (progesterone +/- estrogen)** if fresh ET planned, start after collection		
* Adequate stim: Transfer						

Fig. 9.1 Sample GnRH agonist downregulation gonadotropin stimulation, "long" protocol. This figure demonstrates a sample long GnRH agonist protocol. *COC* combined oral contraceptive, *GnRHa* GnRH agonist, *GN* gonadotropin(s) stimulation, *US* transvaginal ultrasound, *ET* embryo transfer. Still the first monitoring remains too far out; place it on day 6 of stim. Of note: cycle day 1 may be induced by progesterone and/or estrogen compounds or natural cycle. COC continued for 15 days minimum before starting the GnRH agonist. GnRH agonist should be started 5–7 days prior to stopping COC. Baseline US to confirm adequate downregulation – i.e., no cysts and thin endometrium. Mean desensitization time with agonist in the long protocol is approximately 3 weeks. Duration and initiation of GnRHa before gonadotropin stimulation varies widely. GnRH agonist dose is reduced when gonadotropin therapy begins. Typical protocol: e.g., buserelin 0.5 ml qd → 0.2 ml qd. Lower-dose GnRHa protocol: e.g., Burserelin 0.5 ml qd → 0.05 ml bid. First US done after 5–7 days of stimulation. Fist estradiol level done 3–5 days after commencing stimulation. Monitoring with US and estradiol levels continues every 1–3 days, depending on follicular growth and estradiol levels. Once adequate stimulation is achieved, hCG trigger is given. Collection is planned on average 36 h later. Embryos are then transferred on days 3–5 or frozen

tions in order to achieve similar follicular development compared to daily dosing [31]. To date, data related to the clinical use of depot leuprolide acetate and other long-acting agonists in IVF cycles is sparse.

In women with regular cycles, treatment can be started in the mid-luteal phase determined as 5 days after a spontaneous LH surge [32, 33]. Such a start will result in functional cysts in about 30% of women. Another option for starting of the GnRH agonist is 5 to 7 days prior to stopping combined oral contraceptives (COCs). Starting GnRH treatment while on COCs minimizes the initial flare effect, thereby decreasing the likelihood of the flare causing a wave of follicular development prior to exogenous gonadotropin stimulation [32, 33]. Compared to starting in the luteal phase, starting the GnRH agonist in the follicular phase results in a higher numbers of retrieved oocytes in good responders [34].

Downregulation should be confirmed prior to beginning of gonadotropin stimulation, by the absence of ovarian cysts or follicles greater than 10 mm. As described earlier, evidence is contradictory whether the presence of ovarian cysts significantly reduces pregnancy outcomes. However, there is a risk that patients with functional cysts may be less likely to successfully become pregnant [35].

Once downregulation is accomplished and menses have commenced, gonadotropin treatment is initiated. *Importantly, GnRH agonist treatment is continued during gonadotropin stimulation to prevent premature ovulation.* GnRH agonists can either be continued at the same (e.g., leuprolide acetate 1.0 mg daily) or lower dose (e.g., leuprolide acetate 0.5 mg daily) (of note: patients with PCOS could maintain the full dose of agonist possibly decreasing risk of OHSS). Gonadotropin treatment is begun at doses from 75 to 300 units daily as a subcutaneous injection, which can then be increased (step-up dosing) or decreased (step-down dosing) depending on ovarian response. Starting dose is prescribed based on the patients age, weight, ovarian reserve, and, if available, responses in previous cycles.

Gonadotropins with simultaneous LH and FSH activity (hMG) or only FSH activity (purified urinary FSH (uFSH) or recombinant FSH (rFSH)) can be used (Table 9.4). Initially, stimulation was done with menotropins (human menopausal gonadotropins, hMG), purified extracts from urine of menopausal women, which had both LH and FSH activity. It was subsequently learned that the minimal amounts of endogenous LH that are produced in downregulated patients might be sufficient for normal ovarian steroidogenesis and follicular development. Therefore, additional supplementation of LH may not be necessary [36] unless the patient had hypothalamic amenorrhea. Thereafter, there was a shift in practice toward stimulating with highly purified or recombinant FSH. A number of studies comparing pregnancy and other outcomes of downregulated IVF cycles with different types of gonadotropin stimulation have been published. Results were contradictory, either favoring hMG or only FSH stimulation. Subsequently, the first meta-analysis comparing the effectiveness of hMG vs. recombinant FSH in GnRH agonist cycles was performed. In that meta-analysis they identified that hMG resulted in significantly more clinical pregnancies, but not necessarily ongoing pregnancy or live birth rates, compared to FSH alone [37]. In a more recent systematic review including recent trials, urinary hMG was found to have a 4% increase in live birth rate compared with rFSH in GnRH agonist long protocols [38]. Taken into clinical context, there presently is not strong evidence to support to the superiority of one preparation of gonadotropins over another. Special consideration should be made in certain circumstances, including ovulation induction in patients with hypogonadotropic amenorrhea and PCOS. In the former, without endogenous LH secretion, gonadotropins with LH activity must be used to support follicular development. In the latter group, endogenous LH levels despite GnRH agonist suppression are likely high enough to allow for stimulation with FSH preparations alone.

Most women will require 7–12 days of stimulation, during which response to gonadotropins is monitored via serum estradiol levels and follicle size and count by transvaginal ultrasound (TVUS). Typically, serum estradiol is first assessed after 3 to 5 days of gonadotropin stimulation, to allow for a dose increase if stimulation is inadequate. From there on, patients are monitored with TVUS ± estradiol, every 1–3 days, and gonadotropin doses are adjusted accordingly. Stimulation is continued until there are at least two to three follicles greater than 17 mm in size and several other follicles 14–16 mm in size. Ideally, the retrieval of at least ten oocytes will maximize the cumulative pregnancy rates when frozen embryo transfers are considered as well [39].

Once gonadotropin stimulation is determined to be complete in that there are a sufficient number of mature follicles, gonadotropin stimulation is stopped. Either recombinant or urinary hCG is administered the next day (rhCG 250 mcg sc or uhCG 5000–10,000 units sc), along with the last dose of the GnRH agonist. Both recombinant and urinary forms of hCG are available (Table 9.2), and there is no evidence of superiority of either preparation [40]. The hCG trigger acts to mimic the physiologic LH surge and initiates the ovulatory cascade. Subjects at risk for OHSS 2500 or 3300 IU of hCG can be considered to trigger for the oocyte collection without affecting success rates [41, 42]. Transvaginal ultrasound-guided oocyte retrieval is planned for 36 h (ideally ranging from 32 to 38 h) after hCG administration. If a fresh embryo transfer is planned for 2 to 5 days after oocyte pickup, luteal phase progesterone supplementation, either vaginal or intramuscular, is provided to support the endometrium. If oocyte or embryo freezing is planned, the cycle is considered complete at this time.

The cohort of patients who recruit significantly larger numbers of follicles and have higher estradiol levels are referred to as "high responders." With continued stimulation and ovulation induction, these patients are at increased risk of developing OHSS. Depending on the patient's clinical condition, different options exist to manage the cycle and reduce the risk of OHSS. For patients who are unwell or at significant risk of developing OHSS, cycle cancellation is the safest option. The cycle is cancelled by withholding the hCG trigger and withdrawing all ovarian stimulation. In future cycles, consideration can be given to stimulation with lower doses of gonadotropins in a GnRH antagonist cycle [43] to reduce the risk of OHSS. If cycle cancellation is not feasible, coasting can be done, where gonadotropins are withheld for one or more days prior to the hCG trigger. This allows larger follicles to continue to grow while withdrawing stimulation and preventing further enlargement of medium- or smaller-sized follicles. If coasting continues for five or more days, pregnancy rates are substantially decreased, and consideration should be given to cycle cancellation. Coasting should be stopped when the estradiol levels start to drop. It should be noted that risks of OHSS are increased with coasting as opposed to withholding the hCG and cancelling the cycle. It also should be noted that most recent evidence compared to not coasting and continuation of the IVF cycle finds no decrease in OHSS with coasting [44]. If deemed safe and the patient well enough, the protocol can be continued as planned. However, the transfer will either be delayed until day 5 while monitoring for signs of OHSS or all embryos will be cryopreserved to be transfered in a subsequent treatment cycle. Lastly, in subsequent cycles, GnRH antagonist cycles, using GnRH agonist triggers for ovulation should be the preferred protocol for the patient.

Alternatively, if a patient fails to recruit adequate follicles with controlled ovarian hyperstimulation in the form of a GnRH agonist protocol, they are referred to as a "poor responder." The following have been proposed as changes to their treatments which may improve ovarian response in subsequent cycles: decrease ovarian suppression (i.e., with lower GnRH agonist dosing), increase follicular stimulation (i.e., with higher doses of gonadotropins for longer durations if taking less than 300 IU daily), change in the gonadotropin used (i.e., switch from u/rFSH to hMG to add LH stimulation or add lutropin alpha to better support steroidogenesis), or stop GnRH agonist treatment soon after beginning gonadotropin stimulation. (In this case, after 7 days without suppression, a GnRH antagonist should be initiated). While the aforementioned changes are sensible, adequate evidence is lacking regarding their individual effectiveness in improving ovarian response to stimulation [45].

9.2.2 GnRH Agonist "Flare" Gonadotropin Protocol

The GnRH agonist "flare" gonadotropin protocol is also often referred to as the "short" GnRH agonist protocol. It can be given in the standard manner or with a microdose variation. The development of these protocols stems from the hypothesis that some patients may respond poorly to the long protocol due to the significant suppression achieved using long-term GnRH agonist therapy, which may inhibit ovarian response to exogenous gonadotropins [46, 47], although current evidence suggests that this protocol should not be used in poor responders [44]. In good responders, the flare protocol may result in lower gonadotropin requirements than the standard long protocol.

The short protocols are based on the same principles as the long protocol, with some important differences. Firstly, in the short protocol, the GnRH agonist is begun in the early follicular phase, compared to the mid-luteal start in the long protocol. Secondly, their approach differs in regard to the initial gonadotropin flare shortly after GnRH treatment begins. In the long protocol, the initial flare effect of the GnRH agonist prior to achieving pituitary suppression is associated with unwanted side effects including cyst formation, and gonadotropins are only begun once complete pituitary suppression is achieved, usually after 2 weeks. However, the "flare" protocol takes advantage of the initial flare effect within the first 48 h of GnRH agonist administration, which acts as a stimulus for follicular recruitment and promotes follicular development. After 2 days of agonist treatment, stimulation with exogenous gonadotropins begins and promotes the continuation of follicular growth. During this time, GnRH agonists are continued in order to prevent an endogenous LH surge and premature ovulation. From thereon, the protocol continues as described above in the long protocol. Monitoring of follicular response is the same as above, with either step-up or step-down dosing of gonadotropins depending on ovarian response to stimulation. Once a good response is achieved, hCG trigger, oocyte pickup, and either transfer or freezing proceed as in the long protocol. It should be noted the flare protocol is only effective in women with a functional hypothalamic-pituitary-ovarian axis.

The standard GnRH agonist "flare" protocol (Fig. 9.2) is timed with the patient's menstrual cycle. Full-dose GnRH agonist treatment is given on cycle days 2–4 (e.g., leuprolide acetate 1.0 mg daily sc) and thereafter continued at a reduced (usually half) dose. Gonadotropin stimulation is begun on cycle day 3, typically at lower doses than the long protocol, and dosing is adjusted as needed.

The microdose protocol is similar to the standard "flare" protocol, however, uses lower doses of GnRH agonists (e.g., leuprolide acetate 40 mcg daily). Additionally, 14–21 days of COCs can be given to synchronize the follicles and time collection prior to beginning GnRH agonists. (Fig. 9.3) The logic behind lowering the agonist dose is to reduce ovarian suppression while still inducing a flare effect of endogenous gonadotropins. This is done in the hope of further improving response and pregnancy rates in patients who are poor responders [48, 49].

Compared to the long protocol, the "flare" or short protocols may have lower costs given their shorter duration of treatment and lower gonadotropin requirements in good responder patients. However, unless COCs are used prior to

CD1: Day 1 Menstruation. *Baseline US	**GnRHa**	**GnRHa GN**	**GnRHa**	**GnRHa (reduced dose) GN**	**GnRHa (reduced dose) GN**	**GnRHa (reduced dose) GN**
GnRHa (reduced dose) GN	**GnRHa (reduced dose) GN**	**GnRHa (reduced dose) GN**	**GnRHa (reduced dose) GN**	*Monitoring US & estradiol **GnRHa (reduced dose) ?? GN**	* Adequate stim: **hCG** *Incomplete stim: **GnRHa (reduced dose) GN** *repeat US & estradiol q1-3days	* Adequate stim: --- *Incomplete stim: **GnRHa (reduced dose) GN** *repeat US & estradiol q1-3days
* Adequate stim: Collection ***Luteal phase support (progesterone +/- estrogen)** if fresh ET planned, start after collection			* Adequate stim: Transfer			

Fig. 9.2 GnRH agonist flare sample protocol. Missing GN on day 3, put monitoring on day 6 here and below. This figure demonstrates a sample GnRH agonist flare protocol without oral contraceptives prior. *GnRHa* GnRH agonist, *GN* gonadotropin(s), *US* transvaginal ultrasound, *ET* embryo transfer. Cycle day 1 may be induced by progesterone and/or estrogen compounds (e.g., OCP) or natural cycle

CD1: Day 1 Menstruation. Begin COC	COC	COC	COC	COC	COC	COC
COC	COC	COC	COC	COC	COC	COC
COC	COC	COC	COC	COC	COC	COC
—	—	*Baseline US GnRHa	GnRHa	GnRHa GN	GnRHa GN	GnRHa GN
GnRHa GN	GnRHa GN	GnRHa GN	GnRHa GN	*Monitoring US & estradiol GnRHa ?? GN	*Adequate stim: hCG *Incomplete stim: GnRHa GN *repeat US & estradiol q1-3days	*Adequate stim: --- *Incomplete stim: GnRHa GN *repeat US & estradiol q1-3days
*Adequate stim: Collection *Luteal phase support (progesterone +/- estrogen) if fresh ET planned, start after collection			*Adequate stim: Transfer			

Fig. 9.3 GnRH agonist microdose flare sample protocol. This figure demonstrates a sample GnRH agonist microdose flare protocol with prior COC to coordinate. *COC* combined oral contraceptive, *GnRHa* GnRH agonist, *GN* gonadotropin(s), *US* transvaginal ultrasound, *ET* embryo transfer. Of note: cycle day 1 may be induced by progesterone and/or estrogen compounds (e.g., OCP) or natural cycle. 14–21 days of COC can be used to achieve downregulation. Baseline US to confirm adequate downregulation—i.e., no cysts and thin endometrium. GnRH agonist dose remains the same when gonadotropin therapy begins. Monitoring with US and estradiol levels continues every 1–3 days, depending on follicular growth and estradiol levels. Once adequate stimulation is achieved, hCG trigger is given. Collection is planned on average 36 h later. Embryos are then transferred on days 3–5 or frozen

their start, timing the cycle with the patient's menstruation often poses challenges and inconveniences. In the standard protocol, without ovarian suppression with COCs, treatment failures have been partially attributed to the consequences of a rescued corpus luteum from a previous cycle. With a follicular phase start and no prior suppression, a rise in serum androgen and progesterone levels has been observed and is thought to reduce oocyte quality and subsequent pregnancy rates [50, 51]. With COC suppression and lower doses of GnRH agonists, the microdose protocol theoretically should overcome this issue [52].

9.3 Conclusion

Controlled ovarian hyperstimulation with gonadotropins alone carries a significant risk of cycle cancellation due to premature ovulation. GnRH agonist and antagonist protocols overcome this issue by their effect on the hypothalamic-pituitary-ovarian axis to reduce endogenous hormone secretion. Via the pathways described above, these agents can be used to substantially reduce the rate of premature ovulation, allowing for exogenous ovarian stimulation to achieve a greater number of larger and mature follicles.

In this chapter, we first described the traditional long protocol. The shorter GnRH agonist "flare" protocols (standard and microdose) were later developed in attempt to increase responses and pregnancy rates among poor responders to the standard and popular long protocol. While each have their associated advantages and disadvantages, it is clear that the benefits and outcomes significantly outweigh the disadvantages for most patients.

Multiple comparative studies have shown conflicting results regarding responses and relevant clinical outcomes (pregnancy and live birth rates). The most recent Cochrane review found no conclusive difference in pregnancy or live birth rates between any of the long or short GnRH agonist protocols [53]. However, in our practice and elsewhere in the literature, we still observe that some patients may have higher success rates, specifically likelihood of pregnancy and live birth, using certain protocols. GnRH agonist long cycles are best in poor and moderate responders and should be avoided in patients at risk for OHSS. The flare protocol has fallen out of favor for poor responders and may be used to reduce gonadotropin doses in good responders.

References

1. Conn PM, Crowley WF Jr. Gonadotropin-releasing hormone and its analogues. N Engl J Med. 1991;324(2):93–103.
2. Karten MJ, Rivier JE. Gonadotropin-releasing hormone analog design. Structure-function studies toward the development of agonists and antagonists: rationale and perspective. Endocr Rev. 1986;7(1):44–66.
3. Tarlatzis BC, Kolibianakis EM. GnRH agonists vs antagonists. Best Pract Res Clin Obstet Gynaecol. 2007;21(1):57–65.
4. Schally AV, Arimura A, Baba Y, et al. Isolation and properties of the FSH and LH-releasing hormone. Biochem Biophys Res Commun. 1971;43(2):393–9.
5. Porter RN, Smith W, Craft IL, Abdulwahid NA, Jacobs HS. Induction of ovulation for in-vitro fertilisation using buserelin and gonadotropins. Lancet. 1984;2(8414):1284–5.
6. Smitz J, Devroey P, Braeckmans P, et al. Management of failed cycles in an IVF/GIFT programme with the combination of a GnRH analogue and HMG. Hum Reprod. 1987;2(4):309–14.
7. Diedrich K, Ludwig M, Felberbaum RE. The role of gonadotropin-releasing hormone antagonists in in vitro fertilization. Semin Reprod Med. 2001;19(3):213–20.
8. Shalev E, Leung PC. Gonadotropin-releasing hormone and reproductive medicine. J Obstet Gynaecol Can. 2003;25(2):98–113.
9. Tan SL, Balen A, el Hussein E, et al. A prospective randomized study of the optimum timing of human chorionic gonadotropin administration after pituitary desensitization in in vitro fertilization. Fertil Steril. 1992;57(6):1259–64.
10. Biljan MM, Mahutte NG, Dean N, Hemmings R, Bissonnette F, Tan SL. Pretreatment with an oral contraceptive is effective in reducing the incidence of functional ovarian cyst formation during pituitary suppression by gonadotropin-releasing hormone analogues. J Assist Reprod Genet. 1998;15(10):599–604.
11. Hughes EG, Fedorkow DM, Daya S, Sagle MA, Van de Koppel P, Collins JA. The routine use of gonadotropin-releasing hormone agonists prior to in vitro fertilization and gamete intrafallopian transfer: a meta-analysis of randomized controlled trials. Fertil Steril. 1992;58(5):888–96.
12. Daya S. Gonadotropin releasing hormone agonist protocols for pituitary desensitization in in vitro fertilization and gamete intrafallopian transfer cycles. Cochrane Database Syst Rev. 2000;2:CD001299.
13. Ron-El R, Herman A, Golan A, Raziel A, Soffer Y, Caspi E. Follicle cyst formation following long-acting gonadotropin-releasing hormone analog administration. Fertil Steril. 1989;52(6):1063–6.
14. Firouzabadi RD, Sekhavat L, Javedani M. The effect of ovarian cyst aspiration on IVF treatment with GnRH. Arch Gynecol Obstet. 2010;281(3):545–9.
15. Qublan HS, Amarin Z, Tahat YA, Smadi AZ, Kilani M. Ovarian cyst formation following GnRH agonist administration in IVF cycles: incidence and impact. Hum Reprod. 2006;21(3):640–4.
16. Rizk B, Tan SL, Kingsland C, Steer C, Mason BA, Campbell S. Ovarian cyst aspiration and the outcome of in vitro fertilization. Fertil Steril. 1990;54(4):661–4.
17. Smitz J, Erard P, Camus M, et al. Pituitary gonadotrophin secretory capacity during the luteal phase in superovulation using GnRH-agonists and HMG in a desensitization or flare-up protocol. Hum Reprod. 1992;7(9):1225–9.
18. Jee BC, Suh CS, Kim SH, Kim YB, Moon SY. Effects of estradiol supplementation during the luteal phase of in vitro fertilization cycles: a meta-analysis. Fertil Steril. 2010; 93(2):428–36.
19. Fatemi HM, Popovic-Todorovic B, Papanikolaou E, Donoso P, Devroey P. An update of luteal phase support in stimulated IVF cycles. Hum Reprod Update. 2007;13(6):581–90.
20. Delvigne A, Rozenberg S. Epidemiology and prevention of ovarian hyperstimulation syndrome (OHSS): a review. Hum Reprod Update. 2002;8(6):559–77.
21. Rizk B, Smitz J. Ovarian hyperstimulation syndrome after superovulation using GnRH agonists for IVF and related procedures. Hum Reprod. 1992;7(3):320–7.
22. Mordel N, Schenker JG. Gonadotrophin-releasing hormone agonist and ovarian hyperstimulation syndrome in assisted reproduction. Hum Reprod. 1993;8(12):2009–14.

23. MacDougall MJ, Tan SL, Jacobs HS. In-vitro fertilization and the ovarian hyperstimulation syndrome. Hum Reprod. 1992;7(5):597–600.
24. Ragni G, Vegetti W, Riccaboni A, Engl B, Brigante C, Crosignani PG. Comparison of GnRH agonists and antagonists in assisted reproduction cycles of patients at high risk of ovarian hyperstimulation syndrome. Hum Reprod. 2005;20(9):2421–5.
25. Sunkara SK, Coomarasamy A, Faris R, Braude P, Khalaf Y. Long gonadotropin-releasing hormone agonist versus short agonist versus antagonist regimens in poor responders undergoing in vitro fertilization: a randomized controlled trial. Fertil Steril. 2014;101(1):147–53.
26. Kolibianakis EM, Collins J, Tarlatzis BC, Devroey P, Diedrich K, Griesinger G. Among patients treated for IVF with gonadotrophins and GnRH analogues, is the probability of live birth dependent on the type of analogue used? A systematic review and meta-analysis. Hum Reprod Update. 2006;12(6):651–71.
27. Werner MD, Forman EJ, Hong KH, Franasiak JM, Molinaro TA, Scott RT Jr. Defining the "sweet spot" for administered luteinizing hormone-to-follicle-stimulating hormone gonadotropin ratios during ovarian stimulation to protect against a clinically significant late follicular increase in progesterone: an analysis of 10,280 first in vitro fertilization cycles. Fertil Steril. 2014;102(5):1312–7.
28. El-Nemr A, Bhide M, Khalifa Y, et al. Clinical evaluation of three different gonadotrophin-releasing hormone analogues in an IVF programme: a prospective study. Eur J Obstet Gynecol Reprod Biol. 2002;103(2):140–5.
29. Bastu E, Buyru F, Ozsurmeli M, Demiral I, Dogan M, Yeh J. A randomized, single-blind, prospective trial comparing three different gonadotropin doses with or without addition of letrozole during ovulation stimulation in patients with poor ovarian response. Eur J Obstet Gynecol Reprod Biol. 2016;203:30–4.
30. Dada T, Salha O, Baillie HS, Sharma V. A comparison of three gonadotrophin-releasing hormone analogues in an in-vitro fertilization programme: a prospective randomized study. Hum Reprod. 1999;14(2):288–93.
31. Albuquerque LE, Saconato H, Maciel MC. Depot versus daily administration of gonadotrophin releasing hormone agonist protocols for pituitary desensitization in assisted reproduction cycles. Cochrane Database Syst Rev. 2002;3:CD002808.
32. Meldrum DR, Wisot A, Hamilton F, Gutlay AL, Huynh D, Kempton W. Timing of initiation and dose schedule of leuprolide influence the time course of ovarian suppression. Fertil Steril. 1988;50(3):400–2.
33. Urbancsek J, Witthaus E. Midluteal buserelin is superior to early follicular phase buserelin in combined gonadotropin-releasing hormone analog and gonadotropin stimulation in in vitro fertilization. Fertil Steril. 1996;65(5):966–71.
34. Pellicer A, Simon C, Miro F, et al. Ovarian response and outcome of in-vitro fertilization in patients treated with gonadotrophin-releasing hormone analogues in different phases of the menstrual cycle. Hum Reprod. 1989;4(3):285–9.
35. Segal S, Shifren JL, Isaacson KB, et al. Effect of a baseline ovarian cyst on the outcome of in vitro fertilization-embryo transfer. Fertil Steril. 1999;71(2):274–7.
36. Chappel SC, Howles C. Reevaluation of the roles of luteinizing hormone and follicle-stimulating hormone in the ovulatory process. Hum Reprod. 1991;6(9):1206–12.
37. van Wely M, Westergaard LG, Bossuyt PM, van der Veen F. Effectiveness of human menopausal gonadotropin versus recombinant follicle-stimulating hormone for controlled ovarian hyperstimulation in assisted reproductive cycles: a meta-analysis. Fertil Steril. 2003;80(5):1086–93.
38. Coomarasamy A, Afnan M, Cheema D, van der Veen F, Bossuyt PM, van Wely M. Urinary hMG versus recombinant FSH for controlled ovarian hyperstimulation following an agonist long down-regulation protocol in IVF or ICSI treatment: a systematic review and meta-analysis. Hum Reprod. 2008;23(2):310–5.
39. Poseidon G, Alviggi C, Andersen CY, et al. A new more detailed stratification of low responders to ovarian stimulation: from a poor ovarian response to a low prognosis concept. Fertil Steril. 2016;105(6):1452–3.
40. Youssef MA, Abou-Setta AM, Lam WS. Recombinant versus urinary human chorionic gonadotrophin for final oocyte maturation triggering in IVF and ICSI cycles. Cochrane Database Syst Rev. 2016;4:CD003719.
41. Nargund G, Hutchison L, Scaramuzzi R, Campbell S. Low-dose HCG is useful in preventing OHSS in high-risk women without adversely affecting the outcome of IVF cycles. Reprod Biomed Online. 2007;14(6):682–5.
42. Schmidt DW, Maier DB, Nulsen JC, Benadiva CA. Reducing the dose of human chorionic gonadotropin in high responders does not affect the outcomes of in vitro fertilization. Fertil Steril. 2004;82(4):841–6.
43. Damario MA, Barmat L, Liu HC, Davis OK, Rosenwaks Z. Dual suppression with oral contraceptives and gonadotrophin releasing-hormone agonists improves in-vitro fertilization outcome in high responder patients. Hum Reprod. 1997;12(11):2359–65.
44. D'Angelo A, Brown J, Amso NN. Coasting (withholding gonadotrophins) for preventing ovarian hyperstimulation syndrome. Cochrane Database Syst Rev. 2011;6:CD002811.
45. Pandian Z, McTavish AR, Aucott L, Hamilton MP, Bhattacharya S. Interventions for 'poor responders' to controlled ovarian hyper stimulation (COH) in in-vitro fertilisation (IVF). Cochrane Database Syst Rev. 2010;1:CD004379.
46. Padilla SL, Dugan K, Maruschak V, Shalika S, Smith RD. Use of the flare-up protocol with high dose human follicle stimulating hormone and human menopausal gonadotropins for in vitro fertilization in poor responders. Fertil Steril. 1996;65(4):796–9.
47. Garcia JE, Padilla SL, Bayati J, Baramki TA. Follicular phase gonadotropin-releasing hormone agonist and human gonadotropins: a better alternative for ovulation induction in in vitro fertilization. Fertil Steril. 1990;53(2):302–5.
48. Scott RT, Navot D. Enhancement of ovarian responsiveness with microdoses of gonadotropin-releasing hormone agonist during ovulation induction for in vitro fertilization. Fertil Steril. 1994;61(5):880–5.
49. Schoolcraft W, Schlenker T, Gee M, Stevens J, Wagley L. Improved controlled ovarian hyperstimulation in poor responder in vitro fertilization patients with a microdose follicle-stimulating hormone flare, growth hormone protocol. Fertil Steril. 1997;67(1):93–7.
50. San Roman GA, Surrey ES, Judd HL, Kerin JF. A prospective randomized comparison of luteal phase versus concurrent follicular phase initiation of gonadotropin-releasing hormone agonist for in vitro fertilization. Fertil Steril. 1992;58(4):744–9.
51. Gelety TJ, Pearlstone AC, Surrey ES. Short-term endocrine response to gonadotropin-releasing hormone agonist initiated in the early follicular, midluteal, or late luteal phase in normally cycling women. Fertil Steril. 1995;64(6):1074–80.
52. Surrey ES, Bower J, Hill DM, Ramsey J, Surrey MW. Clinical and endocrine effects of a microdose GnRH agonist flare regimen administered to poor responders who are undergoing in vitro fertilization. Fertil Steril. 1998;69(3):419–24.
53. Siristatidis CS, Gibreel A, Basios G, Maheshwari A, Bhattacharya S. Gonadotrophin-releasing hormone agonist protocols for pituitary suppression in assisted reproduction. Cochrane Database Syst Rev. 2015;11:CD006919.

GnRH Antagonist Protocols

10

Francisco Javier Ruiz Flores
and Juan Antonio García Velasco

10.1 Introduction

The field of human reproduction has seen major improvements in the last few decades. As ovarian stimulation plays an integral part for the treatment of infertility, new protocols using an array of different medications and diverse approaches have appeared.

The first treatments of IVF were based on natural cycles with a spontaneous ovulation, and only a single oocyte was available for retrieval. As soon as the low success rates of IVF in natural cycles were recognized, ovarian stimulation using urinary gonadotropins was adopted to confront this problem. By collecting a higher number of oocytes through ovarian stimulation, the rates of success in IVF cycles increased significantly.

This progress also showed some limitations. Intensive monitoring of the patient was required because ovulation could appear at any hour of the day. Also, premature luteinization and failure to have a more synchronous multiple follicular development were common problems. To confront this, gonadotropin-releasing hormone agonists (GnRHa) were introduced into clinical practice to successfully produce pituitary desensitization to avoid gonadotropin secretion. This happened to be a breakthrough in IVF treatment.

Since then, many stimulation protocols have been introduced into clinical practice. Nowadays highly purified urinary gonadotropins or recombinant gonadotropins are used for follicular development in different protocols. When GnRH agonists are used, a sudden increase in pituitary gonadotropins occurs. Because of this initial flare-up effect, agonists are usually administered in the mid-luteal phase of the previous cycle (better known as the long protocol). This is the oldest and still the most commonly used protocol in clinical practice. A new variation later came into existence known as the short protocol. Agonists are administered in the early follicular phase in an effort to benefit from the initial flare-up effect due to the endogenous FSH release.

Although GnRH agonists are highly effective in IVF treatment, some limitations to their use have been described, such as longer duration of treatment, multiple injections, estrogen-deprivation-associated symptoms, and a requirement for higher doses of gonadotropins for ovarian stimulation with a consequent increase in total costs. Additionally, a potentially serious complication during ovarian stimulation is the ovarian hyperstimulation syndrome (OHSS), which cannot be totally prevented when using GnRH agonist protocols.

During the last few decades, even though many improvements were seen, ovarian stimulation had become increasingly complex, creating a burden not only to the patient but also to the clinician directing the treatment. For these reasons, there was a need in the field to find a simpler approach to ovarian stimulation, with a shorter duration of treatment and decreased costs, that can effectively avoid the most common potentially serious complication: OHSS. To address these complexities in ovarian stimulation without compromising success rates in IVF, GnRH antagonists appeared in clinical practice. The antagonists are started halfway through the gonadotropin stimulation just days before LH surge appears.

All GnRH analogues (agonists and antagonists) prevent the premature LH surge effectively, although the antagonists work by causing an immediate inhibition of gonadotropin release without the flare-up effect.

Although still far from perfect, the antagonists have several advantages over the agonists, and most importantly they seem to have given us an opportunity to make the overall treatment simpler and safer.

F. J. R. Flores
IVI, Abu Dhabi, UAE
e-mail: FranciscoJavier.Ruiz@ivirma.com

J. A. G. Velasco (✉)
Obstetrics and Gynecology at Universidad Rey Juan Carlos, Madrid, Spain

IVI, Madrid, Spain
e-mail: jgvelaso@ivi.es; Juan.Garcia.Velasco@ivi.es

G. N. Allahbadia et al. (eds.), *Textbook of Assisted Reproduction*, https://doi.org/10.1007/978-981-15-2377-9_10

The aim of this chapter is to summarize and describe the different protocols in which GnRH antagonists are used for ovarian stimulation in assisted conception cycles. The latest evidence will be reviewed regarding the effectiveness and safety of their use when compared to agonist protocols.

10.2 GnRH Antagonists: A Brief History

The GnRH antagonists were initially available in the market in 1999 and were aimed at avoiding a premature surge of LH. These new compounds provided an immediate inhibition of gonadotropin release without the flare-up effect, in sharp contrast to the long agonist protocol. This inhibition of gonadotropin release is also reversible and dose-dependent. Their mode of action is through a competitive binding to the pituitary GnRH receptor. This is an important property, as they can be used at any time during the follicular or luteal phase. Discontinuation of antagonist administration leads to a rapid and predictable recovery of the pituitary-gonadal axis.

It was relatively simple to develop safe GnRH agonists for clinical use only by changing one or two amino acids, but it required close to 30 years of trial and error to obtain an antagonist compound with an acceptable pharmacokinetic, safety, and commercial profile [1].

The initial generation of these GnRH antagonists showed adverse allergic reactions due to an induced histamine release, making it difficult for clinical use. For safety reasons, antagonists should have a high therapeutic index (relative potency at inhibiting gonadotropin secretion over relative potency at stimulating histamine release).

In order to minimize the initial adverse effect of histamine release of some GnRH antagonists, new structures with modifications at different positions were synthesized and tested in several biological systems [2].

Regarding the safety profile, the third-generation antagonists were proved to be effective and without the adverse effect of histamine release. The two antagonists approved for clinical use are cetrorelix and ganirelix [3]. Follow-up data related to children born after antagonist use appears to be reassuring. No increased risk of birth defects has been observed [4, 5] (Table 10.1).

Table 10.1 GnRH antagonist advantages compared to agonists

Shorter total cycle duration
Increased patient compliance with reduced physical and emotional stress
Immediate suppression of gonadotropin secretion
Increased safety by allowing ovulation triggering with a GnRH agonist
Flare effect is not present
Decreased gonadotropin dosage
No estrogen-deprivation-associated symptoms

10.3 Antagonist Protocols in Ovarian Stimulation

10.3.1 Single-Dose Protocol

Gonadotropins are started on day 2 or 3 of the menstrual cycle. An initial dose of 3 mg of cetrorelix is injected when serum estradiol levels indicate an appropriate response to stimulation (usually between days 5 and 7). If ovulation triggering is not performed within 4 days after the initial administration, daily doses of 0.25 mg are injected until ovulation triggering [6]. This protocol is usually well tolerated with only mild and transient injection site reactions.

10.3.2 Multiple-Dose Protocol

This is the most commonly used protocol. Gonadotropins are started on day 2 or 3 of the menstrual cycle. An injected daily dose of 0.25 mg of an antagonist is started either on a fixed day or depending on follicular size. These are commonly known as the "fixed" or "flexible" multiple-dose protocol accordingly. In the fixed approach, antagonists are administered on either day 5 or 6 of stimulation (Fig. 10.1). In the flexible approach, antagonists are usually given when the leading follicle reaches 14 mm; the antagonist is then injected daily until ovulation triggering [6] (Fig. 10.2).

The multiple-dose protocol is a simple, safe, and effective regimen for preventing the LH surge. On one side, the fixed approach is simple and requires less monitoring of the cycle, and on the other, the flexible approach advantage relies on the avoidance of unnecessary injections when the risk of the LH surge is minimal, reducing also the total cost of the treatment.

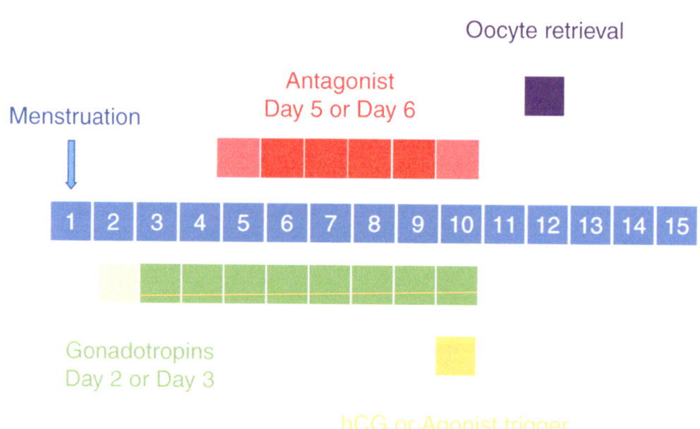

Fig. 10.1 GnRH antagonist protocol: fixed approach

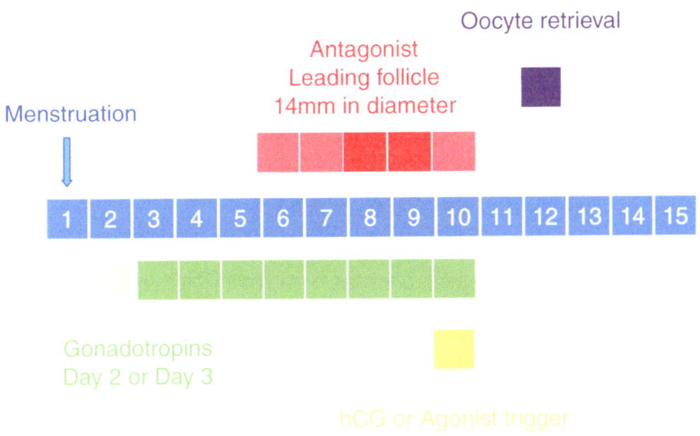

Fig. 10.2 GnRH antagonist protocol: flexible approach

10.3.3 Fixed vs Flexible Approaches

Regarding pregnancy outcomes, two meta-analyses [7, 8] found a trend toward a higher pregnancy and live birth rates in the fixed approach group, although with no statistical significance. In contrast, there were statistically significant reductions in both the number of antagonist ampoules and the amount of gonadotropins used in the flexible approach [7].

10.3.4 Triggering of Ovulation

Urinary human chorionic gonadotropin, commonly referred to as hCG, has been the mainstay of ovulation triggering for the final oocyte maturation. The use of hCG in assisted conception cycles has been directly related to the appearance of OHSS [9]. During ovarian stimulation using a GnRH agonist protocol, hCG for ovulation triggering is used, setting the ground for OHSS to appear. Therefore, an ideal solution would be to completely avoid the use of hCG in patients at high risk of developing the syndrome, such as women with polycystic ovaries, oocyte donors, or patients with a previous history of OHSS. This is where the antagonist protocol has a clear advantage over the agonist protocol. As mentioned before, use of the antagonist protocol has been related to a lower OHSS incidence [10].

Only under a natural cycle or an antagonist cycle a GnRH agonist can be used to induce the final oocyte maturation and acting, at the same time, as a more physiological trigger. By avoiding the administration of hCG, the risk of early OHSS is minimal. The proposal by some authors to shift the practice to antagonist from the usual agonist protocol finds a solid argument in the avoidance of OHSS [11]. Additionally, agonist triggering can be an option for patients who will not continue with a fresh transfer.

It is also important to mention that cases of severe OHSS have been reported in spite of using GnRH agonists for ovulation triggering in antagonist cycles [12].

Agonist triggering can also reduce the chance of pregnancy in fresh autologous cycles when compared to hCG [13]. This is due to the severe luteolysis caused by the agonist triggering [14]. Interestingly, there are reports pointing out the fact that not all patients triggered with an agonist will have severe luteolysis [15]. Several solutions have been proposed to address the issue of a lower pregnancy rate, such as transferring thawed embryos in a later cycle or tailor-made luteal support with low-dose hCG [16–19].

From a clinical point of view, some authors have suggested that luteal support is the variable which affects the pregnancy rate and not the use of the agonist trigger itself [16].

A recent study from our group regarding endometrial gene expression showed that the pattern seen after agonist trigger and modified luteal support adding LH/hCG activity more closely resembles the one seen after hCG triggering [20].

10.3.5 Oral Contraceptive Pill Pretreatment

Oral contraceptive pill (OCP) pretreatment can be given in different situations before ovarian stimulation is started using an antagonist protocol. Cycle scheduling is one of the most common reasons why OCP pretreatment is given, and it helps in equally distributing the workload through the week and avoiding weekend oocyte retrievals.

It has been suggested that this OCP pretreatment may lead to an extended length of treatment, an increased oocyte yield, and a negative impact on the ongoing pregnancy rate (OPR) [21]. Some controversy exists because cycle planning with OCP has shown varying outcomes. A recent meta-analysis showed that OPR was significantly lower in patients with OCP pretreatment [22]. In contrast to these results, a subgroup analysis from previous versions of a systematic review mentioned above [10] showed no difference for OPR or clinical pregnancy rate (CPR). Additionally, in a randomized trial published by our group, similar outcomes were obtained by using OCP pretreatment in antagonist cycles when compared to the long agonist protocol [23].

The different dosing of steroids in OCP presentations, duration of the pill administration, and wash-out period may all account for the different results obtained in previous studies [23].

It also appears that OCP pretreatment does not seem to affect the expression of known genes related to embryo implantation. By evaluating the transcriptomic profile from endometrial biopsies during the expected window of implantation from patients with and without OCP pretreatment, a recent study did not find any difference between both groups [24].

In a recent review article from our group, we discussed that the benefits of cycle scheduling with the pill must be weighed against the drawbacks [25]. When administered for the least amount of days with a wash-out period resembling the natural cycle, OCP pretreatment may not have a negative effect on endometrial receptivity, and assisted conception cycle outcome might be comparable to other protocols like estrogen pretreatment and the long agonist protocol [24].

It is also clear that there is no consensus whether the use of OCP pretreatment in antagonist cycles has a negative effect on live birth rate [25]. Randomized controlled trials that are well designed and adequately powered are required to evaluate the most appropriate approach for OCP pretreatment in antagonist cycles.

10.4 Agonists vs Antagonists: Live Birth Rates and OHSS Risk Comparison

A recent systematic review [10] assessed the effectiveness and safety of GnRH antagonists compared with the standard long protocol of GnRH agonists for ovarian stimulation using artificial reproductive technologies (ART). It is important to mention that older versions of this review presented, to a significant extent, reduced ongoing and clinical pregnancy rates when using antagonists.

Overall, data from the updated systematic review show that by using antagonists as compared to agonists, there is a reduction of OHSS rate without affecting the ongoing pregnancy rate and the probability of a live birth.

These results showed that the antagonist protocol has a better safety profile regarding OHSS compared to the long agonist protocol. It appears that the risk of OHSS in an agonist cycle is approximately 11% while only 6–9% in an antagonist cycle. Also important was the fact that the incidence of severe and moderate OHSS is lower when using the antagonist cycle.

The difficult question to answer after this newly updated review is why the evidence changed toward an improved performance of the antagonist protocol. Some suggestions were added by the authors that may explain the better results, such as an improved learning curve over the last 15 years for the antagonist protocol, optimal patient selection, scheduling of hCG to induce ovulation, whether OCP pretreatment was given, a reduced LH instability, or even other potential bias like a higher number of published works with more favorable outcomes.

There were no differences in miscarriage rate between the use of agonist or antagonist protocol. The use of antagonists also showed a lower number of cancelled cycles related to OHSS.

Another systematic review from 2011 [26] also showed that use of the antagonist protocol was associated with a large reduction in OHSS with no evidence of a difference in live birth rates.

10.5 GnRH Antagonist Protocols in Selected Situations

10.5.1 Poor Response to Ovarian Stimulation

The antagonist protocol is a commonly used approach for poor responders as it offers several advantages. They cause immediate, rapid, and reversible gonadotropin suppression, in contrast to the desensitization and deep suppression seen with the agonist protocol. Different systematic reviews and meta-analyses have tried to prove the value of this approach in poor responders, but the actual effectiveness of the antagonist protocol in poor responders has yet to be demonstrated [27–29].

In the most recent systematic review, the antagonist protocol was compared with the agonist protocol, and no significant difference in the outcome was shown regarding the clinical pregnancy rate (CPR) or number of oocytes retrieved [28].

In a meta-analysis from 2013 comparing as well the antagonist protocol with the agonist protocol, the clinical pregnancy and cycle cancellation rates were similar [29].

A systematic review from 2010 concluded that there is insufficient evidence to support the routine use of any particular intervention for pituitary downregulation, including the use of the antagonist protocol [27].

10.5.2 Expected High Response and Previous History of OHSS

As discussed earlier, because of the possibility of using a GnRH agonist for final oocyte maturation, antagonist protocols should be the regimen of choice in patients with a high risk of OHSS. It can be stated that triggering ovulation with a GnRH agonist without hCG administration almost completely eliminates early OHSS [30].

Oocyte donors can also benefit from the agonist trigger, as it has been shown by various studies in oocyte donation programs in which the incidence of OHSS was significantly reduced or even completely absent [31, 32].

Additionally, due to its powerful preventive effect, the antagonist protocol combined with an agonist trigger should preferentially be used in patients that are not planned for an embryo transfer, such as those undergoing fertility preservation for social reasons. The possibility of severe luteolysis related to agonist triggering is of no concern in these situations.

10.5.3 Fertility Preservation for Oncologic Reasons

Many patients are diagnosed with breast cancer every year, making it the most common malignancy in women. Advances in treatment have contributed to reduced mortality rates, increasing the number of cancer survivor patients. This fact has drawn attention lately, since chemotherapy can have a severe impact on ovarian reserve. Therefore, it has become important to address the issue of fertility preservation for these patients.

After the initial diagnosis, women present with a timeframe of around 6 weeks between surgical treatment and initiation of chemotherapy, making it possible to perform ovarian stimulation for oocyte or embryo cryopreservation, the most commonly used techniques for fertility preservation.

Because of the relatively short period of time before the start of chemotherapy, novel stimulation protocols have come into use with hopes of reducing estradiol levels that otherwise could have potential adverse effects and also others that can be started even in the luteal phase of the menstrual cycle using an antagonist protocol [33–35].

Some studies suggest that using an agonist trigger under an antagonist cycle can improve outcomes as explained by the total number of mature oocytes obtained, cryopreserved embryos available, and a significant reduction in the incidence of OHSS when going through fertility preservation with a breast cancer diagnosis [36].

10.5.4 Long-Acting rFSH

Ovarian stimulation has become a complex treatment and may contribute to a physical and psychological burden on fertility patients and oocyte donors [37]. Current treatment regimens require daily injections of gonadotropins. Current technologies have produced a new molecule, a long-acting rFSH, named corifollitropin alfa (Elonva; MSD, New Jersey, USA). A single injection of this long-acting rFSH can replace the usual seven daily rFSH injections during the first week of ovarian stimulation. When this new compound is used concomitantly with an antagonist protocol, the overall patient experience can be improved significantly by reducing the total number of injections required during ovarian stimulation.

In a recent systematic review [38], the authors concluded that the medium-dose use of long-acting rFSH appears to be a safe treatment option with no difference in benefits or harm compared to daily rFSH in women with unexplained subfertility.

In another study from our group performed in oocyte donors, the degree of treatment satisfaction was evaluated while using corifollitropin alfa. Donors who had undergone a previous cycle with daily rFSH reported a greater satisfaction with the use of corifollitropin alfa under an antagonist protocol, showing that this strategy may reduce treatment burden and increase donor compliance [37] (Table 10.2).

Table 10.2 Selected groups of women who might benefit from GnRH antagonists

Poor responders
Expected high responders
Patients with polycystic ovary syndrome
Oocyte donors
Patients with previous history of OHSS Oncologic patients
Patients undergoing oocyte/embryo vitrification for fertility preservation

10.6 Conclusions

- The GnRH antagonist protocol has comparable live birth rates compared to the long agonist GnRH protocol.
- The GnRH antagonist protocol provides a shorter duration of treatment and is related to reduced total costs.
- There is no clear benefit between the fixed and flexible approaches in the GnRH antagonist protocol regarding pregnancy outcomes.
- There is still no consensus if OCP pretreatment in GnRH antagonist protocols has a negative effect on live birth rates.
- There is a lower incidence of OHSS when using an antagonist protocol, as it provides the option to trigger with a GnRH agonist.
- By using an agonist triggering, early OHSS can almost be completely avoided.
- Agonist triggering is associated with a lower probability of pregnancy due to severe luteolysis, although if a correct luteal support is used, outcomes can be similar to hCG triggering.
- The GnRH antagonist protocol should be the ideal regimen for expected high responders, oocyte donors, women undergoing fertility preservation, and oncologic patients.

References

1. Kumar P, Sharma A. Gonadotropin-releasing hormone analogs: understanding advantages and limitations. J Hum Reprod Sci. 2014 Jul;7(3):170–4. https://doi.org/10.4103/0974-1208.142476.
2. Rivier JE, Porter J, Rivier CL, Perrin M, Corrigan A, Hook WA, Siraganian RP, Vale WW. New effective gonadotropin releasing hormone antagonists with minimal potency for histamine release in vitro. J Med Chem. 1986 Oct;29(10):1846–51.
3. Olivennes F, Alvarez S, Bouchard P, Fanchin R, Salat-Baroux J, Frydman R. The use of GnRH antagonist (cetrorelix) in a single

dose protocol in IVF-embryo transfer: a dose finding study of 3 versus 2mg. Hum Reprod. 1998;13(9):2411–4.
4. Ludwig M, Riethmüller-Winzen H, Felberbaum RE, Olivennes F, Albano C, Devroey P, Diedrich K. Health of 227 children born after controlled ovarian stimulation for in vitro fertilization using the luteinizing hormone-releasing hormone antagonist cetrorelix. Fertil Steril. 2001 Jan;75(1):18–22.
5. Chen H, Wang Y, Lyu Q, Ai A, Fu Y, Tian H, Cai R, Hong Q, Chen Q, Shoham Z, Kuang Y. Comparison of live-birth defects after luteal-phase ovarian stimulation vs. conventional ovarian stimulation for in vitro fertilization and vitrified embryo transfer cycles. Fertil Steril. 2015;103(5):1194–201. e2. https://doi.org/10.1016/j.fertnstert.2015.02.020.
6. Tur-Kaspa I, Ezcurra D. GnRH antagonist, cetrorelix, for pituitary suppression in modern, patient-friendly assisted reproductive technology. Expert Opin Drug Metab Toxicol. 2009 Oct;5(10):1323–36. https://doi.org/10.1517/17425250903279969.
7. Al-Inany H, Aboulghar MA, Mansour RT, Serour GI. Optimizing GnRH antagonist administration: meta-analysis of fixed versus flexible protocol. Reprod Biomed Online. 2005;10:567–70.
8. Kolibianakis EM, Collins J, Tarlatzis BC, Devroey P, Diedrich K, Griesinger G. Among patients treated for IVF with gonadotrophins and GnRH analogues, is the probability of live birth dependent on the type of analogue used? A systematic review and meta-analysis. Hum Reprod Update. 2006;12(6):651–71. Epub 2006 Aug 18
9. Cerrillo M, Rodríguez S, Mayoral M, Pacheco A, Martínez-Salazar J, Garcia-Velasco JA. Differential regulation of VEGF after final oocyte maturation with GnRH agonist versus hCG: a rationale for OHSS reduction. Fertil Steril. 2009;91(4 Suppl):1526–8. https://doi.org/10.1016/j.fertnstert.2008.08.118.
10. Al-Inany HG, Youssef MA, Ayeleke RO, Brown J, Lam WS, Broekmans FJ. Gonadotrophin-releasing hormone antagonists for assisted reproductive technology. Cochrane Database Syst Rev. 2016 Apr 29;4:CD001750. https://doi.org/10.1002/14651858.CD001750.pub4.
11. Griesinger G, Berndt H, Schultz L, Depenbusch M, Schultze-Mosgau A. Cumulative live birth rates after GnRH-agonist triggering of final oocyte maturation in patients at risk of OHSS: a prospective, clinical cohort study. Eur J Obstet Gynecol Reprod Biol. 2010a;149(2):190–4. https://doi.org/10.1016/j.ejogrb.2009.12.030. Epub 2010 Jan 25
12. Fatemi HM, Popovic-Todorovic B, Humaidan P, Kol S, Banker M, Devroey P, García-Velasco JA. Severe ovarian hyperstimulation syndrome after gonadotropin-releasing hormone (GnRH) agonist trigger and "freeze-all" approach in GnRH antagonist protocol. Fertil Steril. 2014 Apr;101(4):1008–11. https://doi.org/10.1016/j.fertnstert.2014.01.019.
13. Youssef MA, Van der Veen F, Al-Inany HG, Mochtar MH, Griesinger G, Nagi Mohesen M, Aboulfoutouh I, van Wely M. Gonadotropin-releasing hormone agonist versus HCG for oocyte triggering in antagonist-assisted reproductive technology. Cochrane Database Syst Rev. 2014;10:CD008046. https://doi.org/10.1002/14651858.CD008046.pub4.
14. Lawrenz B, Ruiz F, Engelmann N, Fatemi HM. Individual luteolysis post GnRH-agonist-trigger in GnRH-antagonist protocols. Gynecol Endocrinol. 2016;26:1–4. https://doi.org/10.1080/09513590.2016.1266325. [Epub ahead of print]
15. Gurbuz AS, Deveer R, Ozcimen N, Ozcimen EE, Lawrenz B, Banker M, Garcia-Velasco JA, Fatemi HM. Absence of luteal phase defect and spontaneous pregnancy in IVF patients despite GnRH-agonist trigger and "freeze all policy" without luteal phase support: a report of four cases. Gynecol Endocrinol. 2016;32(1):18–20. https://doi.org/10.3109/09513590.2015.1110694.
16. Kol S, Humaidan P, Alsbjerg B, Engmann L, Benadiva C, García-Velasco JA, Fatemi H, Andersen CY. The updated Cochrane review 2014 on GnRH agonist trigger: repeating the same errors. Reprod Biomed Online. 2015a Jun;30(6):563–5. https://doi.org/10.1016/j.rbmo.2015.02.009.
17. Fatemi HM, Polyzos NP, van Vaerenbergh I, Bourgain C, Blockeel C, Alsbjerg B, Papanikolaou EG, Humaidan P. Early luteal phase endocrine profile is affected by the mode of triggering final oocyte maturation and the luteal phase support used in recombinant follicle-stimulating hormone-gonadotropin-releasing hormone antagonist in vitro fertilization cycles. Fertil Steril. 2013 Sep;100(3):742–7. https://doi.org/10.1016/j.fertnstert.2013.05.028.
18. Humaidan P, Engmann L, Benadiva C. Luteal phase supplementation after gonadotropin-releasing hormone agonist trigger in fresh embryo transfer: the American versus European approaches. Fertil Steril. 2015 Apr;103(4):879–85. https://doi.org/10.1016/j.fertnstert.2015.01.034.
19. Dosouto C, Haahr T, Humaidan P. Gonadotropin-releasing hormone agonist (GnRHa) trigger - state of the art. Reprod Biol. 2017;S1642-431X(16):30128–0. https://doi.org/10.1016/j.repbio.2017.01.004. [Epub ahead of print] Review
20. Bermejo A, Cerrillo M, Ruiz-Alonso M, Blesa D, Simón C, Pellicer A, Garcia-Velasco JA. Impact of final oocyte maturation using gonadotropin-releasing hormone agonist triggering and different luteal support protocols on endometrial gene expression. Fertil Steril. 2014b;101(1):138–46. e3. https://doi.org/10.1016/j.fertnstert.2013.09.033.
21. Smulders B, van Oirschot S, Farquhar C, Rombauts L, Kremer J. Oral contraceptive pill, progestogen or estrogen pre-treatment for ovarian stimulation protocols for women undergoing assisted reproductive techniques. Cochrane Database Syst Rev. 2010:CD006109.
22. Griesinger G, Kolibianakis EM, Venetis C, Diedrich K, Tarlatzis B. Oral contraceptive pretreatment significantly reduces ongoing pregnancy likelihood in gonadotropin-releasing hormone antagonist cycles: an updated meta-analysis. Fertil Steril. 2010b;94:2382–4.
23. Garcia-Velasco JA, Bermejo A, Ruiz F, Martinez-Salazar J, Requena A, Pellicer A. Cycle scheduling with oral contraceptive pills in the GnRH antagonist protocol vs the long protocol: a randomized, controlled trial. Fertil Steril. 2011 Sep;96(3):590–3. https://doi.org/10.1016/j.fertnstert.2011.06.022.
24. Bermejo A, Iglesias C, Ruiz-Alonso M, Blesa D, Simón C, Pellicer A, García-Velasco J. The impact of using the combined oral contraceptive pill for cycle scheduling on gene expression related to endometrial receptivity. Hum Reprod. 2014a Jun;29(6):1271–8. https://doi.org/10.1093/humrep/deu065.
25. Garcia-Velasco JA, Fatemi HM. To pill or not to pill in GnRH antagonist cycles: that is the question! Reprod Biomed Online. 2015 Jan;30(1):39–42. https://doi.org/10.1016/j.rbmo.2014.09.010.
26. Gilliam ML. Gonadotrophin-releasing hormone antagonists for assisted reproductive technology. Obstet Gynecol. 2011 Sep;118(3):706–7. https://doi.org/10.1097/AOG.0b013e31822bbbb2.
27. Pandian Z, McTavish AR, Aucott L, Hamilton MP, Bhattacharya S. Interventions for 'poor responders' to controlled ovarian hyper stimulation (COH) in in-vitro fertilisation (IVF). Cochrane Database Syst Rev. 2010;1:CD004379. https://doi.org/10.1002/14651858.CD004379.pub3.
28. Jeve YB, Bhandari HM. Effective treatment protocol for poor ovarian response: a systematic review and meta-analysis. J Hum Reprod Sci. 2016;9(2):70–81. https://doi.org/10.4103/0974-1208.183515.
29. Xiao J, Chang S, Chen S. The effectiveness of gonadotropin-releasing hormone antagonist in poor ovarian responders undergoing in vitro fertilization: a systematic review and meta-analysis. Fertil Steril. 2013;100(6):1594–601.e1-9. https://doi.org/10.1016/j.fertnstert.2013.08.024.
30. Fatemi HM, Garcia-Velasco J. Avoiding ovarian hyperstimulation syndrome with the use of gonadotropin-releasing hormone agonist trigger. Fertil Steril. 2015 Apr;103(4):870–3. https://doi.org/10.1016/j.fertnstert.2015.02.004.

31. Bodri D, Guillén JJ, Galindo A, Mataró D, Pujol A, Coll O. Triggering with human chorionic gonadotropin or a gonadotropin-releasing hormone agonist in gonadotropin-releasing hormone antagonist-treated oocyte donor cycles: findings of a large retrospective cohort study. Fertil Steril. 2009 Feb;91(2):365–71. https://doi.org/10.1016/j.fertnstert.2007.11.049.
32. Bodri D, Guillén JJ, Trullenque M, Schwenn K, Esteve C, Coll O. Early ovarian hyperstimulation syndrome is completely prevented by gonadotropin releasing-hormone agonist triggering in high-risk oocyte donor cycles: a prospective, luteal-phase follow-up study. Fertil Steril. 2010;93(7):2418–20. https://doi.org/10.1016/j.fertnstert.2009.08.036.
33. Kuang Y, Chen Q, Hong Q, Lyu Q, Ai A, Fu Y, Shoham Z. Double stimulations during the follicular and luteal phases of poor responders in IVF/ICSI programmes (Shanghai protocol). Reprod Biomed Online. 2014 Dec;29(6):684–91. https://doi.org/10.1016/j.rbmo.2014.08.009.
34. Sönmezer M, Türkçüoğlu I, Coşkun U, Oktay K. Random-start controlled ovarian hyperstimulation for emergency fertility preservation in letrozole cycles. Fertil Steril. 2011;95(6):2125.e9-11. https://doi.org/10.1016/j.fertnstert.2011.01.030.
35. Bedoschi GM, de Albuquerque FO, Ferriani RA, Navarro PA. Ovarian stimulation during the luteal phase for fertility preservation of cancer patients: case reports and review of the literature. J Assist Reprod Genet. 2010 Aug;27(8):491–4. https://doi.org/10.1007/s10815-010-9429-0.
36. Reddy J, Turan V, Bedoschi G, Moy F, Oktay K. Triggering final oocyte maturation with gonadotropin-releasing hormone agonist (GnRHa) versus human chorionic gonadotropin (hCG) in breast cancer patients undergoing fertility preservation: an extended experience. J Assist Reprod Genet. 2014 Jul;31(7):927–32. https://doi.org/10.1007/s10815-014-0248-6.
37. Requena A, Cruz M, Collado D, Izquierdo A, Ballesteros A, Muñoz M, García-Velasco JA. Evaluation of the degree of satisfaction in oocyte donors using sustained-release FSH corifollitropin α. Reprod Biomed Online. 2013 Mar;26(3):253–9. https://doi.org/10.1016/j.rbmo.2012.11.015.
38. Pouwer AW, Farquhar C, Kremer JA. Long-acting FSH versus daily FSH for women undergoing assisted reproduction. Cochrane Database Syst Rev. 2015 Jul 14;7:CD009577. https://doi.org/10.1002/14651858.CD009577.pub3.
39. Kolibianakis EM, Venetis CA, Kalogeropoulou L, Papanikolaou E, Tarlatzis BC. Fixed versus flexible gonadotropin-releasing hormone antagonist administration in in vitro fertilization: a randomized controlled trial. Fertil Steril. 2011;95:558–62.
40. Papanikolaou EG, Pados G, Grimbizis G, Bili E, Kyriazi L, Polyzos NP, et al. GnRH-agonist versus GnRH-antagonist IVF cycles: is the reproductive outcome affected by the incidence of progesterone elevation on the day of HCG triggering? A randomized prospective study. Hum Reprod. 2012;27:1822–8.
41. Doody K, Devroey P, Gordon K, Witjes H, Mannaerts B. LH concentrations do not correlate with pregnancy in rFSH/GnRH antagonist cycles. Reprod Biomed Online. 2010;20:565–7.
42. Griesinger G, Shapiro DB, Kolibianakis EM, Witjes H, Mannaerts BM. No association between endogenous LH and pregnancy in a GnRH antagonist protocol: part II, recombinant FSH. Reprod Biomed Online. 2011;23:457–65.
43. Escudero E, Bosch E, Crespo J, Simón C, Remohí J, Pellicer A. Comparison of two different starting multiple dose gonadotropin-releasing hormone antagonist protocols in a selected group of in vitro fertilization-embryo transfer patients. Fertil Steril. 2004;81:562–6.
44. Hamdine O, Broekmans FJ, Eijkemans MJ, Lambalk CB, Fauser BC, Laven JS, et al. Early initiation of gonadotropin-releasing hormone antagonist treatment results in a more stable endocrine milieu during the mid- and late-follicular phases: a randomized controlled trial comparing gonadotropin-releasing hormone antagonist initiation on cycle day 2 or 6. Fertil Steril. 2013;100:867–74.
45. Copperman AB, Benadiva C. Optimal usage of the GnRH antagonists: a review of the literature. Reprod Biol Endocrinol. 2013 Mar 15;11:20. https://doi.org/10.1186/1477-7827-11-20.
46. Gómez R, Soares SR, Busso C, Garcia-Velasco JA, Simón C, Pellicer A. Physiology and pathology of ovarian hyperstimulation syndrome. Semin Reprod Med. 2010 Nov;28(6):448–57. https://doi.org/10.1055/s-0030-1265670.
47. Martinez MC, Ruiz FJ, García-Velasco JA. GnRH-agonist triggering to avoid ovarian hyperstimulation syndrome: a review of the evidence. Curr Drug Targets. 2013 Jul;14(8):843–9.
48. Selman H, Rinaldi L. Effectiveness of corifollitropin alfa used for ovarian stimulation of poor responder patients. Int J Women's Health. 2016;8:609–15.
49. Kol S, Breyzman T, Segal L, Humaidan P. 'Luteal coasting' after GnRH agonist trigger – individualized, HCG-based, progesterone-free luteal support in 'high responders': a case series. Reprod Biomed Online. 2015b Dec;31(6):747–51. https://doi.org/10.1016/j.rbmo.2015.09.001.

Corifollitropin Alfa in Ovarian Stimulation

11

Martina Kollmann, Panagiotis Drakopoulos, and Christophe Blockeel

11.1 Introduction

Protocols to induce a monofollicular or multifollicular response in women undergoing controlled ovarian stimulation (COS) commonly rely on follicular stimulating hormone (FSH) injections. Some decades ago, the purification of gonadotrophin from human menopausal urine, which contained FSH and luteinizing hormone (LH), has been described [1]. The use of specific monoclonal antibodies, which bind FSH or LH molecules in human menopausal gonadotrophin (hMG), leads to the availability of urinary (u) FSH. Further purification of hMG minimized the activity of LH by immunoaffinity chromatography and resulted in a higher purified FSH.

A next step was the development of recombinant (rFSH) by transfecting genes into Chinese hamster ovary (CHO) cells which then produce functional molecules [2, 3]. It has been shown that rFSH preparations have analog biological characteristics to those of uFSH preparations [4–8]. In the 1990s the first rFSH products were licensed for marketing, and they are now widely used for infertility treatment. Similar to uFSH, rFSH has to be administered by daily injections to reach steady FSH levels [9].

FSH, LH, human chorionic gonadotropin (hCG), and thyroid stimulating hormone (TSH) belong to a family of glycoproteins that are heterodimers of two subunits (α- and β-subunit). All four hormones have the same α-subunit. The β-subunit is different and determines the biological specificity of each hormone. LH and hCG have a quite similar β-subunit. The unique difference is a carboxy-terminal peptide (CTP) extension of the hCG β-subunit. Studies found that this carboxy-terminal peptide is the key for the long terminal half-life of hCG (24 hours) as compared with that of LH (2 h) [10].

The first reports on the design of a long-acting FSH agonist were published in 1992 [11, 12]. By coupling the CTP of the β-subunit of hCG to the FSH β-subunit, the long-acting FSH (FSH-CTP) was created. Therefore researchers used site-directed mutagenesis and gene transfer techniques [11, 12]. Other attempts to create a longer-acting FSH molecule were made by generating a covalently bound fusion protein containing the common α- and FSH β-subunits separated by the hCG β-CTP, by introducing additional sequences containing potential glycosylation sites at the N-terminus of the FSH α-subunit or by fusion with the constant region fragment domain of immunoglobulin G1 [13–19]. The latter is still subject of further investigation.

11.2 Daily vs Once-a-Week FSH Injection: Mode of Action, Pharmacokinetics, and Pharmacodynamics

(Phase 1–2 trials)

The recombinant fusion protein FSH-CTP, which is called corifollitropin alfa, is again produced by CHO cells. Corifollitropin alfa is composed of four N-linked carbohydrate chains (α52, α78, β7, and β24) and four O-linked carbohydrate chains at the CTP (β115, β121, β126, and β132). The in vivo half-life of corifollitropin is 3–4 times longer than the wild-type FSH, due to the O-linked carbohydrate chains at the CTP [11, 12, 20]. In vitro assembly, secretion, or stimulation of steroidogenesis is not significantly affected by the added CTP sequences [11]. Fares et al. determined the half-life of wild-type FSH and the chimeras after intravenous

The authors consider that the first two authors should be regarded as joint first authors

M. Kollmann
Division of Obstetrics and Maternal Fetal Medicine, Department of Obstetrics and Gynecology, Medical University of Graz, Graz, Austria

P. Drakopoulos · C. Blockeel (✉)
Centre for Reproductive Medicine, Universitair Ziekenhuis Brussel, Vrije Universiteit Brussel, Brussels, Belgium

Department of Obstetrics & Gynaecology, School of Medicine of the University of Zagreb, Zagreb, Croatia
e-mail: christophe.blockeel@uzbrussel.be

G. N. Allahbadia et al. (eds.), *Textbook of Assisted Reproduction*, https://doi.org/10.1007/978-981-15-2377-9_11

(IV) injection of 10 international units (IU) of dimers in immature female rats' in vivo [11]. The biopotencies were examined by investigating ovarian weight augmentation and granulosa cell aromatase induction. Chimera-treated rats were found to have significantly increased ovarian weight and 3–5-fold increased estrogen production by granulosa cells as compared with wild-type FSH treated rats [11]. The group further examined the derivative containing two CTP units (FSH-CTP_2) but found no significant difference between the FSH-CTP and FSH-CTP_2 [11]. Granulosa cell differentiation and follicle ovulatory potential with FSH-CTP and FSH-CTP_2 were compared [12]. Immature female rats were given FSH or the agonist injections at 0 and 24 hours injections following estrogen-priming. 48 h later, 1.0 and 3.0 IU/day FSH-CTP or FSH-CTP_2 treated rats had up to 2.5-fold increase in ovarian weight, whereas a higher dose (10 IU/day) of wild-type FSH was associated with a 1.8-fold stimulation [12]. Granulosa cell aromatase activity and LH receptor induction were almost increased by a factor of 10 with FSH-CTPs as compared with wild-type FHS. Granulosa cell aromatase activity and LH receptor content were increased in a dose-dependent manner between doses of 1 and 10 IU of FSH-CTP [12]. They further tested the ovulatory potential of ovarian follicles and showed that a single injection of FSH-CTP adequately stimulated follicle maturation, and ovulation could be induced by hCG 52 hours later. On the contrary, while a single 10 IU injection of wild-type FSH was inadequate to increase ovulatory potential, the same total dose of wild-type FSH, administered as four 2.5-IU injections 12 h apart, was similarly effective as FSH-CTP [12]. Authors conclude that sustained blood levels of FSH in stimulating follicle maturation seem to be more important than the total dose of FSH. Additionally, the study revealed that subcutaneous (s.c.) and intraperitoneal (i.p.) administration provided similar ovulatory potential [12].

The first report of human exposure to FSH-CTP (corifollitropin alpha, Org 36,286) was published in 2001 by Bouloux et al. [21]. Thirteen hypogonadotrophic hypogonadal male subjects received 15 μg FSH-CTP four times with an interval of around 4 weeks between each injection. The elimination half-life ($t_{1/2}$) of FSH-CTP was increased 2–3 times compared to rFSH [21]. In an open-label trial, Duijkers and colleagues investigated the pharmacokinetic and pharmacodynamic properties of FSH-CTP (corifollitropin alpha, Org 36,286) in healthy female volunteers [22]. A single dose of 15, 30, and 60 μg FSH-CTP was injected s.c. to 24 subjects, and 7 of these 24 subjects were subsequently treated with a single dose of 120 μg FSH-CTP. Maximum FSH-CTP concentrations were reached between 36 and 48 h after injection and $t_{1/2}$ ranged from 60 to 75 h [22]. Those findings were dose independent within the dose range tested. The maximum serum concentration of corifollitropin alpha increased with the dose injected [22]. The first live birth after ovarian stimulation using FSH-CTP was reported in 2003 [23]. To investigate whether a low dosage of corifollitropin alfa could be administered for ovulation induction in anovulatory patients, a trial was conducted in women with World Health Organization group II anovulatory infertility [24]. A single low dose of corifollitropin was able to induce one or more follicles to grow up to ovulatory sizes, but the anovulatory status was not reversed because the incidence of subsequent (mono)ovulations was low [24].

Two phase II trials of corifollitropin alfa have been performed in women undergoing ovarian stimulation for IVF or ICSI using single doses of 120–240 μg [20] and of 60–180 μg [25]. The first study randomized 98 subjects to receive a single dose of 120 μg, 180 μg, and 240 μg corifollitropin alfa (FSH-CTP) or to start daily fixed doses of 150 IU rFSH [20]. Patients who received a single dose of corifollitropin alfa continued 1 week after injection with fixed doses of 150 IU rFSH until the day of hCG administration. $T_{1/2}$ for all three FSH-CTP doses tested was approximately 65 hours. No differences were detected between the four groups in regard to the number of follicles of at least 11 mm, 15 mm, and 17 mm, respectively, at the day of triggering final oocyte maturation [20]. The median duration of stimulation was 10 days in the corifollitropin alfa groups and 9 days in the daily rFSH group. A premature LH rise occurred with a similar incidence in all groups. The mean number of recovered oocytes recovered per started cycle tended to be higher in subjects treated with corifollitropin compared with rFSH-treated subjects. However, equal numbers of embryos were available for embryo transfer [20]. In a study performed by the "Corifollitropin Alfa Dose-finding Study Group," women undergoing controlled ovarian stimulation for IVF or ICSI were randomized to a single dose of 60 μg, 120 μg, and 180 μg corifollitropin alfa (FSH-CTP) or to start daily fixed doses of 150 IU rFSH [25]. Similar to the previous study, 150 IU rFSH injections daily were given to the corifollitropin group after 1 week until hCG administration. Patients received gonadotropin releasing hormone (GnRH) antagonists from stimulation day 5 until triggering final oocyte maturation [25]. Maximum serum concentrations of corifollitropin alfa were dose-proportional within the range 60–180 μg. Mean $t_{1/2}$ was 65–66 hours and dose independent. The study reports that the corifollitropin alfa exposure showed an inverse relationship with body weight. Body weight was found to be an important covariate of clearance and volume of distribution. On day 8, the mean number of follicles ≥11 mm showed a dose-related increase ($p < 0.001$) and was 6.8 (standard deviation [26] 4.4), 10.1 (6.1), and 12.8 (7.5) in the 60, 120, and 180 μg groups, respectively. The number of cumulus–oocyte complexes recovered points also to a clear dose–response relationship ($p < 0.0001$), being 5.2 (5.5), 10.3 (6.3) and 12.5 (8.0) in the three dose groups, respectively. Ongoing pregnancy rates per started cycle were 15, 16, 14, and 14% in the 60, 120, 180 μg, and 150 IU groups, respectively.

11.3 Corifollitropin Alpha and Ovarian Stimulation (Phase 3 and 4 Trials)

11.3.1 Normal Responders

Large randomized trials in women with normal ovarian response demonstrated good reproductive outcomes following stimulation with corifollitropin alfa. In particular, the Engage [27], Ensure [28], and Pursue [29] trials conducted in women undergoing ovarian stimulation in a GnRH antagonist protocol showed that corifollitropin alfa was equivalent or non-inferior to rFSH in terms of number of oocytes retrieved, pregnancy, and live birth rates. Furthermore, recent data derived from individual patient meta-analysis including the aforementioned RCTs and cumulated data from over 3.000 patients demonstrated that corifollitropin alfa resulted in one additional oocyte, after adjusting for relevant confounders such as age and BMI [30]. However, although the higher oocyte yield was not associated with a higher pregnancy rate, it is a finding that certainly merits caution for clinical practice.

In conclusion, a single dose of corifollitropin alfa for the first 7 days of ovarian stimulation has a similar efficacy compared with seven daily injections of rFSH and may result in one additional oocyte.

11.3.2 Poor Responders

In order to investigate the efficacy of this new gonadotropin in women with poor ovarian response, preliminary, pilot studies have been conducted in this special infertile population. However, although administration of corifollitropin alfa followed by the administration of hMG in an antagonist protocol may indeed offer benefits in terms of pregnancy rates in women <40 years fulfilling the Bologna criteria, results remain low for older women regardless of the protocol used [31–33]. Moreover, the use of a single injection of corifollitropin alfa in an antagonist setting in women with poor ovarian response, who usually represent patients undergoing multiple cycles of IVF, may help in reducing the burden associated with treatment and therefore the dropout rate.

11.3.3 High Responders: Risk for OHSS

Ovarian hyperstimulation syndrome (OHHS) is a potentially lethal iatrogenic complication of ovarian stimulation. Even if the introduction of GnRH antagonist protocol was a landmark in assisted reproduction, given that OHSS rate could be significantly decreased by GnRH antagonist use [34], mild to moderate OHSS may still occur. However, results from the previous RCTs are reassuring, showing that the incidence of OHSS remains low and similar between corifollitropin alfa and rFSH [30]. In addition, even if the previous studies included normal responders and excluded women with known risk factors for low or high response, there is evidence that ongoing pregnancy rates of patients showing high response following administration of corifollitropin alfa are not affected [35]. Furthermore, high response as reflected by a higher number of oocytes retrieved is associated with increased cumulative live birth rates, which is the most meaningful outcomes for infertile patients [36].

The "freeze-all" strategy with the segmentation of IVF treatment, mainly with the use of a GnRH antagonist protocol, GnRH agonist triggering, the cryopreservation of embryos, and frozen-warmed embryo transfer in a subsequent cycle, is an alternative and effective option to virtually eliminate OHSS [37].

11.4 Predictors of Ovarian Response to Corifollitropin Alfa

A number of biomarkers have been used to predict response to ovarian stimulation, with AMH being reported the best predictor [38]. While there is an extensive literature in ovarian response prediction by AMH, only three studies in predicting ovarian response of women stimulated with corifollitropin alfa have been reported [39–41]. Based on these results, AMH was the best predictor to discriminate patients with high (more than18 oocytes) or low response (less than 6 oocytes) in a fixed GnRH antagonist protocol, demonstrating high sensitivity and specificity. It seems that patients with an AMH between 0.9 and 2.6 ng/ml measured in the GenII AMH assay are highly unlikely to demonstrate an extreme response to corifollitropin alfa.

11.5 Safety Aspects

No antibodies against FSH-CTP or CHO-derived proteins could have been identified, and measurements of local tolerance demonstrated that s.c. administration is well tolerated. No increase in intensity of injection-site responses was observed after repeated exposure to FSH-CTP [20–22, 25]. During phase I studies, no serious adverse events (SAE) were observed and none of the subjects discontinued the investigations due to adverse events (AE) [21, 22]. Reported adverse events across phase II trials were bleeding after oocyte retrieval, ectopic pregnancy, OHSS, headache, and pelvic pain [20, 25]. A meta-analysis of four RCTs reports that OHSS incidence varied from 5 to 6% in the FSH-CTP group and from 1 to 8% in the rFSH group (odds ratio [OR] 1.27, 95% confidence interval [CI] 0.72–2.22) [42].

11.6 Conclusion

IVF and ICSI treatment adds to a significant physical, psychological, and emotional burden in infertile patients, and psychological distress is one of the main reasons for discontinuation of fertility treatment [43–47]. Hence, a more simplified treatment approach helps those couples enormously, and the development of a single injection which can initiate and sustain multiple follicular growth for an entire week can reduce the burden of infertility treatment. Corifollitropin alfa is an effective treatment option for potential normal responder patients undergoing controlled ovarian stimulation with GnRH antagonist co-treatment for IVF or ICSI [27, 42].

References

1. Donini P, Puzzuoli D, Montezemolo R. Purification of Gonadotrophin from human menopausal urine. Acta Endocrinol. 1964;45:321–8.
2. Keene JL, Matzuk MM, Otani T, Fauser BC, Galway AB, Hsueh AJ, et al. Expression of biologically active human follitropin in Chinese hamster ovary cells. J Biol Chem. 1989;264(9):4769–75.
3. Matzuk MM, Boime I. Mutagenesis and gene transfer define site-specific roles of the gonadotropin oligosaccharides. Biol Reprod. 1989;40(1):48–53.
4. Mannaerts B, de Leeuw R, Geelen J, Van Ravestein A, Van Wezenbeek P, Schuurs A, et al. Comparative in vitro and in vivo studies on the biological characteristics of recombinant human follicle-stimulating hormone. Endocrinology. 1991;129(5):2623–30.
5. Hård K, Mekking A, Damm JB, Kamerling JP, de Boer W, Wijnands RA, et al. Isolation and structure determination of the intact sialylated N-linked carbohydrate chains of recombinant human follitropin expressed in Chinese hamster ovary cells. Eur J Biochem. 1990;193(1):263–71.
6. de Leeuw R, Mulders J, Voortman G, Rombout F, Damm J, Kloosterboer L. Structure-function relationship of recombinant follicle stimulating hormone (Puregon). Mol Hum Reprod. 1996;2(5):361–9.
7. Olijve W, de Boer W, Mulders JW, van Wezenbeek PM. Molecular biology and biochemistry of human recombinant follicle stimulating hormone (Puregon). Mol Hum Reprod. 1996;2(5):371–82.
8. Mannaerts B, Shoham Z, Schoot D, Bouchard P, Harlin J, Fauser B, et al. Single-dose pharmacokinetics and pharmacodynamics of recombinant human follicle-stimulating hormone (org 32489*) in gonadotropin-deficient volunteers. Fertil Steril. 1993;59(1):108–14.
9. Schoot DC, Harlin J, Shoham Z, Mannaerts BM, Lahlou N, Bouchard P, et al. Recombinant human follicle-stimulating hormone and ovarian response in gonadotrophin-deficient women. Hum Reprod. 1994;9(7):1237–42.
10. Matzuk MM, Hsueh AJ, Lapolt P, Tsafriri A, Keene JL, Boime I. The biological role of the carboxyl-terminal extension of human chorionic gonadotropin [corrected] beta-subunit. Endocrinology. 1990;126(1):376–83.
11. Fares FA, Suganuma N, Nishimori K, LaPolt PS, Hsueh AJ, Boime I. Design of a long-acting follitropin agonist by fusing the C-terminal sequence of the chorionic gonadotropin beta subunit to the follitropin beta subunit. Proc Natl Acad Sci U S A. 1992;89(10):4304–8.
12. LaPolt PS, Nishimori K, Fares FA, Perlas E, Boime I, Hsueh AJ. Enhanced stimulation of follicle maturation and ovulatory potential by long acting follicle-stimulating hormone agonists with extended carboxyl-terminal peptides. Endocrinology. 1992;131(6):2514–20.
13. Ben-Menahem D, Boime I. Converting heterodimeric gonadotropins to genetically linked single chains: new approaches to structure activity relationships and analogue design. Trends Endocrinol Metab. 1996;7(3):100–5.
14. Sugahara T, Sato A, Kudo M, Ben-Menahem D, Pixley MR, Hsueh AJ, et al. Expression of biologically active fusion genes encoding the common alpha subunit and the follicle-stimulating hormone beta subunit. Role of a linker sequence. J Biol Chem. 1996;271(18):10445–8.
15. Klein J, Lobel L, Pollak S, Ferin M, Xiao E, Sauer M, et al. Pharmacokinetics and pharmacodynamics of single-chain recombinant human follicle-stimulating hormone containing the human chorionic gonadotropin carboxyterminal peptide in the rhesus monkey. Fertil Steril. 2002;77(6):1248–55.
16. Perlman S, van den Hazel B, Christiansen J, Gram-Nielsen S, Jeppesen CB, Andersen KV, et al. Glycosylation of an N-terminal extension prolongs the half-life and increases the in vivo activity of follicle stimulating hormone. J Clin Endocrinol Metab. 2003;88(7):3227–35.
17. Dumont JA, Low SC, Peters RT, Bitonti AJ. Monomeric fc fusions: impact on pharmacokinetic and biological activity of protein therapeutics. BioDrugs. 2006;20(3):151–60.
18. Low SC, Nunes SL, Bitonti AJ, Dumont JA. Oral and pulmonary delivery of FSH-fc fusion proteins via neonatal fc receptor-mediated transcytosis. Hum Reprod. 2005;20(7):1805–13.
19. Klein J, Lobel L, Pollak S, Lustbader B, Ogden RT, Sauer MV, et al. Development and characterization of a long-acting recombinant hFSH agonist. Hum Reprod. 2003;18(1):50–6.
20. Devroey P, Fauser BC, Platteau P, Beckers NG, Dhont M, Mannaerts BM. Induction of multiple follicular development by a single dose of long-acting recombinant follicle-stimulating hormone (FSH-CTP, corifollitropin alfa) for controlled ovarian stimulation before in vitro fertilization. J Clin Endocrinol Metab. 2004;89(5):2062–70.
21. Bouloux PM, Handelsman DJ, Jockenhövel F, Nieschlag E, Rabinovici J, Frasa WL, et al. First human exposure to FSH-CTP in hypogonadotrophic hypogonadal males. Hum Reprod. 2001;16(8):1592–7.
22. Duijkers IJ, Klipping C, Boerrigter PJ, Machielsen CS, De Bie JJ, Voortman G. Single dose pharmacokinetics and effects on follicular growth and serum hormones of a long-acting recombinant FSH preparation (FSH-CTP) in healthy pituitary-suppressed females. Hum Reprod. 2002;17(8):1987–93.
23. Beckers NG, Macklon NS, Devroey P, Platteau P, Boerrigter PJ, Fauser BC. First live birth after ovarian stimulation using a chimeric long-acting human recombinant follicle-stimulating hormone (FSH) agonist (recFSH-CTP) for in vitro fertilization. Fertil Steril. 2003;79(3):621–3.
24. Balen AH, Mulders AG, Fauser BC, Schoot BC, Renier MA, Devroey P, et al. Pharmacodynamics of a single low dose of long-acting recombinant follicle-stimulating hormone (FSH-carboxy terminal peptide, corifollitropin alfa) in women with World Health Organization group II anovulatory infertility. J Clin Endocrinol Metab. 2004;89(12):6297–304.
25. Group CAD-fS. A randomized dose-response trial of a single injection of corifollitropin alfa to sustain multifollicular growth during controlled ovarian stimulation. Hum Reprod. 2008;23(11):2484–92.
26. Aad G, Abajyan T, Abbott B, Abdallah J, Abdel Khalek S, Abdelalim AA, et al. Observation of associated near-side and away-side long-range correlations in sqrt[s(NN)]=5.02 TeV proton-lead collisions with the ATLAS detector. Phys Rev Lett. 2013;110(18):182302.
27. Devroey P, Boostanfar R, Koper NP, Mannaerts BM, Ijzerman-Boon PC, Fauser BC, et al. A double-blind, non-inferiority RCT

comparing corifollitropin alfa and recombinant FSH during the first seven days of ovarian stimulation using a GnRH antagonist protocol. Hum Reprod. 2009;24(12):3063–72.
28. Corifollitropin alfa Ensure Study G. Corifollitropin alfa for ovarian stimulation in IVF: a randomized trial in lower-body-weight women. Reprod Biomed Online. 2010;21(1):66–76.
29. Boostanfar R, Shapiro B, Levy M, Rosenwaks Z, Witjes H, Stegmann BJ, et al. Large, comparative, randomized double-blind trial confirming noninferiority of pregnancy rates for corifollitropin alfa compared with recombinant follicle-stimulating hormone in a gonadotropin-releasing hormone antagonist controlled ovarian stimulation protocol in older patients undergoing in vitro fertilization. Fertil Steril. 2015;104(1):94–103.e1
30. Griesinger G, Boostanfar R, Gordon K, Gates D, McCrary Sisk C, Stegmann BJ. Corifollitropin alfa versus recombinant follicle-stimulating hormone: an individual patient data meta-analysis. Reprod Biomed Online. 2016;33(1):56–60.
31. Polyzos NP, De Vos M, Corona R, Vloeberghs V, Ortega-Hrepich C, Stoop D, et al. Addition of highly purified HMG after corifollitropin alfa in antagonist-treated poor ovarian responders: a pilot study. Hum Reprod. 2013;28(5):1254–60.
32. Polyzos NP, Corona R, Van De Vijver A, Blockeel C, Drakopoulos P, Vloeberghs V, et al. Corifollitropin alfa followed by hpHMG in GnRH agonist protocols. Two prospective feasibility studies in poor ovarian responders. Gynecol Endocrinol. 2015;31(11):885–90.
33. Polyzos NP, Devos M, Humaidan P, Stoop D, Ortega-Hrepich C, Devroey P, et al. Corifollitropin alfa followed by rFSH in a GnRH antagonist protocol for poor ovarian responder patients: an observational pilot study. Fertil Steril. 2013;99(2):422–6.
34. Mourad S, Brown J, Farquhar C. Interventions for the prevention of OHSS in ART cycles: an overview of Cochrane reviews. Cochrane Database Syst Rev. 2017;1:CD012103.
35. Fatemi HM, Doody K, Griesinger G, Witjes H, Mannaerts B. High ovarian response does not jeopardize ongoing pregnancy rates and increases cumulative pregnancy rates in a GnRH-antagonist protocol. Hum Reprod. 2013;28(2):442–52.
36. Drakopoulos P, Blockeel C, Stoop D, Camus M, de Vos M, Tournaye H, et al. Conventional ovarian stimulation and single embryo transfer for IVF/ICSI. How many oocytes do we need to maximize cumulative live birth rates after utilization of all fresh and frozen embryos? Hum Reprod. 2016;31(2):370–6.
37. Blockeel C, Drakopoulos P, Santos-Ribeiro S, Polyzos NP, Tournaye H. A fresh look at the freeze-all protocol: a SWOT analysis. Hum Reprod. 2016;31(3):491–7.
38. Broer SL, Dolleman M, van Disseldorp J, Broeze KA, Opmeer BC, Bossuyt PM, et al. Prediction of an excessive response in in vitro fertilization from patient characteristics and ovarian reserve tests and comparison in subgroups: an individual patient data meta-analysis. Fertil Steril. 2013;100(2):420–9. e7
39. Polyzos NP, Tournaye H, Guzman L, Camus M, Nelson SM. Predictors of ovarian response in women treated with corifollitropin alfa for in vitro fertilization/intracytoplasmic sperm injection. Fertil Steril. 2013;100(2):430–7.
40. Lerman T, Depenbusch M, Schultze-Mosgau A, von Otte S, Scheinhardt M, Koenig I, et al. Ovarian response to 150 microg corifollitropin alfa in a GnRH-antagonist multiple-dose protocol: a prospective cohort study. Reprod Biomed Online. 2017;34(5):534–40.
41. Oehninger S, Nelson SM, Verweij P, Stegmann BJ. Predictive factors for ovarian response in a corifollitropin alfa/GnRH antagonist protocol for controlled ovarian stimulation in IVF/ICSI cycles. Reprod Biol Endocrinol. 2015;13:117.
42. Mahmoud Youssef MA, van Wely M, Aboulfoutouh I, El-Khyat W, van der Veen F, Al-Inany H. Is there a place for corifollitropin alfa in IVF/ICSI cycles? A systematic review and meta-analysis. Fertil Steril. 2012;97(4):876–85.
43. Boivin J, Takefman JE. Impact of the in-vitro fertilization process on emotional, physical and relational variables. Hum Reprod. 1996;11(4):903–7.
44. Olivius C, Friden B, Borg G, Bergh C. Psychological aspects of discontinuation of in vitro fertilization treatment. Fertil Steril. 2004;81(2):276.
45. Olivius C, Friden B, Borg G, Bergh C. Why do couples discontinue in vitro fertilization treatment? A cohort study. Fertil Steril. 2004;81(2):258–61.
46. Rajkhowa M, McConnell A, Thomas GE. Reasons for discontinuation of IVF treatment: a questionnaire study. Hum Reprod. 2006;21(2):358–63.
47. Brandes M, van der Steen JO, Bokdam SB, Hamilton CJ, de Bruin JP, Nelen WL, et al. When and why do subfertile couples discontinue their fertility care? A longitudinal cohort study in a secondary care subfertility population. Hum Reprod. 2009;24(12):3127–35.

12 Transdermal Delivery Systems in Medically Assisted Reproduction

Herbert Zech and Maximilian Murtinger

Controlled ovarian stimulations (COS) are integral parts of most infertility treatments. Several pharmaceuticals are administered via needles. Painless transdermal drug administration represents an attractive alternative to subcutaneous injections—especially for the patients. Needle puncture might be considered to be mild but is often suggested as painful, and for individuals with a high degree of needle phobia, the injection represents an insurmountable obstacle. But even patients who are not afraid of injections need a high level of self-conquest when it comes to self-injecting which is quite common in COS. Moreover, self-injecting bears the danger of incorrect drug administration associated with medical waste and subsequent suboptimal outcomes. Additionally, there is a risk of infection in the case of needle reuse or non-sterile handling. Oral drug administration instead is often not applicable due to PH-dependent decomposition, inactivation and enzymatic cleavage in the gastrointestinal tract, a lack of absorption due to the intestinal barrier and finally the first-pass effect of the liver which could mean that the drug might be prematurely metabolized into inactive products. Though the idea of TDD systems is very innovative, it is definitely not a new one. Almost 90 years ago, Marshall Lockhart had patented a need-free injection device for "jet injection" [1]. However, TDD technology has only really attracted attention in recent years due to high demand and the enormous technical progress made in this field.

12.1 Injection of Fertility Drugs

Fertility drugs encompass various substances including aromatase inhibitors, ovarian stimulation and anti-ovulation drugs, trigger shot substances, downregulation drugs and luteal phase support medications. Most of those drugs are administered either subcutaneously or intramuscularly over an extended period (Table 12.1). This issue will mostly focus on IVF medications administered mainly by traditional injections.

For example, in a gonadotropin releasing hormone agonist (GnRHa) scheme, the pituitary downregulation begins in the luteal phase (usually on day 20–23 of a regular cycle) by injections of GnRH analogues. This can be performed either in the form of daily subcutaneous injections (SCI) or depot injections or using a nasal spray. However, beside irritations of the mucosa of the nasopharynx, the pituitary response to intranasal buserelin applications was often found to be ineffective [2]. For ovarian stimulation, recombinant follicle-stimulating hormone/luteinizing hormone (FSH/LH) preparations or human menopausal gonadotropin (HMG) which encompass urinary FSH/LH isoforms are administered subcutaneously or IM. These drugs are applied to induce multifollicular growth in a conventional IVF therapy and cannot be absorbed orally. Thus, to date, administration by injection cannot be replaced. In a conventional GnRHa long protocol, HMG is usually administered for an average period of 12 days. However, the injection dose required varies from one woman to another and from one cycle to another depending on the woman's age, body weight and ovarian response.

The peptide hormone human chorionic gonadotropin (hCG) mimics the natural LH surge and is usually administered for final trigger ovulation in a GnRH agonist scheme (long or short protocol) or in clomiphene cycles. It releases the egg during ovulation. Thus, hCG is given for final oocyte maturation (meiosis). Human chorionic gonadotropin must be administered as SCI or IM injections.

In a GnRH antagonist protocol, the trigger shot can also be performed—beside using hCG—with GnRH analogues, SCI or IM injections such as leuprorelin (Lupron). Triggering with GnRH analogues in a GnRH antagonist scheme might be indicated for patients with a high risk of developing ovarian hyperstimulation syndrome (OHSS).

Proper luteal function is essential to achieve embryo implantation and an intact pregnancy. However, it is well

H. Zech · M. Murtinger (✉)
IVF Centers, Bregenz, Austria
e-mail: m.murtinger@ivf.at

G. N. Allahbadia et al. (eds.), *Textbook of Assisted Reproduction*, https://doi.org/10.1007/978-981-15-2377-9_12

Table 12.1 Overview of some fertility drugs being administered

Substance	Brand names	Route of administration	Systematic name (IUPAC)	Molecular function	Molecular mass/molar mass[a]
Most common medications in infertility treatment					
Downregulation					
Buserelin	Metrelef® Suprefact® CinnaFact®	SCI/nasally	(2S)-N-[(2S)-1-[[(2S)-1-[[(2S)-1-[[(2S)-1-[[(2R)-1-[[(2S)-1-[[(2S)-5-(diaminomethylideneamino)-1-[(2S)-2-(ethylcarbamoyl) pyrrolidin-1-yl]-1-oxopentan-2-yl]amino]-4-methyl-1-oxopentan-2-yl] amino]-3-[(2-methylpropan-2-yl) oxy]-1-oxopropan-2-yl] amino]-3-(4-hydroxyphenyl)-1-oxopropan-2-yl]amino]-3-hydroxy-1-oxopropan-2-yl] amino]-3-(1H-indol-3-yl)-1-oxopropan-2-yl] amino]-3-(1H-imidazol-5-yl)-1-oxopropan-2-yl]-5-oxopyrrolidine-2-carboxamide	Analogue of gonadotropin-releasing hormone suppressing FSH and LH prior stimulation	1239.42 g/Mol
Triptorelin	Decapeptyl® Diphereline™- Gonapepty®l	IM	5-oxo-D-prolyl-L-histidyl-Ltryptophyl-L-seryl-Ltyrosyl-3-(1H-indol-2-yl)-L-alanylleucyl-L-arginyl-L-prolylglycinamide	Analogue of gonadotropin-releasing hormone suppressing FSH and LH prior stimulation	1311.5 g/Mol
Ovarian stimulating drugs					
Human menopausal gonadotropin (hMG) urinary FSH rFSH	Menogon® Merional® Menopur® Fostimon®	IM/SCI	Mixture of different gonadotropins (FSH/LH)	Stimulates the growth and recruitment of immature follicles Luteinizing hormone (LH) initiates follicular growth or triggers ovulation	Follicle-stimulating hormone (FSH): 35.5 kDa LH: Approx. 30 kDa
Aromatase inhibitor					
Lentrozole	Femara®	Orally	4,4′-((1H-1,2,4-triazol-1-yl) methylene)dibenzonitrile		285.303 g/Mol
Selective oestrogen receptor modulator					
Clomiphene (citrate)	Clomid®	Orally	(E,Z)-2-(4-(2-chloro-1,2-diphenylethenyl) phenoxy)-N,N-diethyl-ethanamine	Oestrogen receptor modulating, induction of ovulation	406 or 598.10 g/Mol, respectively
Anti-ovulation					
Cetrorelix acetate	Cetrotide®	SCI	Acetyl-D-3-(2′-naphtyl)-alanine-D-4-chlorophenylalanine-D-3-(3′-pyridyl)- alanine-L-serine-L-tyrosine-D-citrulline-L-leucine-L-arginine-L-proline-D-alanine-amide	GnRH antagonist	1431.06 g/Mol
Ganirelix acetate	Antagon™		(2S)-1-[(2S)-2-[[(2S)-2-[[(2R)-2-[[(2R)-2-[[(2S)-2-[[(2R)-2-[[(2R)-2-[[(2R)-2-acetamido-3-naphthalen-2-ylpropanoyl] amino]-3-(4-chlorophenyl) propanoyl]amino]-3-pyridin-3-ylpropanoyl]amino]-3-hydroxypropanoyl] amino]-3-(4-hydroxyphenyl) propanoyl]amino]-6-[bis(ethylamino) methylideneamino]hexanoyl] amino]-4-methylpentanoyl] amino]-6-[bis(ethylamino) methylideneamino]hexanoyl]-N-[(2R)-1-amino-1-oxopropan-2-yl] pyrrolidine-2-carboxamide	Prevention of premature ovulation	1570.4 g/Mol

Table 12.1 (continued)

Most common medications in infertility treatment					
Substance	Brand names	Route of administration	Systematic name (IUPAC)	Molecular function	Molecular mass/ molar mass[a]
Trigger shot (induction of ovulation)					
Human chorionic gonadotropin (hCG)	Predalon®, Novarel®, Ovidrel®, Pregnyl®, Profasi®, Chorigon®, Choron-10®	SCI / IM			Approx. 26 kDa
Busrelin [b]	See downregulation				
Decapeptyl[b]	See downregulation				
Luteal phase support					
Progesterone	Pro-gest®, Prontogest®, Prometrium®, Crinone®	IM/vaginally	Pregn-4-ene-3,20-dione		314.46 g/Mol

[a]Molar mass is given in g/mol, molecular mass is given in Dalton (Da), 1 kDa = 1.66 × 10–21 g
[b]in GnRH antagonist scheme only
SCI, subcutaneous injection; *IM*, intramuscular

established that luteal function is compromised in COS cycles [3]. To avoid luteal phase defects, mostly progesterone (P) is administered orally, vaginally or by IM [4]. Nevertheless, the effectiveness of orally administered progesterone is clearly inferior to its intramuscular or vaginal administration [5], while the best results can still be obtained by injecting P (Agolutin, Prontogest).

12.2 The Skin as a Natural Barrier

As mentioned earlier, TDD is mostly limited due to the functional nature of the skin. Beside water resistance, thermoregulation, storage and sensory functions, the human skin has a protective function representing an anatomical barrier for pathogens, certain radiations and harmful chemical agents. The human skin consists of the *epidermis*, the *dermis* and the *hypodermis*. What is most important here is that the outermost sublayer (*strata*) of the *epidermis*, the *stratum corneum* (SC), forms the main barrier to penetration (Fig. 12.1). The thickness of the SC varies throughout the body (10–40 μm). SC represents a two-compartment system consisting of (1) 12–200 cell layers of death corneocytes, containing the fibrous structural protein keratin and (2) the intercellular matrix, predominantly composed of neutral lipids that determine its hydrophobic character.

In principle, there are two (or three, when considering the follicular route) possibilities of TDD: (1) through the skin either intercellular through the intercellular space or (2) transcellular (Fig. 12.2). The effectiveness of noninvasive TDD is also determined by the use of potent enhancers (see transdermal patches, sprays and gels).

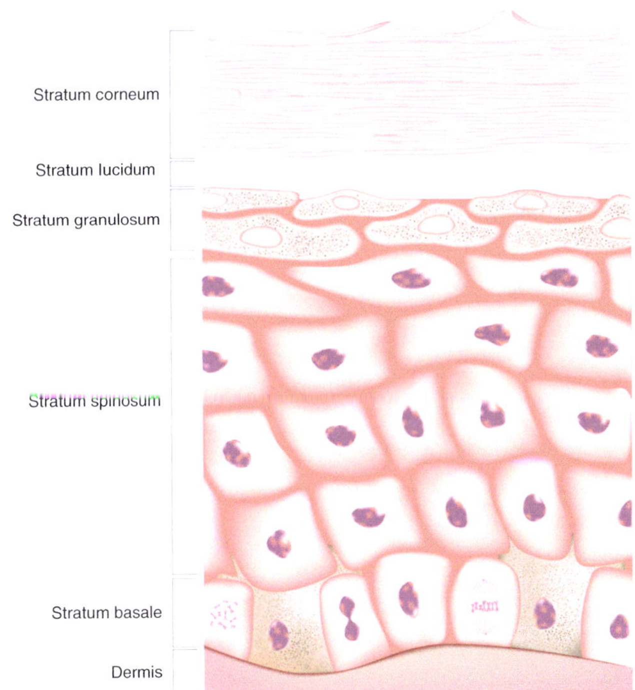

Fig. 12.1 Schematic diagram of the human epidermis

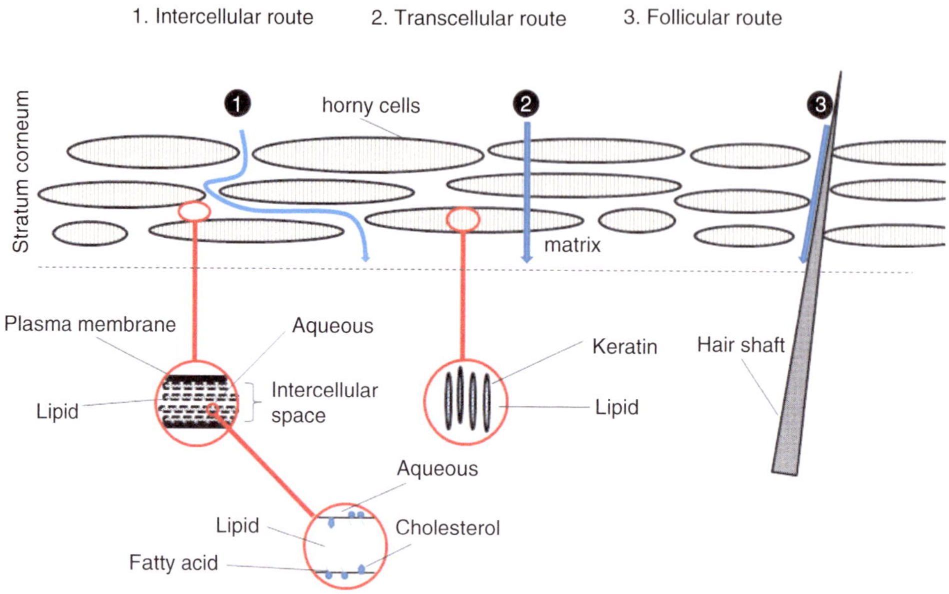

Fig. 12.2 Simplified scheme of the SC and route diagram of transdermal drug penetration

12.3 Factors Affecting the Skin Permeation

As a matter of fact, TDD within the scope of medically assisted reproduction (MAR) is still limited. This is due to various reasons. First, reproductive medicine is a relatively new medical research field and has only gained in importance during the last two decades, however, with a strong increasing tendency with respect to global demand. Second, TDD is usually restricted to the application of a few substances depending on their molecular weight (ideally <0.6 kDa or even lower), a high lipophilicity and, last but not least, their ability to be effective at relative low and variable doses. Most importantly, the drug must not contain any irritant substances or cause an immune (allergic) response in the skin. The success of TDD also depends on the route of permeation. And one of the biggest challenges of TDD systems is—without any doubt—the inter- and intra-individual variations in the skin penetration of the drug, up to 45% [6].

12.4 The Advantage of Transdermal Drug Delivery in MAR

The greatest advantage of TDD is its noninvasive nature and the associated easiness of self-medication. Noninvasive or minimally invasive transdermal drug administration is undoubtedly an interesting alternative to SCI injections. However, in regard to TDD systems for IVF drugs, the published data are still limited (Table 12.2). Most studies cover TDD of the steroids testosterone (T) and oestrogen (E2.). These substances are lipophilic with low molecular weight and thus much more comfortable for TDD.

Embryo implantation is limited to proper endometrial buildup. Although the role of E2 in regulating endometrial growth remains still elusive, it is required to build up a sufficiently thick endometrium. The E2 administration is mainly indicated in clomiphene cycles due to the E2 antagonist properties of clomiphene.

In fact, the first IVF drugs administered by TDD were E2 and T.

E2 and T are, however, small molecules and have low molecular weight. These facts facilitated the development of transdermal E2 and T delivery systems [7]. One big advantage of TDD of E2 compared to other administration routes is the avoidance of metabolization and inactivation in the intestine and liver [8]. Meanwhile, there are dozens of review articles published in the Medline database concerning the TDD of E2, indicating the importance of this issue. A recently published RCT compared the IVF outcome of oral and transdermal E2 administration in frozen-thawed embryo transfer [9]. Although there was a significant difference in E2 concentration on the day of P administration, pregnancy rates were similar for those two administration routes.

Androgens such as T have been shown to play a key role in the physiology of the ovaries. Recently, attempts have been made to improve ovarian response in patients who are found to be poor responders by androgen supplementation including dehydroepiandrosterone (DHEA) and T [10]. Whether or not and to what extent this approach can be really purposeful is beyond the scope of this chapter, but in fact, TDD of T is gaining more and more importance [11]. Within the scope of T administration, there are more studies in the medical database using TDD of T instead of oral application.

Table 12.2 Published applications of TDD systems related to ART

Author	PMID	Application system	Substance	Brand
Bosdou et al., (2016)	26,956,551	Gel	Testosterone	Tostran®
Davar et al., (2016)	27,141,464	Transdermal patch	Oestrogen	Not given
Malinovskaja et al., (2014)	25,173,088	Iontophoresis	Leuprorelin	Smopex®
Kim et al., (2014)	25,949,183	Gel	Testosterone	Testogel®
Zech et al., (2011)	21,497,348	Laser-assisted (Er/YAG laser)	Urinary FSH	P.L.E.A.S.E.® laser microporation device
Ata et al., (2011)	21,495,800	Transdermal patch	Oestrogen	Climara®
Kim et al., (2011)	20,801,436	Gel	Testosterone	Testogel®
Fábregues et al., (2009)	19,054,777	Transdermal patch	Testosterone	Androderm®
Solnica et al., (2009)	19,356,750	JET	rFSH	Biojector® 2000
Lavery et al., (2008)	18,166,182	JET	rFSH	J-tip needle-free injection system
Serna et al., (2008)	18,191,847	Transdermal patch	Oestrogen	Estraderm matrix®
Massin et al. (2006)	16,476,678	Gel	Testosterone	Not given
Balasch et al., (2006)	16,517,559	Transdermal patch	Testosterone	Androderm®

PIMD PubMed identifier

Progesterone (P) administration is crucial in IVF/COS for subsequent luteal phase support. In regard to TDD, however, very few studies have been published leading to highly controversial results. Mostly, the bioavailability of P is low and highly variable, most probably due to cutaneous metabolization by the enzyme 5α-reductase to 5α-dihydroprogesterone [12]. For all other fertility drugs, TDD is mostly experimental, too. TDD for administering therapeutic peptides such as triptorelin is an interesting subject. However, implementation of TDD is still hampered by the high molecular size of the active compounds, especially in the case of TDD for peptides and proteins. Several studies have investigated TDD for GnRH analogues. At present, however, they mostly refer to animal studies and in vitro systems [13, 14].

In the past, however, the results turned out to be somewhat sobering. This might be due to the fact that e.g. there are currently no commercially available transdermal progesterone application systems for IVF [7]. Additionally, due to proteases in the skin layers, opsonization and agglutination, free peptides are often not stable without some modifications or the usage of additives [15]. However, enhancing additives, in turn, might negatively influence drug stability [16] or drug efficiency.

TDD of ovarian stimulation hormones might be regarded as one of the most prestigious issues due to the high molecular weight of gonadotropins and the risk of losing structural integrity and thus protein function. Due to short half-life (and rapid metabolic clearance) of administered gonadotropins, daily administrations are required. Facing the fact that the stratum corneum is an almost insurmountable barrier for high molecular weight substances, a minimal invasive technique is, without any doubt, indispensable for transdermal peptide and protein delivery. In fact, the development of new generation TDD systems even allowed the transdermal pass of proteins using a novel and innovative laser technology [17]. Recently, the first pregnancy after IVF involving COS with TDD of urinary FSH using a laser microporation-based TDD technology was achieved [18]. This approach might end up revolutionizing COS processes in MAR.

12.5 Systems for (Improved) Transdermal Delivery Systems

Current efforts to improve TDD involve the alternation of drug composition or molecular changes to the active substance to enhance skin permeability without altering medical efficacy and the development of sophisticated innovations in the area of TDD systems. Meanwhile, several skin-permeabilizing techniques have been described and investigated, and a confusing number of combined methods and protocols are known to us today. The most commonly used methods and approaches are given in Table 12.3 and are described briefly below.

12.5.1 Transdermal Patches, Sprays and Gels and Enhancers

One of first TDD systems was a 3-day patch for scopolamine to treat motion sickness (Novartis Consumer Health, Parsippany, NJ). The system was approved for use in the United States in 1979 [19]. In transdermal patches the drug is usually stored in a reservoir that is surrounded on one side by an impermeable backside and an adhesive for skin contact on the other [20]. This system, however, is limited to extremely stable lipophilic and low-molecular drugs such as E2 or T that are effective even at low doses and/or

Table 12.3 Overview of the (dis)advantages of different TDD systems

Type of TDD	Time-consuming	Invasive	Intact stratum corneum mandatory	Painful	Applicable for high molecular mass drugs	Risk of impairment of surrounding tissue	Drug release control
Patches/gels/sprays	Yes	No	No	No	No	No	Poor
Enhancers	Yes	No	No	No	Extremely limited	No	Poor
JET injection	No	Minimal	No	Sometimes	Yes	Yes	Poor
Microneedles	No	Minimal	No	No	Yes	No	Good
Electroporation	No	Minimal	Yes	Sometimes	Limited	Yes	Fair
Iontophoresis	Yes	Minimal	Yes	Sometimes	Limited	Yes	Fair
Sonophoresis	Yes	Minimal	Yes	Sometimes	Limited	Yes	Fair
Laser-assisted TDD (P.L.E.A.S.E®)	No	Minimal	No	No	Yes	No	Excellent

with varying TDD. The same holds true for other simple, non-skin perforating systems such as liquid sprays and gels. In such systems transdermal drug passage takes place in a passive way.

In order to expand the scope of application to other, less skin permeable substances, the second generation of TDD systems contain(ed) (bio-)chemical enhancers to alter the skin permeability especially of the SC. An optimal enhancer should work rapidly and its effect should be reproducible. Meanwhile, there are hundreds of enhancers and thousands of combination preparations known to increase skin permeability—in general, amphiphilic substances with saturated carbon rings or chains [21]. The best known chemical enhancers are urea, propylene glycol (PG), Azone (1-dodecy lazacycloheptan-2-one), SEPA I (2-nonyl-1,3-dioxolane) or SLS (sodium lauryl sulphate). The problem with enhancers is that they must considerably increase the permeability of the SC without having skin-irritating, allergic or even toxic side effects. However, for many chemical enhancers, the underlying mechanisms of action have often remained unclear, and, in consequence, some hazardous side effects have still remained unclarified. Newer generations of enhancers such as liposomes or microemulsions do not only enhance the TDD but additionally increase the solubilization and partitioning of the drug. The use of biochemical enhancers is still experimental. They encompass special peptides, also known as peptide facilitators with pore-forming properties—a new approach in TDD [22].

12.5.2 Pressure-Driven JET Injections

Beside the application of transdermal patches, this technique is the most ancient technique. For several vaccinations, jet injectors have been used for decades. The principle behind it is quite simple: the drugs (liquid or solid formulations) are administered to the skin by high pressure accelerators, for example by using compressed N_2 or CO_2 from a reservoir. In consequence, a high-velocity jet (>100 m/s) penetrates the skin. Interestingly, despite their long-term use, jet injections mostly failed to replace conventional needle injection. The most limiting factor is the inconsistency of penetration, probably due to the skin's mechanical properties that vary from one person to another [23]. Additionally, relatively strong inflammations and bleedings might occur owing to the application [24]. And, in addition, needle-free JET injections are not always pain-free.

A few studies have investigated this TDD system for gonadotropin administration [25, 26]. Although authors reported no differences in regard to the COS outcome, the patients' comfort elucidated by questionnaire was not superior in the group using a needle-free JET injection system (Biojector® 2000) compared to patients using standard needles for gonadotropin administration [25]. This finding and the lack of further studies on this TDD technique emphasize the weaknesses of this system. Moreover, although the application of the Biojector® 2000 device was deemed safe, the pharmaceutical company Roche has withdrawn its application for antiretroviral drug administration to US regulatory authorities. Before, the application of this device was found to cause long-lasting nerve pain in a few patients [27].

12.5.3 Microneedles

In contrast to needles (cannulas), microneedles are only minimally invasive. The use of microneedles (MN) is—due to their shortness - almost painless, since MN only reach the deeper layer of the epidermis but not the dermal nerve endings. MN can be applied as solid (used for pretreatment of the skin followed by the application of a topical cream), coated MN (where the drug is coated over the MN surface), hollow MN (for infusion of higher quantities) and dissolving MN. MN can be made of metal (mainly for solid MN). Their production is quite easy. Silicon has also been used for MN; however, silicon-based MN are expensive and often brittle. Additionally, silicon is not the best material in terms of biocompatibility. Dissolving MN consists of biodegradable polymers such as polylactic acid (PLA), polyglycolic acid (PGA), polycarbonate or many others. Thereby, the dissolvable MN encapsulates the drug (reviewed in [28]).This kind of MN even allows a fairly well-controlled drug release that is determined by the dissolving rate of the MN [29]. The field of biopolymer microstructures is a rapidly growing segment, and the approaches for dissolvable MN are promising. Several MN are now commercially available for vaccination or glucose monitoring in diabetes patients.

12.5.4 Electrical TDD Techniques

Electrical TDD encompasses two techniques: electroporation and Iontophoresis.

12.5.4.1 Electroporation

Electroporation (EP) increases the permeability of the SC by the application of short voltage pulses (µsec—msec). This technique is well known in molecular biological laboratories, e.g. for transfecting cells with DNA, short oligonucleotides or iRNA. For TDD, however, higher voltages (> 50 V) are required. The efficacy of EP-based TDD additionally depends on the shape, amplitude, duration and number of electric pulses, as well as on the distance between electrodes [30]. The mechanism behind this is the disruption of membranes and the formation of aqueous pores in the lipid bilayers and the reversible membrane disruption of the SC. Electroporation has been successfully applied for TDD of even high molecular weight substances including proteins, peptides, polysaccharides and oligonucleotides. One disadvantage consists in the fact that skin properties may change at high voltages. The result might be a nonlinear dependence of influx and voltage.

12.5.4.2 Iontophoresis

TDD by iontophoresis encompasses the application of a low-density current and low

voltage (~0.1–1.0 mA/cm^2) via an electrical circuit constituted by two drug reservoirs

(positively and negatively charged chambers or anode and cathode, respectively) deposited on the skin surface. The suggested mode of action consists of electroosmosic and electrophoretic or electromigratic effects. The human skin has an isoelectric point of approximately pH 4.5. At a higher pH value, carboxy groups are ionized (COO^-). This results in the attraction and movement of small cations. In final consequence, uncharged molecules are also carried by this flow. Uncharged molecules are moved via this electro-osmosic effect only; however, this force is quite ineffective. Thus, drugs must either have ionic charges or have to be solved in an ionic carrier substance. Ions having the same polarity as the stimulating electrode are repelled into the skin (electrophoretic effect). The advantage of Iontophoresis is the lack of adverse effects in short-term use. Currently, Iontophoresis is mainly used for TDD of lidocaine for local anaesthesia. The iontophoretic TDD, however, is only sufficient for charged molecules [28] and is therefore restricted to molecules with a molecular weight of less than ~10–15 kDa [31]. Additionally, the drawback of this technique is the occasional occurrence of skin irritations and pain caused by the effects of Iontophoresis which are not restricted to the SC [32].

12.5.5 Sonophoresis

This technique can be divided according to the ultrasound (US) used in (1) "high frequency (3–10 MHz) or diagnostic US," (2) "medium frequency" (0.7–3 MHz) or "therapeutic US" and 3) "low frequency" (18 to 100 KHz) or conveniently in cavitating and non-cavitating sonophoresis.

12.5.5.1 Non-cavitating Sonophoresis

Ultrasound (US) is able to disrupt the lipid structure of the SC. The effect is, however, limited to lipophilic substances with a relatively small molecular weight. Using higher-frequency US bears the danger of damaging the deeper tissues.

12.5.5.2 Cavitating Sonophoresis

US is also known to induce oscillating cavities at the skin surface. In consequence, the SC is disrupted, and thus, skin permeability is increased without damaging deeper tissue layers: Cavitation, however, can only be achieved by low-frequency (<1 MHz) US and is directly correlated to US intensity. This enhanced passive transdermal drug transport can increase TDD for substances up to tens of kDa [17]. Other advantages are a strictly controlled TDD without destroying the skin integrity. The disadvantages of this procedure can be found in the fact that it is time-consuming and the results are not always promising. Additionally, irritation and burning of the skin have been reported.

12.5.6 Laser-Assisted TDD

There is no question that the laser-based TDD technologies are the latest, most innovative and most promising approaches in this field. The principle of this technique is based on the laser-based thermal ablation of the SC in terms of micro-pores. The challenge presented by TDD of high molecular substances and controlled drug release can be mastered much better thanks to this technique. However, the first generation of laser-based TDD technology was ineffective due to imprecise SC ablation, meaning more skin irritations, coagulation or inadequate microporation, and, in consequence, limited TDD and drug uptake (Fig. 12.3). However, for laser-assisted TDD, the controllable microporation in depth and size is mandatory. Meanwhile, many types of lasers with a broad wavelength range are commercially available. But in fact, only a few of them are actually suitable for SC ablation. For example, near-infrared (NIR) or CO_2 lasers have only little skin absorption effect compared to erbium-doped yttrium aluminium garnet (Er/YAG) laser systems [32]. Pantec Biosolutions AG (Ruggell, Liechtenstein) has developed a "Precise Laser Epidermal System" (P.L.E.A.S.E.®) device containing a diode-pumped fractional (Er/YAG) laser. This technology was patented in 2009. The P.L.E.A.S.E.® laser can emit short pulses of radiation at the excitation wavelength of H_2O at approximately 2.940 nm. In consequence, laser pulses heat the skin surface causing the H_2O molecules to evaporate rapidly, thereby creating micropores with a diameter of ~200 μm in the epidermis by thermolysis. The advantage of this system consists in its short energy pulse which is shorter than the thermal relaxation time of H_2O. Thus, thermal damage of the surrounding tissue can be extremely minimized or even avoided [20, 33]. In contrast to conventional (Er/YAG) laser systems that typically ablate a 7 mm spot on the skin, this technical innovation generates patterns of identical micropores with diameters of 100–150 μm [33]. Moreover, modifications of laser-induced micropores in terms of depth, diameter and the density of micropores allow perfect adaption to different drugs used as well as an optimal drug release control (Fig. 12.3). This high variability allows a broad range of applications. Besides some aesthetic applications, the P.L.E.A.S.E.® technology enables needle-free vaccination, different diagnostic applications, immunological applications, the intradermal delivery of biological compounds and many other fields of application (Fig. 12.4). This is documented by various publications [34–37]. Most importantly, this technique was successfully applied for the TDD of peptides and even proteins without losing their structural integrity and function [38, 39].

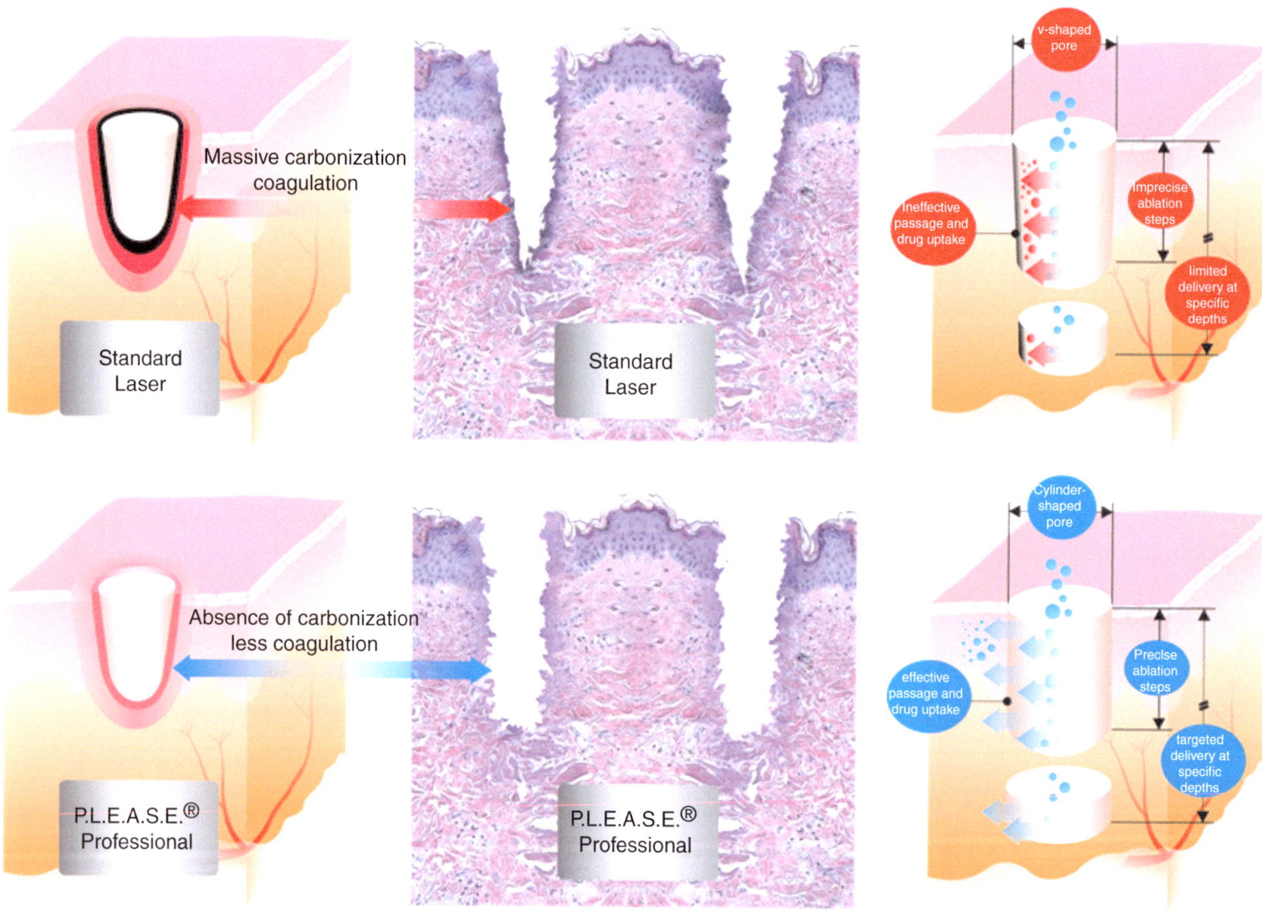

Fig. 12.3 Ablation by a standard laser and P.L.E.A.S.E.® technology compared. The P.L.E.A.S.E.® technology allows a precise cylinder-shaped skin ablation and effective drug delivery at different depth. (Courtesy of Pantec Biosolutions AG)

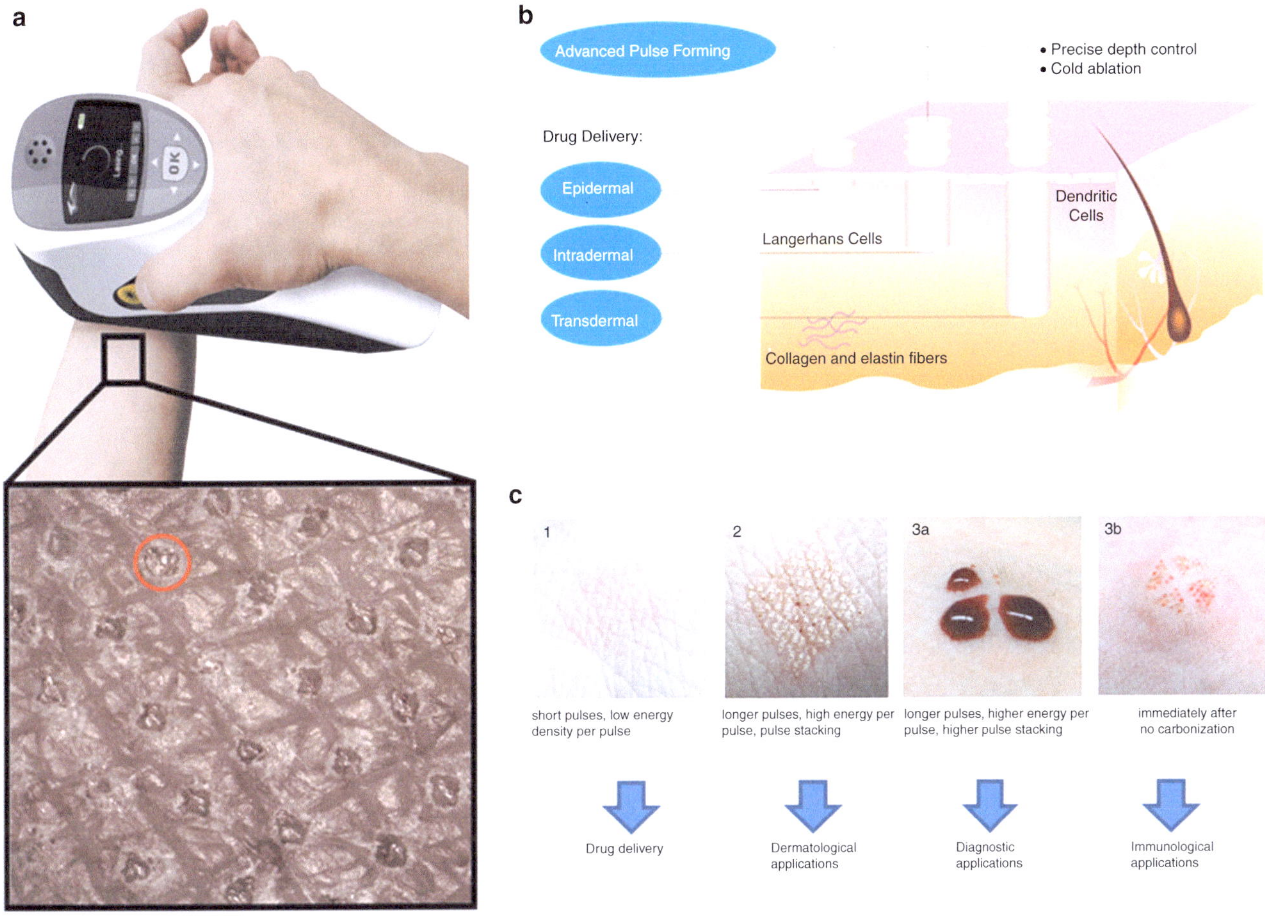

Fig. 12.4 Different applications of P.L.E.A.S.E.® technology by varying parameter settings. (**a**) Demonstration of simple application of the P.L.E.A.S.E.® device. Lower graph demonstrates magnification of the skin. Dark spots represent laser-induced micropores. Cycled in red shows a micropore. (**b**) Schematic drawing of microporation with different depth by the P.L.E.A.S.E.® technology. (**c**) Variation of parameter setting allows different scopes of applications. (Courtesy of Pantec Biosolutions AG)

The P.L.E.A.S.E.® technology enables even the TDD of high molecular weight drugs—up to approximately 150 kDa. In fact, the P.L.E.A.S.E.® system was the first reported laser-assisted TDD system enabling successful COS by transdermal administration of high molecular weight gonadotropins that resulted in a pregnancy after oocyte puncture, IVF and subsequent embryo transfer [18]. The first laser-induced TDD of prednisone, a corticosteroid, has also been achieved using the P.L.E.A.S.E.® technology [40]. Although this drug is rather used for the treatment of various inflammatory and autoimmune diseases, prednisone therapies are sometimes MAR-related as prednisone is reported to sometimes attenuate the risks of embryo implantation failure and miscarriage.

The P.L.E.A.S.E.® technology was also proven to be effective for TDD of triptorelin in terms of bioavailability and safety aspects and has meanwhile completed clinical phase I [34].

12.5.7 Others

We know a number of other TDD systems, but they do not really play a role in clinical practice, inasmuch as either they have hazardous effects on health, are not efficient and are too expensive or they still have not passed developmental and test phase. However, one of them should be discussed briefly, namely a system involving the use of nanocarriers (NC), as this technique might gain some importance in the future. NC have a size of 10–1000 nm. They can be administered by all routes including TDD. They are suggested to be undetectable by the immune system. NC encompass nanoparticles, nanocapsules, nanoemulsions, dendrimers and liposomes. Within the last years, huge advances in the development of NC have been made [41]. However, potential side effects are still unclear. In addition, most NC (jet) are still not suitable for TDD.

12.6 Outlook and Conclusions

MAR is associated with (sometimes) painful injections of fertility drugs. In most IVF patients, injections evoke negative associations. The self-administration by needle injections also bears the danger of inadequate drug application. There is undoubtedly an overriding requirement for improving and facilitating drug application in MAR as part of the optimization of the entire therapy. Thus, needle-free TDD of fertility drugs should be the overarching goal. Although TDD in MAR is a new topic and still finds itself at an experimental stage (with the exception of a few applications), there are some promising approaches. The next generations of laser-assisted TDD devices, such as the scanning fractional laser ablation systems, are undoubtedly the most innovative and most promising approaches. With their flexibility in regard to the control of drug release kinetics by modulation of the number of micropores, their depth and size, a precise, reliable and painless TDD can be obtained even for high molecular weight drugs, while at the same time taking into account individual skin conditions. Even though amazing progress has been made in other TDD systems, the new laser devices are the only approaches not subject to any limitations in terms of size, charge and stability of the drug.

References

1. Lockhart, M. U.S. Patent No. 69,199, Mar 16 1936. [Internet] [cited 2016 Dec 15]. Available from: https://www.google.com/patents/US2322244?dq=US+69,199+injection&hl=de&sa=X&ved=0ahUKEwiyj6_NofbQAhULuRQKHbLMBSYQ6AEIHTAA
2. Zech NH, Zech M, Baldauf S, Comploj G, Murtinger M, Spitzer D, et al. Ovarian stimulation in ART–unwinding pressing issues. Minerva Ginecol. 2015;67:127–47.
3. Tavaniotou A, Smitz J, Bourgain C, Devroey P. Ovulation induction disrupts luteal phase function. Ann N Y Acad Sci. 2001;943:55–63.
4. Practice Committee of American Society for Reproductive Medicine in collaboration with Society for Reproductive Endocrinology and Infertility. Progesterone supplementation during the luteal phase and in early pregnancy in the treatment of infertility: an educational bulletin. Fertil Steril. 2008;90(5 Suppl):S150–3.
5. Ghanem ME, Al-Boghdady LA. Luteal phase support in ART: an update, enhancing success of assisted reproduction, Prof. Atef Darwish (Ed.), InTech, 2012. p.155–72.
6. Southwell D, Barry BW, Woodford R. Variations in permeability of human skin within and between specimens. Int J Pharm. 1984;18:299–309.
7. Connell MT, DeCherney AH, Hill MJ. Recent advances in the development of transdermal delivery systems for treatment of infertility. Research and Reports in Transdermal Drug Delivery. 2015;4:1–7.
8. Kopper NW, Gudeman J, Thompson DJ. Transdermal hormone therapy in postmenopausal women: a review of metabolic effects and drug delivery technologies. Drug Des Devel Ther. 2009;2:193–202.
9. Davar R, Janati S, Mohseni F, Khabazkhoob M, Asgari S. A comparison of the effects of transdermal estradiol and estradiol Valerate on endometrial receptivity in frozen-thawed embryo transfer cycles: a randomized clinical trial. J Reprod Infertil. 2016;17:97–103.
10. Fábregues F, Peñarrubia J, Creus M, Manau D, Casals G, Carmona F, et al. Transdermal testosterone may improve ovarian response to gonadotrophins in low-responder IVF patients: a randomized, clinical trial. Hum Reprod. 2009;24:349–59.
11. Luo S, Li S, Li X, Qin L, Jin S. Effect of pretreatment with transdermal testosterone on poor ovarian responders undergoing IVF/ICSI: a meta-analysis. Exp Ther Med. 2014;8:187–94.
12. Haukkamaa M, Laurikka-Routti M, Heikinheimo O. Transdermal absorption of the progestin ST-1435: therapeutic serum steroid concentrations and high excretion of the steroid in saliva. Contraception. 1991;44:269–76.
13. Schuetz YB, Naik A, Guy RH, Vuaridel E, Kalia YN. Transdermal iontophoretic delivery of triptorelin in vitro. J Pharm Sci. 2005;94:2175–82.
14. Bachhav YG, Kalia YN. Stability of triptorelin in the presence of dermis and epidermis. Int J Pharm. 2009;378:149–51.
15. Bruno BJ, Miller GD, Lim CS. Basics and recent advances in peptide and protein drug delivery. Ther Deliv. 2013;4:1443–67.
16. Nicoli S, Rimondi S, Colombo P, Santi P. Physical and chemical enhancement of transdermal delivery of triptorelin. Pharm Res. 2001;18:1634–7.
17. Bachhav YG, Heinrich A, Kalia YN. Controlled intra- and transdermal protein delivery using a minimally invasive erbium:YAG fractional laser ablation technology. Eur J Pharm Biopharm. 2013;84:355–64.
18. Zech NH, Murtinger M, Uher P. Pregnancy after ovarian superovulation by transdermal delivery of follicle-stimulating hormone. Fertil Steril. 2011;95:2784–5.
19. Antor MA, Uribe AA, Erminy-Falcon N, Werner JG, Candiotti KA, Pergolizzi JV, et al. The effect of transdermal scopolamine for the prevention of postoperative nausea and vomiting. Front Pharmacol. 2014;5:55.
20. Prausnitz MR, Langer R. Transdermal drug delivery. Nat Biotechnol. 2008;26:1261–8.
21. Karande P, Jain A, Ergun K, Kispersky V, Mitragotri S. Design principles of chemical penetration enhancers for transdermal drug delivery. Proc Natl Acad Sci U S A. 2005;102:4688–93.
22. Kim YC, Late S, Banga AK, Ludovice PJ, Prausnitz MR. Biochemical enhancement of transdermal delivery with magainin peptide: modification of electrostatic interactions by changing pH. Int J Pharm. 2008;362:20–8.
23. Schramm J, Mitragotri S. Transdermal drug delivery by jet injectors: energetics of jet formation and penetration. Pharm Res. 2002;19:1673–9.
24. Williams J, Fox-Leyva L, Christensen C, Fisher D, Schlicting E, Snowball M, et al. Hepatitis a vaccine administration: comparison between jet-injector and needle injection. Vaccine. 2000;18:1939–43.
25. Solnica A, Oh C, Cho MM, Loughlin JS, McCulloh DH, McGovern PG. Patient satisfaction and clinical outcome after injecting gonadotropins with use of a needle-free carbon dioxide injection system for controlled ovarian hyperstimulation for in vitro fertilization. Fertil Steril. 2009;92:1369–71.
26. Lavery SA, El-Shawarby SA, Turner C, Trew G. The J-tip needle-free injection system in controlled ovarian hyperstimulation in in vitro fertilization: a pilot study. Fertil Steril. 2008;90:1969–72.
27. Carter M. Roche abandon Biojector 2000 for T-20 administration. NAM Publications [Internet] 2007 Oct [cited 2016 Dec 15]. Available from: http://www.aidsmap.com/Roche-abandon-Biojector-2000-for-T-20-administration/page/1428514/
28. Schoellhammer CM, Blankschtein D, Langer R. Skin permeabilization for transdermal drug delivery: recent advances and future prospects. Expert Opin Drug Deliv. 2014;11:393–407.
29. Demuth PC, Garcia-Beltran WF, Ai-Ling ML, Hammond PT, Irvine DJ. Composite dissolving microneedles for coordinated control of

antigen and adjuvant delivery kinetics in transcutaneous vaccination. Adv Funct Mater. 2013;23:161–72.
30. Ita K. Perspectives on transdermal electroporation. Pharmaceutics. 2016;8(1)
31. Kalluri H. Banga AK transdermal delivery of proteins. AAPS PharmSciTech. 2011;12:431–41.
32. Prausnitz MR. The effects of electric current applied to the skin: a review for transdermal drug delivery. Adv Drug Deliv Rev. 1996;18:395–425.
33. Li Y, Guo L, Wei L. Laser ablation-enhanced transdermal drug delivery. Photonics and Lasers in Medicine. 2013;2:315–22.
34. Pantec Biosolutions AG. [Internet] [cited 2016 Dec 15]. Available from: http://www.pantec-biosolutions.com/en/home
35. Bach D, Weiss R, Hessenberger M, Kitzmueller S, Weinberger EE, Krautgartner WD, et al. Transcutaneous immunotherapy via laser-generated micropores efficiently alleviates allergic asthma in Phl p 5-sensitized mice. Allergy. 2012;67:1365–74.
36. Weiss R, Hessenberger M, Kitzmüller S, Bach D, Weinberger EE, Krautgartner WD, et al. Transcutaneous vaccination via laser microporation. J Control Release. 2012;162:391–9.
37. Haering N, Boehler C, Barlas K, Dertinger S, Strohal R. The combination of fractionated erbium:YAG laser skin Microporation and topical Imiquimod is a new, safe and efficient strategy for the treatment of actinic keratosis and basal cell carcinoma: report of two pilot studies. J Dermatologic Res Therapy. 2015;1:7–18.
38. Bachhav YG, Kalia YN. Development and validation of a rapid high performance liquid chromatography method for the quantification of exenatide. Biomed Chromatogr. 2011;25:838–42.
39. Bachhav YG, Kalia YN. Development and validation of an analytical method for the quantification of cytochrome c in skin transport studies. Biomed Chromat. 2010;24:732–6.
40. Yu J, Bachhav YG, Summer S, Heinrich A, Bragagna T, Boehler C, et al. Using controlled laser-microporation to increase transdermal delivery of prednisone. J Control Release. 2010;148:e71–3.
41. Patel A, Patel M, Yang X, Mitra AK. Recent advances in protein and peptide drug delivery: a special emphasis on polymeric nanoparticles. Protein Pept Lett. 2014;21:1102–20.

Ovulation Induction for the Woman with Hypogonadotropic Hypogonadism

13

Sezcan Mumusoglu, Pinar Tokdemir Calis, and Gurkan Bozdag

13.1 Introduction

Hypogonadotropic hypogonadism is a condition in which the testis or ovary could not produce sex hormones due to functional or anatomical disorders in pituitary or hypothalamus. It should be noted that gonads are not typically affected but coincidental cases might be expected.

The incidence of hypogonadotropic hypogonadism varies from 1/3000 to 1/4000, and males have a three- to fivefold risk of prevalence than female cohort [1]. Among women suffering from anovulatory infertility, 5–10% of them have been assigned as hypogonadotropic hypogonadism. The clinical presentation generally consists of delayed puberty, primary or secondary amenorrhea, and hence infertility. Although there is a great effort for the diagnosis and management of women with polycystic ovary syndrome (PCOS) in the available literature, there is substantially less consensus not only for the diagnostic criterion but also for the management in hypogonadotropic hypogonadism, particularly for the aspect of infertility. As already addressed by the British Fertility Society, the management protocols for WHO group I are "non-standardized" and "scarce" [2].

13.2 Definition

WHO group I anovulation reflects a heterogeneous group of patients in which three subgroups might be stratified as previously defined by the British Fertility Society. *(a) Hypothalamic amenorrhea* (HA) refers to a condition due to excessive exercise, weight loss, or chronic diseases. Generally, there is secondary amenorrhea with more significantly depressed levels of LH than FSH concentration. Under ultrasonography, polycystic ovary morphology might be noted in certain rate of those women [3]. *(b) Hypogonadotropic hypogonadism (HH)* is primarily due to congenital GnRH deficiency related with >25 gene polymorphism and thus forms a heterogeneous clinical condition. Acquired causes include trauma, tumor, radiation, chemotherapy, or infiltrative diseases. In clinical presentation, uterus and ovaries are small. Primary or secondary amenorrhea and delay or absence of puberty might be encountered due to underlying reason. *(c) Hypopituitarism (HP)* defined conditions when production or secretion of pituitary hormones is affected. Tumors, infiltrative diseases, and Sheehan's syndrome are known conditions related with hypopituitarism. Notably, growth hormone (GH) appears to be more affected than thyroid-stimulating hormone (TSH) and adrenocorticotropic hormone (ACTH) in patients with HP [4].

13.3 Infertility Treatment

13.3.1 Lifestyle Management

A lifestyle management should be initially recommended in patients with HA. Multidisciplinary management should be undertaken with dietician and psychiatry. Although there is no clearly defined body weight to restore menstrual regularity, a mean increase in weight around 9% was associated with treatment success, while it was around 2% in women who failed to ovulate in a study including 18 professional athletes suffering from HA. Of interest, restoration of menstruation had taken over 1 year to recover even after those women had achieved a target weight gain (15 ± 2.6 months) [5]. Similarly, there are also unsuccessful attempts to define a high accurate threshold for menstrual restoration with regard to fat mass or leptin concentration [6].

For anovulation associated with excessive exercise and physical stress, we have to remember the fact that corticotrophin-releasing hormone (CRH) plays an important

S. Mumusoglu · G. Bozdag (✉)
Department of Obstetrics and Gynecology, Hacettepe University School of Medicine, Ankara, Turkey
e-mail: gbozdag@hacettepe.edu.tr

P. T. Calis
Department of Obstetrics and Gynecology, Gazi University School of Medicine, Ankara, Turkey

G. N. Allahbadia et al. (eds.), *Textbook of Assisted Reproduction*, https://doi.org/10.1007/978-981-15-2377-9_13

role on hypothalamus-pituitary-ovarian axis. Nevertheless, physical and emotional stress may activate instant increase in CRH that stimulates pituitary secretion of adrenocorticotrophic hormone (ACTH). Hence, increased secretion of glucocorticosteroids inhibits secretion of GnRH and finally gonadotrophins [7]. In patients who are candidate for exercise-related anovulation, limiting exercise level and optimizing calorie intake should be initially considered which will result in decreased CRH levels and restoration of hypothalamus-pituitary-ovarian axis activates [7].

13.3.2 GnRH Pumps

For pharmacological treatment, gonadotropin-releasing hormone (GnRH) pumps could be an option in patients with intact pituitary gland. Pulsatile GnRH treatment is generally preferred in patients with congenital HH. In women with HA who failed to conceive after lifestyle management, utilization of GnRH pump is also a valid option before advanced treatment [8]. Inducing mono-follicular development with maintaining physiological estradiol levels is the goal of pulsatile GnRH therapy. Commercially, it might be applied via subcutaneous, intramuscular, nasal, or intravenous routes. Of the available approaches, subcutaneous route appears to be feasible and practical with a slower sustained rise in FSH and LH [2]. When various intervals were tested among 20 patients with HA who had been treated over 41 cycles with GnRH pumps, the best outcome of ovulation and pregnancy rate was achieved with a 90 or 120 min of intervals [9]. Commonly, the starting dose of GnRH analogue is 15 μg for subcutaneous route. If the follicle development does not occur (>10 mm), increasing the dose of GnRH analogue by 5 μg or adding exogenous gonadotropin is recommended.

The success rate is generally reported to be 25% per cycle with GnRH pumps and even be better than induction with exogenous gonadotropins [10]. In a randomized controlled trial [11], 30 consecutive patients with HA and polycystic ovary syndrome (PCOS) were induced with either GnRH pump or exogenous gonadotropins (75 IU FSH + 75 IU rec LH). The ovarian responses were comparable (73% vs. 60%), but clinical pregnancy rate was reported to be significantly higher in favor of pulsatile GnRH treatment (46% vs. 15%). Since that study population was heterogeneous with its limited sample size, we need more data to decide which strategy is superior and should be offered in the first step in that group of women.

The major side effect related with its clinical application includes skin reactions and antibody formation. In addition, it might be more expensive in commercially available countries when compared with exogenous gonadotropin therapy.

13.3.3 Ovulation Induction with Exogenous Gonadotropins

Ovulation induction with exogenous gonadotropins might be preferred as an alternative approach in patients with WHO group I anovulation. With respect to the theory of 2-cell and 2-gonadotropin, there appears a necessity to supply LH activity with addition to stimulation with FSH [12]. According to initial studies on basic reproductive endocrinology [2, 13], whereas LH activity induces the production of androgens from circulating cholesterol in theca cells, FSH is essential to convert androgen precursors to estrogens within granulosa cells by inducing aromatase enzyme activity. Stimulation with only FSH yields less follicular development and serum estradiol concentration but much higher gonadotropin requirement and lower ovulation rates when compared with LH supplementation. Hence, both preclinical and clinical findings appear to be concordant with each other and propose a need for LH activity particularly in LH-depleted women [2].

The potential sources of LH activity might be human chorionic gonadotropin (hCG) or recombinant technology. Whereas hCG is produced from a α subunit including 92 amino acids and β chain made of 145 amino acids with 8 glycosylation sites, LH presents diversity with a β chain formed by 121 amino acids and 3 glycosylation sites. Although they share the same receptor (LHCGR), there might be functional differences at receptor level with regard to three pathways analyzed in in vitro cell lines (Fig. 13.1).

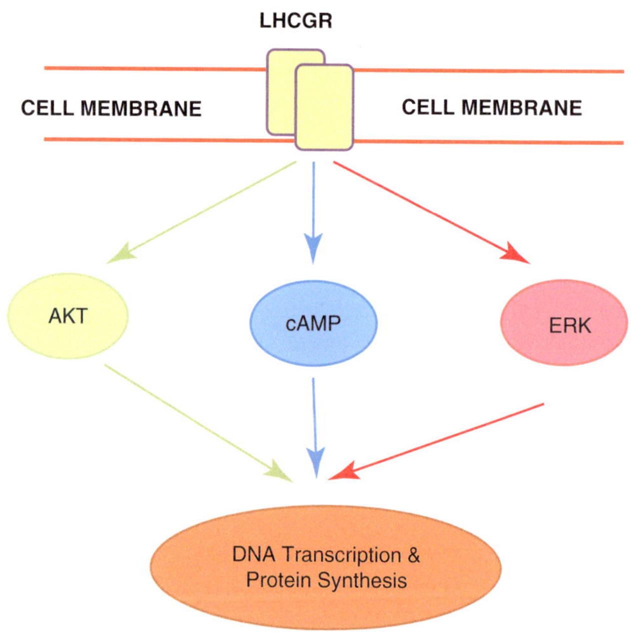

Fig. 13.1 Post-receptor pathways of LHCGR receptor

For the ***cAMP*** pathway, whereas biopotency of HCG is five times higher, LH action is six times faster, and hGLCs become refractory to a continuous LH stimulation over 24 h [14]. With regard to ***ERK*** and ***AKT*** pathways, LH is more potent and faster than hCG, and high doses of hCG seem to inhibit the AKT pathway [14]. The gene expression levels of LH/hCG receptor gene in granulosa cells and genes involved in biosynthesis of cholesterol and steroids might present also diversity when stimulated with either LH or hCG [15].

Although significant difference exists between LH and hCG activity at molecular and functional level, most of the available studies had evaluated women undergoing treatment with human menopausal gonadotrophin (hMG). According to a systematic review [16], pregnancy rate per cycle is around 25%, and miscarriage rate is similar with women diagnosed as unexplained infertility. However, multiple pregnancy rate is approximately 30% which warrants need for low dose of gonadotropin use. Particularly in women with a polycystic ovary appearance, 75 IU of daily gonadotropin might be preferred, but 150 IU might be a better choice when there is no visible antral follicle under ultrasonography. Weekly increments might be considered in patients with no exceeding follicle in diameter of >10 mm for a given dose. To avoid multi-follicular development, monitoring with ultrasonography of the cycle is also recommended by the British Fertility Society to enhance efficacy and safety [2]. Ovarian hyperstimulation syndrome has been generally reported with less than 1% [17] of all cases.

Instead of hMG, recombinant LH might be also preferred with addition to recombinant FSH supplementation. In a randomized controlled trial including 38 women [18], patients were stratified for the dose of LH supplementation as 0 IU, 25 IU, 75 IU, or 225 IU in addition to 150 IU FSH for all. Participants undergoing 75 IU LH with 150 IU FSH had the highest chance of optimal response as defined by presence of ≥1 follicle exceeding 17 mm in diameter and estradiol level of >400 pg/ml on the day of triggering with hCG. For the comparison of highly purified hMG versus FSH and recombinant LH supplementation with a 2:1 ratio, there is only one randomized controlled trial including small number of patients (n = 35) in women with HH [19]. Following a total of 70 cycles, FSH and LH combination yielded similar ovulation rate (88% vs. 70%, p = 0.11) but higher pregnancy rates (55.6% vs. 23.3%, p = 0.01) when compared with highly purified hMG. However, one should be cautious about small sample size and lack of validation with further studies.

Growth Hormone Supplementation

The utilization of growth hormone (GH) in women with HH was first described by Homburg et al. and offered as a new approach to ovulation induction [20]. The authors reported that the addition of biosynthetic GH (24 IU on alternate days) to hMG improved ovarian responsiveness in seven patients who were previously hMG resistant [20]. Growth hormone reduced both the duration of treatment and daily hMG requirement. Subsequent reports documented increased circulating levels of insulin-like growth factor concentrations that act as a mediator of GH itself [21]. GH supplementation can be most beneficial for women with a surgical, pathological, or medically induced dysfunction of GH kinetics [22]. Although there is no dose-finding study for GH, use of 12–24 IU per cycle generally has resulted in an adequate ovarian response. In patients with pan-hypopituitarism, it might be commenced 2 to 4 months before ovarian stimulation cycle and continued until the day of pregnancy test [23]. However, pregnancy rates in hypopituitary patients might be still worse than those in HH and HA patients [2].

Luteal Phase Support in Ovulation Induction Cycles

According to an updated systematic review and meta-analysis [24], progesterone luteal phase support is beneficial to patients undergoing ovulation induction with gonadotropins in intrauterine insemination cycles. However, there is paucity of data for the necessity of luteal phase support either in the form of progesterone or with estrogen, particularly for patients with HH undergoing ovarian stimulation. For patients treated with a GnRH pulsatile pump, early studies indicate its sufficiency when administered throughout luteal phase [25]. Progesterone support in the form of vaginal preparation or intramuscular injections might be also preferred, even though a prospective comparative study is not available [2].

13.3.4 Assisted Reproductive Technologies

Women with WHO group I anovulation achieve cumulative pregnancy rates between 30 and 96% with ovulation induction (OI) alone [10, 26]. Yet, assisted reproductive technologies (ART) are still required for a substantial proportion of these women due to failure of OI and/or intrauterine insemination or the presence of other indications, e.g., tubal obstruction or male factor. Within the context of ART, the key point in individualization in women with HH is the presence of intact pituitary function (HA, HH, or HP).

13.3.4.1 Induction of Multiple Follicular Developments

In contrast to OI alone, the goal of OI in ART cycle is to achieve multi-follicular development. Since there is paucity of data with regard to OI protocols in ART cycles in patients with HH, we will discuss some unanswered questions in this field.

Pretreatment Before Ovulation Induction (e.g., Oral Contraceptive Pill, Rec LH)

Due to lack of gonadotropin and low estrogen levels in women with HH, particularly with congenital HH, shorter uterine length and a smaller uterine cross-sectional area have been reported [27]. Pretreatment with oral contraceptive pill (OCP) for 2 or 3 months prior to ovarian stimulation cycles has been widely adopted in congenital HH patients as a standard protocol. It is assumed that OCP could change the hypo-estrogenic environment or increase endometrial development and receptivity. It was also speculated that pretreatment with OCP might reduce total gonadotropin consumption by stimulating gonadotropin receptor formation in granulosa cells [28]. Nonetheless, there is no comparative study to suggest routine pretreatment with OCP before ART cycles. Actually, ovarian stimulation can be started either randomly during amenorrhea or following the withdrawal bleeding with OCP.

As a matter of fact, vast majority of women with HH in reproductive age already use OCP not only for inducing compatible development of the breasts and genitalia but also to maintain cyclic menstrual bleeding and sense of femininity required for emotional and sexual well-being [29].

Recently, a new pretreatment protocol with rec LH has been proposed [30]. Pretreatment with rec LH (300 IU s.c.) for 7 days significantly decreased the mean threshold (daily effective) FSH dose and the requirement of total FSH doses to induce follicular maturation, appropriate serum estradiol (E_2) level, and endometrial thickness.

Ovarian Reserve Test

Briefly, there are two regulation steps of folliculogenesis in ovary: (1) FSH-independent initial recruitment and (2) FSH-dependent cyclic recruitment. The first step (initial recruitment) begins immediately after birth [31], and the second step (cyclic recruitment) starts at puberty with activation of pulsatile secretion of FSH. Follicle-stimulating hormone-deficient hypophysectomized women present with the absence of large antral follicles [32]. Therefore, antral follicle count (AFC) is not a good predictor of ovarian response in HH patients to tailor the starting dose of gonadotropin. Since anti-Müllerian hormone (AMH) is secreted from granulosa cells of secondary, preantral, and small antral follicles <4 mm in diameter [33], it may be a better predictor of ovarian response.

Recently, in ART cycle of 12 patients with congenital HH, positive correlations were observed between serum AMH levels and number of follicles >14 mm and > 17 mm on the day triggering ovulation, serum peak E_2 levels, metaphase II oocytes, and number of high-quality embryos [34]. Those results suggest that AMH might be used as marker of ovarian response in patients with congenital HH undergoing ART. Even though most women with congenital HH have normal serum AMH levels, still some females with severe congenital HH might coincidentally suffer from AMH deficiency [35]. In those women, AMH is unlikely to be an accurate prognostic factor of ovarian response. This is very relevant for clinical practice, since decreased AMH levels in female women with congenital HH and severe GnRH deficiency may be erroneously interpreted as a decrease in ovarian reserve and therefore a reduced chance of success [35].

Individualization of Gonadotropin Starting Dose

It is very important to adjust starting dose of FSH not only for the optimal response but also to prevent complications associated with OI. Conventional ovulation induction protocol in women with HH for mono-follicular development is a "low-dose step-up protocol" with a starting dose of 75 IU hMG (human menopausal gonadotropin). However, the goal of induction of ovulation in ART is totally different, and exogenous gonadotropins are used to ensure the maintenance of a suprathreshold level during the time of follicle selection for the multi-follicular development. We suggest that FSH starting dose should be at least between 150 and 225 IU in women with HH. FSH starting dose could also be tailored according to AMH level and response to previous ovulation induction, as quoted previously [34].

Luteinizing Hormone Supplementation

As mentioned above, although FSH alone can induce follicular growth in the total absence of LH, the growing follicles will have developmental deficiencies such as abnormally low production of E_2 and inability to luteinize and rupture in response to an hCG stimulus. As a result of low E_2 level, the outcome of the cycle might be threatened with thin and potentially non-receptive endometrium [18, 36, 37].

The amount of LH activity necessary for normal follicle and oocyte development is unknown, but it is likely low, as only <1% of LH receptors need to be occupied to allow normal steroidogenesis [38]. Serum LH "threshold" level to provide adequate LH support to FSH-induced follicular development is >1.2 IU/L. Subcutaneous co-administration of 75 IU rec LH with rec FSH is safe and effective in inducing follicular development in women with profound gonadotropin deficiency [37]. It is clear that LH supplementation is mandatory in patients with HH. However, there is a "LH ceiling" theory suggesting inhibition of follicular growth when the certain level of LH is exceeded [39]. According to "LH ceiling" theory, the utilization of increasing rec LH doses in the follicular phase decrease the number of growing follicles [18].

There is no randomized controlled trial (RCT) comparing the efficacy of different LH sources such as hMG, hMG-HP, or rec LH in ART cycle of women with HH. Although not conducted in ART cycles, according to one small ($n = 35$) open-labeled RCT, the pregnancy rate of rec FSH/rec LH (150 IU/75 IU) for OI is superior to hMG-HP (150 IU) in women with HH (55.6% vs. 23.3%, $p = 0.01$, respectively) [19]. Those results might suggest that it is reasonable to use rec LH separately with adjunct to rec FSH in patients with HH in ART cycles to tailor the rec LH dose per se with staying under the "LH ceiling" level.

Growth Hormone Supplementation

It is noteworthy that GH co-stimulation could be employed in ART cycles particularly in patients with GH deficiency and women suffering from HP. GH regulates the IGF-I or IGFBP-3 levels and may play a role in the growth of the follicle [21]. GH appears to selectively increase the sensitivity of the dominant follicle to FSH, facilitating mono-follicular growth [40]. GH treatment in women with low GH levels increases the sensitivity of the ovaries to gonadotropin stimulation [40].

Many women with GH deficiency suffer from subfertility and require assisted reproductive technologies to conceive [41]. GH supplementation yields more oocytes and higher fertilization and pregnancy rates in poor responder women with HH [22].

Pituitary Suppression

Pituitary suppression with GnRH analogues to prevent an endogenous LH surge is an integral component of controlled ovarian stimulation (COS) protocols. In the absence of pituitary suppression, premature luteinization occurs in up to 25% of stimulation cycles in women with an intact hypothalamic-pituitary-gonadal axis leading to cycle cancellation and severely compromised outcomes [42]. Of interest, in 2009, it has been shown that pretreatment with rLH/rhCG could evoke unambiguous elevations in serum levels of endogenous LH during FSH in patients with congenital HH and intact pituitary function [30]. Moreover, 10–22% of patients with congenital HH may have lifetime reversal of disease [29]. Both unambiguous elevation of endogenous LH and high reversal rates (previously underestimated) in women with HH and intact pituitary function support the suppression of pituitary with GnRH agonist/antagonist for the prevention of premature ovulation in ART cycles. We recently have tested whether gonadotropin-releasing hormone (GnRH) analogues were beneficial in women with HH in a retrospective multicenter cohort study. Fifty-seven women with congenintal HH (CHH) were included, GnRH antagonists were given to 19, and 13 were stimulated with the long GnRH agonist protocol, while 25 were not given pituitary suppression at all. Women without pituitary suppression achieved significantly higher embryo implantation rates (21.6 vs. 52.6%, $p = 0.03$), and higher live birth rate per cycle (25.0 vs. 40.0%, $p = 0.26$), albeit the latter was short of statistical significance [43].

13.3.4.2 Monitoring the Cycle and Triggering Final Oocyte Maturation

Ultrasonography is warranted for monitoring follicular growth and endometrial thickness in women with HH. A measurement of E2 for adjusting gonadotropin dose or for the timing of triggering of ovulation is not a requirement. Ovulation triggering with hCG based on endometrial thickness and follicular growth is associated with improved pregnancy rates. Serial ultrasound examinations used alone are safe and highly efficient [44].

13.3.4.3 Luteal Phase Support

It is obvious that luteal phase support (LPS) with progesterone is mandatory in agonist or antagonist OI cycles for ART with fresh embryo transfer [45]. Threefold higher mid-luteal serum progesterone levels (25–30 ng/ml) are required for sustained implantation in ART cycles compared to natural conception cycle [46]. Unfortunately, there is scarce of data for the LPS in ART cycles of the women with HH.

Different LPS protocols were used in OI alone cycles without ART: (1) pulsatile GnRH administration either in a same or in a decreased pulse frequency in follicular phase [25]; (2) 400–800 mg of vaginal progesterone or 100 mg intramuscular (i.m.) progesterone; and (3) subcutaneous (s.c.) hCG (1500–2500 IU, twice a week).

Intramuscular progesterone (75–100 mg/d), progesterone vaginal gel (twice a day), and estrogen plus progesterone via either vaginal or intramuscular injection were given in ART cycles with fresh embryo transfer (Table 13.1). These trials reported at least similar success rate in women with HH compared to patients with tubal factor, male factor, and unexplained infertility [47–49]. Since patients supported with progesterone alone have comparable pregnancy rates when compared with various group of controls, there is no evidence in favor of adding estrogen after embryo transfer in women with HH [43].

13.3.4.4 Success Rates of ART Cycles

There are six studies in the literature investigating outcomes in patients with HH compared the control group patients with tubal factor [43, 47, 50, 51], male factor [49], and unexplained infertility [48] (Table 13.1). All of them presented similar pregnancy outcomes compared to controls with longer stimulation duration and higher gonadotropin consumption. Only one of them reported higher cancellation rate in patients with HH [50].

Table 13.1 Studies comparing successes rate of assisted reproductive technology cycles in between patient with hypogonadotropic hypogonadism and control group with various infertility reasons

Author, year	Cycles, HH vs. control (n)	Gonadotropin dose, type	Control group	Luteal phase support
Ulug, (2005)	58 vs. 116	450–600, hMG	Tubal factor	Progesterone 100 mg/d, i.m.
Kumbak, (2006)	27 vs. 39	300–600, hMG	Unexplained	Progesterone 75 mg/d, i.m.
Yildirim, (2010)	13 vs. 20	NA	Tubal factor	NA
Ghaffari, (2013)	81 vs. 89	NA	Tubal factor	NA
Yilmaz, (2015)	33 vs. 47	300–450, hMG	Male factor	Vaginal progesterone gel, 2 × 1
Mumusoglu, (2017)	57 vs. 114	225–600, hMG or r-FSH + r-LH	Tubal factor	Progesterone alone or estrogen+progesterone

HH hypogonadotropic hypogonadism; *NA* not available

13.4 Conclusion

This chapter can be summarized as follows:

- WHO group I anovulation is a rare condition but consists of heterogeneous groups of patients including hypothalamic amenorrhea (HA), hypogonadotropic hypogonadism (HH), and hypopituitarism (HP).
- In women with HA, initially lifestyle changes including limiting exercise and restoration of body weight, under the control of endocrinologist, dietician, and psychiatrist with a multidisciplinary approach, should be recommended. Ovulation induction with pharmacological treatment should be offered after optimization of body weight.
- Gonadotropin-releasing hormone (GnRH) pump is a valid option in patients with intact pituitary gland (HH, HA). However, GnRH pumps are not available in many countries due to high cost.
- Regarding ovulation induction treatment with gonadotropins, either hMG or rec FSH plus rec LH (with optimum 75 IU) might be preferred. Particularly in women with a polycystic ovary appearance, 75 IU of daily gonadotropin might be used, but 150 IU might be a feasible dose when no antral follicle was observed under ultrasonography.
- Growth hormone (GH) depletion might be relevant in patients with HP. In patients with HP, GH might be commenced 2 to 4 months before ovarian stimulation cycle and continued until the day of pregnancy test.
- There is lack of data with regard to necessity of luteal phase support in OI cycles with HH.
- ART is needed following OI and/or intrauterine insemination failure or in the presence of other indications, e.g., tubal obstruction or male factor.
- In terms of controlled ovarian stimulation in ART, we suggest that FSH starting dose should be between 150 and 225 IU in women with HH. Starting dose of gonadotropin could also be tailored according to AMH level and response to previous ovulation induction. Since limited data suggest that pituitary suppression with GnRH analogues might lead to lower implantation rates, we do not recommended routine use of GnRH analogues in patients with CHH.
- Ultrasonography is warranted for monitoring follicular growth and endometrial thickness in women with HH.
- Optimal approach and dose of progesterone supplementation for luteal phase in ART are not clear.
- At least similar success rate in ART cycle was reported in women with HH when compared to patients with tubal factor, male factor, and unexplained infertility.

References

1. Seminara SB, Hayes FJ, Crowley WF Jr. Gonadotropin-releasing hormone deficiency in the human (idiopathic Hypogonadotropic Hypogonadism and Kallmann's syndrome): pathophysiological and genetic considerations. Endocr Rev. 1998;19(5):521–39.
2. Yasmin E, Davies M, Conway G, Balen A, British FS. British fertility society. 'Ovulation induction in who type 1 anovulation: guidelines for Practice'. Produced on behalf of the Bfs policy and practice committee. Hum Fertil (Camb). 2013;16(4):228–34.
3. Sum M. Warren Mp. Hypothalamic amenorrhea in young women with underlying polycystic ovary syndrome. Fertil Steril. 2009;92(6):2106–8.
4. Kk H. Consensus guidelines for the diagnosis and treatment of adults with Gh deficiency ii: a statement of the Gh research society in association with the European society for pediatric endocrinology, Lawson Wilkins society, European society of endocrinology, Japan Endocrine Society, and Endocrine Society of Australia. Eur J Endocrinol. 2007;157(6):695–700.
5. Arends JC, Cheung MY, Barrack M, Nattiv A. Restoration of menses with nonpharmacologic therapy in college athletes with menstrual disturbances: a 5-year retrospective study. Int J Sport Nutr Exerc Metab. 2012;22(2):98–108.
6. Grinspoon S, Gulick T, Askari H, Landt M, Lee K, Anderson E, et al. Serum Leptin levels in women with anorexia nervosa. J Clin Endocrinol Metab. 1996;81(11):3861–3.
7. Wade GN, Jones JE. Neuroendocrinology of nutritional infertility. Am J Physiol Regul Integr Comp Physiol. 2004;287(6):R1277–96.
8. Homburg R, Kilborn J, West C. Jacobs Hs. Treatment with pulsatile luteinizing hormone-releasing hormone modulates Folliculogenesis

in response to ovarian stimulation with exogenous gonadotropins in patients with polycystic ovaries. Fertil Steril. 1990;54(4):737–9.
9. Letterie GS, Coddington CC, Collins RL, Merriam GR. Ovulation induction using S.C. pulsatile Gonadotrophin-releasing hormone: effectiveness of different pulse frequencies. Hum Reprod. 1996;11(1):19–22.
10. Martin KA, Hall JE, Adams JM, Crowley WF Jr. Comparison of exogenous gonadotropins and pulsatile gonadotropin-releasing hormone for induction of ovulation in Hypogonadotropic amenorrhea. J Clin Endocrinol Metab. 1993;77(1):125–9.
11. Dubourdieu S, Freour T, Dessolle L, Barriere P. Prospective, randomized comparison between pulsatile Gnrh therapy and combined gonadotropin (Fsh+Lh) treatment for ovulation induction in women with hypothalamic amenorrhea and underlying polycystic ovary syndrome. Eur J Obstet Gynecol Reprod Biol. 2013;168(1):45–8.
12. Short RV. Steroids in the follicular fluid and the corpus Luteum of the Mare. A 'Two-cell Type' theory of ovarian steroid synthesis. J Endocrinol. 1962;24:59–63.
13. Couzinet B, Lestrat N, Brailly S, Forest M, Schaison G. Stimulation of ovarian follicular maturation with pure follicle-stimulating hormone in women with gonadotropin deficiency. J Clin Endocrinol Metab. 1988;66(3):552–6.
14. Casarini L, Lispi M, Longobardi S, Milosa F, La Marca A, Tagliasacchi D, et al. Lh and Hcg action on the same receptor results in quantitatively and qualitatively different intracellular Signalling. PLoS One. 2012;7(10):E46682.
15. Jeppesen JV, Kristensen SG, Nielsen ME, Humaidan P, Dal Canto M, Fadini R, et al. Lh-receptor gene expression in human Granulosa and cumulus cells from Antral and Preovulatory follicles. J Clin Endocrinol Metab. 2012;97(8):E1524–31.
16. Messinis IE. Ovulation induction: a mini review. Hum Reprod. 2005;20(10):2688–97.
17. Fluker MR, Urman B, Mackinnon M, Barrow SR, Pride SM, Yuen B. Exogenous gonadotropin therapy in World Health Organization groups I and ii ovulatory disorders. Obstet Gynecol. 1994;83(2):189–96.
18. Recombinant Human Luteinizing Hormone (Lh) To Support Recombinant Human Follicle-Stimulating Hormone (Fsh)-Induced Follicular Development In Lh- And Fsh-Deficient Anovulatory Women: a Dose-Finding Study. The European recombinant human Lh study group. J Clin Endocrinol Metab. 1998;83(5):1507–14.
19. Carone D, Caropreso C, Vitti A, Chiappetta R. Efficacy of different gonadotropin combinations to support ovulation induction in who type I anovulation infertility: clinical evidences of human recombinant Fsh/human recombinant Lh in a 2:1 ratio and highly purified human menopausal gonadotropin stimulation protocols. J Endocrinol Investig. 2012;35(11):996–1002.
20. Homburg R, Eshel A, Abdalla HI, Jacobs HS. Growth hormone facilitates ovulation induction by Gonadotrophins. Clin Endocrinol. 1988;29(1):113–7.
21. Homburg R, West C, Ostergaard H. Jacobs Hs. Combined growth hormone and gonadotropin treatment for ovulation induction in patients with non-responsive ovaries. Gynecol Endocrinol. 1991;5(1):33–6.
22. Homburg R, Ostergaard H. Clinical applications of growth hormone for ovarian stimulation. Hum Reprod Update. 1995;1(3):264–75.
23. Salle A, Klein M, Pascal-Vigneron V, Dousset B, Leclere J, Weryha G. Successful pregnancy and birth after sequential Cotreatment with growth hormone and gonadotropins in a woman with Panhypopituitarism: a new treatment protocol. Fertil Steril. 2000;74(6):1248–50.
24. Green KA, Zolton JR, Schermerhorn SM, Lewis TD, Healy MW, Terry N, et al. Progesterone luteal support after ovulation induction and intrauterine insemination: an updated systematic review and meta-analysis. Fertil Steril. 2017.
25. Filicori M, Flamigni C, Meriggiola MC, Cognigni G, Valdiserri A, Ferrari P, et al. Ovulation induction with pulsatile gonadotropin-releasing hormone: technical modalities and clinical perspectives. Fertil Steril. 1991;56(1):1–13.
26. Aboulghar MA, Mansour R, Serour GI, Ramzy AM. Successful treatment of infertile women with hypothalamic primary and secondary protracted Amenorrhoea using Gonadotrophin releasing hormone analogue and human menopausal Gonadotrophin. Hum Reprod. 1990;5(5):557–60.
27. Tsilchorozidou T, Conway GS. Uterus size and ovarian morphology in women with isolated growth hormone deficiency, Hypogonadotrophic Hypogonadism and hypopituitarism. Clin Endocrinol. 2004;61(5):567–72.
28. Lobb DK, Soliman SR, Daya S, Younglai EV. Steroidogenesis in luteinized Granulosa cell cultures varies with follicular priming regimen. Hum Reprod. 1998;13(8):2064–7.
29. Boehm U, Bouloux PM, Dattani MT, De Roux N, Dode C, Dunkel L, et al. Expert consensus document: european consensus statement on congenital Hypogonadotropic Hypogonadism--pathogenesis, diagnosis and treatment. Nat Rev Endocrinol. 2015;11(9):547–64.
30. Balasch J, Fabregues F, Carmona F, Casamitjana R, Tena-Sempere M. Ovarian luteinizing hormone priming preceding follicle-stimulating hormone stimulation: clinical and endocrine effects in women with long-term Hypogonadotropic Hypogonadism. J Clin Endocrinol Metab. 2009;94(7):2367–73.
31. Durlinger AL, Gruijters MJ, Kramer P, Karels B, Ingraham HA, Nachtigal MW, et al. Anti-Mullerian hormone inhibits initiation of primordial follicle growth in the mouse ovary. Endocrinology. 2002;143(3):1076–84.
32. Schoot DC, Coelingh Bennink HJ, Mannaerts BM, Lamberts SW, Bouchard P, Fauser BC. Human recombinant follicle-stimulating hormone induces growth of Preovulatory follicles without concomitant increase in androgen and estrogen biosynthesis in a woman with isolated gonadotropin deficiency. J Clin Endocrinol Metab. 1992;74(6):1471–3.
33. Weenen C, Laven JS, Von Bergh AR, Cranfield M, Groome NP, Visser JA, et al. Anti-Mullerian hormone expression pattern in the human ovary: potential implications for initial and cyclic follicle recruitment. Mol Hum Reprod. 2004;10(2):77–83.
34. Sonmezer M, Ozmen B, Atabekoglu CS, Papuccu EG, Ozkavukcu S, Berker B, et al. Serum anti-Mullerian hormone levels correlate with ovarian response in idiopathic Hypogonadotropic Hypogonadism. J Assist Reprod Genet. 2012;29(7):597–602.
35. Deubzer B, Weber K, Lawrenz B, Schweizer R, Binder G. Anti-Mullerian hormone deficiency in girls with congenital multiple pituitary hormone deficiency. J Clin Endocrinol Metab. 2014;99(6):E1045–9.
36. Loumaye E. Ovarian stimulation: is exogenous Lh necessary in all patients? Gynecol Obstet Fertil. 2002;30(11):890–5.
37. Shoham Z, Smith H, Yeko T, O'brien F, Hemsey G, O'dea L. Recombinant Lh (Lutropin Alfa) for the treatment of Hypogonadotrophic women with profound Lh deficiency: a randomized, double-blind, placebo-controlled, proof-of-efficacy study. Clin Endocrinol. 2008;69(3):471–8.
38. Chappel SC, Howles C. Reevaluation of the roles of luteinizing hormone and follicle-stimulating hormone in the ovulatory process. Hum Reprod. 1991;6(9):1206–12.
39. Hillier SG. Current concepts of the roles of follicle stimulating hormone and luteinizing hormone in Folliculogenesis. Hum Reprod. 1994;9(2):188–91.
40. De Boer J, Van Der Meer M, Van Der Veen E, Schoemaker J. Growth hormone (Gh) substitution in Hypogonadotropic, Gh-deficient women decreases the follicle-stimulating hormone threshold for Monofollicular growth. J Clin Endocrinol Metab. 1999;84(2):590–5.

41. De Boer J, Schoemaker J, Van Der Veen E. Impaired reproductive function in women treated for growth hormone deficiency during childhood. Clin Endocrinol. 1997;46(6):681–9.
42. Hayden C. Gnrh analogues: applications in assisted reproductive techniques. Eur J Endocrinol. 2008;159(Suppl 1):S17–25.
43. Mumusoglu S, Ata B, Turan V, Demir B, Kahyaoglu I, Aslan K, et al. Does pituitary suppression affect live birth rate in women with congenital Hypogonadotrophic Hypogonadism undergoing intra-cytoplasmic sperm injection? A Multicenter Cohort Study. Gynecol Endocrinol. 2017;33(9):728–32.
44. Shoham Z, Di Carlo C, Patel A. Conway Gs, Jacobs Hs. Is it possible to run a successful ovulation induction program based solely on ultrasound monitoring? The importance of endometrial measurements. Fertil Steril. 1991;56(5):836–41.
45. Van Der Linden M, Buckingham K, Farquhar C, Ja K, Metwally M. Luteal phase support for assisted reproduction cycles. Cochrane Database Syst Rev. 2015;7:Cd009154.
46. Yding Andersen C, Vilbour AK. Improving the luteal phase after ovarian stimulation: reviewing new options. Reprod Biomed Online. 2014;28(5):552–9.
47. Ulug U, Ben-Shlomo I, Tosun S. Erden Hf, Akman Ma, Bahceci M. the reproductive performance of women with Hypogonadotropic Hypogonadism in an in vitro fertilization and embryo transfer program. J Assist Reprod Genet. 2005;22(4):167–71.
48. Kumbak B, Kahraman S. Women with Hypogonadotropic Hypogonadism: cycle characteristics and results of assisted reproductive techniques. Acta Obstet Gynecol Scand. 2006;85(12):1453–7.
49. Yilmaz S. Ozgu-Erdinc as, Yumusak O, Kahyaoglu S, Seckin B, Yilmaz N. the reproductive outcome of women with Hypogonadotropic Hypogonadism undergoing in vitro fertilization. Syst Biol Reprod Med. 2015;61(4):228–32.
50. Yildirim G, Ficicioglu C, Attar R, Akcin O, Tecellioglu N. Comparison of reproductive outcome of the women with Hypogonadotropic Hypogonadism and tubal factor infertility. Clin Exp Obstet Gynecol. 2010;37(2):120–2.
51. Ghaffari F, Arabipoor A. Lankarani Nb, Etminan Z, Tehraninejad Es. Assisted reproductive technique outcomes in Hypogonadotropic Hypogonadism women. Ann Saudi Med. 2013;33(3):235–40.

Ovarian Stimulation Using Oral Therapy Protocols for the Ovulatory Patient Undergoing Intrauterine Insemination

14

Jamie P. Dubaut and La Tasha B. Craig

Clomiphene citrate was originally approved for ovulation induction in anovulatory patients [1]. Since then, the use of oral agents such as clomiphene and letrozole has been extended to include ovulation augmentation in ovulatory women: to increase the number of dominant follicles produced in a single cycle. This "superovulation" (SO) in combination with intrauterine insemination (IUI) increases the number of oocytes and motile sperm in the fallopian tubes and results in an increased probability that one or more conceptions will occur each cycle. A patient must have at least one patent fallopian tube and her partner have an adequate sperm sample or donor sperm in order to consider this treatment. The effect of SO-IUI on pregnancy rates in ovulatory women is modest, but oral SO-IUI is less costly, exposes the woman to less risks, and is less invasive than gonadotropin SO with IUI (GnSO-IUI) or in vitro fertilization (IVF) and should be considered before pursuing these more aggressive treatments. This chapter focuses on the oral medications used for SO-IUI, the indications, side effects, and risks of this treatment, as well as the pregnancy and delivery rates.

14.1 SO-IUI Technique

14.1.1 Medications

The primary oral medications that have been utilized for SO-IUI in ovulatory women include clomiphene, a selective estrogen receptor modulator (SERM), and letrozole, an aromatase inhibitor. Other SERMs and aromatase inhibitors have been used less frequently for ovulation induction in anovulatory women, and there is little data regarding use of these medications in ovulatory women.

J. P. Dubaut · L. T. B. Craig (✉)
Department of Obstetrics and Gynecology, University of Oklahoma Health Sciences Center, Oklahoma City, OK, USA
e-mail: latasha-craig@ouhsc.edu

Clomiphene was first reported to induce ovulation in 1961 [1]. It is a SERM that has both estrogen agonist and antagonist activity [2]. However, the primary mechanism resulting in superovulation in ovulatory women is through binding and blocking of the estrogen receptor at the level of the hypothalamus. The perception of a low estrogen state results in an increase in circulating follicle-stimulating hormone (FSH), resulting in selection of more than one dominant follicle to ovulate [3]. The multi-follicular development in ovulatory women is usually modest resulting in two to three follicles [4, 5]. Clomiphene is an estrogen receptor antagonist at the level of the uterus and may decrease endometrial thickness, impair endometrial development, and alter cervical mucus secretion [6]. Clomiphene is approved by the US Food and Drug Administration for ovulatory dysfunction rather than the indication discussed in this chapter.

Letrozole selectively inhibits the activity of intracellular aromatase activity, thereby inhibiting the conversion of androgens to estrogens. This decreases local and circulating levels of estrogen. As with clomiphene, the hypothalamus perceives low estrogen and increases gonadotropin production from the anterior pituitary [7]. The intraovarian androgen increase may sensitize the ovary to FSH [8]. It has been shown in an animal model that letrozole results in less detrimental effects on the endometrium based on markers of receptivity [9]. However, clinically, endometrial thickness has not been shown to be consistently greater in patients taking letrozole compared with clomiphene [10]. Of note, letrozole is not approved by the US Food and Drug Administration for the indication of fertility treatment.

Both medications are dosed for 5 days beginning on cycle days 2–5. The medication should be started before a single dominant follicle has been selected, in order to achieve multi-follicular development. Therefore, in women with shorter cycles, consider starting the medication on cycle days 2 or 3. The dosing to achieve multi-follicular development is variable in ovulatory women. In most patients, consider starting with either clomiphene 100 mg or letrozole 5 mg starting on cycle day 3 [11]. It is advisable not to routinely

G. N. Allahbadia et al. (eds.), *Textbook of Assisted Reproduction*, https://doi.org/10.1007/978-981-15-2377-9_14

increase the dose of oral agents in ovulatory SO-IUI without ultrasound monitoring due to the risk of multiple gestation. However, if monofollicular development is noted on transvaginal ultrasound in an ovulatory patient undergoing oral SO-IUI, the medication dose is increased in the subsequent cycle (clomiphene 150 mg or letrozole 7.5 mg), to a maximum of clomiphene 150 mg or letrozole 10 mg daily. If more than three follicles are expected to ovulate, then it is recommended to cancel the cycle and decrease the dose in the subsequent cycle, depending on the patient's age, couple's length of infertility, and previous fertility treatment (Fig. 14.1).

14.1.2 Timing of the IUI

Timing the insemination can be accomplished by one of two monitoring methods: (1) the female partner uses home urinary ovulation predictor kits (OPKs) to detect the natural luteinizing hormone (LH) surge that occurs shortly before ovulation and leads to release of the oocyte; or (2) the female partner undergoes transvaginal ultrasound (US) monitoring of follicular development followed by an injection of hCG (5000 to 10,000 units) to mimic the natural LH surge and result in ovulation approximately 36–40 h after the injection. For women who have no difficulty detecting the LH surge using OPKs, at-home urine tests are a less expensive, less invasive, and an equally efficacious method to time IUI compared to US-hCG monitoring [12]. Lewis et al. found no statistical difference in pregnancy rates in subjects randomized to US-hCG monitoring versus OPKs for up to three cycles of CC-IUI (11.1% versus 12.9%, respectively). However, 31% of patients in the OPK group dropped out of the study compared to 11% in the US-hCG group. The most common reason noted was non-detection of the LH surge in 17 of 58 women [13]. Both false negatives and false positives can result in poorly timed IUI or no IUI. False positives are more likely to occur in women with a higher baseline LH level including those with decreased ovarian reserve [14]. When women choose OPKs to time IUI, we recommend daily testing in the early afternoon, starting cycle day 10. The LH surge is most likely to begin early in the morning but unable to be detected by urine until midday. An OPK performed early afternoon will detect >70% of positive surges that will begin that day [15]. Once a patient has a positive OPK, we generally perform the insemination within 24 h. When women have difficulty detecting the LH surge, we recommend US-hCG monitoring.

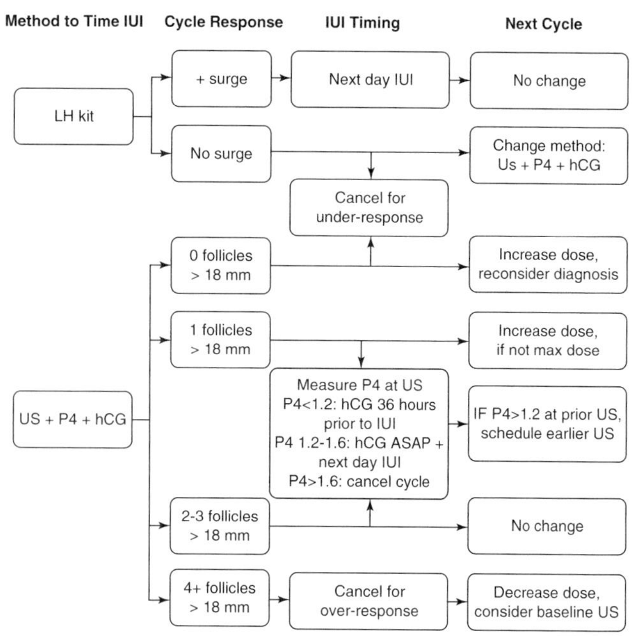

Fig. 14.1 Practical guide to oral superovulation with intrauterine insemination in ovulatory women. *LH* luteinizing hormone, *IUI* intrauterine insemination, *US* transvaginal ultrasound, *P4* progesterone, *hCG* human chorionic gonadotropin

With the goal of multi-follicular development when an ovulatory patient undergoes SO-IUI, ultrasound monitoring can ensure that the patient is on the correct dose of medication and that the endometrium is sufficiently thickened. At our institution, the patient is generally scheduled for transvaginal US between cycle days 10 to 14 (earlier if they report shorter menstrual cycles or have decreased ovarian reserve). HCG is typically administered when at least one follicle is ≥18 mm. Using the rule of thumb that follicles grow approximately 2 mm per day once they are greater than or equal to 12 mm, we will sometimes have the patient wait an extra day to take the hCG injection in order to increase the likelihood that two to three follicles will ovulate. One study randomized patients to hCG administration early (lead follicle >16 mm) versus late (lead follicle >18 mm) and found no difference in clinical or ongoing pregnancy rates (11.9 vs 12.1%, 11.0 vs 8.6%, respectively) [16]. However, another study reported larger mean follicle size at trigger in conception cycles using CC-IUI compared to cycles without conception (20.4 mm vs 18.9 mm) [17].

Ultrasound monitoring alone may not be enough to detect a premature LH surge before the patient injects hCG and schedules IUI. Approximately 30% of patients will have a spontaneous LH surge prior to administering hCG if relying solely on ultrasound [18, 19]. Additionally, serum estradiol levels in combination with US are not predictive of a premature LH surge [20]. Serum progesterone level, on the other hand, may be indicative of premature LH surge. A progesterone >1.1 on day of hCG injection was associated with lower pregnancy rates in GnSO-IUI (gonadotropin superovulation-IUI) cycles when IUI was timed 36 h after hCG [21]. We routinely draw serum progesterone levels on the day of US monitoring. If the progesterone level is <1.2 ng/ml, the patient is instructed to take 10,000 units hCG intramuscular or subcuticular at a time that facilitates the IUI to be performed approximately 36 h later [12]. If the progesterone level is between 1.2 and 1.6 ng/ml, the patient is instructed to take hCG as soon as possible and schedule IUI for the next morning.

14.1.3 Endometrial Appearance

A landmark retrospective cohort study described pregnancy rates by endometrial thickness and pattern (unilinear, trilinear) in IUI for ovulatory infertility [22]. No pregnancies occurred in cycles with endometrial thickness < 6 mm, and ongoing pregnancy rates were significantly lower in cycles with endometrial thickness 6–8.9 mm (6.9%) compared to 9 mm or greater (12.6%). However, a meta-analysis of 17 RCTs and 6 cohort studies on endometrial thickness in IUI pregnancies did not confirm these findings. The meta-analysis found that clomiphene was associated with a thinner endometrium than gonadotropins (mean difference − 0.33 mm, 95% CI −0.64 to −0.01); however, endometrial thickness was not significantly different in pregnant versus nonpregnant cycles [10]. If the endometrium is thin on clomiphene, then we have the patient take letrozole in the subsequent cycle. We do not recommend cycle cancellation based on endometrial pattern.

14.1.4 After the IUI

Following the IUI, clinics have patients rest for varying amounts of time. There have been conflicting results from RCTs that evaluated whether immobilization following IUI for a short period of time improved pregnancy rates. Some studies have found higher pregnancy rates in those randomized to recumbence after IUI, with 10–20 min of recumbence compared to 0–5 min [23, 24]. However, a large, RCT with uniform treatment protocol found no difference between 15 min immobilization compared to immediate ambulation in pregnancy or live birth rates [25]. After a 5-min period of immobilization, we recommend no restrictions on physical or sexual activity.

Luteal supplementation with progesterone is not routinely used following clomiphene or letrozole cycles. A recent systematic review and meta-analysis concluded that clinical pregnancy rates were not statistically different when progesterone was taken in the luteal phase in cycles with clomiphene or letrozole compared to no progesterone medication, in contrast to gonadotropin-IUI cycles [26].

A home pregnancy test should be performed 14–15 days following IUI if the patient has not started her menstrual cycle. We do not routinely perform baseline ultrasounds between cycles unless other issues arise, like hyperstimulation or premature ovulation in the previous cycle.

14.2 Indications for So-IUI

As stated previously, the goal of SO-IUI treatment in ovulatory patients is to combine an increased numbers of oocytes with increased number of motile sperm in close proximity at the appropriate time, which may quicken the time to pregnancy. This strategy may overcome subtle ovulatory defects, bypass any potential underlying or clomiphene-related cervical factors, and maximize the chance of fertilization and subsequent pregnancy. Indications for this treatment include unexplained infertility, endometriosis, decreased ovarian reserve, mild to moderate male factor infertility, and therapeutic donor insemination.

14.2.1 Unexplained Infertility

Up to 30% of couples will have no identifiable cause for their infertility after completing the diagnostic evaluation, which includes confirmation of ovulation, at least one patent fallopian tube, and an adequate semen analysis Dodson [27]. Unexplained infertility may be better understood as subfertility, in that the couple's chance for pregnancy with expectant management is lower than normal, but not absent. In research studies, the definition of unexplained infertility varies greatly including the cutoff for a "normal" semen analysis, as well as inclusion of women with endometriosis or diminished ovarian reserve. Treatment options for couples with unexplained infertility include expectant management, SO with oral agents, or gonadotropins with or without IUI and IVF [28]. No RCT has attempted to examine all treatment options to date, so decision-making relies on best evidence from less definitive studies. Patient values, cost, and likelihood of success all factor into tailoring treatment to a particular couple.

A landmark article by Guzick et al. in 1998 aggregated data from multiple trials to give the best estimates for the efficacy of the different treatment options for unexplained infertility. This article is often cited to counsel patients on their per cycle pregnancy rates for various treatment options. After adjustments were made for study quality, this review reported expectant management was associated with 1.3–4.1% pregnancy rate per cycle, clomiphene or IUI alone slightly increased the pregnancy rates, and clomiphene with IUI increased it more to 8.3% [29] (Fig. 14.2). The numbers are concrete and intuitive, though their use may oversimplify and overestimate our certainty of the effectiveness of clomiphene, IUI, and clomiphene-IUI. Furthermore, this review did not include letrozole or letrozole-IUI, which are commonly used in today's practice. The success rates for IVF have certainly improved since this article was published. However, the pregnancy rates per cycle remain similar for less aggressive treatment options.

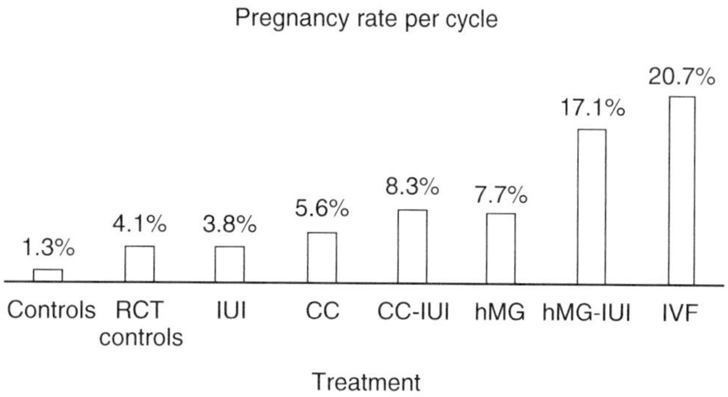

Fig. 14.2 Per cycle pregnancy rates in couples with unexplained infertility based on the article by Guzick et al. [29]. *RCT* randomized controlled trial, *IUI* intrauterine insemination, *CC* clomiphene citrate, *hMG* human menopausal gonadotropin, *IVF* in vitro fertilization

The validated Hunault model to predict live birth with expectant management of unexplained infertility was developed from a Dutch and Canadian population of 2459 couples [30]. Female age < 32 years, prior pregnancy, duration of infertility <2 years, and progressive motility >40% are favorable prognostic factors. An online calculator is available [31] which uses these factors and predicts probability of live birth in the first year of expectant management. If the predicted live birth is >40% within 1 year, it is recommended the couple consider expectant management [32]. Newer models with more variables have been developed, but they have not been externally validated [33]. Although expectant management may be acceptable to some couples due to its negligible cost and avoidance of treatment-associated risks, other couples may wish to move on to more proactive treatment options [34].

Prescribing clomiphene with timed intercourse for unexplained infertility is low cost, widely available, and has been common practice for decades. However, a 2010 Cochrane review concluded that there was not a significant difference in pregnancy rate per cycle compared to expectant management or placebo, though moderate heterogeneity between trials was noted [35]. Based on three fairly homogenous RCTs published between 1983 and 1990, the 2006 ASRM Practice Committee Opinion "Treatment of Unexplained Infertility" suggests the overall number of couples needed to treat with clomiphene (with timed intercourse) for one additional pregnancy is 40 (95% CI 20–202) [36]. A multicenter RCT published in 2008 from the United Kingdom for unexplained infertility (including some mild male factor and endometriosis) compared expectant management (natural cycle-timed intercourse; n = 193), CC-timed intercourse (n = 194), and natural cycle-IUI timed by OPKs (n = 193) for up to 6 months. The cumulative live birth rates were not significantly different between the three groups [34].

CC-IUI has been found to be superior to both expectant management and natural cycle-IUI. In one study of patients with unexplained infertility or surgically treated endometriosis, CC-IUI was found to have a statistically higher clinical pregnancy rate per cycle than expectant management (9.5% versus 3.3%, respectively; $p < 0.05$) [37]. A randomized controlled trial found that the pregnancy rate per cycle in patients with unexplained infertility was significantly higher at 26.1% per cycle with clomiphene-IUI (n = 23 cycles), compared to 5% for natural cycle-IUI (n = 20 cycles) [38]. The rigor of these findings has been questioned in the intervening years, largely due to the small size, study design, and absence of live birth outcome per couple in these studies [39]. A recent randomized controlled trial with a pragmatic study design demonstrated live birth rate was indeed higher in couples randomized to 3 months oral SO-IUI compared to 3 months expectant management for unexplained infertility. In this larger study, 31% of 101 couples in the SO-IUI and 9% of the 100 couples in the expectant management group had live births [40].

A few recent studies have included letrozole-IUI in comparison with CC-IUI. A randomized controlled trial in Canada compared letrozole 7.5 mg-IUI (n = 115 cycles) to clomiphene 100 mg-IUI (n = 123 cycles) and found similar pregnancy rates per cycle (11.5% versus 8.9%, respectively) but a higher miscarriage rate with clomiphene [41]. An Egyptian randomized controlled trial comparing letrozole 5 mg-IUI to clomiphene 100 mg-IUI (with luteal progesterone) found similar, but strikingly high pregnancy rates per cycle (18.2% versus 19.3% in 400 and 404 cycles, respectively), with an ongoing pregnancy rate per cycle of 15.5% and 16.3%, respectively [42]. Another Egyptian study randomized patients to extended dose letrozole (2.5 mg cycle days 1–9) or clomiphene 100 cycle days 3–7, both with IUI, and found statistically higher pregnancy rate per cycle with letrozole compared to clomiphene (19.0% versus 11.4%, respectively; $p = 0.03$) and ongoing pregnancy rate per cycle of 16.6% versus 9.5%, respectively [43]. However, this study dosed letrozole for 10 days, rather than 5.

A landmark trial from the Reproductive Medicine Network entitled Assessment of Multiple Intrauterine Gestations from Ovarian Stimulation (AMIGOS) aimed to determine if letrozole resulted in a lower rate of multiple gestations than the current standard ovulation methods of clomiphene or gonadotropins. In this partially blinded, multicenter RCT, couples were randomized to letrozole 5 mg-IUI, clomiphene 100 mg-IUI, or gonadotropin-IUI for unexplained infertility up to four cycles [11]. In subsequent cycles, the dose could be adjusted to obtain two to three dominant follicles. Clinical pregnancy rates per cycle were not statistically different between letrozole-IUI (n = 906 cycles) and CC-IUI (n = 887 cycles) groups (7.3% versus 9.6%, respectively) nor were live birth rates different (6.2% versus 7.9%, respectively). There was no significant difference in pregnancy loss or the rate of multiple gestations (13% letrozole versus 9% clomiphene). GnSO-IUI cycles had a significantly higher clinical pregnancy rate (13.6%) and live birth rate (12.3%) than either oral agent. However, 32% of GnSO-IUI pregnancies were multiples, including 9.3% triplets [11]. Based on the currently available research, clomiphene and letrozole appear equally efficacious for unexplained infertility couples when combined with IUI.

14.2.2 Male Factor

Many studies of unexplained infertility included subjects that could be considered to have mild to moderate male factor infertility based on the cutoffs used. For example, the AMIGOS trial included couples if the male had at least five million total motile sperm in the ejaculate [11]. The few studies specifically evaluating IUI efficacy in male factor infertility are also difficult to interpret due to heterogeneity in inclusion criteria and limitations of the semen analysis. The general acceptance of IUI as treatment for male factor infertility stems from reports of higher pregnancy rates with IUI than natural intercourse or intracervical insemination [44]. Studies specifically examining oral SO-IUI for male factor infertility are limited. A retrospective review of 356 IUI cycles found no statistical difference in per cycle pregnancy rates in natural cycle-IUI 3% (3/94), letrozole-IUI 3% (1/39), CC-IUI 7.5% (8/107), and GnSO-IUI 6% (7/116) [45]. Of note, the average female age in this study was 38. Despite limited evidence, it seems reasonable to stimulate mild multi-follicular development in male factor infertility treated with IUI.

14.2.3 Age-Related Infertility/Decreased Ovarian Reserve

As with IVF, pregnancy rates in SO-IUI cycles are clearly linked to female age. A cohort study in the United States of 2351 CC-IUI cycles showed a progressively decreasing pregnancy rate per cycle with increasing female age: 11.5% age < 35, 9.2% in 35–37 year olds, 7.3% in 38–40 year olds, 4.3% in 41–42 year olds, and 1% women greater than 42 years old [46]. A retrospective study from the United Kingdom analyzed 699 IUI cycles with or without superovulation in women 38–40 years old with unexplained infertility and suggested a higher per cycle pregnancy rate (PR) and live birth rate (LBR) in natural-IUI cycles (PR 12.0% LBR 7.5%) compared to GnSO-IUI (PR 8.2% LBR 3.5%) and CC-IUI cycles (PR 9.3% LBR 2.1%) [47], leading to questions about the benefit of superovulation in older women. However, the retrospective nature of the study indicates concern for selection bias within which poorer prognosis patients may have been prescribed more aggressive treatment.

Part of letrozole's effect may be through upregulation and sensitization of FSH receptors, by increasing intrafollicular androgens [8]. This has led to the addition of letrozole to gonadotropin-IUI cycles [48] and IVF for women with diminished ovarian reserve [49]. More definitive research in letrozole-IUI for age-related or other DOR is lacking.

The AMIGOs study required a FSH ≤12 IU/L and age ≤ 40 years old, but did not exclude patients based on AMH [11]. AMH was measured as part of the trial, and after multivariate analysis adjustment, AMH was not associated with pregnancy outcome [50]. Overall, the data supports the consensus that AMH is a better marker for oocyte quantity rather than quality and therefore has a larger impact on therapies where high oocyte number is associated with improved pregnancy rate, like IVF [51].

14.2.4 Donor Sperm

Patients undergoing therapeutic donor IUI are not necessarily considered infertile. Therefore, it is reasonable to consider natural cycle-donor IUI for the first three to six treatment cycles unless the patient has oligo-ovulation. However, the cost of donor IUI is substantial, and it is common for patients to undergo superovulation in hopes of increasing pregnancy rates per cycle. Several cohort studies have shown no difference in pregnancy rates between natural cycle-donor IUI and CC-donor IUI cycles. A large retrospective study of 1056 cycles in 261 patients demonstrated a pregnancy rate per cycle of 13% (natural-donor IUI), 7.2% (CC-donor IUI), and 11% (GnSO-donor IUI) cycles [52]. However, without randomization or a standardized protocol, better prognosis candidates were likely concentrated in the natural cycle group. A smaller study of 216 donor IUI cycles in 101 patients used a standardized approach of 3 natural cycles followed by 3 cycles with clomiphene and then 3 cycles of gonadotropins, showing per cycle pregnancy rates of 13%, 10%, and 21%, respectively. The increase for GnSO-donor IUI was statistically significant [53]. The design of three natural cycles first selects out those with the best prognosis from subsequent groups, as they achieve a pregnancy, with the lowest risk of multiple pregnancy. One retrospective cohort of ovulatory patients compared CC-donor IUI to letrozole-IUI. Comparing CC-donor IUI to letrozole-donor IUI, there were no statistically significant differences in live birth rate per cycle (16.5% vs 11.5%, respectively) or cumulative live birth rate after three cycles (36.6% vs 27.7%, respectively) [54]. Stimulation with oral agents as first line for donor insemination remains common practice, but may not increase pregnancy rates while increasing the risk for multiple gestations.

14.2.5 Endometriosis

It is certain that there is overlap in the diagnosis and study of endometriosis and unexplained infertility. For example, the protocol for the AMIGOs trial included patients with stage I/II endometriosis (stage III/IV excluded), but laparoscopy was not required as part of the workup [11]. With waning use of laparoscopy in the workup of infertility, undiagnosed endometriosis will undoubtedly continue to be included in unexplained infertility trials.

Few have studied oral SO-IUI specifically for endometriosis-related infertility. An Egyptian RCT reported similar per cycle clinical pregnancy rate in letrozole-IUI (5 mg) and CC-IUI (100 mg) in surgically treated stage I/II endometriosis (15.9% versus 14.5%, respectively; $p = 0.82$) [55].

14.2.6 Number of Treatment Cycles

In addition to cumulative cost and likelihood of success with IUI, aspects to consider when recommending number of treatment cycles include point of diminishing returns and availability of more efficacious options. A retrospective multicenter cohort study in the Netherlands is consisting of 3714 couples who underwent 15,303 IUI cycles, 51% of which included clomiphene. Couples underwent up to nine cycles with IUI with a 41.2% cumulative ongoing pregnancy rate. Of all the pregnancies, nearly half occurred in the first three cycles of treatment, and 75% of the pregnancies occurred in the first six cycles. However, ongoing pregnancy rate per cycle did not drop lower than 4.4% in each of the first nine cycles [56]. Based on this and previous literature, we recommend couples to undergo three to four cycles of SO-IUI and then consult with the provider to discuss whether to continue oral SO-IUI up to six cycles total versus move on to more aggressive and more costly treatment options. Based on the fast track and standard treatment trial (FAST-T) and the forty and older treatment trial (FORT-T), we typically recommend the couple to move on to IVF (rather than GnSO-IUI) [57, 58]. When patients cannot afford to move on to IVF even when recommended, we allow up to nine cycles of oral SO-IUI, but we counsel patients on the decrease in per cycle pregnancy rates in successive cycles.

14.3 Risks of So-IUI

14.3.1 Side Effects

Clomiphene and letrozole result in central misperception that estrogen levels are low, so it is not unexpected that vasomotor symptoms are reported; recent trials have reported hot flashes in 30.9% of CC cycles and 16.8% of letrozole cycles [11].

Transient mood changes are also common in CC treatment cycles, but this is harder to quantify in the literature. A recent review cited five case reports of CC-associated psychosis with a common feature of paranoia; symptoms stopped when the drug was withdrawn, and the review suggests that transient psychosis may be underreported, given that mood changes are expected [59]. Clomiphene has mydriatic action, and vision changes are reported in 1–3% of patients taking CC [11, 60], including blurred vision, double vision, scotomata, and light sensitivity. Most cases are transient; however, permanent scotomata, light sensitivity, and visual hallucinations have been documented in case reports [61, 62]. If vision changes are noted, CC should be discontinued and letrozole considered as an alternative. Clomiphene and letrozole both have other side effects such as headaches, bloating, nausea, dizziness, fatigue, and joint pain [11]. Letrozole is associated with more intra-menstrual bleeding, which could be due to low estrogen despite oocyte maturation, but this is anecdotal.

Bleeding from contact with the cervix is a relatively common and benign side effect of IUI [63]. The IUI procedure rarely results in a pelvic infection [64, 65]. The AMIGOs study reported pyosalpinx in one patient in the GnSO-IUI arm of the study [11].

14.3.2 Multiple Gestations

Despite aiming for two to three follicles to ovulate, >85% of patients that conceive have a single IUP after oral medications and IUI [11]. However, where there is multi-follicular development, there is an increased risk of multiple pregnancies. Non-IVF fertility treatment (including gonadotropins) also appeared to increase monozygotic twinning rates [66].

Most multiple pregnancies resulting from clomiphene are twins; however, higher-order multiple pregnancies occur in approximately 1% of CC-induced pregnancies [60]. Of 2369 pregnancies in the clinical trials for FDA approval of CC, 7.98% were multiples, 6.9% were twins, 0.5% were triplets, 0.3% were quadruplets, and 0.1% were quintuplets. A sextuplet pregnancy was reported outside the original trials, and the most recent case report of quintuplets cites five others in the literature [67].

The AMIGOs trial was designed to test the hypothesis that letrozole may have a lower multiple pregnancy rate than clomiphene or gonadotropins in unexplained infertility [68]. If letrozole had a lower multiple pregnancy rate, it might have become the oral agent of choice, even if pregnancy rates were mildly reduced. However, the outcome of the AMIGOs trial did not validate the earlier cohort studies. Multiple gestation was present in 9.4% (8/85) of clinical clomiphene pregnancies and 13.4% (9/57) of clinical pregnancies conceived after letrozole, which was not significant ($p = 0.44$) [11]. High-order multiple pregnancies after letrozole have occasionally been reported, the most extreme being a sextuplet pregnancy in an anovulatory patient treated with 7.5 mg of letrozole [69].

The goal of infertility therapy is a healthy pregnancy, and the likelihood of achieving this goal is highest with a singleton gestation. The risks of multiple gestation are numerous, serious, and in high prevalence. Preterm delivery (<37 weeks), very preterm delivery (<32 weeks), neonatal morbidity, neonatal mortality, and intrauterine fetal death are increased in multiple pregnancies [70, 71]. Maternal morbidity is also higher, partly due to increase in risk factors including gestational diabetes, preeclampsia, and cesarean delivery [70, 71].

14.3.3 Pregnancy/Perinatal Outcomes

Miscarriage rates are similar between clomiphene and letrozole [11, 72]. The AMIGOs trial found rates of first trimester loss in letrozole-IUI of 29.4% (25/85) compared to 26.4% (28/106) in CC-IUI cycles. Second and third trimester losses were 1.2% (1/85) and 2.8% (3/106), respectively [11].

Congenital anomalies, low birth weight, and small for gestational age have been associated with infertility treatments including IUI and IVF, but this association is difficult to isolate as subfertility itself is associated with these outcomes [73, 74]. A large cohort study in Denmark did suggest that CC-IUI was associated with higher rates of low birth weight and small for gestational age compared to naturally conceived infants [75]. Larger published studies have not verified this finding [76], and the AMIGOs trial found no significant differences in congenital anomalies [11].

14.3.4 Ovarian Cancer: Invasive and Borderline

There is no meaningful increased risk of borderline ovarian tumors or invasive ovarian cancer with infertility treatment including clomiphene [77, 78].

14.3.5 Ovarian Hyperstimulation Syndrome

Severe ovarian hyperstimulation syndrome (OHSS) is an exceedingly rare complication of clomiphene use [79]. Letrozole does not increase the chance of OHSS and indeed has been studied as treatment of OHSS caused by IVF [80]. However, symptoms on the spectrum of mild OHSS were reported in AMIGOs trial in both clomiphene and letrozole groups (abdominal/pelvic pain, 30.5% and 36.1%; bloating, 16.8% and 18.6%; nausea, 14.1% & 16.8%, respectively). Patients undergoing SO-IUI cycles with oral agents can be reassured that while bloating, abdominal/pelvic pain, and nausea can occur, they are very unlikely to develop severe OHSS.

14.4 Conclusion

The use of clomiphene or letrozole in ovulatory women undergoing intrauterine insemination is more effective than expectant management, natural cycle-IUI, or oral SO-timed intercourse. Clomiphene or letrozole with IUI is modestly effective and relatively inexpensive treatment with demonstrated safety. The risk with the most impact is multiple gestations. Randomized controlled trials comparing all available treatment options for unexplained infertility, in particular, are needed in order to better counsel patients on the success of treatment while taking into account the time, cost, and side effects.

References

1. Greenblatt RB, Barfield WE, Jungck EC, Ray AW. Induction of ovulation with MRL/41. Preliminary report Jama. 1961;178:101–4.
2. Clark JH, Markaverich BM. The agonistic-antagonistic properties of clomiphene: a review. Pharmacol Ther. 1981;15(3):467–519.
3. Kerin JF, Liu JH, Phillipou G, Yen SS. Evidence for a hypothalamic site of action of clomiphene citrate in women. J Clin Endocrinol Metab. 1985;61(2):265–8.
4. Randall JM, Templeton A. Transvaginal sonographic assessment of follicular and endometrial growth in spontaneous and clomiphene citrate cycles. Fertil Steril. 1991;56(2):208–12.
5. Fisher SA, Reid RL, Van Vugt DA, Casper RF. A randomized double-blind comparison of the effects of clomiphene citrate and the aromatase inhibitor letrozole on ovulatory function in normal women. Fertil Steril. 2002;78(2):280–5.
6. Massai MR, de Ziegler D, Lesobre V, Bergeron C, Frydman R, Bouchard P. Clomiphene citrate affects cervical mucus and endometrial morphology independently of the changes in plasma hormonal levels induced by multiple follicular recruitment. Fertil Steril. 1993;59(6):1179–86.
7. Requena A, Herrero J, Landeras J, Navarro E, Neyro JL, Salvador C, et al. Use of letrozole in assisted reproduction: a systematic review and meta-analysis. Hum Reprod Update. 2008;14(6):571–82.
8. Pritts EA. Letrozole for ovulation induction and controlled ovarian hyperstimulation. Curr Opin Obstet Gynecol. 2010;22(4):289–94.
9. Bao SH, Sheng SL, Peng YF, Lin QD. Effects of letrozole and clomiphene citrate on the expression of HOXA10 and integrin alpha v beta 3 in uterine epithelium of rats. Fertil Steril. 2009;91(1):244–8.
10. Weiss NS, van Vliet MN, Limpens J, Hompes PGA, Lambalk CB, Mochtar MH, et al. Endometrial thickness in women undergoing IUI with ovarian stimulation. How thick is too thin? A systematic review and meta-analysis. Hum Reprod. 2017;32(5):1009–18.
11. Diamond MP, Legro RS, Coutifaris C, Alvero R, Robinson RD, Casson P, et al. Letrozole, gonadotropin, or clomiphene for unexplained infertility. N Engl J Med. 2015;373(13):1230–40.

12. Cantineau AE, Janssen MJ, Cohlen BJ, Allersma T. Synchronised approach for intrauterine insemination in subfertile couples. Cochrane Database Syst Rev. 2014;12:Cd006942.
13. Lewis V, Queenan J Jr, Hoeger K, Stevens J, Guzick DS. Clomiphene citrate monitoring for intrauterine insemination timing: a randomized trial. Fertil Steril. 2006;85(2):401–6.
14. Anderson RA, Eccles SM, Irvine DS. Home ovulation testing in a donor insemination service. Hum Reprod. 1996;11(8):1674–7.
15. Khattab AF, Mustafa FA, Taylor PJ. The use of urine LH detection kits to time intrauterine insemination with donor sperm. Hum Reprod. 2005;20(9):2542–5.
16. da Silva AL, Arbo E, Fanchin R. Early versus late hCG administration to trigger ovulation in mild stimulated IUI cycles: a randomized clinical trial. Eur J Obstet Gynecol Reprod Biol. 2012;164(2):156–60.
17. Shalom-Paz E, Marzal A, Wiser A, Hyman J, Tulandi T. Does optimal follicular size in IUI cycles vary between clomiphene citrate and gonadotrophins treatments? Gynecol Endocrinol. 2014;30(2):107–10.
18. Cantineau AE, Cohlen BJ. The prevalence and influence of luteinizing hormone surges in stimulated cycles combined with intrauterine insemination during a prospective cohort study. Fertil Steril. 2007;88(1):107–12.
19. Antaki R, Dean NL, Lapensee L, Racicot MH, Menard S, Kadoch IJ. An algorithm combining ultrasound monitoring and urinary luteinizing hormone testing: a novel approach for intrauterine insemination timing. J Obstet Gynaecol Can. 2011;33(12):1248–52.
20. Cunha-Filho JS, Kadoch J, Righini C, Fanchin R, Frydman R, Olivennes F. Premature LH and progesterone rise in intrauterine insemination cycles: analysis of related factors. Reprod Biomed Online. 2003;7(2):194–9.
21. Requena A, Cruz M, Pacheco A, Garcia-Velasco JA. Ongoing pregnancy rates in intrauterine insemination are affected by late follicular-phase progesterone levels. Fertil Steril. 2015;104(4):879–83.
22. Dickey RP, Olar TT, Taylor SN, Curole DN, Harrigill K. Relationship of biochemical pregnancy to pre-ovulatory endometrial thickness and pattern in patients undergoing ovulation induction. Hum Reprod. 1993;8(2):327–30.
23. Saleh A, Tan SL, Biljan MM, Tulandi T. A randomized study of the effect of 10 minutes of bed rest after intrauterine insemination. Fertil Steril. 2000;74(3):509–11.
24. Custers IM, Flierman PA, Maas P, Cox T, Van Dessel TJ, Gerards MH, et al. Immobilisation versus immediate mobilisation after intrauterine insemination: randomised controlled trial. BMJ (Clinical research ed). 2009;339:b4080.
25. van Rijswijk J, Caanen MR, Mijatovic V, Vergouw CG, van de Ven PM, Lambalk CB, et al. Immobilization or mobilization after IUI: an RCT. Hum Reprod. 2017;32(11):2218–24.
26. Green KA, Zolton JR, Schermerhorn SM, Lewis TD, Healy MW, Terry N, et al. Progesterone luteal support after ovulation induction and intrauterine insemination: an updated systematic review and meta-analysis. Fertil Steril. 2017;107(4):924–33.
27. Dodson WC, Whitesides DB, Hughes CL Jr, Easley HA 3rd, Haney AF. Superovulation with intrauterine insemination in the treatment of infertility: a possible alternative to gamete intrafallopian transfer and in vitro fertilization. Fertil Steril. 1987;48(3):441–5.
28. Gunn DD, Bates GW. Evidence-based approach to unexplained infertility: a systematic review. Fertil Steril. 2016;105(6):1566–74. e1
29. Guzick DS, Sullivan MW, Adamson GD, Cedars MI, Falk RJ, Peterson EP, et al. Efficacy of treatment for unexplained infertility. Fertil Steril. 1998;70(2):207–13.
30. Hunault CC, Habbema JD, Eijkemans MJ, Collins JA, Evers JL, te Velde ER. Two new prediction rules for spontaneous pregnancy leading to live birth among subfertile couples, based on the synthesis of three previous models. Hum Reprod. 2004;19(9):2019–26.
31. Calculate the probability of a spontaneous ongoing pregnancy within 1 year (leading to live birth). Available from: https://www.freya.nl/probability.php.
32. van der Steeg JW, Steures P, Eijkemans MJ, Habbema JD, Hompes PG, Broekmans FJ, et al. Pregnancy is predictable: a large-scale prospective external validation of the prediction of spontaneous pregnancy in subfertile couples. Hum Reprod. 2007;22(2):536–42.
33. Bensdorp AJ, van der Steeg JW, Steures P, JDF H, PGA H, PMM B, et al. A revised prediction model for natural conception. Reproductive biomedicine online. 2017;34(6):619–26.
34. Bhattacharya S, Harrild K, Mollison J, Wordsworth S, Tay C, Harrold A, et al. Clomifene citrate or unstimulated intrauterine insemination compared with expectant management for unexplained infertility: pragmatic randomised controlled trial. BMJ (Clinical research ed). 2008;337:a716.
35. Hughes E, Brown J, Collins JJ, Vanderkerchove P. Clomiphene citrate for unexplained subfertility in women. Cochrane Database Syst Rev. 2010;1:CD000057.
36. Effectiveness and treatment for unexplained infertility. Fertil Steril. 2006;86(5 Suppl 1):S111–4.
37. Deaton JL, Gibson M, Blackmer KM, Nakajima ST, Badger GJ, Brumsted JR. A randomized, controlled trial of clomiphene citrate and intrauterine insemination in couples with unexplained infertility or surgically corrected endometriosis. Fertil Steril. 1990;54(6):1083–8.
38. Arici A, Byrd W, Bradshaw K, Kutteh WH, Marshburn P, Carr BR. Evaluation of clomiphene citrate and human chorionic gonadotropin treatment: a prospective, randomized, crossover study during intrauterine insemination cycles. Fertil Steril. 1994;61(2):314–8.
39. Veltman-Verhulst SM, Hughes E, Ayeleke RO, Cohlen BJ. Intrauterine insemination for unexplained subfertility. Cochrane Database Syst Rev. 2016;2:Cd001838.
40. Farquhar CM, Liu E, Armstrong S, Arroll N, Lensen S, Brown J. Intrauterine insemination with ovarian stimulation versus expectant management for unexplained infertility (TUI): a pragmatic, open-label, randomised, controlled, two-Centre trial. Lancet (London, England). 2018;391(10119):441–50.
41. Al-Fozan H, Al-Khadouri M, Tan SL, Tulandi T. A randomized trial of letrozole versus clomiphene citrate in women undergoing superovulation. Fertil Steril. 2004;82(6):1561–3.
42. Badawy A, Elnashar A, Totongy M. Clomiphene citrate or aromatase inhibitors for superovulation in women with unexplained infertility undergoing intrauterine insemination: a prospective randomized trial. Fertil Steril. 2009;92(4):1355–9.
43. Fouda UM, Sayed AM. Extended letrozole regimen versus clomiphene citrate for superovulation in patients with unexplained infertility undergoing intrauterine insemination: a randomized controlled trial. Reprod Biol Endocrinol. 2011;9:84.
44. Ford WC, Mathur RS, Hull MG. Intrauterine insemination: is it an effective treatment for male factor infertility? Baillieres Clin Obstet Gynaecol. 1997;11(4):691–710.
45. Luco SM, Agbo C, Behr B, Dahan MH. The evaluation of pre and post processing semen analysis parameters at the time of intrauterine insemination in couples diagnosed with male factor infertility and pregnancy rates based on stimulation agent. A retrospective cohort study. Eur J Obstet Gynecol Reprod Biol. 2014;179:159–62.
46. Dovey S, Sneeringer RM, Penzias AS. Clomiphene citrate and intrauterine insemination: analysis of more than 4100 cycles. Fertil Steril. 2008;90(6):2281–6.
47. Kalu E, Thum MY, Abdalla H. Intrauterine insemination in natural cycle may give better results in older women. J Assist Reprod Genet. 2007;24(2–3):83–6.
48. Bedaiwy MA, Shokry M, Mousa N, Claessens A, Esfandiari N, Gotleib L, et al. Letrozole co-treatment in infertile women 40 years old and older receiving controlled ovarian stimulation and intrauterine insemination. Fertil Steril. 2009;91(6):2501–7.

49. Garcia-Velasco JA, Moreno L, Pacheco A, Guillen A, Duque L, Requena A, et al. The aromatase inhibitor letrozole increases the concentration of intraovarian androgens and improves in vitro fertilization outcome in low responder patients: a pilot study. Fertil Steril. 2005;84(1):82–7.
50. Hansen KR, He AL, Styer AK, Wild RA, Butts S, Engmann L, et al. Predictors of pregnancy and live-birth in couples with unexplained infertility after ovarian stimulation-intrauterine insemination. Fertil Steril. 2016;105(6):1575–83. e2
51. Brodin T, Hadziosmanovic N, Berglund L, Olovsson M, Holte J. Antimullerian hormone levels are strongly associated with live-birth rates after assisted reproduction. J Clin Endocrinol Metab. 2013;98(3):1107–14.
52. Ferrara I, Balet R, Grudzinskas JG. Intrauterine insemination with frozen donor sperm. Pregnancy outcome in relation to age and ovarian stimulation regime. Hum Reprod. 2002;17(9):2320–4.
53. Lashen H, Afnan M, Kennefik A. Early resort to ovarian stimulation improves the cost-effectiveness of a donor insemination programme. Hum Reprod. 1999;14(8):1983–8.
54. El Hachem H, Antaki R, Sylvestre C, Kadoch IJ, Lapensee L, Bouet PE. Clomiphene citrate versus Letrozole for ovarian stimulation in therapeutic donor sperm insemination. Gynecol Obstet Investig. 2016;82(5):481–6.
55. Abu Hashim H, El Rakhawy M, Abd EI. Randomized comparison of superovulation with letrozole vs. clomiphene citrate in an IUI program for women with recently surgically treated minimal to mild endometriosis. Acta Obstet Gynecol Scand. 2012;91(3):338–45.
56. Custers IM, Steures P, Hompes P, Flierman P, van Kasteren Y, van Dop PA, et al. Intrauterine insemination: how many cycles should we perform? Hum Reprod. 2008;23(4):885–8.
57. Goldman MB, Thornton KL, Ryley D, Alper MM, Fung JL, Hornstein MD, et al. A randomized clinical trial to determine optimal infertility treatment in older couples: the forty and over treatment trial (FORT-T). Fertil Steril. 2014;101(6):1574–81.e1-2.
58. Reindollar RH, Regan MM, Neumann PJ, Levine BS, Thornton KL, Alper MM, et al. A randomized clinical trial to evaluate optimal treatment for unexplained infertility: the fast track and standard treatment (FASTT) trial. Fertil Steril. 2010;94(3):888–99.
59. Seeman MV. Transient psychosis in women on clomiphene, bromocriptine, domperidone and related endocrine drugs. Gynecol Endocrinol. 2015;31(10):751–4.
60. Research CfDEa. Approval package for Clomid 2012. Available from: https://www.accessdata.fda.gov/drugsatfda_docs/nda/2012/016131Orig1s026.pdf.
61. Purvin VA. Visual disturbance secondary to clomiphene citrate. Arch Ophthalmol. (Chicago, Ill: 1960). 1995;113(4):482–4.
62. Venkatesh R, Gujral GS, Gurav P, Tibrewal S, Mathur U. Clomiphene citrate-induced visual hallucinations: a case report. J Med Case Rep. 2017;11(1):60.
63. Thijssen A, Creemers A, Van der Elst W, Creemers E, Vandormael E, Dhont N, et al. Predictive value of different covariates influencing pregnancy rate following intrauterine insemination with homologous semen: a prospective cohort study. Reprod Biomed Online. 2017;34(5):463–72.
64. Sacks PC, Simon JA. Infectious complications of intrauterine insemination: a case report and literature review. Int J Fertil. 1991;36(6):331–9.
65. Broder S, Sims C, Rothman C. Frequency of postinsemination infections as reported by donor semen recipients. Fertil Steril. 2007;88(3):711–3.
66. Derom C, Vlietinck R, Derom R, Van den Berghe H, Thiery M. Increased monozygotic twinning rate after ovulation induction. Lancet (London, England). 1987;1(8544):1236–8.
67. Tallon N, Case A. Quintuplets: a rare event following clomiphene citrate therapy. J Obstet Gynaecol Can. 2012;34(3):217.
68. Diamond MP, Mitwally M, Casper R, Ager J, Legro RS, Brzyski R, et al. Estimating rates of multiple gestation pregnancies: sample size calculation from the assessment of multiple intrauterine gestations from ovarian stimulation (AMIGOS) trial. Contemp Clin Trials. 2011;32(6):902–8.
69. Warraich G, Vause TD. First reported case of sextuplets conceived via letrozole for ovulation induction. Fertil Steril. 2015;103(2):535–6.
70. Multiple gestation associated with infertility therapy: an American Society for Reproductive Medicine Practice Committee opinion. Fertil Steril. 2012;97(4):825–34.
71. Practice Bulletin No. 169 summary: multifetal gestations: twin, triplet, and higher-order multifetal pregnancies. Obstet Gynecol. 2016;128(4):926–8.
72. Mitwally MF, Biljan MM, Casper RF. Pregnancy outcome after the use of an aromatase inhibitor for ovarian stimulation. Am J Obstet Gynecol. 2005;192(2):381–6.
73. Sagot P, Bechoua S, Ferdynus C, Facy A, Flamm X, Gouyon JB, et al. Similarly increased congenital anomaly rates after intrauterine insemination and IVF technologies: a retrospective cohort study. Hum Reprod. 2012;27(3):902–9.
74. Hayashi M, Nakai A, Satoh S, Matsuda Y. Adverse obstetric and perinatal outcomes of singleton pregnancies may be related to maternal factors associated with infertility rather than the type of assisted reproductive technology procedure used. Fertil Steril. 2012;98(4):922–8.
75. Malchau SS, Loft A, Henningsen AK, Nyboe Andersen A, Pinborg A. Perinatal outcomes in 6,338 singletons born after intrauterine insemination in Denmark, 2007 to 2012: the influence of ovarian stimulation. Fertil Steril. 2014;102(4):1110–6.e2.
76. Pavone ME, Bulun SE. Clinical review: the use of aromatase inhibitors for ovulation induction and superovulation. J Clin Endocrinol Metab. 2013;98(5):1838–44.
77. Pfeifer S, Butts S, Dumesic D, Fossum G, Gracia C, La Barbera A, et al. Fertility drugs and cancer: a guideline practice Committee of the American Society for reproductive medicine. Fertil Steril. 2016;106(7):1617–26.
78. Bjornholt SM, Kjaer SK, Nielsen TS, Jensen A. Risk for borderline ovarian tumours after exposure to fertility drugs: results of a population-based cohort study. Hum Reprod. 2015;30(1):222–31.
79. Chow KK, Choo HT. Ovarian hyperstimulation syndrome with clomiphene citrate. Case report. Br J Obstet Gynaecol. 1984;91(10):1051–2.
80. He Q, Liang L, Zhang C, Li H, Ge Z, Wang L, et al. Effects of different doses of letrozole on the incidence of early-onset ovarian hyperstimulation syndrome after oocyte retrieval. Syst Biol Reprod Med. 2014;60(6):355–60.

Ovarian Stimulation Using Gonadotropins Protocols for Ovulatory Patient Undergoing IUI

15

Shayne Plosker

15.1 Intrauterine Insemination: From Origins to Current Practice

Human intrauterine insemination (IUI) was first described by Marion Sims in 1866. He achieved 1 pregnancy, resulting in a miscarriage, in 55 inseminations performed on 6 women. In the early part of the twentieth century, a variety of insemination routes were proposed, including intratubal insemination with an insufflator, intra-abdominal insemination, injection of sperm into the pouch of Douglas, placement of sperm in a cup overlying the cervix, injecting donor sperm into the seminal vesicles of the husband for subsequent intercourse, intravaginal insemination, intracervical insemination, and IUI. Prior to the development of procedures to separate sperm from semen, IUI was limited by concerns about endometritis, salpingitis, peritonitis, and severe uterine contractions induced by the inseminate [1]. Indications for artificial insemination included abnormal sperm count, immunologic infertility, unexplained infertility, cervical factor infertility, endometriosis, and erectile dysfunction [2].

Louise Brown, the world's first IVF baby, was born on July 25, 1978. Much less heralded, 2 months earlier, Glass and Ericsson published their study of 67 cycles of IUI in 19 couples in which motile sperm were separated from non-motile sperm and semen by being passed through a liquid albumin column. IUI was timed using temperature charting, without the use of fertility drugs. Although no pregnancies resulted, no clinically apparent infections occurred, and the procedure was well-tolerated [3]. In 1984, Sher and colleagues launched the concept of coupling ovulation induction with IUI (OI-IUI). They described the use of gonadotropins and HCG trigger, followed by intrauterine insemination of motile sperm separated from semen using the swim-up technique and suspended in Hams F-10 solution. Five pregnancies were achieved in 14 couples [4]. Thereafter, paralleling the accelerated use and development of assisted reproductive technologies, IUI metamorphosed from a relatively uncommon procedure to a ubiquitous treatment for women with subfertility. By 2003, an estimated 232,601 gonadotropin-IUI cycles were performed in the United States, more than double the amount of IVF cycles during that year [5]. If one factors in expanded utilization of fertility services since 2003, and the likelihood that even more oral ovulation induction-IUI cycles than gonadotropin-IUI cycles are performed, it is possible that currently more than 500,000 IUI cycles are performed in the United States annually. The exponential expansion in the use of OI-IUI can be attributed to the development of sperm washing procedures which reduce the risk of infection and intense uterine contractions, to increased familiarity with fertility drug administration in the IVF era by increased numbers of reproductive endocrinologists, and to a desire to reduce the cost of infertility treatment for couples with subfertility compared with IVF.

The rationale for ovulation induction with intrauterine insemination was, and remains, based on the assumption that the likelihood of conception will increase if multiple fertilizable oocytes can be recruited in a treatment cycle and if motile sperm can be introduced directly into the uterine cavity at the time of ovulation in order to bypass the cervical mucus barrier and be placed closer to the oocytes [6]. Empirically, a common treatment algorithm evolved, in which IUI treatment was initiated in conjunction with clomiphene citrate (CC). If pregnancy was not achieved after several CC-IUI cycles, then gonadotropins were introduced in conjunction with IUI (GT-IUI). If, after several GT-IUI cycles, pregnancy had not occurred, then IVF was advised.

S. Plosker (✉)
Department of Obstetrics and Gynecology, University of South Florida Morsani College of Medicine, Tampa, FL, USA
e-mail: splosker@health.usf.edu

G. N. Allahbadia et al. (eds.), *Textbook of Assisted Reproduction*, https://doi.org/10.1007/978-981-15-2377-9_15

15.2 What Is the Role for IUI, and IUI with Gonadotropins, in 2019?

Recently, the role for IUI in the treatment of subfertility has been challenged. In 2013, in its clinical guideline of fertility assessment and treatment, the UK National Institute for Health and Care Excellence (NICE) recommended that IUI not be offered to couples with subfertility and that these couples be triaged directly to IVF after 2 years of expectant management [7]. The effectiveness of GT-IUI, specifically, has also been challenged, with one investigator describing gonadotropin therapy as "a 20th century relic" [8, 9].

Cycle fecundity rates in IUI treatment cycles are modest at best, generally in the 8%–12% per cycle range for CC-IUI [10, 11] and in the 9%–20% range for GT-IUI [11]. The preponderance of data suggests that GT-IUI treatment yields higher pregnancy rates than CC-IUI treatment [12], but this has not been observed universally. One trial of 618 GT-IUI cycles in treatment-naïve patients [13] and a second trial involving 439 GT-IUI cycles in patients who failed to conceive with CC-IUI [8] both reported cycle fecundity rates in the 9%–10% range, similar to fecundity rates reported for CC-IUI.

The true benefit of IUI to couples with subfertility is difficult to ascertain because pregnancies achieved with IUI cannot be attributed to the treatment with absolute certainty. There is always a chance that a successful pregnancy has occurred coincidentally with treatment, rather than as a result of treatment, since a significant number of subfertile couples ultimately conceive even in the absence of a treatment intervention. A multi-center Canadian trial found a live birth rate of 21.2% and a 36-month cumulative live birth rate of 33.3% among 562 untreated couples with unexplained infertility who were referred to academic infertility centers [14]. A Dutch study of couples with subfertility in the primary care setting found a cumulative live birth rate of 53% without treatment [15]. A multi-center Dutch trial of 253 couples, randomized to GT-IUI or to 6 months of expectant management, showed no difference in pregnancy (33% vs 32%) and ongoing pregnancy rates (23% vs 27%) between the 2 arms [16]. In contrast, a recent New Zealand study of 201 couples randomized to IUI in combination with clomiphene citrate or letrozole, or to expectant management, demonstrated a benefit to OI-IUI. In this trial, the cumulative live birth rate after three cycles of treatment was 31%, compared to 9% in the expectant management group [17].

As IVF has improved over the years, the gap between pregnancy rates after IVF vs GT-IUI is widening in favor of IVF. In 1993, the all-age delivery rate per fresh oocyte retrieval in the United States was 18.3%, similar to pregnancy rates reported per GT-IUI cycle [18]. By 2015 the all-age delivery rate per fresh oocyte retrieval was 28% (https://www.cdc.gov/art/reports/2015/fertility-clinic.html), and the cumulative live birth rate per retrieval was 54% in women less than age 35, 40% in women in the 35–37 age group, and 26% in the 38–40 (www.sartcorsonline.com/rptCSR_PublicMultYear.aspx?reportingYear=2015).

Concern about high-order multiple gestations (HOMP) caused by gonadotropin treatment was first expressed nearly 40 years ago, when Schenker et al. stated that gonadotropin-induced multiple gestations "must be regarded as a complication in light of their frequent association with maternal morbidity and their higher rate of pregnancy wastage [19]". As IVF has become increasingly efficient, the recommended number of embryos to transfer has declined [20], leading to a sharp drop in the occurrence of HOMP resulting from IVF. The relative contribution of GT-IUI to HOMP has exceeded that of IVF since 2003, and the gap continues to widen. Kulkarni and colleagues estimated that GT-IUI accounted for 45% of all HOMP in the United States in 2011, whereas IVF accounted for 32%. GT-IUI and IVF contributed similarly to twin gestations, accounting for 19% and 17%, respectively, in 2011 [21]. More recently, with the expanded use of preimplantation genetic screening and single embryo transfers, twin pregnancy rates in IVF, and the contribution of IVF to all twin pregnancies, have also started to decline [22, 23].

A recent trial from the United Kingdom randomized 207 subfertile couples to either three cycles of GT-IUI at a low fixed gonadotropin dose of 75 IU daily (101 couples) or one cycle of IVF (106 couples). Twenty-five singleton live births were achieved in the GT-IUI arm (24.7% per couple), and 33 singleton live births were achieved in the IVF arm (31.1% per couple). The multiple pregnancy rate in the GT-IUI group was 13.8%, and the multiple pregnancy rate in the IVF group was 8.3%, but this difference was not statistically significant. The live birth rates per initiated GT-IUI cycle were 8.9% for cycle 1, 7.1% for cycle 2, and 4.3% for cycle 3. Seventeen couples conceived and delivered spontaneously (8.2% of couples), 12 while awaiting IVF and 5 while awaiting or between GT-IUI cycles. The trial was terminated prematurely when the National Health Service ceased to cover IUI [24]. The results of this study delineate the debate about the role of GT-IUI in 2018. One conclusion from the study could be that three cycles of GT-IUI is equivalent, or nearly equivalent, to one IVF treatment cycle and thus should be offered to patients as a reproductive choice. On the other hand, given the similar live birth rates between spontaneous conceptions during untreated cycles and live birth rates per GT-IUI cycle, one could conclude that expectant management while awaiting IVF is an equivalent, and more economic, choice.

The Fast Track and Standard Treatment Trial (FASTT) randomized 503 treatment-naïve couples with subfertility, in whom the female partner was between the ages of 21 and 39, into a conventional treatment arm (247 couples randomized,

200 couples followed the treatment protocol) and an accelerated treatment arm (256 couples randomized, 217 couples followed the treatment protocol). Conventional treatment involved up to three CC-IUI cycles, followed by up to three GT-IUI cycles, followed by up to six IVF cycles. Accelerated treatment involved up to three CC-IUI cycles, followed by direct triage to up to six IVF attempts, bypassing GT-IUI. Time to pregnancy (hazard ratio [HR], 1.25; 95% CI, 1.00–1.56; log rank $P = 0.045$) and estimated median time to pregnancy (8 months vs 11 months) were shorter in the accelerated treatment group. For the first 11 months after randomization into the trial, the pregnancy rate was higher in the accelerated treatment arm (Fig. 15.1). The live birth + ongoing pregnancy rate per couple was similar in the two groups (75% in the conventional group vs 78% in the accelerated group). Charges per delivery in the accelerated group ($61,553 per delivery; 95% CI, $54,075–$ 69,489) were $10,000 lower than they were in the conventional group ($71,399 per delivery; 95% CI, $60,168–$ 84,490). The FASTT found no added benefit to GT-IUI treatment and recommended triage to IVF if CC-IUI failed to achieve pregnancy [8].

An area of consideration could be the role of GT-IUI in older reproductive age women and women with diminished ovarian reserve. The FORT-T trial randomized 154 subfertile couples, in which the women were 38–42 years old, to two cycles of CC-IUI followed by IVF, two cycles of GT-IUI followed by IVF, or immediate IVF. Cumulative clinical pregnancy rates were 21.6% in the CC-IUI group, 17.3% in the GT-IUI group, and 49.0% in the immediate IVF group. 84% of all live-born infants resulted from IVF. The investigators concluded that immediate IVF was a feasible first treatment choice in this age group and that for those couples who did not wish to initiate treatment with IVF, GT-IUI conferred no advantage over CC-IUI [10]. A secondary analysis of the FASTT and FORT-T identified a subset of 18 women between the ages of 21 and 42 with elevated FSH in the 10–15 mIU/ml range and elevated estradiol >40 pg/ml, in whom no live births occurred after IUI but who had a 33% live birth rate after IVF, suggesting that IUI was futile in this subset and that immediate triage to IVF should be considered [25].

One unanswered question regards the effectiveness of GT-IUI in older reproductive age women with good ovarian reserve. SART IVF data suggests that the risk of triplets is exceedingly low in women greater than age 38 undergoing IVF, regardless of the number of embryos transferred [26, 27]. In the absence of PGS, transfer of up to 3–5 embryos is recommended in this age group during IVF treatment, depending on embryonic stage and patient age, to increase

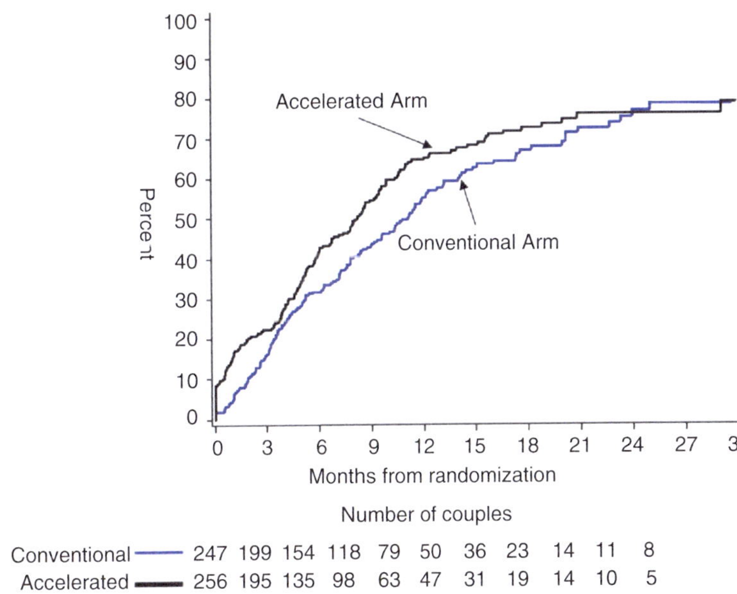

Time Period (m)	Hazard Ratio	95% CI		P-value
≤ 3	1.52	1.02	2.28	0.04
> 3 to 11	1.40	1.03	1.90	0.03
> 11	1.60	1.34	1.06	0.08

Fig. 15.1 The Fast Track and Standard Treatment Trial. (From Reindollar, R.H., et al., *A randomized clinical trial to evaluate optimal treatment for unexplained infertility: the fast track and standard treatment (FASTT) trial*. Fertil Steril, 2010. 94(3): p. 888–99, with permission)

the likelihood of implantation [20]. Similarly, in a series of 561 GT-IUI cycles in women between the ages of 38 and 43, no triplet or higher multiple gestations occurred, and the twin pregnancy rate at 10% was less than half the twin pregnancy rates in women who were 37 years or younger [5, 28]. Analogous to a "heavy" embryo transfer in IVF, aggressive gonadotropin stimulation for IUI may optimize pregnancy rates, with little or no risk for HOMP.

In summary, in 2019, GT-IUI treatment for subfertility may be limited to patients who do not wish IVF, cannot afford IVF, and/or have government-sponsored or private insurance health benefits which cover IUI but not IVF. A trial to compare GT-IUI to IVF for women of ages 38–42 with good ovarian reserve may be warranted.

15.3 Predictors of GT-IUI Outcomes and Risk Factors for Multiple Gestation

Non-IVF use of gonadotropins, such as for GT-IUI, accounted in large part for the 76% increase in twin pregnancies from 1980 to 2009 and the 400% increase in triplet pregnancies from 1980 to 1998 [5, 21]. An estimated 32,000 multiple gestations, including 3000 triplet or greater gestations, were estimated to have occurred from non-IVF ovulation induction in 2004 [29]. Several large GT-IUI series have reported clinical pregnancy rates of 13%–14.5%, twin pregnancy rates of 16%–20% of achieved clinical pregnancies, and high-order multiple pregnancy rates of 5.7%–6.1% of achieved clinical pregnancies [28, 30, 31]. Thus, the goal of increasing the chances for pregnancy by increasing the number of available fertilizable oocytes through GT stimulation must be balanced by the inherently increased risk of multiple gestation, and HOMP, as the number of available oocytes increases.

Intuitively, it could be anticipated that an increasing number of mature follicles would result in higher pregnancy rates. In fact, the available data is more complex. In a series of 381 consecutive IUI cycles, we found a significant increase in pregnancy rate when two follicles ≥16 mm in diameter were recruited compared to when one mature follicle was recruited, but pregnancy rates did not increase further (range 12%–14%) in the presence of three or four mature follicles [6]. In a series of 1650 GT-IUI cycles, similar live birth rates (range 13.2%–15.7%) were observed whether one, two, three, or more than three follicles ≥14 mm were recruited [32]. In a large single-center series of 4067 GT-IUI cycles, follicle diameters ≥14 mm, ≥ 16 mm, or ≥ 18 mm were not significantly associated with pregnancy rate [28]. Moreover, the number of mature follicles did not predict HOMP in three large series of 1781–4067 GT-IUI cycles [28, 30, 31]. Dickey et al. have found that pregnancy rates are linked to the number of follicles ≥12 mm in diameter, and HOMP are linked to the number of follicles >10 mm in diameter, rather than the number of mature follicles [28].

Pregnancy rates vary inversely with the treatment cycle number. Dickey et al., and we, found similar pregnancy rates in the 14%–16% range in the first two IUI cycles, 10%–11% in cycle 3, and less than 10% per cycle beyond the third IUI attempt [6, 28]. In a prospective observational study of 594 couples with unexplained infertility, the cycle fecundity rate was 16.4%, and the cumulative pregnancy rate was 39.2% after three GT-IUI treatment cycles. The cycle fecundity rate dropped to 5.6% among the 91 women who continued GT-IUI treatment for cycles 4–6, and the cumulative pregnancy rate increased by only an additional 9.3% to 48.5% by cycle 6 [33]. A fourth trial did not identify a decline in cycle fecundity until the fifth GT-IUI cycle [34]. The substantial drop in pregnancy rate per cycle after three GT-IUI attempts provides rationale for the typical recommendation to move on to IVF after three failed GT-IUI cycles.

Pregnancy rates with GT-IUI are decreased in women of advanced reproductive age [6, 10, 28]; hence the recommendation to proceed directly to IVF as a first-line treatment exists in women with advanced reproductive age, particularly those with diminished ovarian reserve [10, 25].

Several large series have consistently identified the following predictors of HOMP in GT-IUI treatment: the number of small or mid-size follicles on the day of HCG, younger age, estradiol level on the day of HCG, and treatment cycle [28, 30, 31]. For example, Dickey et al. found that, for age < 32 years, the presence of 3–6 follicles ≥10 mm was associated with a HOMP risk of 6%. If more than seven follicles ≥10 mm were present, the HOMP rate jumped to 20%. Corresponding HOMP rates in the 32–37 age group were 5% and 12%. No HOMP occurred in women age 38 or older. Women in the 32–37 age group with seven follicles >10 mm were at greater risk of triplets if their estradiol exceeded 1000 pg/ml. During a second GT-IUI cycle, HOMP only occurred if seven or more follicles were present, and no HOMP occurred in the third GT-IUI treatment cycle or beyond [28]. In Tur et al.'s analysis, the probability of HOMP in a woman less than age 32, with an estradiol >862 pg/ml and ≥ 5 follicles greater than 10 mm in diameter, was 19%. By comparison, a woman > age 32, with an estradiol <862 pg/ml and three or fewer follicles greater than 10 mm in diameter, had a probability of HOMP of only 3.3% [30]. Gleicher et al. found that the risk of high-order multiple pregnancy was significantly increased with an estradiol >1385 pg/ml, or with seven or more follicles on the day of HCG administration [31].

The risk of HOMP may be increased in Clomid-naïve patients undergoing GT-IUI. Dickey et al. compared outcomes from 918 GT-IUI cycles in 551 women who had previously failed Clomid-IUI to outcomes from 1459 GT-IUI cycles in 908 Clomid-naïve women in a retrospective study. The patients were < age 38. The pregnancy rate per cycle was 22% in the Clomid-naïve patients, 20% in women who had previously failed 1–4 Clomid-IUI cycles, and 4% in women who had previously failed ≥5 prior Clomid-IUI cycles. HOMP with GT-IUI treatment was 9% in the Clomid-naïve group, 7.5% with a history of one prior Clomid-IUI cycle, and 6% after two prior Clomid-IUI cycles. No HOMP, but 36 (19%) clinical pregnancies, occurred during 187 GT-IUI treatment cycles of women who had previously attempted 3 or 4 Clomid-IUI cycles [35]. These findings advocate for three cycles of oral ovulation induction-IUI before moving on to GT-IUI.

Several studies have reported decreased pregnancy rates when GT-IUI is undertaken in the presence of tubal factor or peri-adnexal adhesions [6, 28, 36]. In contrast to these findings, a Taiwanese study compared GT-IUI outcomes in 133 women with unilateral obstruction on HSG to 570 women with bilateral tubal patency. Clinical pregnancy rate per cycle was 17.3% in the unilateral tubal occlusion group and 18.9% in the bilateral tubal patency group, a difference that was not significant [37].

Some investigators have found the success of GT-IUI to be decreased with endometriosis [6, 38, 39], and in endometriosis with tubal factor [28], but others have not [36, 38]. One trial showed equivalent pregnancy rates among women with unexplained infertility and women with prior laparoscopic surgical treatment of minimal or mild endometriosis undergoing GT-IUI [40].

15.4 Treatment and Stimulation Strategies to Optimize Pregnancy Rates and Minimize Multiple Gestation

Considering predictors for success in GT-IUI, and risk factors for multiple gestation and HOMP, Dickey has recommended several strategies for GT-IUI treatment. These include (1) striving to achieve mono-follicular or double follicular ovulation, including use of low-dose gonadotropins 37.5 IU–75 IU daily for up to six cycles; (2) avoiding GT-IUI in the initial cycles of treatment, in favor of oral medications with IUI; (3) in women age < 38, canceling in the presence of three or more follicles ≥10 mm–12 mm; (4) starting gonadotropins after stimulation day 7; (5) not canceling cycles in women greater than age 38 given low risk of HOMP in this age group; (6) recognizing risk factors for HOMP including estradiol greater than 1000 pg/ml, age < 32, presence of seven or more pre-ovulatory follicles in the 10 mm–12 mm range, and low BMI; and (7) triaging patients at risk for HOMP to IVF [5].

McClamrock et al. have similarly recommended that high-dose GT therapy for IUI be abandoned, in favor of oral agents and/or low-dose gonadotropins [41].

An alternative to canceling GT-IUI cycles demonstrating excessive follicle recruitment has been to reduce supernumerary follicles by transvaginal ultrasound-guided aspiration prior to IUI, using a procedure similar to transvaginal oocyte retrieval. In a small series of 26 IUI cycles, transvaginal aspiration was undertaken on the day of HCG administration to reduce the number of follicles ≥15 mm from a mean of 4.5 follicles to not more than 3 follicles. Additionally, follicles <15 mm in diameter were aspirated. Seven singleton pregnancies (27% per cycle), and no multiple pregnancies, occurred [42]. A much larger series from Germany compared outcomes of 226 GT-IUI cycles performed during the years 1989–1992 to outcomes of 257 GT-IUI cycles performed during the years 1992–2006, before and after a policy of transvaginal aspiration of supernumerary follicles on the day of IUI was introduced, leaving the three largest follicles intact but aspirating all others. Cycle fecundity rates (20.4% vs 20.5%) were not different comparing the two eras, but multiple pregnancy rates fell from 20% to 9%. Aspirations occurred in 45% of GT-IUI cycles [43]. While this approach may be clinically effective in reducing multiples, given the need for rapid planning of a procedure, the invasiveness of the intervention, the cost, and the limited efficacy of IUI, it may not practical to introduce this intervention to the workflow in 2019.

In its committee opinion on multiple gestation associated with infertility therapy, the American Society for Reproductive Medicine acknowledges the potential benefits of low-dose gonadotropin stimulation, and of pre-ovulatory transvaginal aspiration of supernumerary follicles. However, unlike Dickey and McClamrock, the ASRM states "in the absence of any established predictors for multiple pregnancies in OI and SO cycles, it is not possible to propose valid guidelines for reducing the rate of multiple gestations." The ASRM opinion further states "regardless of which medication or stimulation regimen is used, it may not be possible to eliminate entirely the risk of multiple gestation associated with OI or SO" [44].

What is the optimal gonadotropin dose and administration frequency for GT-IUI in women less than age 38 with normal ovarian reserve? Given that pregnancy rates [6, 28, 32], and HOMP rates [28, 30, 31], correlate poorly, if at all, with the number of mature follicles recruited, a reasonable approach might be to stimulate with the lowest possible gonadotropin dose capable of achieving recruitment of 1–2 dominant follicles. At the stage where 1–2 dominant follicles, and not more than 3 dominant follicles, have been recruited and HCG administration is contemplated, the final decision about whether or not to move forward could be made after assessing other factors such as patient age, number of follicles in the >10 mm in the intermediate range, estradiol concentration, cycle number, BMI, number of prior oral ovulation induction-IUI cycles, and number of prior GT-IUI cycles. Intuitively, one would expect that cycle contributors to HOMP, such as number of follicles in the intermediate range and estradiol concentration, might be minimized at the lowest effective gonadotropin dose.

A recent Cochrane Review found that alternate-day gonadotropins at doses ranging from 50 IU to 150 IU every other day yielded very low pregnancy rates. Only four pregnancies occurred in 97 women identified from two studies [12, 45, 46]. One of the trials randomized 32 women to receive recombinant FSH 50 IU daily and 34 women to receive recombinant FSH 50 IU every other day and found a 30% pregnancy rate in the daily FSH group vs a 3% pregnancy rate in the alternating day treatment arm [45]. This would suggest that a gonadotropin administration frequency of every other day is inadequate and that daily gonadotropin administration is preferable.

At the other extreme, Dodson et al. were the first group to report results from a reasonably large series, in which they performed 148 cycles of GT-IUI on 85 couples, excluding women with ovulatory factor. They used an initial gonadotropin dose of 225 IU of HMG. Twenty-one clinical pregnancies were achieved in 136 cycles, all within the first two treatment cycles, for a pregnancy rate per cycle of 15%. The multiple pregnancy rate was 29%, including five sets of twins and one set of triplets. This report alerted clinicians to the high prevalence of multiple gestation at a dose of 225 IU and pointed to the need to assess the effectiveness of lower doses of gonadotropins [36].

In determining optimal gonadotropin dosage, the Cochrane Review pooled data from two trials involving a total of 297 patients in which a gonadotropin dose of 150 IU was compared with a gonadotropin dose of 75 IU. There was no difference in pregnancy rates between the two doses (OR 1.2, 95% CI 0.69–1.9), but the higher dose was associated with a significantly greater risk of ovarian hyperstimulation syndrome (OR 5, 95% CI 1.6–20) [12]. Data from studies in which the initial gonadotropin dose is 150 IU or greater report twin pregnancy rates in the 15%–20% range and HOMP in the 6%–9% range [28, 30, 31]. In comparison, data from studies in which the initial gonadotropin dose is 37.5 IU–75 IU report clinical pregnancy rates per cycle in the 9%–14% range and multiple pregnancy rates ranging from 6.5% to 9.5% [47–49]. Only one HOMP was reported in 3219 GT-IUI cycles in one series, and no HOMP in 1259 GT-IUI cycles in a second series using low-dose gonadotropins [45, 47].

Taken together, the data provides rationale to the assertion that an optimal dose of gonadotropin for GT-IUI cycles is in the range of 37.5 IU–75 IU daily. Figure 15.2 depicts a possible decision tree for determining when to proceed, and when to cancel, a GT-IUI cycle in order to avoid HOMP.

15.5 Adjuncts to Gonadotropins in GT-IUI Treatment: GNRH Analogs and Luteal Phase Progesterone

The introduction of GnRH analogs to IVF gonadotropin ovulation induction protocols heralded a significant improvement in IVF outcomes. The risk of cycle cancelation decreased, the average number of oocytes per retrieval increased, oocyte retrievals could be scheduled at a predetermined time, and the pregnancy rate per initiated IVF cycle increased [50]. Unlike in IVF, incorporating GnRH agonists into GT-IUI protocols is not beneficial, and may be detrimental. A Cochrane Review of four randomized controlled trials pooling 415 couples concluded that pregnancy rates per couple were significantly lower, and multiple preg-

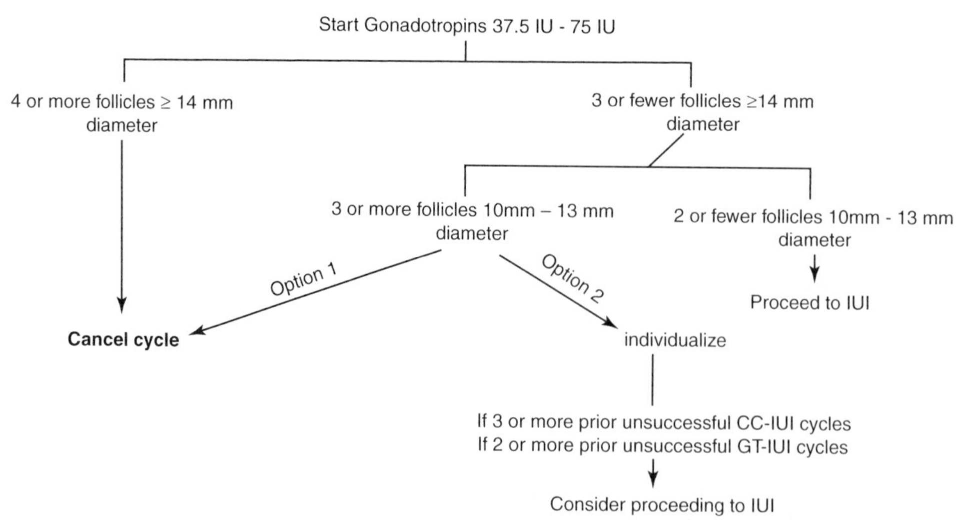

Fig. 15.2 Decision tree for determining when to proceed, and when to cancel, a GT-IUI cycle in order to avoid HOMP

nancy rates were significantly higher, when a GnRH agonist was added to GT-IUI [12]. Data to support the addition of GnRH antagonists to GT-IUI treatment is similarly lacking. Most individual trials, and a pooled analysis, have not demonstrated a significant improvement in pregnancy rates with the introduction of a GnRH antagonist [12, 51–53], with only one randomized controlled trial suggesting a higher pregnancy rate per couple when a GnRH antagonist is introduced [54]. In the absence of GnRH analogs, HCG administration is generally recommended in GT-IUI when the lead follicle approaches a diameter of 16 mm–18 mm, a little earlier than with IVF where the minimum diameter at HCG is usually 18 mm or more.

Luteal phase progesterone supplementation is a fundamental component of IVF treatment protocols. The luteal phase of stimulated IVF cycles is abnormal, particularly when GnRH analogues are used. Etiologies of accelerated luteolysis during IVF stimulation could include prolonged pituitary suppression when GnRH agonists are used and suppression of pituitary LH secretion in the early luteal phase due to negative feedback from supra-physiologic levels of gonadal steroids in both GnRH agonist and antagonist cycles [55]. Gonadotropin stimulation for IUI may similarly be associated with an inadequate luteal phase due to negative feedback from supra-physiologic estradiol. A recent meta-analysis was able to pool data from six randomized controlled trials of GT-IUI with or without luteal phase support, permitting an evaluation of 2220 IUI cycles. Clinical pregnancies per cycle (RR 1.44 [95% CI 1.18–1.75]), live births per cycle (RR 1.59 [95% CI 1.24–2.04]), clinical pregnancies per patient (RR 1.56 [95% CI 1.21–2.02]), and live births per patient (RR 1.77 [95% CI 1.30–2.42]) were all increased with exogenous luteal phase progesterone support. The estimated number needed to treat to achieve one additional pregnancy was 11 [56].

Summary GT-IUI has a modest, limited, success rate but contributes disproportionately to high-order multiple pregnancies (HOMP). As IVF has become increasingly more successful, and single embryo transfer rates have increased, the gap between IVF and GT-IUI success rates and HOMP rates has widened in favor of IVF. Low-dose daily gonadotropin regimens confer pregnancy rates that approach those of high-dose regimens and may provide a means of reducing HOMP rates. Luteal phase progesterone support may improve GT-IUI results. Women age 38 or older, particularly with diminished ovarian reserve, may benefit from immediate triage to IVF. GT-IUI is likely to assume an increasingly marginal role as the efficiency of IVF increases.

References

1. Hanson FM, Rock J. Artificial insemination with husband's sperm. Fertil Steril. 1951;2(2):162–74.
2. Byrd W, et al. Treatment of refractory infertility by transcervical intrauterine insemination of washed spermatozoa. Fertil Steril. 1987;48(6):921–7.
3. Glass RH, Ericsson RJ. Intrauterine insemination of isolated motile sperm. Fertil Steril. 1978;29(5):535–8.
4. Sher G, et al. In vitro sperm capacitation and transcervical intrauterine insemination for the treatment of refractory infertility: phase I. Fertil Steril. 1984;41(2):260–4.
5. Dickey RP. Strategies to reduce multiple pregnancies due to ovulation induction. Fertil Steril. 2009;91(1):1–17.
6. Plosker SM, Jacobson W, Amato P. Predicting and optimizing success in an intra-uterine insemination programme. Hum Reprod. 1994;9(11):2014–21.
7. Clinical guideline [CG156]:Fertility problems: assessment and treatment (2013) [cited 2018 January 29]; Available from: https://www.nice.org.uk/guidance/CG156.
8. Reindollar RH, et al. A randomized clinical trial to evaluate optimal treatment for unexplained infertility: the fast track and standard treatment (FASTT) trial. Fertil Steril. 2010;94(3):888–99.
9. Reindollar RH, Goldman MB. Gonadotropin therapy: a 20th century relic. Fertil Steril. 2012;97(4):813–8.
10. Goldman MB, et al. A randomized clinical trial to determine optimal infertility treatment in older couples: the forty and over treatment trial (FORT-T). Fertil Steril. 2014;101(6):1574–81. e1-2
11. Practice Committee of the American Society for Reproductive, M., Effectiveness and treatment for unexplained infertility. Fertil Steril. 2006;86(5 Suppl 1, 4):S111.
12. Cantineau, E.P.A. and B.J. Cohlen, Ovarian stimulation protocols (anti-oestrogens, gonadotrophins with and without GnRH agonists/antagonists) for intrauterine insemination (IUI) in women with subfertility. Cochrane Database Syst Rev, 2011(6).
13. Guzick DS, et al. Efficacy of superovulation and intrauterine insemination in the treatment of infertility. National Cooperative Reproductive Medicine Network. N Engl J Med. 1999;340(3):177–83.
14. Collins JA, Burrows EA, Wilan AR. The prognosis for live birth among untreated infertile couples. Fertil Steril. 1995;64(1):22–8.
15. Snick HK, et al. The spontaneous pregnancy prognosis in untreated subfertile couples: the Walcheren primary care study. Hum Reprod. 1997;12(7):1582–8.
16. Steures P, et al. Intrauterine insemination with controlled ovarian hyperstimulation versus expectant management for couples with unexplained subfertility and an intermediate prognosis: a randomised clinical trial. Lancet. 2006;368(9531):216–21.
17. Farquhar, C.M., et al., Intrauterine insemination with ovarian stimulation versus expectant management for unexplained infertility (TUI): a pragmatic, open-label, randomised, controlled, two-Centre trial. Lancet, 2017.
18. Assisted reproductive technology in the United States and Canada. 1993 results generated from the American Society for Reproductive Medicine/Society for Assisted Reproductive Technology Registry. Fertil Steril. 1995;64(1):13–21.
19. Schenker JG, Yarkoni S, Granat M. Multiple pregnancies following induction of ovulation. Fertil Steril. 1981;35(2):105–23.
20. Practice Committee of the American Society for Reproductive Medicine. Electronic address, A.a.o. and T. Practice Committee of the Society for assisted reproductive, Guidance on the limits to the number of embryos to transfer: a committee opinion. Fertil Steril. 2017;107(4):901–3.
21. Kulkarni AD, et al. Fertility treatments and multiple births in the United States. N Engl J Med. 2013;369(23):2218–25.
22. European, I.V.F.M.C.f.t.E.S.o.H.R, et al. Assisted reproductive technology in Europe, 2012: results generated from European registers by ESHRE. Hum Reprod. 2016;31(8):1638–52.
23. Berkovitz A, et al. Predictors of twin pregnancy after ovarian stimulation and intrauterine insemination in women with unexplained infertility. Hum Fertil (Camb). 2017;20(3):200–3.
24. Nandi A, et al. Intrauterine insemination with gonadotropin stimulation or in vitro fertilization for the treatment of unex-

plained subfertility: a randomized controlled trial. Fertil Steril. 2017;107(6):1329–35. e2
25. Kaser DJ, et al. When is clomiphene or gonadotropin intrauterine insemination futile? Results of the fast track and standard treatment trial and the forty and over treatment trial, two prospective randomized controlled trials. Fertil Steril. 2014;102(5):1331–7. e1
26. Stern JE, et al. Optimizing the number of blastocyst stage embryos to transfer on day 5 or 6 in women 38 years of age and older: a Society for Assisted Reproductive Technology database study. Fertil Steril. 2009;91(1):157–66.
27. Stern JE, et al. Optimizing the number of cleavage stage embryos to transfer on day 3 in women 38 years of age and older: a Society for Assisted Reproductive Technology database study. Fertil Steril. 2009;91(3):767–76.
28. Dickey RP, et al. Risk factors for high-order multiple pregnancy and multiple birth after controlled ovarian hyperstimulation: results of 4,062 intrauterine insemination cycles. Fertil Steril. 2005;83(3):671–83.
29. Dickey RP. The relative contribution of assisted reproductive technologies and ovulation induction to multiple births in the United States 5 years after the Society for Assisted Reproductive Technology/American Society for Reproductive Medicine recommendation to limit the number of embryos transferred. Fertil Steril. 2007;88(6):1554–61.
30. Tur R, et al. Risk factors for high-order multiple implantation after ovarian stimulation with gonadotrophins: evidence from a large series of 1878 consecutive pregnancies in a single Centre. Hum Reprod. 2001;16(10):2124–9.
31. Gleicher N, et al. Reducing the risk of high-order multiple pregnancy after ovarian stimulation with gonadotropins. N Engl J Med. 2000;343(1):2–7.
32. Ghesquiere SL, et al. Relationship between follicle number and (multiple) live birth rate after controlled ovarian hyperstimulation and intrauterine insemination. Am J Obstet Gynecol. 2007;197(6):589. e1–5
33. Aboulghar M, et al. Controlled ovarian hyperstimulation and intrauterine insemination for treatment of unexplained infertility should be limited to a maximum of three trials. Fertil Steril. 2001;75(1):88–91.
34. Nulsen JC, et al. A randomized and longitudinal study of human menopausal gonadotropin with intrauterine insemination in the treatment of infertility. Obstet Gynecol. 1993;82(5):780–6.
35. Dickey RP, et al. Clomiphene citrate intrauterine insemination (IUI) before gonadotropin IUI affects the pregnancy rate and the rate of high-order multiple pregnancies. Fertil Steril. 2004;81(3):545–50.
36. Dodson WC, et al. Superovulation with intrauterine insemination in the treatment of infertility: a possible alternative to gamete intrafallopian transfer and in vitro fertilization. Fertil Steril. 1987;48(3):441–5.
37. Lin MH, et al. Treatment of infertile women with unilateral tubal occlusion by intrauterine insemination and ovarian stimulation. Taiwan J Obstet Gynecol. 2013;52(3):360–4.
38. Ahinko-Hakamaa K, Huhtala H, Tinkanen H. Success in intrauterine insemination: the role of etiology. Acta Obstet Gynecol Scand. 2007;86(7):855–60.
39. Omland AK, et al. Artificial insemination by husband in unexplained infertility compared with infertility associated with peritoneal endometriosis. Hum Reprod. 1998;13(9):2602–5.
40. Werbrouck E, et al. No difference in cycle pregnancy rate and in cumulative live-birth rate between women with surgically treated minimal to mild endometriosis and women with unexplained infertility after controlled ovarian hyperstimulation and intrauterine insemination. Fertil Steril. 2006;86(3):566–71.
41. McClamrock HD, Jones HW Jr, Adashi EY. Ovarian stimulation and intrauterine insemination at the quarter centennial: implications for the multiple births epidemic. Fertil Steril. 2012;97(4):802–9.
42. Albano C, et al. Avoidance of multiple pregnancies after ovulation induction by supernumerary preovulatory follicular reduction. Fertil Steril. 2001;76(4):820–2.
43. De Geyter C, De Geyter M, Nieschlag E. Low multiple pregnancy rates and reduced frequency of cancellation after ovulation induction with gonadotropins, if eventual supernumerary follicles are aspirated to prevent polyovulation. J Assist Reprod Genet. 1998;15(3):111–6.
44. Practice Committee of American Society for Reproductive, M. Multiple gestation associated with infertility therapy: an American Society for Reproductive Medicine Practice Committee opinion. Fertil Steril. 2012;97(4):825–34.
45. Ragni G, et al. GnRH antagonists and mild ovarian stimulation for intrauterine insemination: a randomized study comparing different gonadotrophin dosages. Hum Reprod. 2004;19(1):54–8.
46. Hughes EG, Collins JA, Gunby J. A randomized controlled trial of three low-dose gonadotrophin protocols for unexplained infertility. Hum Reprod. 1998;13(6):1527–31.
47. Papageorgiou TC, et al. Low dose recombinant FSH treatment may reduce multiple gestations caused by controlled ovarian hyperstimulation and intrauterine insemination. BJOG. 2004;111(11):1277–82.
48. Ragni G, et al. Preventing high-order multiple pregnancies during controlled ovarian hyperstimulation and intrauterine insemination: 3 years' experience using low-dose recombinant follicle-stimulating hormone and gonadotropin-releasing hormone antagonists. Fertil Steril. 2006;85(3):619–24.
49. Peeraer K, et al. Low-dose human menopausal gonadotrophin versus clomiphene citrate in subfertile couples treated with intrauterine insemination: a randomized controlled trial. Hum Reprod. 2015;30(5):1079–88.
50. Hughes EG, et al. The routine use of gonadotropin-releasing hormone agonists prior to in vitro fertilization and gamete intrafallopian transfer: a meta-analysis of randomized controlled trials. Fertil Steril. 1992;58(5):888–96.
51. Lambalk CB, et al. Treatment with the GnRH antagonist ganirelix prevents premature LH rises and luteinization in stimulated intrauterine insemination: results of a double-blind, placebo-controlled, multicentre trial. Hum Reprod. 2006;21(3):632–9.
52. Williams RS, et al. A randomized, multicenter study comparing the efficacy of recombinant FSH vs recombinant FSH with Ganirelix during superovulation/IUI therapy. Am J Obstet Gynecol. 2004;191(2):648–51. Discussion 651-3
53. Jain S, Majumdar A. Impact of gonadotropin-releasing hormone antagonist addition on pregnancy rates in gonadotropin-stimulated intrauterine insemination cycles. J Hum Reprod Sci. 2016;9(3):151–8.
54. Gomez-Palomares JL, et al. Timing ovulation for intrauterine insemination with a GnRH antagonist. Hum Reprod. 2005;20(2):368–72.
55. Fatemi HM, et al. An update of luteal phase support in stimulated IVF cycles. Hum Reprod Update. 2007;13(6):581–90.
56. Green KA, et al. Progesterone luteal support after ovulation induction and intrauterine insemination: an updated systematic review and meta-analysis. Fertil Steril. 2017;107(4):924–33. e5

Hyperprolactinemia: Effect on Reproduction, Diagnosis, and Management

16

Kathleen O'Leary

16.1 Prolactin Physiology

Hyperprolactinemia has many etiologies and is one of the most common causes of amenorrhea, accounting for up to 15–30% of cases. Prolactin (PRL) is encoded by a single gene on chromosome 6 and is a 199-amino acid polypeptide hormone, 23.4 kDa in size, synthesized and secreted mainly by lactotroph cells of the anterior pituitary gland. It comprises five coding exons with 40% homology to growth hormone gene and is also similar to placental lactogen [1]. The prolactin receptors are included as members of the cytokine receptor superfamily, distributed throughout the immune system [2]. Several biologic forms of PRL exist due to various post-translation modifications, including cleavage, phosphorylation, polymerization, glycosylation, and degradation [3]. These include the "little" monomeric form (the most active and non-glycosylated, 85–95%), the low-activity dimeric "big" form (50–60 kDa, 5–15%), and the inactive tetrameric "big big" form (macroprolactin, 150–170 kDa, <1%) [3–5]. Differences in splicing and protein modification of the PRL hormone create the structural diversity of PRL molecules, and it is assumed that the bigger forms of PRL have diminished bioactivity due to decreasing receptor-binding affinity caused by glycosylation [1]. PRL is expressed in sources other than the pituitary, such as the T lymphocytes, brain, skin fibroblasts, adipose tissue, breast, endometrial decidua, prostate, and even neoplastic cells. Decidual PRL has been proposed to affect the functional changes of the endometrium from the time of implantation to delivery by silencing genes that are detrimental to pregnancy [1, 3]. The majority of circulating PRL is of pituitary origin.

The main role of PRL is stimulation of lactation in the postpartum period, but PRL has many other diverse physiologic functions that include immunomodulation, angiogenesis, growth, synergism with steroid hormones, integumentary functions, and osmoregulation [6]. The secretion of PRL is episodic with an increase of secretion observed 60–90 minutes after sleep begins, increasing during REM sleep with highest concentrations noted between 2:00 and 5:00 a.m. [5]. Normal PRL is regulated by many stimulatory and inhibitory factors. Dopamine (prolactin-inhibiting factor) binding to the D2 receptors of pituitary lactotroph cell membranes is the main inhibitory factor of PRL and is secreted into the portal circulation by the arcuate and paraventricular nuclei of the hypothalamus. Other neuropeptides and hormones act as prolactin-releasing factors, such as thyrotropin-releasing hormone (TRH), estradiol, oxytocin, epidermal growth factor, vasopressin, GnRH, angiotensin II, vasoactive intestinal polypeptide, and dopamine antagonists [3, 7–9]. The amount of prolactin in the serum is also affected by kidney clearance. The factors influencing PRL secretion are listed in Table 16.1.

PRL promotes milk biosynthesis and maintains lactation in the postpartum period. The increased estrogen production during pregnancy causes lactotroph cells to proliferate, increasing PRL secretion starting around 8 weeks' gestation. During pregnancy, prolactin levels rise from the normal level of 10–25 ng/mL to a peak of 200–400 ng/mL at term, a tenfold increase in PRL [8, 10]. The increased PRL with other hormones, such as estradiol, progesterone, placental lactogen, insulin, and cortisol, causes mammary gland growth. While estrogen enhances breast development, it blunts the effects of PRL on lactation during pregnancy. Progesterone also inhibits full lactation during pregnancy [8]. The fall of serum estrogens and progesterone to non-pregnant levels after delivery results in the initiation of lactation [8]. One week postpartum, serum prolactin declines 50% (to about 100 ng/mL) in postpartum breastfeeding women. During breastfeeding, nipple stimulation by the suckling infant causes a short-term twofold rise in PRL production, based on a neuro-humoral mechanism, which is important for milk production [7, 8]. Prolactin levels normalize within 6 months after delivery in breastfeeding mothers and return to normal within a few weeks in non-nursing women.

K. O'Leary (✉)
Institute for Reproductive Health, Cincinnati, OH, USA

G. N. Allahbadia et al. (eds.), *Textbook of Assisted Reproduction*, https://doi.org/10.1007/978-981-15-2377-9_16

Table 16.1 Factors affecting prolactin secretion

Category	Increase	Decrease
Physiologic	Pregnancy Luteal phase Nipple stimulation Nursing Exercise Sleep Eating High-protein diet Hypoglycemia Seizures Stress Surgery Sex Neonatal	
Endocrine/autocrine/paracrine factors	*Prolactin-releasing factors (PRFs):* Estradiol TRH Oxytocin Epidermal growth factor Growth hormone-releasing hormone GnRH Vasoactive intestinal polypeptide Angiotensin II Histidine Serotonin Prolactin-releasing peptide	*Prolactin-inhibiting factors (PIFs)* Dopamine GABA GnRH-associated protein (GAP)
Pharmacologic	Antipsychotics/neuroleptics Risperidone Phenothiazines Haloperidol Antidepressants Tricyclic antidepressants Monoamine oxidase inhibitors Serotonin reuptake inhibitors Benzodiazepines Amphetamines Opiates/opioid peptides Morphine Heroin Cocaine Dopaminergic blockers Metoclopramide Domperidone Cisapride Antihistamines H2 blockers Intravenous cimetidine Antihypertensives Verapamil Methyldopa Reserpine Licorice	Dopamine agonists Bromocriptine Cabergoline Levodopa Pergolide Apomorphine
Pathologic Pituitary	Prolactinomas Other secretory or non-secretory tumors Acromegaly Lymphocytic hypophysitis Trauma Surgery Radiation Empty sella syndrome Histiocytosis X Cushing's disease	
Hypothalamic	Craniopharyngioma Meningioma Germinoma Sarcoidosis Eosinophilic granuloma Pituitary stalk section Rathke's cleft cyst Metastasis Infiltration Trauma Encephalitis	
Systemic conditions	Chronic renal disease Primary hypothyroidism Polycystic ovary syndrome Cirrhosis Renal cell carcinoma Polycystic kidney disease Bronchogenic carcinoma Addison's disease Epilepsy Chronic uremia Ectopic production	
Neurogenic	Herpes zoster Chest trauma or burns (intercostal nerves stimulation) Post-thoracic surgery Cervical spine lesions Malignant ovarian teratoma	
Idiopathic	Macroprolactinemia Pseudocyesis	

16.2 Effect of Hyperprolactinemia on the Reproductive System

Although PRL does not appear to play a direct physiologic role in the regulation of gonadal function, hyperprolactinemia can cause hypogonadotropic hypogonadism in men and women. The exact mechanism of disruption of gonadal function is not fully defined, but there appears to be alteration of the hypothalamic-pituitary-gonadal axis. In women, pulsatile secretion of FSH and LH is decreased through suppression of GnRH, and the midcycle LH surge is suppressed. The decrease in the amplitude and frequency of the LH pulses and the decrease in FSH concentration affect Graafian follicle development, leading to anovulatory cycles. The suppression of LH secretion also affects the luteal phase by disrupting steroidogenesis in granulosa cells [5]. In addition, hyperprolactinemia has direct effects on the ovary by stimulating expression of type II 3B-hydroxysteroid dehydrogenase, which is the final step in progesterone biosynthesis and increases IGF-II secretion [11]. Hyperprolactinemia indirectly causes an imbalance of lipid metabolism, an increase in ACTH and adrenal androgens, disruptions of insulin secretion, and a decrease in sex hormone-binding globulin [5]. This elevation of androgens affects the developmental competence of the oocyte [5].

Depending on the serum level of prolactin, first there is a shortening of the luteal phase (20–50 ng/mL). This is due to the poor pre-ovulatory follicular development and decreased progesterone secretion and premature regression of the corpus luteum; thus high PRL is considered luteolytic [5, 8, 12]. Anovulation, oligomenorrhea or amenorrhea, and infertility can occur with moderate levels of hyperprolactinemia (50–100 ng/mL). Serum prolactin levels over 100 ng/mL can cause frank hypogonadism by significantly affecting ovarian follicles and causing low estrogen levels and resultant clinical symptoms of vasomotor symptoms, vaginal atrophy, dyspareunia, lowered libido, disturbances of the arousal phase and orgasm, and osteopenia [5]. Other symptoms include hirsutism and acne. Delayed puberty and primary amenorrhea and even growth arrest can occur if hyperprolactinemia occurs before menarche [3]. Only about one-third of women with hyperprolactinemia exhibit galactorrhea. This may be because breast milk production requires estrogen, and hyperprolactinemia often results in anovulation or more severe hypogonadotropic hypogonadism with low serum estrogen levels.

While hyperprolactinemia mostly affects younger women of reproductive age and its incidence decreases with age, menopausal women may have symptoms of hyperprolactinemia, including obesity, lipid abnormalities, or insulin resistance [5]. Bone fractures are more common in women with hyperprolactinemia in menopause due the effects on bone mineralization and osteoblast proliferation [5].

In men, most recent data suggest that PRL stimulates testicular functions [6]. PRL increase LH receptors, cellular morphology, steroidogenesis, and androgen function in Leydig cells [6]. PRL increases lipids and spermatocyte-spermatid changes in germ cells [6]. PRL also has a role in sexual responsiveness in men [6]. Hyperprolactinemia can cause decreased testosterone and decreased spermatogenesis. The decreased testosterone may cause decreased libido, impotence (16%), oligospermia (11%), infertility, decreased muscle mass and body hair, anemia, and, rarely, gynecomastia and galactorrhea [6, 13, 14]. Prostate volume is decreased in hyperprolactinemic men, presumably due to decreased testosterone [3].

Decreased bone mineral density can occur in both sexes and occurs in 25% of women diagnosed with hyperprolactinemia [9]. Bone loss and progressive atherosclerosis can also occur in both men and women due to altered body composition with increased body fat and reduced lean mass as well as the indirect decrease in estrogen secretion [7]. Behavioral and mood changes can also occur with chronic hyperprolactinemia [14]. Patients with sellar or parasellar lesions that are the cause of hyperprolactinemia may present with symptoms of headaches or vision loss in addition to the symptoms of hypogonadism.

16.3 Etiologies of Hyperprolactinemia

Hyperprolactinemia can be identified in up to 10% of the population and in 5% of patients who present with infertility [7, 9]. In reproductive-age women 25–34 years, the annual incidence of hyperprolactinemia is reported to be 23.9 per 100,000 person years [9]. There are many conditions that cause hyperprolactinemia (Table 16.1). Physiological etiologies include pregnancy, lactation, intercourse, exercise, stress, and sleep. Pathological causes of hyperprolactinemia include renal disease and hepatic cirrhosis—conditions that decrease clearance of prolactin—renal and lung cancers, and endocrinopathies such as primary hypothyroidism, polycystic ovary syndrome (up to 30%), and primary adrenocortical insufficiency. Hypothyroidism causes hyperprolactinemia by the compensatory increase in the hypothalamic thyrotropin-releasing hormone, which stimulates secretion of prolactin. Neurogenic stimulation caused by chest wall injury or severe burns can also cause hyperprolactinemia. Pharmacologic causes of hyperprolactinemia reduce hypothalamic secretion of dopamine, cause antagonistic effects on D2 receptors, or have an inhibitory effect on the enzyme that converts L-dopa to dopamine [15]. These are mainly antipsychotic medications (such as risperidone) and neuroleptic drugs. Others include antidepressants, antiemetics, opiates, H2-receptor blockers, antihypertensives, and calcium channel blockers. Sellar lesions, such as prolactinomas or other pituitary adenomas and infiltrative conditions, induce hyperprolactinemia by compressing the pituitary stalk and damaging the dopaminergic neurons [16]. Hypothalamic-pituitary stalk damage can also occur with craniopharyngiomas, granulomas, Rathke's cleft cysts, and other tumors.

Pituitary tumors are common and found in 12% of pituitary glands at autopsy. They can have a diverse range of hormonal and growth activity [9]. Prolactinomas are the most common hormone-secreting pituitary tumors, comprising 40% of all pituitary tumors, and are found in approximately half of patients with hyperprolactinemia. Prolactinomas are composed mainly of lactotrophs, which secrete prolactin and can occasionally secrete other hormones, such as growth hormone, an important clinical distinction as treatment options will differ [16].

Prolactinomas are characterized by size. Microadenomas, found in 1% of women age 20–40, measure less than 10 mm; macroadenomas measure 10 mm or larger in diameter [3]. Most men present with macroadenomas, often with associated neurologic symptoms, which may reflect diagnostic delay [13]. These tumors are usually found in the lateral wings of the anterior pituitary but rarely can infiltrate the surrounding tissue. Because prolactinomas can extend outside of the sella, these tumors cause hyperprolactinemia by interrupting dopamine delivery from the hypothalamus to the pituitary, causing a loss of the tonic inhibitory release of prolactin. A macroadenoma may expand out of the sella to impinge on structures such as the optic chiasm resulting in symptoms such as severe headaches and ophthalmoplegia, due to entrapment of cranial nerves III, IV, V_1 V_2, and V1 [16]. Serum prolactin is usually proportional to tumor burden. Prolactinomas are rarely hereditary but can occur as part of the multiple endocrine neoplasia (MEN) syndrome in 20% of patients diagnosed with MEN type 1 [3, 13]. The incidence of a microadenoma enlarging to a macroadenoma is low, 3–7% [16], and the risk of enlargement during pregnancy is also very low. However, tumor growth of macroadenomas is up to 25% in pregnancy [13].

Macroprolactinemia is implicated as a major cause of hyperprolactinemia (in up to 46% of cases of hyperprolactinemia in a retrospective analysis) and occurs in 3.7% of the general population [5, 7]. It is a heterogeneous, benign, and usually asymptomatic condition with many different causes [9]. IgG complexes bind the 23 kDa prolactin molecule, especially anti-PRL autoantibodies, and form a large macroprolactin complex. The resulting molecular mass of over 150 kDA can increase the circulating serum PRL, likely by delayed clearance of prolactin. The complexes are immunologically detectable but not usually biologically active, as the polymer cannot interact with the prolactin receptor. However, a small proportion of patients may have clinical symptoms of hyperprolactinemia such as galactorrhea or oligomenorrhea [9]. This is thought due to intermittent dissociation of monomeric PRL from the low affinity, high capacity IgG antibody [17]. Alternatively, this could be due coincidental findings or another etiology such as polycystic ovary syndrome. In certain instances, a patient may have both hyperprolactinemia and macroprolactinemia [5, 18].

Up to 30% of etiologies of hyperprolactinemia are classified as "idiopathic" because no etiology has been determined [4]. In many cases, small prolactinomas may be present that are too small to be detected radiologically [3]. Long-term follow-up in these patients found that many have normal PRL levels (30%), while 10–15% will develop an increase in PRL over baseline [3].

16.4 Diagnosis of Hyperprolactinemia

In most laboratories, normal serum prolactin levels are less than 25 ng/mL in women and less than 20 ng/mL in men. Slight elevations of less than twofold could reflect a stressful phlebotomy and should be repeated to prevent otherwise costly imaging [8]. Most secondary causes and macroprolactinemia induce mild elevations of prolactin from 25 to 100 ng/mL. Hypothalamic damage or pituitary stalk compression typically causes prolactin levels of 100–150 ng/mL. Prolactin levels often correspond to prolactin size, but symptoms do not correspond well with prolactin levels. A macroadenoma will usually have a prolactin level of over 200 ng/mL [3]. The prolactin level is rarely above 250 ng/mL if a non-prolactin-secreting tumor is present. In cases of large pituitary tumors with only mild hyperprolactinemia, prolactin should be repeated with dilutions to rule out the "hook effect," which artifactually lowers the lab value [3, 16]. Levels higher than 250 ng/ML may suggest a macroadenoma. However some drugs such as risperidone or phenothiazines can induce prolactin to levels higher than 200 ng/ML, indicating overlap between different conditions causing hyperprolactinemia [19].

A thorough medical history may help provide clues for determining whether physiological, pharmacologic, or pathological etiologies are causing hyperprolactinemia. The physical exam should be focused on evidence of hypothyroidism, hypogonadism, systemic disease like renal or hepatic failure, and visual field defects. A thorough history and exam are important, because pituitary incidentaloma can be found in 10% of pituitary MRI in normal patients [15]. Depending on the medical and physical exam, the next step in diagnostic approach is a lab and radiologic evaluation. Because PRL is secreted in a pulsatile fashion, a single elevated value if obtained in the morning, 2–3 hours after awaking and in a fasting state, is recommended, although the Endocrine Society states that an atraumatic venipuncture performed at any time of the day is adequate to diagnose hyperprolactinemia [9]. Since macroprolactinemia can occur in up to 20% of patients with hyperprolactinemia, it should be measured in all asymptomatic patients by precipitation of the sample with polyethylene glycol (PEG) [19]. Macroprolactinemia should also be evaluated if the patient has an atypical clinical picture or conflicting PRL results in distinct assays [15]. Macroprolactinemia is present when the recovery of monomeric PRL following treatment with PEG is less than 40%

[17]. In patients with symptoms of hyperprolactinemia or a known macroadenoma but in which PRL is within the normal range or is only mildly elevated, further evaluation with lab dilutional measurements (1100) of the original sample should be performed to rule out a "hook effect" which is an assay artifact when high serum prolactin levels saturate antibodies in the two-site immunoradiometric assay [9]. This will help distinguish between a large macroadenoma and a large nonfunctioning tumor [19].

After the diagnosis of hyperprolactinemia, other labs such as thyroid function tests, liver panel, and kidney function tests should be considered [19]. A pregnancy test should be obtained in all reproductive-age women. In amenorrheic women, follicle-stimulating hormone should be obtained to rule out primary ovarian insufficiency [13]. Testosterone should be measured in men with hyperprolactinemia. Once hyperprolactinemia is diagnosed and secondary causes ruled out, imaging of the pituitary fossa should be performed with T1-weighted MRI with gadolinium to rule out a pituitary tumor, pituitary stalk lesion, hypothalamic tumors, granulomas, or other lesions, especially if there are neurologic symptoms present [18]. Microprolactinomas often appear to be hypointense compared to the bright pituitary gland and usually do not distort the pituitary shape [3]. Often, microadenomas may not be seen on the MRI, suggesting that the lesion is less than 2 mm in diameter or that the patient has lactotroph hyperplasia [18]. Larger macroadenomas have a variable enhancement with gadolinium and appear to cause the inferior portion of the pituitary stalk to be distorted [3]. It is also important to rule out acromegaly. Growth hormone (GH) is a prolactogen, so galactorrhea in a patient with a pituitary adenoma and elevated prolactin could be secondary to a growth hormone-secreting tumor (somatotropinoma); treatment with a dopamine agonist would decrease serum prolactin, but undiagnosed acromegaly could cause irreversible consequences from continued somatotropinoma growth [3, 16]. Importantly, in patients who are found to have a lesion in the pituitary or hypothalamus, it is possible that partial or complete hypopituitarism may be present, and a complete evaluation of the other pituitary hormones and pituitary-adrenal axis may be necessary [18].

In patients with drug-induced hyperprolactinemia, a repeat measurement 72 hours after discontinuation of the drug can be considered unless it is a psychotropic medication [19]. Antipsychotics should only be stopped or changed under the supervision of the psychiatrist. A pituitary MRI should be considered if the drug cannot be discontinued or if the onset of the symptoms does not coincide with initiation of the drug.

Other diagnostic elements to consider are visual field tests or pituitary function tests, especially in the presence of a macroadenoma or if the lesion compresses the optic chiasm [19]. Bone density tests should be considered if long-term hypogonadism has been present. A semen analysis should be obtained in men [6].

16.5 Treatment

Once physiological and pathological causes of hyperprolactinemia have been discerned, treatment options are decided based on the patient's symptoms and treatment goals. Medical therapy is the first line of therapy to achieve eugonadism by restoring ovarian function, normalizing both cyclical estrogen production and ovulation, suppressing lactation, and preventing further reductions in bone mineral density [18]. An important treatment goal is to also control tumor growth in patients with prolactinomas [7]. Dopamine agonists are first-line treatment to reduce prolactin levels and tumor size by absorbing lactotroph cell cytoplasm and limiting cell multiplication, causing tumor shrinkage [3, 10]. Asymptomatic patients or patients with microadenomas do not necessarily need treatment as 93% of microadenomas do not enlarge over a 4- to 6-year period [3].

Cabergoline, an ergot and selective D2 agonist, is the most favorable dopamine agonist due to its long half-life, tolerability, and efficacy. The long duration of action is due to its higher affinity for lactotroph dopamine receptor binding sites, slow elimination from pituitary tissue, and extensive enterohepatic recycling [3, 7, 9]. The starting dose is 0.25–0.5 mg/week, slowly increased to normalize PRL (mean dose 0.5–1 mg/week) [19]. At dose of 0.5 mg per week in 95% of patients with microadenomas and at a dose of 1 mg per week in 80% of patients with macroadenomas, hypogonadism can be reversed and prolactinoma size decreased [7, 9]. A placebo-controlled study showed that cabergoline in doses of 0.125–1 mg twice weekly for 1–2 years resulted in restoration of menses in 82% of patients [9]. Another retrospective study of over 400 patients showed benefit of cabergoline in 92% of patients with either a microadenoma or idiopathic hyperprolactinemia [9]. While there have been no clinical trials directly comparing the tumor shrinkage effects of the different dopamine agonists, various studies show that cabergoline decreases pituitary tumor size by 90% versus 50% with bromocriptine in two-thirds of patients [9].

Bromocriptine, a semisynthetic ergot derivative and a D2-selective dopamine agonist and D1 antagonist, was the first drug introduced to treat hyperprolactinemia. Bromocriptine is an inexpensive and effective alternative to cabergoline, although multiple daily doses may be required to be therapeutic (2.5–15 mg/day) because of its short half-life [7]. Bromocriptine is often associated with gastrointestinal side effects, such as nausea, vomiting, constipation, and reflux [19]. It may also cause nasal congestion, postural hypotension, and lightheadedness, or dizziness [3, 19]. Higher doses up to 20–30 mg/daily are often not tolerated due to the side effects. Bromocriptine should be taken with a meal and may be used intravaginally if patients are intolerant of taking it orally.

Women with microadenomas causing menstrual disturbances, such as amenorrhea, can be treated with an oral contraceptive pill as an alternative to dopamine agonist or if they do not wish to conceive or if they have minimal galactorrhea and wish to prevent bone loss [7]. Importantly, no randomized controlled trials have compared treatment with a dopamine agonist versus oral contraceptive in this context, but it does not appear that microadenomas increase in size after 2 years of treatment with oral contraceptive treatment [9, 13]. The low incidence of tumor growth during pregnancy (when estrogen levels are elevated) also further supports that oral contraceptive therapy is a safe option. PRL levels should still be checked annually in these women, and caution should be used in women who have macroadenomas [10].

Once a dopamine agonist is initiated, the patient should be followed with repeat prolactin measurements starting 1 month after therapy to help guide dosing adjustments to achieve normoprolactinemia and resolution of hypogonadism symptoms. An MRI should be repeated in 1 year if prolactin levels continue to increase despite therapy or if new symptoms develop (or sooner, at 3 months, if there is a known macroadenoma) [9]. Visual field testing is recommended for patients with macroadenomas that may impinge the optic chiasm [9]. MRIs should be performed annually in patients with macroprolactinomas. Bone mineral density tests should be repeated if the baseline tests showed osteopenia.

Patients who do not tolerate or respond to medications may need transsphenoidal surgical resection of a prolactinoma. Patients have a 75% cure rate for surgical removal of microadenomas but only a 26% long-term success rate for macroadenomas [3]. Surgical results depend on the initial tumor size, prolactin levels, and experience of the surgeon [3, 19]. Most recurrences occur within 3 years [19]. Dopamine agonists are not definitive therapy for nonfunctioning pituitary adenomas. Adenomas that secrete both growth hormone and prolactin should be treated with transsphenoidal surgery or a long-acting somatostatin analog [16].

Dopamine agonist therapy provides effective improvement of clinical symptoms in most patients. Eighty percent of macroadenomas may decrease in size with treatment [18]. However, recurrence of symptoms or regrowth can occur within months of stopping dopamine agonists, ranging from 26 to 69% [9]. The higher the level of prolactin and the larger the pituitary tumor at the time of diagnosis correlates with the risk of recurrence [9]. Dopamine agonist treatment can be decreased after 2–3 years of normal prolactin levels and no evidence of residual tumor on MRI and may be stopped if serum prolactin has been normal after a period of 1 year at the reduced dose. If dopamine agonists are stopped, monitoring for symptoms of recurrence and prolactin levels should be checked monthly for 3 months for the first year and annually afterward for at least 5 years, especially if a patient has a macroadenoma [9, 19]. If prolactin levels again increase above normal range, an MRI may be indicated. Even without tumor regrowth, up to 28% of patients may develop symptoms of hypogonadism, which suggests the importance of long-term monitoring [9]. It is reasonable to discontinue therapy after a patient has reached menopause in women with microadenomas or idiopathic hyperprolactinemia since the protection of ovarian function is no longer needed [3, 5]. Estrogen hormone therapy can be considered if bone mineral density is a concern as long as PRL level and pituitary adenoma size is monitored [18].

Because men often have a more indolent course, many present to clinicians with large macroadenomas and very elevated prolactin levels, which may affect treatment. Men often already have compression symptoms such as diplopia or vision loss or significant hypogonadism, including erectile dysfunction. Sperm counts can be affected if the patient has gone for several years without treatment. However, sperm count and motility and normal sexual function has resulted after 6 months of treatment with cabergoline in some studies [6, 9].

Men respond well to dopamine agonists, unless hypogonadism has occurred for many years. While the restoration of ovarian function occurs in almost 90% of women, the testicular function in males may be less completely restored, with up to 50% of patients requiring testosterone replacement therapy despite an adequate reduction of serum prolactin [18]. Further, sperm counts that do not improve with dopamine agonists may require human chorionic gonadotropin for fertility. Sexual problems, such as erectile dysfunction, may not fully improve with a dopamine agonist and testosterone until the prolactin level has returned to the normal range [3].

In a small subset of patients and for reasons not entirely known (possibly due to a decreased number of D2 receptors on lactotroph cells), standard doses of dopamine agonists do not result in tumor shrinkage or normoprolactinemia. If maximum doses of dopamine agonists are used and not successful in reducing the tumor by 50%, the patient is noted to have a dopamine agonist-resistant prolactinoma [9]. Macroadenomas and males are more likely to be resistant to treatment [9]. Resistance to dopamine agonist therapy at standard doses may also be reflected in continued infertility. Caution must be used if increasing cabergoline to maximal doses (such as 11 mg/week), as there have been incidences of cardiac valvular regurgitation at doses higher than 3 mg daily as in Parkinson's patients [9]. The valvular disease appears to be due to serotonin receptor agonism leading to fibromyoblast proliferation by cabergoline [3, 13]. Monitoring patients with periodic echocardiography is recommended if using high-dose cabergoline (over 2 mg/week) or after 5 years of treatment [9, 19, 20]. Referral to an experienced pituitary surgeon for transsphenoidal surgery in symptomatic patients who are resistant or intolerant to maximum doses of dopamine agonists is recommended. Post-operative risks include hypopituitarism, cerebrospinal fluid leak, and diabetes insipidus [9]. Surgically treated dopamine agonist-resistant tumors may recur in 7–50% of patients [3, 9]. Radiotherapy is another option for malignant or medically resistant prolactinomas but may take decades for tumors to respond to treatment [9].

For patients with pharmacologic-induced hyperprolactinemia who are symptomatic, the recommendation is assessment of the advantages and disadvantages of continuing the medication. If possible, discontinuation of the medication or substitution of another drug with less dopamine agonist properties can be attempted. Antipsychotic drugs should not be stopped without consultation and supervision by the treating physician. A dopamine agonist should only be added to antipsychotic-induced hyperprolactinemia with extreme caution as exacerbation of the underlying psychiatric disorder can occur [9]. Asymptomatic patients with drug-induced hyperprolactinemia do not need treatment, but there are reports of women with decreased bone density who have antipsychotic-induced hyperprolactinemia [9]. In symptomatic patients where the medication cannot be stopped, women can be treated with estrogens and men with testosterone to prevent long-term effects of hypogonadism [19].

For women trying to conceive, hyperprolactinemia occurs in 30–40% and has been shown to act as an aromatase inhibitor and can affect follicular fluid steroid metabolism [12, 17]. High PRL disrupts follicular maturation and corpus luteum function and may even reduce fertilization [12]. Some have suggested that hyperprolactinemia can affect the immune system and has opened the door to many studies investigating the neuroendocrine-immune axis (such as the role of natural killer cells) and primary infertility or recurrent pregnancy loss [2]. Further high-quality studies are needed to determine the relationship between hyperprolactinemia and recurrent loss [21]. However, dopamine agonists remain the first line of treatment in women hoping to conceive. Ovulation rates achieved by dopamine agonist treatment only are about 80–90% if hyperprolactinemia is the only cause for anovulation [21, 22]. There is question over management of infertile patients who have elevated levels of PRL who are otherwise asymptomatic, a condition termed "asymptomatic incidental hyperprolactinemia" [12]. Little is known about the initiation of dopamine agonists during ovarian stimulation in in vitro fertilization (IVF) in this situation, but neither cabergoline nor bromocriptine seems to have a deleterious effect on IVF outcomes [12] and may even improve responses in women considered poor responders [12]. If reproductive hormone levels remain low with persistent hyperprolactinemia even after maximal doses of dopamine agonists, injectable gonadotropins replacement therapy may be needed to treat the hypogonadism symptoms [13]. Women with microadenomas can be cycled on and off dopamine agonists to allow for subsequent pregnancies [3].

16.6 Hyperprolactinemia and Pregnancy

While there is no evidence of increased adverse outcomes, such as miscarriage, ectopic pregnancy, trophoblastic disease, birth defects, multiples, or preterm delivery, associated with dopamine agonists in pregnancy, pregnant women with microadenomas should stop bromocriptine or cabergoline, because the risk of tumor expansion is low (less than 3%) and the drugs do cross the placenta [9, 10, 22]. However, the growth of a macroadenoma in pregnancy is possible in up to 31% of patients, so continued use of bromocriptine (which has been studied more extensively than cabergoline in pregnancy) is advised or reinitiation of bromocriptine if previously discontinued [9, 11]. If clinical evidence for tumor growth, such as visual field defects or worsening headaches, develops while a patient is on bromocriptine, MRI without gadolinium is recommended with possible referral for possible pituitary surgery [11]. Preconception counseling for patients with macroadenomas that have not responded to dopamine agonist therapy should include consideration of surgical resection before pregnancy [9], which has shown to limit macroadenoma growth to about 5% [10]. However, patients should be informed that post-procedural risks include hypopituitarism with resulting pituitary hormone deficiencies necessitating fertility treatment with injectable gonadotropins to conceive [9].

Patients with prolactinomas should be clinically assessed every trimester during pregnancy, but formal visual testing is not needed in the absence of compressive symptoms unless a known macroadenoma is present. Obtaining serum prolactin levels during pregnancy is not recommended because prolactin levels increase tenfold by term [3, 9, 10]. Also, physiologic changes to the pituitary gland during pregnancy includes lactotroph hyperplasia and volume increase due to estrogen stimulation from the placenta. The increase in prolactin levels does not accurately correspond with activity or size of prolactinoma [9]. Routine MRIs should not be obtained during pregnancy with microadenomas or macroadenomas unless compressive symptoms develop. If mass effect symptoms develop during pregnancy, dopamine agonist therapy with bromocriptine can be initiated or referral for surgical treatment. There are no studies comparing dopamine agonist therapy to surgical resection in this circumstance in pregnancy.

Women can breastfeed their infant postpartum, but if she plans to do this, treatment with dopamine agonists is not recommended since the resulting decrease in PRL would disrupt lactation. There is no evidence that breastfeeding causes pituitary tumor enlargement [3]. Pregnancy may have a favorable effect on a prolactinoma in that PRL levels are lower after delivery and remission of hyperprolactinemia has been reported in up to 37% of women [3, 10]. However, a woman with a macroadenoma should restart dopamine agonist therapy after pregnancy, unless breastfeeding is planned.

References .

1. Nawroth F. Hyperprolactinaemia and the regular menstrual cycle in asymptomatic women: should it be treated during therapy for infertility? Reprod Biomed Online. 2005;11(5):581–8.
2. Triggianese P, Perricone C, Perricone R, De Carolis C. Prolactin and natural killer cells: evaluating the neuroendocrine-immune axis in women with primary infertility and recurrent spontaneous abortion. Am J Reprod Immunol. 2015;73:56–65.
3. Strauss JF, Barbieri RL. Yen and Jaffe's reproductive endocrinology: Physiology, pathophysiology, and clinical management. Philadelphia, PA: Saunders/Elsevier; 2009.
4. Lu C, Hsieh C. The importance of measuring macroprolactin in the differential diagnosis of hyperprolactinemic patients. Kaohsiung J Med Sci. 2012;28:94–9.
5. Palubska S, Adamiak-Godlewska A, Winkler I, Romanek-Piva K, Rechberger T, Gogacz M. Hyperprolactinemia-a problem in patients from the reproductive period to the menopause. Menopause Rev. 2017;16(1):1–7.
6. Bolyakov A, Paduch DA. Prolactin in men's health and disease. Curr Opin Urol. 2011;21:527–34.
7. Capozzi A, Scambia G, Pontecorvi A, Lello A. Hyperprolactinemia: pathophysiology and therapeutic approach. Gyncol Endocrinol. 2015;31(7):506–10.
8. Fritz MA, Speroff L. Clinical gynecologic endocrinology and infertility. 8th ed. Philadelphia: Lippincott Williams and Wilkins; 2011.
9. Melmed S, Casanueva FF, Hoffman AR, Kleinberg DL, Montori VM, Schlechte JA, Wass JAH. Diagnosis and treatment of hyperprolactinemia: an endocrine society clinical practice guideline. J Clin Endocrinol Metab. 2011;96(2):273–88.
10. Shibli-Rahhal A, Schlechte J. Hyperprolactinemia and infertility. Endocrinol Metab Clin N Am. 2011;40:837–46.
11. Molitch ME. Prolactinoma in pregnancy. Best Pract Res Clin Endocrinol Metab. 2011;25:885–96.
12. Bahceci M, Sismanoglu A, Ulug U. Comparison of cabergoline and bromocriptine in patients with asymptomatic incidental hyperprolactinemia undergoing ICSI-ET. Gynecol Endocrinol. 2010;26(7):505–8.
13. Klibanski A. Clinical practice. Prolactinomas. N Eng J Med. 2010;362:1219–26.
14. Wong-Anuchit C. Clinical management of antipsychotic-induced hyperprolactinemia. Perspect Psychiatr Care. 2016;52:145–52.
15. Glezer A, Bronstein MD. Approach to the patient with persistent hyperprolactinemia and negative sellar imaging. J Clin Endocrinol Metab. 2012;97(7):2211–6.
16. Gardner DG, Shoback D. Greenspan's basic and clinical endocrinology. 8th ed. New York: McGraw-Hill; 2007.
17. Thirunavakkarasu K, Dutta P, Sridhar S, Dhaliwal L, Prashad GRV, Gainder S, Sachdva N, Bhansali A. Macroprolactinemia in hyperprolactinemic infertile women. Encocrine. 2013;44:750–5.
18. Davis JR. Prolactin and reproductive medicine. Curr Opin Obstet Gynecol. 2004;16:331–7.
19. Rabinovich IH, Gomez RC, Mouriz MG, Garcia-Agullo DO. Clinical guidelines for diagnosis and treatment of prolactinoma and hyperprolactinemia. Endocrinol Nutr. 2013;60(6):308–19.
20. Nachtigall LB. Cabergoline for hyperprolactinemia: getting to the heart of it. Endocrine. 2017;57:3.
21. Chen H, Fu J, Huang W. Dopamine agonists for preventing future miscarriage in women with idiopathic hyperprolactinemia and recurrent miscarriage history. Cochrane Database Syst Rev. 2016;7:1–25.
22. Berinder K, Hulting A, Granath F, Hirschberg AL, Akre O. Parity, pregnancy and neonatal outcomes in women treated for hyperprolactinemia compared with a control group. Clin Endocrinol. 2007;67:393–7.

Natural Cycle IVF/Modified Natural Cycle IVF and Natural Cycle IVF/IVM

17

Justin Tan and Seang Lin Tan

17.1 Chapter Objectives

1. Appreciate the historical milestones of in vitro fertilization (IVF) development.
2. Identify the major types of ovarian stimulation during IVF:
   (a) Controlled ovarian hyperstimulation IVF (COH-IVF)
   (b) Natural cycle IVF (NC-IVF)
   (c) Modified natural cycle IVF (MNC-IVF)
   (d) Mild stimulation IVF
3. Recognize the rationale and indications for NC-IVF.
4. Identify the benefits and reproductive outcomes of NC-IVF vs. COH-IVF.
5. Understand the limitations and alternatives to NC-IVF vs. COH-IVF.
6. Future advancements and implications.

17.2 Background

17.2.1 Definitions

Infertility is defined as the failure of a couple of reproductive age to conceive after at least 12 months of regular intercourse without contraception, affecting 15–20% of couples trying to conceive [1]. More specifically, **primary infertility** occurs in a couple who have never had a child, while **secondary infertility** is failure to conceive following a previous pregnancy. In the last 40 years, numerous improvements to assisted reproductive technologies (ARTs) have been developed, especially for in vitro fertilization (IVF), greatly improving the chances of achieving pregnancy and live births.

17.2.2 Brief History of IVF

The field of assisted reproductive technologies (ARTs) began to take shape in the late nineteenth century, starting with the first systematic approach to human artificial insemination (AI) performed by the nineteenth-century surgeon-gynecologist Dr. J. Marion Sims at the Women's Hospital in New York [1]. Although his findings from 55 fresh intrauterine inseminations (IUIs) resulted in only one pregnancy that ended in miscarriage, his revolutionary approach to female infertility with an emphasis on treatment was well ahead of his time, albeit rife with ethical controversies as he experimented on vulnerable populations without informed consent [2]. The first successful AI resulting in live birth occurred in 1884 when Dr. William Pancoast of the Jefferson Medical College in Philadelphia used donor sperm from one of his medical students (unbeknownst to the patient) to perform the IUI—after he found the husband's semen to be deficient in sperm. Despite the success of this case, the lack of informed consent would be completely unacceptable today. With the exception of IUI and rudimentary microscopic semen analysis, fertility treatment in the late nineteenth to early twentieth centuries still mostly consisted of gynecological operations.

As the understanding of human physiology, embryology, and reproductive endocrinology flourished in the early to mid-twentieth century, so did the advancements in ART and laboratory techniques in cell culture. In 1934, biologists Gregory Pincus and Ernst Vinzenz Enzmann attempted the first "in vitro" fertilization (IVF) with rabbits. Although their attempt resulted in a successful pregnancy, further analysis revealed that fertilization had actually occurred in vivo, rather than in vitro, as they had implanted immature eggs

J. Tan (✉)
Department of Obstetrics and Gynecology, BC Women's Hospital, Vancouver, BC, Canada

S. L. Tan
Department of Obstetrics and Gynecology, McGill University, Montreal, QC, Canada

OriginElle Fertility Clinic and Women's Health Centre, Montreal, QC, Canada

McGill Reproductive Centre, Montreal, QC, Canada

G. N. Allahbadia et al. (eds.), *Textbook of Assisted Reproduction*, https://doi.org/10.1007/978-981-15-2377-9_17

into the rabbit's uterus without sufficient exposure to sperm. It wasn't until 1951, when Colin Austin from Australia and Min Chueh Chang from the Worcester Foundation in the United Sates independently demonstrated that spermatozoa and oocytes need to mature through certain stages before they develop the capacity to fertilize. By 1959, Chang clearly demonstrated that in vitro fertilization of rabbit oocytes and subsequent uterine transfer were indeed capable of pregnancy and live birth of a rabbit. Not only did this seminal study propel IVF to the forefront of ART and embryology research, but the successes of IVF in an animal model suggested that the same procedure might be possible in humans.

In 1944, obstetrician-gynecologist Dr. John Rock first successfully fertilized a human egg outside of the body [3]. Due to the societal hesitancy toward ARTs and embryology research at the time, the fertilized embryos were never implanted in humans. Nonetheless, Rock demonstrated that a successful IVF technique in humans was within reach. The first human pregnancy achieved through IVF was achieved by Alan Trounson, John Leeton, and Carl Wood of Monash University in 1973, although it resulted in a biochemical pregnancy. Around the same time, English physiologist Dr. Robert Edwards began research on the genetics of human oocyte maturation and fertilization of oocytes in vitro [4]. Shortly after, Dr. Patrick Steptoe, an obstetrician-gynecologist who practiced laparoscopic retrieval of human oocytes, collaborated with Edwards in 1966 on human IVF development—combining laboratory innovation with clinical application. Although their initial efforts resulted in an ectopic pregnancy, they finally succeeded in the first IVF baby, Louise Joy Brown, who was born in England on July 25, 1978, using an unstimulated natural cycle IVF [5]. As the news resounded throughout the world and paved the way for IVF to take center stage for infertility treatment, Edwards would go on to receive the 2010 Nobel Prize in Medicine for their contributions to the field.

As human IVF moved from an experimental laboratory procedure to established clinical practice for infertile couples in the 1980s, many scientists and physicians from around the world sought to optimize the IVF ovulatory cycle protocol through incorporating exogenous hormones like clomiphene citrate (CC) and human menopausal hormone (hMG) to stimulate folliculogenesis. The rationale was that inducing a cohort of follicles to mature would increase the yield of oocyte retrieval, therefore improving the chances of creating embryos for transfer [6]. Alan Trounson and Howard Jones pioneered the use of these hormones in a regimen referred to as controlled ovarian hyperstimulation (COH) in order to increase the yield of oocytes retrieved [7, 8]. Similarly, gonadotropin-releasing hormone (GnRH) agonists and antagonists enhanced protocols [9–14] by improving oocyte quality on retrieval and minimize complications and risks such as premature ovulation, ovarian hyperstimulation syndrome, and multiple gestations [15]. By the 1990s, the sophistication of IVF protocols has led to the expansion of treatment options and improved pregnancy outcomes. These include new recombinant injectable gonadotropin agents, in vitro maturation and fertilization for women with poor ovarian response [16], and cryopreservation of embryos for subsequent uterine transfer. Cryopreservation and vitrification of oocytes and embryos meant that women do not have to repeat the full fertility treatment cycle when implantation of a fresh embryo fails. Furthermore, Gianpiero Palermo and his team helped couples better overcome male factor infertility from defective sperm function with the development of intracytoplasmic sperm injection (ICSI) in 1991. Procedural sophistication such as the advent of transvaginal ultrasound aspiration of oocytes made egg retrieval more tolerable and less invasive for patients [17].

While historic IVF live birth rates were less than 16% per transfer, current clinics report live birth rates of up to 25% per cycle for women under 40 years [9]. In 2012, an estimated total of 5 million babies were born around the world as a result of ART, with around 1.5 million cycles being performed each year globally. The demand for IVF and other ARTs has seen a dramatic increase in the last decade, due to a combination of delayed childbearing and increased accessibility to infertility treatment. While ART-assisted births account for 2–3% of all births in Europe, only 0.7% of all births in the United States are the result of ARTs. The impact of IVF on the patient's health, her pregnancy, and her infant has some researchers begin to question the safety of ARTs [10]. IVF pregnancies have been well documented to be of higher risk than those from spontaneous conception, resulting in significantly higher odds of perinatal mortality, preterm delivery, low birth weight, and small for gestational age babies [10].

A successful IVF cycle entails the balance between optimizing egg retrieval to create high-quality embryos for uterine transfer while minimizing the exposure of the patient to the risks of excessive ovarian stimulation. The current conventional IVF approach for an infertile couple is the controlled ovarian hyperstimulation IVF (COH-IVF), where a cocktail of fertility medications to stimulate follicular growth and maturation aim to maximize the yield of oocytes retrieved from each cycle. The introduction of COH-IVF led to it becoming the standard ovarian stimulation method because of the improved birth rates. In this chapter we explore the rationale, outcomes, limitations, and alternatives to COH-IVF by focusing on the "natural cycle IVF" (NC-IVF), where the patient is brought through an unstimulated cycle with minimal to no medication before oocyte retrieval and uterine transfer of a single embryo—just like how Louise Brown was conceived. While NC-IVF intends to lower the incidence of ovarian stimulation side effects, success rates were low secondary to unpredictable luteinizing hormone (LH) surges which resulted in premature ovulation and cycle cancelations. Yet, in context of a patient who cannot tolerate or prefers minimal ovarian stimulation due to side effects or financial restrictions, NC-IVF may be preferable choice. Whereas some scientists and physicians aim to find the right protocol that best simulates the physiologic ovulatory cycle while tailoring to the patient's needs and wishes, others are trying to compare whether ovarian stimulation affects embryo quality and perinatal outcomes. Needless to say, the reconsideration of NC-IVF in personalized clinical practice may reshape the future of ART development and convention.

17.3 Types of Ovarian Stimulation Protocols

17.3.1 Controlled Ovarian Hyperstimulation (COH)

A successful IVF cycle depends on the optimization of egg retrieval for generating high-quality embryos and minimizing the patients' exposure to excessive ovarian stimulation. The aim of exogenous hormones in COH is to initiate the maturation of a group of follicles while preventing premature spontaneous ovulation which would result in cycle cancelation. Therefore, all COH protocols comprise the following three components:

1. Stimulation of multiple follicles through oral or injectable exogenous gonadotropins (CC, hMG, recombinant FSH, etc.)
2. Additional therapy with either GnRH agonist or antagonists to prevent premature ovulation through pituitary axis suppression
3. Triggering of final oocyte maturation about 34–36 hours prior to oocyte retrieval when the follicles are 17 mm in diameter, with human chorionic gonadotropin (hCG) or GnRH agonist
4. Transvaginal oocyte retrieval via ultrasound-guided aspiration under mild sedation

COH increases oocyte yield and thus the potential for having multiple embryos, facilitating preimplantation genetic screening and cryopreservation of surplus embryos, improving the success rates, and minimizing repeated gonadotropin exposure if there was pregnancy failure [11] (Table 17.1). Segmented IVF, where oocyte retrieval and frozen-thaw embryo transfers are performed in separate cycles, is thought to improve implantation success through luteal phase support of the endometrium and makes the initial cycle more tolerable for the patient. Use of exogenous hormone regimens, however, also means increased costs and complications for the patient. Most patients initially use oral medications such as clomiphene and letrozole for ovarian stimulation through dampening of the negative feedback of endogenous estrogen on the hypothalamus-pituitary axis. Although pregnancy rates are higher with injectable hormones such as recombinant follicle stimulation hormone (rFSH) and hMG, they do confer a higher risk of multiple gestation, ovarian hyperstimulation syndrome (OHSS), costs, and monitoring time [12].

Table 17.1 Types in vitro fertilization (IVF) cycle stimulation protocols

Terminology	Aim	Methodology
Classical natural cycle IVF	Single oocyte	No medication, hCG at 17–18
Classical modified natural cycle IVF	Single oocyte	hCG at 17–18 mm, antagonist from 14 mm and FSH/hMG add-back
Early stimulation, early trigger modified natural cycle IVF/IVM	1–125 oocytes (some MII, some GV)*	FSH day 4, 6, 8 hCG when lead follicle 14 mm
Mild IVF	2–7 oocytes	Low-dose FSH/hMG + antagonists or oral compounds
Conventional IVF	≥8 oocytes	Agonist or antagonist conventional FSH/hMG dose

COH controlled ovarian hyperstimulation, *hCG* human chorionic gonadotropin, *FSH* follicle-stimulating hormone, *hMG* human menopausal gonadotropin

*From Dahan MH, Ata B, Rosenberg R, Chunh JT, Son WY, Tan SL. Collection of 125 oocytes in an in vitro maturation cycle using a new oocyte collection technique. J Obstet Gynaecol Can. 2014; 36:900–3, with permission

17.3.2 Mild Stimulation IVF (MS-IVF)

MS-IVF is a gentler form of COH-IVF where a lower daily dose of gonadotropins (i.e., FSH, hMG) is given for a shorter duration in a flexible GnRH-antagonist cycle. Oral antiestrogens (CC, letrozole) may also be used either alone or in combination with gonadotropins [13]. The clinical significance of MS-IVF revolves around the concept that gentler follicular stimulation would improve oocyte quality at retrieval. Although FSH dose is directly correlated with the number of oocytes recovered, the number of good-quality blastocysts was not found to have a similar relationship with gonadotropin dose. Essentially, the blastocyst-oocyte ratio and fertilization rate showed an inverse relationship with the magnitude of ovarian stimulation [14]. Furthermore, the cumulative pregnancy outcomes of MS-IVF versus COH-IVF were found to be similar, despite less oocytes or embryos being available with MS-IVF [13].

17.3.3 Natural Cycle IVF and Variants

Natural differs from COH-IVF and MS-IVF in that little to no hormone treatments are administered to stimulate folliculogenesis. Rather, clinicians rely on the monitoring of follicular maturation by measuring their size and structure. When the follicle reaches an estimated size of 15–20 mm, final maturation of the oocyte can either be anticipated before spontaneous ovulation or induced by administering ovulation triggers like subcutaneous hCG [18]. The oocyte is then retrieved by follicle aspiration under transvaginal ultrasound guidance, similar to that of COH-IVF. There are several types of natural cycle IVF:

1. Unstimulated NC-IVF
   - When a follicle approaches maturity (approximately 10–12 mm in diameter), the oocyte retrieval date is anticipated. hCG is administered to trigger ovulation when follicle is about 18–20 mm in size, or when the serum estradiol rises [19]. In the case of premature spontaneous LH surge (measured in urine), either cycle cancelation or earlier oocyte retrieval occurs [17].
2. Modified natural cycle IVF (MNC-IVF)
   - For MNC-IVF, a short course (2–6 days) of gonadotropins is given for follicular stimulation. Daily GnRH antagonist injections are used to suppress premature ovulation after a short period of ovarian stimulation or when the largest follicle reaches a diameter of 14 mm.
   - Similar to COH-IVF, hCG is given to trigger oocyte maturation when the leading follicle reaches a size of 15–20 mm, but only one fully matured oocyte is retrieved.
   - Luteal phase support is required despite immediate recovery of the pituitary after cessation of the GnRH antagonist [20].

17.4 Rationale, Indications, and Potential Risks for Natural Cycle IVF

The main differences between NC-IVF and COH-IVF arise as a consequence of not using gonadotropin agents for ovarian stimulation. Patients undergoing COH-IVF increased risk of multiple gestation pregnancies than in NC-IVF [21]. Multiple gestations are associated with a high risk of prematurity, causing considerable morbidity and mortality in neonates [22]. Women undergoing COH-IVF cycles may also experience OHSS in up to 10% of cases [23]. OHSS is a serious and sometimes life-threatening iatrogenic adverse effect as a result of prolonged gonadotropin therapy. NC-IVF and MNC-IVF reduce this risk by minimizing exposure time to ovarian stimulation. This also results in a less physically and emotionally demanding, less time-consuming procedure. Since no resting cycle is needed following a failed cycle, patients can undergo back-to-back cycles to increase cumulative success rates [19]. Finally, for couples with male factor subfertility, which comprises 20% of all causes of infertility [24], NC-IVF may be more appropriate to minimize the physical, psychological, and financial burden that comes with COH-IVF for the couple [11]. NC-IVF is also a desirable alternative from conventional COH-IVF for women with poor ovarian response or a history of failed stimulated IVF cycles. These patients may have low anti-Mullerian hormone (AMH) and high FSH or have had a poor response to fertility drugs previously. For financially restricted couples, NC-IVF is less costly overall, up to 97.5% less than the least expensive conventional IVF cycle [25, 26]. Even when comparing ovulatory cycles used in conjunction with IUI, unstimulated cycles were statistically significantly less costly than stimulated cycles [26].

17.5 Benefits and Outcomes

Although pregnancy rate per NC-IVF cycle does not match that of COH-IVF, cumulative pregnancy rates are similar. Nargund and colleagues compared cumulative outcome of successive cycles of NC-IVF with COH-IVF [18]. They reported a cumulative probability of pregnancy of 46% and live birth rate of 32%. It seems a series of NC-IVF should be offered as an alternative to COH-IVF [18]. Decreased cost of drugs and monitoring can render NC-IVF more affordable than conventional treatment. In that same study, they calculated that even a series of NC-IVF cycles cost only 23% of one stimulated cycle, suggesting that it may be a cost-effective alternative to conventional IVF [18].

Despite mimicking maternal normal physiology, perinatal outcomes are worse for families that have undergone IVF cycles than that of spontaneous conception. For example, lower birth weights and an increased risk of preterm birth were found in a recent prospective analysis of over 60,000 singleton stimulated IVF live births [27]. Pelinck in 2010 also found a correlation between these adverse perinatal outcomes with ovarian hyperstimulation and higher oocyte count [28]. Interestingly, infants conceived by unstimulated or natural IVF have a lower risk of being low birth weight than infants conceived by stimulated IVF [29]. This risk, however, did not remain significant after adjusting for gestation age at birth. More recent retrospective studies examining the effects of exogenous gonadotropins on embryo quality showed that cleavage capacity and objective qualitative assessment of resulting embryos were not affected by hormonal stimulation. Neither the cleavage rate of oocytes nor the early cleavage stage morphology of embryos differed between stimulated and natural IVF cycles [30]. However, the same study did not assess the effects of gonadotropin administration on post-implantation embryonic development, which could still contribute to perinatal outcomes. Overall, these findings seem to suggest that the contributing difference in reproductive outcomes between COH-IVF and NC-IVF seems to be mostly due to the difference in oocyte numbers.

17.6 Limitations and Alternatives

One potential disadvantage of NC-IVF includes a higher cycle cancelation rate due to unpredictability of premature LH surges. Furthermore, because only one dominant follicle develops into an oocyte when retrieved, there is a lower chance of successful embryo transfer. The utility of preimplantation genetic screening is also limited due to a limited pool of embryos formed. While the MNC-IVF employs the use of short-term gonadotropins and GnRH antagonists to prevent premature ovulation, oocyte yield is still minimal, with 1–2 eggs retrieved per cycle. When compared with conventional COH-IVF, where there are well-established therapy regimens with a long track record of success rates, NC-IVF has lower live birth rates (LBR) per cycle after fresh embryo transfer, depending on the provider experience and the clinical factors of each individual patient [31]. The lower LBR per cycle may mean that it could be potentially more time-consuming and require more effort for a couple to reach successful pregnancy [11, 25, 32]. With LBR as low as 7% per cycle, this is the most significant reason against attempting NC-IVF for many patients.

One alternative to address the issue of low oocyte yield and premature ovulation is through the combination of NC-IVF with in vitro maturation (IVM), where follicles are retrieved at 14 mm and oocytes are matured in the laboratory. Benefits include a much higher oocyte yield and the ability to perform genetic screening and embryo cryopreservation for a subsequent transfer. However, this could potentially be more resource intensive, utilizing other adjunctive ARTs such as ICSI after IVM. A few studies have also assessed the risk of congenital abnormalities and adverse obstetrical outcomes for NC-IVF and IVM versus COH-IVF and found no differences between the two modalities [33]. Interestingly, a smaller retrospective study in 2010 found that embryos derived from IVM oocytes that matured more than 48 hours after retrieval had higher chromosomal abnormality rates than those that matured within 24 hours or matured in vivo [34]. The use of IVM in ART is still an active area of research and innovation, ever since Dr. Edwards began his research on human oocyte maturation in his lab.

Mild stimulation IVF has also been explored as an alternative to both COH and NC-IVF, as a way to combine the strengths of each modality. While MS-IVF has comparable reproductive outcomes with COH-IVF, it is associated with a more favorable safety profile, with higher perinatal birth weights and higher patient satisfaction [13]. One MS-IVF cycle also yields a higher oocyte count than that of NC-IVF, increasing the chances for successful embryo transfer, and allows for genetic screening and cryopreservation. With a lower dose of gonadotropins, patients are at a lower risk for OHSS and thrombosis, making MS-IVF a more suitable, accessible alternative for both couples and IVF providers [35]. Emerging economic analyses for MS-IVF have additionally shown its cost-saving impact on clinical practice, where a multicenter randomized controlled trial demonstrated the considerable savings accrued through lowering gonadotropins doses while maintaining comparable pregnancy outcomes.

17.7 Future Advancements

When cryopreservation techniques were first developed in the 1990s, the procedure was largely experimental and reserved mostly for embryo storage. The more recent innovation of "vitrification" or flash-freezing has significantly improved the freeze quality, making egg-freezing a potential way to preserve fertility [36]. This expansion of "social oocyte cryopreservation" in recent years has been largely due to the increased number of couples who delay childbearing for a multitude of personal, professional, financial, and psychological reasons [37]. In the early 2010s, the Society for Assisted Reproductive Technology (SART) announced that oocyte cryopreservation was no longer an experimental procedure but cautioned against the use of egg-freezing to defer age-related fertility decline. The data on its efficacy, safety, and cost-effectiveness were limited for healthy women of reproductive age. For a couple undergoing conventional COH-IVF, one can see the potential harms, adverse effects, and financial costs of the process on the patient. On the other hand, a woman seeking to freeze her eggs using NC-IVF can achieve similar success with lower costs, health risks, and emotional and physical burden as no drugs are used in the process. Future analysis and trials should be conducted to illustrate the impact of unstimulated IVF cycles on the acceptability of social egg-freezing [38].

17.8 Conclusion

NC-IVF combines the body's natural process of folliculogenesis and endometrial development with the precision of oocyte retrieval at maturity and improved laboratory techniques in order to optimize oocyte embryo quality within a less physically demanding treatment cycle. While pregnancy rates can be as low as 6% per cycle, the cumulative rate after several repeated cycles is comparable to one conventional COH-IVF cycle, especially for poor-responder women to fertility medication. Whereas direct benefits of NC-IVF include no risk of OHSS and multiple gestation, minimal side effects, and less financial burden, cycle cancelation rates are higher due to unpredictable premature ovulation. As such, more frequent intrusive monitoring may be warranted for the patient to prevent this [11]. In addition, there are no surplus eggs or embryos for use in future transfers should the current cycle fail.

To date, no large-scale randomized controlled trials exist that directly compares NC-IVF with standard COH-IVF, with primary outcomes focusing on cumulative live birth rates, the number of treatment cycles per woman necessary to reach live birth, adverse effects, and treatment costs of the drugs. Other alternative IVF protocols, such as MNC-IVF and MS-IVF, should be investigated in the same matter, with the data analysis geared toward a clear comparison in reproductive outcomes per woman [11].

The natural cycle IVF aims to achieve quality over quantity of oocytes and embryos while making the process more affordable for couples. The accessibility of IVF treatments, and ARTs in general, can only be realized by reducing the costs and complications [39]. In the four decades since Louise Brown was born, ART innovation has only accelerated, aided by new technologies and bedside techniques to better understand and preserve human fertility—both in vivo and in vitro.

References

1. Ombelet W, Van Robays J. Artificial insemination history: hurdles and milestones. Facts Views Vis Obgyn. 2015;7(2):137–43.
2. Wall LL. The medical ethics of Dr J Marion Sims: a fresh look at the historical record. J Med Ethics. 2006;32(6):346–50.
3. Rock J, Menkin MF. In vitro fertilization and cleavage of human ovarian eggs. Science. 1944;100(2588):105–7.
4. Edwards RG. Maturation in vitro of human ovarian oocytes. Lancet. 1965;286(7419):926–9.
5. Steptoe PC, Edwards RG. Reimplantation of a human embryo with subsequent tubal pregnancy. Lancet. 1976;1(7965):880–2.
6. Dellenbach P, Nisand I, Moreau L, Feger B, Plumere C, Gerlinger P. Transvaginal sonographically controlled follicle puncture for oocyte retrieval. Fertil Steril. 1985;44(5):656–62.
7. Trounson AO, Leeton JF, Wood C, Webb J, Wood J. Pregnancies in humans by fertilization in vitro and embryo transfer in the controlled ovulatory cycle. Science. 1981;212(4495):681–2.
8. Jones HW, Jones GS, Andrews MC, Acosta A, Bundren C, Garcia J, et al. The program for in vitro fertilization at Norfolk**Presented at the thirty-eighth annual meeting of the American fertility society, March 20 to 24, 1982, Las Vegas. Nevada Fertility and Sterility. 1982;38(1):14–21.
9. Naaktgeboren N, Devroey P, Traey E, Wisanto A, Van Steirteghem AC. Success of in vitro fertilization and embryo transfer in relation to the causes of infertility. Acta Eur Fertil. 1985;16(4):281–7.
10. Jackson RA, Gibson KA, Wu YW, Croughan MS. Perinatal outcomes in singletons following in vitro fertilization: a meta-analysis. Obstet Gynecol. 2004;103(3):551–63.
11. Allersma T, Farquhar C, Cantineau AE. Natural cycle in vitro fertilisation (IVF) for subfertile couples. Cochrane Database Syst Rev. 2013;8:CD010550.
12. Gallos ID, Eapen A, Price MJ, Sunkara S, Macklon NS, Bhattacharya S, et al. Controlled ovarian stimulation protocols for assisted reproduction: a network meta-analysis. Cochrane Database of Syst Rev. 2017;(3). Art. No.: CD012586. https://doi.org/10.1002/14651858.CD012586.
13. Nargund G, Datta AK, Fauser B. Mild stimulation for in vitro fertilization. Fertil Steril. 2017;108(4):558–67.
14. Arce JC, Andersen AN, Fernandez-Sanchez M, Visnova H, Bosch E, Garcia-Velasco JA, et al. Ovarian response to recombinant human follicle-stimulating hormone: a randomized, antimullerian hormone-stratified, dose-response trial in women undergoing in vitro fertilization/intracytoplasmic sperm injection. Fertil Steril. 2014;102(6):1633–40. e5.
15. Frydman R, Cornel C, de Ziegler D, Taieb J, Spitz IM, Bouchard P. Prevention of premature luteinizing hormone and progesterone rise with a gonadotropin-releasing hormone antagonist, Nal-Glu, in controlled ovarian hyperstimulation. Fertil Steril. 1991;56(5):923–7.
16. Corbett S, Shmorgun D, Claman P. Reproductive endocrinology infertility C, special C. The prevention of ovarian hyperstimulation syndrome. J Obstet Gynaecol Can. 2014;36(11):1024–33.
17. LE Zayed F, Cooke ID. Natural cycle in-vitro fertilization in couples with unexplained infertility: impact of various factors on outcome. Hum Reprod. 1997;12(11):2402–7.
18. Nargund G, Waterstone J, Bland J, Philips Z, Parsons J, Campbell S. Cumulative conception and live birth rates in natural (unstimulated) IVF cycles. Hum Reprod. 2001;16(2):259–62.
19. Pelinck MJ, Hoek A, Simons AH, Heineman MJ. Efficacy of natural cycle IVF: a review of the literature. Hum Reprod Update. 2002;8(2):129–39.
20. Ho JR, Paulson RJ. Modified natural cycle in in vitro fertilization. Fertil Steril. 2017;108(4):572–6.
21. Elsner CW, Tucker MJ, Sweitzer CL, Brockman WDW, Morton PC, Wright G, et al. Multiple pregnancy rate and embryo number transferred during in vitro fertilization. Am J Obstet Gynecol. 1997;177(2):350–7.
22. Elster N. Less is more: the risks of multiple births. Fertil Steril. 2000;74(4):617–23.
23. Beerendonk CC, van Dop PA, Braat DD, Merkus JM. Ovarian hyperstimulation syndrome: facts and fallacies. Obstet Gynecol Surv. 1998;53(7):439–49.
24. Jarow JP, Sharlip ID, Belker AM, Lipshultz LI, Sigman M, Thomas AJ, et al. Best practice policies for male infertility. J Urol. 2002;167(5):2138–44.
25. Aanesen A, Nygren KG, Nylund L. Modified natural cycle IVF and mild IVF: a 10 year Swedish experience. Reprod Biomed Online. 2010;20(1):156–62.
26. Pashayan N, Lyratzopoulos G, Mathur R. Cost-effectiveness of primary offer of IVF vs. primary offer of IUI followed by IVF (for IUI failures) in couples with unexplained or mild male factor subfertility. BMC Health Serv Res. 2006;6:80.
27. Sunkara SK, La Marca A, Seed PT, Khalaf Y. Increased risk of preterm birth and low birthweight with very high number of oocytes following IVF: an analysis of 65 868 singleton live birth outcomes. Hum Reprod. 2015;30(6):1473–80.
28. Pelinck MJ, Keizer MH, Hoek A, Simons AH, Schelling K, Middelburg K, et al. Perinatal outcome in singletons after modified natural cycle IVF and standard IVF with ovarian stimulation. Eur J Obstet Gynecol Reprod Biol. 2010;148(1):56–61.

29. Mak W, Kondapalli LA, Celia G, Gordon J, DiMattina M, Payson M. Natural cycle IVF reduces the risk of low birthweight infants compared with conventional stimulated IVF. Hum Reprod. 2016;31(4):789–94.
30. Ziebe S, Bangsboll S, Schmidt KL, Loft A, Lindhard A, Nyboe AA. Embryo quality in natural versus stimulated IVF cycles. Hum Reprod. 2004;19(6):1457–60.
31. Walls ML, Ryan JP, Keelan JA, Hart R. In vitro maturation is associated with increased early embryo arrest without impairing morphokinetic development of useable embryos progressing to blastocysts. Hum Reprod. 2015;30(8):1842–9.
32. Claman P, Domingo M, Garner P, Leader A, Spence JEH. Natural cycle in vitro fertilization-embryo transfer at the University of Ottawa: an inefficient therapy for tubal infertility*. Fertil Steril. 1993;60(2):298–302.
33. Buckett WM, Chian RC, Holzer H, Dean N, Usher R, Tan SL. Obstetric outcomes and congenital abnormalities after in vitro maturation, in vitro fertilization, and intracytoplasmic sperm injection. Obstet Gynecol. 2007;110(4):885–91.
34. Zhang XY, Ata B, Son WY, Buckett WM, Tan SL, Ao A. Chromosome abnormality rates in human embryos obtained from in-vitro maturation and IVF treatment cycles. Reprod Biomed Online. 2010;21(4):552–9.
35. Youssef MA, van Wely M, Al-Inany H, Madani T, Jahangiri N, Khodabakhshi S, et al. A mild ovarian stimulation strategy in women with poor ovarian reserve undergoing IVF: a multicenter randomized non-inferiority trial. Hum Reprod. 2017;32(1):112–8.
36. Oktay K, Cil AP, Bang H. Efficiency of oocyte cryopreservation: a meta-analysis. Fertil Steril. 2006;86(1):70–80.
37. Argyle CE, Harper JC, Davies MC. Oocyte cryopreservation: where are we now? Hum Reprod Update. 2016;22(4):440–9.
38. ETFo E, Law DW, de Wert G, Pennings G, Shenfield F, et al. Oocyte cryopreservation for age-related fertility loss. Hum Reprod. 2012;27(5):1231–7.
39. Frydman R, Nargund G. Mild approaches in assisted reproduction--better for the future? Fertil Steril. 2014;102(6):1540–1.

Unconventional Ovarian Stimulation for Medically Assisted Reproduction

18

Sule Yildiz and Baris Ata

Ovarian stimulation for assisted reproductive technology (ART) or medically assisted reproduction (MAR) aims to provide multiple oocytes available for in vitro fertilization since the chances of a live birth increase in parallel to the number of oocytes [1, 2]. Multifollicular development is achieved by maintaining follicle-stimulating hormone (FSH) levels above the threshold required to drive growth of FSH-sensitive follicles. The spontaneous luteinizing hormone (LH) surge is suppressed by the use of gonadotropin-releasing hormone (GnRH) analogues to prevent ovulation before oocyte retrieval, and oocyte maturation is triggered with either human chorionic gonadotropin (hCG) or a GnRH agonist, depending on the stimulation protocol.

Traditionally, exogenous gonadotropin stimulation is started at the beginning of follicular phase to ensure the growth of the cohort of antral follicles, which are recruited during the luteo-follicular transition. This enables OR at the end of follicular phase and in vitro embryo development during the early luteal phase. Thus, embryo development is synchronized with endometrial development, transition to the secretory phase, and importantly with the implantation window, enabling fresh embryo transfer. However, with the advent of successful vitrification, a fresh embryo transfer is not considered mandatory on certain occasions, including total cryopreservation to prevent ovarian hyperstimulation syndrome and to increase the chances of a live birth in hyper-responders, women undergoing preimplantation genetic testing (PGT), or when the intent is to use the oocytes/embryos in the future for fertility preservation for a medical or social indication.

S. Yildiz
Department of Obstetrics and Gynecology, Koc University Hospital, Istanbul, Turkey

B. Ata (✉)
Division of Reproductive Endocrinology and Infertility, Department of Obstetrics and Gynecology, Koç University School of Medicine, Istanbul, Turkey

Department of Obstetrics, Gynecology and Reproductive Sciences, Yale University School of Medicine, New Haven, CT, USA
e-mail: barisata@ku.edu.tr

It is realized that multiple waves of antral follicles develop during one menstrual cycle rather than a single recruitment episode during the follicular phase [3]. This understanding has brought about the concepts of starting ovarian stimulation at any time during a menstrual cycle, dubbed as "random-start stimulation" and ovarian stimulation during the luteal phase. The wave theory provides the rationale for ovarian stimulation during the luteal phase. In a natural cycle, the dominant follicle formed in the final wave of the inter-ovulatory interval reaches ovulation, and the other waves are anovulatory [3]. However, follicles that are recruited during the anovulatory waves have the potential to reach ovulation when exposed to FSH stimulation, enabling random-start stimulation [4].

While random-start stimulation was initially used for fertility preservation in women with cancer [5, 6], encouraging results have been reported with luteal phase-start ovarian stimulation in healthy women undergoing MAR [7, 8]. Stimulating the ovaries twice during one menstrual cycle has also been used to rapidly accumulate embryos for women with a low ovarian reserve. The first round of stimulation is commenced in the follicular phase with the use of a GnRH antagonist to suppress the LH surge, usually a GnRH agonist is used to trigger final oocyte maturation, and the second round of stimulation is initiated after OR [7]. Since the endogenous progesterone secreted by the corpora lutea can suppress endogenous LH production, the second round of stimulation in the luteal phase stimulation can be done without using GnRH antagonist in many cases. However, ovarian stimulation in the luteal phase can take longer (on average 1.5 days), require more gonadotropins (on average 817 IU), but can provide higher number of mature oocytes [8–10]. Blastocyst development from the oocytes collected in the luteal phase seems similar with oocytes collected from stimulation in the follicular phase. Ubaldi et al. reported that 42% and 54% of 42 women, with an average age of 39 years who underwent double stimulation, had at least one euploid blastocyst following stimulation in the follicular and luteal phases, respectively. These

G. N. Allahbadia et al. (eds.), *Textbook of Assisted Reproduction*, https://doi.org/10.1007/978-981-15-2377-9_18

blastocysts seem to be similarly likely to be euploid and provide similar pregnancy rates when transferred in a subsequent cycle [10, 11]. Limited data on obstetric outcome of and congenital anomalies in pregnancies derived from frozen-thawed transfer of embryos derived from luteal phase stimulation ovaries suggest similar results with follicular phase oocyte retrievals [12]. Chen et al. reported the obstetric outcomes of 587 children born from luteal phase stimulation and compared with 1257 children born from frozen-thawed embryo transfers following conventional MAR cycles and 216 children from mild ovarian stimulation cycles. Gestational age, birth weight and length, and early neonatal death rates were comparable. Likewise, the incidence of live-birth defects were similar among the three groups: 1.02% in the luteal stimulation, 0.64% in the short GnRH-a protocol, and 0.46% in the mild ovarian-stimulation group. Prevalence of congenital anomalies were also similar between the three groups.

References

1. Sunkara SK, Rittenberg V, Raine-Fenning N, Bhattacharya S, Zamora J, Coomarasamy A. Association between the number of eggs and live birth in IVF treatment: an analysis of 400 135 treatment cycles. Hum Reprod. 2011;26:1768–74.
2. Polyzos NP, Drakopoulos P, Parra J, Pellicer A, Santos-Ribeiro S, Tournaye H, Bosch E, Garcia-Velasco J. Cumulative live birth rates according to the number of oocytes retrieved after the first ovarian stimulation for in vitro fertilization/intracytoplasmic sperm injection: a multicenter multinational analysis including approximately 15,000 women. Fertil Steril. 2018;110:661–670e1.
3. Baerwald AR, Adams GP, Pierson RA. Ovarian antral folliculogenesis during the human menstrual cycle: a review. Hum Reprod Update. 2012;18:73–91.
4. Sonmezer M, Turkcuoglu I, Coskun U, Oktay K. Random-start controlled ovarian hyperstimulation for emergency fertility preservation in letrozole cycles. Fertil Steril. 2011;95:2125e9–11.
5. Cakmak H, Rosen MP. Random-start ovarian stimulation in patients with cancer. Curr Opin Obstet Gynecol. 2015;27:215–21.
6. Kim JH, Kim SK, Lee HJ, Lee JR, Jee BC, Suh CS, Kim SH. Efficacy of random-start controlled ovarian stimulation in cancer patients. J Korean Med Sci. 2015;30:290–5.
7. Kuang Y, Chen Q, Hong Q, Lyu Q, Ai A, Fu Y, Shoham Z. Double stimulations during the follicular and luteal phases of poor responders in IVF/ICSI programmes (Shanghai protocol). Reprod Biomed Online. 2014;29:684–91.
8. Kuang Y, Hong Q, Chen Q, Lyu Q, Ai A, Fu Y, Shoham Z. Luteal-phase ovarian stimulation is feasible for producing competent oocytes in women undergoing in vitro fertilization/intracytoplasmic sperm injection treatment, with optimal pregnancy outcomes in frozen-thawed embryo transfer cycles. Fertil Steril. 2014;101:105–11.
9. Boots CE, Meister M, Cooper AR, Hardi A, Jungheim ES. Ovarian stimulation in the luteal phase: systematic review and meta-analysis. J Assist Reprod Genet. 2016;33:971–80.
10. Liu C, Jiang H, Zhang W, Yin H. Double ovarian stimulation during the follicular and luteal phase in women >/=38 years: a retrospective case-control study. Reprod Biomed Online. 2017;35:678–84.
11. Ubaldi FM, Capalbo A, Vaiarelli A, Cimadomo D, Colamaria S, Alviggi C, Trabucco E, Venturella R, Vajta G, Rienzi L. Follicular versus luteal phase ovarian stimulation during the same menstrual cycle (DuoStim) in a reduced ovarian reserve population results in a similar euploid blastocyst formation rate: new insight in ovarian reserve exploitation. Fertil Steril. 2016;105:1488–1495e1.
12. Chen H, Wang Y, Lyu Q, Ai A, Fu Y, Tian H, Cai R, Hong Q, Chen Q, Shoham Z, Kuang Y. Comparison of live-birth defects after luteal-phase ovarian stimulation vs. conventional ovarian stimulation for in vitro fertilization and vitrified embryo transfer cycles. Fertil Steril. 2015;103:1194–1201e2.

Endocrine Monitoring of Controlled Ovarian Stimulation for Medically Assisted Reproduction

19

Paula Celada, Elena Labarta, and Ernesto Bosch

19.1 Introduction

Since the first in vitro fertilization (IVF) birth in 1978, assisted reproductive techniques (ART) have evolved, and the use of natural cycles was very soon replaced by ovarian stimulation protocols to optimize the results of the technique. The main goal of controlled ovarian stimulation (COS) is to obtain a large number of mature oocytes that can be fertilized resulting in a cohort of embryos. This strategy has substantially increased pregnancy rates in patients because more oocytes are obtained per cycle and, presumably, a greater embryo selection for transfer becomes possible [1].

This technique involves the use of drugs to force the production of oocytes; as a consequence, there is an alteration of the ovarian cycle.

It is important to understand ovarian function and related hormonal changes in order to correctly manage treatments.

19.2 Hormonal Assessment Prior to a Cycle of Ovarian Stimulation

19.2.1 Biomarkers of Ovarian Response

Patients requiring IVF treatment are heterogeneous; therefore, it is important to make a good pretreatment assessment. Among the parameters to take into account for the prognosis of a cycle of IVF, those that have shown to have a greater impact on cycle outcome are age, body mass index (BMI), and the state of ovarian function.

Ovarian response to COS can now be predicted with a high degree of accuracy using two biomarkers that estimate the ovarian reserve: antral follicle count (AFC) and anti-Müllerian hormone (AMH) level in serum. Depending on the expected ovarian response to stimulation, the objectives of the treatment can be defined in advance, providing more reliable information to the patient about the prognosis and facilitating counselling about the process. On the other hand, clinicians can adopt therapeutic strategies specific to each patient, selecting a personalized protocol [2] (Table 19.1).

Serum AMH measurement has been observed to be highly predictive of ovarian response; furthermore, it has been positively related to the probability of newborn once adjusted for age [3].

It has been postulated that AMH can be determined at any point in the cycle, without affecting its values; however, AMH values can be artificially diminished due to the prior intake of anovulatory, either orally, transdermally, or vaginally. This decrease is directly related to the dose and the time of administration [4]. It has also been observed that AMH is significantly decreased in patients undergoing endometriosis surgery [5]. In contrast, patients with polycystic ovarian syndrome (PCOS) have higher AMH levels than control patients, or even than patients with polycystic ovaries appearance, but without a diagnosis of PCOS [6].

19.2.2 Other Hormonal Factors That May Influence the Ovarian Response

The response of a particular patient to COS is fundamentally conditioned by the ovarian reserve and age. However, there are other hormonal factors that can influence this response. It is important to evaluate these parameters before starting treatment.

19.2.2.1 Age

Ovarian aging involves endocrinological changes that influence the response to a COS cycle. Serum FSH levels increase at the beginning of the follicular phase, and this event may lead to accelerated folliculogenesis, which in the context of a COS cycle for IVF will result in an asynchronous follicular growth.

P. Celada · E. Labarta · E. Bosch (✉)
Instituto Valenciano de Infertilidad, València, Spain
e-mail: ernesto.bosch@ivi.es

G. N. Allahbadia et al. (eds.), *Textbook of Assisted Reproduction*, https://doi.org/10.1007/978-981-15-2377-9_19

Table 19.1 Correlation between serum AMH levels and the number of Metaphase II oocytes obtained with stimulation (internal data IVI Valencia)

AMH Gen II (pMol/L)	AMH-Roche (pMol/L)	Median (pp 25–75)	Mean ± SD	95% CI	Min-Max
<0.57	**0.1–0.8**	1.5 (0–2)	1.8 ± 1.5	1.4–2.2	0–7
0.57–1.0	**0.8–1.5**	2 (2–3)	3.1 ± 3.0	1.5–4.6	0–13
1.1–1.5	**1.5–2.0**	3 (2–5)	2.9 ± 2.2	1.8–3.9	0–7
1.6–2.0	**2.1–3.0**	4 (2.5–6)	4.1 ± 2.1	3.2–5.2	0–8
2.1–5.0	**3.1–5.0**	4 (2–7)	4.7 ± 2.7	3.8–5.6	0–11
5.1–7.5	**5.1–6.0**	6 (4–9)	6.8 ± 4.0	5.8–7.9	0–21
7.6–10.0	**6.0–8.0**	7 (5–9)	7.6 ± 4.1	6.0–9.1	1–17
10.1–15.0	**8.1–12.0**	8 (5–9)	7.7 ± 3.2	6.4–8.8	2–15
15.1–20.0	**12.0–15.0**	8 (5–10)	8.0 ± 3.8	6.4–9.7	2–18
20.1–30.0	**15.1–22.5**	13 (9–16)	12.4 ± 4.7	10.1–14.6	5–22
>30	**>22.5**	21 (17–23)	19.3 ± 5.9	15.3–23.2	7–29

However, this is not the only hormonal change in these patients. In late reproductive age, there is a decrease in basal androgen levels occurring despite the maintenance of sex hormone binding globulin levels (SHBG). In addition to this hypoandrogenic condition, follicular capability for inducing androstenedione synthesis after rFSH administration is significantly impaired in older patients compared with younger reproductive-aged patients, whereas estradiol (E2) secretion is preserved by increased aromatase function [7].

19.2.2.2 Basal Levels of Androgens

Both ovary and adrenal gland contribute to androgen production in women with normal reproductive function. Androgens play an important role in ovarian functioning as they stimulate pre-antral and antral follicle growth and are the precursors for estradiol synthesis following FSH receptor stimulation to promote granulosa cell proliferation. The synthesis of androgens in the follicle is induced by the luteinizing hormone (LH). Patients with low androgen levels would hypothetically benefit from LH administration during ovarian stimulation, which could explain the better results observed in patients older than 35 years who used this gonadotrophin in IVF treatments. Our group proposed a study to test this hypothesis whose results showed a great pregnancy rate in patients who received LH during stimulation when their testosterone levels were low, whereas no differences were observed in patients with normal or high testosterone levels. Thus basal levels of androgens could constitute an appropriate biomarker to determine the suitability for LH administration during ovarian stimulation.

19.2.2.3 Basal Levels of Gonadotropins

It is necessary to evaluate the basal levels of gonadotropins because ovarian reserve markers such as AMH or antral follicles count are normal in patients with hypogonadotropic hypogonadism. However, it has been demonstrated that these patients need the administration of LH during ovarian stimulation in order to obtain an adequate estrogen production and therefore a correct oocyte maturation and a good endometrial proliferation [8]. Stimulation with FSH alone in these cases can lead to follicular development but not to an adequate oocyte maturation, hence the importance of knowing the basal levels of gonadotrophins to choose a correct protocol.

Otherwise basal FSH levels increase on days 2–4 on the menstrual cycle with advancing age, so high levels have been associated with both poor ovarian stimulation and the failure to conceive.

However, a single elevated FSH value in women <40 years of age may not predict a poor response to stimulation or failure to achieve pregnancy due to the variability in FSH levels. Given the inter-assay variability of FSH, the cut-off point selected by an IVF program ideally should be based on its own data or on data from studies using the same FSH assay [9].

19.2.2.4 Hyperinsulinism

The production of E2 and progesterone (P) is significantly increased during FSH stimulation when elevated levels of insulin are present [10]. In a situation of hyperinsulinism, presumably there is a better response to COS and therefore an increased risk of (ovarian hyperstimulation syndrome) OHSS.

19.2.2.5 Hyperprolactinemia

Prolactin (PRL) influences the hypothalamus-pituitary-ovary axis as far as levels of PRL are related in a dose-dependent manner to the LH production. However, very low (<5 ng/mL) or very high (≥500 ng/mL) levels of PRL result in an increased LH production under GnRH stimulus [11]. It is important to know the basal levels of PRL before proceeding to COS cycle, since the response to stimulation may fluctuate.

19.2.2.6 Gonadotropin Receptor Polymorphisms

In recent years, several studies correlating the presence of gonadotropin receptor polymorphisms with the response to ovarian stimulation have been published. The normal phenotype of FSH receptor is aspargine/aspargine (Asn/Asn), and a heterozygous polymorphism Asn/Serine (Ser) and homozygous (Ser/Ser) are distinguished. It was observed that, although there were no differences in AMH levels in the three groups, patients with Asn/Asn phenotype required fewer FSH doses during the stimulation cycle and those with Ser/Ser phenotype required the most doses [12].

As for the LH receptor, a higher incidence of polymorphism (31.8%) was found in women who required high doses of FSH than in those requiring intermediate doses (6.8%). No case of polymorphism was observed in patients who responded well to low doses of FSH [13].

19.2.2.7 Thyroid Dysfunction

An association of thyroid function and ART success has been widely studied. Although hyperthyroidism and hypothyroidism have been associated with infertility, pregnancy loss, and other adverse obstetrical and fetal outcomes, the effects of subclinical hypothyroidism on reproduction are not very well known. Indeed, the findings regarding implantation success may be different from those that have adverse outcomes.

Some studies suggest that untreated subclinical hypothyroidism (TSH level > 4.5 mIU/L, with normal free thyroxine levels) negatively impacts the implantation rate after ART [14].

Regarding pregnancy losses the results remain controversial. Since previous studies reported higher risk of pregnancy loss in women with subclinical hypothyroidism, a prospective study of 1228 women with a history of pregnancy loss found no association between preconception subclinical hypothyroidism and miscarriage [15].

A threshold of 2.5 mIU/L TSH has been commonly used to start thyroid hormone treatment in many ART programs. This is to maintain the Endocrine Society's suggested TSH levels of <2.5 mIU/L during the first trimester. Few studies have evaluated whether thyroid hormone replacement for women with TSH levels between 2.5 mIU/L and the upper limit of normal affects implantation or miscarriage rates after IVF. One large prospective study reported that the rate of spontaneous pregnancy loss was significantly lower among pregnant women with TSH levels less than 2.5 mUI/L compared with those with TSH level between 2.5 and 5 mIU/ml [16]. Other studies have failed to reproduce similar findings; on the contrary they failed to show an association between TSH levels and IVF outcomes including pregnancy, live birth, or miscarriage rates [17, 18].

Available evidence does not suggest that thyroid autoimmunity curbs implantation, but different studies reported conflicting results regarding the association with miscarriage [14, 15].

19.2.3 Hormonal Evaluation Prior to COS

Based on the above, the following endocrine evaluation is recommended prior to a COS.

- Minimum: FSH + E2, AMH, PRL, TSH, free T4
- In certain cases: Testosterone, sex hormone binding globulin (SHBG), insulin/glycemia, FSH/LH receptor polymorphisms, 17-alpha-hydroxyprogesterone

19.3 Endocrine Monitoring in COS for IVF

Controlled ovarian stimulation is an important factor that determines the success of IVF cycles. The aim of the stimulation is to procure a good number of mature oocytes, resulting in an adequate number of embryos that can be transferred or frozen for the future use. Monitoring these cycles is essential to maximize success through collecting an ideal number of oocytes while maintaining a low rate of complication such as an ovarian hyperstimulation syndrome (OHSS) or detecting a poor response.

Ultrasound imaging of the ovarian response to gonadotropins and hormone analysis are the most commonly methods used in clinics to control the cycle. However, the role of intensive monitoring combining both techniques, ultrasound and hormonal serum levels, is controversial; there is no evidence that combined monitoring is more efficacious than monitoring by ultrasound alone with regard to the number of oocytes retrieved and clinical pregnancy rates [19].

Despite the above, in this chapter we describe how useful it is to measure serum hormone levels involved in folliculogenesis and endometrial receptivity.

Endocrine monitoring is essential to:

- Monitor follicular growth and evaluate the progression of the stimulation
- Adjust daily gonadotropin therapy for each patient
- Predict the optimal day for the induction of the ovulation
- Avoid the major complication of OHSS
- Improve implantation rates by avoiding fresh embryo transfer if necessary

19.3.1 Gonadotropin During Controlled Ovarian Stimulation

According to the two-cell model, both FSH and LH are required for promoting follicular growth and differentiation.

While it is clear that hormonal assay cannot reflect adequately the biologic activity of gonadotropins, over the last decades, its measurement performed to understand the contribution to folliculogenesis has allowed the assessment of the supplementation of FSH and LH required in ART cycles.

19.3.1.1 Follicular-Stimulating Hormone (FSH)

FSH plays a role in recruitment, selection, and dominance of follicles during the follicular phase. Two important concepts can explain this process: "FSH threshold" and "FSH window."

In 1978 Brown describes that it is necessary a certain amount of FSH secretion to induce the follicular growth, defined as the "FSH threshold" [20]. However, this threshold seems to vary for each follicle, even those of the same cohort. Follicles with an FSH threshold below plasma levels will not grow.

The concept of an open gate or "FSH window" was introduced by Braid after few years [21].

A follicle continues growth as long as the FSH level is above its growth threshold. The number of days that serum FSH levels are above the threshold determines the number of follicles that will be activated.

In a natural cycle, the gradual increase of FSH involves a negative feedback of ovarian hormones on the pituitary, causing a progressive decrease in FSH secretion; as a consequence, a follicle is selected, and the others undergo atresia, contributing to the dominance of the follicle.

Using the FSH threshold and the FSH window, it is easy to explain why FSH is the main therapeutic agent to control folliculogenesis. Increasing FSH in the early stage of the cycle is a key factor for the follicular recruitment process; thus, exogenous FSH is crucial in COS cycles to induce a multiple follicular development.

The FSH dose should be higher than the threshold of the least FSH-sensitive follicles, and these levels have to be maintained until the final stage of follicular development, resulting in multiple follicles at the time of trigger.

Despite the importance of the FSH level to recruit follicles, the determination of plasma FSH levels during COS doesn't provide any benefit in adjusting the dose of gonadotropin to improve the ovarian response due to its variability.

A plateau of serum FSH is obtained after 5 consecutive days of injections due to the long elimination half-life of the FSH molecule (30–35 hours). This FSH accumulation lasts for 5 days after cessation of exogenous administration. Furthermore, after an intramuscular or subcutaneous dose, plasma FSH levels can rise moderately during 4–8 hours, which cannot reflect the bioactivity of the molecule [22].

Moreover, there is a poor correlation between plasma FSH levels and the FSH threshold as plasma FSH levels are similar in patients with multiple follicular recruitment and patients who did not recruit follicles [23].

Resultantly, serum FSH measurement during stimulation is not justified since it does not provide any benefit in adjusting doses or prognosis results.

19.3.1.2 Luteinizing Hormone (LH)

Physiologically, the LH acts synergistically with FSH in both folliculogenesis and steroidogenesis. FSH induces the expression of LH receptors and enables its action.

On one hand, LH acts on the theca cells ensuring the production of androgens during the follicular phase. Androgens are aromatized to E2 by the granulosa cells. LH induces a dose-dependent production of E2, which is necessary to ensure endometrial preparation for embryo implantation. The term "LH threshold" refers to the minimum LH level required for pregnancy [24]. However, the determination of plasma LH levels is not helpful for an accurate assessment of the LH threshold as low endogenous serum LH levels during ovarian stimulation for IVF are not associated with a decreased probability of ongoing pregnancy [25].

On the other hand, LH participates in the control of granulosa cells' function. It has been observed that high doses of LH have a negative influence on follicular development because of the suppression of granulosa cells' proliferation, resulting in atresia of less mature follicles [26].

The use of gonadotrophins with LH activity in ovarian stimulation continues to be a topic of debate.

It is accepted that it does not generate any benefit in the general patient population. However, the most recent evidence shows significantly better results when used in patients older than 35 years [27] and poor responders [28]. The mechanism of action by which LH can improve the results in these subpopulations could be due to the restoration of the follicular microenvironment, which would result in a better oocyte and embryonic quality and a better endometrial receptivity, associated with lower levels of P at the end of the stimulation.

19.3.2 Steroid Hormones

Unlike gonadotrophins, steroid hormones are commonly evaluated during COS since they directly reflect the biological activity of the gonadotropins on the ovary. Serum E2 levels are useful to evaluate follicular maturity before triggering ovulation. Measuring P levels helps to evaluate early increases, before triggering. Steroids are also involved in the implantation process, which is crucial in determining the outcome of assisted reproductive technology treatments.

19.3.2.1 Estradiol (E2)

Serum E2 levels are correlated to the stage of follicular development. The amount of estrogen produced by the dominant follicle increases as it grows, and there is a linear correlation between follicular diameter and E2 levels [29].

The total serum E2 at a given moment in the cycle reflects the state of maturity of all follicles present at that time.

Therefore, monitoring E2 during ovarian stimulation is useful to predict the response, but, even if ovarian response can be identified early in the cycle, the optimum levels of E2 are not defined because of the diversity of protocols.

- In the GnRH agonist long protocol, downregulation is indicated by serum E2 levels below 50 pg/ml. An increase of E2 levels after 6 days of gonadotrophins is defined as optimal response since these levels increase by 50% per day. Low serum E2 values after the first few days of stimulation have been associated with poor outcome and higher cancelation rates. Thus, a better outcome of in vitro fertilization may be expected when serum E2 starts early in the cycle and adopts a moderate growth rate [30]. A plateau in plasma E2 for more than 3 days suggests a poor response.
- In GnRH antagonist protocols, plasma E2 levels are higher before the addition of the GnRH antagonist to control the LH surge. After that, E2 levels may decrease or remain the same, but these variations do not compromise the cycle outcome. The E2 value does not help to adjust the dose of gonadotropins after administration of the antagonist.

In good outcome cycles, E2 continued to rise until hCG was administered, but in nonpregnant cycles, E2 plateaued on the day before hCG administration, which suggests that luteinization or atresia of the more advanced follicles had commenced spontaneously.

The levels of E2 reached at the time of hCG administration are more relevant than the slope's increase. A value of 100–200 pg/ml per dominant follicle suggests adequate response [31].

Furthermore, a high serum E2 concentration on the day of hCG trigger has been suggested as a predictor of OHSS. The E2 level threshold above which there is a considerable risk of OHSS varies widely among different studies. Most of the studies selected an E2 of 3000 pg/ml as threshold; however, applying this E2 threshold would have only predicted 1/3 of the total OHSS cases [32, 33].

Some studies suggest that the number of follicles on the day of hCG administration is a better predictor of severe OHSS than E2 levels. Papanikolaou et al. [33] revealed that the predictive value of the threshold of ≥13 follicles ≥11 mm on the day of hCG (85.5% sensitivity; 69% specificity) was statistically significantly superior to the optimal threshold of 2560 ng/L for E2 concentrations (53% sensitivity, 77% specificity) in identifying patients at risk for OHSS. Recently, a retrospective analysis of combined data from three trials found that the optimal threshold of follicles ≥11 mm on the day of hCG to identify patients at risk of moderate and severe OHSS was 19, while E2 levels were less prognostic of OHSS than the number of follicles ≥11 mm [34].

Number of follicles is probably a better predictor of OHSS than E2 levels because OHSS develops due to vascular endothelial growth factor production of the follicles rather than their E2 production [33].

Serum Estradiol and Endometrial Receptivity

It is well known from basic studies that the success of embryonic implantation relies on a perfect dialogue between good-quality embryos and a receptive endometrium.

The aim of COS is to recruit more follicles. As a consequence, the ovary produces supraphysiologic levels of steroid hormones, inducing relevant changes in endometrial receptivity. These changes are detrimental, since uterine receptivity deteriorates during COS compared with hormone replacement therapy and natural cycles [35].

Some studies have demonstrated that there was a poor IVF outcome in high-responder patients compared with normal-responder patients treated with gonadotrophins and GnRH analogues.

Simon et al. [36] showed that E2 concentrations above 3000 pg/ml the day of HCG administration have a deleterious effect on implantation, not only in high-responder patients but also in normal-responder patients (Fig. 19.1). It has been proposed that high E2 levels impair endometrial receptivity instead of oocyte quality because fertilization rate and embryo cleavage (until day 2) in patients with a high response were normal. Indeed, the quality of embryos and the implantation rate in recipients of embryos derived from oocytes of high responders are similar to those in normal responders.

However, other authors have failed to find an association between high E2 levels on the day of hCG administration and a harmful effect on pregnancy outcomes [37, 38]. Due to the controversy in this regard, a well-designed prospective

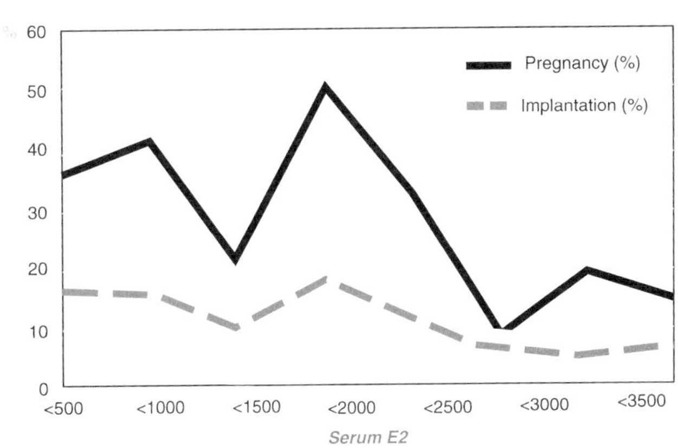

Fig. 19.1 Serum E2 and IVF outcome

study is needed to establish the degree of endometrial advancement related to the serum E2 levels.

19.3.2.2 Progesterone (P)

Despite an effective suppression of endogenous gonadotrophins by GnRH analogues, a small increment in serum progesterone levels has been reported in 5–30% of COS cycles before HCG administration [39–42].

The origin of this premature elevation of serum P cannot be explained by luteinization of granulosa cells, since endogenous LH levels are low due to suppression by GnRH analogues. Besides LH and P levels do not seem to be related since the observed increases in P at the end of the follicular phase were not accompanied by increase in LH [39]. Some studies have shown a positive correlation between P levels and the administered FSH dose [43] as well with a longer stimulation period [39]. In a retrospective study performed in a total of 4032 COS cycles in our center, a multivariate analysis highlighted that higher daily FSH dose was the factor most closely related to serum P elevation [44].

Otherwise, P increase is correlated with a high ovarian response, as it was demonstrated recently that patients with high E2 concentrations and a great number of follicles on the day of hCG have significantly higher P concentrations [45, 46].

Whether serum P elevation on the day of hCG administration is associated with ongoing pregnancy rate is debatable. However, it has been widely demonstrated to have a negative impact on embryo implantation and therefore on cycle outcome [37, 42, 45].

Although P increase has been subject of multiple studies in recent years, the cutoff point beyond which high these increases could affect clinical data remains controversial. Our group has reported that serum P level ≥ 1.5 ng/ml on the last day of COS leads to a significant decrease in the ongoing pregnancy rate, irrespective of the GnRH analogue used for pituitary downregulation [44]. Nevertheless, it seems that in high responders the detrimental threshold could be higher [46–48]. In these patients the negative impact of premature P elevation has less of an impact on pregnancy rate than other patients. Probably the negative effect of elevated P is outweighed by other factors with a positive effect in high responders. They may have better and faster developing embryos, which can keep up with endometrial advancement due to premature P elevation [49].

Serum Progesterone and Endometrial Receptivity

Progesterone plays an important role during luteal phase, particularly in creating decidualization changes needed for implantation and progression of pregnancy.

The mechanism underlying the deleterious effect of an elevated P level is related to the endometrial receptivity rather than oocyte quality [50]. It has been proposed that in COS cycles, there is an abnormal accelerated endometrial maturation due to the exposure to supraphysiological concentrations of P in the late follicular phase of IVF cycles [51]. This endometrial advancement anticipates the window of implantation, in which the endometrial epithelium acquires a functional ability to support blastocyst adhesion [52, 53].

In order to investigate whether the worse IVF outcomes in the presence of P elevation on the day of hCG administration are due to impaired endometrial receptivity, Labarta et al. [54] analyzed the endometrial gene expression profiles of young healthy oocyte donors with different serum P levels. They reported that women with late follicular phase P levels ≥1.5 ng/ml had substantially different gene expression profiles than women with normal P levels.

Based on these results, it is recommended to monitor P levels, especially during late follicular phase of a COS cycle. It is advisable to vitrify all the embryos for a deferred transfer when P is elevated, because P elevation does not seem to affect frozen-thawed transfer of embryos obtained in the index cycle [47, 55].

19.4 Conclusions

Adequate monitoring of COS is essential. Endocrine characteristics of ART cycles depend largely on the drugs used to achieve COS. It is clear that FSH therapy is mandatory in every stimulation cycle, but assessment of serum FSH values is not sufficiently predictive of the adequacy of FSH supply to be routinely determined. Furthermore, there is no evidence that serum LH measurements could help detect patients who might need the addition of some LH during ART cycles.

Nevertheless, steroid measurement could be helpful to control stimulation. As we have described in this chapter, too high E2 and an early P increase have an impact on cycle outcome.

On the one hand, although the growing follicles can be visualized by ultrasound, E2 production by granulosa cells also reflects the maturation of oocytes. Combined monitoring has been almost universally practiced. Some studies postulated that E2 monitoring is not essential since mature oocyte yield was not improved over monitoring follicle size alone [56]. However, Orvieto [31] suggest that serum E2 level per oocyte is predictive of pregnancy rate per cycle. Moreover, even if combined monitoring with E2 levels does not improve cycle outcome, it would still be valuable until it is proven that OHSS can be avoided without hormonal monitoring [19].

Regarding serum P levels, its measurement helps us to determine an early increase, before triggering, which has a negative impact on endometrial receptivity. If this event occurs, it is recommended to vitrify all the embryos and defer the transfer to a subsequent cycle where endometrial receptivity will not be compromised by elevated P as in the stimulated cycle.

References

1. Templeton A, Morris JK. Reducing the risk of multiple births by transfer of two embryos after in vitro fertilization. N Engl J Med. 1998 Aug 27;339(9):573–7.
2. La Marca A, Sunkara SK. Individualization of controlled ovarian stimulation in IVF using ovarian reserve markers: from theory to practice. Hum Reprod Update. 2014 Jan–Feb;20(1):124–40.
3. Holte J. Antimüllerian hormone levels are strongly associated with live-birth rates after assisted reproduction. J Clin Endocrinol Metab. 2013;98:1107–14.
4. Kallio S, Puurunen J, Ruokonen A, Vaskivuo T, Piltonen T, Tapanainen JS. Antimüllerian hormone levels decrease in women using combined contraception independently of administration route. Fertil Steril. 2013;99:1305–10.
5. Streuli I, de Ziegler D, Gayet V, Santulli P, Bijaoui G, de Mouzon J, et al. In women with endometriosis anti-Müllerian hormone levels are decreased only in those with previous endometrioma surgery. Hum Reprod. 2012;27:3294–303.
6. Homburg R, Ray A, Bhide P, Gudi A, Shah A, Timms P, et al. The relationship of serum anti-Mullerian hormone with polycystic ovarian morphology and polycystic ovary syndrome: a prospective cohort study. Hum Reprod. 2013;28:1077–83.
7. Davison SL, Bell R, Donath S, Montalto JG, Davis SR. Androgen levels in adult females: changes with age, menopause, and oophorectomy. J Clin Endocrinol Metab. 2005;90:3847–53.
8. The European Recombinant Human LH Study Group. Recombinant human luteinizing hormone (LH) to support recombinant human follicle-stimulating hormone (FSH)-induced follicular development in LH- and FSH-deficient anovulatory women: a dose-finding study. J Clin Endocrinol Metab. 1998;83:1507–14.
9. Practice Committee of the American Society for Reproductive Medicine. Testing and interpreting measures of ovarian reserve: a committee opinion. Fertil Steril. 2015 Mar;103(3):e9–e17.
10. Willis D, Mason H, Gilling-Smith C, Franks S. Modulation by insulin of follicle-stimulating hormone and luteinizing hormone actions in human granulosa cells of normal and polycystic ovaries. J Clin Endocrinol Metab. 1996;81:302–9.
11. Hodson DJ, Townsend J, Tortonese DJ. Characterization of the effects of prolactin in gonadotroph target cells. Biol Reprod. 2010;86:1046–55.
12. Alviggi C, Humaidan P, Ezcurra D. Hormonal, functional and genetic biomarkers in controlled ovarian stimulation: tools for matching patients and protocols. Reprod Biol Endocrinol. 2012;10:9.
13. Alviggi C, Clarizia R, Pettersson K, Mollo A, Humaidan P, Strina I, et al. Suboptimal response to GnRHa long protocol is associated with a common LH polymorphism. Reprod Biomed Online. 2009;18:9–14.
14. Fox C, Morin S, Jeong JW, Scott RT Jr, Lessey BA. Local and systemic factors and implantation: what is the evidence? Fertil Steril. 2016 Apr;105(4):873–84.
15. Plowden TC, Schisterman EF, Sjaarda LA, Zarek SM, Perkins NJ, Silver R, et al. Subclinical hypothyroidism and thyroid autoimmunity are not associated with fecundity, pregnancy loss, or live birth. J Clin Endocrinol Metab. 2016 Jun;101(6):2358–65.
16. Negro R, Schwartz A, Gismondi R, Tinelli A, Mangieri T, Stagnaro-Green A. Increased pregnancy loss rate in thyroid antibody negative women with TSH levels between 2.5 and 5.0 in the first trimester of pregnancy. J Clin Endocrinol Metab. 2010;95:E44–8.
17. Green KA, Werner MD, Franasiak JM, Juneau CR, Hong KH, Scott RT Jr. Investigating the optimal preconception TSH range for patients undergoing IVF when controlling for embryo quality. J Assist Reprod Genet. 2015 Oct;32(10):1469–76.
18. Jin L, Wang M, Yue J, Zhu GJ, Zhang B. Association between TSH level and pregnancy outcomes in euthyroid women undergoing IVF/ICSI: a retrospective study and meta-analysis. Curr Med Sci. 2019 Aug;39(4):631–7.
19. Kwan I, Bhattacharya S, Kang A, Woolner A. Monitoring of stimulated cycles in assisted reproduction (IVF and ICSI). Cochrane Database Syst Rev. 2014 Aug 24;8:CD005289.
20. Brown JB. Pituitary control of ovarian function--concepts derived from gonadotrophin therapy. Aust N Z J Obstet Gynaecol. 1978 Feb;18(1):46–54.
21. Baird DT. A model of follicular selection and ovulation: lessons from superovulation. Steroid Biochem. 1987;27(1–3):15–23.
22. Hugues JN, Cédrine-Durnerin I. Endocrine characteristics of ART cycle. In: Gardner DK, Weissman A, Colin M, Howles CM, Shoham Z, editors. Textbook of assisted reproductive technologies: Laboratory and clinical perspectives. 3rd ed. London: Informa Healthcare; 2009. p. 511–28.
23. Schoemaker J, van Weissenbruch MM, Scheele F, van der Meer M. The FSH threshold concept in clinical ovulation induction. Baillieres Clin Obstet Gynaecol. 1993 Jun;7(2):297–308.
24. The European Recombinant Human LH Study Group. Recombinant human luteinizing hormone (LH) to support recombinant human follicle-stimulating hormone (FSH)-induced follicular development in LH- and FSH-deficient anovulatory women: a dose-finding study. J Clin Endocrinol Metab. 1998 May;83(5):1507–14.
25. Kolibianakis EM, Collins J, Tarlatzis B, Papanikolaou E, Devroey P. Are endogenous LH levels during ovarian stimulation for IVF using GnRH analogues associated with the probability of ongoing pregnancy? A systematic review. Hum Reprod Update. 2006 Jan–Feb;12(1):3–12.
26. Loumaye E, Engrand P, Shoham Z, Hillier SG, Baird DT. Clinical evidence for an LH 'ceiling' effect induced by administration of recombinant human LH during the late follicular phase of stimulated cycles in World Health Organization type I and type II anovulation. Hum Reprod. 2003 Feb;18(2):314–22.
27. Hill MJ, Levens ED, Levy G, Ryan ME, Csokmay JM, DeCherney AH, et al. The use of recombinant luteinizing hormone in patients undergoing assisted reproductive techniques with advanced reproductive age: a systematic review and meta-analysis. Fertil Steril. 2012;97:1108–14.
28. Lehert P, Kolibianakis EM, Venetis CA, Schertz J, Saunders H, Arriagada P, et al. Recombinant human follicle-stimulating hormone (r-hFSH) plus recombinant luteinizing hormone versus r-hFSH alone for ovarian stimulation during assisted reproductive technology: systematic review and meta-analysis. Reprod Biol Endocrinol. 2014;20:12–7.
29. Loumaye E, Engrand P, Howles CM, O'Dea L. Assessment of the role of serum luteinizing hormone and estradiol response to follicle-stimulating hormone on in vitro fertilization treatment outcome. Fertil Steril. 1997 May;67(5):889–99.
30. Dirnfeld M, Lejeune B, Camus M, Vekemans M, Leroy F. Growth rate of follicular estrogen secretion in relation to the outcome of in vitro fertilization and embryo replacement. Fertil Steril. 1985 Mar;43(3):379–84.
31. Orvieto R, Zohav E, Scharf S, Rabinson J, Meltcer S, Anteby EY, et al. The influence of estradiol/follicle and estradiol/oocyte ratios on the outcome of controlled ovarian stimulation for in vitro fertilization. Gynecol Endocrinol. 2007 Feb;23(2):72–5.

32. Aboulghar M. Prediction of ovarian hyperstimulation syndrome (OHSS). Estradiol level has an important role in the prediction of OHSS. Hum Reprod. 2003 Jun;18(6):1140–1.
33. Papanikolaou EG, Pozzobon C, Kolibianakis EM, Camus M, Tournaye H, Fatemi HM, et al. Incidence and prediction of ovarian hyperstimulation syndrome in women undergoing gonadotropin-releasing hormone antagonist in vitro fertilization cycles. Fertil Steril. 2006;85:112–20.
34. Griesinger G, Verweij PJ, Gates D, Devroey P, Gordon K, Stegmann BJ, et al. Prediction of ovarian hyperstimulation syndrome in patients treated with corifollitropin alfa or rFSH in a GnRH antagonist protocol. PLoS One. 2016 Mar 7;11(3):e0149615.
35. Paulson RJ, Sauer MV, Lobo RA. Embryo implantation after human in vitro fertilization: importance of endometrial receptivity. Fertil Steril. 1990 May;53(5):870–4.
36. Simón C, Cano F, Valbuena D, Remohí J, Pellicer A. Clinical evidence for a detrimental effect on uterine receptivity of high serum oestradiol concentrations in high and normal responder patients. Hum Reprod. 1995 Sep;10(9):2432–7.
37. Kosmas IP, Kolibianakis EM, Devroey P. Association of estradiol levels on the day of hCG administration and pregnancy achievement in IVF: a systematic review. Hum Reprod. 2004;19:2446–53.
38. Kyrou D, Popovic-Todorovic B, Fatemi HM, Bourgain C, Haentjens P, Van Landuyt L, et al. Does the estradiol level on the day of human chorionic gonadotrophin administration have an impact on pregnancy rates in patients treated with rec-FSH/GnRH antagonist? Hum Reprod. 2009 Nov;24(11):2902–9.
39. Bosch E, Valencia I, Escudero E, Crespo J, Simón C, Remohí J, et al. Premature luteinization during gonadotropin-releasing hormone antagonist cycles and its relationship with in vitro fertilization outcome. Fertil Steril. 2003 Dec;80(6):1444–9.
40. Silverberg KM, Burns WN, Olive DL, Riehl RM, Schenken RS. Serum progesterone levels predict success of in vitro fertilization/embryo transfer in patients stimulated with leuprolide acetate and human menopausal gonadotropins. J Clin Endocrinol Metab. 1991;73:797–803.
41. Edelstein MC, Seltman HJ, Cox BJ, Robinson SM, Shaw RA, Muasher SJ. Progesterone levels on the day of human chorionic gonadotropin administration in cycles with gonadotropin-releasing hormone agonist suppression are not predictive of pregnancy outcome. Fertil Steril. 1990;54:853–7.
42. Ubaldi F, Albano C, Peukert M, Riethmuller-Winzen H, Camus M, Smitz J, et al. Subtle progesterone rise after the administration of the gonadotrophin-releasing hormone antagonist cetrorelix in intracytoplasmic sperm injection cycles. Hum Reprod. 1996;11:1405–7.
43. Filicori M, Cognigni GE, Pocognoli P, Tabarelli C, Spettoli D, Taraborrelli S, et al. Modulation of folliculogenesis and steroidogenesis in women by graded menotrophin administration. Hum Reprod. 2002;17:2009–15.
44. Bosch E, Labarta E, Crespo J, Simón C, Remohí J, Jenkins J, et al. Circulating progesterone levels and ongoing pregnancy rates in controlled ovarian stimulation cycles for in vitro fertilization analysis of over 4000 cycles. Hum Reprod. 2010;25:2092–100.
45. Kyrou D, Al-Azemi M, Papanikolaou EG, Donoso P, Tziomalos K, Devroey P, et al. The relationship of premature progesterone rise with serum estradiol levels and number of follicles in GnRH antagonist/recombinant FSH-stimulated cycles. Eur J Obstet Gynecol Reprod Biol. 2012;162:165–8.
46. Griesinger G, Mannaerts B, Andersen CY, Witjes H, Kolibianakis EM, Gordon K. Progesterone elevation does not compromise pregnancy rates in high responders: a pooled analysis of in vitro fertilization patients treated with recombinant follicle-stimulating hormone/gonadotropin-releasing hormone antagonist in six trials. Fertil Steril. 2013;100:1622.
47. Xu B, Li Z, Zhang H, Jin L, Li Y, Ai J, et al. Serum progesterone level effects on the outcome of in vitro fertilization in patients with different ovarian response: an analysis of more than 10,000 cycles. Fertil Steril. 2012;97:1321.
48. Requena A, Cruz M, Bosch E, Meseguer M, García-Velasco JA. High progesterone levels in women with high ovarian response do not affect clinical outcomes: a retrospective cohort study. Reprod Biol Endocrinol. 2014;12:69.
49. Fatemi HM, Doody K, Griesinger G, Witjes H, Mannaerts B. High ovarian response does not jeopardize ongoing pregnancy rates and increases cumulative pregnancy rates in a GnRH-antagonist protocol. Hum Reprod. 2013 Feb;28(2):442–52.
50. Melo M, Meseguer M, Garrido N, Bosch E, Pellicer A, Remohí J. The significance of premature luteinization in an oocyte-donation programme. Hum Reprod. 2006 Jun;21(6):1503–7.
51. Papanikolaou EG, Bourgain C, Kolibianakis E, Tournaye H, Devroey P. Steroid receptor expression in late follicular phase endometrium in GnRH antagonist IVF cycles is already altered, indicating initiation of early luteal phase transformation in the absence of secretory changes. Hum Reprod. 2005;20:1541–7.
52. Horcajadas JA, Sharkey AM, Catalano RD, Sherwin JRA, Domínguez F, Burgos LA, et al. Effect of an intrauterine device on the gene expression profile of the endometrium. J Clin Endocrinol Metab. 2006;91:3199–207.
53. Bourgain C, Devroey P. The endometrium in stimulated cycles for IVF. Hum Reprod Update. 2003;9:515–22.
54. Labarta E, Martínez-Conejero JA, Alamá P, Horcajadas JA, Pellicer A, Simón C, et al. Endometrial receptivity is affected in women with high circulating progesterone levels at the end of the follicular phase: a functional genomics analysis. Hum Reprod. 2011 Jul;26(7):1813–25.
55. Venetis CA, Kolibianakis EM, Bosdou JK, Tarlatzis BC. Progesterone elevation and probability of pregnancy after IVF: a systematic review and meta-analysis of over 60 000 cycles. Hum Reprod Update. 2013 Sep-Oct;19(5):433–57.
56. Vandekerckhove F, Gerris J, Vansteelandt S, De Sutter P. Adding serum estradiol measurements to ultrasound monitoring does not change the yield of mature oocytes in IVF/ICSI. Gynecol Endocrinol. 2014 Sep;30(9):649–52.

20 Ovulation Triggers

Esra Bulgan Kılıçdağ and Erhan Şimşek

Ovulation is the release of a viable oocyte from a selected mature follicle in the menstrual cycle. Monthly ovulation and menses, unless pregnancy occurs, is the rule for proper and regular cycle of a woman. Normally one egg is released each month in humans; but occasionally, two and very rarely more can be ovulated in one menstrual cycle. Timing and process of ovulation are regulated by extensive interactions of various hormones and peptides functional in the reproductive system. Therefore, a thorough knowledge of menstrual cycle physiology is essential for understanding ovulation triggers. Ovulation triggers are advocated as a surrogate for the endogenous LH surge to achieve better control of the timing of ovulation in stimulated assisted reproductive technology (ART) cycles. Multifollicular development and resultant excess amount of steroid hormone production and the agents for prevention of premature luteinization suppress the endogenous LH surge. Suppression of endogenous gonadotropins both by GnRH analogues and supraphysiologic steroid hormone levels results in defective luteal phase and demise of corpora lutea and decreased chances of pregnancy and/or increased rates of miscarriages. Controlled ovarian stimulation (COS) protocols inevitably require luteal phase support to maintain live birth rates.

Increasing estrogen production from the growing follicle is thought to elicit the LH surge. This surge triggers the resumption of meiosis and eventually results in expulsion of the oocyte from the ovarian follicle. After the selection of dominant follicle, estrogen levels produced by this follicle rises to 150–200 pg/ml as its diameter reaches 20 mm or more. The critical event which initiates LH surge is the elevated estrogen levels for a critical period of time which starts a surge on the hypophyseal LH by positive central feedback [1].

E. B. Kılıçdağ (✉)
Department of Obstetrics and Gynecology,
Division of Reproductive Endocrinology and IVF Unit,
Baskent University Faculty of Medicine, Adana, Turkey

E. Şimşek
Baskent University Faculty of Medicine, Adana, Turkey

Human chorionic gonadotropin (hCG) is traditionally used as the LH surrogate to induce final oocyte maturation. Final oocyte maturation is a crucial step in in vitro fertilization, usually achieved with a single bolus of 5000–10000 IU hCG given approximately 36 hours before oocyte retrieval. This approach carries a potential risk of ovarian hyperstimulation syndrome (OHSS) in susceptible women. Furthermore, the severity of OHSS is proportional to the amount of follicles and corpora lutea obtained after ovarian stimulation. OHSS might be even life-threatening for otherwise healthy young women on in vitro fertilization (IVF) treatment. Therefore, identification of risk factors, use of milder ovarian stimulation protocols, withholding hCG, and withholding follicle stimulating hormone (FSH) doses (coasting) were the mainstay of therapy for years to prevent OHSS. After popularization of GnRH antagonist stimulation protocols, OHSS prevention became easier by substituting the long-acting hCG trigger by a single injection of a GnRH agonist. Research introduces promising new agents like kisspeptin for more physiologic ovulation trigger mimics and even lower OHSS incidence. This chapter will describe various methods used to trigger final oocyte maturation and advancement and alternatives of ovulation trigger agents and their use in clinical practice.

20.1 hCG Trigger

hCG is a glycoprotein hormone produced primarily by the trophoblast, and it sustains the production of progesterone from the corpus luteum which is indispensable for implantation. Structurally, the hCG molecule has two subunits (alpha and beta), and the alpha subunit is similar to the alpha subunits of LH, FSH, and TSH. hCG bolus injection was used for final oocyte maturation for many years as the standard of care. During IVF treatment, 5000–10000 IU hCG has been routinely used to trigger final oocyte maturation and resumption of meiosis prior to oocyte retrieval as the standard. hCG

G. N. Allahbadia et al. (eds.), *Textbook of Assisted Reproduction*, https://doi.org/10.1007/978-981-15-2377-9_20

has the same effect of luteinizing hormone (LH) but with a longer half-life around 4–5 days. The long half-life of hCG increases the risk of OHSS in susceptible patients due to its sustained luteotropic effect. hCG triggering of ovulation in combination with the luteal supra-physiological estradiol (E) and progesterone (P) levels in COS cycles suppresses endogenous LH secretion by the pituitary. LH deficiency in early luteal phase results in disruption of luteal phase, and unless supported by exogenous luteotropic agents, pregnancy rates are poor. Significantly longer half-life of hCG causes very low luteal LH levels due to inhibitory effects on the pituitary. Therefore corpus luteum function relies entirely on LH-like activity of exogenously administered hCG at the time of ovulation [2]. Around the time of implantation, exogenous progesterone support is obligatory until embryo produces enough hCG for adequate secretion of progesterone by corpus luteum. Therefore, defective luteal phase of hCG-triggered COS cycles is supported by hCG at the early stage and by progesterone thereafter, both of which are indispensable for luteal phase support in hCG-triggered COS protocol.

The combination of ovarian stimulation by gonadotropins after GnRH agonist-induced pituitary downregulation and hCG as final oocyte maturation trigger carries a risk of OHSS especially in susceptible patients. The prolonged half-life of hCG provides excellent pregnancy rates but supports survival of multiple corpora lutea, resulting in an increased risk of OHSS. Early OHSS is almost exclusively due to prolonged LH activity as seen after hCG trigger. Thirty-eight hours-long half-life of hCG results in prolonged stimulation of LH receptors, i.e., over a week [3, 4]. Long half-life of hCG leads two types of derangement in the stimulation cycle. First, risk of OHSS due to multiple corpora lutea formation and secondly, luteal insufficiency around the time of implantation after the end of hCG stimulation.

hCG can cause moderate-severe OHSS in 15.3% of patients undergoing IVF treatment [5]. In high-risk patients, such as women with polycystic ovarian syndrome (PCOS), the risk of severe OHSS is increased fivefold [6]. Moreover, the risks of late pregnancy complications including prematurity and low birth weight are increased in women affected by OHSS in early pregnancy [7]. Several measures can be taken to prevent OHSS. Withholding hCG injection, lowering the dose of hCG, coasting, total freeze of all embryos, and preventative measures during oocyte pickup such as macromolecule infusion in high-risk patients are some of these measures [3], but none of those approaches are as effective as GnRH agonist use for ovulation trigger. The introduction of the GnRH agonist trigger after widespread use of GnRH antagonists in ovulation induction curbed OHSS incidence.

20.2 GnRH Agonist Trigger

GnRH agonist triggering was introduced in the early 1990s [8, 9] but its use was hampered by the long GnRH agonist protocol being commonly used for pituitary downregulation in ART cycles. After the introduction of GnRH antagonist for the prevention of early LH surge, GnRH agonist triggering enjoyed a renewed interest.

In general, affinity of GnRH analogues for the GnRH receptor is 2–50 times of that of endogenous GnRH [10, 11]. A bolus of GnRH agonist displaced GnRH antagonists from the GnRH receptors and caused the release of both LH and FSH from the gonadotropic cells of the anterior pituitary.

The simultaneous FSH surge may have some physiologic functions, yet the exact role of the mid-cycle FSH is not known. FSH, among other actions, promotes nuclear maturation, i.e., resumption of meiosis [12]. This might have contributed to the collection of more mature oocytes after a GnRHa trigger compared with hCG trigger as reported in some studies [13, 14]. However, this is not confirmed across all studies. While the natural mid-cycle LH surge has three phases, i.e., ascent, plateau, and decline, lasting for a total of 48 hours, a GnRH agonist-induced surge consists of only two phases without a plateau and lasts for 24–36 hours [8] (Fig. 20.1). This relatively short-lived LH and FSH surge is inadequate to support corpus luteum functions properly. Moreover, some in vitro studies suggest that GnRH agonist can have direct apoptotic effects on granulosa cells [15, 16]. GnRH agonist trigger causes corpus luteum dysfunction and premature corpus luteum demise. Therefore initial studies reported unacceptably high rates of miscarriage [2]. The observation of increased risk of miscarriage due to inadequate luteal function led to freezing all embryos after a GnRHa trigger,

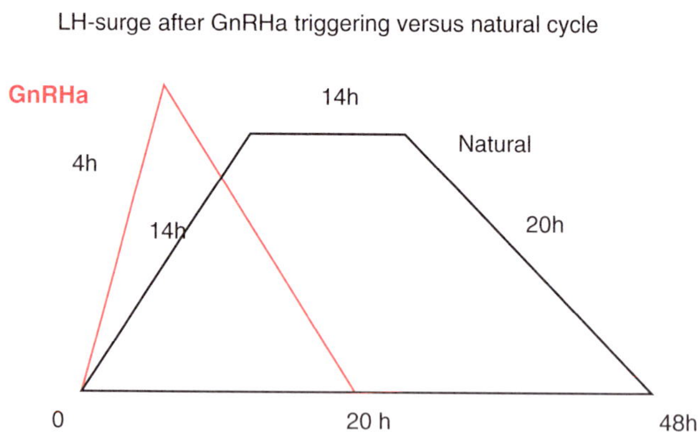

Fig. 20.1 Differences in LH surge after GnRH agonist triggering when compared with a natural cycle. (From Humaidan P, Kol S. GnRH agonist for triggering of final oocyte maturation: time for a change of practice? Human Reproduction Update, Volume 17, Issue 4, July–August 2011, 510–524, with permission)

followed by frozen-thawed embryo transfer in subsequent cycles, dubbed as cycle segmentation. Thus, GnRHa trigger when used for women at risk of developing OHSS is commonly followed by a "freeze all" policy.

Few cases of OHSS are still reported following a GnRH agonist trigger and are most probably related to unexpected mutations or polymorphisms of the GnRH, FSH, or LH receptors [10].

GnRH agonist trigger was suggested to have some advantages other than OHSS risk reduction. In some but not all studies, GnRH analogue trigger was shown to increase the number of metaphase-two (MII) oocytes and two pronuclear (2PN) embryos available for cryopreservation in cancer patients undergoing ovarian stimulation for fertility preservation. Pereira et al. have retrospectively showed that approximately three more MII oocytes and 2PN embryos were available for cryopreservation in the GnRH agonist trigger group [13]. It is also suggested that GnRH agonist administration after the use of GnRH antagonist in an ART cycle brings about true benefits for implantation, since the antagonists block endometrial GnRH receptors, supposedly worsening endometrial function. Once a GnRH agonist, which has much higher affinity for the receptors than GnRH antagonists, is administered, the latter is displaced from endometrial receptors, possibly improving endometrial receptivity [17, 18]. Another advantage of GnRH agonists is tolerability. Compared with the hCG trigger, GnRHa trigger is associated with less fluid accumulation in the cul-de-sac, reduced ovarian volume and discomfort, and, thus, a higher patient convenience [1, 19, 20].

Empty follicle syndrome, i.e., failure to collect mature oocytes, has been reported following GnRH agonist trigger. However, empty follicle syndrome rates were similar with GnRH agonist and hCG triggers (3.5% vs 3.1%, respectively) [21].

Dissociation of the trigger and luteal phase support, allowing individualization of luteal support according to ovarian response, can be regarded as another advantage of the GnRH agonist trigger. GnRH agonist trigger allows "exogenous progesterone-free luteal phase protocol," which relies solely on endogenous progesterone driven by repeated GnRH agonist injections providing LH-like or luteinizing activity for corpora lutea [22]. This would provide relief for women by eliminating vaginal discharge and the need for painful progesterone injections [14]. However, more studies are needed to confirm its effectiveness.

GnRH agonist trigger is the best available ovulation trigger for egg donors and for women undergoing fertility preservation since they do not have a fresh embryo transfer and the concerns regarding luteal phase after GnRHa trigger become irrelevant.

20.3 Combined Approaches: Dual Trigger

Combination of hCG with a GnRH agonist for final oocyte maturation is dubbed as "dual trigger" and was introduced by Shapiro et al. as a solution to prevent OHSS while maintaining pregnancy/live birth rates in high responders [23, 24].

Theoretically, dual trigger combines the advantages of both GnRHa and hCG trigger. First of all, a lower dose of hCG is used to decrease the risk of OHSS while maintaining some support for corpora lutea. Meanwhile the GnRH agonist causes endogenous LH and FSH surges, providing additional but short-lived stimulus for oocyte maturation. However, these potential advantages are questionable especially as far as OHSS risk is concerned [18].

20.3.1 Double Trigger

A modification of the "dual trigger" (hCG+ GnRH agonist) is the so-called Double trigger (hCG + GnRH agonist at different times). The dual trigger is first described in a woman who was given a GnRH agonist injection 40 hours before oocyte pickup and hCG 6 hours after this GnRH agonist injection [25]. Two small case series observed a significant improvement in mature/MII oocytes yield with a reasonable clinical pregnancy rate [26, 27]. The "double trigger," which consists of the co-administration of GnRH agonist and hCG for final oocyte maturation 40 and 34 hours prior to OPU, respectively, differs from the "dual trigger" by the additional prolongation of the time between ovulation triggering and oocyte pickup. This later prolongation may explain the beneficial effect in terms of both oocyte maturation and pregnancy rate.

20.3.2 New Options in Ovulation Trigger: Kisspeptin

Kisspeptin (Kp) is a neuropeptide produced in the ventral hypothalamus and is the major positive modulator of GnRH release. Kisspeptin neurons are located in arcuate nucleus and preoptic area in the hypothalamus, and these neurons are in direct contact with GnRH neurons which express kisspeptin receptors. In humans, the KiSS1 gene is translated into a 145-amino acid-long precursor, which is cleaved into a C-terminally amidated 54-amino acid peptide, called Kp54 [28, 29]. Additional cleavage causes shorter peptides like Kp10, but Kisspeptin-54 is a key regulator of the human reproductive axis [30]. Kisspeptins play crucial roles in onset of puberty and ovulatory functions in mammals [31]. Kisspeptin receptor, KISS1R, is a member of G-protein coupled receptor superfamily. KISS1R activation causes calcium influx into the cell. Kisspeptin system is also crucial for normal reproductive function and fertility. A loss-of-function mutation in KISS1R leads to hypogonadotropic hypogonadism and infertility in humans [32].

Jayasena et al. reported first ovulation trigger study with Kp54 in 53 normal responder women. They reported 23% ongoing pregnancy rate with no case of OHSS [33]. The first two clinical phase 2 trials of kisspeptin trigger in women at risk of OHSS were reported by same group. They were able to collect at least one mature oocyte from 95% of patients [34]. Single injection of Kp54 caused a relatively short-lived LH surge of 12–14 hours in duration. The same group performed another phase 2 study to observe whether repeated doses of Kp54 provided better oocyte yield. Two doses of Kp54 were given 10 hours apart to 62 patients at risk of OHSS after stimulation. Patients were randomized to either single or two doses of Kp54, and the oocyte yield, number of follicles >14 mm, and number of oocytes retrieved were compared. The proportion of patients achieving an oocyte yield of ≥60% was improved from 45% in the single kisspeptin-54 group to 71% in the double kisspeptin-54 group ($P = 0.042$). There were one moderate early OHSS in the single-dose group and one late OHSS in the two doses of Kp54 group. Despite the study population being at high risk of developing OHSS, a second dose of kisspeptin-54 did not increase the occurrence of excessive ovarian response or OHSS [35]. Studies of Abbara et al. have showed that kisspeptin family might present a good alternative for oocyte maturation in patients at risk for OHSS. However, the luteal phase is severely defective after the kisspeptin trigger, even more than it is following GnRHa trigger. This is because the triggered LH surge is significantly shorter and has a lower amplitude; thus, the total gonadotropin release is substantially reduced compared with the GnRHa trigger. Therefore luteal phase support should be adapted to these conditions after kisspeptin trigger [36].

References

1. Engmann L, Siano L, Schmidt D, Nulsen J, Maier D, Benadiva C. GnRH agonist to induce oocyte maturation during IVF in patients at high risk of OHSS. Reprod Biomed Online. 2006;13(5):639–44.
2. Humaidan P, Ejdrup Bredkjær H, Bungum L, et al. GnRH agonist (buserelin) or hCG for ovulation induction in GnRH antagonist IVF/ICSI cycles: a prospective randomized study. Hum Reprod. 2005;20(5):1213–20.
3. Ezcurra D, Humaidan P. A review of luteinising hormone and human chorionic gonadotropin when used in assisted reproductive technology. Reprod Biol Endocrinol. 2014;12(1):95.
4. HOFF JD, QUIGLEY ME, YEN SSC. Hormonal dynamics at Midcycle: a reevaluation*. J Clin Endocrinol Metab. 1983;57(4):792–6.
5. Toftager M, Bogstad J, Bryndorf T, et al. Risk of severe ovarian hyperstimulation syndrome in GnRH antagonist versus GnRH agonist protocol: RCT including 1050 first IVF/ICSI cycles. Hum Reprod. 2016;31(6):1253–64.
6. Seyhan A, Ata B, Polat M, Son W-Y, Yarali H, Dahan MH. Severe early ovarian hyperstimulation syndrome following GnRH agonist trigger with the addition of 1500 IU hCG. Hum Reprod. 2013;28(9):2522–8.
7. Courbiere B, Oborski V, Braunstein D, Desparoir A, Noizet A, Gamerre M. Obstetric outcome of women with in vitro fertilization pregnancies hospitalized for ovarian hyperstimulation syndrome: a case-control study. Fertil Steril. 2011;95(5):1629–32.
8. Itskovitz J, Boldes R, Levron J, Erlik Y, Kahana L, Brandes JM. Induction of preovulatory luteinizing hormone surge and prevention of ovarian hyperstimulation syndrome by gonadotropin-releasing hormone agonist*. Fertil Steril. 1991;56(2):213–20.
9. Suda T, Balakier H, Powell W, Casper RF. Use of gonadotropin-releasing hormone agonist to trigger follicular maturation for in vitro fertilization. J Clin Endocrinol Metab. 1990;71(4):918–22. https://doi.org/10.1210/jcem-71-4-918.
10. Dosouto C, Haahr T, Humaidan P. Gonadotropin-releasing hormone agonist (GnRHa) trigger – state of the art. Reprod Biol. 2017;17(1):1–8.
11. Beckers T, Bernd M, Kutscher B, Kühne R, Hoffmann S, Reissmann T. Structure-function studies of linear and cyclized peptide antagonists of the GnRH receptor. Biochem Biophys Res Commun. 2001;289(3):653–63.
12. Zelinski-Wooten MB, Hutchison JS, Hess DL, Wolf DP, Stouffer RL. Follicle stimulating hormone alone supports follicle growth and oocyte development in gonadotrophin-releasing hormone antagonist-treated monkeys. Hum Reprod. 1995;10(7):1658–66.
13. Pereira N, Kelly AG, Stone LD, et al. Gonadotropin-releasing hormone agonist trigger increases the number of oocytes and embryos available for cryopreservation in cancer patients undergoing ovarian stimulation for fertility preservation. Fertil Steril. 2017;108(3):532–8.
14. Humaidan P, Alsbjerg B. GnRHa trigger for final oocyte maturation: is HCG trigger history? Reprod Biomed Online. 2014;29(3):274–80.
15. Ranta T, Knecht M, Kody M, Catt KJ. GnRH receptors in cultured rat granulosa cells: mediation of the inhibitory and stimulatory actions of GnRH. Mol Cell Endocrinol. 1982;27(2):233–40.
16. Takekida S, Deguchi J, Samoto T, Matsuo H, Maruo T. Comparative analysis of the effects of gonadotropin-releasing hormone agonist on the proliferative activity, apoptosis, and steroidogenesis in cultured porcine granulosa cells at varying stages of follicular growth. Endocrine. 2000;12(1):61–8.
17. Schachter M, Friedler S, Ron-El R, et al. Can pregnancy rate be improved in gonadotropin-releasing hormone (GnRH) antagonist cycles by administering GnRH agonist before oocyte retrieval? A prospective, randomized study. Fertil Steril. 2008;90(4):1087–93.
18. de Oliveira SA, Calsavara VF, Cortés GC. Final oocyte maturation in assisted reproduction with human chorionic gonadotropin and gonadotropin-releasing hormone agonist (dual trigger). JBRA Assist Reprod. 2016;20(4):246–50.
19. Garcia-Velasco JA, Motta L, López A, Mayoral M, Cerrillo M, Pacheco A. Low-dose human chorionic gonadotropin versus estradiol/progesterone luteal phase support in gonadotropin-releasing hormone agonist-triggered assisted reproductive technique cycles: understanding a new approach. Fertil Steril. 2010;94(7):2820–3.
20. Cerrillo M, Rodríguez S, Mayoral M, Pacheco A, Martínez-Salazar J, Garcia-Velasco JA. Differential regulation of VEGF after final oocyte maturation with GnRH agonist versus hCG: a rationale for OHSS reduction. Fertil Steril. 2009;91(4 Suppl):1526–8.
21. Castillo JC, Garcia-Velasco J, Humaidan P. Empty follicle syndrome after GnRHa triggering versus hCG triggering in COS. J Assist Reprod Genet. 2012;29(3):249–53.

22. Kol S, Humaidan P, Itskovitz-Eldor J. GnRH agonist ovulation trigger and hCG-based, progesterone-free luteal support: a proof of concept study. Hum Reprod. 2011;26(10):2874–7.
23. Shapiro BS, Daneshmand ST, Garner FC, Aguirre M, Thomas S. Gonadotropin-releasing hormone agonist combined with a reduced dose of human chorionic gonadotropin for final oocyte maturation in fresh autologous cycles of in vitro fertilization. Fertil Steril. 2008;90(1):231–3.
24. Griffin D, Benadiva C, Kummer N, Budinetz T, Nulsen J, Engmann L. Dual trigger of oocyte maturation with gonadotropin-releasing hormone agonist and low-dose human chorionic gonadotropin to optimize live birth rates in high responders. Fertil Steril. 2012;97(6):1316–20.
25. Beck-Fruchter R, Weiss A, Lavee M, Geslevich Y, Shalev E. Empty follicle syndrome: successful treatment in a recurrent case and review of the literature. Hum Reprod. 2012;27(5):1357–67.
26. Zilberberg E, Haas J, Dar S, Kedem A, Machtinger R, Orvieto R. Co-administration of GnRH-agonist and hCG, for final oocyte maturation (double trigger), in patients with low proportion of mature oocytes. Gynecol Endocrinol. 2015;31(2):145–7.
27. Haas J, Zilberberg E, Dar S, Kedem A, Machtinger R, Orvieto R. Co-administration of GnRH-agonist and hCG for final oocyte maturation (double trigger) in patients with low number of oocytes retrieved per number of preovulatory follicles--a preliminary report. J Ovarian Res. 2014;7:77.
28. Pinilla L, Aguilar E, Dieguez C, Millar RP, Tena-Sempere M. Kisspeptins and reproduction: physiological roles and regulatory mechanisms. Physiol Rev. 2012;92(3):1235–316.
29. Beltramo M, Decourt C. Towards new strategies to manage livestock reproduction using kisspeptin analogs. Theriogenology. September 2017;112:2. https://doi.org/10.1016/j.theriogenology.2017.08.026.
30. Clarke SA, Dhillo WS. Kisspeptin across the human lifespan: evidence from animal studies and beyond. J Endocrinol. 2016;229(3):R83–98.
31. Seminara SB, Messager S, Chatzidaki EE, et al. The GPR54 gene as a regulator of puberty. N Engl J Med. 2003;349(17):1614–27.
32. de Roux N, Genin E, Carel J-C, Matsuda F, Chaussain J-L, Milgrom E. Hypogonadotropic hypogonadism due to loss of function of the KiSS1-derived peptide receptor GPR54. Proc Natl Acad Sci U S A. 2003;100(19):10972–6.
33. Jayasena CN, Abbara A, Comninos AN, et al. Kisspeptin-54 triggers egg maturation in women undergoing in vitro fertilization. J Clin Invest. 2014;124(8):3667–77.
34. Abbara A, Jayasena CN, Christopoulos G, et al. Efficacy of Kisspeptin-54 to trigger oocyte maturation in women at high risk of ovarian Hyperstimulation syndrome (OHSS) during in vitro fertilization (IVF) therapy. J Clin Endocrinol Metab. 2015;100(9):3322–31.
35. Abbara A, Clarke S, Islam R, et al. A second dose of kisspeptin-54 improves oocyte maturation in women at high risk of ovarian hyperstimulation syndrome: a phase 2 randomized controlled trial. Hum Reprod. 2017;32(9):1915–24.
36. Thomsen L, Humaidan P. Ovarian hyperstimulation syndrome in the 21st century: the role of gonadotropin-releasing hormone agonist trigger and kisspeptin. Curr Opin Obstet Gynecol. 2015;27(3):210–4.

The Art of Anesthesia in Medically Assisted Reproduction

21

Marjorie Gloff, Melissa Kreso, and Stewart Lustik

The field of ART has advanced at an incredible rate, and as a result, the field of anesthesia as it pertains to ART has been required to match pace. Improvements in the ultrasound technology have morphed the oocyte retrieval procedure from very invasive into one that is now accomplished under ultrasound guidance transvaginally. This has enabled the procedure to be performed routinely in ambulatory centers and even in properly equipped offices. The importance of patient safety and efficiency in this setting is paramount, as there is increasing focus on decreasing length of stay as well as postanesthetic side effects, such as postoperative nausea, vomiting, and excessive sedation. The objectives of this chapter include presenting standards for maintaining patient safety in the field of anesthesiology; presenting medications commonly used in ART and reviewing mechanisms of action and safety; presenting standard definitions used in the field of anesthesiology with regard to depth of sedation; and presenting some routine techniques for anesthesia and analgesia in a patient undergoing ART.

21.1 Basics of Anesthesia

It is important to understand the types of anesthesia available for ART. To do this, it is vital to understand the levels of sedation and the various combinations of techniques that have been successful in these types of procedures. Table 21.1 outlines the various types of anesthesia as well as benefits and risks of each that can be offered to patients for various ART procedures [1].

Local anesthesia is what is referred to when anesthesia is provided by the use of local anesthetics alone. A common example of a local anesthetic technique pertaining to ART would be a paracervical block. Despite no direct cervical involvement with transvaginal ultrasound-guided oocyte retrieval, there has been evidence that paracervical blocks can reduce the abdominal pain associated with this procedure [2]. There have been studies to look at patient satisfaction with sedation alone and sedation with local anesthesia. For example, Ng et al. showed that patient's satisfaction improved substantially when paracervical block was combined with a sedative. However, in cases of strict local anesthesia, the absence of sedation is unlikely to be well tolerated. When most studies look at the success of a particular anesthetic technique over local anesthesia, the patients have generally been given a premedication. For example, a study by Christiaens et al. looked at a comparison of ART performance after oocyte retrieval with general anesthesia versus paracervical block only. However, upon analysis of the meth ods, the patients were provided a premedication anxiolytic, therefore incorrectly calling it a local-only procedure. Care needs to be exercised when interpreting the studies and the various techniques [2].

Neuraxial anesthesia is what is referred to when an anesthesiologist places a spinal or epidural. Spinal anesthesia involves injecting local anesthetics with or without opioid or other adjunct medications in the intrathecal space, whereas epidural anesthesia involves injection into the epidural space. The anesthesiologist can control the amount of motor and sensory blockade with the dosage and concentration of local anesthetics provided. While generally referred to as neuraxial anesthesia, spinals and epidurals can also be considered a form of regional anesthesia. In an early approach to ART, oocyte retrieval was performed via a transvesicular approach requiring the bladder to be distended with saline to optimize the ultrasonic images of the ovaries. This was a very stimulating transabdominal injection which required the needle to

M. Gloff
Department of Anesthesiology and Perioperative Medicine, University of Rochester, Rochester, NY, USA

M. Kreso
Departments of Anesthesiology and Perioperative Medicine, University of Rochester Medical Center, School of Medicine and Dentistry, Rochester, NY, USA

S. Lustik (✉)
Department of Anesthesiology, University of Rochester, Rochester, NY, USA
e-mail: stewart_lustik@urmc.rochester.edu

G. N. Allahbadia et al. (eds.), *Textbook of Assisted Reproduction*, https://doi.org/10.1007/978-981-15-2377-9_21

Table 21.1 Common types of anesthesia and risks and benefits for a patient undergoing ART

Type of anesthesia	Definition	Benefits	Risks
Local anesthesia	Use of local anesthetics alone	Generally quicker time to discharge, no need for an anesthesiologist, low chance for post-op nausea/vomiting, no need for NPO	Full recall of events, patient anxiety may make procedure challenging, patient may move during procedure
Neuraxial anesthesia (i.e., spinal or epidural anesthesia/analgesia)	Use of local anesthetics +/− adjuncts in the epidural or intrathecal space	Dense anesthesia can be obtained, motor blockade prevents movement, no absolute need for sedatives	Longer time to discharge is possible, urinary retention, rarer but possible risks include: post-dural puncture headache, neuraxial hematoma, nerve injury, transient neurologic symptoms (TNS)
Light sedation	Also known as anxiolysis	Maintenance of airway reflexes, responds appropriately to verbal commands, generally quicker recovery, lower risk of Post Operative Nausea and Vomiting (PONV) (but not zero)	Recall of event, patient may move during procedure`
Moderate sedation	A drug-induced depression in consciousness; patient can respond appropriately to verbal +/− tactile stimulation	Able to tolerate more stimulating procedures, generally quick recovery	Can easily slip into deep sedation or general anesthesia; patient may have recall of event; patient may move during procedure; PONV risk
Deep sedation	A drug-induced depression in consciousness where with repeated painful stimulation, the patient will respond appropriately	Able to tolerate stimulating procedures, recall is less likely	May need airway support, can easily slip into general anesthesia, patient may move during the procedure
General anesthesia	Unarousable to painful stimulation	Low risk of recall, can impose paralysis, able to tolerate the most stimulating of procedures	Likely will need airway support, PONV can be more pronounced

From the Practice Guidelines for Sedation and Analgesia by Non-Anesthesiologists, An Updated Report by the American Society of Anesthesiologists Task Force on Sedation and Analgesia by Non-Anesthesiologists. Anesthesiology 2002; 96:1004–17, with permission

traverse an overdistended bladder with concomitant external bladder pressure from the ultrasound probe. Epidural anesthesia was found to be particularly effective in the care of these patients [3]. However, with the standardization of the transvaginal ultrasound and transvaginal collection, neuraxial anesthesia has fallen out of favor for ART. Yet, it is still safe and effective and may be the anesthetic of choice in distinct clinical scenarios, such as in patients with severe obstructive sleep apnea.

The American Society of Anesthesiologists (ASA) has defined the spectrum of sedation as follows [1]:

Light sedation is also known as anxiolysis. This is a drug-induced state during which patients can respond appropriately to verbal commands. By definition, airway reflexes, ventilation, and cardiovascular support are unaffected.

Moderate sedation (colloquially called "conscious sedation") is the state that results when the patient has a drug-induced depression of consciousness during which the patient will respond purposefully when provided verbal commands or a combination of verbal commands and light tactile stimulation. Another key feature of moderate sedation is that airway reflexes are maintained and no interventions to maintain a patent airway are required.

Deep sedation is the depth of anesthesia where a patient cannot be easily aroused. If a patient is provided repeated or painful stimulation, however, she will have a purposeful response. Purposeful, by definition, is a response that is not a reflex withdrawal response. With deep sedation, the patient may require assistance maintaining a patent airway, and spontaneous ventilation may be inadequate.

General anesthesia is the depth of anesthesia where patients become unarousable to painful stimulation. The patient may or may not need assistance ventilating, but frequently they do.

Notice, the term monitored anesthesia care (or MAC) is not a defined term on the sedation spectrum because MAC does not correlate to an anesthetic depth. MAC simply means any anesthetic prescribed by an anesthesiologist or certified anesthesia care provider.

Regardless of the type of anesthesia a patient receives, the American Society of Anesthesiologists has specific guidelines for preoperative fasting to help prevent pulmonary aspiration in the perioperative period (Table 21.2). These guidelines pertain to any patient undergoing an elective procedure where upper airway protective reflexes have a reasonable risk of being impaired. This can occur during all anesthetic types listed above except local anesthetic only [4].

When providing anesthesia, it is vitally important to monitor the patient according to ASA standards and to ensure that all needed safety equipment to deal with any serious

Table 21.2 Guidelines for preoperative fasting and the use of pharmacologic agents to reduce the risk of pulmonary aspiration

Food type	Fasting guidelines prior to procedure
Clears (e.g., water, sodas, apple juice)	2+ hours
Light meal (e.g., toast and a clear liquid, nonhuman milk)	6+ hours
Solids (e.g., heavy, fatty, fried, or protein-based food)	8+ hours

From "Practice Guidelines for Preoperative Fasting and the Use of Pharmacologic Agents to Reduce the Risk of Pulmonary Aspiration: Application to Healthy Patients Undergoing Elective Procedures." Updated Report by the American Society of Anesthesiologists Committee on Standards and Practice Parameters. Anesthesiology 2011; 114:495–511, with permission

complications is available. The ASA requires that for all patients undergoing anesthesia, monitors to ensure adequacy of oxygenation, ventilation, circulation, and temperature must be used. It is required to have monitors such as a pulse oximeter, capnography, ECG, blood pressure monitoring, and thermometers available. There also needs to be a backup supply of oxygen available. In addition, safety equipment such as a bed safety strap to ensure safe positioning, a bag-valve mask to assist ventilation, airway equipment such as appropriate laryngoscopes, endotracheal tubes (ETTs), laryngeal mask airways (LMAs), and oral and nasal airways need to be within reach. It is also important to have a code cart stocked with appropriate medications as well as a defibrillator to ensure adequate treatment in the rare but potentially fatal case of cardiovascular collapse. Pictures of a working oocyte retrieval procedure room, with required equipment, are shown.

No anesthetic technique has been described as being ultimately superior to the others, and furthermore, it is hard to decipher meaningful information from many of the studies since the anesthetic and surgical techniques are so varied. Much of the early literature utilized laparoscopic techniques for oocyte retrieval followed by transvesicular ultrasound-guided retrievals, both of which have fallen out of favor. As a result of the emerging field of ART, much of the earlier literature evaluated the safety standards of common medications used for anesthesia for oocyte retrieval. In these studies, the retrieval, fertilization, cleavage, and implantation rates were evaluated along with the concentration of medication found in the serum and follicular fluids at various times of exposure. More recent studies have shifted to evaluating the shorter- acting medications and techniques because of the new emphasis on efficiency and patient satisfaction. With this armamentarium of information, an anesthesiologist aims to select the appropriate agents for these procedures and administer them in a technique that will maximally benefit the patient and surgeon. Benefits of each medication should be weighed against potential risks. Optimally, the prescription for an anesthetic will decrease nausea, provide good analgesia, decrease motor involvement, ensure hemodynamic stability, and ensure a rapid recovery while balancing the hypothetical risk of lower pregnancy rates.

21.2 Medications

21.2.1 Local Anesthetics

As discussed above, the use of local anesthetics is highly effective for periprocedural pain tolerance, for reduction in the amount of other anesthetic agents required and improved side-effect profile.

21.2.1.1 Lidocaine

Lidocaine is an amide local anesthetic. It has a relatively short duration of action and is a good choice for paracervical block for ART.

Experience in Humans Human studies include a study of 46 women whom received 50 mg of lidocaine in the form of a paracervical block and 46 women who did not. There was no statistical difference in lidocaine concentration between follicles containing oocytes that were fertilized and those that were not. Fertilization, cleavage, and pregnancy rates did not differ significantly either in these two groups; however there is no mention in this paper on the anesthetic method of analgesia utilized in the group not receiving a paracervical block [5]. It is also common to provide a bolus dose of IV lidocaine while administering propofol, to lessen the pain associated with injection. Therefore, additive dosing of the IV and paracervical lidocaine should be considered.

Ng et al. studied 152 double-blinded women undergoing transvaginal ultrasound-guided oocyte retrieval to various doses of lidocaine to elicit the minimally effective dose for paracervical blockade. The women were matched demographically and all ranked pain to IV insertion and transvaginal ultrasonography similarly, suggesting similar baseline pain tolerance. The paracervical lidocaine doses compared were 10 ml 0.5% lidocaine; 10 ml 1% lidocaine; and 10 ml 1.5% lidocaine. There were no differences in the pain during the procedure and no differences for the first 4 hours postoperatively. Thus, lidocaine, while a useful adjunct to women undergoing oocyte retrieval, can be minimized without sacrificing pain control [6].

21.2.1.2 Benzodiazepines

This class of medication is useful for anxiolysis and anterograde memory loss. Midazolam and diazepam have been used for decades in ART and are considered safe. Midazolam is the most frequently utilized benzodiazepine for ART given its relatively short half-life and relative comfort and familiarity among healthcare providers. There are many studies that evaluate midazolam with respect to safety and tolerability. Some of these studies are summarized below.

Experience in Animals In a two-cell mouse embryo study, embryos were co-cultured with increasing concentrations of midazolam to determine any effects on development. Midazolam did not produce any inhibitory effects on in vitro two-cell blastocyst embryo development up to and including a concentration of 12,500 ng/mL. A second set of experiments in the same study included simulating conditions of human ovum exposure to midazolam in follicular fluids during egg retrieval. This was injected intraperitoneally into mice about 10–13 hours before ovulation and was found not to impair fertilization. Doses up to 500-fold normal did not inhibit fertilization. In fact, in both sets of experiments, midazolam appeared to accelerate embryo development [7].

Experience in Humans Midazolam is found in the follicular fluid in women undergoing ART. One study looked at 15 women who were given a single dose of 0.1 mg/kg midazolam. While this dose is quite high for anxiolysis, it isn't unreasonable; in this study, a 50 kg person would be provided 5 mg intravenously. The amount of drug found in follicular fluid was significantly smaller compared to plasma levels and had a slow rise peaking at 25 minutes whereas the plasma levels of the drug peaked at around 5 minutes and then exponentially decreased. Pregnancy rates were not affected in this study. Although this was a very small investigation, it does suggest that depending on the length of the ART procedure itself, the drug amount found in the follicular fluid should be less in faster procedures relative to slower ones [8].

A survey questioned 30 women who received a combination of midazolam and a continuous remifentanil infusion were compared to 30 women who received a continuous infusion of propofol- and fentanyl-based anesthetic for oocyte retrieval. Common unwanted experiences in the midazolam/remifentanil group included muscular rigidity (13%), itching (20%), patient motion (37%), and recall of the procedure (70%). The survey found that four patients would refuse this type of anesthetic for subsequent procedures due to the perceived discomfort and recall. While this may have been mitigated by an increased dose of midazolam, there is a dose-dependent synergistic effect of respiratory depression when combined with opioids or propofol that is important to consider. Interestingly, three surgeons also opted against this type of anesthetic for future procedures because of patient movement. In contrast, all of the patients and surgeons in the propofol/fentanyl group thought the overall conditions were satisfactory and would have this type of anesthesia administered again. This was despite the need to increase support to facemask (spontaneous) ventilation more frequently in this group and even advance to manual ventilation in 57% of patients. This study highlights that there are different and effective anesthetic methods for performing oocyte retrievals. Balancing various side effects with the patient's and surgeon's wishes is vitally important to ensure satisfaction among all parties [9].

21.2.1.3 Propofol

Propofol is a 2,6-diisopropylphenol which is a short-acting intravenous anesthetic that can cause moderate sedation in lower doses and unconsciousness at higher doses. It also is an excellent antiemetic. It has a rapid onset of action and also exhibits rapid recovery secondary to redistribution into the tissues given its lipophilicity and therefore large volume of distribution.

Propofol is a helpful adjunct to both general anesthesia and anesthesia that falls on the spectrum of sedation. It is vital to understand the implications prior to using this medication. Many people attempt to utilize propofol with a sedation plan in mind, but very easily and quickly a patient's anesthetic depth can move into the general anesthesia range. A study looked at 50 patients scheduled for oocyte retrieval utilizing a fentanyl and propofol anesthetic. The thought was that patients undergoing oocyte retrieval could potentially need a deeper propofol-based anesthetic since there can be a high level of anxiety with this procedure and there is unreliable coverage by local anesthesia for both needle insertion and repeated ovarian puncture. Bispectral index values and modified Ramsey sedation scores were recorded during the retrieval in this study. Moderate sedation was found during the first 5–10 minutes of the oocyte retrieval, but thereafter in ALL patients, deep sedation or general anesthesia was achieved. This was quantified by the modified observer's assessment of alertness/sedation scale, BIS scores, and lack of response to painful stimulation. It is highly likely that many research studies are underestimating the level of sedation used during oocyte retrievals [10]. If an anesthesia service is not directly responsible for providing anesthesia for patients, then it is prudent that the deepest level of sedation achieved remains at a level where the patient can maintain verbal contact the entire time. It is also important to know what your institution's policy is for procedural use of propofol by non-anesthesiologists.

Experience in Animals Propofol is found in the murine follicular fluid. Early animal studies showed a dose- and time-dependent effect of propofol on the fertilization of mouse oocytes while in vitro development of fertilized oocytes remained normal [11]. Varying concentrations of propofol (0.1–10 ug/mL) were studied in the mouse model to evaluate the effect of concentration on the ability of the oocytes to mature in vitro. There was a notable reduction in maturation rate when mouse oocytes were exposed to concentrations higher than 10ug/mL of propofol for 30 minutes. However, all mature oocytes had similar fertilization and cleavage rates compared to controls [12]. In another mouse study, adverse effects of concentration (0.01–10 ug/ml) and duration (1 hour) of propofol exposure on oocyte fertilization were examined. Oocytes exposed to concentrations at 0.4ug/ml or higher had a significant decrease in fusion rates. The oocytes that could be fertilized showed no differences in their ability to form pronuclei and no differences in the extrusion of the polar body. They also looked at embryos exposed to different concentrations of propofol 0.01–10ug/ml for 14 hours and saw no difference in blastocyst formation rates [13]. This raises the possibility of a potentially harmful effect of propofol at higher concentrations when administered for longer periods of time.

Experience in Humans Propofol is widely used for ART but can have potential negative implications. Propofol given as a single bolus is less likely to continuously accumulate in the follicular fluid, as compared to continuous infusions. This effect is secondary to the redistribution properties of propofol. In one small study of 20 women, a single dose of propofol 2.5 mg/kg was found to have no effect on cleavage rate, which was approximately 70%. In fact, the oocytes that failed to cleave in this study were surrounded by follicular fluid containing significantly less propofol than those that did cleave. In this study, propofol blood concentrations were the highest between the 8th and 11th minutes with a ratio of propofol concentration in the follicular fluid/blood of 0.2 ± 0.11 [14]. Comparatively, propofol accumulation was demonstrated in oocytes over time in nine women receiving propofol infusions at ten mg/kg/hr. (166 mcg/kg/min) with one to two 20 mg propofol boluses during the procedures. Venous blood was sampled every 15 minutes up to 45 minutes (corresponding to the longest aspiration time). Each patient had a minimum of ten oocytes aspirated. It was found that serum blood levels did not correlate exactly with increases in follicular fluid, but there was significant correlation with duration of infusion and the increase in the propofol concentration of the last follicle. In this small study, follicular fluid concentrations of propofol were well below serum propofol levels. One hypothesis for this finding is that ovarian tissue and or the follicular wall may cause a barrier to the equilibration of propofol between serum and follicular fluid [15]. In another study of 30 women, propofol concentration in follicular fluid was assessed after a 2 mg/kg initial bolus followed by an infusion of 10 mg/kg/hr (166 mcg/kg/min). These patients also received a single 0.5 mg dose of alfentanil. This study also showed that the follicular fluid rise in concentration also correlates to duration of infusion. From these studies it was determined that follicular fluid most likely lies in the deep peripheral compartment of the three-compartment open model for propofol. The process of propofol transfer from blood to follicular fluid was very slow with a clearance ratio of 6%. However, this study only took 2–4 arterial blood samples per patient, so estimations of pharmacokinetic models for propofol concentrations in follicular fluid could not be completed [16].

21.2.1.4 Etomidate

Etomidate, an imidazole derivative, has been less well studied for its role in ART. Etomidate is a medication, much like propofol, that is generally administered by credentialed providers such as anesthesiologists. In 1987, Fragen et al. showed that etomidate inhibits adrenocortical steroidogenesis [17]. That same year, a study evaluated eight patients undergoing laparoscopic oocyte retrieval. These patients were randomized to etomidate versus thiopental induction groups followed by isoflurane maintenance. In the etomidate group, a sharp decrease in plasma concentrations of 17beta-oestradiol, 17OH-progesterone, and testosterone levels was found within 10 minutes of induction. This was followed by a gradual return to baseline levels. Thiopental did not show this decrease. While the study size was small, it can still be hypothesized that etomidate interferes with the endocrine function of the ovary in addition to that of the adrenal glands [18].

21.2.1.5 Ketamine

Ketamine is a unique anesthetic in that it provides good analgesia while also providing a dissociative anesthesia. This is unlike any other anesthetic on the market today.

Experience in Humans One study randomized 50 women to receive either a midazolam-ketamine sedation technique for egg retrieval or a general anesthetic technique with propofol, fentanyl, and isoflurane. This study, although small, showed no differences between the two groups for number of oocytes obtained, fertilization rates, implantation rates, nor pregnancy rates [19].

21.2.1.6 Opioids

Opioids are a staple to any balanced anesthetic plan. Fraught with side effects, they are still widely used and depended upon for adequate procedural and post-procedural pain control. In an attempt to improve tolerability and clearance, there are now multiple formulations and delivery options which can impact duration of action and therefore safety and tolerability.

21.2.1.7 Fentanyl

Fentanyl is a very potent opioid with a fairly short duration of action when administered IV (0.5–1 hour). It can be used systemically, in the epidural space and in the intrathecal space. Fentanyl has been used for years in ART and considered safe and effective. Its side-effect profile and duration of action make it particularly useful for efficient care in the ambulatory setting.

In a study looking at 15 patients that were given a single dose of 1 ug/kg fentanyl, fentanyl was found in the follicular fluid of oocytes. The amount of drug found in follicular fluid was significantly small compared to plasma levels and had a slow rise which again suggests that shorter procedures will have less accumulation of fentanyl in follicular fluid. Fentanyl also works in a three-compartment model of distribution. In this study there was no impact on pregnancy outcomes although this was not the primary intent of the study [8].

21.2.1.8 Alfentanil

Alfentanil, much like fentanyl, has a quick onset and short duration of action (0.5–1 hour). These properties make this a useful agent for the balanced anesthetic management of ART patients. Of note, it also is found in the follicular fluid. The accumulation of alfentanil in the follicular fluid confirms that the follicular fluid belongs to the scarcely perfused or shallow compartment in the three-compartment model of pharmacokinetics [20], with a slow rate of equilibration compared with the central compartment. The ratio of serum to follicular fluid concentrations was about 10:1 at 15 minutes after the initial bolus injection of alfentanil. There is evidence that about 10% of serum alfentanil is unbound to serum proteins and able to diffuse into peripheral tissues and fluids. Since the follicular fluid proteins do not include alpha-l-acid glycoprotein that is related to the binding of alfentanil, the amount of alfentanil detected in the follicular fluid may reflect the free fraction of alfentanil [21].

Experience in Humans Studies to evaluate the pharmacokinetics of alfentanil have been performed in women undergoing oocyte retrieval. One study evaluated 14 ASA 1 patients undergoing ART with an anesthetic induced by 15 mcg/ml of alfentanil and 2 mg midazolam initially. Patients were maintained with nitrous oxide and with additional boluses of 0.5 mg alfentanil and midazolam (up to 4 mg total). These patients showed a tenfold difference in serum levels (higher) relative to follicular fluid levels at the same time points. This was similar when propofol was utilized for maintenance [21]. This study also evaluated serum and follicular alfentanil levels in 13 patients given a single dose of 10 ug/kg alfentanil. Alfentanil was found in follicular fluid with the similar pattern slowly rising at progressively longer time points. The peak ratio of alfentanil (1:40) in follicular fluid was lower relative to fentanyl (1:10). There is no evidence to suggest that this impacts pregnancy outcomes [22]. In another study evaluating the tolerability of alfentanil, 36 women were randomized into either an alfentanil 0.025 mg/kg group or a fentanyl 0.0025 mg/kg group. It was found that time to induction was shorter in the alfentanil group and patients were less drowsy at the end of the procedure relative to the fentanyl group [23].

21.2.1.9 Remifentanil

Remifentanil is an ultrashort-acting opioid agent that is metabolized by nonspecific tissue esterases. Given its incredibly short duration of action, it is generally provided by continuous infusion. Remifentanil does not appear to be harmful in ART procedures.

Experience in Humans One retrospective study compared 548 similar (except for age) infertile women. One group was provided a paracervical lidocaine block for anesthesia, while the other half was anesthetized using a paracervical lidocaine block with the adjunct of a continuous remifentanil infusion. The paracervical block-only group's average age was 34.8. This is compared to the remifentanil group's average age of 35.9 years. Because of the higher age in the remifentanil group, these women received a high dose of gonadotropin on average to reach an equivalent ovarian response as the no remifentanil group. Interestingly, the number of oocytes retrieved in the remifentanil group was higher, and the quality of the oocytes was not deteriorated. Since the perceived ovarian response was intended to be similar despite the extra gonadotropin stimuli (to make up for the difference in ages), possibly the better pain control allowed for more oocytes to be retrieved. It is reasonable to assume that remifentanil does not appear to affect the quality of oocytes retrieved [24]. Anesthesia generally requires a balance between sedative agents, anxiolytic agents, and local anesthetics. A study evaluating 40 patients broken into 2 even groups compared remifentanil sedation alone versus remifentanil in combination with a paracervical block. It was discovered that there are higher concentrations of plasma remifentanil at the time of second ovarian puncture in the remifentanil-only group relative to combining this with a paracervical block. This illustrates that anesthetics can be used more sparingly when combining medications that work via different mechanisms of action [25].

21.2.1.10 Buprenorphine

Buprenorphine is becoming more popular as the epidemic of opioid tolerance and dependence increases. Buprenorphine is a partial opioid agonist that in higher doses can function as an opioid antagonist. While buprenorphine is not routinely used for specific procedural pain management in practice, it is important to account for how a patient may respond differently to anesthesia if she is already on these medications. Generally, it would be considered safe to continue opioid partial agonists and antagonists during this fairly short ambulatory procedure. However, it would be pertinent to ensure that there is access to medications for pain control that are not in the opioid class. It would also be pertinent to consider consulting with an anesthesiologist regarding the periprocedural pain and anesthetic management of these patients.

Experience in Animals An animal study utilized buprenorphine as a longer-acting opioid for more optimal pain control in 33 rodents undergoing ART. The opioid addition to the anesthesia regimen showed no obvious effect on the number of embryo implantations, and it was noted that stimuli led to less heart rate and blood pressure elevations [26].

21.2.1.11 Nonsteroidal Anti-inflammatory Agents

Ketorolac and diclofenac are effective analgesics especially for alleviating cramping pain after oocyte retrievals and are commonly used adjuvants for anesthesia in ART. Both of these medications have potent COX1 and COX2 inhibitory activity. It was previously thought that this action would negatively impact implantation due to this inhibitory effect on prostaglandin synthesis. The studies, summarized below however, have not shown this to be the case.

Experience in Animals In the mouse model, NSAID use was studied specifically looking at yield and birth rate in 99 surgical sets. Multimodal analgesia utilizing opioid and NSAIDs did not positively or negatively impact the ability to create novel lines of transgenic mice by blastocyst transfer [27]. Another animal study randomized a total of 96 mice to receive an opioid, an NSAID, or saline. No significant difference was seen in the pregnancy rates or live birth rates in any group [28].

Experience in Humans A retrospective study conducted by Mesen et al. evaluated 454 women undergoing fresh transfers over a 7-year period. Approximately one fifth of these patients received ketorolac immediately after oocyte retrieval. The pregnancy rate in both groups was approximately 50%, and the implantation rate and live birth rate between the two groups was not statistically different. Not surprisingly, patients who received the NSAID had improved pain scores in recovery (visual analog scale (VAS) = 2) compared to their counterparts (VAS = 5). A likely explanation for this comes from the pharmacokinetics of ketorolac. Ketorolac has a half-life of 4–7 hours, and only 2% of the drug remains in the body after 24 hours. Implantation occurs typically 6–8 days post-retrieval. By this time, ketorolac has long been metabolized away. Also, now with the more widespread use of frozen transfers, ketorolac is even more convincingly safe [29].

Diclofenac was also investigated with respect to ART outcomes and pain scores. Kailasam et al. assembled a randomized prospective double-blind study of 381 assisted conception cycles. Two groups were established and consisted of 187 women who received 100 mg of diclofenac via suppository at the end of the procedure and 194 women who received nothing. The number of women progressing to embryo transfer was 185 and 190, respectively. Implantation rates were found to be 25.3% in the diclofenac group and 21.6% in the non-diclofenac group. Pregnancy occurred in 38.9% of women in the diclofenac group and 32.6% in the non-diclofenac group. These rates were not statistically different. However there were reduced pain scores in the group receiving diclofenac prior to discharge, and this reached statistical significance. The use of diclofenac reduced pain scores without compromising fertility outcomes [30].

21.2.1.12 Antiemetic Agents

While key to a smooth anesthetic, antiemetic agents are not without potential risk. Some antiemetics have been associated with elevations in plasma and or follicular fluid prolactin concentrations, an effect that has been associated with impaired follicular maturation, steroidogenesis, ovulation, and corpus luteum function. Drugs that have induced hyperprolactinemia rapidly like droperidol and metoclopramide cause impairment of the ovarian follicle maturation and corpus luteum function, and thus should not be used [31]. Ondansetron and dexamethasone are two standard antiemetics used for postoperative nausea prophylaxis that appear to be safe in ART.

21.2.1.13 Nitrous Oxide

Nitrous oxide is one of the oldest anesthetics still in use. It has an excellent safety profile and works to both cause amnesia and to treat acute pain. There has been concern documented that nitrous oxide is teratogenic.

Experience in Animals Warren et al. studied the effects of nitrous oxide in mouse embryo development. This study looked specifically at nitrous oxide administered to embryos at various time points prior to expected cleavage. They showed that zygotes exposed to nitrous oxide close to the expected time of cleavage did indeed have deleterious effects on further development. For instance, only 4.7% of zygotes that were exposed to nitrous oxide at 0–1 hour prior to expected cleavage went on to complete division versus 77% of controls. These stats improved with time out from the expected cleavage [32].

21.2.1.14 Volatile Anesthetics

Volatile anesthetics (i.e., inhalational anesthetics such as isoflurane and sevoflurane) have largely fallen out of favor with the push toward performing ART in office-based settings. A balanced anesthetic with propofol, benzodiazepines, local anesthetics, and short-acting opioids is an efficient anesthetic that is well tolerated and has been shown to have minimal risk to the oocytes and the patient. The use of volatile anesthetics also requires an anesthesia machine, which is expensive and potentially unavailable in office locations.

Despite that, there could be a situation where a volatile-based general anesthetic would be indicated. There is little literature that evaluates the safety of volatile anesthetics in oocyte retrieval.

Experience in Humans Early in the development and establishment of oocyte retrieval techniques, Hayes et al. evaluated 276 women patients who had presented for IVF over a 3.5-year span. These procedures were all performed under laparoscopic conditions and therefore under a combination of thiopental, nitrous oxide, isoflurane, fentanyl, and succinylcholine for induction and maintenance of general anesthesia. Interestingly, the average time for anesthesia exposure to oocytes was 36.8 ± 16.7 minutes with a range of 5–99 minutes – considerably longer than current practice. This study showed that oocytes retrieved from the second ovary had significantly less chance of cleavage compared to their maturity matched counterpart from the first ovary. The group concluded that perhaps length of anesthesia, the CO_2 pneumoperitoneum or some combination of the two resulted in these findings [33].

21.2.1.15 Alternative Techniques and Multimodal Analgesia

Much research has looked at the role of acupuncture in ART. Acupuncture techniques have been described as an additional multimodal method of analgesia during oocyte retrieval procedures. In a study comparing remifentanil to acupuncture techniques including electro- and auricular acupuncture, patients had reduced pain intensity and reduced consumption of remifentanil during their procedures with the addition of electroacupuncture. However, all patients requested a remifentanil PCA in this study, so this seemed to be insufficient at providing sole analgesia. Electroacupuncture seems like a good additive therapy in facilities where this is possible but likely not sufficient for analgesia alone [34]. For instance, VAS pain scores were significantly higher at oocyte aspiration in a study out of Sweden randomizing patients to an electroacupuncture/paracervical block technique relative to a paracervical/alfentanil technique [35]. Humaidan et al. have also found this effect but noted the time to discharge from their facility was found to be 8 minutes shorter with the acupuncture technique [36].

21.3 Associated Conditions and Effect on Anesthesia

21.3.1 Hyperprolactinemia

Historically there has been great interest on studying the effects anesthetics on prolactin levels. Hyperprolactinemia has been found to impair ovarian follicle maturation as well as corpus luteum function [31]. Stress-related increases in prolactin can be seen in surgical procedures. There is some evidence to suggest that this may be increased with both total IV anesthetics and volatile anesthetics such as sevoflurane [37]. Bromocriptine has been used successfully in women undergoing ART. Bromocriptine (a prolactin inhibitor) 1 hour prior to the procedure has been shown to decrease serum prolactin levels and also decrease the level of prolactin in follicular fluid hormone concentrations. Fertilization and pregnancy rates were not affected by administration of bromocriptine. Prevention of hyperprolactinemia may improve embryonic cleavage rates after IVF [38]. However, routine oocyte retrieval procedures are so short in duration, and this is not routinely used in practice.

21.3.2 Ovarian Hyperstimulation Syndrome

Ovarian hyperstimulation syndrome can range from mild to severe and can be life-threatening. The syndrome in its severe form is classified by fluid shifts that can be extensive resulting in ascites, pleural effusions, pericardial effusions, electrolyte abnormalities, renal impairment, and profound hypovolemia. While it is still uncertain, there is some evidence to suggest that a mutation in the FSH receptor can lead to this process [39]. Regardless, performing procedures in these patients with sedation needs to be approached very carefully as their pathophysiology makes arrhythmia, profound hypotension, hypoxemia, and aspiration much more likely. Careful monitoring in a hospital should occur – even for routine procedures such as a paracentesis – to insure hemodynamic stability and adequate resuscitation. If a procedure needs sedation, it would not be unreasonable to consult with an anesthesiologist in this scenario.

21.3.3 Patient Characteristics

No matter what the technique, each patient deserves to have their needs met on an individualized basis. Patient characteristics certainly do play a role into optimizing analgesia and safety. It is so imperative that each patient be screened for comorbidities that may complicate their perioperative and anesthetic care. A screening paradigm should be developed collaboratively between the reproductive endocrinologist and the anesthesiologist as there is no nationally accepted patient exclusion/inclusion criteria for office-based or ambulatory anesthesia centers. It cannot be highlighted enough that each patient be deemed appropriate to have anesthesia in the planned setting. Office-based anesthesia has by definition minimal ancillary resources physically present. It is poor patient care to have oocyte retrievals canceled for predictable reasons on the day of the procedure because of poor planning and communication. This can have serious downstream implications on the ART cycle and on the patient.

Given the nature of all the energy expended prior to getting to the point of egg retrieval, it is predictable that women present with anxiety, sometimes severe. In a study where 150 women undergoing oocyte retrieval were divided into 2 groups based on their anxiety assessed by the VAS scoring system, patients in the high-anxiety group required more propofol for their induction, and overall required a larger dose of propofol for sedation relative to the low-anxiety group. Similarly context-sensitive half time was longer in the high-anxiety group. Interestingly, patients with higher anxiety also tended to have a higher postoperative pain score. This study highlights that a patient's level of anxiety should be taken into account when determining the dosing and the agents to administer for oocyte retrieval [40].

21.4 Conclusions

The primary goals when choosing an anesthetic technique are to alleviate pain during the procedure and minimize recovery time afterward. One should utilize medications with minimal adverse effects. There have been myriad techniques described in the literature, which range from a paracervical block to general anesthesia. Although the average type of anesthesia has changed with time and the invention of the transvaginal ultrasound probe, there are pros and cons to using each type. Sedation and analgesia embrace a continuum ranging from minimal sedation all the way to general anesthesia.

References

1. The American Society of Anesthesiologists Task Force on Sedation and Analgesia by Non-Anesthesiologists. Practice guidelines for sedation and analgesia by non-anesthesiologists. Anesthesiology. 2002;96(4):1004–17.
2. Ng EHY, et al. A prospective, randomized, double-blind and placebo-controlled study to assess the efficacy of paracervical block in the pain relief during egg collection in IVF. Hum Reprod. 1999;14(11):2783–7.
3. Kogosowski A, et al. Epidural block: a preferred method of anesthesia for ultrasonically guided oocyte retrieval. Fertil Steril. 1987;47(1):166–8.
4. American Society of Anesthesiologists Committee on Standards and Practice Parameters. Practice guidelines for preoperative fasting and the use of pharmacologic agents to reduce the risk of pulmonary aspiration: application to healthy patients undergoing elective procedures: an updated report by the American society of anesthesiologists committee on standards and practice parameters. Anesthesiology. 2011;114(3):495.
5. Wikland M, et al. The concentration of lidocaine in follicular fluid when used for paracervical block in a human IVF-ET programme. Hum Reprod. 1990;5(8):920–3.
6. Ng EHY, Miao B, Ho PC. A randomized double-blind study to compare the effectiveness of three different doses of lignocaine used in paracervical block during oocyte retrieval. J Assist Reprod Genet. 2003;20(1):8–12.
7. Swanson RJ, Leavitt MG. Fertilization and mouse embryo development in the presence of midazolam. Anesth Analg. 1992;75(4):549–54.
8. Soussis I, et al. Follicular fluid levels of midazolam, fentanyl, and alfentanil during transvaginal oocyte retrieval. Fertil Steril. 1995;64(5):1003–7.
9. Casati A, et al. Anaesthesia for ultrasound guided oocyte retrieval: midazolam/remifentanil versus propofol/fentanyl regimens. Eur J Anaesthesiol. 1999;16(11):773–8.
10. Circeo L, et al. Prospective, observational study of the depth of anesthesia during oocyte retrieval using a total intravenous anesthetic technique and the Bispectral index monitor. Fertil Steril. 2011;96(3):635–7.
11. Depypere HT, Dhont, M, de Sutter P, Vanderkerchkhove D. Abstracts of the 7th annual Meeting of the ESHRE and the 7thWorld congress on IVF and Assisted Procreations, Paris, June–July 19991, Institut de Medicine de la Reproduction Marseille, France. Human Reproduction, Oxford University Press. 1991;6(s1):151.
12. Alsalili M, Thornton S, Fleming S. The effect of the anaesthetic, Propofol, on in-vitro oocyte maturation, fertilization and cleavage in mice. Hum Reprod. 1997;12(6):1271–4.
13. Tatone C, et al. An evaluation of propofol toxicity on mouse oocytes and preimplantation embryos. Hum Reprod. 1998;13(2):430–5.
14. Palot M, et al. Propofol in general anesthesia for Ivf (by vaginal and transurethral route)-follicular fluid Concentration and cleavage rate. J Am Soc Anesth. 1988;69(3A):A573.
15. Coetsier T, et al. Propofol anaesthesia for ultrasound guided oocyte retrieval: accumulation of the anaesthetic agent in follicular fluid. Hum Reprod. 1992;7(10):1422–4.
16. Christiaens F, et al. Propofol concentrations in follicular fluid during general anaesthesia for transvaginal oocyte retrieval. Hum Reprod. 1999;14(2):345–8.
17. Fragen RJ, Weiss HW, Molteni A. The effect of Propofol on adrenocortical Steroidogenesis A comparative study with etomidate and thiopental. J Am Soc Anesth. 1987;66(6):839–41.
18. Heytens L, et al. Effects of etomidate on ovarian steroidogenesis. Hum Reprod. 1987;2(2):85–90.
19. Ben-Shlomo I, et al. Midazolam/ketamine sedative combination compared with fentanyl/propofol/isoflurane anaesthesia for oocyte retrieval. Hum Reprod. 1999;14(7):1757–9.
20. Cascone S, et al. Pharmacokinetics of Remifentanil: a three-compartmental modeling approach. Transl Med UniSa. 2013;7:18.
21. Shapira SC, et al. Use of alfentanil for in vitro fertilization oocyte retrieval. J Clin Anesth. 1996;8(4):282–5.
22. Soussis I, et al. Follicular fluid levels of midazolam, fentanyl, and alfentanil during transvaginal oocyte retrieval. Fertil Steril. 1995;64(5):1003–7.
23. Shapira SC, Magora F, Katzenelson R, Laufer N. Fentanyl vs. Alfentanil for in vitro fertilization. Harefuah. 1991;121:17–8.
24. Milanini MN, et al. Local anesthesia versus intravenous infusion of remifentanil for assisted reproductive technologies. A retrospective study. Minerva Ginecol. 2008;60(3):203–7.
25. Gunaydin B, et al. Remifentanil versus remifentanil with paracervical block on plasma remifentanil concentrations and pulmonary function tests for transvaginal ultrasound-guided oocyte retrieval. J Opioid Manag. 2006;3(5):267–72.
26. Krueger KL, Fujiwara Y. The use of buprenorphine as an analgesic after rodent embryo transfer. Lab Animal. 2008;37(2):87.
27. Parker JM, et al. Effects of multimodal analgesia on the success of mouse embryo transfer surgery. J Am Assoc Lab Anim Sci. 2011;50(4):466–70.
28. Goulding DR, et al. The effects of perioperative analgesia on litter size in Crl: CD1 (ICR) mice undergoing embryo transfer. J Am Assoc Lab Anim Sci. 2010;49(4):423–6.
29. Mesen TB, et al. The effect of ketorolac on pregnancy rates when used immediately after oocyte retrieval. Fertil Steril. 2013;100(3):725–8.
30. Kailasam C, et al. Safety and effectiveness of diclofenac sodium in assisted reproduction treatment: a randomized prospective double-blind study. Reprod Biomed Online. 2008;16(5):724–9.

31. Kauppila A, et al. Metoclopramide-induced hyperprolactinemia impairs ovarian follicle maturation and Corpus luteum function in women*. J Clin Endocrinol Metabol. 1982;54(5):955–60.
32. Warren JR, Shaw B, Steinkampf MP. Effects of nitrous oxide on preimplantation mouse embryo cleavage and development. Biol Reprod. 1990;43(1):158–61.
33. Hayes MF, et al. Effect of general anesthesia on fertilization and cleavage of human oocytes in vitro. Fertil Steril. 1987;48(6):975–81.
34. Sator-Katzenschlager SM, et al. Auricular electro-acupuncture as an additional perioperative analgesic method during oocyte aspiration in IVF treatment. Hum Reprod. 2006;21(8):2114–20.
35. Gejervall A-L, et al. Electro-acupuncture versus conventional analgesia: a comparison of pain levels during oocyte aspiration and patients' experiences of Well-being after surgery. Hum Reprod. 2005;20(3):728–35.
36. Humaidan P, Stener-Victorin E. Pain relief during oocyte retrieval with a new short duration electro-acupuncture technique—an alternative to conventional analgesic methods. Hum Reprod. 2004;19(6):1367–72.
37. Marana E, et al. Neuroendocrine stress response in gynecological laparoscopy: TIVA with propofol versus sevoflurane anesthesia. J Clin Anesth. 2010;22(4):250–5.
38. Sopelak VM, et al. Bromocriptine inhibition of anesthesia-induced hyperprolactinemia: effect on serum and follicular fluid hormones, oocyte fertilization, and embryo cleavage rates during in vitro fertilization. Fertil Steril. 1989;52(4):627–32.
39. Delbaere A, et al. New insights into the pathophysiology of ovarian hyperstimulation syndrome. What makes the difference between spontaneous and iatrogenic syndrome? Hum Reprod. 2004;19(3):486–9.
40. Hong J-Y, Jee YS, Luthardt FW. Comparison of conscious sedation for oocyte retrieval between low-anxiety and high-anxiety patients. J Clin Anesth. 2005;17(7):549–53.

Embryo Transfer

22

Richard Thomas Russell and Daphne Chong

Successful implantation of embryos remains the most crucial and least successful step in assisted reproduction. Success depends on the selection of a high-quality chromosomally competent embryo, replaced in a synchronized and receptive endometrium, in the least traumatic process possible. Embryo transfer (ET) is therefore one of the most critical steps in the IVF process, and implantation success is known to correlate with the ease of transfer [1, 2]. Training in the ET technique is variable, with many clinicians performing very few embryo transfers before going 'live'.

ET is a relatively easy to learn and hardly 'unlearned' procedure with training individualized and monitored. The reader may be surprised that proficiency is usually achieved by procedure number 15 [3]. However, several studies have demonstrated variability in IVF pregnancy rates dependent on the clinician performing the ET [4–6].

Varying techniques of ET have been reported [7]. This chapter aims to cover some of the key elements in affording success.

22.1 Pre-Embryo Transfer

22.1.1 Acupuncture

Acupuncture is increasingly practised as part of the IVF process, and whilst there is a wealth of literature to look at, the trials are often poorly conceived with varying acupuncture techniques and treatments advocated. Dating back over 3000 years of Chinese tradition, the practice involves insertion of fine needles through the skin to modulate hormones, alter energy flow (chi), improve uterine blood flow and reduce stress.

There have been several randomized controlled trials (RCTs) demonstrating the benefits of acupuncture [8–12]. The trial by Qu et al. demonstrated higher implantation, clinical and live birth rates in the auricular acupuncture groups [10], whilst Westergaard et al. demonstrated a higher clinical pregnancy rate in patients who had acupuncture on the day of ET (39% versus 24%) compared to those that had no acupuncture [12]. A subsequent meta-analysis of seven trials also demonstrated improved clinical pregnancy rates (odds ratio (OR) 1.65, 95% CI 1.27–2.14) and live birth rates (OR 1.91, CI 1.39–2.64) when acupuncture was given in combination with ET [13].

By contrast, several RCTs have shown no benefit of acupuncture [14–21], including meta-analyses [22]. Although acupuncture is widely practised, there is insufficient evidence, at present, to recommend it as part of routine IVF protocol.

22.1.2 Anaesthesia

Pain experienced by patients at ET has been reported to be independently associated with significantly lower pregnancy rate [23], leading to studies invested in assessing efforts to minimize patients' discomfort. Only one large comparative trial has looked at the effect of anaesthesia for ET and found no beneficial impact [24]. The routine use of anaesthesia during ET is not generally recommended considering the potential complications; however, there are certain situations where it could be considered, e.g. difficult previous procedures, vaginismus, psychosexual issues or transmyometrial ETs. It is worth considering that although general anaesthesia is not recommended, neither is there any evidence of reduced pregnancy outcomes with its use.

22.1.3 Antibiotics

It is common sense that a clinical or possibly subclinical endometrial infection may result in lower implantation rates, as similarly observed in patients with chronic endometritis.

R. T. Russell (✉) · D. Chong
The Hewitt Fertility Centre, Liverpool Women's NHS Foundation Trust Hospital, Liverpool, UK
e-mail: rtrussell@doctors.org.uk

G. N. Allahbadia et al. (eds.), *Textbook of Assisted Reproduction*, https://doi.org/10.1007/978-981-15-2377-9_22

Although the use of prophylactic broad-spectrum antibiotics around the time of ET has successfully demonstrated a reduction in bacteria isolated from the catheter tip post-transfer, it did not confer an improvement in clinical or live birth rates [25].

22.1.4 Cleaning the Cervix

It is generally considered that cleaning the cervix is beneficial prior to ET. It has been suggested that cervical mucus may impede the passage of embryo through the tip of the catheter and may even pull the embryos back in to the catheter from the site of expulsion.

It has been postulated that traversing cervical mucus could introduce subclinical infection along with the embryo. Furthermore, some might argue that removing mucus might stimulate uterine contractility or bleeding that may negatively impact on pregnancy outcomes. However, there is very little evidence in the literature to draw from as cervical cleaning is essentially considered accepted practice. In a large RCT, clinical pregnancy rates (39.2% study vs 22.6% controls, *P*, 0.001) and live birth rates (33.6% study vs 17.4% controls, $P < 0.001$) favoured removal of cervical mucus [26], with similar results also observed in another non-randomized study [27].

22.1.5 Uterine Relaxants

Uterine contractility is associated with reduced IVF success. Increased contractility has been linked to ovarian stimulation as well as induced contractility should the ET catheter touch the uterine fundus [28, 29]. A few observational studies have suggested a benefit of atosiban (an inhibitor of the hormones oxytocin and vasopressin) around the time of ET. However, a large multicentre RCT reported no difference following the use of uterine relaxants in terms of implantation, pregnancy, miscarriage or ectopic pregnancy rate [30]. Similar studies have looked at the role of beta2-adrenergic agonists (terbutaline and ritodrine) used during controlled ovarian stimulation, with no difference in pregnancy, implantation and miscarriage rates [31]. We await the results of an ongoing double-blinded RCT assessing the effect of nifedipine as a smooth muscle relaxant on improving outcome of ET [32].

22.2 Embryo Transfer

22.2.1 Type of Catheter

There are numerous ET catheters available; they are most commonly ascribed as a soft or firm catheter. The latter is not commonly used in today's practice as firm catheters are traditionally recognized as having poorer IVF outcomes. This is supported by a meta-analysis by the American Society for Reproductive Medicine (ASRM), which demonstrated higher pregnancy rates with soft catheters compared with firm catheters (RR 1.36, 95%CI 1.16–1.59) [33].

There is a significant amount of data comparing differing types of soft catheters with no difference in implantation, pregnancy or live birth rates noted [33]. Therefore, it appears that no soft catheter is superior.

22.2.2 Deposition of the Embryo at Transfer

The exact position to deposit the embryo has yet to be explicitly defined, although data is emerging to show that there may be a better 'area' within the uterus. It is generally accepted that touching the uterine fundus with the catheter tip should be avoided, as this can initiate uterine contractility that may expel the embryo. If this practice takes place, then significantly reduced pregnancy rates will result.

There are a number of good-quality RCTs that have attempted to identify the optimal location of embryo deposit. One RCT examined three different placement locations, 1.0, 1.5 and 2.0 cm from the fundus. Significantly higher implantation rates were observed for embryos deposited between 1.5 and 2.0 cm compared to 1.0 cm, and statistically higher pregnancy rates were reported when the selected location was at 2.0 cm compared with 1.0 cm from the fundus [34]. When placement was compared between <1.0 and 1–1.5 cm, both implantation and pregnancy rates were higher in the latter group [35].

Two additional RCTs compared dividing placement between the upper and lower half of the uterine cavity [36] and compared the 2.0 cm point from the fundus versus the uterine cavity midpoint [37]. However, neither study reported a difference in implantation and pregnancy rates.

All of the available evidence suggests the highest pregnancy rates are associated with embryo placement in the upper or middle third of the uterine cavity, at least 1.0 cm away from the fundus [34, 35, 37–41].

Embryo migration post-ET has also ignited recent research interest. In a novel study, a 3D ultrasound assessment of the embryo 'flash' was assessed at 1, 5 and 60 minutes after ET (remembering that the 'flash' appears as an area of white pixilation on the ultrasound monitor, relating to the air bubble that is injected along with the bolus containing the embryo; Fig. 22.1). Within 60 minutes of the ET, 76.4% of the embryo flashes migrated towards the fundus, 12.4% migrated towards the cervix, and 11.2% remained static. There was no significant association between the embryo position at 1 and 5 minutes. At 60 minutes, the pregnancy and implantation rates with the embryo flashes located less

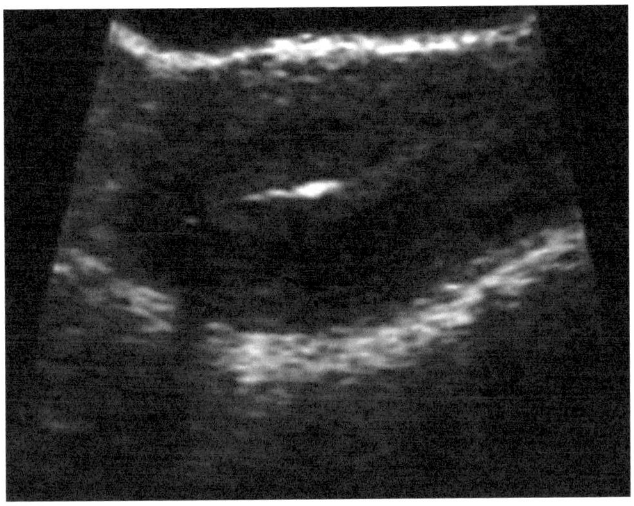

Fig. 22.1 Ultrasound at the time of embryo transfer. The white 'flash' appears as an area of white pixilation on the ultrasound monitor, relating to the air bubble that is injected along with the bolus containing the embryo. (From Allahbadia G, Merchant R, Gahdhi G, et al. Ultrasound-guided ETs or Clinical Touch ETs, in Allahbadia GN, Chillik CF, ed., Human Embryo Transfer. New York: Springer, 2015, with permission)

than 15 mm from the fundus were significantly higher than those located more than 15 mm from the fundus (46.5% vs 32.8% and 25.8 vs 18.2%, respectively, $P < 0.05$). The pregnancy and implantation rates when the embryo flash was seen moving towards the cervix were significantly lower (25% and 15%) compared with those that were static or moving towards the fundus [42].

During ET, it is sometimes necessary to switch from a soft catheter to a more rigid outer catheter to navigate a difficult cervix. This may confer increased bleeding and trauma which may affect success. A study by Abdelmassih et al. demonstrated a significantly lower pregnancy rate (57% vs 43%, $P = 0.0054$) when the outer sheath did not go beyond the internal os at ET [43].

Some practitioners 'pause' the ET procedure once the embryo has been dispelled from the catheter and before withdrawing the catheter from the uterus. It is thought that this slight delay may reduce contractility of the uterus and allow the embryo to settle. Two RCTs have attempted to address this issue, but neither study suggested a difference in pregnancy rates comparing either a 30 second or 60 second delay versus immediate catheter withdrawal [44, 45].

22.2.3 Ultrasound-Guided Embryo Transfer

Traditionally, embryos were transferred into the uterine cavity using the 'clinical touch' method, which was essentially a 'blind' procedure relying on the clinician's tactile sense to judge when the ET catheter was in the correct position. Some clinicians then transferred the embryos at a fixed distance from the external os (~6 cm). However, this approach did not account for the variability in anatomy in terms of cervical and uterine lengths and uterine positions. As such, the 'clinical touch' method was generally considered unreliable, with suboptimal catheter placement in more than half of cases, such that the catheter could indent or embed in the endometrium [44].

The use of ultrasound guidance to facilitate ET is one of the most studied aspects of the overall process. Direct visualization of the catheter is thought to assist navigation of the cervix with less trauma, to allow deposition of the embryo within the uterus to enable a higher pregnancy rate. Patients also tend to feel reassured that they have witnessed the process for themselves. Evidence from a number of RCTs is available, with several meta-analyses confirming improved implantation, clinical or ongoing pregnancy and live birth rates with ultrasound-guided ET compared with 'clinical touch' techniques ([46–51]). The latest meta-analysis involving nearly 6000 patients suggested an ongoing pregnancy/live birth rate (OR 1.47, 95%CI 1.20–1.65) in favour of ultrasound-guided ET versus 'clinical touch' [52]. Other studies have similarly demonstrated improved outcomes with ETs of frozen-thawed embryos and from programmed cycles utilizing donor oocytes [53, 54]. A number of studies have looked at the role of ultrasound guidance with difficult procedures, with two studies suggesting a benefit [54, 55].

Transvaginal ultrasound for ET has also been investigated. The rationale is that this will provide greater clarity of pelvic images, resulting in more accurate embryo placement as well as higher expertise in optimal performance capture [56–59]. However, proven superiority of the technique is lacking, although it is appreciated that the procedure is better tolerated by the patient due to not filling the bladder, albeit with longer procedural times [58, 59]. In the authors' experience, a transvaginal guided ET is a worthwhile technique provided an appropriate ET catheter is used and the resolution of the ultrasound monitor is suitably high. At the time of writing, there is at least one RCT ongoing looking at this specific use along with live 4D ultrasound guidance.

Although Sarevlos et al. found no improvement in pregnancy rates when comparing 2D with 3D ET [60], the further advancement in ultrasound has led Gergely et al. to propose utilizing live transabdominal 4D ultrasound guidance when replacing the embryos in a study involving over 5000 patients. The technique involved mapping the point of maximal implantation potential (the MIP point) utilizing live 3D and 4D imaging of the endometrial cavity. This study showed an increase in the pregnancy rate by 10.04% with a reduction in incidence of ectopic pregnancy from 1.82 to 0.49% [61].

22.2.4 Velocity of Embryo Injection

The velocity with which an embryo is expelled from the catheter and how it affects implantation are difficult to gauge.

Large inter- and intra-observer injection speeds have been noted even in the most experienced practitioners [62]. In the hands of an embryologist, the velocity speeds of syringe expulsion may be more controlled, as they are used to micro-manipulating gametes; however, the authors do not know of any studies to support this suggestion. A number of studies have attempted to standardize injection speeds by using a 'pump-regulated embryo transfer' (PRET) device. Use has also been supported by a RCT which confirmed less variance in embryo positioning when compared with manual injection, as assessed by ultrasound measurement [63].

22.2.5 Retained Embryos After Attempted Embryo Replacement

The rate of embryo retention in the ET catheter has been reported at 7.5%; however, immediate re-transfer of the embryo in the same or a replacement catheter has consistently demonstrated maintenance in implantation and clinical pregnancy rates [64].

22.3 Post-Embryo Transfer

Bed rest is one of the most common practices following ET despite a lack of scientific evidence. The idea postulates that if patients are kept supine post-ET, this position may prevent premature expulsion of the embryos by either lowering uterine contractility or the effect of gravity.

Periods of rest for as long as 24 hours have been suggested, but commonly 20–120 minutes are observed in practice. However, three systematic reviews have failed to demonstrate any benefits comparing immediate ambulation versus bed rest [65–67]. It is worth noting the RCT by Gaikwad et al. that suggested that live birth rates were significantly higher in the 'no bed rest group' compared with the '10 minutes bed rest group' (56.7% versus 41.6%, $p = 0.02$), for the first time suggesting that bed rest might cause relative harm in terms of success rates [68]. The findings were even more striking given that this study was performed in recent years benefiting from more current success rates and population demographics similar to present-day patients undergoing fertility treatments.

In a novel study of over 600 patients, prevention of embryo expulsion following ET was attempted by exerting gentle mechanical pressure on the cervix using the vaginal speculum for a period of 7 minutes after. The clinical pregnancy rates were significantly higher in the study group versus the control group (67% vs 48%; OR 1.39; 95% CI 1.11–1.74); however, it does not appear that this has been widely introduced into practice [69].

22.4 Other Considerations

22.4.1 Transmyometrial Embryo Transfer

A difficult ET has been reported in 5–7% of patients undergoing IVF treatment [70]. All clinicians at some point will encounter an attempted ET where it is impossible to navigate the cervix and gain entry to the uterine cavity, most often due to anatomical/pathological reasons such as congenital cervical stenosis or previous trachelectomy. In these instances, alternative routes of embryo replacement can be considered, principally via the transmyometrial route or replacement of the embryo via the fallopian tubes.

Transmyometrial transfer was first described in 1993 [71], but is very infrequently used due to fear of potential trauma of the endometrium and myometrium which can herald bleeding and junctional zone contractions which are believed to decrease the chance of implantation [72]. In a study comparing very difficult transcervical embryo replacements with transmyometrial replacements, the pregnancy rates were very similar (33% vs 25%, respectively) without any major complications. In fact, the success of both procedures was comparable to national databases comparing routine ET success. The results were also generally in keeping with other studies [71, 73, 74].

The ability of a tubal transfer of embryos to result in a live birth was reported in 1986 with early reports suggesting superiority of zygote intra-fallopian tube (ZIFT) transfer compared with transcervical embryo replacement [75]. However, with the development of softer ET catheters and higher-resolution ultrasound, ZIFT is a procedure that has lost favour. Nowadays, ZIFT and TET (Tubal Embryo Transfer) may be reserved for patients in whom it is not possible to cannulate the cervix.

Most retrospective studies show an increased pregnancy rate with ZIFT [76, 77]. Many non-randomized studies have also reported higher pregnancy rates for tubal transfers of embryos than for intrauterine ETs [78, 79]. In the largest uncontrolled study, the SART registry has consistently demonstrated higher pregnancy rates with tubal transfers than with uterine transfers in the last decade, with a superior clinical pregnancy rate per retrieval (37.5% vs 31.1%) and per transfer (40.1% vs 33.3%) [80].

Whilst ZIFT has commonly been associated with replacement of pronuclear and cleavage-stage embryos, successful pregnancy has been reported following the tubal transfer of blastocysts, although in the authors' experience, transfer of a day 4 embryo seems most appropriate. The risks of the procedure are essentially those of a routine laparoscopy although the hyperstimulated ovaries often make the pelvis more difficult to navigate and may confer a higher risk of intraperitoneal bleeding should any of the haemorrhagic follicles rupture through accidental puncture. Some studies also report a trend towards increased risk of ectopic pregnancies with ZIFT [81, 82]. Mechanical dilatation of the cervix at the time of oocyte retrieval has been described and may result in a technically easier ET; however, it does not always yield good pregnancy rates [83, 84].

22.5 Conclusion

This chapter has discussed the main considerations for ET. Before an ET takes place, a patient may decide to have acupuncture or even anaesthesia or uterine relaxants to help abate any stress. At the time of the procedure, attention should be paid to cleaning the cervix and the choice of the most appropriate catheter to gain access to the uterus with minimal trauma. The advantages of ultrasound guidance have been discussed together with the need to consider the site and speed of embryo deposition. Despite our best efforts, sometimes an embryo may be retained after the ET, yet provided the embryo is quickly and carefully reloaded by the embryologist, then the chances of pregnancy do not appear to be compromised. ET is the final part of the IVF process and is thus a critical step. Providing a careful methodical approach with an experienced team will offer the best chance for people undergoing the ET procedure. Furthermore, future technology, such as 4D ultrasound, may further improve the chance of successful treatment.

References

1. Mains L, Van Voorhis BJ. Optimizing the technique of embryo transfer. Fertil Steril. 2010;94(3):785–90.
2. Brown J, Buckingham K, Abou Setta AM, Buckett W. Ultrasound versus 'clinical touch' for catheter guidance during embryo transfer in women. Cochrane Database Syst Rev. 2010;1:CD006107.
3. Lopez MJ, Garcia D, Rodriguez A, Colodron M, Vassena R, Vernaeve V. Individualized embryo transfer training: timing and performance. Hum Reprod. 2014;29(7):1432–7.
4. Angelini A, Brusco GF, Barnocchi N, El-Danasouri I, Pacchiarotti A, Selman HA. Impact of physician performing embryo transfer on pregnancy rates in an assisted reproductive program. J Assist Reprod Genet. 2006;23(7–8):329–32.
5. Hearns-Stokes RM, Miller BT, Scott L, Creuss D, Chakraborty PK, Segars JH. Pregnancy rates after embryo transfer depend on the provider at embryo transfer. Fertil Steril. 2000;74(1):80–6.
6. Karande VC, Morris R, Chapman C, Rinehart J, Gleicher N. Impact of the "physician factor" on pregnancy rates in a large assisted reproductive technology program: do too many cooks spoil the broth? Fertil Steril. 1999;71(6):1001–9.
7. Toth TL, Lee MS, Bendikson KA, Reindollar RH. Embryo transfer techniques: an American Society for Reproductive Medicine survey of current Society for Assisted Reproductive Technology practices. Fertil Steril. 2017;107(4):1003–11.
8. Domar AD, Meshay I, Kelliher J, Alper M, Powers RD. The impact of acupuncture on in vitro fertilization outcome. Fertil Steril. 2009;91(3):723–6.
9. Paulus WE, Zhang M, Strehler E, El-Danasouri I, Sterzik K. Influence of acupuncture on the pregnancy rate in patients who undergo assisted reproduction therapy. Fertil Steril. 2002;77(4):721–4.
10. Qu F, Zhang D, Chen LT, Wang FF, Pan JX, Zhu YM, et al. Auricular acupressure reduces anxiety levels and improves outcomes of in vitro fertilization: a prospective, randomized and controlled study. Sci Rep. 2014;4:5028.
11. Rashidi BH, Tehrani ES, Hamedani NA, Pirzadeh L. Effects of acupuncture on the outcome of in vitro fertilisation and intracytoplasmic sperm injection in women with polycystic ovarian syndrome. Acupunct Med: J British Medical Acupunct Soc. 2013;31(2):151–6.
12. Westergaard LG, Mao Q, Krogslund M, Sandrini S, Lenz S, Grinsted J. Acupuncture on the day of embryo transfer significantly improves the reproductive outcome in infertile women: a prospective, randomized trial. Fertil Steril. 2006;85(5):1341–6.
13. Manheimer E, Zhang G, Udoff L, Haramati A, Langenberg P, Berman BM, et al. Effects of acupuncture on rates of pregnancy and live birth among women undergoing in vitro fertilisation: systematic review and meta-analysis. BMJ. 2008;336(7643):545–9.
14. Andersen D, Lossl K, Nyboe Andersen A, Furbringer J, Bach H, Simonsen J, et al. Acupuncture on the day of embryo transfer: a randomized controlled trial of 635 patients. Reprod Biomed Online. 2010;21(3):366–72.
15. Craig LB, Rubin LE, Peck JD, Anderson M, Marshall LA, Soules MR. Acupuncture performed before and after embryo transfer: a randomized controlled trial. J Reprod Med. 2014;59(5–6):313–20.
16. Madaschi C, Braga DP, Figueira Rde C, Iaconelli A Jr, Borges E Jr. Effect of acupuncture on assisted reproduction treatment outcomes. Acupunct Med: J British Med Acupunct Soc. 2010;28(4):180–4.
17. Moy I, Milad MP, Barnes R, Confino E, Kazer RR, Zhang X. Randomized controlled trial: effects of acupuncture on pregnancy rates in women undergoing in vitro fertilization. Fertil Steril. 2011;95(2):583–7.
18. Smith C, Coyle M, Norman RJ. Influence of acupuncture stimulation on pregnancy rates for women undergoing embryo transfer. Fertil Steril. 2006;85(5):1352–8.
19. Ethics Committee of the American Society for Reproductive Medicine. Transferring embryos with genetic anomalies detected in preimplantation testing: an ethics committee opinion. Fertil Steril. 2017;107(5):1130–5.
20. So EW, Ng EH, Wong YY, Lau EY, Yeung WS, Ho PC. A randomized double blind comparison of real and placebo acupuncture in IVF treatment. Hum Reprod. 2009;24(2):341–8.
21. So EW, Ng EH, Wong YY, Yeung WS, Ho PC. Acupuncture for frozen-thawed embryo transfer cycles: a double-blind randomized controlled trial. Reprod Biomed Online. 2010;20(6):814–21.
22. Cheong YC, Dix S, Hung Yu Ng E, Ledger WL, Farquhar C. Acupuncture and assisted reproductive technology. Cochrane Database Syst Rev. 2013;7:CD006920.
23. Saravelos SH, Wong AW, Kong GW, Huang J, Klitzman R, Li TC. Pain during embryo transfer is independently associated with clinical pregnancy in fresh/frozen assisted reproductive technology cycles. J Obstet Gynaecol Res. 2016;42(6):684–93.
24. van der Ven HH, Jeyendran RS, Al-Hasani S, Tunnerhoff A, Hoebbel K, Diedrich K, et al. Glass wool column filtration of human semen: relation to swim-up procedure and outcome of IVF. Hum Reprod. 1988;3(1):85–8.
25. Kroon B, Hart RJ, Wong BM, Ford E, Yazdani A. Antibiotics prior to embryo transfer in ART. Cochrane Database Syst Rev. 2012;3:CD008995.

26. Moini A, Kiani K, Bahmanabadi A, Akhoond M, Akhlaghi A. Improvement in pregnancy rate by removal of cervical discharge prior to embryo transfer in ICSI cycles: a randomised clinical trial. Aust N Z J Obstet Gynaecol. 2011;51(4):315–20.
27. Eskandar MA, Abou-Setta AM, El-Amin M, Almushait MA, Sobande AA. Removal of cervical mucus prior to embryo transfer improves pregnancy rates in women undergoing assisted reproduction. Reprod Biomed Online. 2007;14(3):308–13.
28. Montoya-Botero P, Polyzos NP. The endometrium during and after ovarian hyperstimulation and the role of segmentation of infertility treatment. Best Pract Res Clin Endocrinol Metab. 2018;33(1):61–75.
29. Zhu L, Che HS, Xiao L, Li YP. Uterine peristalsis before embryo transfer affects the chance of clinical pregnancy in fresh and frozen-thawed embryo transfer cycles. Hum Reprod. 2014;29:1238–43.
30. Ng EH, Li RH, Chen L, Lan VT, Tuong HM, Quan S. A randomized double blind comparison of atosiban in patients undergoing IVF treatment. Hum Reprod. 2014;29(12):2687–94.
31. Pinheiro OL, Cavagna M, Baruffi RL, Mauri AL, Petersen C, Franco JG Jr. Administration of beta2-adrenergic agonists during the peri-implantation period does not improve implantation or pregnancy rates in intracytoplasmic sperm injection (ICSI) cycles. J Assist Reprod Genet. 2003;20(12):513–6.
32. Ng KK, Rozen G, Stewart T, Agresta F, Polyakov A. A double-blinded, randomized, placebo-controlled trial assessing the effects of nifedipine on embryo transfer: study protocol. Medicine (Baltimore). 2017;96(51):e9194.
33. Practice Committee of the American Society for Reproductive Medicine. Performing the embryo transfer: a guideline. Fertil Steril. 2017;107(4):882–96.
34. Coroleu B, Barri PN, Carreras O, Martinez F, Parriego M, Hereter L, et al. The influence of the depth of embryo replacement into the uterine cavity on implantation rates after IVF: a controlled, ultrasound-guided study. Hum Reprod. 2002;17(2):341–6.
35. Pacchiarotti A, Mohamed MA, Micara G, Tranquilli D, Linari A, Espinola SM, et al. The impact of the depth of embryo replacement on IVF outcome. J Assist Reprod Genet. 2007;24(5):189–93.
36. Franco JG Jr, Martins AM, Baruffi RL, Mauri AL, Petersen CG, Felipe V, et al. Best site for embryo transfer: the upper or lower half of endometrial cavity? Hum Reprod. 2004;19(8):1785–90.
37. Kwon H, Choi DH, Kim EK. Absolute position versus relative position in embryo transfer: a randomized controlled trial. Reprod Biol Endocrinol. 2015;13:78.
38. Oliveira JB, Martins AM, Baruffi RL, Mauri AL, Petersen CG, Felipe V, et al. Increased implantation and pregnancy rates obtained by placing the tip of the transfer catheter in the central area of the endometrial cavity. Reprod Biomed Online. 2004;9(4):435–41.
39. Cavagna M, Contart P, Petersen CG, Mauri AL, Martins AM, Baruffi RL, et al. Implantation sites after embryo transfer into the central area of the uterine cavity. Reprod Biomed Online. 2006;13(4):541–6.
40. Tiras B, Polat M, Korucuoglu U, Zeyneloglu HB, Yarali H. Impact of embryo replacement depth on in vitro fertilization and embryo transfer outcomes. Fertil Steril. 2010;94(4):1341–5.
41. Cenksoy PO, Ficicioglu C, Yesiladali M, Akcin OA, Kaspar C. The importance of the length of uterine cavity, the position of the tip of the inner catheter and the distance between the fundal endometrial surface and the air bubbles as determinants of the pregnancy rate in IVF cycles. Eur J Obstet Gynecol Reprod Biol. 2014;172:46–50.
42. Saravelos SH, Wong AW, Chan CP, Kong GW, Cheung LP, Chung CH, et al. Assessment of the embryo flash position and migration with 3D ultrasound within 60 min of embryo transfer. Hum Reprod. 2016;31(3):591–6.
43. Abdelmassih VG, Neme RM, Dozortsev D, Abdelmassih S, Diamond MP, Abdelmassih R. Location of the embryo-transfer catheter guide before the internal uterine os improves the outcome of in vitro fertilization. Fertil Steril. 2007;88(2):499–503.
44. Martinez F, Coroleu B, Parriego M, Carreras O, Belil I, Parera N, et al. Ultrasound-guided embryo transfer: immediate withdrawal of the catheter versus a 30 second wait. Hum Reprod. 2001;16(5):871–4.
45. Sroga JM, Montville CP, Aubuchon M, Williams DB, Thomas MA. Effect of delayed versus immediate embryo transfer catheter removal on pregnancy outcomes during fresh cycles. Fertil Steril. 2010;93(6):2088–90.
46. Woolcott R, Stanger J. Potentially important variables identified by transvaginal ultrasound-guided embryo transfer. Hum Reprod. 1997;12(5):963–6.
47. Sallam HN, Sadek SS. Ultrasound-guided embryo transfer: a meta-analysis of randomized controlled trials. Fertil Steril. 2003;80(4):1042–6.
48. Abou-Setta AM, Mansour RT, Al-Inany HG, Aboulghar MM, Aboulghar MA, Serour GI. Among women undergoing embryo transfer, is the probability of pregnancy and live birth improved with ultrasound guidance over clinical touch alone? A systemic review and meta-analysis of prospective randomized trials. Fertil Steril. 2007;88(2):333–41.
49. Buckett WM. A meta-analysis of ultrasound-guided versus clinical touch embryo transfer. Fertil Steril. 2003;80(4):1037–41.
50. Teixeira DM, Dassuncao LA, Vieira CV, Barbosa MA, Coelho Neto MA, Nastri CO, et al. Ultrasound guidance during embryo transfer: a systematic review and meta-analysis of randomized controlled trials. Ultrasound Obstet Gynecol. 2015;45(2):139–48.
51. Brown J, Buckingham K, Buckett W, Abou-Setta AM. Ultrasound versus 'clinical touch' for catheter guidance during embryo transfer in women. Cochrane Database Syst Rev. 2016;3:CD006107.
52. Barrie A, Homburg R, McDowell G, Brown J, Kingsland C, Troup S. Examining the efficacy of six published time-lapse imaging embryo selection algorithms to predict implantation to demonstrate the need for the development of specific, in-house morphokinetic selection algorithms. Fertil Steril. 2017;107(3):613–21.
53. Coroleu B, Barri PN, Carreras O, Martinez F, Veiga A, Balasch J. The usefulness of ultrasound guidance in frozen-thawed embryo transfer: a prospective randomized clinical trial. Hum Reprod. 2002;17(11):2885–90.
54. Lindheim SR, Cohen MA, Sauer MV. Ultrasound guided embryo transfer significantly improves pregnancy rates in women undergoing oocyte donation. Int J Gynaecol Obstet. 1999;66(3):281–4.
55. Kan AK, Abdalla HI, Gafar AH, Nappi L, Ogunyemi BO, Thomas A, et al. Embryo transfer: ultrasound-guided versus clinical touch. Hum Reprod. 1999;14(5):1259–61.
56. Anderson RE, Nugent NL, Gregg AT, Nunn SL, Behr BR. Transvaginal ultrasound-guided embryo transfer improves outcome in patients with previous failed in vitro fertilization cycles. Fertil Steril. 2002;77(4):769–75.
57. Kojima K, Nomiyama M, Kumamoto T, Matsumoto Y, Iwasaka T. Transvaginal ultrasound-guided embryo transfer improves pregnancy and implantation rates after IVF. Hum Reprod. 2001;16(12):2578–82.
58. Bodri D, Colodron M, Garcia D, Obradors A, Vernaeve V, Coll O. Transvaginal versus transabdominal ultrasound guidance for embryo transfer in donor oocyte recipients: a randomized clinical trial. Fertil Steril. 2011;95(7):2263-8–2268.e1.
59. Revelli A, Rovei V, Dalmasso P, Gennarelli G, Racca C, Evangelista F, et al. Large randomized trial comparing transabdominal ultrasound-guided embryo transfer with a technique based on uterine length measurement before embryo transfer. Ultrasound Obstet Gynecol. 2016;48(3):289–95.
60. Saravelos SH, Kong GW, Chung JP, Mak JS, Chung CH, Cheung LP, et al. A prospective randomized controlled trial of 3D versus

2D ultrasound-guided embryo transfer in women undergoing ART treatment. Hum Reprod. 2016;31(10):2255–60.
61. Gergely R. 3D/4D Ultrasound guided embryo transfer targeting maximal implantation potential (MIP) point increases pregnancy rate, reduces complications. Reprod Med Online. 2010;20(S3 Suppl):S7-S.
62. Groeneveld E, de Leeuw B, Vergouw CG, Visser OW, Lambers MJ, Heymans MW, et al. Standardization of catheter load speed during embryo transfer: comparison of manual and pump-regulated embryo transfer. Reprod Biomed Online. 2012;24(2): 163–9.
63. Caanen MR, van der Houwen LE, Schats R, Vergouw CG, de Leeuw B, Lambers MJ, et al. Embryo transfer with controlled injection speed to increase pregnancy rates: a randomized controlled trial. Gynecol Obstet Investig. 2016;81(5):394–404.
64. Oraif A, Hollet-Caines J, Feyles V, Rebel M, Abduljabar H. Do multiple attempts at embryo transfer affect clinical pregnancy rates? J Obstet Gynaecol Can. 2014;36(5):406–7.
65. Botta G, Grudzinskas G. Is a prolonged bed rest following embryo transfer useful? Hum Reprod. 1997;12(11):2489–92.
66. Amarin ZO, Obeidat BR. Bed rest versus free mobilisation following embryo transfer: a prospective randomised study. BJOG. 2004;111(11):1273–6.
67. Purcell KJ, Schembri M, Telles TL, Fujimoto VY, Cedars MI. Bed rest after embryo transfer: a randomized controlled trial. Fertil Steril. 2007;87(6):1322–6.
68. Gaikwad S, Garrido N, Cobo A, Pellicer A, Remohi J. Bed rest after embryo transfer negatively affects in vitro fertilization: a randomized controlled clinical trial. Fertil Steril. 2013;100(3): 729–35.
69. Mansour R. Minimizing embryo expulsion after embryo transfer: a randomized controlled study. Hum Reprod. 2005;20(1):170–4.
70. Wood C, McMaster R, Rennie G, Trounson A, Leeton J. Factors influencing pregnancy rates following in vitro fertilization and embryo transfer. Fertil Steril. 1985;43(2):245–50.
71. Kato O, Takatsuka R, Asch RH. Transvaginal-transmyometrial embryo transfer: the Towako method; experiences of 104 cases. Fertil Steril. 1993;59(1):51–3.
72. Biervliet FP, Lesny P, Maguiness SD, Robinson J, Killick SR. Transmyometrial embryo transfer and junctional zone contractions. Hum Reprod. 2002;17(2):347–50.
73. Ghazzawi IM, Al-Hasani S, Karaki R, Souso S. Transfer technique and catheter choice influence the incidence of transcervical embryo expulsion and the outcome of IVF. Hum Reprod. 1999;14(3):677–82.
74. Khairy M, Shah H, Rajkhowa M. Transmyometrial versus very difficult transcervical embryo transfer: efficacy and safety. Reprod Biomed Online. 2016;32(5):513–7.
75. Devroey P, Braeckmans P, Smitz J, Van Waesberghe L, Wisanto A, Van Steirteghem A, et al. Pregnancy after translaparoscopic zygote intrafallopian transfer in a patient with sperm antibodies. Lancet. 1986;1(8493):1329.
76. Hammitt DG, Syrop CH, Hahn SJ, Walker DL, Butkowski CR, Donovan JF. Comparison of concurrent pregnancy rates for in-vitro fertilization--embryo transfer, pronuclear stage embryo transfer and gamete intra-fallopian transfer. Hum Reprod. 1990;5(8):947–54.
77. Pool TB, Ellsworth LR, Garza JR, Martin JE, Miller SS, Atiee SH. Zygote intrafallopian transfer as a treatment for nontubal infertility: a 2-year study. Fertil Steril. 1990;54(3):482–8.
78. Boldt J, Schnarr P, Ajamie A, Ketner J, Bonaventura L, Colver R, et al. Success rates following intracytoplasmic sperm injection are improved by using ZIFT vs IVF for embryo transfer. J Assist Reprod Genet. 1996;13(10):782–5.
79. Hurst BS, Tucker KE, Guadagnoli S, Awoniyi CA, Schlaff WD. Transcervical gamete and zygote intrafallopian transfer. Does it enhance pregnancy rates in an assisted reproduction program? J Reprod Med. 1996;41(11):867–70.
80. No Authors. Assisted reproductive technology in the United States 1996 results generated from the American society for reproductive medicine/society for assisted reproductive technology registry. Fertil Steril. 1999;71(5):798–807.
81. Habana AE, Palter SF. Is tubal embryo transfer of any value? A meta-analysis and comparison with the Society for Assisted Reproductive Technology database. Fertil Steril. 2001;76(2):286–93.
82. Clayton HB, Schieve LA, Peterson HB, Jamieson DJ, Reynolds MA, Wright VC. Ectopic pregnancy risk with assisted reproductive technology procedures. Obstet Gynecol. 2006;107(3):595–604.
83. Groutz A, Lessing JB, Wolf Y, Azem F, Yovel I, Amit A. Comparison of transmyometrial and transcervical embryo transfer in patients with previously failed in vitro fertilization-embryo transfer cycles and/or cervical stenosis. Fertil Steril. 1997;67(6):1073–6.
84. Groutz A, Lessing JB, Wolf Y, Yovel I, Azem F, Amit A. Cervical dilatation during ovum pick-up in patients with cervical stenosis: effect on pregnancy outcome in an in vitro fertilization-embryo transfer program. Fertil Steril. 1997;67(5):909–11.

Part III

Medically Assisted Reproduction Under Special Circumstances

23 Surgical Sperm Retrieval and MicroTESE

Ivor Cullen and Asıf Muneer

Surgical sperm retrieval (SSR) techniques are surgical methods that are used to retrieve mature spermatozoa from the epididymides or testicles of azoospermic men seeking fertility treatment using intracytoplasmic sperm injection (ICSI). The sperm can either be used fresh or be cryopreserved for use in future ICSI cycles [1]. The use of non-ejaculated sperm combined with ICSI has now become an established procedure for couples where the male is azoospermic in order to father their own biological offspring [2].

Nowadays, microdissection testicular sperm extraction (microTESE) allows successful assisted reproduction treatments (ART) for many previously untreatable patients with non-obstructive azoospermia.

In contrast to obstructive azoospermia (OA), where there is an obstruction within the reproductive tract, non-obstructive azoospermia (NOA) is characterized by a complete absence of spermatozoa in semen because of minimal or no spermatogenesis. Possible aetiologies include genetic disorders such as sex chromosome abnormalities, translocation and microdeletions of the Y-chromosome (AZFa, b, c), cryptorchidism, testicular torsion, radiotherapy and exposure to toxins [3]. Approximately 1% of all men, 60% of all azoospermic men and 10% of infertile men are affected by testicular failure as a result of NOA [4, 5]. The histologic patterns associated with NOA include Sertoli cell-only syndrome (SCOS), maturation arrest (MA), hypospermatogenesis and sclera-hyalinosis.

Different options are available for obtaining viable spermatozoa in these patients: fine needle aspiration (FNA), conventional testicular sperm extraction (cTESE) and microdissection TESE (microTESE). Testicular spermatozoa can be retrieved in some NOA men because of the existence of isolated foci of active spermatogenesis.

23.1 History

In 1999, Schlegel et al. [6] reported on a novel microsurgical technique to perform TESE, known as microTESE. Prior to this, a variety of surgical approaches had been used to undertake the sperm retrieval. The most common of these is a conventional testicular sperm extraction (cTESE), which is a random procedure whereby small samples of testicular tissue are obtained from the testis via multiple stab incisions through the tunica albuginea. cTESE was described for obstructive azoospermia by Schoysman et al. [7] as well as Craft et al. [8] and then later used for NOA (Silber et al. [9] and Devroey et al. [10]).

Schlegel's concept was simple: seminiferous tubules with Sertoli cells only (SCO) are deemed to be thinner than tubules containing spermatogenic cells. The difference between the larger and smaller tubules is not visible without optical magnification. With microTESE, the tunica albuginea is opened, followed by an examination of the testicular tissue at 20–25× magnification using an operating microscope. This allows identification of the larger and more opaque tubules which are more likely to contain active spermatogenesis. Another benefit of microTESE is that the technique allows the opportunity to better identify sub-tunical vessels, thereby reducing the risk of testicular devascularization.

In Schlegel's hands, this technique of microTESE resulted in an improvement of sperm retrieval rates from 45% to 63% [11].

I. Cullen
University Hospital Waterford, Waterford, Ireland

Blackrock Clinic, Dublin, Ireland

A. Muneer (✉)
Department of Urology and NIHR Biomedical Research Centre, University College London Hospitals NHS Foundation Trust, London, UK

Division of Surgery and Interventional Science, University College London, London, UK
e-mail: asif.muneer@nhs.net

G. N. Allahbadia et al. (eds.), *Textbook of Assisted Reproduction*, https://doi.org/10.1007/978-981-15-2377-9_23

23.2 MicroTESE Versus Conventional TESE

Conventional TESE (cTESE) consists of random stab incisions through the tunica albuginea of the testis followed by multiple sampling of extruded seminiferous tubules. This can result in atrophy and devascularization of the surrounding testicular tissue. This effect, together with the intratesticular bleeding and parenchymal fibrosis, can result in impaired spermatogenesis and compromise the endocrine function of the testis.

MicroTESE is more selective and removes much smaller amounts of testicular tissue. This is important for testicular function, particularly if a man already has testicles of smaller than normal size, associated with infertility. In addition, the identification of avascular regions in the tunica albuginea minimizes the chance of vascular injury. Multifocal sampling from different regions of the testicle may increase the possibility of detecting spermatozoa when compared with cTESE.

It is well established that men with NOA can still have some focal areas of spermatogenesis within the testicles, whereas others have complete absence of germ cells and/or full block of maturation of spermatozoa within the tubules. Contrary to expectations, a histological diagnosis of Sertoli cell-only syndrome (SCOS) may indeed still be associated with areas of focal spermatogenesis [12].

MicroTESE has advantages and disadvantages compared with other open surgical methods. Implementation of microTESE in a clinical ART setting requires the availability of an operating room equipped with a top-quality operating microscope located next door to the IVF laboratory. Moreover, microTESE is a labour-intensive procedure that requires microsurgical expertise as well as urological training in scrotal and testicular surgery.

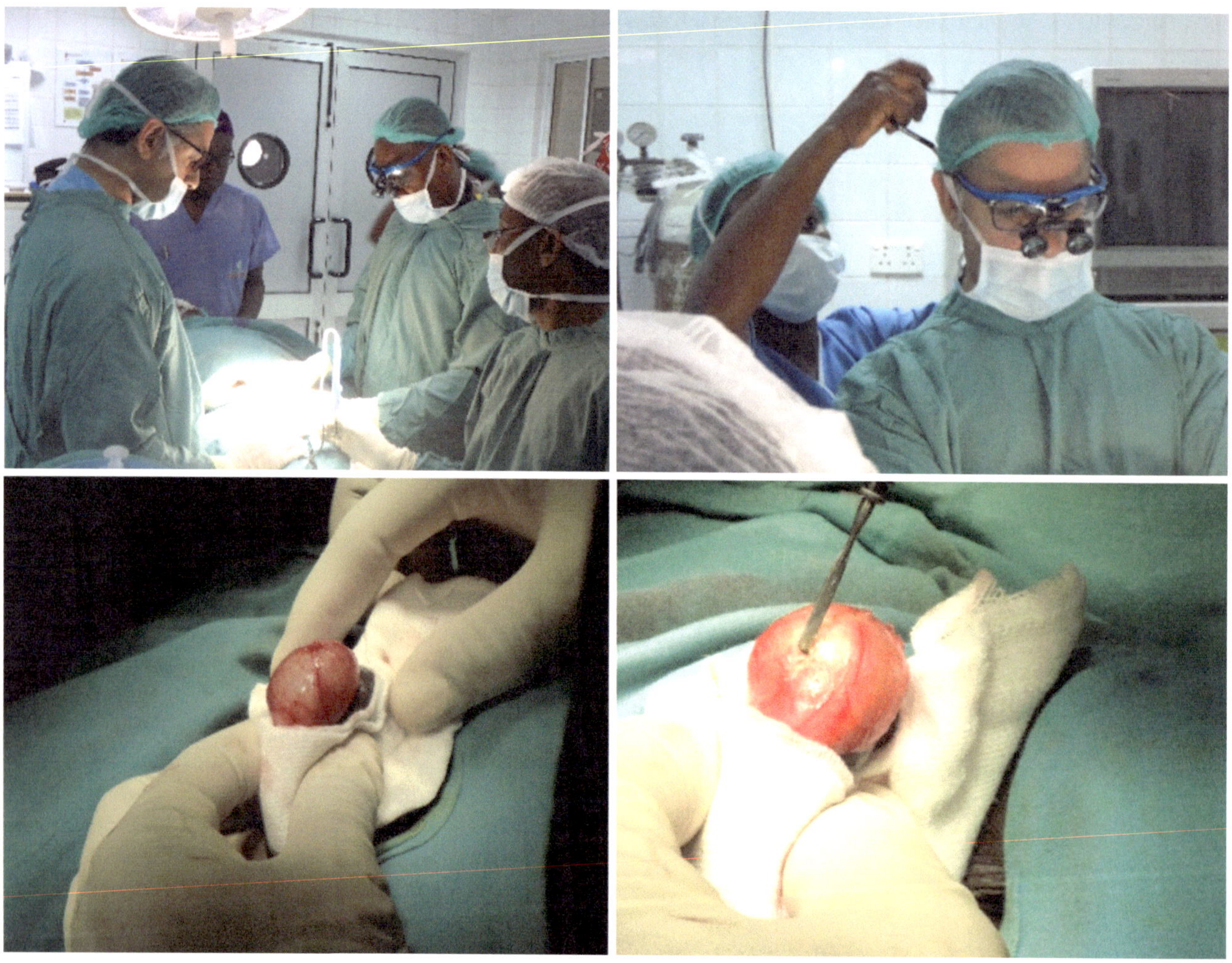

Fig. 23.1 The microTESE operation involves using a midline raphe incision in the scrotum approximately 3–5 cm in length, depending on the size of the testicles (Courtesy of the Lister Hospital and Fertility Centre, Accra, Ghana)

23.3 Technical Aspects

MicroTESE should commence on the more favourable testis/larger volume testicle if this is applicable. The surgeon moves to the contralateral testis in all cases of negative sperm retrieval, in order to maximize the chance of success.

The microTESE operation involves using a midline raphe incision in the scrotum approximately 3–5 cm in length, depending on the size of the testicles. This provides access into the right and left hemiscrotum to deliver each testicle through the incision. The testis and its overlying layers are then incised, and the tunica vaginalis is opened to deliver the testicle (Figs. 23.1 and 23.2).

A single equatorial incision covering approximately 270° of the circumference of each testicle is performed parallel to the tunical blood vessels using 6–8X magnification. A couple of haemostats are then attached to the tunica which allows the testicular parenchyma to be exposed.

A small testicular biopsy is taken and placed into Bouin's solution so that a pathological diagnosis can be obtained as well as confirmation of azoospermia should no sperm are successfully retrieved. A 5mm^3 biopsy yields a sufficient number of tubules (<50 cross sections) to perform an adequate quantitative analysis for performing a Johnsen's score [13] to evaluate spermatogenesis and also to rule out any concomitant neoplasia or pre-malignant intratubular germ cell neoplasia (ITGCN).

Sertoli cell-only syndrome (SCOS) is characterized by tubules lined with Sertoli cells and devoid of germ cells. Maturation arrest (MA) is defined as an absence of mature spermatozoa, despite normal early stages of spermatogenesis. Normal spermatogenesis is defined as the presence of tubules exhibiting all stages of spermatogenesis up to mature sperm.

Dissection of the testicular parenchyma is undertaken at ×16–25 magnification searching for the best seminiferous tubules (STs), which are more likely to contain germ cells, as originally described by Schlegel. Microsurgical dissection between the lobules in an avascular plane allows most of the regions in the testicle to be examined.

If enlarged tubules are not seen, or the tubules appear homogenous within a lobule, then microsurgical biopsies of the lobules can be performed and examined for the presence of sperm within the theatre setting. This can be repeated until each testicle has been sampled.

The tunica albuginea is closed using continuous or interrupted sutures (4/0 or 5/0). Following haemostasis, the tunica vaginalis is then closed in a running fashion using absorbable sutures followed by a layered closure of the dartos and skin.

A spermatic cord nerve block is a useful adjunct to ensure post-operative analgesia.

Patients are generally able to be discharged home on the same day of surgery. Bed rest and application of ice packs over the scrotum are recommended for the first 48 hours. Patients should be instructed to remove the scrotal dressing after 24 hours.

The use of a scrotal support is recommended for 72 hours post-operatively. Patients should be instructed to abstain from sports activities, heavy lifting and sexual intercourse for 21 days and need to be informed of the likelihood of scrotal swelling, ecchymosis at the wound site and mild discomfort that usually subsides within approximately 1 week. Scrotal ultrasound is indicated in cases of complications.

Sterile handling conditions under a laminar flow cabinet must be used during all laboratory steps. MicroTESE fragments are examined under stereomicroscopy [14]. Firstly, a 23-gauge needled-tuberculin syringe can be used to remove

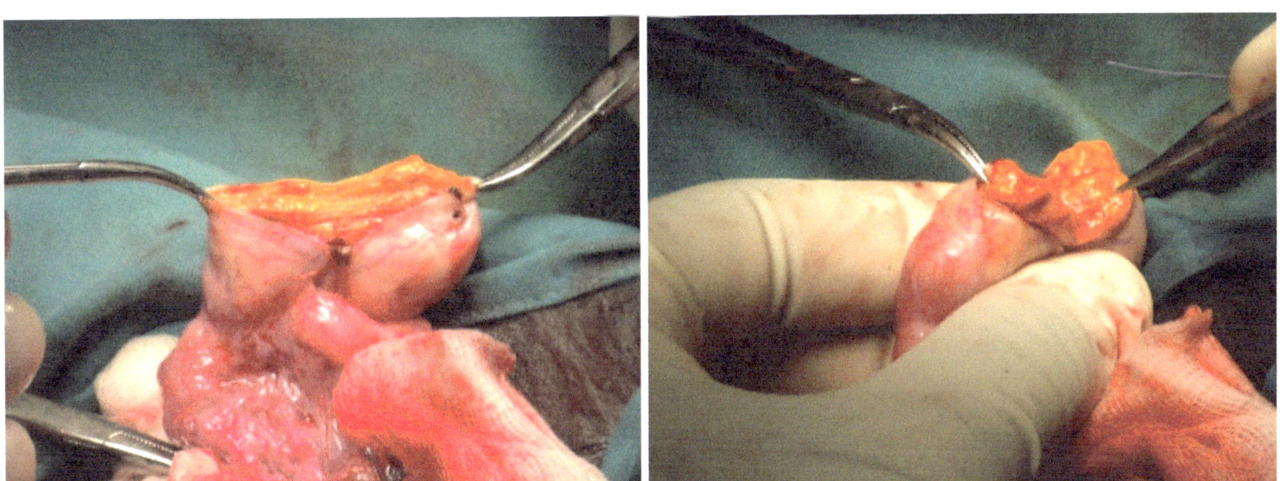

Fig. 23.2 The testis and its overlying layers are incised and the tunica vaginalis is opened to deliver the testicle (Courtesy of the Lister Hospital and Fertility Centre, Accra, Ghana)

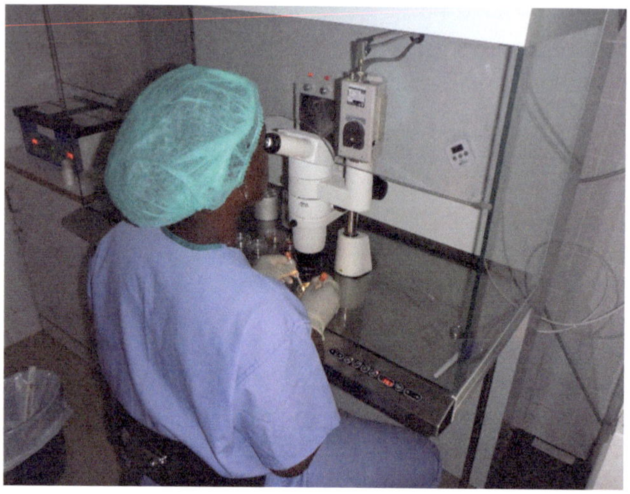

Fig. 23.3 Processing the tubules prior to determining tubule diameter using a digital imaging system (Courtesy of the Lister Hospital and Fertility Centre, Accra, Ghana)

any blood clots from the tissue and to disperse the STs [15]. Then the specimens are transferred to dishes containing fresh sperm handling buffered culture medium where they are dissected and 'minced' in order to release sperm into the medium. The medium can then be examined using an inverted microscope.

The diameter of the tubules may be determined using a digital imaging system (CIVA, Hamilton Thorne, USA) attached to the inverted microscope. For this, the operator captures the images of individual ST at ×100 magnification (Fig. 23.3).

Measurements are taken in microns from edge to edge of the most dilated tubules, and the larger ones from each patient are considered for analysis. Subsequently, mechanical mincing of the STs is carried out using two needled-tuberculin syringes (one is used to hold the tubules in place at the bottom of the dish, while the other squeezes and opens the tubules).

This step is repeated until no intact tubules are seen. Homogenates are then examined on a warm-staged inverted microscope at ×200–400 magnification to confirm the presence of sperm. If multiple microTESE specimens are received, all described steps are repeated.

It is recommended that a minimum of two laboratory technicians/embryologists are involved in processing the microTESE specimens: one to mince the tubules under stereomicroscopy and the other to search for spermatozoa under the inverted microscope.

Optimally, the surgeon can then be informed when sperm are found on initial examination. If sperm are not observed after initial microscopic examination, extensive mechanical processing and searching must be undertaken. For this, cell suspensions are diluted with sperm medium and centrifuged at ×300 g for 7 minutes. The supernatants are discarded, and the pellets should be resuspended in approximately 0.2 mL of sperm handling buffered culture medium. It is beneficial for the culture medium temperature to be maintained in the range of 32–37 °C during sperm handling and processing to optimize sperm motility.

23.4 Success Rates for Sperm Retrieval

Within the literature, sperm retrieval rates for microTESE in cases of NOA range from 35% to 77% [15–18]. More importantly, controlled series have demonstrated that microTESE performs better than conventional sperm extraction (cTESE) or percutaneous aspirations (TESA), in terms of obtaining viable sperm (Table 23.1).

Okada et al. [19] performed a retrospective comparative study of patients undergoing conventional TESE and micro-TESE. Forty-six patients, including 22 patients with OA and 24 with NOA, underwent conventional TESE. Another 100 patients, including 26 with OA and 74 with NOA, underwent microTESE. Conventional TESE was performed via three small 5 mm incisions in the tunica albuginea. Sperm recovery rates were compared, as were complication rates assessed by ultrasonographic and endocrinological evaluations. For the OA cases, the sperm recovery rate was 100% for each procedure, as expected. However, for the NOA cases, sperm were recovered in 16.7 and 44.6% by conventional and microTESE, respectively ($p = 0.0271$).

Deruyver et al. [20] performed a systematic review to compare the efficacy and safety of microTESE with cTESE in men with NOA. The primary outcome was sperm retrieval rate (SRR). Secondary outcomes were clinical predictors of sperm retrieval as well as complication rate. A total of seven studies were included in the final analysis. Overall, the SRR was significantly higher in the microTESE group (42.9–63%) compared with the cTESE group (16.7–45%) in five of these studies. A sub-analysis of the SRR according to testicular histology was available in four of the selected articles. MicroTESE in men with SCOS and hypospermatogenesis carried a small but significant more favourable outcome according to, respectively, two and one of the studies. There was a variable correlation of serum FSH and testicular volume with a positive outcome. However, fewer complications were observed on ultrasound examination after microTESE.

To date, there are still no absolute preoperative predictive factors for successful SRR in NOA. FSH and testosterone levels, together with testes volume, reflect global testicular

Table 23.1 Comparison of sperm retrieval rates (SRRs)

Authors	Overall SRR (%) cTESE (*n*) microTESE (*n*)	SRR in SCO (%) cTESE (*n*) microTESE (*n*)	SRR in maturation arrest (%) cTESE (*n*) microTESE (*n*)	SRR in hypospermatogenesis (%) cTESE (*n*) microTESE (*n*)
Schlegel (1999)	45 ($n = 22$) 63 ($n = 27$)			
Amer et al. (2000)	30 ($n = 100$ testes) 47 ($n = 100$ testes)[a]			
Okada et al. (2002)	16.7 ($n = 24$) 44.6 ($n = 74$)[a]	6.3 ($n = 16$) 33.9 ($n = 56$)[a]	37.5 ($n = 8$) 75 ($n = 12$)	
Tsujimura et al. (2002)	35.1 ($n = 37$) 42.9 ($n = 56$)	13 ($n = 23$) 22.5 ($n = 40$)	0 ($n = 1$) 75 ($n = 4$)	76.9 ($n = 13$) 100 ($n = 12$)
Ramasamy et al. (2005)	32 ($n = 83$) 57 ($n = 460$)[a]	29 ($n = 24$) 41 ($n = 237$)	20 ($n = 10$) 44 ($n = 62$)	50 ($n = 14$) 81 ($n = 73$)[a]
Ghalayini et al. (2011)	38.2 ($n = 68$) 56.9 ($n = 65$)[a]	6.2 ($n = 32$) 26.9 ($n = 26$)[a]	27.3 ($n = 11$) 36.4 ($n = 11$)	84 ($n = 25$) 92.9 ($n = 28$)
Mean SRR weighed by sample size	33 54	14 37	27 49	73 85

From Deruyver Y, Vanderschueren D, Van der Aa F. Outcome of microdissection TESE compared with conventional TESE in non-obstructive azoospermia: a systematic review. Andrology. 2013;2(1):20–24, with permission

[a]Statistically significant ($p < 0.05$)

function and not the presence of a site of normal sperm production within a dysfunctional testis [21]. By contrast, testicular histopathology results confer a better prognostic value compared with the aforesaid markers. SRRs by microTESE are significantly higher in hypospermatogenesis (93%) compared with MA (64%) and SCOS (20%) [22]. This observation indicates that sperm production is distributed in a heterogeneous pattern within the testis and histologic assessment of a single testicular fragment is limited in its ability to determine the presence of rare foci of sperm production in NOA [22].

Greater tubule diameter in cases of successful retrievals has been corroborated by a report in which the mean maximal diameter of sperm-containing ST was significantly higher than non-sperm-containing tubules (298 vs. 225 microns, $P > 0.0001$) [23]. This study showed that the best sensitivity and specificity for a positive result on SR were obtained at a cut-off level of 250 microns [23].

Although in some small series and anecdotal reports, elevated FSH levels are postulated to reduce successful outcome for microTESE procedures, it is questionable whether serum FSH levels are really predictive for successful sperm retrieval. A large retrospective study by Ramasamy et al. [21] demonstrated that the chances of sperm retrieval are just as common for NOA men with elevated FSH levels than for men with lower FSH levels.

Success at obtaining testicular sperm by microTESE has shown to be comparable among different aetiologies such as cryptorchidism, varicocele, orchitis, genetic, radio-/chemotherapy and idiopathic [24–26].

Medical therapy to enhance endogenous testosterone levels prior to SR has been suggested to optimize the retrieval rates in men with NOA [27]. The rationale of such intervention relies on the fact that most men with NOA have testes of reduced volume, which is associated with decreased testosterone production and hypogonadism.

Adequate levels of intratesticular androgenic bioactivity are essential to sustain spermatogenesis that might be compromised in NOA [28]. Indeed, aromatase inhibitors, clomiphene citrate and hCG have been successfully used to boost testosterone production in men with NOA and nonmosaic Klinefelter syndrome (KS). Indeed, it has been shown that SR rates were increased by 1.4-fold in KS men who responded to medical therapy [29].

Despite being greatly anticipated in men with NOA who will be halted in their attempt to conceive due to the absence of testicular sperm on retrieval, medical treatment is still under investigation [28]. In a recent retrospective study on the role of optimizing testosterone before microTESE in men with NOA, Reifsnyder et al. evaluated 736 individuals and concluded that hormonal therapy had no impact on retrieval rate [27]. As such, a definitive conclusion cannot yet be drawn on the role of medical therapy in NOA. This dilemma will only be resolved if randomized trials are undertaken, for different subsets of men with NOA in whom intratesticular androgenic activity is measured.

23.5 Sperm Retrieval Rates After Failed TESE

MicroTESE has been shown to be successful in approximately one-third of previous failed retrievals by other methods. Tsujimura and colleagues reported a SRR of 45% obtained with salvage microTESE performed after previous failed conventional TESE [30].

Similarly Kalsi et al. looked at 58 men with NOA who had previously undergone either single/multiple TESE or TESA with no sperm found [31]. Spermatozoa were successfully retrieved in 27 men by microTESE (46.5%). When the various histological subtypes were analysed, patients with a diagnosis of SCOS [14/35 (40%)] and maturation arrest [4 of 11 (36%)] had lower SRRs than those in the hypospermatogenesis group [9 of 12 (75.0%)] ($P < 0.05$). Interestingly preoperative serum testosterone correlated with the microTESE outcome.

23.6 ICSI Success Rates: Fresh Versus Frozen Sperm

Studies have reported conflicting findings with regard to the reproductive potential of fresh and frozen-thawed testicular sperm from men with NOA [32–35].

While some investigators have suggested impaired fertilization [33], embryo development [34] and implantation [35] using frozen testicular sperm compared with fresh, others could not find significant differences in these parameters [36].

In a meta-analysis of 10 studies involving 825 cycles, fertilization rates remained similar, but implantation rates were significantly higher (by 73%) when ICSI was performed with fresh rather than frozen-thawed testicular sperm [35].

However, ongoing pregnancy rates in the aforementioned study were not negatively affected by the state of testicular sperm used for ICSI, that is, fresh or frozen-thawed (relative risk [RR], 0.88; 95% confidence interval [CI], 0.58–1.33).

23.7 MicroTESE and ICSI: Take-Home Baby Rates

ICSI success is reduced when using sperm retrieved from men with NOA compared to sperm from ejaculated semen and from men with OA [37]. ICSI results in significantly lower fertilization and implantation rates, and birth rates are also lower following ICSI for NOA vs. OA (19% vs. 28%) [38].

In longitudinal studies including patients with NOA as defined by testicular histopathology, only one out of seven NOA patients embarking for microTESE and ICSI will successfully father their genetically own child [39]. Nevertheless, it must be emphasized that this is a population of men that prior to microTESE/ICSI had zero chance of paternity.

23.8 Complications

MicroTESE allows the identification of testicular vessels under the tunica albuginea, and these can be avoided when performing the incision. Microsurgery also allows preservation of intratesticular blood supply. This reduces the chance of complications due to haematoma formation and testicular devascularization, which is more likely to occur in cases of cTESE [40, 41]. In addition, cTESE may lead to removal of comparatively excessive amounts of testicular tissue, which may jeopardize androgen production and limit the chances of a repeat SSR. This factor is important for men with NOA, since they usually have small and highly dysfunctional testicles.

The testicular blood supply penetrates the tunica albuginea and runs under the tunica before penetrating between the septa and lobules of seminiferous tubules. As these are end arteries, any injury to these blood vessels may cause devascularization of a segment of the testicle. Schlegel et al. looked at severe complications after testicular biopsy in the pre-microTESE era and reported on two cases of complete testicular atrophy in a series of 64 patients [42].

They reported that 82% of the patients who underwent a TESE procedure had intratesticular abnormalities on ultrasound as long as 3 months following surgery. Most of the lesions seemed to disappear 6 months after the procedure, leaving only linear scars visible on ultrasound.

Schill et al. evaluated the risk of testicular damage from testicular biopsies that were carried out during cTESE in infertile men [43]. This group found that endocrine testicular function and testicular size were not impaired after testicular biopsy when compared with preoperative data. However, they did note that in the NOA population, rates of subnormal testosterone were higher post-operatively than preoperatively (12 of 26 patients had subnormal testosterone values before TESE; 14 of 39 patients had subnormal levels afterwards).

Similarly, Manning et al. described a decrease in serum testosterone levels following cTESE in patients with NOA for up to 1 year after the procedure [44]. It is therefore reasonable to conclude that patients with NOA show an increased risk of androgen deficiency following cTESE and recommend long-term follow-up in this group of patients.

Everaert and colleagues looked at the endocrine implications of microTESE in 48 patients with NOA [45]. Patients with de novo androgen deficiency were asked to perform a second blood analysis, where all blood samples were taken between 8 and 10 am. Their minimum reference value for testosterone was 280 ng/dl. Biochemical androgen deficiency was diagnosed if testosterone levels in serum were below the reference value on two occasions. 8.9% (4 out of 45) of the patients had serum testosterone levels below the reference range at the preoperative evaluation (280 ng/dl). Hormonal follow-up was available on 31 patients. Serum testosterone levels were on average 10% lower at follow-up compared to preoperative levels ($p < 0.05$). 16.1% (5 out of 31) of the patients were found to have a de novo androgen deficiency at follow-up. Among the eight patients of whom a clinical evaluation was available during post-operative follow-up, no symptoms or signs of androgen deficiency were noted. These patients all had also normal testosterone levels both preoperatively and at the follow-up visit (433 ± 99 ng/dl) (paired t-test: $p > 0.05$). Interestingly, no significant correlations were found between serum testosterone and the male age or testicular volume.

Komori et al. also demonstrated no significant endocrine changes after microTESE. This group recorded serum testosterone concentrations and the presence of antisperm antibodies (ASA) 12 months after cTESE or microTESE [46], of 13 patients undergoing cTESE and 12 patients undergoing microTESE. Serum total and free testosterone concentrations were evaluated preoperatively and at 1, 6 and 12 months following the procedure. Serum ASAs were also evaluated before and 12 months after TESE. Serum total and free testosterone concentrations in all patients in both groups showed no significant post-operative decrease. A comparison between the two groups of serum total and free testosterone concentrations showed no significant difference (total testosterone, $p = 0.2477$; free testosterone, $p = 0.3098$). No incidence of new ASA formation was identified in the study.

Takada et al. investigated the endocrine implications of microTESE on patients ($n = 69$) with NOA and KS [47]. The overall SRR was 50.7%. The endocrinological data was evaluated before and 3, 6, and 12 months following surgery. The mean serum total testosterone level in patients with hypospermatogenesis decreased post-operatively but recovered by 12 months. The mean serum total testosterone level in the patients with KS also decreased post-operatively but had recovered to only 50% of the baseline value at 12 months after microTESE.

Isikawa et al. also demonstrated a significant post-operative decrease in serum testosterone following micro-TESE in men with KS [48]. Mean testosterone levels significantly decreased an average of 30–35% vs. baseline when assessed 1, 3, 6, 9 and 12 months post-operatively. However, mean testosterone levels returned to 75% of the preoperative level after 18 months.

It is therefore important that patients are informed on the long-term consequences of microTESE, including the potential for androgen deficiency necessitating testosterone replacement therapy in the future. However, before starting hormone replacement therapy, it seems advisable to wait for about 1 year after the surgery, since some degree of spontaneous recovery may occur [44].

23.9 MESA

Microsurgical-guided sperm acquisition has also been applied in epididymal sperm retrievals. The goal of microsurgical epididymal sperm aspiration (MESA) is to identify and open a single epididymal tubule in order to aspirate a sperm-rich, red blood cell-free fluid that can be used for ICSI. In contrast to microTESE, MESA is indicated for cases of OA.

MESA was first described in 1985 [49]. This surgical technique requires exposure of the testicle through a 2–3 cm scrotal incision. The epididymal tunica is incised, and a single enlarged tubule is then selected. The epididymal tubule is dissected and opened with sharp microsurgical scissors. The fluid that flows out of the tubule is aspirated with the aid of a silicone tube or a needle attached to a tuberculin syringe. The aspirate is flushed into a tube containing warmed sperm handling buffered medium, which is transferred to the laboratory for microscopic examination.

MESA can be repeated at a different site on the same epididymis (from the cauda to caput regions) and/or the contralateral epididymis until motile sperm are retrieved [50].

A single MESA procedure usually enables retrieval of a large number of high-quality sperm that can be used for ICSI or cryopreservation for subsequent ICSI attempts [51, 52]. However, if MESA fails to retrieve motile sperm, TESA or TESE can be performed as part of the same procedure.

When compared to traditional TESE or PESA, MESA has been reported to be an excellent option for sperm retrieval in men with congenital bilateral absence of the vas deferens (CBAVD) [53]. The technique can also be employed at the time of an epididymovasostomy which allows 'backup' sperm to be obtained for cryopreservation. This also confirms that the tubule being used for the anastomosis has viable sperm within it.

23.10 OncoTESE

In view of the high cure rates for testicular germ cell tumours (TGCTs) and malignant lymphomas, increasing clinical importance is attached to preserving fertility. High-dose cytotoxic chemotherapy may cause long-term infertility. Thus, the standard procedure for fertility preservation is cryopreservation of ejaculated spermatozoa before undergoing potentially gonadotoxic therapy [54]. However, it should be noted that impairment of spermatogenesis may have already occurred before any chemotherapy has commenced in a significant proportion of young patients with a TGCT [55]. Furthermore, some patients may be azoospermic prior to treatment due to various factors (see below).

The mechanisms underlying the cancer-related impairment to spermatogenesis are poorly understood [56]. The following causes have been postulated and investigated:

1. Disorders of urogenital development and/or primary endocrine dysfunction [56].
2. The presence of contralateral testicular pathology (atrophy or unclassified intratubular germ cell neoplasia).
3. Possible tumour-related factors including endocrine activity of β-human chorionic gonadotropin (hCG), elevated concentrations of total serum estradiol and serum estradiol not bound to sex-hormone-binding globulin and blocking of multiple enzymes necessary for steroidogenesis [56]. It is assumed that tumour-derived hCG stimulates estradiol production in 'normal' testicular tissue but not in tumour tissue and that the resulting high estradiol levels then impair spermatogenesis [57].

A further mechanism under discussion is enhanced aromatization and in situ oestrogen production in Leydig cells of the non-neoplastic testis and in interstitial or stromal cells of the tumour in patients with NS [57]. Moreover, ASAs have also been detected in germ cell tumour patients [58].

Emotional stress has also been discussed as another factor contributing towards reduced fertility of tumour patients. This impairment of spermatogenesis is reversible in some cases after surgical treatment [59].

Evidence of a carcinoma-induced alteration of spermatogenesis is also supported by studies demonstrating that the sole removal and/or successful treatment of germ cell cancer is associated with an improvement of spermatogenesis in at least some of the patients [59].

Schrader et al. proposed a new strategy for cryopreservation of spermatozoa in azoospermic men, via spermatozoa retrieval at the time of orchidectomy. This has been termed 'oncoTESE' [60]. When performing the contralateral testicular biopsy to exclude an intratubular germ cell neoplasia, a part of the specimen from all azoospermic patients is cryopreserved in a fashion analogous to TESE. This ensures sperm extraction before spermatogenesis is additionally compromised by cytotoxic therapy. Moreover, TESE does not require an additional intervention if performed during the contralateral testicular biopsy.

MicroTESE appears to be the optimum strategy for men with coexistent NOA and testicular cancer, particularly at the time of radical orchiectomy [61]. OncoTESE can be performed on the non-malignant testicular tissue, separate from the malignant lesion in men with NOA and testicular cancer. This is particularly relevant in those men with NOA and bilateral testicular cancer, absent contralateral testicle and atrophic contralateral testicle.

23.11 Conclusion, Commentary and Future Directions

The treatment of NOA has undergone many recent advances [11]. Surgical extraction of spermatozoa from focal areas of sperm production in men with NOA has been a primary challenge to the successful treatment of these patients. Using a microsurgical approach, sperm retrieval is effective in 56% of men with NOA, and pregnancy is possible in 45% of couples once sperm are retrieved. The microTESE approach seems to be safer than other sperm retrieval approaches and has a specific application for subsets of men with NOA.

In a recent correspondence with the journal *Andrology*, Professor Song has highlighted the broad range of reported success rates for microTESE and suggested that the real-world experience of many urologists often results in lower success rates than the ranges reported [62]. Song proposed that specific changes are needed to the reporting and analyses of microTESE studies and calls for a need for standardization so that definitions are explicit. For example, 'successful microTESE' may be defined broadly by some as the isolation of any form of an elongated spermatid, rather than isolation of viable mature sperm suitable for ICSI. Song proposed that the procedure be considered 'successful' only if viable sperm suitable for ICSI are obtained. While the identification and processing of spermatogonia, round spermatids and/or elongating spermatids may be relevant and important, especially in the future, such data should be reported in a separate category.

In agreement with Song's recommendations, SRR compared within specific groups, e.g. from NOA patients with elevated serum FSH, could be one effective way to objectively compare the results. Furthermore, microTESE data for cryptozoospermia perhaps should be excluded from the overall outcome data reported, since a higher chance of sperm retrieval can be expected because ongoing spermatogenesis has already been proven in these patients. Finally, we suggest reporting units exclude azoospermia patients with normal FSH and normal testis size who have not undergone testis biopsy showing impaired spermatogenesis. If these patients are not excluded, OA might be included in outcome reporting resulting in higher reported SRRs.

Looking to the future, multiphoton microscopy has been applied successfully to differentiate normal from abnormal spermatogenesis in an ex vivo rodent model, and encouraging preliminary results have been reported in humans [63, 64]. Confocal fluorescence microscopy has also been used in a murine model of microTESE [65]. Although the latter offers the advantage of rapid in vivo detection of sperm in the ST, a concern might be the use of fluorescein to label sperm may limit the translation of this method to the clinical setting.

Lastly, full-field optical coherence tomography, which uses a safe light source with no apparent detrimental effect on sperm quality, was recently described as a useful tool to facilitate real-time visualization of spermatogenesis in an ex vivo rodent SCO model [66]. Thus, the aforesaid methods have the potential to be coupled with the operating microscope and aid in microTESE.

References

1. Gil-Salom M, Romero J, Rubio C, Ruiz A, Remohi J, Pellicer A. Intracytoplasmic sperm injection with cryopreserved testicular spermatozoa. Mol Cell Endocrinol. 2000;169(1–2):15–9.
2. Belva F, De Schrijver F, Tournaye H, Liebaers I, Devroey P, Haentjens P, et al. Neonatal outcome of 724 children born after ICSI using non-ejaculated sperm. Hum Reprod. 2011;26(7):1752–8.
3. Ezeh U. Beyond the clinical classification of azoospermia: opinion. Hum Reprod. 2000;15(11):2356–9.
4. Gudeloglu A, Parekattil S. Update in the evaluation of the azoospermic male. Clinics. 2013;68(S1):27–34.
5. Su LM, Palermo GD, Goldstein M, Veeck LL, Rosenwaks Z, Schlegel PN. Testicular sperm extraction with intracytoplasmic sperm injection for nonobstructive azoospermia: testicular histology can predict success of sperm retrieval. J Urol. 1999;161(1):112–6.
6. Schlegel P. Testicular sperm extraction: microdissection improves sperm yield with minimal tissue excision. Hum Reprod. 1999;14:131–5.
7. Schoysman R, Vanderzwalmen P, Nijs M, Segal-Bertin C, Geerts L, Van de Casseye M. Successful fertilization by testicular spermatozoa in an in-vitro fertilization programme. Human Reproduction. 1993;8:1339–40.
8. Craft I, Bennett V, Nicholson N. Fertilizing ability of testicular spermatozoa. Lancet. 1993;342:864.
9. Silber S, Nagy Z, Liu J. The use of epididymal and testicular spermatozoa for intracytoplasmic sperm injection: the genetic implications for male infertility. Hum Reprod. 1995;10:2031–43.
10. Devroey P, Liu J, Nagy Z, Goossens A, Tournaye H, Camus M, Van Steirteghem A, Silber S. Pregnancies after testicular sperm extraction and intracytoplasmic sperm injection in non-obstructive azoospermia. Hum Reprod. 1995;10:1457–60.
11. Schlegel P. Nonobstructive Azoospermia: a revolutionary surgical approach and results. Semin Reprod Med. 2009;27(02):165–70.
12. Donoso P, Tournaye H, Devroey P. Which is the best sperm retrieval technique for non-obstructive azoospermia? A systematic review. Hum Reprod Update. 2007;13(6):539–49.
13. Johnsen SG. Testicular biopsy score count – a method for registration of spermatogenesis in human testes: normal values and results in 335 hypogonadal males. Hormones. 1970;1:2–25.
14. Esteves S, Raj D, Ramakrishnan S, Singh S, Ashraf M. Microdissection testicular sperm extraction as an alternative for sperm acquisition in the most difficult cases of Azoospermia: technique and preliminary results in India. J Human Reprod Sci. 2013;6(2):111.
15. Esteves SC, Verza S Jr. PESA/TESA/TESE sperm processing. In: Nagy ZP, Varghese AC, Agarwal A, editors. Practical manual of *in vitro* fertilization: advanced methods and novel devices. 1st ed. New York: Springer; 2012. p. 207–20.
16. Silber SJ. Microsurgical TESE and the distribution of spermatogenesis in non-obstructive azoospermia. Hum Reprod. 2000;15:2278–84.
17. Esteves SC, Miyaoka R, Agarwal A. Sperm retrieval techniques for assisted reproduction. Int Braz J Urol. 2011;37:570–83.
18. Carpi A, Sabanegh E, Mechanick J. Controversies in the management of nonobstructive azoospermia. Fertil Steril. 2009;91:963–70.
19. Okada H, Dobashi M, Yamazaki T, Hara I, Fujisawa M, Arakawa S, et al. Conventional versus microdissection testicular sperm extraction for nonobstructive azoospermia. J Urol. 2002;168(3):1063–7.
20. Deruyver Y, Vanderschueren D, Van der Aa F. Outcome of microdissection TESE compared with conventional TESE in non-obstructive azoospermia: a systematic review. Andrology. 2013;2(1):20–4.
21. Ramasamy R, Lin K, Gosden L, Rosenwaks Z, Palermo G, Schlegel P. High serum FSH levels in men with nonobstructive azoospermia does not affect success of microdissection testicular sperm extraction. Fertil Steril. 2009;92(2):590–3.
22. Verza S, Esteves SC. Microsurgical versus conventional single-biopsy testicular sperm extraction in nonobstructive azoospermia: a prospective controlled study. Fertil Steril. 2011;96:S53.
23. Verza ESC. Computer-assisted objective evaluation of sperm-containing seminiferous tubule in testicular sperm retrievals. Fertil Steril. 2012;98:S242.
24. Schiff JD, Palermo GD, Veeck LL, Goldstein M, Rosenwaks Z, Schlegel PN. Success of testicular sperm injection and intracytoplasmic sperm injection in men with Klinefelter syndrome. J Clin Endocrinol Metab. 2005;90:6263–7.
25. Chan PT, Palermo GD, Veeck LL, Rosenvacks Z, Schlegel PN. Testicular sperm extraction combined with intracytoplasmic sperm injection in the treatment of men with persistent azoospermia postchemotherapy. Cancer. 2001;92:1632–7.
26. Raman JD, Schlegel PN. Testicular sperm extraction with intracytoplasmic sperm injection is successful for the treatment of nonobstructive azoospermia associated with cryptorchidism. J Urol. 2003;170:1287–90.
27. Reifsnyder JE, Ramasamy R, Husseini J, Schlegel PN. Role of optimizing testosterone before microdissection testicular sperm extraction in men with nonobstructive azoospermia. J Urol. 2012;188:532–6.
28. Esteves SC. Editorial comment. J Urol. 2012;188:536–7.
29. Ramasamy R, Ricci JA, Palermo GD, Gosden LV, Rosenwaks Z, Schlegel PN. Successful fertility treatment for Klinefelter's syndrome. J Urol. 2009;182:1108–13.
30. Tsujimura A, Miyagawa Y, Takao T, Takada S, Koga M, Takeyama M, et al. Salvage microdissection testicular sperm extraction after failed conventional testicular sperm extraction in patients with nonobstructive azoospermia. J Urol. 2006;175(4):1446–9.
31. Kalsi JS, Shah P, Thum Y, Muneer A, Ralph DJ, Minhas S. Salvage micro-dissection testicular sperm extraction; outcome in men with non-obstructive azoospermia with previous failed sperm retrievals. BJU Int. 2015 Sep;116(3):460–5.
32. Schlegel PN, Liotta D, Hariprashad J, Veeck LL. Fresh testicular sperm from men with nonobstructive azoospermia works best for ICSI. Urology. 2004;64:1069–71.
33. Dafopoulos K, Griesinger G, Schultze-Mosgau A, Orief Y, Schöpper B, Nikolettos N, et al. Factors affecting outcome after ICSI with spermatozoa retrieved from cryopreserved testicular tissue in non-obstructive azoospermia. Reprod Biomed Online. 2005;10:455–60.
34. Konc J, Kanyó K, Cseh S. The effect of condition/state of testicular spermatozoa injected to the outcome of TESE-ICSI-ET cycles. Eur J Obstet Gynecol Reprod Biol. 2008;141:39–43.
35. Nicopoullos JD, Gilling-Smith C, Almeida PA, Norman-Taylor J, Grace I, Ramsay JW. Use of surgical sperm retrieval in azoospermic men: a meta-analysis. Fertil Steril. 2004;82:691–701.

36. Niederberger C. Do not let technician biases fool you: frozen sperm from any azoospermic man is as good as fresh for ICSI and easier for the couple. Urology. 2004;64:1072–4.
37. Ghanem M, Bakr N, Elgayaar M, El Mongy S, Fathy H, Ibrahim A. Comparison of the outcome of intracytoplasmic sperm injection in obstructive and non-obstructive azoospermia in the first cycle: a report of case series and meta-analysis. Int J Androl. 2005;28(1):16–21.
38. Vernaeve V, Tournaye H, Osmanagaoglu K, Verheyen G, Van Steirteghem A, Devroey P. Intracytoplasmic sperm injection with testicular spermatozoa is less successful in men with nonobstructive azoospermia than in men with obstructive azoospermia. Fertil Steril. 2003;79(3):529–33.
39. Vloeberghs V, Verheyen G, Haentjens P, Goossens A, Polyzos N, Tournaye H. How successful is TESE-ICSI in couples with non-obstructive azoospermia? Hum Reprod. 2015;30(8):1790–6.
40. Amer M, Ateyah A, Hany R, Zohdy W. Prospective comparative study between microsurgical and conventional testicular sperm extraction in non-obstructive azoospermia: follow-up by serial ultrasound examinations. Hum Reprod. 2000;15(3):653–6.
41. Practice Committee of the American Society for Reproductive Medicine. Sperm retrieval for obstructive azoospermia. Fertil Steril. 2006;86(5 Suppl 1):S115–20.
42. Schlegel PN, Su L. Physiologic consequences of testicular sperm extraction. Hum Reprod. 1997;12:1688–92.
43. Schill T, Bals-Pratsch M, Kupker W, Sandmann J, Johannison R, Diederich K. Clinical and endocrine follow-up of patients after testicular sperm extraction. Fertil Steril. 2003;79:281–6.
44. Manning M, Junemann K, Alken P. Decrease in testosterone blood concentrations after testicular sperm extraction for intracytoplasmic sperm injection in azoospermic men. Lancet. 1998;352:37.
45. Everaert K, De Croo I, Kerckhaert W, Dekuyper P, Dhont M, Van der Elst J, et al. Long term effects of micro-surgical testicular sperm extraction on androgen status in patients with non obstructive azoospermia. BMC Urol. 2006;6:9.
46. Komori K, Tsujimura A, Miura H, Shin M, Takada T, Honda M, et al. Serial follow-up study of serum testosterone and antisperm antibodies in patients with non-obstructive azoospermia after conventional or microdissection testicular sperm extraction. Int J Androl. 2004;27(1):32–6.
47. Takada S, Tsujimura A, Ueda T, Matsuoka Y, Takao T, Miyagawa Y, et al. Androgen decline in patients with nonobstructive azoospermia after microdissection testicular sperm extraction. Urology. 2008;72(1):114–8.
48. Ishikawa T, Yamaguchi K, Chiba K, Takenaka A, Fujisawa M. Serum hormones in patients with nonobstructive azoospermia after microdissection testicular sperm extraction. J Urol. 2009;182(4):1495–9.
49. Temple-Smith PD, Southwick GJ, Yates CA, Trounson AO, de Kretser DM. Human pregnancy by in vitro fertilization (IVF) using sperm aspirated from the epididymis. J In Vitro Fert Embryo Transf. 1985;2(3):119–22.
50. Esteves SC, Agarwal A, Gardner DK, BRMB R, Falcone T, editors. Sperm retrieval techniques Human assisted reproductive technology: future trends in laboratory and clinical practice. 1st ed. Cambridge: Cambridge University Press; 2011. p. 41–53.
51. Van Peperstraten A, Proctor ML, Johnson NP, Philipson G. Techniques for surgical retrieval of sperm prior to ICSI for azoospermia. Cochrane Database Syst Rev. 2006;3:CD002807.
52. Schroeder-Printzen I, Zumbe J, Bispink L, Palm S, Schneider U, Engelmann U, et al. Microsurgical epididymal sperm aspiration: aspirate analysis and straws available after cryopreservation in patients with non-reconstructable obstructive azoospermia. Hum Reprod. 2000;15(12):2531–5.
53. Jungwirth A, Giwercman A, Tournaye H, Diemer T, Kopa Z, Dohle G, et al. European Association of Urology guidelines on male infertility: the 2012 update. Eur Urol. 2012;62(2):324–32.
54. Schrader M, Müller M, Sofikitis N, Straub B, Miller K. Testicular sperm extraction in azoospermic cancer patients prior to treatment—a new guideline? Hum Reprod. 2002;17(4):1127–8.
55. Petersen P, Giwercman A, Skakkebaek N, Rorth M. Gonadal function in men with testicular cancer. J Urol. 1998;160(6):2291.
56. Morrish D, Venner P, Siy O, Barron G, Bhardwaj D, Outhet D. Mechanisms of endocrine dysfunction in patients with testicular cancer. JNCI J Natl Cancer Inst. 1990;82(5):412–8.
57. Nakazumi H. Estrogen metabolism and impaired spermatogenesis in germ cell tumors of the testis. J Clin Endocrinol Metab. 1996;81(3):1289–95.
58. Guazzieri S, Lembo A, Ferro G, Artibani W, Merlo F, Zanchetta R, et al. Sperm antibodies and infertility in patients with testicular cancer. Urology. 1985;26(2):139–42.
59. Fosså S, Theodorsen L, Norman N, Aabyholm T. Recovery of impaired pretreatment spermatogenesis in testicular cancer**Supported by the Norwegian Cancer Society, Oslo. Norway Fertil Steril. 1990;54(3):493–6.
60. Schrader M, Mller M, Sofikitis N, Straub B, Krause H, Miller K. "Onco-tese": testicular sperm extraction in azoospermic cancer patients before chemotherapy—new guidelines? Urology. 2003;61(2):421–5.
61. Haddad N, Al-Rabeeah K, Onerheim R, Zini A. Is ex vivo microdissection testicular sperm extraction indicated for infertile men undergoing radical orchiectomy for testicular cancer? Case report and literature review. Fertil Steril. 2014;101(4):956–9.
62. Song S. It is time for a more standardized approach to identifying surgical outcome of non-obstructive azoospermia. Andrology. 2017;5(3):401–2.
63. Ramasamy R, Sterling J, Fisher ES, Li PS, Jain M, Robinson BD, et al. Identification of spermatogenesis with multiphoton microscopy: an evaluation in a rodent model. J Urol. 2011;186:2487–92.
64. Najari BB, Ramasamy R, Sterling J, Aggarwal A, Sheth S, Li PS, et al. Pilot study of the correlation of multiphoton tomography of ex vivo human testis with histology. J Urol. 2012;188:538–43.
65. Smith RP, Lowe GJ, Kavoussi PK, Steers WD, Costabile RA, Herr JC, et al. Confocal fluorescence microscopy in a murine model of microdissection testicular sperm extraction to improve sperm retrieval. J Urol. 2012;187:1918–23.
66. Ramasamy R, Sterling J, Manzoor M, Salamoon B, Jain M, Fisher E, et al. Full field optical coherence tomography can identify spermatogenesis in a rodent sertoli-cell only model. J Pathol Inform. 2012;3:4.

Surgical Management of Endometriosis

24

Jorge F. Carrillo and Yolianne Lozada-Capriles

Endometriosis is a condition where endometrial glands and stroma are found outside the uterine cavity, frequently at the ovarian fossa, ovaries, fallopian tubes, and the cul-de-sac. Sometimes it can involve intraabdominal or pelvic organs like the bowel, bladder, and ureter, endopelvic fascia components like the uterosacral ligaments, the rectovaginal septum, and in rare occasions extra-abdominal organs, such as the lung and pleura.

The exact prevalence or incidence is difficult to estimate, but is thought to affect 7–10% of female population [1]. It is thought to have a prevalence between 20 and 50% among patients with infertility [2, 3]. Endometriosis is found in 30% of chronic pelvic pain patients who undergo laparoscopy [4]. A retrospective study by Mowers et al. revealed that of 9622 patients who underwent laparoscopic or abdominal hysterectomy for benign indications, 15.2% had endometriosis. This same study also showed that only 21% of patients with chronic pelvic pain had endometriosis and among patients with a preoperative diagnosis of suspected endometriosis, only 42% had pathology-confirmed disease [5].

Although patients are not always symptomatic, they usually present in their reproductive age with dysmenorrhea, infertility, pelvic mass, deep dyspareunia, or organ-specific symptoms like dysuria, dyschezia, or hemoptysis [6, 7]. Empirical medical therapy may be started if there is a clinical suspicion; however the final diagnosis can only be made with histological confirmation [8]. There is data suggesting that a visual diagnosis of endometriosis has a positive predictive value of 45% [9]. Endometriosis has many different forms of visual presentation. Thus, the surgeon must be familiar with these patterns to decide which lesions to biopsy (Table 24.1, Fig. 24.1).

Table 24.1 Appearances of endometriosis

1. Red raspberries	2. Purple raspberries
3. Blueberries	4. Blebs
5. Peritoneal pockets	6. Whitish scar tissue
7. Stellate scar tissue	8. Strawberry-colored lesions
9. Red vesicles	10. White vesicles
11. Clear vesicles	12. Powder burns
13. Peritoneal windows	14. Yellow-brown patches
15. Brown-black patches	16. Adhesions
17. Clear polypoid lesions	18. Red polypoid lesions
19. Red flame-like lesions	20. Black puckered spots
21. White plaques with black puckers	22. Chocolate cysts

The current classification by the American Society for Reproductive Medicine is surgical and unfortunately does not correlate with the clinical presentation of this condition.

Surgery is an important therapy available to offer patients who are suspected to have or have been diagnosed with endometriosis. Who, when, how, and how much are just a few of the many questions a gynecologic surgeon should ask themselves before offering surgical treatment for this condition. For example, when treated surgically, it has always been the thought that aggressively treating most endometriosis lesions would improve patient's symptoms. Nonetheless, there is recent data suggesting that patients with stage 3 or 4 endometriosis have better response rates in their pain symptoms when compared to patients with stage 1–2 disease [10]. There are many aspects to consider when offering a surgical approach to a patient with suspected or confirmed endometriosis whether it is for pain or fertility indications.

In this chapter, we will discuss these points and the current surgical management of this interesting and complex condition.

J. F. Carrillo (✉)
Department of Obstetrics and Gynecology, University of Central Florida, Orlando, FL, USA
e-mail: jorge_carrillo@urmc.rochester.edu

Y. Lozada-Capriles
Department of Obstetrics and Gynecology, University of Puerto Rico, Medical Sicences Campus, San Juan, PR, USA

G. N. Allahbadia et al. (eds.), *Textbook of Assisted Reproduction*, https://doi.org/10.1007/978-981-15-2377-9_24

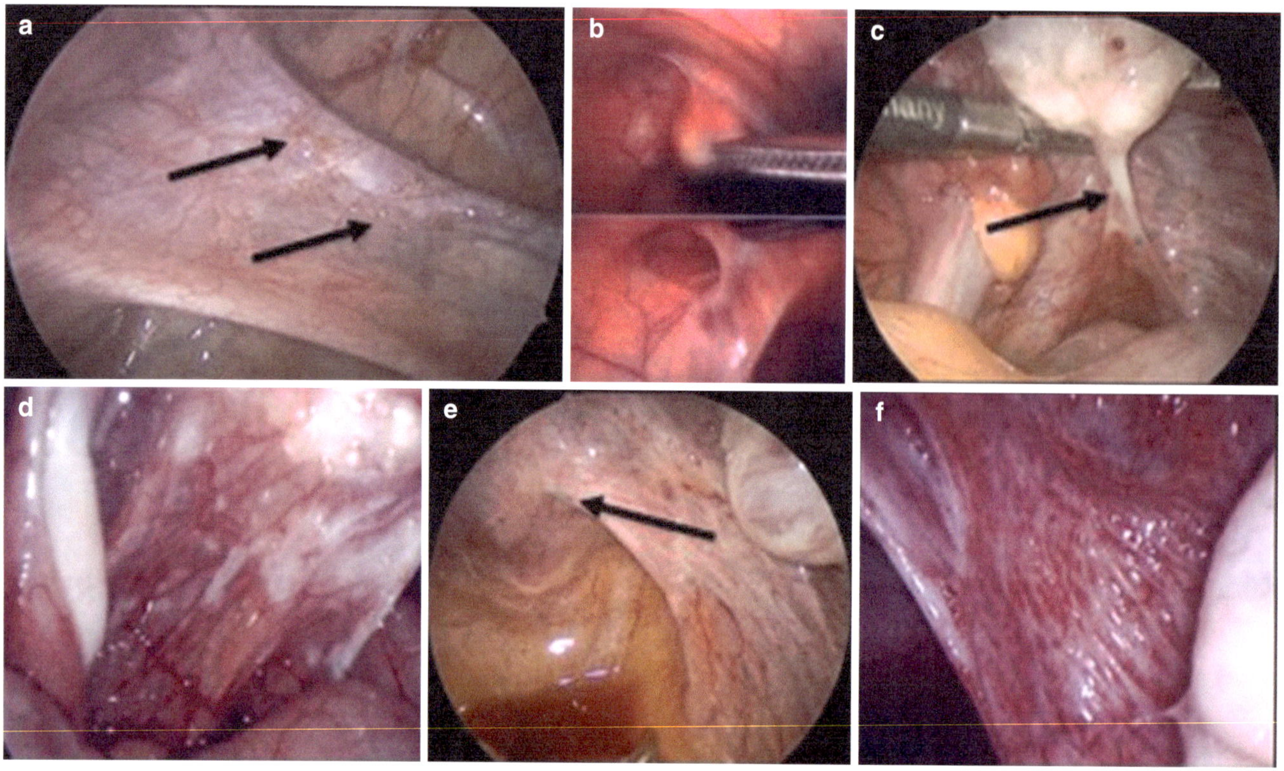

Fig. 24.1 Some appearances for endometriosis. (**a**) Clear vesicles, (**b**) peritoneal defects/pockets, (**c**) adhesions, (**d**) white lesions, (**e**) powder burn lesions, (**f**) cribiform peritoneal lesions

24.1 Surgical Considerations

When to perform surgery on a patient with suspected or confirmed endometriosis is a very important decision to make, especially if one of the indications is chronic pelvic pain. A comprehensive history and physical exam must be performed. The most common indications for a surgical approach are persistent pain despite hormonal suppression, any contraindication for medical management, an adnexal mass, some infertility related reasons, and to confirm diagnosis, among others (Table 24.2).

Table 24.2 Criteria for surgical management of endometriosis

Appropriate candidate	Non-candidate
1. Failed/contraindicated medical treatment	1. Incomplete evaluation
2. Establish diagnosis	2. Multiple non-effective surgeries
3. Adnexal masses	3. Postmenopausal
4. Infertility	
5. Deep infiltrative endometriosis (bowel, bladder involvement)	

Preoperative evaluation with imaging such as ultrasound or magnetic resonance might be helpful to identify pelvic masses and deep infiltrative lesions of the bladder, rectovaginal septum, or bowel. The main goal with a surgical approach is to remove/ablate endometriosis lesions and to restore normal anatomy, and depending on the patient's desire, this should be achieved by sparing fertility. It is important for the surgeon to be conscious that, as mentioned before, because endometriosis staging does not correlate with symptoms, one should be prepared to manage distorted anatomy and lesions invading organs such as the bladder, rectum, and ureter, among others. Being cautious and self-aware of her or his own surgical skills should permit the surgeon to decide if the complexity of the surgery allows appropriate achievement of goals or if the patient should be referred to a specialized center. Inadequate procedures or failure to recognize and treat lesions can lead to persistent symptoms.

24.2 Techniques

24.2.1 Laparotomy Versus Laparoscopy

The advantages of laparoscopic surgery versus laparotomy are very well known and have been described; recovery time and cost are just a few of them. A laparoscopic approach is

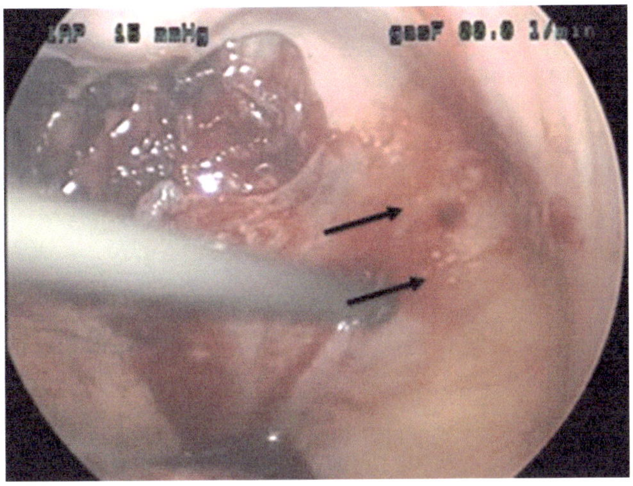

Fig. 24.2 This is how lesions can be enhanced after "painting" them with blood. We use the suction to spread blood over the lesions or suspected area

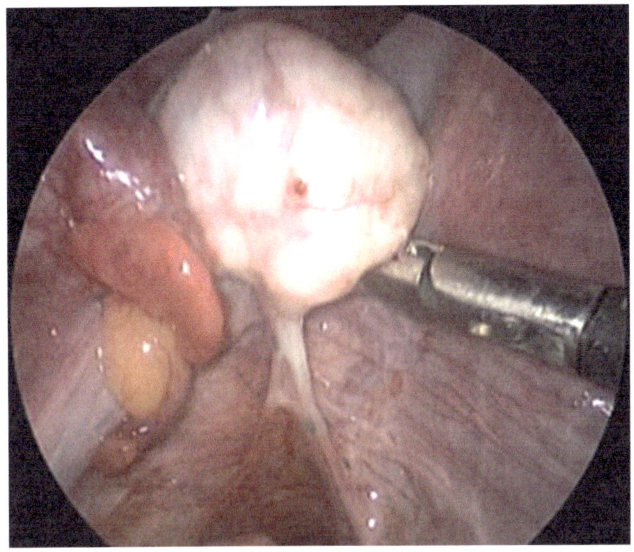

Fig. 24.3 Technique to expose ovarian fossa, with Maryland forceps; the ovarian ligament is grasped proximally, and the instrument tip is rotated clockwise, rotating the ovary

considered routine for the diagnosis and removal of endometriosis [8, 11, 12]. Having said this, laparoscopy and laparotomy are equally effective in treating endometriosis pelvic pain [13]. Laparoscopy provides a better visualization of lesions that otherwise would go unnoticed, and "near contact" laparoscopy allows about an eightfold magnification. Techniques used at our institution include "zoom in, zoom out" and "blood painting" (Fig. 24.2) in which blood is used to enhance elevated borders of lesions implanted at the peritoneum in the cul-de-sac or the pelvic side walls [8].

A thorough survey of the pelvis and abdomen should take place at the beginning of the procedure, and it should be performed in a systematic fashion. This is especially important in patients with chronic pelvic pain. We start at the insertion of the left round ligament and then inspect the anterior cul-de-sac, followed by the insertion of the right round ligament. After this, the uterus is anteverted, and a Maryland forceps is used to grasp one of the utero-ovarian ligaments and rotate the tips to expose the ovarian fossa. This allows excellent visualization of the ovary, the pelvic sidewall, the ipsilateral ureter, and uterosacral ligament. Following this, we inspect the posterior cul-de-sac. In a similar fashion, the contralateral ovarian fossa and pelvic side wall are explored (Fig. 24.3). Lastly, the sigmoid and the appendix are also visualized and inspected; this is important since appendiceal endometriosis has been reported in 2–4% of patients with endometriosis [14]. If a "peritoneal pocket" is visualized, this is inspected down to its base because lesions will be frequently found inside. The purpose of performing a systematic inspection is to avoid missing lesions at less frequent areas. At our institution, we document the exact area in which endometriosis lesions are found, and we describe the appearance of the lesion so there is a comparison if a repeat surgery is needed. Sometimes extensive disease and very distorted anatomy necessitate converting a laparoscopic procedure to open, depending on the goal of the surgery.

24.2.2 Ablation Versus Excision

Ablation refers to the destruction of lesions with electrosurgical techniques, laser vaporization, or ultrasonic scalpel. By excision we refer to the dissection of lesions away from normal tissue, generally using the laparoscopic scissors. A recent systematic review from the Cochrane Collaboration evaluating laparoscopic surgery for endometriosis revealed that laparoscopic surgery (with either ablation or excision) reduced overall pain associated with minimal and moderate endometriosis, when compared to just diagnostic laparoscopy at 6 and 12 months. It was also found that laparoscopic treatment of minimal or moderate endometriosis improves pregnancy and live birth in couples with infertility [15]. When both ablation and excision were compared, it was found that they had similar effects in reducing pain [15, 16]. We should be mindful of the invasive nature of endometriosis when we are treating lesions. Sometimes it is not enough to ablate the lesion due to the depth of infiltration. When deep infiltrative endometriosis is found, the tactile feedback provided by conventional laparoscopy could be useful; a "sand paper" or "rough" consistency is perceived, and once the abnormal tissue is removed, this area should feel "smooth." At our institution, we excise lesions and often use laparoscopic scissors without energy to dissect the peritoneum away from the sub-peritoneal fat to avoid bleeding (Fig. 24.4). This technique is especially use-

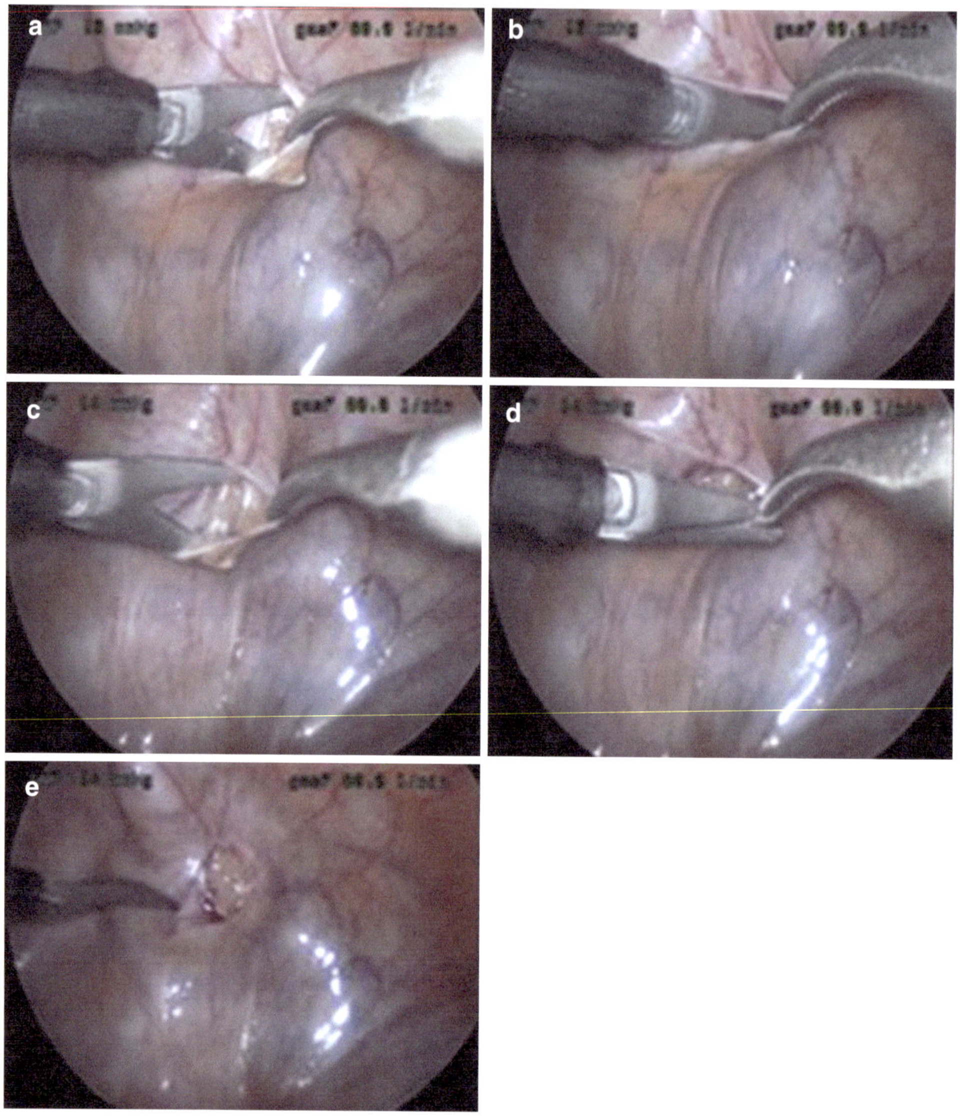

Fig. 24.4 Excision of endometriosis lesion. (**a**) With a grasper elevate the lesion, and with scissors incise the peritoneum. (**b**, **c**) Use a "poke and open" technique to dissect the subperitoneal fat to avoid bleeding. (**d**) Finish incision around the lesion. (**e**) Area of peritoneum excised

ful when the lesions are near to vital organs such as the ureter or blood vessels.

24.2.3 Neurectomies

Pelvic neurectomies have been described since the late 1800s. These procedures were developed with the thought of interrupting ascending pathway of sensory fibers from the uterus and cervix. They are offered when patients with dysmenorrhea or endometriosis have poor response to medical therapy and desire a fertility-sparing procedure. There are essentially two procedures described: uterine nerve ablation (UNA) and presacral neurectomy (PSN).

UNA gained popularity in the 1960s. In 1985, the first laparoscopic UNA (LUNA) was described [17]. The procedure consisted of transecting a segment of the uterosacral ligaments, from their insertion into the cervix (1 cm in length and depth). Four prospective randomized trials and a Cochrane review concluded that LUNA has no role in the treatment of chronic pelvic pain and should not be performed for endometriosis-related pelvic pain [17–20].

The superior hypogastric plexus or presacral nerve is a neurologic plexus formed primarily by sympathetic (T12–L2) and visceral afferent fibers. It is located in the interiliac triangle at the level of L4–L5–S1 vertebral bodies. Anteriorly, this plexus nerve is covered by preperitoneal fat and parietal peritoneum. Posteriorly, it is in relation to the left common iliac vein (at the superior end of it), the middle sacral artery, and the anterior longitudinal ligament of the spine. It then divides into two inferior hypogastric plexuses which will receive the pelvic splanchnic nerves or nervi erigentes coming from S2, S3, and S4, adding parasympathetic fibers to form the three plexuses that will innervate the blad-

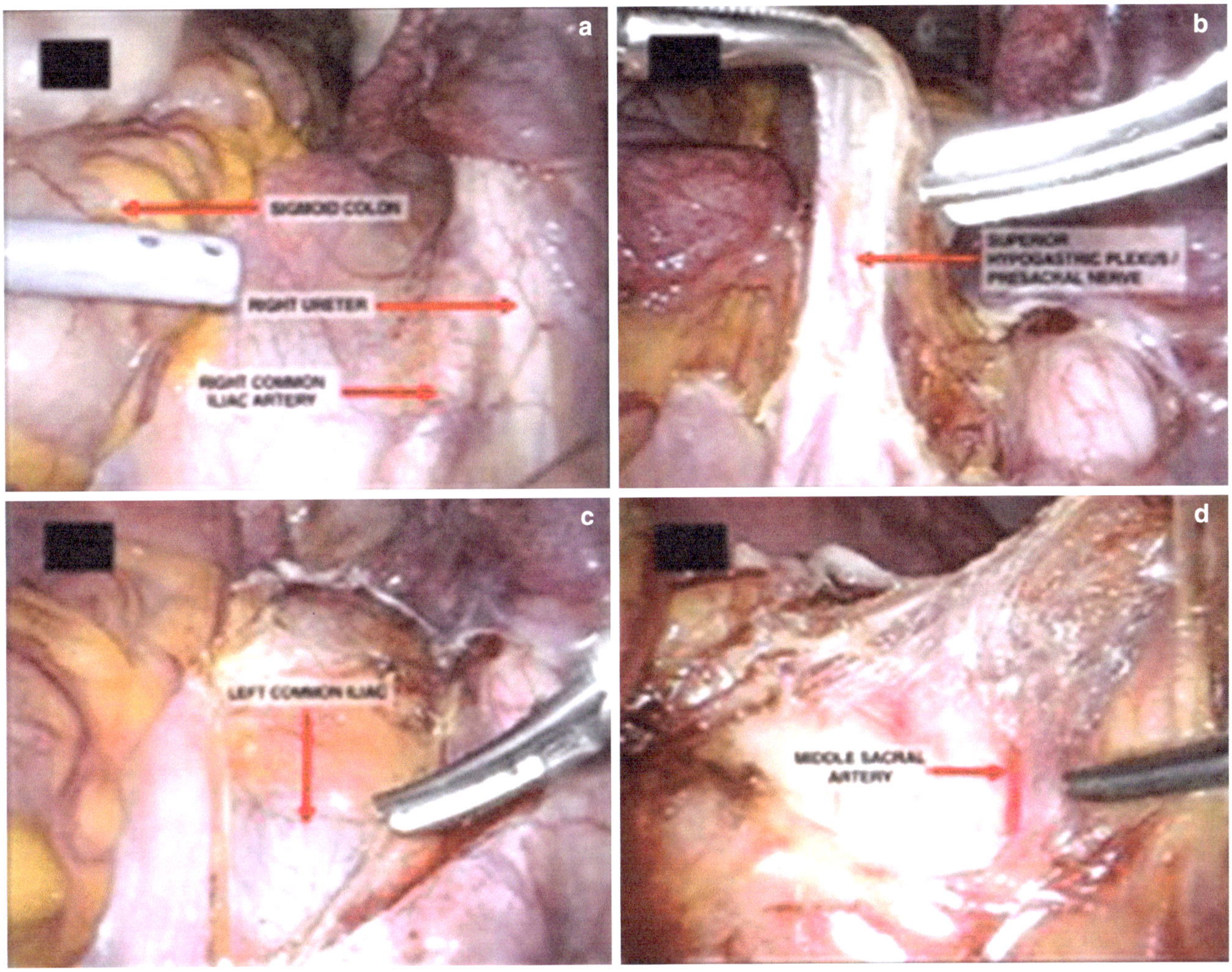

Fig. 24.5 Presacral neurectomy. (**a**) Landmarks to identify. (**b**) Superior hypogastric plexus. (**c**) Left common iliac identified. (**d**) Middle sacral artery identified

der, uterus-vagina (Frankehauser's plexus), and rectum [21, 22]. By transecting the presacral nerve, one can interrupt this pathway between the uterus and the central nervous system. Before starting a laparoscopic PSN (LPSN), the surgeon needs to identify all the structures of the interiliac triangle. The sigmoid colon is retracted laterally exposing the space. The promontory is identified and the bifurcation of the aorta visualized. The left common iliac vein is identified. The right ureter is the right limit of the dissection, and the inferior mesenteric artery is the left border. Then the parietal peritoneum is incised at the interiliac triangle; this incision can be vertical or horizontal and is extended just below the bifurcation. The peritoneum is dissected off the peritoneal fat. At our institution, we prefer to use the ultrasonic scalpel, but bipolar or monopolar energy can be used for dissection as well. The anterior longitudinal ligament should be exposed, taking care during dissection around the left common iliac to avoid injuries and to ensure proper resection of the neurologic fibers. The specimen should be sent to pathology to confirm presence of neural tissue (Fig. 24.5). In the same Cochrane review cited previously, it was found that LPSN combined with surgical treatment for endometriosis was more beneficial than surgical treatment of endometriosis only, in cases where midline pelvic pain was described [20]. When LPSN was performed for primary dysmenorrhea, success rates of 80% have been reported; when it was performed for pelvic pain associated with endometriosis, success rates ranged from 73 to 94% in decreasing pain [23]. At out institution, patients undergo a CT-guided hypogastric nerve block before being considered for a LPSN. This ensures that interruption of these nerve fibers will be effective in alleviating their pain. Associated complications are low, but could be very serious due to the surgical area and the vascular relations leading to catastrophic injuries. Also, by disrupting the neurologic pathway, visceral side effects can present, the most frequent one being severe constipation (14.3%), followed by urinary urgency (4.8%) [24, 25].

24.3 Endometrioma Management

Endometriomas are ovarian cysts that arise from the endometrial tissue located at their inner wall. These cysts contain dark thick fluid resembling old blood, frequently described as "chocolate cysts," that are usually adherent to the ovarian cortex and surrounding organs, such as the bowel, ureter, peritoneum, fallopian tubes, uterus, and uterosacral ligaments. It is thought that endometriomas can present in 17–44% of patients with endometriosis [26]. Their size can range from 1 to >15 cm size [27]. Patients may complain of pelvic pain, and the pelvic exam could reveal an adnexal mass and limited uterine mobility. A transvaginal pelvic ultrasound is the best imaging modality to make the diagnosis with a sensitivity and specificity of almost 90% [26]. Ultrasound findings typically describe a unilocular ovarian cyst with a ground-glass appearance. Among surgical treatments for endometriomas, excision of the cyst wall with stripping seems to be superior in terms of endometrioma recurrence and pelvic pain symptoms and increase conception rates when compared to fenestration with ablation/coagulation [10, 26]; it also provides a final diagnosis. Proper excision technique of an endometrioma requires training and experience to minimize ovarian trauma and potential impact of ovarian function. Regarding the technique, it is very important to identify the relevant anatomical structures nearby, like the fallopian tube, infundibulopelvic ligament, or ureter to name some. If lysis of adhesions needs to be performed, it should be done taking care to identify these structures, as the ovary is frequently adherent to other organs such as the uterus, bowel, or pelvic side wall. We usually plan our first ovarian incision by making very small, superficial punctures in a linear fashion along the ovarian cortex. Then, we use scissors with blunt and sharp dissection to "connect the dots." This results in a longitudinal incision that reveals the cyst capsule. The ovarian cortex is grasped and peeled from the cyst wall. Sometimes, drainage of the cyst is necessary to gain better visualization, definition of the dissection planes, and more adequate control of the tissue. The use of injected diluted vasopressin into the space between the cyst and the ovarian cortex has been described, with findings suggesting a reduction in operating times and ovarian damage to ovarian reserve (by reducing the loss of healthy ovarian tissue and use of cautery on it); but more studies are needed to further investigate these effects [27, 28]. There is conflicting data about the impact on infertility after cystectomy. On one hand, there are some studies that reveal increase of spontaneous pregnancy (20–60%) after laparoscopic treatment of endometriomas, while others concluded there was no significant difference [26]. Multiple reviews discussing the impact of cystectomy on ovarian reserve and anti-Müllerian hormone (AMH) levels have concluded that a reduction in levels for up to 9 months postoperatively is common. Factors that should be taken into consideration when planning surgery for infertility purposes and the impact in ovarian function are baseline AMH level, the size of the endometrioma (removal of larger cysts can present with larger incidental removal of healthy ovarian tissue), and previous cystectomies [26].

24.4 Lysis of Adhesions

It is common to encounter intraperitoneal adhesions in women with endometriosis [29]. It is well known that adhesions can occur spontaneously, but often are the consequence of peritoneal trauma or inflammation. With endometriosis, the inflammatory process from the endometrial implants could lead to this. There is controversy regarding whether adhesions are a cause of pain or not, but adhesions could compromise fertility by affecting ovaries or fallopian tubes. The presence of dense adhesions can add difficulty and risks to a planned surgical procedure. We do not recommend treatment of all adhesions, and it is our practice to only treat adhesions that are thought to be affecting fertility, the ones that are necessary to treat when performing a specific procedure (endometrioma resection, hysterectomy), if they are dense and vascular, compromising viscera, or if they are suspicious of being a cause of pain based on location. When adhesions are identified, and treated surgically, either liquid or solid barrier agents could be used to try to prevent recurrence or de novo formation, including lactated Ringer's, 4% icodextrin, hyaluronic acid and ferric ion, HAL-C bioresorbable membrane, hydrogel, expanded polytetrafluoroethylene, hyaluronic acid and carboxymethylcellulose, or oxidized regenerated cellulose, among others [10].

24.5 Deep Infiltrative Endometriosis

Deep infiltrative endometriosis (DIE) refers to the presence of endometriotic lesions that invade the peritoneal surface by at least 5 mm in depth [30]. It can extend into the retroperitoneal space or into the wall of abdominopelvic organs such as the bladder and bowel (Fig. 24.6). Patients may be asymptomatic, have nonspecific symptoms such as chronic pelvic pain, or present with organ-specific symptomatology like dysuria, hematuria, constipation, or rectal bleeding. In some patients, it can be severely debilitating [31, 32].

Deep infiltrative endometriosis is less likely to respond adequately to medical or hormonal treatment. Many studies have shown that excision is the standard of care for these

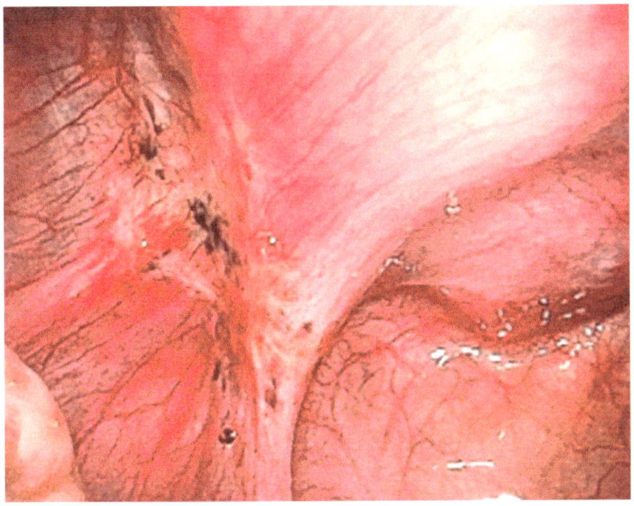

Fig. 24.6 Deep infiltrating endometriosis lesions found along left uterosacral ligament

patients as it improves postoperative pain scores and recurrence rates. Extensive knowledge and comprehension of the retroperitoneal spaces and anatomy is essential for the gynecologic surgeon who will treat advanced endometriosis.

The retroperitoneal spaces include paravesical, paravaginal, pararectal, retrorectal, vesicovaginal, rectovaginal, and retropubic spaces [33]. The gynecologic surgeon must be familiar with the three surgical layers that are found within the pelvic sidewall:

- First layer: contains the ureter on the parietal peritoneum
- Second layer: contains the internal iliac artery and its branches
- Third layer: includes the external iliac vessels and the obturator bundle

Complete excision of DIE often requires dissection into these planes. Various techniques that facilitate retroperitoneal entry and dissection have been described. The surgeon must always start at an area where there is no distortion of the anatomy. This will make it easier to identify surrounding structures and avoid inadvertent injuries.

In the presence of severe pelvic adhesions or disease, access to the retroperitoneum may be gained at the level of the pelvic brim. The peritoneum lateral to the infundibulopelvic ligament is grasped and tented upward. A small superficial incision is made parallel to the ovarian vessels using scissors. Monopolar energy may be used for this step. If the procedure is being performed laparoscopically, carbon dioxide will enter the retroperitoneal space and help develop the avascular planes. This aids in the separation of the medial and lateral leaves of the peritoneum. Access can also be obtained by transecting the round ligament and separating the broad ligament into anterior and posterior leaves and gaining access to the base of the broad ligament.

Table 24.3 Tips and tricks for DIE dissection

Tips and tricks for DIE dissection
• Comprehensive understanding of retroperitoneal anatomy, spaces, and surgical planes
• Begin dissection at "clean" areas where anatomy is not distorted
• Initial peritoneal incision should be superficial and small
• Allow carbon dioxide (in laparoscopy) to aid in developing surgical planes
• The suction-irrigator is helpful for blunt dissection and hydrodissection
• Maintain philosophy of "every millimeter counts"
• Techniques for blunt dissection include traction-countertraction, gentle "wiping, or teasing" of tissue
• The tip of the scissors or dissectors can be used for "push-and-spread" or "poke-and-open" techniques

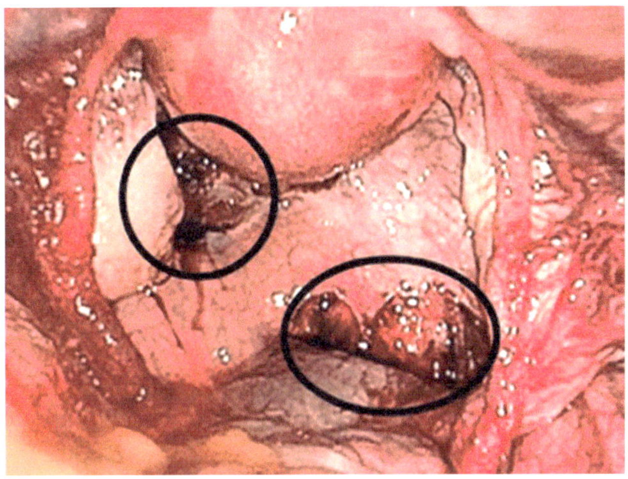

Fig. 24.7 Appearance of posterior cul-de-sac after resection of lesions using a combination of blunt and sharp dissection and monopolar energy

Once within this space, the surgeon must always be aware of the surroundings, keeping in mind that "every millimeter counts" will prevent the surgeon from being too aggressive or making large cuts. Techniques like gentle "wiping" of the tissues, "push and spread," or "poke and open" can be used for dissection of the areolar avascular tissue that surrounds the retroperitoneal structures. Always trying to dissect vascular structures and ureters in a parallel fashion to their axis will avoid potential transection or injuries. "Traction-countertraction" can be extremely helpful for resection of endometriosis and deep lesions as it facilitates definition and identification of tissue planes (Table 24.3). During this dissection, vital structures like the iliac vessels, ureters, psoas muscles, and obturator nerve should be exposed and safeguarded when relevant (Fig. 24.7).

24.6 Urinary Tract Endometriosis

Urinary tract endometriosis (UTE) refers to presence of endometriotic disease in the bladder, ureters, urethra, or kidneys. The occurrence has been reported to range from 0.3 to 12% among women with endometriosis. The bladder accounts for 80% of these cases, followed by the ureters (14%) and the kidneys and urethra comprising the remainder of them. Bladder and ureteral endometriosis rarely coexist [31, 34, 35].

24.6.1 Bladder

Endometriosis affecting the bladder causes urinary symptoms in approximately one-third of women, while the rest may be asymptomatic. The symptoms typically mimic those of a urinary tract infection or interstitial cystitis. Contrary to popular belief, hematuria is only present in 20 to 30% of affected women. This is because bladder nodules do not commonly penetrate through the mucosa [36]. The first imaging modality used for diagnosis is the transvaginal ultrasound (Fig. 24.8). MRI and three-dimensional ultrasound may also be helpful, but further studies are needed to establish which one has superior sensitivity and specificity [37, 38].

Treatment of bladder endometriosis should aim for complete removal of the lesion. Laparoscopic partial cystectomy is considered the treatment of choice and has a low recurrence rate. The cystoscopic approach has been described, but given that most lesions are not transmural, it has a high rate of incomplete resection and bladder perforation.

When there is a known bladder lesion or nodule, the case should begin with a cystoscopy to assess for involvement of the mucosal layer and the distance from the nodule to the ureteral orifices and trigone. Ureteral stents are recommended to facilitate identification of the ureteral orifices during partial cystectomy or in cases where ureteral reimplantation is warranted. Reimplantation is often required when the nodule is within 2 cm of the interureteric ridge.

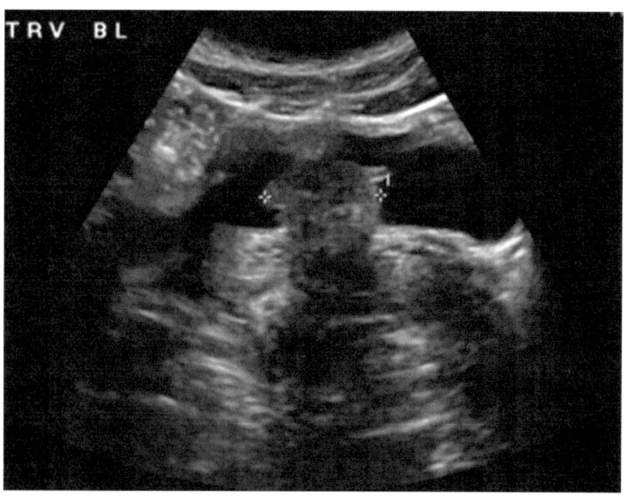

Fig. 24.8 Appearance of a 2.7 cm endometriosis nodule in the posterior wall of the bladder

Backfilling the bladder with normal saline, sterile milk, or methylene blue helps delineate the lesion and begin dissection. Monopolar cutting energy is used to incise the peritoneum around the nodule. Blunt and sharp dissection is used until the base of the nodule is reached while the layers of the bladder are identified. The surgeon should avoid using energy to cut the mucosa. It is important to leave adequate margins. The defect is repaired in two layers using 2–0/3–0 delayed absorbable suture. An indwelling Foley catheter is left in place for approximately 7 days (5–14); after which, a cystogram is performed to ensure integrity of the repair.

Most lesions are found at the bladder dome and can be resected without much difficulty. However, lesions in the trigone may be technically more challenging and are associated with more bothersome postoperative sequelae.

24.6.2 Ureters

Ureteral endometriosis is not usually accompanied by urinary symptoms. More frequently, nonspecific symptoms such as pelvic, back, or flank pain are reported. Essentially, two types of ureteral disease have been described: extrinsic and intrinsic. *Extrinsic disease* is caused by endometriosis that is external and compresses the ureter by causing fibrosis of the overlying peritoneum or uterosacral-cardinal complex. *Intrinsic disease*, which is less common, refers to disease that invades the muscularis or mucosa. The most serious complication that can arise from ureteral involvement is hydronephrosis and loss of kidney function. The left ureter is more frequently affected; bilateral disease is only encountered in 10% of cases [39].

The specific surgical approach will depend on the type and extent of disease as well as the surgeon's skills. Routine ureteral stenting may facilitate the procedure and is recommended albeit not mandatory. Ureterolysis alone is sufficient for the treatment of extrinsic disease in almost 90% of patients. The dissection begins at the pelvic brim and continues caudally toward the bladder. The aim is to fully free the ureter from restrictive lesions while removing any endometriotic nodules encountered along the dissection. In contrast, intrinsic disease may necessitate resection of the ureter with ureteroureterostomy or ureteroneocystostomy.

In any of these cases, consultation with a urologist to plan a joint approach is reasonable and an advisable course of action. Patients should be counseled that the reoperation rate can be as high as 3.9% [34]. Complications arising from urinary tract endometriosis include fistula formation (rates vary depending on exact location and extent of disease), bleeding requiring blood transfusion, and altered urinary function such as neurogenic bladder.

24.7 Bowel Endometriosis

The most common site of extragenital endometriosis is the bowel. Chronic pelvic pain, constipation, and dyschezia are the symptoms more frequently reported, which are frequently cyclical [40]. Imaging studies that can be helpful in providing information are the transvaginal and transrectal ultrasounds. MRI is also widely used due to a high sensitivity and specificity. Colonoscopy is not routinely recommended as lesions that penetrate the mucosa are unusual. It may be useful, however, to exclude a neoplasm or to assess for stenosis if suspected.

Techniques for treating bowel endometriosis are basically divided into three categories [41]:

- *Shaving* – only applied for lesions that do not invade beyond the serosa. Electrosurgery or laser may be used.
- *Discoid full-thickness excision* – for lesions that penetrate beyond the serosa. The lesion and surrounding bowel are removed in "full thickness." The defect is then repaired in two layers.
- *Segmental resection* – reserved for larger or multifocal lesions, lesions causing stenosis or sigmoid involvement. Decision to perform primary anastomosis or diversion depends on location of disease. Consultation with a colorectal surgeon is recommended.

Surgical treatments are tailored to size and location of the lesion(s) as described in Table 24.4.

Table 24.4 Tips and tricks for DIE dissection 4. Treatment for endometriosis affecting bowel

Size	Treatment	
<3 cm	Shaving or discoid resection	
>3 cm (or more than 50% of circumference)	Segmental resection with anastomosis	
Distance from anal verge	*Treatment*	*Most common complications*
<5 cm	May require temporary ileostomy/colostomy	RV fistula (up to 10%) Urinary retention/bladder dysfunction
>5 cm	Segmental resection with anastomosis	RV fistula (up to 2.7%) Anastomotic leakage (1.6%) Abscess (0.3%)

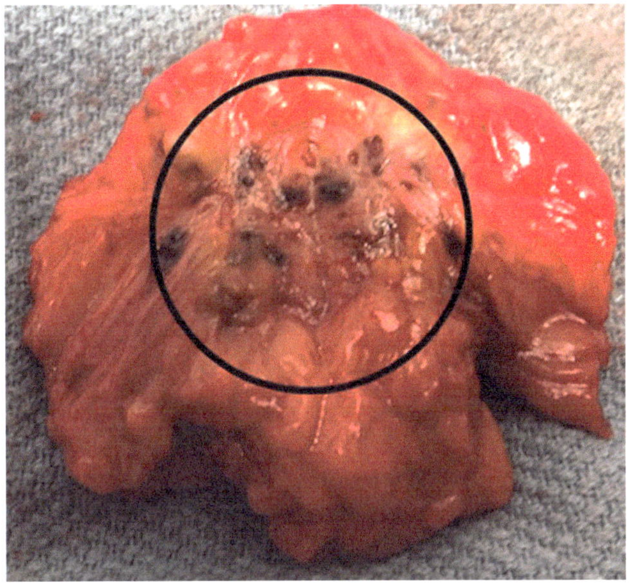

Fig. 24.9 Abdominal wall endometrioma removed from a cesarean section incision in a 36-year-old female with a history of one prior cesarean delivery

24.8 Extra-pelvic Endometriosis

Some of the extra-pelvic sites of endometriosis are the abdominal wall (AWE), diaphragm, lungs, and nervous system. AWE has been described in laparotomy scars and trocar site incisions. Cases of isolated umbilical endometriosis without a prior incision have also been reported. The most common presenting symptom is a palpable, painful abdominal mass. Surgical resection ensuring adequate margins is the mainstay of treatment. Large nodules in the umbilicus may require umbilical reconstruction. Consultation with a plastic surgeon should be considered if extensive reconstruction is anticipated (Fig. 24.9).

24.9 Conservative Versus Extirpative Surgery: The Role of Hysterectomy

Conservative surgery refers to procedures that are fertility-sparing. These include excision or ablation of implants, cystectomy, adhesiolysis, and, in some cases, unilateral oophorectomy. This should be the first-line option for women who opt for surgical management of endometriosis. In contrast, definitive therapy refers to hysterectomy with or without oophorectomy. This modality should be reserved for patients with persistent symptoms who have completed childbearing and have failed medical treatment and conservative surgery. Preoperative counseling should include higher potential intraoperative complications, known adverse health effects of early menopause, potential need to hormone replacement, and possibility of regret. It is of vital importance that other chronic pelvic pain-associated conditions are diagnosed and adequately treated prior to performing extirpative surgery. Among the benefits of hysterectomy are a high rate of satisfaction and a significantly lower reoperation rate. Shakiba et al. reported that women who had conservative laparoscopy versus those who had hysterectomy with bilateral salpingo-oophorectomy had reoperation rates at 7 years of 59 vs 8%, respectively. For patients who had hysterectomy with one or both ovaries preserved, this rate was 24 and 22% [42]. Patients who opt for a supracervical hysterectomy should be counseled on the 10% rate of future trachelectomy [43].

24.10 Role of Robotic Surgery

The benefits of conventional laparoscopic surgery over laparotomy have been well-established. In recent years, attention has been turned to robotic-assisted technology. Few studies have assessed the advantage of robotic surgery in endometriosis cases. Available data suggests that robot-assisted laparoscopy is safe and effective for the treatment of endometriosis, especially in cases of advanced disease. Overall operative time appears to be longer with the use of the robot, with no difference in terms of blood loss, complication rate, or outcomes [44, 45].

24.11 Postoperative Considerations

Postoperative medical therapy is recommended for women who are not actively seeking pregnancy. Long-term medical suppression (6–24 months) appears to be more effective at reducing symptom recurrence and the need for repeat surgery than short-term therapy (3 months or less). The use of combined oral contraceptives or the levonorgestrel-releasing intrauterine device seems to have the most benefit. However, any of the known alternatives may be used (i.e., gonadotropin-releasing hormone analogues, danazol, progestin-only pills).

Hormone replacement therapy (HRT) may be indicated for reproductive-aged women who undergo definitive surgery with removal of both ovaries to decrease health-related adverse effects of early surgical menopause. HRT is also indicated to treat menopausal symptoms such as hot flashes, night sweats, sleep disturbance, and sexual dysfunction. The addition of HRT does not seem to be associated with an increased risk of symptom or disease recurrence [46, 47].

24.12 Conclusions

The decision to operate on a patient with endometriosis should be based on her symptoms and her desire for future fertility. When surgery is performed for pain symptoms, a detailed history and physical exam is key to potentially discover other conditions that are not likely to respond to surgery. Self-awareness of surgical skills is crucial to offer a safe procedure, and when needed an interdisciplinary approach should be considered. Review of postoperative expectations is very important to avoid frustrations due to undesired outcomes.

References

1. Parazzini F, Esposito G, Tozzi L, Noli S, Bianchi S. Epidemiology of endometriosis and its comorbidities. Eur J Obstet Gynecol Reprod Biol. 2016;S0301–2115(16):30172–5.
2. Balasch J, Creus M, Fabregues F, Carmona F, Ordi J, Martinez-Roman S, et al. Visible and non-visible endometriosis at laparoscopy in fertile and infertile women and in patients with chronic pelvic pain: a prospective study. Hum Reprod. 1996;11:387–91.
3. Meuleman C, Vandenabeele B, Fieuws S, Spiessens C, Timmerman D, D'Hooghe T. High prevalence of endometriosis in infertile women with normal ovulation and normospermic partners. Fertil Steril. 2009;92:68–74.
4. Howard FM. The role of laparoscopy in the evaluation of chronic pelvic pain: pitfalls with a negative laparoscopy. J Am Assoc Gynecol Laparosc. 1996;4(1):85.
5. Mowers EL, Lim CS, Skinner B, et al. Prevalence of endometriosis during abdominal or laparoscopic hysterectomy for chronic pelvic pain. Obstet Gynecol. 2016;127(6):1045–53.
6. Sinaii N, Plumb K, Cotton L, et al. Differences in characteristics among 1000 women with endometriosis based on extent of disease. Fertil Steril. 2008;89:538.
7. Vercellini P, Vigano P, Somigliana E, Fedele L. Endometriosis: pathogenesis and treatment. Nat Rev Endocrinol. 2014;10:261.
8. Howard FM. Surgical treatment of endometriosis. Obstet Gynecol Clin N Am. 2011 Dec;38(4):677–86.
9. Walter AJ, Hentz JG, Magtibay PM, et al. Endometriosis: correlation between histologic and visual findings at laparoscopy. Am J Obstet Gynecol. 2001;184:1407–11.
10. Flyckt R, Kim S, Falcone T. Surgical management of endometriosis in patients with chronic pelvic pain. Semin Repod Med. 2017 Jan;35(1):54–64.
11. Ahmad GD, O'Flynn H, Duffy JM, Phillips K, Watson A. Laparoscopic entry techniques. Cochrane Database Syst Rev. 2012;2:CD006583.
12. Somigliana E, Vigano P, Barbara G, Vercellini P. Treatment of endometriosis-related pain: options and outcomes. Front Biosci. 2009;1:455–65.
13. Dunselamn GA, Vermeulen N, Becker C, et al. ESHRE guideline: management of women with endometriosis. Hum Reprod. 2014;29:400.
14. Gustofson KF, Kim N, Liu S, Stratton P. Endometriosis and the appendix: a case series and comprehensive review of the literature. Fertile Steril. 2006;86:298.
15. Duffy JM, Arambage K, Correa FJ, et al. Laparoscopic surgery for endometriosis. Cochrane Database Syst Rev. 2014;(4):CD011031. Published 2014 Apr 3. https://doi.org/10.1002/14651858.CD011031.pub2.

16. Feste JR. Laser laparoscopy: a new modality. J Reprod Med. 1985;30:413–7.
17. Vercellini P, Aimi G, Busacca M, Apolone G, Uglieti A, Crosignani PG. Laparoscopic uterosacral ligament transection for dysmenorrhea associated with endometriosis: results of a randomized, control trial. Fertl Steril. 2003;80(2):310–9.
18. Lee T, Yang L. Pelvic denervation procedures: a current reappraisal. Int J Gynaecol Obstet. 2008 Jun;101(3):304–8.
19. Latthe PM, Proctor ML, Farquhar CM, Johnson N, Khan KS. Surgical interruption of pelvic nerve pathways in dysmenorrhea: a systematic review of effectiveness. Acta Obstet Gynecol Scand. 2007;86(1):4–15.
20. Proctor ML, Latthe PM, Farquhar CM, Khan KS, Johnson NP. Surgical interruption of pelvic nerve pathways for primary and secondary dysmenorrhea. Cochrane Database Syst Rev. 2005;19(4):CD001896.
21. Willard F, Schuenke M. The neuroanatomy of female pelvic pain. In: Pain in women a clinical guide. Berlin: Springer Science+Business Media; 2013. p. 17–58. https://doi.org/10.1007/978-1-4419-7113-5_2.
22. Shoja MM, Sharma A, Mirzayan N, Groat C, Watanabe K, Loukas M, Tubbs RS. Neuroanatomy of the female abdominopelvic region: a review with application to pelvic pain syndromes. Clin Anat. 2013 Jan;26(1):66–76. https://doi.org/10.1002/ca.22200. Epub 2012 Nov 23.
23. Lee R, Stone K, Magelssen D, Belts R, Benson W. Presacral neurectomy for chronic pelvic pain. Obstet Gynecol. 1986;68:517–21.
24. Nezhat C, Nezhat F. A simplified method of laparoscopic presacral neurectomy for treatment of central pelvic pain due to endometriosis. Br J Obstet Gynaecol. 1992;99:659–63.
25. Zullo F, Palomba S, Zupi E, Russo T, Morelli M, Capiello F, et al. Effectiveness of presacral neurectomy in women with severe dysmenorrheal caused by endometriosis who were treated with laparoscopic conservative surgery: a 1 year prospective randomized double blinded controlled trial. Am J Obstet Gynecol. 2003;189:5–10.
26. Cranney R, Condus G, Reid S. An update on the diagnosis, surgical management, and fertility outcomes for women with endometrioma. Acta Obstet Gynecol Scand 2017 Jun;96(6):633–643. https://doi.org/10.1111/aogs.13114. Epub 2017 Mar 11.
27. Qiong-Zhen R, Ge Y, Deng Y, Qian ZH, Zhu WP. Effect of vasopressin injection technique in laparoscopic excision of bilateral ovarian endometriomas on ovarian reserve: prospective randomized study. J Minim Invasive Gynecol. 2014 Mar–Apr;21(2):266–71.
28. Ghafarnejad M, Akrami M, Davari-Tanha F, Adabi K, Nekuie S. Vasopressin effect on operation time and frequency of electrocauterization during laparoscopic stripping of ovarian endometriomas: a randomized controlled clinical trial. J Reprod Infertil. 2014 Oct;15(4):199–204.
29. Parker JD, Sinaii N, Segars JH, et al. Adhesion formation after laparoscopic excision of endometriosis and lysis of adhesions. Fertil Steril. 2005;84:1457.
30. King C, Lum D. Techniques in minimally invasive surgery for advanced endometriosis. Curr Opin Obstet Gynecol. 2016;28(4):316–22.
31. Nezhat C, Falik R, McKinney S, et al. Pathophysiology and management of urinary tract endometriosis. Nat Rev Urol. 2017;14(6):359–72.
32. Nezhat C, Hajhosseini B. King Louise. Laparoscopic management of bowel endometriosis: predictors of severe disease and recurrence. J Society Laparoendoscopic Surgeons. 2011;15(4):431–8.
33. Rogers R, Pasic R. Pelvic retroperitoneal dissection: a hands-on primer. J Minim Invasive Gynecol. 2017;24(4):546–51.
34. Cavaco-Gomes J, Martinho M, Gilabert-Aguilar J, et al. Laparoscopic management of ureteral endometriosis. Eur J Obstet Gynecol Reprod Biol. 2017;210:94–101.
35. Kolodzeij A, Krajewski W, Dolowy L, et al. Urinary tract endometriosis. Urol J. 2015;12(4):2213–7.
36. Liu C, Peresic D, Samadi D, et al. Robotic-assisted laparoscopic partial bladder resection for the treatment of infiltrating endometriosis. J Minim Invasive Gynecol. 2008;15(6):745–8.
37. Nisenblat V, Bossuyt PM, Farquhar C, et al. Imaging studies for the non-invasive diagnosis of endometriosis. Cochrane Database Syst Rev. 2016;26(2):CD009591.
38. Hoyos LR, Johnson S, Puscheck E. Endometriosis and imaging. Clin Obstet Gynecol. 2017;60(3):503–16.
39. Seracchioli R, Mabrouk M, Manuzzi L, et al. Importance of retroperitoneal ureteric evaluation in cases of deep infiltrating endometriosis. J Minim Invasive Gynecol. 2008;15(4):435–9.
40. Soto E, Catenacci M, Bedient C, et al. Assessment of long-term bowel symptoms after segmental resection of deeply infiltrating endometriosis: a matched cohort study. J Minim Invasive Gynecol. 2016;23(5):753–9.
41. Alabiso G, Alio L, Arena S, et al. How to manage bowel endometriosis: the ETIC approach. J Minim Invasive Gynecol. 2015;22(4):517–29.
42. Shakiba K, Bena JF, McGill KM, et al. Surgical treatment of endometriosis: a 7-year follow-up on the requirement for further surgery. Obstet Gynecol. 2008;111(6):1285–92.
43. Martin D. Hysterectomy for treatment of pain associated with endometriosis. J Minim Invasive Gynecol. 2006;13:566–72.
44. Nezhat C, Stevens A, Balassiano E, et al. Robotic-assisted laparoscopy vs conventional laparoscopy for the treatment of advanced stage endometriosis. J Minim Invasive Gynecol. 2013;22(1):40–4.
45. Nezhat C, Lewis M, Kotikela S, et al. Robotic versus standard laparoscopy for the treatment of endometriosis. Fertil Steril. 2010;94(7):2758–60.
46. Frishman G, Salak J. Conservative surgical management of endometriosis in women with pelvic pain. J Minim Invasive Gynecol. 2006;13(6):546–58.
47. Anpalagan A, Condous G. Is there a role for use of levonorgestrel intrauterine system in women with chronic pelvic pain? J Minim Invasive Gynecol. 2008;15(6):663–6.

25 Elective Surgical Removal of Hydrosalpinges

Laura C. Gemmell and Jeffrey M. Goldberg

This chapter aims to discuss the optimal surgical management of hydrosalpinges. The chapter will begin with a discussion on the diagnosis and impact of hydrosalpinges on IVF success rates before paying particular attention to various surgical treatment options. Important preoperative considerations, surgical procedures, and postoperative success rates are included. Evidence for the efficacy of these treatment options, as well as potential alternative treatments, will close the chapter.

25.1 Background

Up to a third of female factor infertility is due to tubal disease [1]. Hydrosalpinx is a distally occluded fallopian tube filled with fluid that may be asymptomatic or result in infertility or chronic pelvic pain. Hydrosalpinges are generally due to a prior episode of salpingitis, most commonly from gonorrhea or chlamydia. Other causes of pelvic inflammation such as appendicitis or endometriosis may also lead to distal tubal occlusion as can a prior ectopic pregnancy. Hydrosalpinges can be treated surgically to improve fertility.

25.2 Investigating Tubal Patency

At the present time, nonsurgical assessment of tubal anatomy and patency in the subfertile patient is best assessed by a hysterosalpingogram (HSG) [2]. HSG involves the transcervical injection of X-ray contrast medium while observing the flow of contrast though the fallopian tubes under fluoroscopic visualization. As a first-line diagnostic tool that is relatively non-invasive, HSG not only investigates tubal patency but also may provide therapeutic effect. This is likely due to flushing mucus plugs and/or debris from the proximal tubal lumen, though the exact mechanism is unknown. A recent meta-analysis reports higher live birth rates and ongoing pregnancy in patients that underwent HSG [3]. The same meta-analysis noted higher pregnancy rates with oil-soluble contrast media compared to no HSG, whereas pregnancy rates with water-soluble contrast vs no HSG were not different. However, studies comparing HSGs performed using oil vs water-soluble contrast found comparable pregnancy rates.

Information obtained from the hysterosalpingogram can help with diagnosis and appropriate therapy. For example, the potential for neosalpingostomy can be estimated based on the diameter of the hydrosalpinx and the presence of mucosal folds. Fimbrial phimosis appears as a distally dilated tube with free spill and may be amenable to laparoscopic fimbrioplasty. Salpingitis isthmica nodosa is best diagnosed by HSG, and post-spill loculation of contrast is suggestive of peritubal adhesions.

Although the negative predictive value of HSG is relatively high [4], it is important for clinicians to be aware that a positive HSG is by no means definitive, especially for proximal tubal occlusion. A prospective study of 360 infertile women found that over 60% of patients with a finding of proximal tubal occlusion on HSG will be patent on a second HSG 1 month later [5]. This is likely due to functional spasm of the utero-tubal ostium. Even the direct visualization of bilateral occlusion during laparoscopy is not 100 percent definitive, as spontaneous pregnancies after this finding have been reported [6].

Tubal patency can also be investigated using hysterosalpingo-contrast sonography (HyCoSy) [7]. Saline or albumin containing small bubbles is injected through a transcervical catheter, and the echogenic medium is observed to traverse the tubes and enter the peritoneal cavity by

L. C. Gemmell
Case Western Reserve University School of Medicine, Cleveland, OH, USA

J. M. Goldberg (✉)
Reproductive Endocrinology and Infertility, Department of Obstetrics and Gynecology, Cleveland Clinic, Cleveland, OH, USA
e-mail: goldbej@ccf.org

G. N. Allahbadia et al. (eds.), *Textbook of Assisted Reproduction*, https://doi.org/10.1007/978-981-15-2377-9_25

transvaginal ultrasonography. It has the advantages of avoiding ionizing radiation exposure and also provides information about the myometrium and ovaries. However, it lacks the anatomic details of the tubal lumen seen with HSG, and there is no evidence of a therapeutic effect.

25.3 Hydrosalpinx and Poor IVF Outcome

Women with unilateral or bilateral hydrosalpinges have significantly decreased implantation and pregnancy rates following in vitro fertilization and embryo transfer (IVF-ET) compared to patients without hydrosalpinges [8]. Two meta-analyses have explored these associations [9, 10].

The first meta-analysis included 13 published reports and 10 abstracts, none of which were prospective in design. IVF-ET cycles without hydrosalpinx (n = 5569) and with hydrosalpinx (n = 1144) were compared. Results indicated that both implantation and clinical pregnancy rates were reduced by 50% in patients with a hydrosalpinx. In addition, the presence of a hydrosalpinx appeared to increase the risk of pregnancy loss, as the abortion rate was increased 2.3 fold (95% CI: 1.6–3.5) [9]. The second meta-analysis, published a year later, included many of the same studies (nine published studies and five abstracts) and similarly concluded that hydrosalpinx during IVF-ET was associated with a reduced (i) pregnancy rate (OR: 0.64; 95% CI: 0.56–0.74), (ii) implantation rate (8.5% vs. 13.7% in the non-hydrosalpinx group), and (iii) delivery rate (13.4% vs. 23.4% in the non-hydrosalpinx group) [10].

Several theories exist to explain the negative impact of hydrosalpinges on IVF outcomes. The proximal end of the hydrosalpinx is usually open, and thus immunologic mediators, toxic debris, and excess fluid may enter the uterine cavity. The fluid may have a direct embryotoxic effect, decrease endometrial receptivity (via decreased beta-3 integrin, HOXA10, VEGF, and/or vascular perfusion) [11–14], or mechanically flush the embryo from the uterus prior to implantation. Whatever the mechanism may be, it is clear that surgical intervention in patients with hydrosalpinges before IVF improves pregnancy rates and outcomes.

25.4 Surgical Management of Hydrosalpinges Prior to IVF

25.4.1 Salpingectomy

A Cochran meta-analysis of three randomized controlled trials (RCTs) with 395 patients compared IVF clinical pregnancy rates with and without prior laparoscopic salpingectomy and reported that salpingectomy restored the IVF pregnancy rate back to normal, OR 2.31 (CI 1.48–3.62) [15]. Salpingectomy involves removal of the fallopian tube. The procedure is typically performed laparoscopically with a 5 mm laparoscopic port in each lower quadrant and a 10 mm port in the umbilicus to extract the tube from the abdominal cavity. The surgeon may begin proximally or distally. The proximal tube and mesosalpinx are coagulated and divided. This can be accomplished with whatever modality is preferred such as bipolar graspers and scissors, harmonic scalpel, or vessel sealing devices such as LigaSure (Covidien, Minneapolis). During this coagulation, it is important to stay as close to the tube as possible to limit the chance of compromising the ovarian blood supply resulting in diminished ovarian reserve. However, a randomized controlled trial challenged this by finding no significant differences in ovarian reserve between this technique and wide excision of the mesosalpinx [16]. The tube is removed through the 10 mm umbilical port while observing through the laparoscope in one of the lower quadrant 5 mm ports. The abdomen is irrigated, and the vascular pedicles are checked for hemostasis, while the insufflation pressure is reduced. Postoperatively, patients may undergo IVF once menses resume.

25.4.2 Tubal Ligation

Laparoscopic tubal ligation may be performed in cases where extensive pelvic adhesions make salpingectomy not only technically difficult but also risky to the patient. Given that hydrosalpinges may exert their adverse effects on fertility outcome via communication with the uterine cavity, proximal tubal ligation can interrupt this mechanism. However, there is a theoretical concern that this may cause the hydrosalpinges to dilate further and cause pain. It is therefore recommended that the hydrosalpinx be fenestrated as fully as possible. If one does accept that salpingectomy has the potential to diminish ovarian reserve, tubal ligation should eliminate or, at least, minimize the risk. However, a prospective cohort study of 134 cycles found no significant difference in anti-mullerian hormone (AMH) or ovarian response to stimulation for IVF in patients who underwent salpingectomy vs proximal tubal occlusion [17]. A RCT compared salpingectomy (n = 50) to bipolar tubal ligation (n = 50 and 15 patients with untreated hydrosalpinges) [18]. In addition to confirming no significant difference in response to controlled ovarian hyperstimulation for IVF as above, there were no differences between the number of eggs and embryos obtained. Furthermore, the clinical pregnancy and live birth rates were not different between salpingectomy and tubal ligation, but both treatments were significantly better than the untreated control group [18]. Table 25.1 summarizes the RCTs of salpingectomy vs untreated hydrosalpinges (control), tubal ligation vs control, and salpingectomy vs tubal ligation [15]. The outcome is the IVF clinical pregnancy rate.

Table 25.1 RCTs of salpingectomy vs untreated hydrosalpinges (control), tubal ligation vs control, and salpingectomy vs tubal ligation

	Studies/patients	OR (95% CI)
Salpingectomy vs control	3/395	2.3 (1.48, 3.62)
Tubal ligation vs control	2/209	4.7 (2.17, 10.01)
Salpingectomy vs ligation	2/228	1.3 (0.76, 2.14)

25.4.3 Hysteroscopic Proximal Tubal Occlusion

For patients who are poor surgical candidates for even laparoscopic tubal ligation, hysteroscopic proximal tubal occlusion can be accomplished with the Essure device (Bayer, Whippany, NJ). However, the trailing coils within the endometrial cavity have the hypothetical risk of an IUD-like effect on the endometrial cavity. A non-randomized study found no difference in clinical pregnancy rate with IVF in patients who underwent prior laparoscopic tubal ligation or hysteroscopic proximal tubal occlusion. Unfortunately, the spontaneous abortion rate was double with Essure, 50% vs 25%, and the live birth rate was lower, 23.8% vs 32.1% [19]. A subsequent RCT between tubal ligation and Essure also reported that the spontaneous abortion rate with Essure was double [20]. This study also noted that the implantation rate, clinical pregnancy, and live birth rates with tubal ligation were approximately twice those with Essure, 16.7% vs 38.3%, 31.0% vs 58.1%, and 21.4% vs 46.5%, respectively. Thus, it appears that IVF outcomes following hysteroscopic proximal tubal occlusion with the Essure device are not different from those with untreated hydrosalpinges [20].

25.4.4 Salpingostomy

Another option for managing hydrosalpinges prior to IVF is laparoscopic distal neosalpingostomy. A nonrandomized study looked at IVF pregnancy rates in patients with hydrosalpinges treated with salpingectomy vs salpingostomy [21]. Of the 24 patients treated with bilateral salpingectomy, 11 conceived for a 47.8% pregnancy rate. The pregnancy rate in the 22 patients following salpingostomy was 45.5%. In addition, 10/34 (29.4%) conceived spontaneously after salpingostomy alone. The effect of salpingostomy on fertility outcome was recently explored by a systematic review and meta-analysis. Twenty-two observational studies with 2810 patients were included. All patients had undergone salpingostomy as treatment for hydrosalpinx and attempted natural conception. The reported pooled natural clinical pregnancy rate from this cohort was 27% [22]. This low rate may be attributed to significant heterogeneity in numerous clinical aspects such as surgical technique, surgeons' experience, duration of follow-up, and, most importantly, the degree of tubal damage. Studies that stratified outcomes based on the extent of disease reported that in those classified as having mild disease, pregnancy rates were 58–77% compared to 0–22% in those with severe tubal disease who had higher ectopic pregnancy rates as well [23]. Table 25.2 summarizes the pros and cons of salpingectomy vs salpingostomy prior to IVF.

Table 25.2 The pros and cons of salpingectomy vs salpingostomy prior to IVF

Salpingectomy	Salpingostomy
Proven efficacy in RCTs	Limited data
Can't conceive without IVF	Spontaneous conception is possible
May decrease ovarian reserve	May reocclude. Ectopic risk
For moderate—severe hydrosalpinges	For mild hydrosalpinges

Salpingostomy should be considered first-line treatment in relatively young patients with no other significant infertility factors and good prognosis mild hydrosalpinges. Although there is no standard scoring system for grading hydrosalpinges, good prognosis features include tubal dilation <3 cm, no more than mild adnexal adhesions, thin pliable tubal walls, mucosal folds on HSG, and normal appearing endosalpinx upon opening of the tube [24]. Patients should be consented for both salpingostomy and salpingectomy, as the final decision is made upon direct visualization of the tube during laparoscopy. Preoperative intravenous antibiotics should be routinely administered to avoid stimulating a chronic salpingitis infection.

Neosalpingostomy is performed laparoscopically using microsurgical technique. The precepts of microsurgical technique are attention to gentle tissue handling, irrigation to prevent tissue desiccation, meticulous hemostasis, avoiding foreign body contamination, and use of fine non-reactive sutures placed without undue tension to prevent tissue ischemia. An orogastric tube and indwelling Foley catheter are placed at the start of every laparoscopic procedure to reduce the risk of trocar injuries. A uterine manipulator with chromotubation capability is also inserted. Our preference is to place the laparoscope through a 5 mm umbilical port and insert an additional 5 mm laparoscopic port in each lower quadrant.

The neosalpingostomy begins with complete excision of all adhesions and transcervical chromotubation to confirm patency of the proximal tubes. The distal mesosalpinx is injected with dilute vasopressin (20 units in 100 mL of injectable saline) to improve hemostasis. The vasoconstriction reduces bleeding and limits the need for electrosurgery with the potential for thermal injury. During neosalpingostomy, the distal end of the hydrosalpinx is incised using a unipolar needle with cutting current. Thermal spread is minimized due to the high power density at the needle tip. The incision is opened widely to assess the endosalpinx for normal tubal mucosa and to fully evert the edges of the opened

Table 25.3 Comparison between scissors and suture and unipolar needle Bruhat and suture

	PR	IUP	Ectopic
Scissors, suture $n = 26$	9 (35%)	5 (19%)	4 (15%)
Unipolar needle, Bruhat $n = 27$	13 (48%)	10 (37%)	3 (11%)
Unipolar needle, suture $n = 29$	15 (52%)	14 (48%)	1 (3%)

tube. The newly created flaps are maintained in the everted position by suturing them to the adjacent tubal serosa with 4–0 delayed absorbable suture using intracorporeal knot tying. Both the surgeon and assistant together complete the knot tying, eliminating the need for a third ancillary laparoscopic port. To facilitate passage of the needle through the 5 mm port, the suture end of the SH needle may be straightened using hemostats to form a "ski." Transcervical chromopertubation with dilute indigo carmine or methylene blue dye is performed through the uterine manipulator to document tubal patency. Lastly, Interceed (Ethicon, Somerville, NJ), a self-adhering absorbable sheet of oxidized regenerated cellulose, is placed over the tube to aid in the prevention of postoperative adhesions. Utilizing the unipolar needle to open the tube and sutures to keep the tube open has been shown to yield higher intrauterine pregnancy rates compared to using scissors to open the tube and the Bruhat technique of using thermal energy to evert the tubal flaps (Table 25.3) [25].

Postoperative considerations focus on time before attempting conception and ectopic pregnancy precautions. Typically, patients are instructed to wait two cycles prior to attempting conception. If a patient is not pregnant within 6 months of attempting conception, tubal patency should be reassessed using HSG. If reocclusion were apparent on imaging, salpingectomy prior to IVF would be recommended. In a very small percentage of patients where IVF is not an option, repeat operations for distal occlusions may be considered, although success rates are very low in this cohort [26]. Patients are also thoroughly counseled regarding the risk and symptoms of ectopic pregnancy and are instructed to call immediately with a positive pregnancy test.

25.5 Nonsurgical Options

In cases where salpingectomy is not practical or safe, transvaginal ultrasound-guided aspiration of hydrosalpinges at oocyte retrieval may provide an alternative option. A retrospective study with 34 patients noted that aspiration of the hydrosalpinges improved IVF implantation and clinical and ongoing pregnancy rates vs untreated hydrosalpinges [27]. Another retrospective study with 48 patients could not confirm a benefit to aspiration [28]. A more recent RCT with 66 hydrosalpinges patients found that aspiration increased the biochemical pregnancy rate compared to the untreated control group, but there was no significant difference in implantation, clinical pregnancy, or spontaneous abortion rates [29]. This study also treated those in the aspiration group with a 3-day course of oral antibiotics. An uncontrolled retrospective study treated 17 hydrosalpinges patients with doxycycline for a week before and after oocyte retrieval and noted that the live birth rate was similar to patients undergoing IVF without hydrosalpinges [30]. The obvious limitations of this study preclude making any conclusions regarding the effectiveness of antibiotic treatment.

In the RTC above, 30.8% of the aspirated hydrosalpinges had re-accumulated within 2 weeks, though it did not appear to affect the IVF success rates [29]. A subsequent study performed sclerotherapy in 123 patients by injecting 98% ethanol into the aspirated hydrosalpinges for 5–10 min [31]. Despite this, 21.7% of the hydrosalpinges recurred. The implantation, clinical pregnancy, and live birth rates were no different whether or not the hydrosalpinges recurred compared to a non-hydrosalpinx control group. All three groups were significantly higher than the untreated hydrosalpinx group [31]. This treatment option warrants further investigation. Obviously, only hydrosalpinges that are visible by ultrasonography are amenable to sclerotherapy. This opens the ongoing debate as to whether hydrosalpinges that are not visible by ultrasonography have the same detrimental effect as those that are seen. Thus, there are no data to guide the decision regarding the necessity to treat mild hydrosalpinges seen only on HSG prior to IVF.

25.6 Summary

Evidence suggests that women with unilateral or bilateral hydrosalpinges prior to IVF-ET have reduced pregnancy outcomes. Surgical management in the form of laparoscopic neosalpingostomy is considered first-line treatment for good prognosis patients. Salpingectomy or tubal ligation procedures are recommended for all other patients with hydrosalpinges. Essure placement is indicated only in high-risk surgical patients but may negate the benefit of treating hydrosalpinges. Insufficient data exists on the efficacy of transvaginal aspiration, with or without sclerotherapy, at the time of oocyte retrieval to make any conclusions with confidence.

References

1. Honore GM, Holden AE, Schenken RS. Pathophysiology and management of proximal tubal blockage. Fertil Steril. 1999;71(5):785–95.
2. Optimal evaluation of the infertile female. Fertil Steril. 2006;86(5 Suppl 1):S264–7.
3. Mohiyiddeen L, Hardiman A, Fitzgerald C, Hughes E, Mol BW, Johnson N, et al. Tubal flushing for subfertility. Cochrane Database Syst Rev. 2015;2015(5):Cd003718.

4. Evers JL, Land JA, Mol BW. Evidence-based medicine for diagnostic questions. Semin Reprod Med. 2003;21(1):9–15.
5. Dessole S, Meloni GB, Capobianco G, Manzoni MA, Ambrosini G, Canalis GC. A second hysterosalpingography reduces the use of selective technique for treatment of a proximal tubal obstruction. Fertil Steril. 2000;73(5):1037–9.
6. Mol BW, Collins JA, Burrows EA, van der Veen F, Bossuyt PM. Comparison of hysterosalpingography and laparoscopy in predicting fertility outcome. Hum Reprod. 1999;14(5):1237–42.
7. Hamed HO, Shahin AY, Elsamman AM. Hysterosalpingo-contrast sonography versus radiographic hysterosalpingography in the evaluation of tubal patency. Int J Gynaecol Obstet. 2009;105(3):215–7.
8. Murray DL, Sagoskin AW, Widra EA, Levy MJ. The adverse effect of hydrosalpinges on in vitro fertilization pregnancy rates and the benefit of surgical correction. Fertil Steril. 1998;69(1):41–5.
9. Zeyneloglu HB, Arici A, Olive DL. Adverse effects of hydrosalpinx on pregnancy rates after in vitro fertilization-embryo transfer. Fertil Steril. 1998;70(3):492–9.
10. Camus E, Poncelet C, Goffinet F, Wainer B, Merlet F, Nisand I, et al. Pregnancy rates after in-vitro fertilization in cases of tubal infertility with and without hydrosalpinx: a meta-analysis of published comparative studies. Hum Reprod. 1999;14(5):1243–9.
11. Mukherjee T, Copperman AB, McCaffrey C, Cook CA, Bustillo M, Obasaju MF. Hydrosalpinx fluid has embryotoxic effects on murine embryogenesis: a case for prophylactic salpingectomy. Fertil Steril. 1996;66(5):851–3.
12. Strandell A, Lindhard A. Why does hydrosalpinx reduce fertility? The importance of hydrosalpinx fluid. Hum Reprod. 2002;17(5):1141–5.
13. Daftary GS, Taylor HS. Hydrosalpinx fluid diminishes endometrial cell HOXA10 expression. Fertil Steril. 2002;78(3):577–80.
14. Savaris RF, Pedrini JL, Flores R, Fabris G, Zettler CG. Expression of alpha 1 and beta 3 integrins subunits in the endometrium of patients with tubal phimosis or hydrosalpinx. Fertil Steril. 2006;85(1):188–92.
15. Johnson N, van Voorst S, Sowter MC, Strandell A, Mol BW. Surgical treatment for tubal disease in women due to undergo in vitro fertilisation. Cochrane Database Syst Rev. 2010;2010(1):Cd002125.
16. Venturella R, Morelli M, Lico D, Di Cello A, Rocca M, Sacchinelli A, et al. Wide excision of soft tissues adjacent to the ovary and fallopian tube does not impair the ovarian reserve in women undergoing prophylactic bilateral salpingectomy: results from a randomized, controlled trial. Fertil Steril. 2015;104(5):1332–9.
17. Ni L, Sadiq S, Mao Y, Cui Y, Wang W, Liu J. Influence of various tubal surgeries to serum antimullerian hormone level and out come of the subsequent IVF-ET treatment. Gynecol Endocrinol. 2013;29(4):345–9.
18. Kontoravdis A, Makrakis E, Pantos K, Botsis D, Deligeoroglou E, Creatsas G. Proximal tubal occlusion and salpingectomy result in similar improvement in in vitro fertilization outcome in patients with hydrosalpinx. Fertil Steril. 2006;86(6):1642–9.
19. Ozgur K, Bulut H, Berkkanoglu M, Coetzee K, Kaya G. ICSI pregnancy outcomes following hysteroscopic placement of Essure devices for hydrosalpinx in laparoscopic contraindicated patients. Reprod Biomed Online. 2014;29(1):113–8.
20. Dreyer K, Lier MC, Emanuel MH, Twisk JW, Mol BW, Schats R, et al. Hysteroscopic proximal tubal occlusion versus laparoscopic salpingectomy as a treatment for hydrosalpinges prior to IVF or ICSI: an RCT. Hum Reprod. 2016;31(9):2005–16.
21. Chanelles O, Ducarme G, Sifer C, Hugues JN, Touboul C, Poncelet C. Hydrosalpinx and infertility: what about conservative surgical management? Eur J Obstet Gynecol Reprod Biol. 2011;159(1):122–6.
22. Chu J, Harb HM, Gallos ID, Dhillon R, Al-Rshoud FM, Robinson L, et al. Salpingostomy in the treatment of hydrosalpinx: a systematic review and meta-analysis. Hum Reprod. 2015;30(8): 1882–95.
23. Nackley AC, Muasher SJ. The significance of hydrosalpinx in in vitro fertilization. Fertil Steril. 1998;69(3):373–84.
24. Role of tubal surgery in the era of assisted reproductive technology: a committee opinion. Fertil Steril. 2015;103(6):e37–43.
25. Oh ST. Tubal patency and conception rates with three methods of laparoscopic terminal neosalpingostomy. J Am Assoc Gynecol Laparosc. 1996;3(4):519–23.
26. The American Fertility Society classifications of adnexal adhesions, distal tubal occlusion, tubal occlusion secondary to tubal ligation, tubal pregnancies, mullerian anomalies and intrauterine adhesions. Fertil Steril. 1988;49(6):944–55.
27. Van Voorhis BJ, Sparks AE, Syrop CH, Stovall DW. Ultrasound-guided aspiration of hydrosalpinges is associated with improved pregnancy and implantation rates after in-vitro fertilization cycles. Hum Reprod. 1998;13(3):736–9.
28. Sowter MC, Akande VA, Williams JA, Hull MG. Is the outcome of in-vitro fertilization and embryo transfer treatment improved by spontaneous or surgical drainage of a hydrosalpinx? Hum Reprod. 1997;12(10):2147–50.
29. Hammadieh N, Coomarasamy A, Ola B, Papaioannou S, Afnan M, Sharif K. Ultrasound-guided hydrosalpinx aspiration during oocyte collection improves pregnancy outcome in IVF: a randomized controlled trial. Hum Reprod. 2008;23(5):1113–7.
30. Hurst BS, Tucker KE, Awoniyi CA, Schlaff WD. Hydrosalpinx treated with extended doxycycline does not compromise the success of in vitro fertilization. Fertil Steril. 2001;75(5):1017–9.
31. Zhang WX, Jiang H, Wang XM, Wang L. Pregnancy and perinatal outcomes of interventional ultrasound sclerotherapy with 98% ethanol on women with hydrosalpinx before in vitro fertilization and embryo transfer. Am J Obstet Gynecol. 2014;210(3): 250.e1–5.

Lateral Metroplasty and Hysteroscopic Uterine Septum Surgery

26

Ian Waldman and Stephanie J. Estes

26.1 Chapter Objectives

At the end of this chapter, the reader will be able to identify characteristics of a T-shaped and septate uterus. The reader will also understand the current literature on surgical treatment focused on achieving optimal pregnancy outcomes for these uterine anomalies.

26.2 Uterine Physiology: T-Shaped and Septate Uteri

26.2.1 General Embryology

The paramesonephric ducts are the embryologic origin of the uterus and are created by the midline fusion of the mullerian ducts by the tenth week of gestation. Typical developmental milestones include uterine canalization by the 22nd week of gestation with formation of the endometrial cavity that will then be ready for implantation and the carrying of a gestation once pubarche occurs [1].

Normal growth and development of the uterus does not always occur which can result in mullerian anomalies such as uterine agenesis or hypoplasia, unicornuate uterus, bicornuate uterus, uterine didelphys, septate uterus, arcuate uterus, T-shaped uterus, or other unclassified abnormalities. The prevalence of uterine malformations in the general population is approximately 2–4% [2, 3]; however, in the patients with infertility or recurrent pregnancy loss, the frequency of a uterine anomaly increases to 8.0% and 25%, respectively [4, 5]. Traditionally, a septate uterus is the most common form of mullerian abnormalities and is approximately 35% of cases when evaluating the combined population of fertile and infertile women (Fig. 26.1) [6]. In a study of 1089 women without a history of infertility or recurrent pregnancy loss, the prevalence of septate uterus was 3% and arcuate uterus was 5% [7]. The prevalence of a "T"-shaped uterus is more difficult to ascertain as it has been most commonly associated with fetal diethylstilbestrol (DES) exposure in utero which was discontinued in the 1970s [8, 9].

The "T"-shaped uterus is primarily seen in those women whose mothers' were treated between 1950 and 1957 with DES, a potent non-steroidal estrogen to prevent preterm labor. At least 4 million women, and subsequently their fetuses, were exposed to DES in utero prior to its discontinuation after determining it had a mild carcinogenic effect and a potent teratogenic effect [10]. In a study of 267 DES exposed women, it was found that 69% demonstrated an abnormality of the reproductive tract. Of those with an abnormal finding, the "T"-shaped uterus occurred in 89% and was the most common anomaly found [11]. Uterine anomalies such as a T-shaped uterus (19%), hypoplastic uterus (13%), and T-shaped/hypoplastic uterus (30%) have been described [12]. Fortunately, none of the "third-

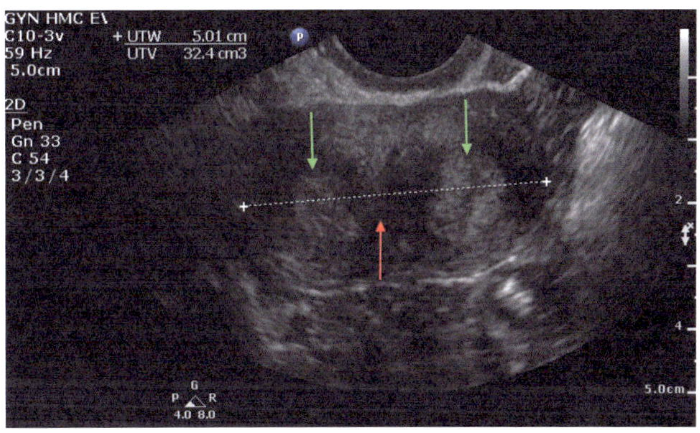

Fig. 26.1 Transvaginal ultrasound transverse view of uterine septum. Dotted line indicates uterine width. Green arrows designate the endometrial cavities. Red arrow notes the area of the uterine septum

I. Waldman
Department of Obstetrics and Gynecology, Penn State Milton S. Hershey Medical Center, Hershey, PA, USA

S. J. Estes (✉)
Division of Reproductive Endocrinology and Infertility, Department of Obstetrics and Gynecology, Penn State Health, Hershey, PA, USA
e-mail: sestes@pennstatehealth.psu.edu

G. N. Allahbadia et al. (eds.), *Textbook of Assisted Reproduction*, https://doi.org/10.1007/978-981-15-2377-9_26

generation" daughters of women exposed to DES were found to have the changes that were usually associated with DES exposure making the carryover effects of in utero DES exposure unlikely [13].

The mullerian duct is the embryologic origin of the female reproductive tract, and once differentiation occurs, the homeobox (Hox) and wingless-type MMTV integration site (Wnt) gene signaling pathways are likely linked to normal female reproductive tract development [14]. In mouse models, the primary Hox genes involved in this process include Hoxa9 (oviduct), Hoxa10 (uterine mesenchyme), Hoxa11 (posterior uterus and cervix), and Hoxa13 (cervix and upper vagina) [15]. Mutations in these genes have been found to have subsequent anomalies, and there exists a synergistic and overlapping gene expression for the different Hox genes [14]. Abnormalities related to Hox genes are a theoretical cause of mullerian anomalies found in humans. All of the genetic and molecular mechanisms causing uterine anomalies have not yet been elucidated, but continued study could one day result in targeted gene therapy.

26.2.2 T-Shaped Uterus

The exact pathophysiology of the "T"-shaped morphology is not known. In DES cases, inhibition of Wnt5a, Wnt7a, Hoxa10, and Hoxa11 genes are probable targets as they are important in development of the uterotubal junction, stratification of the uterine epithelium, organization of uterine muscle layers, and uterine adenogenesis, which are all aberrant in the DES-exposed fetus [14, 16]. Abnormal uterine morphology has been replicated utilizing Hox and Wnt null mice. Wnt7a has been shown to be necessary to the maintenance of Hoxa10 and Hoxa11 expression, and lack of Wnt7a expression results in a thin, small uterus lacking glands [17]. In a DES-exposed mouse model, this caused a shift in Hoxa9 resulting in downregulation of Hoxa10 and Hoxa11 which subsequently expressed the phenotypic malformations of the reproductive tract consistent with aberrant uterine transformation [18].

In a meta-analysis evaluating DES-exposed patients, there was found to be a tenfold increase in ectopic pregnancy (5% vs 0.05%), doubling of spontaneous abortion rate (24% vs 13%), doubling of preterm delivery (14% vs. 7%), and a decrease in live birth rate (76% vs. 92%) compared to age-matched controls [19]. Physiologically, several explanations have been found to account for these poor pregnancy outcomes in those patients who had been exposed to DES. There was found to be decreased endometrial thickness in the luteal phase making early embryo support lacking, increased impedance through the uterine arteries thereby decreasing uterine perfusion and making it difficult to sustain the increase blood flow necessary to maintain a pregnancy, higher rates of autoimmune disease (such as antiphospholipid syndrome) found in women exposed to DES, and multiple altered immune responses [20–22].

26.2.3 Septate Uterus

The septate uterus is formed from a complete or partial lack of resorption of the septum between the two fused mullerian ducts. Candidate genes in cohorts with septate uteri have been noted for Hoxa10, Hoxa11, and Hoxa13 variants. In a prospective observational study, Zhu et al. evaluated the presence of Hoxa10, empty spiracles homeobox 2 (EMX2), and tenascin-M (TENM1) in patients with a partial uterine septum and infertility [23]. Significantly increased expression of Hoxa10 compared to controls and a significantly decreased expression of both EMX2 and TENM1 in the mid-secretory endometrium suggest their involvement in uterine septum formation and other mullerian anomalies. Another potential gene of interest is the hepatocyte nuclear factor 1B (HNF1B). HNF1B has been implicated in familial syndromes with congenital absence of the uterus and subsequently in variable uterine malformations with HNF1B heterozygous mutations [24]. HNF1B is primarily seen in those syndromic patients who also have a coexistent renal anomaly but is of interest for continued research in those with isolated uterine malformations.

The physiology of the septate uterus contributes to potential adverse pregnancy outcomes in situations such as recurrent pregnancy loss. The rationale for pregnancy loss is felt, in part, to be secondary to the septal implantation site which does not contain the necessary physiologic requirements due to inadequate vascularization of the septum to support pregnancy [25]. A uterine septum can lead to a variation in basal state that can negatively affect embryonic or placental implantation [26, 27]. In the past, others opined that a septum could result in irregular uterine contractions that alter sperm migration and transport [28]. Another possible etiology may be a defect in messenger RNA (mRNA) expression in vascular endothelial growth factor (VEGF) receptors. Raga et al. found, in a prospective observational study, the mRNA expressions of VEGF receptors were significantly lower in the endometrium overlying the septum compared to the normal lateral uterine side walls [29].

26.3 Classification of Uterine Anomalies

Diagnosis by the American Fertility Society criterion (ASRM) [30] or European Society of Human Reproduction and Embryology-European Society for Gynaecological Endoscopy (ESHRE-ESGE) has been proposed [31] in the search for an all-encompassing useful and facile categorization of female genital tract anomalies [32]. Subclassifications for the American Fertility Society Classes V and VI uterine anomalies have been suggested as well [33]. Classification regarding structural anatomy is critical for standardization, not only for clarifying treatment intervention and their outcomes but also for communication between providers and ultimately prognosis counseling for patients.

The American Fertility Society (AFS) created a classification system that was published in 1988. This categorizes a T-shaped uterus as a *Group VII* DES Drug-related anomaly and a septate uterus (partial or complete) within a *Group V* designation with the depth of the external fundal indentation no greater than 1 cm and internal fundal indentation ≥1.5 cm. An arcuate uterus is separately listed in *Group VI* and is described as an internal fundal indentation of ≥1 cm and ≤1.5 cm [30].

The European Society of Human Reproduction and Embryology (ESHRE)/European Society for Gynaecological Endoscopy (ESGE) system was published in 2013 to account for the known anomalies that were not included in the AFS system and eliminate the subjective diagnosis of septate uterus by the AFS criteria [34, 35]. This classification reports a T-shaped uterus a *Class I* (dysmorphic) uterus. The septate uterus is *Class II* which incorporates all cases with normal fusion and abnormal absorption of the midline septum. The diagnosis of a septate uterus occurs with an internal fundal indentation greater than 50% of the uterine wall, if the depth of the external intercornual cleft is less than 50%. No specific measurement, as in millimeters of thickness, is utilized [36].

The primary issue with the ESHRE-ESGE criteria for diagnosis of septate uteri is the significantly higher frequency of diagnosis compared to the AFS criteria (RR 2.74), thereby increasing the likelihood of potential unnecessary therapy and associated morbidity [34]. This is emphasized by noting that 16 of the 44 patients diagnosed with septate uteri by the ESHRE-ESGE criteria had internal fundal indentations less than 1 cm in this prospective trial and therefore would not have met ASRM criteria [34]. Multiple authors have come forward with a variety of other classification strategies. One example is the Tompkins Index (the height of the defect/length of the interostia line) with a value more than 25% considered to be a septate or bicornuate uterus rather than an arcuate uterus [37]. Also, some have used an angle less than 75 degrees between the uterine horns to suggest a septate uterus and an angle >105 degrees to be a bicornuate uterus [38]. Until various classification systems are studied in relationship to outcomes, they will not encompass their full potential. In the meantime, clearly describing the uterine anomaly is the best practice.

The anatomical description can begin with an initial evaluation with transvaginal 2D ultrasound as a valuable first-line tool given its ease of accessibility, low cost, noninvasive nature, and acceptable accuracy. Sonohysterography or transvaginal 3D ultrasonography have improved sensitivity in addition to specificity and predictive values, but MRI provides complete detailed images of the mullerian duct anomalies for complex anomalies and is consistently superior in evaluating the vaginal and cervix anatomy (Fig. 26.2) [39, 40].

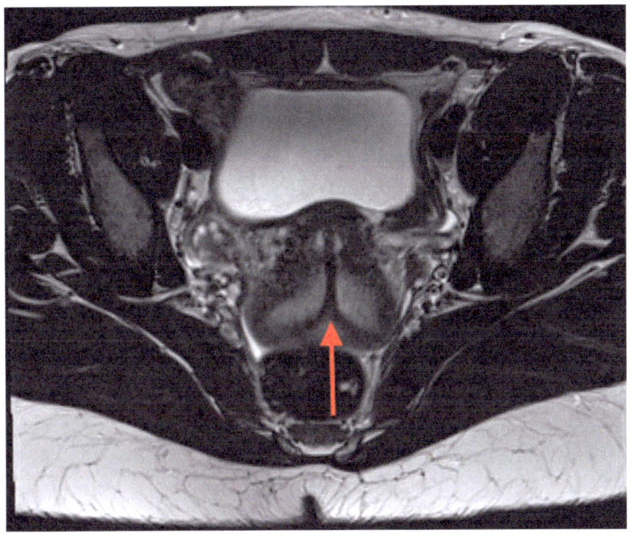

Fig. 26.2 MRI of complete uterine septum. Red arrow runs parallel to complete uterine septum which extends from the uterine fundus to the cervix

26.4 Uterine Cavity Surgical Procedures

Pre-operative preparation with gonadotropin-releasing hormone analogues, testosterone analogues (danazol), or oral contraceptive agents is not necessary [41], but it is helpful to schedule the procedure in the follicular phase (day 5 to 10 is optimal) to decrease the interference of a thickening endometrium. A fluid management system is essential so that fluid overload and electrolyte abnormalities can be avoided. Transvaginal hysteroscopic metroplasty is preferable to the abdominal route in terms of decreased morbidity, blood loss, and hospital stay [42]. Additionally, reproductive outcomes are excellent, and there is no need for cesarean delivery [42–45]. Laparoscopic guidance has been reported, especially in the case of a complete septate uterus, but often ultrasound guidance is sufficient [46].

26.5 Hysteroscopic Lateral Metroplasty

Historically, hysteroscopic lateral metroplasty has been described for a T-shaped uterus, especially in relation to the diethylstilbestrol (DES) exposure. Nagel et al. first reported on the lateral metroplasty technique in DES exposed cases and also included three out of eight patients who did not have DES exposure but were found to have a T-shaped uterus [47]. One patient had recurrent pregnancy loss, one had recurrent pregnancy loss with secondary infertility, and one had primary infertility. After hysteroscopic metroplasty, two of the three patients had live births. The third patient was found to also have a hydrosalpinx with adhesions at laparoscopy and did not conceive [47].

Various instrumentation has be utilized to perform lateral metroplasty including, electrocautery (monopolar hook, monopolar knife, bipolar devices) and rigid scissors. The goal is to normalize the triangular shape of the uterine cavity with incisions that do not damage the uterine myometrium, and this technique was achieved for both Katz et al., who surgically treated 8 T-shaped uteri, and Giacomucci et al., who described 17 (out of 352 cases) T-shaped uteri in patients with 2 or more pregnancy losses [48, 49]. Garbin et al. treated 24 women with hysteroscopic lateral metroplasty with a depth of incision not to exceed 7 mm [50]. Di Spiezio et al. described non-DES-exposed women with T-shaped uteri characterized by two-thirds uterine corpus and one-third cervix with abnormal lateral wall shape in the setting of a normal uterine outline [51]. The outpatient procedure performed involved incisions on not only the lateral uterine walls but also the anterior and posterior uterine walls from the fundus to the isthmus [51]. This technique was utilized in 30 women with T-shaped or tubular-shaped uteri that had history of primary infertility after exclusion of other infertility factors. Seventeen women became pregnant after metroplasty with a live birth rate of 71% [35]. A summary of hysteroscopic metroplasty for patients with a T-shaped uterus is shown (Table 26.1).

In a poster abstract from the 24th World Congress on Ultrasound in Obstetrics and Gynecology, the role of hysteroscopic lateral metroplasty in a narrow normal appearing uterine cavity prior to IVF/ICSI cycle was prospectively evaluated. Fifty-seven patients who had a prior IVF/ICSI failed cycle had a 3D ultrasound with measurements obtained at the fundus and at 1 cm below the fundus. Then, 29 patients underwent hysteroscopic lateral metroplasty and 28 underwent diagnostic hysteroscopy. Pregnancy rate following surgical correction was 48% compared to 21% in the diagnostic hysteroscopy group [53]. Full publication of this data in manuscript format with peer-review has not yet been found.

In a review of 1402 subfertile women with congenital uterine anomalies undergoing assisted reproduction, only 1 T-shaped uterus was identified [54]. Therefore, the prevalence of this type of uterine anomaly may be too low to accurately evaluate outcomes in a clinical trial, and given that DES exposure will no longer create a cohort of patients acquiring this anomaly, the numbers are not expected to rise. However, the few reports on lateral metroplasty in patients with poor reproductive outcomes suggest that with minimal intervention by skilled hysteroscopists, there may be possible improvement in uterine remodeling and subsequent pregnancy/live birth rates.

26.6 Hysteroscopic Uterine Septum Resection/Division/Transection

Hysteroscopic transection of the uterine septum has been performed with electrocautery (loops and needle electrode), scissors, laser energy, and even with hysteroscopic mechanical tissue removal devices. The key factors to success of the procedure are correct timing (early follicular phase) and adequate visualization. Hysteroscopic fluid must flow continuously and clear the cavity to allow visualization of the bilateral tubal ostia as a guide to complete septum division. Alternatively, transabdominal ultrasound guidance can prove beneficial, especially in the setting of uterine septa that extends to the cervix. Others utilize transrectal ultrasonography [55]. Antibiotic prophylaxis is not indicated [56].

The septoplasty technique involves incising the septum equidistant between the anterior and posterior uterine walls and continuing in the midline toward the fundus. Ultrasound guidance can assist with identifying the extent of the uterine septum division (Fig. 26.3), and ultrasound-guided hysteroscopic metroplasty surgeries need less re-intervention than those without guidance (39% vs. 18%, respectively) [57]. As one is nearing the normal uterine musculature, bleeding will increase. Once both tubal ostia are visualized in line with the septum resection line, the procedure is complete.

In the authors' experience, hysteroscopic septum division can also easily be accomplished with the routine use of a standard hysteroscope that would typically be used with a hysteroscopic morcellator [(e.g., Myosure (Hologic, Marlborough, Massachusetts) or Truclear (Medtronic, New Haven, CT)]. Urologic semirigid scissors are placed down the hysteroscope to provide the dissection necessary (Figs. 26.4 and 26.5). While these scissors are not as rigid as those with an operative hysteroscope (i.e., Olympus or Storz), this technique requires less set-up and less dilation, which can augment the ease of the procedure. Also, there is no cautery which is potentially a benefit to decreasing adhesive disease. Saline is used as the distention media. While report of uterine septum resection with the disposable hysteroscopic morcellator component has been described in a video abstract [58], we do not find the side cutting window to be an effective means of true septum division. The goal is to have a normal cavity with a residual septum length <1 cm in length for the internal fundal indentation.

Office hysteroscopic metroplasty has also been successfully performed with careful case selection and when the septum does not extend to the cervix [33, 59]. Bettocchi et al. described the characteristics that are found to be associated with identifying the septum-myometrium interface which is

Table 26.1 Hysteroscopic metroplasty review for T-shaped/hypoplastic uterus cases

Author, year (ref)	Patients, n	DES exposure	Type of surgery	Surgical procedure	Adhesion prevention	Outcome
Nagel, 1993 [47]	8	Yes (5 of 8)	Laparoscopy/ hysteroscopic metroplasty with 6.2 mm 0 degree hysteroscope; rigid scissors	Continued incision until cavity had assumed a smooth straight line from the lower uterine cavity to the tubal ostium or until bleeding was vigorous	Intracavitary balloon (5 mL) combined with conjugated equine estrogens at 2.5 mg two times per day for 25 days with medroxyprogesterone acetate 10 mg/day for the last 5 days	–2/5 DES patients conceived and had live births –2/3 patients not exposed to DES conceived and had live births
Katz, 1996 [49]	8	Yes (4 of 8)	Resectoscope; "cutting electrode"	Uterine side walls incised until a normal triangular uterine cavity was achieved with intraoperative HSG	IUD combined with estradiol valerate 4 mg for 11 days followed by estradiol valerate 4 mg with norgestrel 0.5 mg for 10 days	–No term deliveries in 11 preoperative pregnancies –2/4 DES patients conceived and had live births –1/3 patients not exposed to DES conceived and had live birth
Garbin, 1998 [50]	24	Yes (15 of 24)	Resectoscope; monopolar hook	Hook introduced to uterine horn and incision from fundus to isthmus perpendicular to the lateral wall of the uterus (2 to 3 incisions in the same groove)	Silastic sheet and 50 µg ethinyl estradiol for 2 months followed by 15 tablets of 50 µg ethinyl estradiol and 2.5 mg Lynestrenol	–8/15 with previous pregnancies became pregnant (7/8 term delivery) –5/9 with previous infertility became pregnant (3 term deliveries, 1 preterm, 1 ectopic)
Giacomucci, 2011 [48]	17	No (History of 2 pregnancy losses)	26-F hysteroscope; 0 degree knife with monopolar energy	Incision of lateral wall of the uterine cavity to obtain triangular-shaped cavity	None	–21 pregnancies with 66.7% pregnancy rate –Term delivery rate 66.6% (no term pregnancies prior to metroplasty)
Fernandez, 2011 [52]	97	Yes 63/97	26-F resectoscope; monopolar hook or bipolar (Versapoint)	Depth of incision does not exceed 5–7 mm	Sequential estroprogestative combination for 2 months (50 µg ethinyl estradiol)	–No term deliveries preoperatively in 78 pregnancies –48/97 became pregnant after surgery (28 term, 8 preterm, 5 ectopic, 16 miscarriage)
Di Spiezio, 2015 [51]	30	No	Size "5" hysteroscope, 30 degree; 5 Fr bipolar twizzle electrode	HOME-DU technique: two incisions on the fibro-muscular constriction rings in the isthmic area of the uterine side wall, incisions on anterior and posterior wall from fundus to the isthmus; depth not to exceed 5–6 mm	Polyethylene oxide sodium carboxymethylcellulose gel (intercoat gel)	–17/30 became pregnant –11/17 term delivery –9/22 term delivery rate for infertility patients –3/5 live births for patients with recurrent pregnancy loss

advantageous to consider in the office setting as (1) the color of the cut tissue due to the fibrosis of the septum was white, with myometrium being pink; (2) the septum has no vessels until the border with the myometrium is reached; and (3) the septum has no sensitive innervation, and the onset of pain occurs when myometrium is reached [59]. Counseling

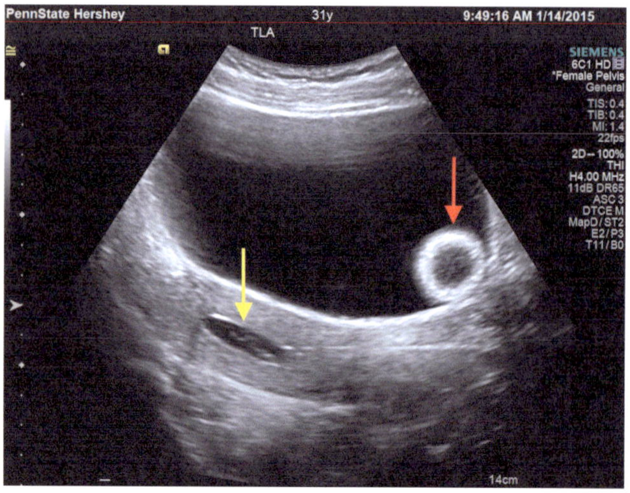

Fig. 26.3 Intraoperative transabdominal ultrasound guidance for uterine surgery. The red arrow indicates the Foley catheter balloon within the bladder. The yellow arrow points to the endometrial cavity in sagittal view distended by normal saline during hysteroscopy

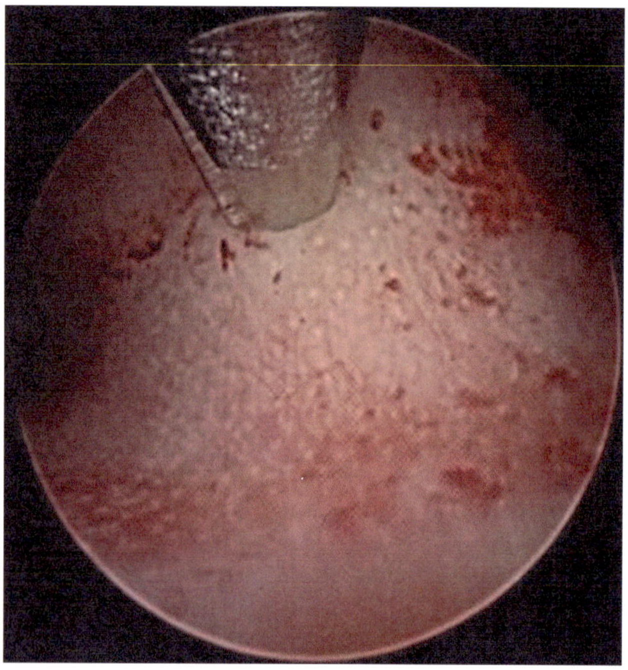

Fig. 26.4 Hysteroscopic view of 2 cm uterine septum with scissors in place to start metroplasty

patients about the possible need for a staged procedure with resection of larger septi is also prudent. Complications are low for hysteroscopic metroplasty but can include bleeding, infection, uterine perforation, and adhesions [33].

The optimal waiting time for subsequent attempt at conception after hysteroscopic metroplasty is not absolutely known, but based on office hysteroscopic inspection, it appears that 1–2 months results in a well-healed endometrium [60]. Follow-up second look office hysteroscopy can confirm normalization of the uterine cavity. There is still

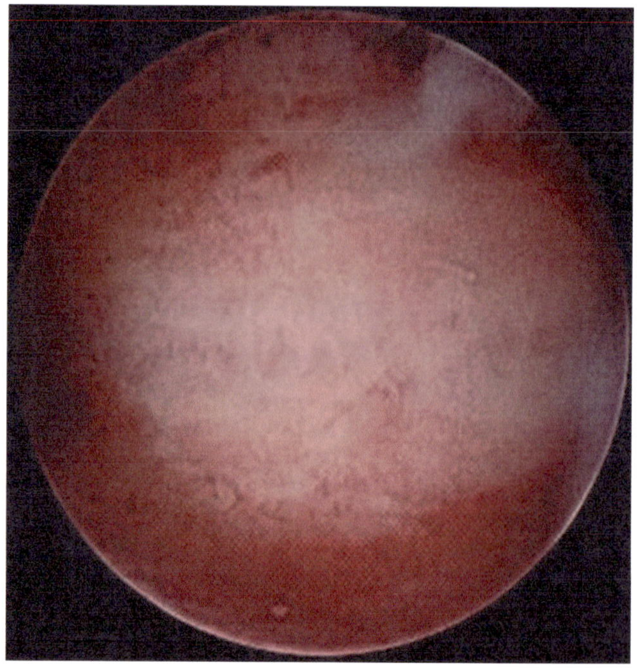

Fig. 26.5 Hysteroscopic view of postsurgical resection of uterine septum

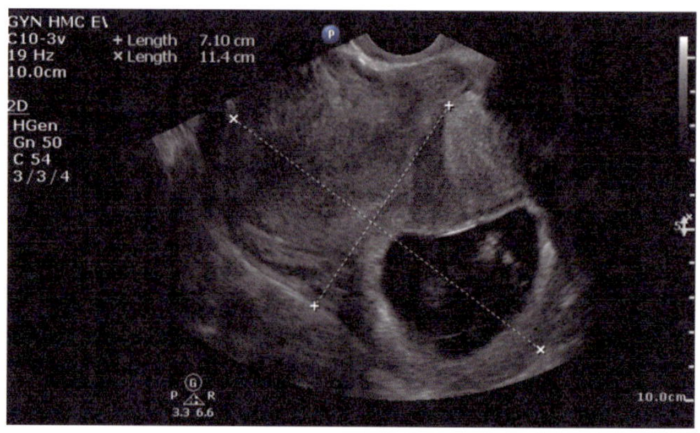

Fig. 26.6 Septate uterus with left sided pregnancy

controversy among practitioners on whether to offer hysteroscopic metroplasty to women with uterine septa or wait until miscarriage/pregnancy failure has occurred (Fig. 26.6) [4, 61, 62].

26.7 Adhesion Prevention for Hysteroscopic Metroplasty

Adhesion development after traumatic injury to the uterine cavity has been previously characterized and is also known as Asherman syndrome, a name acquired in 1948 from Joseph Asherman who organized the description of this condition [63]. Asherman syndrome can include symptoms such as amenorrhea, hypomenorrhea, subfertility, recurrent pregnancy loss, or a history related to abnormal placentation along with the presence of intrauterine adhesions by hysteroscopy and/or histologically confirmed intrauterine fibrosis [63, 64]. If no symptoms are present, then the term asymptomatic intrauterine adhesions is the most appropriate terminology [64]. Multiple classification systems for intrauterine adhesions have been created [30, 65, 66]. The modified version of the classification system originally described by March et al. is noted in Table 26.2 [66, 67]. Also, a proposed clinicohysteroscopic scoring system based on a retrospective review of both hysteroscopic and clinical data of 42 patients suggests that tubular uterine cavities with the inability to visualize both tubal ostia and sclerotic atrophic endometrium are the most severe findings, especially in the setting of amenorrhea or infertility. But the prognostic value of this specific scoring system has not been validated [65].

Historically, between 5 and 25% of women develop adhesions after uterine septum transection [68]. In a prospective, randomized trial, approximately 7% of women developed intrauterine adhesions after uterine septum resection and 45% after hysteroscopic removal of multiple fibroids [38]. Yang et al. observed in retrospective data that adhesiolysis of centrally located adhesions in the uterine cavity had a lower number of postoperative interventions compared to adhesions at the cornua, cervico-isthmic region or if the adhesions occluded part of the uterine cavity [69]. If intrauterine adhesions are more severe, then pregnancy rate is lower compared to mild intrauterine adhesions (20% vs. 81.5%) [70]. Additionally, the type and locations of adhesions such as AFS classification IV (extensive dense adhesions with occlusion of part of the uterine cavity other than cervico-isthmic region) and II (central type adhesions at the uterine cornua) have lower pregnancy rates than central adhesions in the middle area of the uterine cavity or those at the cervico-isthmic region [70].

Experience from the largest women's hospital in China reported on 357 patients that underwent hysteroscopic adhesiolysis with 334 (93.6%) having complete restoration of a normal uterine cavity. A 7 mm hysteroscope with microscissors was utilized for most cases with Versapoint bipolar system (Gynecare, Ethicon, NJ) used for the remaining cases. Postoperative hormonal therapy was given with estradiol 4 mg/day for 7 days, 3 mg/day for 7 days, and then estradiol valerate 2 mg/day and medroxyprogesterone acetate 10 mg/day for 7 days which was repeated for 2 months. The extent of preoperative adhesive disease was related to the conception rate after surgery. For mild intrauterine adhesions, 61% conceived; however, for severe intrauterine adhesions, only 25% conceived. Moderate adhesions were associated with a 53% conception rate. In those who conceived, miscarriage rate was approximately 9%, and term delivery occurred in 84% [71]. Prevention of intrauterine adhesions is therefore of utmost importance in reproductive surgery.

Table 26.2 Classification of intrauterine adhesions

Intrauterine adhesions	Characterization of adhesions
Minimal	< ¼ of uterine cavity involved; thin or filmy adhesions; ostial areas and upper fundus minimally involved or clear
Moderate	¼ to ¾ of uterine cavity involved; no agglutination of walls; adhesions only; ostial areas and upper fundus only partially occluded
Severe	> ¾ of uterine cavity involved; agglutination of walls or thick bands; ostial areas and upper cavity occluded

Modified from Robinson JK, Colimon LM, Isaacson KB. Postoperative adhesiolysis therapy for intrauterine adhesions (Asherman's syndrome). Fertil Steril. 2008;90(2):409–14, with permission

Multiple methods have been attempted to reduce or prevent intrauterine adhesion formation. Initially, the postoperative use of an IUD (intrauterine device) was utilized for the purpose of separating the endometrial surfaces [67, 72, 73]. In a recent retrospective unblinded study, oxidized regenerated cellulose adhesion barrier (Interceed) has been wrapped around a circular inert IUD and inserted into the uterine cavity for adhesion prevention [74]. The authors conclude that fewer operations to achieve an adhesion-free uterine cavity were necessary (3 versus 4; p-value = 0.0010); however, there was no significant difference in menstrual dysfunction, pregnancy rate, or live birth rate. Additionally, all patients in both groups also received oral estradiol valerate 5 mg twice daily for 28 days from day 5 postoperatively [74].

Yu et al. evaluated 238 women who specifically underwent uterine septum resection. One of three adjuvant therapies was given according to surgeon preference; these options included estradiol valerate/medroxyprogesterone acetate regimen for 3 months versus Copper T-380 IUD for 3 months versus a 16-F Foley balloon insertion with 4 ml of saline which was removed after 5 days versus no treatment (control). Office hysteroscopy performed 1 month later revealed intrauterine adhesions to be present in 22% (estrogen/progestin), 29% (copper IUD), 27% (Foley), and 24% (control) of the cases. At the time of the second look hysteroscopy, lysis of adhesions could be performed with the tip of the hysteroscope. Another hysteroscopy 3 months from the initial surgery demonstrated decreased rates of adhesions at 0%, 0.1%, 0.1%, and 0.2%, respectively. At both second- and third-look hysteroscopy, the incidence and severity of adhesions was not significantly different between any of the groups [75]. Others have suggested that serial, repeated office hysteroscopic lysis of adhesions every 1–3 weeks after the primary treatment be utilized as the method to maintain the uterine cavity patency postoperatively [66].

Neither IUD nor estrogen prevents intrauterine adhesions after hysteroscopic uterine septum resection according to several authors [76–79]. Specifically, Tonguc et al. randomized women to no treatment, estrogen treatment

(2 mg estradiol valerate and 0.5 mg norgestrel (Cyclo-Progynova: Schering AG, Istanbul, Turkey) once daily for 2 months, a copper IUD (Multiload Cu250, Multilan, Dublin, Ireland), or estrogen with the IUD. Intrauterine adhesion rates status post uterine septum resection using a monopolar dissection electrode were approximately 5% for the control group, 11% for the IUD only group, 12% for the estrogen plus IUD group, and 0% for the estrogen only group. These results were not statistically different between the groups [76]. For those who became pregnant following surgery, pregnancy and miscarriage rates were also similar between groups [76].

Moreover, there is no effect on pregnancy rates after IUD placement and/or estrogen use after hysteroscopic metroplasty [80]. A Cochrane review found that there were no differences in live birth rates between anti-adhesion therapy and no treatment. Anti-adhesion therapy was associated with fewer intrauterine adhesions at second look hysteroscopy; however, the clinical implications of this finding are unclear [81]. AAGL practice guidelines for management of intrauterine synechiae are listed in a practice report and are summarized (Table 26.3) [82].

Table 26.3 Practice guideline for uterine synechiae

Treatment recommendation	Level of evidence
Direct visualization of the uterine cavity at hysteroscopy combined with a tool for adhesiolysis is the treatment of choice	B
Hysteroscopic adhesiolysis by external imaging techniques or laparoscopy does not prevent uterine perforation or improve clinical outcome but may minimize the consequences if perforation occurs	B
Postoperative hormone treatment (estrogen with or without progestin) may reduce the recurrence of adhesions	B
Postoperative uterine cavity assessment after treatment is recommended	B
Expectant management is a reasonable alternative to intervention in selected women with intrauterine adhesions	C
There is no evidence to support blind cervical probing	C
There is no evidence to support blind D&C	C
If extensive adhesive disease is present, treatment should be performed by an expert hysteroscopist	C
Neither progestin-releasing nor copper or T-shaped IUDs nor intrauterine Foley catheter should be used after surgical division of intrauterine adhesions	C
Medications to improve vascular flow to the endometrium should not be used outside of research protocols	C
There is no evidence to support or refute the use of preoperative, intraoperative, or postoperative antibiotic therapy in surgical treatment of intrauterine adhesions	C

Modified from Worldwide AAMIG. AAGL practice report: practice guidelines for management of intrauterine synechiae. J Minim Invasive Gynecol. 2010;17(1):1–7, with permission

26.8 Pregnancy Outcomes

Congenital uterine anomalies are associated with decreased fecundity, increased miscarriage rate, increased preterm birth and low birth rate, malpresentation, C-section, and perinatal morbidity [83].

In regard to septate uteri, a meta-analysis revealed a decrease in clinical pregnancy rate (RR 0.86, $P = 0.009$), increase in first trimester miscarriage (RR 2.89, $P < 0.001$), increase in preterm delivery (RR 2.30, $P < 0.001$), increased fetal malpresentation (RR 6.24, $P < 0.001$), and no difference on second trimester miscarriage rates (RR 2.22, $P = 0.15$) but with subgroup analysis showing an association (RR 3.74, $P = 0.003$) [4]. Other studies have not validated the findings of decreased fertility seen in this meta-analysis [84, 85]. Another meta-analysis found women with septate uteri to have a higher rate of first trimester miscarriages (RR 2.65), increase in preterm delivery (RR 2.11), increase in malpresentation at delivery (RR 4.35), increased rate of intrauterine growth restriction (RR 2.54), increase in placental abruption (RR 4.37), and increase in perinatal mortality (RR 2.43) [86].

Pregnancy rates are improved, and miscarriage rates decrease after uterine septum division [45, 87–90]. The cumulative progression of pregnancy is only 33% when a septate uterus is diagnosed at the time of initial first trimester ultrasound [91]. Pregnancy rates after hysteroscopic septum surgery have been reported at 58% to as high as 89% [92, 93]. Ban-Frangez et al. reported a retrospective matched control study for women who conceived following IVF before hysteroscopic resection of a large or small (1.3–1.5 cm) uterine septum and women who conceived following IVF after hysteroscopic resection for a large or small uterine septum. The miscarriage rate before resection was significantly higher for both large and small uterine septi (odds ratio with 95% CI 25.0 (3.9–160) and 12.1 (3.2–45.8), respectively) [94]. Therefore, in infertility patients undergoing IVF, it seems prudent to offer uterine septum surgery prior to assisted reproductive techniques.

Some authors advocate for hysteroscopic metroplasty for infertility [46, 95]. One abstract noted a prospective cohort study in which 103 infertile women with unexplained infertility and a uterine septum where treated with hysteroscopic metroplasty. In women with a septum larger than ½ of the uterine cavity, pregnancy rates were significantly higher than those with a uterine septum less than ½ of the uterus [95]. This study has not yet come to full publication; therefore, the conclusions cannot be properly evaluated. Others have not found an association of uterine anomalies and infertility [4]. There are no randomized trials to compare outcomes for septoplasty on fertility rate, but many consider the procedure in women with long-standing infertility (evaluation has ruled out other factors), female age than 35 years, for those undergoing laparoscopy and/or hysteroscopy for another reason, or for women who will be undergoing assisted reproduction because of the potential benefit of reduced miscarriage rate and other obstetrical issues [96, 97]. Hysteroscopic metroplasty is a safe procedure, and undergoing this procedure is not associated with any higher risk of adverse obstetric outcomes compared to the general population [98].

Women with an arcuate uterus should be considered a normal variant as this does not increase poor pregnancy outcomes or pregnancy loss [99]. Even when looking at women undergoing assisted reproductive technology, an arcuate uterus is not associated with a reduction in pregnancy rate or increased risk of miscarriage [54]. A meta-analysis showed no difference in clinical pregnancy rate (RR 1.03, $P = 0.51$), first trimester pregnancy loss (RR 1.35, $P = 0.25$), or preterm birth rate (RR 1.53, $P = 0.28$) between women with arcuate uteri and women with normal uteri [4]. This same meta-analysis showed an increase in second trimester miscarriage (RR 2.39, $P = 0.003$) and fetal malpresentation at delivery (RR 2.5, $P < 0.001$) [4], but this is contrasted by another which showed no negative effect on reproductive outcomes [100].

Routine surgical excision for an arcuate uterus is not recommended. Although, interestingly, Detti et al. recently suggest that 5.9 mm become the new subseptation cutoff length above which surgical correction would be warranted. In this prospective cohort study, 76 women with infertility or recurrent pregnancy loss were diagnosed with subseptate uterus by the American Fertility Society criteria. They were evaluated with 3D ultrasound and were age-matched to a group of women with healthy uteri. After hysteroscopic septoplasty, the uterine cavity width in the subseptate group was significantly smaller than preoperative widths and became similar to measurements of the healthy uteri group. One-third of the patients conceived after surgical intervention with 88% (14/16) in the <10 mm subseptation group and 86% (6/7) in the ≥10 mm subseptation group [101].

26.9 Conclusion

This chapter has reviewed the current state of hysteroscopic metroplasty for T-shaped and septate uteri. This technique continues to be a successful and useful treatment for septate uterine configurations; however, the data is more limited on its effectiveness in the setting of lateral metroplasty to improve fertility. Intrauterine adhesion prevention is a main goal of this surgical treatment, and continued research in this area is necessary.

26.10 Question and Answer Section

Questions

1. Which test is a simple, reliable first step for evaluation of uterine anatomy?
   a. Transabdominal ultrasound
   b. Transvaginal ultrasound
   c. Sonohysterogram
   d. MRI
2. Surgery for a T-shaped uterus with lateral metroplasty is expected to do which of the following?
   a. Always cause uterine scarring
   b. Provide a 100% term live birth rate
   c. Decrease menstrual bleeding
   d. None of the above
3. Which method is the most accurate to diagnose intrauterine adhesions?
   a. Hysteroscopy
   b. Hysterosalpingogram
   c. Hysterosonography
   d. Transvaginal ultrasound

Answers

1. B. Transvaginal ultrasound is a reliable, simple, easily accessible test that can begin the assessment of uterine anatomy. Testing with sonohysterogram, hysteroscopy, MRI, or surgical evaluation can be utilized when indicated for further evaluation.
2. D. Lateral metroplasty is not expected to always cause uterine scarring (although this could be a complication of the procedure), guarantee full term delivery, or decreased menstrual bleeding.
3. A. AAGL guidelines state that hysteroscopy is the most accurate method for diagnosis of intrauterine adhesions and should be the investigation of choice when available.

References

1. Speroff L, Fritz MA. Clinical gynecologic endocrinology and infertility. In: Weinberg RW, Murphy J, Pancotti R, Rivera B, editors. . Philadelphia, PA: Lippincott Williams & Wilkins; 2005.
2. Jurkovic D, Gruboeck K, Tailor A, Nicolaides KH. Ultrasound screening for congenital uterine anomalies. Br J Obstet Gynaecol. 1997;104(11):1320–1.
3. Acién P. Incidence of Müllerian defects in fertile and infertile women. Hum Reprod. 1997;12(7):1372–6.
4. Chan YY, Jayaprakasan K, Zamora J, Thornton JG, Raine-Fenning N, Coomarasamy A. The prevalence of congenital uterine anomalies

in unselected and high-risk populations: a systematic review. Hum Reprod Update. 2011;17(6):761–71.
5. Li Y, Phelps A, Zapala MA, MacKenzie JD, MacKenzie TC, Courtier J. Magnetic resonance imaging of Müllerian duct anomalies in children. Pediatr Radiol. 2016;46(6):796–805.
6. Grimbizis GF, Camus M, Tarlatzis BC, Bontis JN, Devroey P. Clinical implications of uterine malformations and hysteroscopic treatment results. Hum Reprod Update. 2001;7(2):161–74.
7. Woelfer B, Salim R, Banerjee S, Elson J, Regan L, Jurkovic D. Reproductive outcomes in women with congenital uterine anomalies detected by three-dimensional ultrasound screening. Obstet Gynecol. 2001;98(6):1099–103.
8. Hammes B, Laitman CJ. Diethylstilbestrol (DES) update: recommendations for the identification and management of DES-exposed individuals. J Midwifery Womens Health. 2003;48(1):19–29.
9. Center for Disease Control. DES Update. https://www.cdc.gov/des/consumers/about/effects_daughters.html. Accessed April 6, 2017.
10. Mittendorf R. Teratogen update: carcinogenesis and teratogenesis associated with exposure to diethylstilbestrol (DES) in utero. Teratology. 1995;51(6):435–45.
11. Kaufman RH, Noller K, Adam E, Irwin J, Gray M, Jefferies JA, et al. Upper genital tract abnormalities and pregnancy outcome in diethylstilbestrol-exposed progeny. Am J Obstet Gynecol. 1984;148(7):973–84.
12. Kaufman RH. Structural changes of the genital tract associated with in utero exposure to diethylstilbestrol. Obstet Gynecol Annu. 1982;11:187–202.
13. Kaufman RH, Adam E. Findings in female offspring of women exposed in utero to diethylstilbestrol. Obstet Gynecol. 2002;99(2):197–200.
14. Mullen RD, Behringer RR. Molecular genetics of Müllerian duct formation, regression and differentiation. Sex Dev. 2014;8(5):281–96.
15. Raines AM, Adam M, Magella B, Meyer SE, Grimes HL, Dey SK, et al. Recombineering-based dissection of flanking and paralogous Hox gene functions in mouse reproductive tracts. Development. 2013;140(14):2942–52.
16. Ma L. Endocrine disruptors in female reproductive tract development and carcinogenesis. Trends Endocrinol Metab. 2009;20(7):357–63.
17. Miller C, Sassoon DA. Wnt-7a maintains appropriate uterine patterning during the development of the mouse female reproductive tract. Development. 1998;125(16):3201–11.
18. Block K, Kardana A, Igarashi P, Taylor HS. In utero diethylstilbestrol (DES) exposure alters Hox gene expression in the developing Müllerian system. FASEB J. 2000;14(9):1101–8.
19. Goldberg JM, Falcone T. Effect of diethylstilbestrol on reproductive function. Fertil Steril. 1999;72(1):1–7.
20. Noller KL, Blair PB, O'Brien PC, Melton LJ, Offord JR, Kaufman RH, et al. Increased occurrence of autoimmune disease among women exposed in utero to diethylstilbestrol. Fertil Steril. 1988;49(6):1080–2.
21. Burke L, Segall-Blank M, Lorenzo C, Dynesius-Trentham R, Trentham D, Mortola JF. Altered immune response in adult women exposed to diethylstilbestrol in utero. Am J Obstet Gynecol. 2001;185(1):78–81.
22. Salle B, Sergeant P, Awada A, Bied-Damon V, Gaucherand P, Boisson C, et al. Transvaginal ultrasound studies of vascular and morphological changes in uteri exposed to diethylstilbestrol in utero. Hum Reprod. 1996;11(11):2531–6.
23. Zhu Y, Luo M, Huang H, Du X, Chen D, Xing Q, et al. HOXA10, EMX2 and TENM1 expression in the mid-secretory endometrium of infertile women with a Müllerian duct anomaly. Reprod Biomed Online. 2016;32(4):388–93.
24. Jacquinet A, Millar D, Lehman A. Etiologies of uterine malformations. Am J Med Genet A. 2016;170(8):2141–72.
25. Fedele L, Dorta M, Brioschi D, Giudici MN, Candiani GB. Pregnancies in septate uteri: outcome in relation to site of uterine implantation as determined by sonography. AJR Am J Roentgenol. 1989;152(4):781–4.
26. Candiani GB, Fedele L, Zamberletti D, De Virgiliis D, Carinelli S. Endometrial patterns in malformed uteri. Acta Eur Fertil. 1983;14(5):311–8.
27. Grimbizis G, Camus M, Clasen K, Tournaye H, De Munck L, Devroey P. Hysteroscopic septum resection in patients with recurrent abortions or infertility. Hum Reprod. 1998;13(5):1188–93.
28. Blum M. Comparative study of serum CAP activity during pregnancy in malformed and normal uterus. J Perinat Med. 1978;6(3):165–8.
29. Raga F, Casañ EM, Bonilla-Musoles F. Expression of vascular endothelial growth factor receptors in the endometrium of septate uterus. Fertil Steril. 2009;92(3):1085–90.
30. The American Fertility Society classifications of adnexal adhesions, distal tubal occlusion, tubal occlusion secondary to tubal ligation, tubal pregnancies, müllerian anomalies and intrauterine adhesions. Fertil Steril. 1988;49(6):944–55.
31. Grimbizis GF, Campo R, On behalf of the Scientific Committee of the Congenital Uterine Malformations (CONUTA) common ESHRE/ESGE working group: Stephan Gordts SB, Marco Gergolet, Vasilios Tanos, T.-C. Li, Carlo De Angelis, A.tilio Di Spiezio Sardo. Clinical approach for the classification of congenital uterine malformations. Gynecol Surg. 2012;9(2):119–29.
32. Grimbizis GF, Campo R. Congenital malformations of the female genital tract: the need for a new classification system. Fertil Steril. 2010;94(2):401–7.
33. Gubbini G, Di Spiezio SA, Nascetti D, Marra E, Spinelli M, Greco E, et al. New outpatient subclassification system for American Fertility Society Classes V and VI uterine anomalies. J Minim Invasive Gynecol. 2009;16(5):554–61.
34. Ludwin A, Ludwin I. Comparison of the ESHRE-ESGE and ASRM classifications of Müllerian duct anomalies in everyday practice. Hum Reprod. 2015;30(3):569–80.
35. Di Spiezio SA, Campo R, Gordts S, Spinelli M, Cosimato C, Tanos V, et al. The comprehensiveness of the ESHRE/ESGE classification of female genital tract congenital anomalies: a systematic review of cases not classified by the AFS system. Hum Reprod. 2015;30(5):1046–58.
36. Grimbizis GF, Gordts S, Di Spiezio SA, Brucker S, De Angelis C, Gergolet M, et al. The ESHRE/ESGE consensus on the classification of female genital tract congenital anomalies. Hum Reprod. 2013;28(8):2032–44.
37. Tompkins P. Comments on the bicornuate uterus and twinning. Surg Clin North Am. 1962;42:1049–62.
38. Sugiura-Ogasawara M, Ozaki Y, Katano K, Suzumori N, Mizutani E. Uterine anomaly and recurrent pregnancy loss. Semin Reprod Med. 2011;29(6):514–21.
39. Marcal L, Nothaft MA, Coelho F, Volpato R, Iyer R. Mullerian duct anomalies: MR imaging. Abdom Imaging. 2011;36(6):756–64.
40. Vallerie AM, Breech LL. Update in Müllerian anomalies: diagnosis, management, and outcomes. Curr Opin Obstet Gynecol. 2010;22(5):381–7.
41. Römer T, Schmidt T, Foth D. Pre- and postoperative hormonal treatment in patients with hysteroscopic surgery. Contrib Gynecol Obstet. 2000;20:1–12.
42. Fayez JA. Comparison between abdominal and hysteroscopic metroplasty. Obstet Gynecol. 1986;68(3):399–403.
43. DeCherney AH, Russell JB, Graebe RA, Polan ML. Resectoscopic management of müllerian fusion defects. Fertil Steril. 1986;45(5):726–8.

44. Daly DC, Maier D, Soto-Albors C. Hysteroscopic metroplasty: six years' experience. Obstet Gynecol. 1989;73(2):201–5.
45. Goldenberg M, Sivan E, Sharabi Z, Mashiach S, Lipitz S, Seidman DS. Reproductive outcome following hysteroscopic management of intrauterine septum and adhesions. Hum Reprod. 1995;10(10):2663–5.
46. Tajiri R, Ueda T, Aoyama Y, Sakuragi T, Tohyama A, Okabe K, et al. Pregnancy after hysteroscopic metroplasty under laparoscopy in a woman with complete septate uterus: a case report. J UOEH. 2015;37(1):17–22.
47. Nagel TC, Malo JW. Hysteroscopic metroplasty in the diethylstilbestrol-exposed uterus and similar nonfusion anomalies: effects on subsequent reproductive performance; a preliminary report. Fertil Steril. 1993;59(3):502–6.
48. Giacomucci E, Bellavia E, Sandri F, Farina A, Scagliarini G. Term delivery rate after hysteroscopic metroplasty in patients with recurrent spontaneous abortion and T-shaped, arcuate and septate uterus. Gynecol Obstet Investig. 2011;71(3):183–8.
49. Katz Z, Ben-Arie A, Lurie S, Manor M, Insler V. Beneficial effect of hysteroscopic metroplasty on the reproductive outcome in a 'T-shaped' uterus. Gynecol Obstet Investig. 1996;41(1):41–3.
50. Garbin O, Ohl J, Bettahar-Lebugle K, Dellenbach P. Hysteroscopic metroplasty in diethylstilboestrol-exposed and hypoplastic uterus: a report on 24 cases. Hum Reprod. 1998;13(10):2751–5.
51. Di Spiezio SA, Florio P, Nazzaro G, Spinelli M, Paladini D, Di Carlo C, et al. Hysteroscopic outpatient metroplasty to expand dysmorphic uteri (HOME-DU technique): a pilot study. Reprod Biomed Online. 2015;30(2):166–74.
52. Fernandez H, Garbin O, Castaigne V, Gervaise A, Levaillant JM. Surgical approach to and reproductive outcome after surgical correction of a T-shaped uterus. Hum Reprod. 2011;26(7):1730–4.
53. Abdel-Naby M, El-Said R. Role of hysteroscopic lateral metroplasty in narrow normal appearing uterine cavity prior to ICSI. Poster abstract, P29.08. 24th World Congress on Ultrasound in Obstetrics and Gynecology.
54. Jayaprakasan K, Chan YY, Sur S, Deb S, Clewes JS, Raine-Fenning NJ. Prevalence of uterine anomalies and their impact on early pregnancy in women conceiving after assisted reproduction treatment. Ultrasound Obstet Gynecol. 2011;37(6):727–32.
55. Ludwin A, Ludwin I, Pityński K, Banas T, Jach R. Role of morphologic characteristics of the uterine septum in the prediction and prevention of abnormal healing outcomes after hysteroscopic metroplasty. Hum Reprod. 2014;29(7):1420–31.
56. Bulletins-Gynecology ACoP. ACOG practice bulletin No. 104: antibiotic prophylaxis for gynecologic procedures. Obstet Gynecol 2009;113(5):1180–1189.
57. Vigoureux S, Fernandez H, Capmas P, Levaillant JM, Legendre G. Assessment of abdominal ultrasound guidance in hysteroscopic metroplasty. J Minim Invasive Gynecol. 2016;23(1):78–83.
58. Malik R, Rizwan S, Rizk B. Resection of uterine septum using the myosure tissue removal system. J Minim Invasive Gynecol. 2015;22(6S):S123.
59. Bettocchi S, Ceci O, Nappi L, Pontrelli G, Pinto L, Vicino M. Office hysteroscopic metroplasty: three "diagnostic criteria" to differentiate between septate and bicornuate uteri. J Minim Invasive Gynecol. 2007;14(3):324–8.
60. Yang JH, Chen MJ, Chen CD, Chen SU, Ho HN, Yang YS. Optimal waiting period for subsequent fertility treatment after various hysteroscopic surgeries. Fertil Steril. 2013;99(7):2092-6.e3.
61. Bosteels J, Weyers S, Puttemans P, Panayotidis C, Van Herendael B, Gomel V, et al. The effectiveness of hysteroscopy in improving pregnancy rates in subfertile women without other gynaecological symptoms: a systematic review. Hum Reprod Update. 2010;16(1):1–11.
62. Kowalik CR, Goddijn M, Emanuel MH, Bongers MY, Spinder T, de Kruif JH, et al. Metroplasty versus expectant management for women with recurrent miscarriage and a septate uterus. Cochrane Database Syst Rev. 2011;6:CD008576.
63. ASHERMAN JG. Traumatic intra-uterine adhesions. J Obstet Gynaecol Br Emp. 1950;57(6):892–6.
64. Yu D, Wong YM, Cheong Y, Xia E, Li TC. Asherman syndrome – one century later. Fertil Steril. 2008;89(4):759–79.
65. Nasr AL, Al-Inany HG, Thabet SM, Aboulghar M. A clinicohysteroscopic scoring system of intrauterine adhesions. Gynecol Obstet Investig. 2000;50(3):178–81.
66. Robinson JK, Colimon LM, Isaacson KB. Postoperative adhesiolysis therapy for intrauterine adhesions (Asherman's syndrome). Fertil Steril. 2008;90(2):409–14.
67. March CM. Intrauterine adhesions. Obstet Gynecol Clin N Am. 1995;22(3):491–505.
68. Chen MY, Edwards VH, Ott DJ, Fayez JA. Hysterosalpingography after hysteroscopic surgery. Abdom Imaging. 1994;19(5):477–80.
69. Yang JH, Chen CD, Chen SU, Yang YS, Chen MJ. The influence of the location and extent of intrauterine adhesions on recurrence after hysteroscopic adhesiolysis. BJOG. 2016;123(4):618–23.
70. Zhao J, Chen Q, Cai D, Duan Z, Li X, Xue X. Dominant factors affecting reproductive outcomes of fertility-desiring young women with intrauterine adhesions. Arch Gynecol Obstet. 2017;295(4):923–7.
71. Chen L, Zhang H, Wang Q, Xie F, Gao S, Song Y, et al. Reproductive outcomes in patients with intrauterine adhesions following hysteroscopic adhesiolysis: experience from the largest women's hospital in China. J Minim Invasive Gynecol. 2017;24(2):299–304.
72. Massouras HG, Coutifaris B, Kalogirou D. Management of uterine adhesions with 'Massouras Duck's Foot' and 'Butterfly' IUDs. Contracept Deliv Syst. 1982;3(1):25–38.
73. Jewelewicz R, Khalaf S, Neuwirth RS, Vande Wiele RL. Obstetric complications after treatment of intrauterine synechiae (Asherman's syndrome). Obstet Gynecol. 1976;47(6):701–5.
74. Cai H, Qiao L, Song K, He Y. Oxidized, regenerated cellulose adhesion barrier plus intrauterine device prevents recurrence after adhesiolysis for moderate to severe intrauterine adhesions. J Minim Invasive Gynecol. 2017;24(1):80–8.
75. Yu X, Yuhan L, Dongmei S, Enlan X, Tinchiu L. The incidence of post-operative adhesion following transection of uterine septum: a cohort study comparing three different adjuvant therapies. Eur J Obstet Gynecol Reprod Biol. 2016;201:61–4.
76. Tonguc EA, Var T, Yilmaz N, Batioglu S. Intrauterine device or estrogen treatment after hysteroscopic uterine septum resection. Int J Gynaecol Obstet. 2010;109(3):226–9.
77. Vercellini P, Fedele L, Arcaini L, Rognoni MT, Candiani GB. Value of intrauterine device insertion and estrogen administration after hysteroscopic metroplasty. J Reprod Med. 1989;34(7):447–50.
78. Assaf A, Serour G, Elkady A, el Agizy H. Endoscopic management of the intrauterine septum. Int J Gynaecol Obstet. 1990;32(1):43–51.
79. Roy KK, Negi N, Subbaiah M, Kumar S, Sharma JB, Singh N. Effectiveness of estrogen in the prevention of intrauterine adhesions after hysteroscopic septal resection: a prospective, randomized study. J Obstet Gynaecol Res. 2014;40(4):1085–8.
80. Nawroth F, Schmidt T, Freise C, Foth D, Römer T. Is it possible to recommend an "optimal" postoperative management after hysteroscopic metroplasty? A retrospective study with 52 infertile patients showing a septate uterus. Acta Obstet Gynecol Scand. 2002;81(1):55–7.
81. Bosteels J, Weyers S, Kasius J, Broekmans FJ, Mol BW, D'Hooghe TM. Anti-adhesion therapy following operative hysteroscopy for treatment of female subfertility. Cochrane Database Syst Rev. 2015;11:CD011110.
82. Worldwide AAMIG. AAGL practice report: practice guidelines for management of intrauterine synechiae. J Minim Invasive Gynecol 2010;17(1):1–7.

83. Vaz SA, Dotters-Katz SK, Kuller JA. Diagnosis and management of congenital uterine anomalies in pregnancy. Obstet Gynecol Surv. 2017;72(3):194–201.
84. Acién P. Reproductive performance of women with uterine malformations. Hum Reprod. 1993;8(1):122–6.
85. Shuiqing M, Xuming B, Jinghe L. Pregnancy and its outcome in women with malformed uterus. Chin Med Sci J. 2002;17(4):242–5.
86. Venetis CA, Papadopoulos SP, Campo R, Gordts S, Tarlatzis BC, Grimbizis GF. Clinical implications of congenital uterine anomalies: a meta-analysis of comparative studies. Reprod Biomed Online. 2014;29(6):665–83.
87. Mollo A, De Franciscis P, Colacurci N, Cobellis L, Perino A, Venezia R, et al. Hysteroscopic resection of the septum improves the pregnancy rate of women with unexplained infertility: a prospective controlled trial. Fertil Steril. 2009;91(6):2628–31.
88. Colacurci N, De Franciscis P, Mollo A, Litta P, Perino A, Cobellis L, et al. Small-diameter hysteroscopy with Versapoint versus resectoscopy with a unipolar knife for the treatment of septate uterus: a prospective randomized study. J Minim Invasive Gynecol. 2007;14(5):622–7.
89. Bendifallah S, Faivre E, Legendre G, Deffieux X, Fernandez H. Metroplasty for AFS Class V and VI septate uterus in patients with infertility or miscarriage: reproductive outcomes study. J Minim Invasive Gynecol. 2013;20(2):178–84.
90. Wang JH, Xu KH, Lin J, Chen XZ. Hysteroscopic septum resection of complete septate uterus with cervical duplication, sparing the double cervix in patients with recurrent spontaneous abortions or infertility. Fertil Steril. 2009;91(6):2643–9.
91. Ghi T, De Musso F, Maroni E, Youssef A, Savelli L, Farina A, et al. The pregnancy outcome in women with incidental diagnosis of septate uterus at first trimester scan. Hum Reprod. 2012;27(9):2671–5.
92. Ghahiry AA, Refaei Aliabadi E, Taherian AA, Najafian A, Ghasemi M. Effectiveness of hysteroscopic repair of uterine lesions in reproductive outcome. Int J Fertil Steril. 2014;8(2):129–34.
93. Fedele L, Arcaini L, Parazzini F, Vercellini P, Di Nola G. Reproductive prognosis after hysteroscopic metroplasty in 102 women: life-table analysis. Fertil Steril. 1993;59(4):768–72.
94. Ban-Frangez H, Tomazevic T, Virant-Klun I, Verdenik I, Ribic-Pucelj M, Bokal EV. The outcome of singleton pregnancies after IVF/ICSI in women before and after hysteroscopic resection of a uterine septum compared to normal controls. Eur J Obstet Gynecol Reprod Biol. 2009;146(2):184–7.
95. Shokeir T, Haroun F. Hysteroscopic metroplasty in women with unexplained primary infertility: a prospective cohort study. J Minim Invasive Gynecol. 2015;22(6S):S6.
96. Homer HA, Li TC, Cooke ID. The septate uterus: a review of management and reproductive outcome. Fertil Steril. 2000;73(1):1–14.
97. Pabuçcu R, Gomel V. Reproductive outcome after hysteroscopic metroplasty in women with septate uterus and otherwise unexplained infertility. Fertil Steril. 2004;81(6):1675–8.
98. Kenda Šuster N, Gergolet M. Does hysteroscopic metroplasty for septate uterus represent a risk factor for adverse outcome during pregnancy and labor? Gynecol Surg. 2016;13:37–41.
99. Salim R, Regan L, Woelfer B, Backos M, Jurkovic D. A comparative study of the morphology of congenital uterine anomalies in women with and without a history of recurrent first trimester miscarriage. Hum Reprod. 2003;18(1):162–6.
100. Lin PC. Reproductive outcomes in women with uterine anomalies. J Womens Health (Larchmt). 2004;13(1):33–9.
101. Detti L, Hickman H, Levi D'Ancona R, Wright AW, Christiansen ME. Relevance of uterine subseptations: what length should warrant hysteroscopic resection? J Ultrasound Med. 2017;36(4):757–65.

Obesity and Medically Assisted Reproduction

27

Stephanie Welsh, Leah D. Whigham, and Steven R. Lindheim

27.1 Chapter Objectives

After reading this chapter, the reader will be able to:

1. Understand the prevalence of obesity and its impacts on health and assisted reproduction outcomes
2. Explain the current knowledge of pathophysiology behind obesity and adverse reproductive outcomes
3. Recognize recommendations for women with obesity seeking assisted reproduction techniques

27.2 Introduction

Overweight and obesity can be defined as excess body weight above a healthy level. Body mass index (BMI) is commonly used to classify individuals using their height and weight. The BMI categories used for identifying overweight and obesity are BMI 25–29.9 kg/m^2 for overweight and BMI $\geq$30 kg/m^2 for obesity (WHO 2008). Sub categories of obesity are class I (BMI 30–34.9 kg/m^2), class II (BMI 35–39.9 kg/m^2), and class III (BMI $\geq$40 kg/m^2) [1].

Excess adiposity is a risk factor for a multitude of diseases, contributing to increased health expenditures and lost productivity. In 2014, the economic costs of obesity in the United States were estimated to be more than $1.4 trillion, including direct and indirect costs [2]. Furthermore, annual medical costs per patient related to obesity have been projected to be more than twice as high for women compared to men ($3610 versus $1150) [3, 4].

The causes of obesity and overweight are multifactorial. A calorie-dense diet and sedentary lifestyle are both associated with obesity, but other contributors include underlying genetic and endocrine disorders, as well as sociocultural and environmental factors [5]. Of the many adverse health effects associated with obesity, reduced fertility in both men and women has a considerable impact. Through complex pathways, obesity contributes to impaired outcomes in both natural and assisted reproduction. This chapter reviews the prevalence, implications, and pathophysiology of obesity and summarizes the consequences of obesity on assisted reproductive technology (ART) outcomes in both females and males.

27.3 The Obesity Epidemic: Prevalence and Implications

Obesity is one of the most common chronic conditions in the United States and globally. Worldwide, over 600 million adults can be classified as obese [6]. According to the National Health and Nutrition Examination Survey, nearly 38% of US adults were classified as obese, and nearly 8% had class III obesity between 2013 and 2014 [7]. The prevalence of obesity and class III obesity is higher among women and, interestingly, between 2005 and 2014, has only increased for women compared to men [8]. Obesity also affects children, as data from Ogden et al. show that obesity impacts 10% of infants and toddlers under 2 years of age and nearly 17% of children and adolescents aged 2 through 19 years [7].

According to the Pregnancy Risk Assessment Monitoring System (PRAMS) 2004–2005 data, which monitors pregnancy-related health behaviors in US women, approximately 23% of women had an overweight pre-pregnancy BMI, and 19% had an obese pre-pregnancy BMI [9]. In addition, the prevalence of obesity was also reported to be higher

S. Welsh
Wright State University Boonshoft School of Medicine, Dayton, OH, USA

L. D. Whigham
Center for Community Health Impact, Department of Health Promotion and Behavioral Sciences, UTHealth School of Public Health El Paso, El Paso, TX, USA

S. R. Lindheim (✉)
Department of Obstetrics and Gynecology, Wright State University, Boonshoft School of Medicine, Dayton, OH, USA
e-mail: steven.lindheim@wright.edu

G. N. Allahbadia et al. (eds.), *Textbook of Assisted Reproduction*, https://doi.org/10.1007/978-981-15-2377-9_27

in African-American women (29.1%) than white (17.4%) and Hispanic (17.4%) women [9].

Obesity increases the risk of adverse health outcomes in every organ system, including increased risk of hypertension, dyslipidemia, coronary heart disease, stroke, diabetes mellitus, and osteoarthritis [10, 11]. Other health risks specific to women with obesity include estrogen-mediated cancers, polycystic ovarian syndrome (PCOS), anovulation, impaired fertility, and impaired reproductive and ART outcomes compared to women of healthy BMI [12, 13].

Obesity is also the most common complication of pregnancy and is associated with increased risks of hypertension, preeclampsia, gestational diabetes, cesarean section, surgical complications, postpartum infection, and hemorrhage [12–15]. Risks to the newborn include macrosomia, microsomia, premature birth, stillbirth, miscarriage, and congenital anomalies including neural tube defects and ventral wall abnormalities [12–15]. Table 27.1 summarizes the obesity-related health risks to mother and child [16, 17].

Table 27.1 Obesity-related health risks to mother and child

Pregnancy-related complications for women with BMI ≥ 30 kg/m^2		
Complication	Odds ratio (OR)	95% CI
Preeclampsia [16]	3.2	1.8–5.8
Gestational diabetes [16]	2.6	2.1–3.4
Fetal macrosomia [16]	2.2	1.6–3.1
Hypertension [16]	2.5	2.1–3.0
Shoulder dystocia [16]	3.6	2.1–6.3
Stillbirth [16]	2.8	1.9–4.7
Pregnancy-related complications for women with BMI ≥ 40 kg/m^2		
Complication	OR	95% CI
Preeclampsia [17]	4.8	4.04–5.74
Gestational diabetes [17]	4.0	3.1–5.2
Large-for-gestational-age infant [17]	3.8	3.5–4.16
Early neonatal death [17]	3.4	2.07–5.63
Hypertension [17]	3.2	2.6–4.0
Shoulder dystocia [17]	3.1	1.86–5.31
Meconium aspiration [17]	2.9	1.6–5.07
Stillbirth [17]	2.8	1.94–4.02
Cesarean delivery [17]	2.7	2.49–2.90
Fetal distress [17]	2.5	2.12–2.99
Birth defects associated with women with BMI ≥ 30 kg/m^2		
Birth defect	OR	95% CI
Ventral wall defects [17]	3.3	1.0–10.3
Neural tube defects [17]	2.7	1.2–6.1
Cardiac defects [17]	2.0	1.2–3.4
Multiple congenital anomalies [17]	2.0	1.0–3.8

27.4 Obesity and Reproductive Pathophysiology

Women with obesity face lower live birth rates following natural and assisted reproduction conception due to a combination of decreased pregnancy and implantation rates and increased rates of miscarriage and pregnancy complications [18–20]. Obesity impacts reproduction through several mechanisms, including oxidative stress, inflammation, and insulin resistance [21]. These pathways lead to dysregulation of the hypothalamus pituitary ovarian (HPO) axis and subsequent oligoovulation and anovulation [21], though obese women with ovulatory cycles also have reduced fecundity [22]. Specifically, Dağ et al. reported that for each unit of BMI over 29 kg/m^2, the probability of pregnancy decreases by 5% [18].

Obesity contributes to insulin resistance and elevated insulin levels, which lead to a variety of negative impacts on the HPO axis, including increased androgen and estrogen production by the ovaries [13, 15, 19, 23, 24]. Excess insulin and androgens also lead to reduced sex hormone binding globulin (SHBG) levels resulting in elevated free sex hormone levels [15, 19, 23, 24].

As an endocrine organ, adipose tissue produces and stores a variety of substances including adipokines, leptin, and adiponectin. In obesity, leptin levels are increased, and adiponectin levels are decreased [10, 13, 19]. The elevated leptin levels are associated with alterations of the HPO axis, including impaired ovarian function and folliculogenesis [19], as leptin directly inhibits steroidogenesis by theca and granulosa cells of the ovary [24]. Decreased adiponectin may lead to increased insulin, which negatively impacts reproduction as previously described [24]. Furthermore, adipocytes store lipid-soluble substances including sex hormones, contributing further to higher androgen levels [15]. Hyperandrogenism has negative effects on ovarian function, leading to menstrual disturbances and anovulation which may be related to altered follicular development [13, 19].

Alterations of the HPO axis include variations in gonadotropin-releasing hormone and increased luteinizing hormone (LH) from the anterior pituitary gland [19, 23], which may impair folliculogenesis [19]. Reduced oocyte quality in obesity may lead to impaired embryo quality and subsequent implantation [13]. In obese women with normal menstrual cycles, the negative effects on implantation are observed as well [19]. In combination with PCOS, which is estimated to be present in 28% to 50% of women with obesity, obesity exacerbates reproductive impairment; both conditions are characterized by hyperleptinemia, hyperandrogenemia, and anovulation [21, 25, 26].

27.5 Obesity and Conventional Therapy Outcomes

27.5.1 Obesity and IVF Outcomes

Many studies suggest that obesity is associated with altered cycle stimulation characteristics and adverse IVF outcomes, including reduced pregnancy and live birth rates [19, 20, 24, 27]. Rates of cycle cancellation are increased with increasing BMI, which may be a result of gonadotropin (Gn) resistance leading to lack of ovarian response [13, 19, 27]. Dokras et al. reported cycle cancellation rates to be as high as 25% in women with BMI ≥40 kg/m^2, compared to 11% in women with healthy BMI (OR = 2.73, 95% CI: 1.49–5.0) [28]. However, this is not a consistent finding, as indicated in a systematic review that found no differences in cycle cancellation (OR = 1.35, 95% CI: 0.99–1.84) or number of oocytes retrieved (weighted mean difference [WMD] = 0.68, 95% CI: 0.11–1.2) between those with a BMI <30 kg/m^2 and ≥30 kg/m^2 [23].

Increased Gn requirements and longer stimulation times have been consistently observed in women with obesity with an inverse relationship between BMI and response to Gn [13, 19, 24] including a systematic review where there was a WMD of more than 200 IU of Gn (95% CI: 149.12–271.05) [23]. It is hypothesized that this may be linked to ovarian Gn resistance in which elevated intrafollicular leptin may inhibit ovarian steroid synthesis [13, 19, 23, 29]. Alternatively, pharmacokinetic properties may lead to reduced absorption and/or increased clearance of Gn in obese women [13, 19, 28, 29].

Follicular asynchrony and lower peak estradiol concentration in those undergoing ovarian stimulation is also more common in women with obesity [13, 19], further suggesting an attenuated ovarian response to Gn stimulation [13, 28, 29]. Shah et al. reported significantly lower peak serum estradiol levels in 1721 first IVF cycles in women with class II obesity (1498 pg/mL) and class III obesity (1361 pg/mL) than in women with healthy BMI (2047 pg/mL) [30]. The number of retrieved oocytes is consistently reduced, as is the oocyte quality. This has been attributed to poor ovarian response or to challenges associated with performing oocyte recovery in obese women [13, 24]. A systematic review reported that the WMD of oocytes recovered in women with BMI ≥25 kg/m^2 was 42% lower (0.58, 95% CI: 0.22–0.94) than in women with BMI <25 kg/m^2 [23]. It is unclear if reduced oocyte quality was due to the increased doses of Gn required in response to obesity, or to obesity itself [13, 19]. It has been postulated that a lipotoxic effect of excess lipid storage in oocytes, resulting in high levels of free fatty acids and reactive oxygen species, may interfere with the function of the meiotic spindles, mitochondria, and endoplasmic reticulum of oocytes [21, 29]. However, other studies have failed to show any adverse effect of obesity on these parameters [23].

Fertilization rates and embryo quality also appear to be adversely impacted [13, 24]. Shah et al. reported that women with a BMI of 35–39.9 kg/m^2 had significantly fewer normally fertilized oocytes than women with healthy BMI (7.6 versus 9.3) [30], and Jungheim et al. reported decreased fertilization rates in women with BMI ≥ 40 kg/m^2 compared to women with healthy BMI (59% versus 69%, $p < 0.03$) [31]. Resulting embryo quality has been reported to be adversely affected, as blastocyst formation rates are almost 15% lower in overweight and obese women compared to women of healthy weight ($p < 0.007$) [32]. As a result of reduced oocyte yield, fertilization rates, and reduced embryo quality, the mean number of embryos transferred and rates of implantation have been reported to be decreased in obese women [13, 33].

27.5.2 Male Obesity and ART

The literature is conflicting regarding the impact of male obesity on fertility in spontaneous reproduction and ART outcomes. Studies suggest that obese men have significantly reduced sperm motility (WMD = −3.72%, 95% CI: −7.11–0.33) and increased DNA fragmentation (WMD = 3.41%, 95% CI: 2.08–4.75) [34]. In contrast, other studies in obese and healthy weight men have shown no differences in sperm parameters including sperm concentration (standardized mean difference = −0.28, 95% CI: −0.65–0.08) [35], total sperm count (median 134 million in groups with BMI 20–24.9 kg/m^2 and BMI >30 kg/m^2), and motility [36].

With respect to ART outcomes, Campbell reviewed 30 studies of male obesity and ART. Significantly higher rate of infertility (failure to conceive after 2years) in men with obesity was noted (OR = −1.66, 95% CI: 1.53–1.79) [34]. Live birth rates per ART cycle have also been reported to be reduced by as much as 35% (OR = 0.65, 95% CI: 0.44–0.97) [34]. In comparison, not all studies have found significant differences in fertility based on male BMI, including a report by Zhu et al. where nearly 8500 couples undergoing IVF failed to show differences in live birth rates in overweight (Adjusted Risk Ratio [ARR] = 1.03, 95% CI: 0.975–1.090) and obese (ARR = 1.00, 95% CI: 0.912–1.104) men compared to men with healthy BMI [37].

27.5.3 Live Birth and Delivery

In spontaneous pregnancy, maternal adiposity increases the risks of adverse pregnancy outcomes, including gestational diabetes, preeclampsia, preterm birth, and neonatal and childhood morbidity [12, 14]. Further, maternal obesity has been reported to increase the risk of fetal (adjusted odds ratio [AOR] = 2.32, 95% CI: 1.64–3.28, $p < 0.001$) and infant death [AOR = 1.97, 95% CI: 1.13–3.45, $p = 0.02$) [38].

With respect to ART, studies also suggest that obese women have higher rates of obstetric complications and miscarriage and lower live birth rates [13, 19]. In a study of 5019 IVF/ICSI cycles, there was a significant association between BMI >30 kg/m^2 and early pregnancy loss (OR = 1.69, 95% CI: 1.13–2.51, $p = 0.003$) [39]. Further, the odds of live birth were 2% lower with each unit of increased BMI (OR = 0.981, 95% CI: 0.967–0.995, $p = 0.009$) [40]. A systematic review of 21 studies by Maheshwari et al. revealed that women with a BMI ≥25 kg/m^2 had a significant reduction in pregnancy rates (OR = 0.71, 95% CI: 0.62–0.81) following IVF and an increase in miscarriage rates (OR = 1.33, 95% CI: 1.06–1.68) [23]. Another systematic review ($n = 33$ studies) also reported decreased clinical pregnancy rates (RR = 0.90, 95% CI: 0.85–0.94, $p < 0.0001$), decreased live birth rates (RR = 0.84, 95% CI: 0.77–0.92, $p = 0.0002$), and increased miscarriage rates (RR = 1.31, 95% CI: 1.18–1.45, $p < 0.0001$) in women with BMI ≥25 kg/m^2 undergoing IVF/ICSI [41]. Moragianni et al. also reported that live births after first ART cycle were 68% lower in women with BMI ≥40 kg/m^2 compared to women with healthy BMI (OR = 0.32, 95% CI: 0.16–0.64) [33].

This is not a consistent finding, as other studies have reported no differences in live birth rates. Dokras et al. reported no differences in delivery rates between women with BMI 25–29.9 kg/m^2 (42.7%), BMI 30–39.9 kg/m^2 (41.95%), and BMI ≥40 kg/m^2 (36.71%) [28]. While the systematic review by Maheshwari et al. reported an increase in miscarriage rates, the authors found no significant association between BMI and live birth rates [23]. Furthermore, another systematic review ($n = 14$ studies) corroborated these findings where no adverse effect of obesity on live birth rate following ART was seen [42]. Outcomes noted in gestational carriers (GC) ($n = 163$) have also revealed no differences in live birth rates per embryo transfer regardless of GC BMI (70% in BMI 20–24.9 kg/m^2, 84% in BMI 25–29.9 kg/m^2, and 75% in BMI 30–35 kg/m^2) [43].

With respect to maternal complications, Dayan et al. reported that obese women undergoing IVF have nearly a sevenfold higher risk of preeclampsia compared to non-obese women following natural conception (OR = 6.7, 95% CI: 3.3–13.8) [44]. However, there are data showing that the risk of complications of ART for women with obesity is similar in women without obesity, including adverse neonatal outcomes requiring mechanical ventilation or admission to the neonatal intensive care unit (AOR = 1.33, 95% CI: 1.11–1.59 in obese and AOR = 1.34, 95% CI: 1.18–1.51 in non-obese) and preterm birth (AOR = 1.06, 95% CI: 0.86–1.31 in obese and AOR = 1.15, 95% CI: 1.00–1.32 in non-obese) [45]. Conflicting data exist regarding live birth and obesity with the exception of preeclampsia, suggesting further work is needed to clarify this issue.

27.5.4 The Egg or the Uterus?

It is still a matter of debate whether impaired outcomes of natural conception or ART are due to reduced oocyte quality or endometrial receptivity [19]. Elevated leptin seen with obesity may negatively impact decidualization, leading to impaired endometrial receptivity, implantation, and placentation [21]. Using egg donation as a model to distinguish between intrauterine and extrauterine factors has yielded conflicting results. Provost et al. reported that clinical pregnancy rates were reduced by 26% (OR = 0.74, 95% CI: 0.59–0.94, $p = 0.013$), and live birth rates were reduced by 36% (OR = 0.64, 95% CI: 0.51–0.81, $p < 0.001$) in recipients with BMI >40 kg/m^2 compared to women of healthy BMI [46]. Comparisons of autologous and donor oocytes in women with obesity revealed that with increasing BMI, failure to achieve clinical pregnancy increased with the use of autologous oocytes in women with class I obesity (AOR = 1.13, 95% CI: 1.05–1.21), but not when donor oocytes were utilized (AOR = 0.99, 95% CI: 0.80–1.24), suggesting an oocyte over endometrial effect [47].

The impact of donor BMI on ART outcomes has also been investigated. Cardozo et al. showed that as BMI of the oocyte donor increased, clinical pregnancy rates significantly decreased (OR = 0.4, 95% CI: 0.1–0.9), and live birth rates (OR = 0.4, 95% CI: 0.2–1.1) trended lower for women with BMI 25.3–34 kg/m^2 [48], suggesting an adverse effect of obesity on the oocyte. Goldman et al. studied the effect of obesity on aneuploidy with preimplantation genetic screening (PGS) and found no adverse impact of aneuploidy from women with BMI ≥30 kg/m^2 (AOR = 0.74, 95% CI: 0.25–2.20) [49].

An increased risk of miscarriage with increasing BMI in the oocyte recipient has been reported (OR = 4.02, 95% CI: 1.53–10.57, $p = 0.005$) [50]; however, this is not a consistent finding by others. Metwally et al. reported no adverse impact (OR = 1.52, 95% CI; 0.88–2.61) [51] as did Styne Gross et al., who reported that the rates of spontaneous loss after egg donation were comparable across BMI groups: 24.5% in women with BMI 21–25 kg/m^2, 10.9% in women with BMI 26–29 kg/m^2, and 29.8% in women with BMI ≥30 kg/m^2 ($p = 0.096$) [52]. Given the conflicting data, more research in needed to elucidate the effect of oocyte recipient BMI on miscarriage risk.

27.6 Recommendations Prior to Conception

While the Institute of Medicine recommends that preconception counseling should encourage women to aim to enter pregnancy with a healthy BMI [53], recent data reports reveal that 26% of women were overweight and 25% obese prior to becoming pregnant [54]. Evidence of an association between weight loss before ART and improved perinatal outcomes is lacking, including the LIFEstyle study which failed to find improvements in women receiving lifestyle intervention prior to infertility treatment compared to those receiving immediate treatment without weight loss [55]. Weight loss in the intervention group was greater than in the control group, as nearly 38% of women in the intervention group lost 5% of body weight, compared to 0% in the control group during the first 6 months [55]. However, 27% of women who received 6 months of lifestyle intervention before 18 months of infertility treatment had live term births of singleton infants, similar to 35% of women who received 24 months of infertility treatment with no lifestyle intervention (OR = 0.77, 95% CI: 0.60–0.99) [55]. Moreover, no significant differences in complications rates between groups were noted [55].

These findings contrast with those of The Treatment of Hyperandrogenism versus Insulin Resistance in Infertile Polycystic Ovary Syndrome (OWL PCOS) trial [56]. Ovulation significantly increased with weight loss followed by clomiphene, compared to oral contraceptives followed by clomiphene or a combination of weight loss and oral contraceptives followed by clomiphene [56]. When compared to women with PCOS who received immediate clomiphene treatment without delay [57], analysis revealed improved live birth rates in women receiving weight loss and delayed infertility treatment compared to immediate treatment (Risk Ratio [RR] = 2.5, 95% CI: 1.3–4.7; $p = 0.01$) [58]. These findings suggest a benefit to delaying fertility treatment until after successful weight loss efforts. However, the benefits of weight loss must be balanced by the adverse effect of time relative to the age of the patient, as fertility is known to decrease with advancing age.

Some studies suggest that even modest reductions of up to 5% of pre pregnancy weight appear to restore ovulation and improve fertility and birth outcomes [13, 19, 23]. The first line therapy for weight loss has always been behavioral modification including reduced calorie diet and increased physical activity. Exercise, even without weight loss, has been shown to significantly improve outcomes in obese women undergoing IVF, with an increase in clinical pregnancy rates (RR = 3.22, 95% CI: 1.53–6.78, $p = 0.002$) and live birth rates (RR = 3.71, 95% CI: 1.51–9.11, $p = 0.004$) in obese women who had regular physical activity compared to those who did not [59]. It's thought that exercise may improve insulin sensitivity and reduce inflammation and oxidative stress, irrespective of weight loss, thus improving reproductive function [59, 60]. Additionally, although exercise does not lead to weight loss in all individuals, it can improve body composition by decreasing fat mass and increasing lean body mass.

Bariatric surgery has also been recommended for women with a BMI ≥40 kg/m^2 or with BMI ≥35 kg/m^2 and comorbidities who have not benefited from non-surgical weight loss attempts [61]. A systematic review of weight loss interventions suggests that bariatric surgery and non-surgical weight loss procedures were more effective for weight loss than comprehensive behavior change and resulted in increased pregnancy and/or live birth rates after ART [62]. However, it is recommended that pregnancy be avoided for 6–12 months after bariatric surgery due to metabolic and nutritional aberrations resulting from the procedure [19]. Even 2 year post-surgery, long-term malabsorption and metabolic derangements may persist and impair reproductive outcomes [63]. Other risks reported include increased risk of small-for-gestational-age infant (OR = 2.2, 95% CI: 1.64–2.95), increased risk of preterm birth between 32 weeks and 36 weeks and 6 days (OR = 1.3, 95% CI: 1.05–1.6), and a trend for increased risks of stillbirth/neonatal death (OR = 2.39, 95% CI: 0.98–5.85, $p = 0.06$) [64]. It is important that patients undergoing bariatric surgery receive long-term follow-up regarding nutrition, physical activity, and psychosocial health in order to ensure that the benefits of surgery are fully realized while minimizing adverse side effects. The risks of surgical and medical weight loss therapies must be weighed with the benefits for each individual patient and carefully considered, given the expense and potential morbidity. Randomized clinical trials are still needed to clarify these issues.

In some cases, IVF clinics have required that treatment be delayed until after weight loss using BMI cutoffs for IVF eligibility. In a 2015 study of 347 US clinics, 35% used a BMI cutoff to allow IVF treatment [65], with commonly cited reasons including requirements for anesthesia and concerns about anesthesia complications [66]. While weight loss may have some benefits in improving fertility in women with increased BMI, it has been acknowledged that weight loss is time-intensive. It is possible that the benefits of weight loss on fertility can be overshadowed by the negative impacts of advancing age. Some argue that age is more important than obesity in predicting successful ART; thus women with obesity should be counseled with this in mind, working closely with patients and a multidisciplinary team to formulate individualized treatment plans based on each patient's unique circumstances [29].

27.7 Conclusion

The health impacts of obesity are numerous and include reduced fertility and impaired outcomes of ART. While conflicting literature exists, it appears that obesity reduces ovulation, increases Gn dose requirements, reduces clinical pregnancy rates after ART, and increases the risk of miscarriage after ART. To avoid potential risks, it is recommended that women with obesity seeking to have children through natural or assisted conception make positive lifestyle changes in regard to diet and exercise. It is not recommended that ART be withheld from women with elevated BMI, but appropriate counseling about increased risks should be given along with referrals for comprehensive weight management. Further research is needed, using consistent BMI cutoffs and prospective research design, to clarify the risks and improve outcomes for women with obesity seeking ART.

References

1. Consultation WE. Waist circumference and waist-hip ratio. Report of a WHO Expert Consultation Geneva: World Health Organization. 2008 Dec:8–11.
2. Waters H, DeVol R. Weighing down America: the health and economic impact of obesity. Available from http://www.milkeninstituteorg/weighingdownamerica
3. Meldrum DR. Introduction: obesity and reproduction. Fertil Steril. 2017 Apr 30;107(4):831–2.
4. Cawley J, Meyerhoefer C. The medical care costs of obesity: an instrumental variables approach. J Health Econ. 2012 Jan 31;31(1):219–30.
5. The Obesity Society Infographic Task Force. Potential contributors to obesity [Internet]. Silver Spring: The Obesity Society; 2015 Nov [cited 2017 May 17]. Available from http://www.obesity.org/obesity/resources/facts-about-obesity/infographics/potential-contributors-to-obesity
6. World Health Organization. Obesity and overweight Fact sheet N°311 [Internet]. 2015 Jan [cited 2015 April 10]. Available from http://www.who.int/mediacentre/factsheets/fs311/en/
7. Ogden CL, Carroll MD, Kit BK, Flegal KM. Prevalence of childhood and adult obesity in the United States, 2011–2012. JAMA. 2014 Feb 26;311(8):806–14.
8. Flegal KM, Kruszon-Moran D, Carroll MD, Fryar CD, Ogden CL. Trends in obesity among adults in the United States, 2005 to 2014. JAMA. 2016 Jun 7;315(21):2284–91.
9. Chu SY, Kim SY, Bish CL. Prepregnancy obesity prevalence in the United States, 2004–2005. Matern Child Health J. 2009 Sep 1;13(5):614–20.
10. Bastien M, Poirier P, Lemieux I, Després JP. Overview of epidemiology and contribution of obesity to cardiovascular disease. Prog Cardiovasc Dis. 2014 Feb 28;56(4):369–81.
11. Stein CJ, Colditz GA. The epidemic of obesity. J Clin Endocrinol Metabol. 2004 Jun 1;89(6):2522–5.
12. American College of Obstetricians and Gynecologists. Ethical issues in the care of the obese woman: Committee Opinion No. 600. Obstet Gynecol 2014;123:1388–93.
13. Bellver J, Busso C, Pellicer A, Remohí J, Simón C. Obesity and assisted reproductive technology outcomes. Reprod Biomed Online. 2006 Dec 31;12(5):562–8.
14. McDonald SD, Han Z, Mulla S, Beyene J. Overweight and obesity in mothers and risk of preterm birth and low birth weight infants: systematic review and meta-analyses. BMJ. 2010 Jul 20;341:c3428.
15. Pasquali R, Pelusi C, Genghini S, Cacciari M, Gambineri A. Obesity and reproductive disorders in women. Hum Reprod Update. 2003 Jul 1;9(4):359–72.
16. Leddy MA, Power ML, Schulkin J. The impact of maternal obesity on maternal and fetal health. Rev Obstet Gynecol. 2008;1(4):170–8.
17. Practice Committee of the American Society for Reproductive Medicine. Obesity and reproduction: an educational bulletin. Fertil Steril. 2008 Nov 30;90(5):S21–9.
18. Dağ ZÖ, Dilbaz B. Impact of obesity on infertility in women. J Turk German Gynecol Assoc. 2015;16(2):111.
19. Brewer CJ, Balen AH. The adverse effects of obesity on conception and implantation. Reproduction. 2010 Sep 1;140(3):347–64.
20. Pasquali R, Patton L, Gambineri A. Obesity and infertility. Curr Opin Endocrinol Diabetes Obes. 2007 Dec 1;14(6):482–7.
21. Broughton DE, Moley KH. Obesity and female infertility: potential mediators of obesity's impact. Fertil Steril. 2017 Mar;11
22. Law DG, Maclehose RF, Longnecker MP. Obesity and time to pregnancy. Hum Reprod. 2007 Feb 1;22(2):414–20.
23. Maheshwari A, Stofberg L, Bhattacharya S. Effect of overweight and obesity on assisted reproductive technology—a systematic review. Hum Reprod Update. 2007 Sep 1;13(5):433–44.
24. Pandey S, Pandey S, Maheshwari A, Bhattacharya S. The impact of female obesity on the outcome of fertility treatment. J Hum Reprod Sci. 2010 May 1;3(2):62.
25. Álvarez-Blasco F, Botella-Carretero JI, San Millán JL, Escobar-Morreale HF. Prevalence and characteristics of the polycystic ovary syndrome in overweight and obese women. Arch Intern Med. 2006 Oct 23;166(19):2081–6.
26. Ehrmann DA. Polycystic ovary syndrome. N Engl J Med. 2005 Mar 24;352(12):1223–36.
27. Luke B, Brown MB, Missmer SA, Bukulmez O, Leach R, Stern JE, et al. The effect of increasing obesity on the response to and outcome of assisted reproductive technology: a national study. Fertil Steril. 2011 Oct 31;96(4):820–5.
28. Dokras A, Baredziak L, Blaine J, Syrop C, VanVoorhis BJ, Sparks A. Obstetric outcomes after in vitro fertilization in obese and morbidly obese women. Obstet Gynecol. 2006 Jul 1;108(1):61–9.
29. Jungheim ES, Travieso JL, Hopeman MM. Weighing the impact of obesity on female reproductive function and fertility. Nutr Rev. 2013 Oct 1;71(suppl 1):S3–8.
30. Shah DK, Missmer SA, Berry KF, Racowsky C, Ginsburg ES. Effect of obesity on oocyte and embryo quality in women undergoing in vitro fertilization. Obstet Gynecol. 2011 Jul 1;118(1):63–70.
31. Jungheim ES, Lanzendorf SE, Odem RR, Moley KH, Chang AS, Ratts VS. Morbid obesity is associated with lower clinical pregnancy rates after in vitro fertilization in women with polycystic ovary syndrome. Fertil Steril. 2009 Jul 31;92(1):256–61.
32. Comstock IA, Kim S, Behr B, Lathi RB. Increased body mass index negatively impacts blastocyst formation rate in normal responders undergoing in vitro fertilization. J Assist Reprod Genet. 2015 Sep 1;32(9):1299–304.
33. Moragianni VA, Jones SM, Ryley DA. The effect of body mass index on the outcomes of first assisted reproductive technology cycles. Fertil Steril. 2012 Jul 31;98(1):102–8.
34. Campbell JM, Lane M, Owens JA, Bakos HW. Paternal obesity negatively affects male fertility and assisted reproduction outcomes: a systematic review and meta-analysis. Reprod Biomed Online. 2015 Nov 30;31(5):593–604.
35. Le W, Su SH, Shi LH, Zhang JF, Wu DL. Effect of male body mass index on clinical outcomes following assisted reproductive technology: a meta-analysis. Andrologia. 2015 Aug;1
36. Thomsen L, Humaidan P, Bungum L, Bungum M. The impact of male overweight on semen quality and outcome of assisted reproduction. Asian J Androl. 2014 Sep 1;16(5):749.
37. Zhu J, Tang W, Mao J, Li J, Zhuang X, Liu P, et al. Effect of male body mass index on live-birth sex ratio of singletons after assisted reproduction technology. Fertil Steril. 2015 Dec 31;104(6):1406–10.
38. Tennant PW, Rankin J, Bell R. Maternal body mass index and the risk of fetal and infant death: a cohort study from the North of England. Hum Reprod. 2011 Apr 5:der052.
39. Fedorcsák P, Dale PO, Storeng R, Ertzeid G, Bjercke S, Oldereid N, et al. Impact of overweight and underweight on assisted reproduction treatment. Hum Reprod. 2004 Nov 1;19(11):2523–8.

40. Bellver J, Ayllón Y, Ferrando M, Melo M, Goyri E, Pellicer A, et al. Female obesity impairs in vitro fertilization outcome without affecting embryo quality. Fertil Steril. 2010 Jan 15;93(2):447–54.
41. Rittenberg V, Seshadri S, Sunkara SK, Sobaleva S, Oteng-Ntim E, El-Toukhy T. Effect of body mass index on IVF treatment outcome: an updated systematic review and meta-analysis. Reprod Biomed Online. 2011 Oct 31;23(4):421–39.
42. Koning AM, Mutsaerts MA, Kuchenbecher WK, Broekmans FJ, Land JA, Mol BW, et al. Complications and outcome of assisted reproduction technologies in overweight and obese women. Hum Reprod. 2012 Feb 1;27(2):457–67.
43. Coyne KD, O'Leary KM, Yaklic JL, Whigham LD, Lindheim SR. Gestational carrier (GC) BMI and reproductive, fetal and neonatal outcomes: are the risks the same with increasing obesity? Fertil Steril. 2014 Sep 1;102(3):e258.
44. Dayan N, Pilote L, Opatrny L, Basso O, Messerlian C, El-Messidi A, et al. Combined impact of high body mass index and in vitro fertilization on preeclampsia risk: a hospital-based cohort study. Obesity. 2015 Jan 1;23(1):200–6.
45. Valent AM, Hall ES, DeFranco EA. The influence of obesity on perinatal outcomes in pregnancies achieved with assisted reproductive technology: a population-based retrospective cohort study. Obstet Med. 2016 Mar;9(1):34–9.
46. Provost MP, Acharya KS, Acharya CR, Yeh JS, Steward RG, Eaton JL, et al. Pregnancy outcomes decline with increasing recipient body mass index: an analysis of 22,317 fresh donor/recipient cycles from the 2008–2010 Society for Assisted Reproductive Technology Clinic Outcome Reporting System registry. Fertil Steril. 2016 Feb 29;105(2):364–8.
47. Luke B, Brown MB, Stern JE, Missmer SA, Fujimoto VY, Leach R. Female obesity adversely affects assisted reproductive technology (ART) pregnancy and live birth rates. Hum Reprod. 2011 Jan 1;26(1):245–52.
48. Cardozo ER, Karmon AE, Gold J, Petrozza JC, Styer AK. Reproductive outcomes in oocyte donation cycles are associated with donor BMI. Hum Reprod. 2016 Feb 1;31(2):385–92.
49. Goldman KN, Hodes-Wertz B, McCulloh DH, Flom JD, Grifo JA. Association of body mass index with embryonic aneuploidy. Fertil Steril. 2015 Mar 31;103(3):744–8.
50. Bellver J, Rossal LP, Bosch E, Zúñiga A, Corona JT, Meléndez F, Gómez E, Simón C, Remohí J, Pellicer A. Obesity and the risk of spontaneous abortion after oocyte donation. Fertil Steril 2003 May 31;79(5):1136–1140.
51. Metwally M, Ong KJ, Ledger WL, Li TC. Does high body mass index increase the risk of miscarriage after spontaneous and assisted conception? A meta-analysis of the evidence. Fertil Steril. 2008 Sep 30;90(3):714–26.
52. Styne-Gross A, Elkind-Hirsch K, Scott RT. Obesity does not impact implantation rates or pregnancy outcome in women attempting conception through oocyte donation. Fertil Steril. 2005 Jun 30;83(6):1629–34.
53. Institute of Medicine. Weight gain during pregnancy: reexamining the guidelines. Washington, DC: National Academies Press; 2009.
54. Branum AM, Kirmeyer SE, Gregory EC. Prepregnancy Body Mass Index by Maternal Characteristics and State: Data From the Birth Certificate, 2014. National vital statistics reports: from the Centers for Disease Control and Prevention, National Center for Health Statistics, National Vital Statistics System. 2016 Aug;65(6):1.
55. Mutsaerts MA, Van Oers AM, Groen H, Burggraaff JM, Kuchenbecker WK, Perquin DA, et al. Randomized trial of a lifestyle program in obese infertile women. N Engl J Med. 2016 May 19;374(20):1942–53.
56. Legro RS, Dodson WC, Kris-Etherton PM, Kunselman AR, Stetter CM, Williams NI, et al. Randomized controlled trial of preconception interventions in infertile women with polycystic ovary syndrome. J Clin Endocrinol Metabol. 2015 Sep 24;100(11):4048–58.
57. Legro RS, Brzyski RG, Diamond MP, Coutifaris C, Schlaff WD, Casson P, et al. Letrozole versus clomiphene for infertility in the polycystic ovary syndrome. N Engl J Med. 2014 Jul 10;371(2):119–29.
58. Legro RS, Dodson WC, Kunselman AR, Stetter CM, Kris-Etherton PM, Williams NI, et al. Benefit of delayed fertility therapy with preconception weight loss over immediate therapy in obese women with PCOS. J Clin Endocrinol Metabol. 2016 May 12;101(7):2658–66.
59. Palomba S, Falbo A, Valli B, Morini D, Villani MT, Nicoli A, et al. Physical activity before IVF and ICSI cycles in infertile obese women: an observational cohort study. Reprod Biomed Online. 2014 Jul 31;29(1):72–9.
60. Luke B. Adverse effects of female obesity and interaction with race on reproductive potential. Fertil Steril. 2017 Apr 30;107(4):868–77.
61. Jensen MD, Ryan DH, Apovian CM, Ard JD, Comuzzie AG, Donato KA, et al. 2013 AHA/ACC/TOS guideline for the management of overweight and obesity in adults. Circulation. 2014 Jun 24;129(25 suppl 2):S102–38.
62. Sim KA, Partridge SR, Sainsbury A. Does weight loss in overweight or obese women improve fertility treatment outcomes? A systematic review. Obes Rev. 2014 Oct 1;15(10):839–50.
63. Legro RS. Effects of obesity treatment on female reproduction: results do not match expectations. Fertil Steril. 2017 Apr 30;107(4):860–7.
64. Johansson K, Cnattingius S, Näslund I, Roos N, Trolle Lagerros Y, Granath F, et al. Outcomes of pregnancy after bariatric surgery. N Engl J Med. 2015 Feb 26;372(9):814–24.
65. Turner-McGrievy GM, Grant BL. Prevalence of body mass index and body weight cut-off points for in vitro fertilization treatment at US clinics and current clinic weight loss strategy recommendations. Hum Fertil. 2015 Jul 3;18(3):215–9.
66. Kaye L, Sueldo C, Engmann L, Nulsen J, Benadiva C. Survey assessing obesity policies for assisted reproductive technology in the United States. Fertil Steril. 2016 Mar 31;105(3):703–6.

28 Polycystic Ovarian Syndrome and Medically Assisted Reproduction

Sezcan Mumusoglu, Mehmet Sipahi, and Gurkan Bozdag

Polycystic ovary syndrome (PCOS) affects 6–10% of women in reproductive age [1]. According to diagnostic criteria used, 55 to 91% of normogonadotropic anovulatory (WHO-II) women have sign and/or symptoms of the PCOS disease [2]. Women with PCOS symptoms are more likely to be sub-fertile when compared to women without PCOS symptoms (26.5 vs. 17.1%, $p < 0.001$) [3]. However at the end, although time to first pregnancy increase, in women with PCOS, lifetime fertility is similar [3, 4].

Lifestyle management with diet and exercise is recommended not only to increase spontaneous ovulation but also for long-term health benefits. For ovulation induction, first-line treatments for PCOS are oral agents such as clomiphene citrate (CC) or aromatase inhibitors (AI). Exogenous gonadotropin injection and surgical intervention such as laparoscopic ovarian drilling are considered as second step of treatment to induce ovulation. With oral agents and exogenous gonadotropin treatment strategies, it is objected to induce a monofollicular growth and ovulation with or without intrauterine insemination. Although ovulation induction with exogenous gonadotropin alone yields ovulation rate of 72%, and pregnancy rates of 45% in women with PCOS [5], assisted reproductive technologies (ART) or medically assisted reproduction (MAR) is still warranted as a third-line treatment option in the remaining, particularly when another factor (e.g., tubal obstruction or oligospermia) exists. However, there are some difficulties with regard to ovarian stimulation in women with PCOS not only to induce a monofollicular response but also to induce multifollicular response [6]. Whereas women with PCOS might be complicated with multifollicular development, cycle cancellation and multiple pregnancy rates during ovulation induction, excessive ovarian response, and OHSS might be troublesome in ovarian stimulation during an MAR cycle despite the close monitoring [7]. In spite of all those difficulties, the reported live birth rate after MAR treatment in women with PCOS is similar to women with unexplained endometriosis and male factor infertility [8].

In the last decade, several strategies have been introduced into MAR treatment to reduce the risks of OHSS and cycle cancellation and to improve the pregnancy rates in women with PCOS [9–12]. In this chapter, we overviewed the available evidence regarding the efficacy and safety of those proposed strategies aiming to improve successes rate of MAR in women with PCOS.

28.1 Strategies on Ovarian Stimulation Protocols

The first concern regarding to ovulation stimulation (OS) protocol might be on the type of GnRH analogue. When gonadotropin-releasing hormone (GnRH) antagonists are compared to agonists, they have advantages such as having no hypo-estrogenic side effects, no flare-up effect, no need to long-term downregulation, and need for less number of gonadotropin during ovarian stimulation. While agonists are effective by desensitizing the receptors over pituitary in long term, antagonists block these receptors directly, therefore affect rapidly. This provides an opportunity to implement antagonists at any time during follicular phase.

GnRH antagonists might be applied in various protocols like multiple fixed-dose (0.25 mg/day—starting on the fifth–seventh day), multiple flexible-dose (0.25 mg/day after the leading follicle reaches 14–15 mm diameter), or single dose (3 mg on the seventh or eighth day). In a recent meta-analysis by Kollmann et al., 1525 women and 582 live birth/ongoing pregnancies were included from 12 randomized controlled trials (RCTs) [6]. This meta-analysis revealed that the use of agonists during ovarian stimulation does not make significant difference in terms of live birth/ongoing pregnancy when

S. Mumusoglu · G. Bozdag (✉)
Department of Obstetrics and Gynecology, Hacettepe University School of Medicine, Ankara, Turkey
e-mail: gbozdag@hacettepe.edu.tr

M. Sipahi
Department of Obstetrics and Gynecology, Giresun University School of Medicine, Merkez/Giresun, Turkey

G. N. Allahbadia et al. (eds.), *Textbook of Assisted Reproduction*, https://doi.org/10.1007/978-981-15-2377-9_28

compared to the use of antagonists (RR = 0.95, 95% CI: 0.84–1.08, I^2 = 0%) with low heterogeneity among the studies (Table 28.1). Notably, with regard to clinical pregnancy (CP) (RR = 1.02, 95% CI: 0.91–1.15, I^2 = 7%) and miscarriages rates (RR = 1.10, 95% CI, 0.73–1.65, I^2 = 19%), there was no significant difference between agonist and antagonist cycles [6]. However, OHSS rate was significantly less in antagonist protocol (n = 11 RCTs), with low-quality evidence (RR = 0.63, 95% CI: 0.49–0.80, I^2 = 1%) [6]. For the selection of ganirelix or cetrorelix, no significant differences were noted by means of clinical pregnancy rate in ICSI cycles between groups in a study enrolling 80 women with PCOS [12].

For the day of GnRH implementation during OS, GnRH antagonists are generally implemented as fixed-day injections on the fifth–seventh day of the stimulation. Starting GnRH antagonists at mid-follicular phase is based on the reason for potential fluctuation of LH levels during follicular phase. Nevertheless, avoiding LH fluctuations might negatively alter endometrial receptivity and hence decrease pregnancy rate [13–15]. Application of a fixed protocol might sustain more physiologic concentrations of LH and estradiol (E_2), which would better synchronize endometrium during the process of embryo transfer and implantation [16]. To establish the proper time to initiate during early follicular phase, a RCT comparing 140 patients with PCOS reported no significant difference for the clinical pregnancy (68.3% vs. 56.5%), implantation (46.2% vs. 35.5%), and miscarriage (7.3% vs. 8.6%) rates when patients commenced GnRH antagonist on the first or later days of stimulation [17]. Another RCT (n = 150) stratifying patients as luteal long GnRH agonist, flexible antagonist and early antagonist also revealed that both biochemical (34.1%, 34%, and 38.3%, respectively, p = 0.9) and clinical pregnancy (34.1%, 29.8%, and 36.2%, respectively, p = 0.8) rates were similar [18]. Another meta-analysis also supports that live birth/ongoing pregnancy rate between early and late starting of GnRH antagonists (RR = 1.16, 95% CI: 0.8–1.6) does not differ, though the quality of available evidence was low [6].

To sum up, GnRH antagonist protocols, irrespective from the type and day of commencement, give a great opportunity to decrease the risk of OHSS without delineating pregnancy rates, even when final maturation is maintained by hCG. Also by giving the opportunity to trigger with a small dose of GnRH agonist, it further decreases the absolute risk of OHSS in antagonist cycles. Therefore, GnRH antagonist appears to be the choice of protocol in patients expected to have excessive response such as in women with PCOS.

28.1.1 Type of Gonadotropin

The choice of exogenous gonadotropin in patients with PCOS has been widely speculated as in every subgroup of patients undergoing ART cycles. Nevertheless, with regard to type of gonadotropin, Kollmann et al. reported no significant difference in terms of live birth/ongoing pregnancy (RR = 1.05, 95% CI: 0.6–1.7) and clinical pregnancy (RR = 0.9, 95% CI: 0.6–1.4) rates when urinary and recombinant FSH (rec-FSH) were compared [6]. Similarly a Cochrane review consisting of 10 RCTs comparing rec-FSH and urinary gonadotropins (Seven RCTs for rec-FSH vs. FSH-HP, 3 RCTs for rec-FSH vs. HMG) failed to present any significant difference for the outcome of live birth (OR = 1.26, 95% CI: 0.80–1.99, I^2 = 0%) or clinical pregnancy (OR = 1.1, 95% CI: 0.8–1.4, I^2 = 0). Additionally, when rec-FSH and urinary gonadotropins were compared for the risk of OHSS (OR = 1.5, 95% CI: 0.8–2.8, I^2 = 0%), consistently no significant difference was observed according to a very low quality of evidence [19]. Supplementation of oral anti-estrogens to exogenous gonadotropin does not bring any superiority with regard to any parameter of success [6].

Theoretically, using LH instead of FSH at the late follicular phase would allow mature follicles to grow while causing atresia of the immature follicles. Considering that, a RCT analyzed 90 patients with PCOS where the control group proceeds with FSH. In the study arm, hCG was added when the leading follicle reached 14 mm in diameter and FSH was ceased. The authors reported no significant difference for clinical pregnancy but higher severe OHSS risk among hCG implemented group (p = 0.019) [11].

For the gonadotropin protocol that might be preferred during an OS protocol, apparently three options are available, namely, step-up, step-down, and a sequential step-up/step-down protocol. Although, a study including 225 women with PCOS reported that sequential protocol was superior to others [20], the meta-analysis by Kollmann et al. did not confirm those findings either for the outcome of live birth/ongoing pregnancy (RR = 1.05, 95% CI: 0.6–1.9) or clinical pregnancy (OR = 0.96, 95% CI: 0.6–1.5) rates (Table 28.1) [6].

In summary, apparently, no type and combination of exogenous gonadotropin is superior with regard to pregnancy. From that point, maintaining the safety with regard to risk of excessive ovarian response in women with PCOS should be the primary concern while deciding the dose and regimen in a given OS cycle.

28.2 Supplementary Treatments During MAR

Metformin has been suggested as a supplement in patients with PCOS to improve pregnancy rates outcome in MAR cycles. It acts as insulin sensitizing from the group of biguanide, which suppresses hyperinsulinemia and over production of androgens in PCOS.

Table 28.1 Latest meta-analysis data evaluating effect of various treatment strategies in ART cycles for the management of risks of ovulation induction in patients with polycystic ovary syndrome (PCOS)

Author, year	Number of trials	Comparison	Primary outcome	Result
Kollmann, 2016	12	GnRH agonist *vs.* antagonist	Ongoing pregnancy/live birth	RR = 0.95, 95% CI: 0.8–1.1, I^2 = 0%
	11	GnRH agonist *vs.* antagonist	OHSS	RR = 0.63, 95% CI: 0.5–0.8, I^2 = 1%
	1	Early vs. late starting of GnRH antagonists	Ongoing pregnancy/live birth	RR = 1.16, 95% CI: 0.8–1.6
	1	Urinary vs. recombinant-FSH	Ongoing pregnancy/live birth	RR = 1.05, 95% CI: 0.6–1.7
	1	Step-up vs. step-down protocol	Ongoing pregnancy/live birth	RR = 1.05, 95% CI: 0.6–1.9
	10	Metformin vs. no treatment	Ongoing pregnancy/live birth	RR = 1.28, 95% CI: 1.01–1.63, I^2 = 22%
	10	Metformin vs. no treatment	OHSS	RR = 0.47, 95% CI: 0.29–0.76, I^2 = 0%
	1	Myo-inositol (MI) vs D-chiro-inositol (DCI)	Clinical pregnancy	RR = 2.86, 95% CI: 1.1–7.2
	1	Triggering ovulation with reduced vs. standard hCG dose	Live birth	RR = 1.54, 95% CI: 0.7–3.2
	1	Triggering ovulation with reduced vs. standard hCG dose	OHSS	RR = 0.53, 95% CI: 0.03–8.1
	1	IVM vs. conventional IVF	Live birth	RR = 1.26, 95% CI: 0.5–2.9
	2	IVM vs. conventional IVF	OHSS	RR = 0.19, 95% CI: 0.01–3.1
Weiss, 2015	10	Urinary (HP-FSH in 3RCT) vs. recombinant-FSH	Live birth	OR = 1.26, 95% CI: 0.8–2.0, I^2 = 0%
	10	Urinary (HP-FSH in 3RCT) vs. recombinant-FSH	OHSS	OR = 1.52, 95% CI: 0.8–2.8, I^2 = 0%
Tso, 2014	5	Metformin vs. placebo or no treatment	Live birth	OR = 1.39, 95% CI: 0.8–2.4, I^2 = 52%
	8	Metformin vs. placebo or no treatment	Clinical pregnancy	OR = 1.52, 95% CI: 1.1–2.1, I^2 = 18%
	8	Metformin vs. placebo or no treatment	OHSS	OR = 0.29, 95% CI: 0.2–0.5, I^2 = 11%
Pundir, 2017	1	Myo-inositol (MI) or D-chiro-inositol (DCI) vs. placebo	Clinical pregnancy	RR = 3.3, 95% CI: 0.4–27.1

RCT randomized controlled trials, *OHSS* ovarian hyperstimulation syndrome, *RR* relative risk, *OR* odds ratio, *GnRH* gonadotropin-releasing hormone, *FSH* follicle-stimulating hormone, *HP* highly purified, *hCG* human chorionic gonadotropin, *IVF* in vitro fertilization, *IVM* in vitro maturation

In a Cochrane meta-analysis of comparing metformin and placebo with 9 RCTs and 816 patients, although higher clinical pregnancy rates (OR = 1.52, 95% CI: 1.1–2.1, I^2 = 18%, 8 RCTs) was observed, there were no significant difference in terms of live birth rates (OR = 1.39, 95% CI: 0.8–2.4, I^2 = 52%, 5 RCTs). However, OHSS was (OR = 0.29, 95% CI: 0.18–0.49, I^2 = 11%, 8 RCTs) significantly less at metformin-implemented group when compared to placebo [11] (Table 28.1). In discordance, another meta-analysis including 10 RCTs and 856 women, the use of metformin during ovarian stimulation found to be more effective with regard to ongoing or live birth rate (RR = 1.28, 95% CI: 1.01–1.63, I^2 = 22%) when compared to placebo but with a low quality of evidence. In means of miscarriage, no significant difference was observed with a very low-quality evidence (RR = 0.78, 95% CI: 0.47–1.29), I^2 = 0%). However, when 891 women were evaluated for the excessive ovarian response and OHSS, risk was less in metformin users than placebo arm with a very low level quality of evidence (RR = 0.47, 95% CI: 0.29–0.76, I^2 = 0%) [6] (Table 28.1). A recent Cochrane overview of the 27 Cochrane reviews also confirmed the risk reduction of OHSS for women with PCOS when metformin was used before or during the ART cycle [21].

Inositol is a naturally formed polyalcohol that has been utilized in women with PCOS due to its insulin-sensitizing effect as in metformin. It has stereoisomers such as myo-inositol (MI) and D-chiro-inositol (DCI). A three-arm RCT comparing MI + melatonin, MI alone, and control group in ART cycles with 526 PCOS patients shows lower results for oocyte (48.2%, 35%, and 38.2%, $p < 0.001$, respectively) and embryo quality (45.7%, 30.4%, and 25.6%, $p < 0.001$, respectively) in controls, whereas there was no difference at clinical pregnancy rates (41.4%, 36.7%, and 31%, respectively) at all [22]. According to a meta-analysis including only one RCT which compares MI and DCI among 84 patients with PCOS, clinical pregnancy rate (RR = 2.86, 95% CI: 1.1–7.2) was observed higher in MI group with very low evidence. No significant difference was observed for the miscarriage rate (OR = 1.33, 95% CI: 0.36–4.97) between groups [6]. A meta-analysis of 10 RCTs by Pundir et al. included a total of 362 women treated with inositol (257 on myo-inositol; 105 on di-chiro-inositol), 179 with placebo, and 60 with metformin. Inositol was associated with significantly improved ovulation rate (RR = 2.3, 95% CI: 1.1–4.7, $I^2 = 75\%$) and increased frequency of menstrual cycles (RR = 6.8, 95% CI: 2.8–16.6, $I^2 = 0\%$) compared to placebo. One study compared the clinical pregnancy rate in inositol-treated patients with placebo (RR = 3.3, 95% CI: 0.4–27.1) (Table 28.1) and one study compared to metformin (RR = 1.5, 95% CI: 0.7–3.1). No studies evaluated live birth, miscarriage rates, and OHSS risk [23].

28.3 Strategies for Triggering the Final Oocyte Maturation

28.3.1 Reduced Versus Standard Dose of hCG

In the ART treatment protocols, human chorionic gonadotropin (hCG) is a standard for triggering final oocyte maturation due to its LH like effect and high efficacy with a low cost. However, as noted, hCG has six- to sevenfold higher biological activity compared to endogenous LH as a result of longer half-life [24]. Nevertheless, hCG administration for final oocyte maturation is the pivotal stimulus for OHSS, by causing exaggerated secretion of vascular endothelial growth factor (VEGF) from the ovary or peritoneal surface. Since the pathophysiology related with OHSS is depended on hCG administration [25], it had been proposed that lower doses of hCG might be associated with lower risks of OHSS [25]. When different doses of hCG such as 2500, 3300, 5000 were compared to 10000 IU within one retrospective study [26] and 1 RCT [26] but with a small sample size, no benefit was shown by lowering the dose of hCG down to 2500 IU with respect to a reduction in OHSS on a high-risk group of patients [6, 27].

28.3.2 Recombinant LH Versus hCG

Due to the short half-life of LH (10 h) compared to hCG (36 h), it has been investigated in two trials without selecting patients with PCOS whether recombinant LH (rec-LH) to reduce the risk of OHSS. Cochrane systematic review of those trials revealed that using rec-LH for final oocyte maturation leads to similar pregnancy and OHSS rates with urinary hCG [28]. However the sample size and quality of the evidence were low.

28.3.3 Agonist Trigger Versus hCG

It has been proposed that the administration of a GnRH agonist instead of hCG at the end of ovarian stimulation induces an endogenous peak in both LH and FSH by a similar way of physiology seen in oocyte maturation during natural cycles [29, 30]. However, due to the short half-life of endogenous LH compared to hCG, luteal phases have been defective (rapid luteolysis), and live birth rates have been significantly lower in agonist-triggered GnRH antagonist cycles when only luteal phase was supported by vaginal progesterone only [31]. Administration of low-dose hCG immediately after oocyte retrieval might rescue the luteal phase [9]. However, it should be noted that the agonist trigger at GnRH antagonist cycles significantly reduces [32, 33] but not totally eliminate the risk of OHSS [34] particularly when low-dose 1500 IU hCG is used to rescue the luteal phase. In a recent RCT conducted in high-risk population as defined by the presence of 15 and 25 follicles >11 mm at the day of triggering, OHSS was noted in 2% vs. 0% of in patients undergoing hCG and agonist plus low-dose hCG (1500 IU) approach [35]. To achieve the goal of OHSS-free clinic, segmentation and freeze-all strategy (without using 1500 hCG) have been proposed when the patients have >25 growing follicles ≥11 mm at the day of triggering [36]. Intensive luteal phase support defined by Engmann et al. as an alternative option of rescuing luteal phase in agonist-triggered cycles with decreasing the risk of OHSS but not altering the pregnancy rates in women with PCOS [30].

In a study comparing GnRH agonist and rhCG for ovulation triggering in 227 PCOS patients, when the segmentation, namely, freeze-all, strategy have been chosen in both groups, OHSS from moderate to severe have not been observed at all in GnRH agonist trigger group (0–37.6%, $p < 0.001$). In addition, mature oocytes (19.1 ± 11.7 vs. 14.1 ± 4.3, $p < 0.001$), fertilized oocytes (15.6 ± 5.6 vs. 11.7 ± 3.6, $p < 0.001$), and top quality cleavage embryos on day 3 (12.9 ± 4.7 vs. 7.5 ± 4.3, $p < 0.001$) were also significantly higher in GnRH agonist-triggered group than hCG-triggered group [37].

To conclude the issue of triggering in high-risk group, it appears that GnRH agonist yields comparable results with respect to pregnancy rates but with a decreased risk of OHSS. However, segmentation should be considered when there is >25 growing follicle ≥11 mm on the day of final maturation without low-dose hCG (1500 IU) supplementation.

28.4 Different Techniques for Oocyte Retrieval

In vitro maturation (IVM) is a technique in which immature oocytes are retrieved transvaginally when they were in the status of antral follicles with an 8–12 mm in diameter. After collection, in vitro conversion from germinal vesicle stage to the stage of metaphase II within 24–52 h before fertilization is aimed in order to avoid supra-physiological steroid levels and associated risk of OHSS [38]. As might be expected, the maturation potential of immature oocyte in in vitro condition is associated with the development status at the time of retrieval from the follicle [39]. Additionally, the presence of a dominant follicle (>14 mm) might also negatively affect the performance of maturation, fertilization, and embryo development of the remaining oocytes that had been retrieved within the same cycle [40].

In a non-comparative study, IVM resulted with 17. 5%of implantation, 40% of pregnancy, and hence 40% of live birth rates [41]. In a retrospective cohort study, pregnancy rates were reported to be 32–44% in IVM and 38–45% in IVF arms, respectively [42]. Another study in which conventional IVF with GnRH agonist OS protocol compared to IVM revealed significantly less mean number of metaphase II oocytes in IVM approach (10.5 ± 6.5 vs. 15.3 ± 8.8, $p < 0.001$); however pregnancy (48% vs. 45%) and live birth rates (29% vs. 27%) were similar [43]. As expected, there was no case of OHSS in IVM arm [43].

Since the data coming from RCTs consistently demonstrated less OHSS risk in patients with PCOS when stimulated with GnRH antagonist protocol compared to GnRH agonist protocol [6, 44], to evaluate the effectiveness of IVM cycles for the OHSS risk, the comparison should be done with the GnRH antagonist protocol. In two available retrospective studies conducted in women with PCOS, Das et al. suggested that IVM has been associated with a lower risk of OHSS and a lower rate of pregnancy than IVF using a GnRH antagonist protocol [38], and Shavit et al. with a small sample size ($n = 61$) reported statistically significant lower implantation rate, numerically lower pregnancy, and live birth rates. For the view of systematic review and meta-analysis, due to the lack of RCT comparing IVM and conventional IVF, Cochrane review has remained inconclusive [45]. However, a more recent meta-analysis by Kollmann et al. including only one RCT [46], but with a small sample size and low quality of evidence ($n = 61$), has reported comparable live birth rates (RR = 1.26, 95% CI: 0.5–2.9) (Table 28.1) [6].

28.4.1 hCG and FSH Priming

Since gonadotropins are essential for the regulation of oocyte growth and maturation, administration of hCG in IVM setting 36 hours prior to oocyte retrieval has been proposed to improve treatment outcome. However the effect of hCG priming on oocyte maturation and developmental competence in IVM cycles has still remained as a matter of debate. In a RCT study comparing maturation rates 32 h after hCG priming, nuclear maturation rates were observed to be higher than control group (55.4% vs. 42.3% $p < 0.001$). No significant difference was observed in clinical pregnancy (37.5% vs. 50.0%), live birth (22.5% vs. 31.0%), and implantation rates (32.9% vs. 32.56%) when hCG primed and non-primed groups were compared [47]. In concordance, a Cochrane review comparing patients with PCOS either primed with 10000 IU hCG ($n = 40$) or not ($n = 42$) revealed no difference for the outcome of clinical pregnancy (OR = 0.60, 95% CI: 0.25–1.45), live birth (OR = 0.65, 95% CI: 0.24–1.74), or miscarriage (OR = 0.75, 95% CI: 0.24–2.39) rates [48]. However, the quality of evidence was low. With regard to various doses of hCG priming (10000 IU vs. 20000 IU), no differences were noted in the number of oocytes collected and rates of oocyte maturation, embryo cleavage, and clinical pregnancy. Of interest, fertilization rates were significantly lower with 20000 when compared to 10000 units of hCG (58.9% vs. 71.7%; $p = 0.03$) [49].

For the view of priming with FSH, a meta-analysis including 2 RCTs and 76 patients with PCOS might be mentioned. According to that, priming with FSH in IVM cycles does not make any significant difference by means of ongoing pregnancy/live birth rates (RR = 1.13 (95% CI, 0.46–2.79), $I^2 = 0\%$). There was no significant difference in observed rates of miscarriage in both arms either but with a very low level of evidence (RR = 5.73, 95% CI: 0.4–90.8) [6].

28.5 Embryo Transfer Strategy in Women with Polycystic Ovary Syndrome

Women with the risk of OHSS who undergo ART have lower rates of late-onset OHSS if the embryo transfer was performed in a frozen cycle instead of a fresh cycle [50]. A recent RCT with a large sample size ($n = 1500$, PCOS) suggested that frozen-embryo transfer (FET) was associated with a significantly higher live birth (49.3% vs. 42.0%, $p = 0.004$), lower miscarriage rate (14.6% vs. 25.0%, $p < 0.001$), and lower incidence of OHSS (1.3% vs. 7.1%,

$p < 0.001$) compared to fresh-embryo transfer [51]. The reason for higher live birth rates in women with frozen-embryo transfer was due to the lower rate of pregnancy loss in the fresh embryo transfer. As a possible explanation for the difference in pregnancy loss and live birth rates between frozen and fresh cycles, it was hypothesized that there may be a differences in endometrial receptivity due to the transfer strategy. On the other hand, higher frequency of preeclampsia (4.4% vs. 1.4%, $p = 0.009$) was reported in frozen-embryo transfer cycles [51].

Of note, the RCT by Chen et al. which was conducted in China, differed from standard practice, the embryos were cryopreserved on day 3 of culture, and multiple embryos were transferred, whereas most programs in the world aiming to cryopreserve on day 5 and transfer a single embryo. In addition, the BMI of the women studied was 24 kg/m^2, which is much lower than the BMI of women with PCOS in other countries [51]. With this respect, it might be early to suggest routine FET in women with PCOS; however it is clear that freeze-all strategy can reduce the risk of OHSS without causing any adverse effects [51].

With regard to preparation of endometrium for frozen-thawed embryo transfer cycles in patients with PCOS, artificial cycle with GnRH agonist suppression is most commonly preferred protocol due to the irregular menstrual cycles in those patients. There is lack of data in patients with PCOS for the comparison of different endometrium preparation protocols. However, a meta-analysis concluded that there is no consistent superiority of any endometrial preparation protocol for FER in unselected infertile patients [52].

28.6 Conclusions

This chapter can be summarized as follows:

- Ovulation induction with GnRH antagonist protocol should be first choice in order to reduce the risk of moderate to severe OHSS in women with PCOS regardless of the type and starting day of GnRH antagonist.
- In women with PCOS, regarding ovulation induction with gonadotropins, either hMG or rec-FSH might be preferred. There is no difference between any type and combination of exogenous gonadotropin with regard to pregnancy rate. Since using hCG for OS might increase the risk of OHSS, it should not be preferred.
- Metformin supplementation during OS seems be relevant in women with PCOS and might reduce the risk of OHSS.
- Myo-inositol, as an insulin-sensitizing agent, might be supplemented in patients with PCOS to restore the menstrual cycles and increase clinical pregnancy rates in ART cycles. That remark is based on limited data, and it should be definitely confirmed with further studies. However, there is lack of data with regard to OHSS prevention.
- In terms of triggering final oocyte maturation in women with PCOS, there is no beneficial effect of lowering the dose of hCG down to 2500 IU with respect to a reduction in OHSS.
- In women with PCOS, triggering final oocyte maturation with GnRH agonist in GnRH antagonist OS protocol yields comparable results with respect to pregnancy rates but with a decreased risk of OHSS when luteal phase was supported either via intensive estrogen and progesterone or hCG (1500 IU rescue) immediately after oocyte retrieval. However, segmentation should be considered when there is >25 growing follicle ≥11 mm in diameter on the day of triggering for final oocyte maturation.
- Although IVM treatment is capable to eliminate the risk of OHSS in patient with PCOS, growing data regarding the safety and success of agonist-triggered cycles have reduced the interest on IVM in the clinical practice.
- Although FET for all strategy is promising, it might be early to suggest routine FET in patients with PCOS. Nevertheless, it is evident that freeze-all strategy can reduce the risk of OHSS without causing any adverse effects.

References

1. Bozdag G, Mumusoglu S, Zengin D, Karabulut E, Yildiz BO. The prevalence and phenotypic features of polycystic ovary syndrome: a systematic review and meta-analysis. Hum Reprod. 2016;31(12):2841–55.
2. Broekmans FJ, Knauff EA, Valkenburg O, Laven JS, Eijkemans MJ, Fauser BC. PCOS according to the Rotterdam consensus criteria: change in prevalence among WHO-II anovulation and association with metabolic factors. BJOG. 2006;113(10):1210–7.
3. Koivunen R, Pouta A, Franks S, Martikainen H, Sovio U, Hartikainen AL, et al. Fecundability and spontaneous abortions in women with self-reported oligo-amenorrhea and/or hirsutism: Northern Finland Birth Cohort 1966 Study. Hum Reprod. 2008;23(9):2134–9.
4. Group ECW. Health and fertility in World Health Organization group 2 anovulatory women. Hum Reprod Update. 2012;18(5):586–99.
5. White DM, Polson DW, Kiddy D, Sagle P, Watson H, Gilling-Smith C, et al. Induction of ovulation with low-dose gonadotropins in polycystic ovary syndrome: an analysis of 109 pregnancies in 225 women. J Clin Endocrinol Metab. 1996;81(11):3821–4.
6. Kollmann M, Martins WP, Lima ML, Craciunas L, Nastri CO, Richardson A, et al. Strategies for improving outcome of assisted reproduction in women with polycystic ovary syndrome: systematic review and meta-analysis. Ultrasound Obstet Gynecol. 2016;48(6):709–18.
7. Nastri CO, Ferriani RA, Rocha IA, Martins WP. Ovarian hyperstimulation syndrome: pathophysiology and prevention. J Assist Reprod Genet. 2010;27(2-3):121–8.
8. Stern JE, Brown MB, Wantman E, Kalra SK, Luke B. Live birth rates and birth outcomes by diagnosis using linked cycles from the SART CORS database. J Assist Reprod Genet. 2013;30(11):1445–50.

9. Humaidan P, Ejdrup Bredkjaer H, Westergaard LG, Yding AC. 1,500 IU human chorionic gonadotropin administered at oocyte retrieval rescues the luteal phase when gonadotropin-releasing hormone agonist is used for ovulation induction: a prospective, randomized, controlled study. Fertil Steril. 2010;93(3):847–54.
10. Ortega-Hrepich C, Stoop D, Guzman L, Van Landuyt L, Tournaye H, Smitz J, et al. A "freeze-all" embryo strategy after in vitro maturation: a novel approach in women with polycystic ovary syndrome? Fertil Steril. 2013;100(4):1002–7.
11. Tso LO, Costello MF, Albuquerque LE, Andriolo RB, Macedo CR. Metformin treatment before and during IVF or ICSI in women with polycystic ovary syndrome. Cochrane Database Syst Rev. 2014;11:CD006105.
12. Al-Inany HG, Youssef MA, Aboulghar M, Broekmans F, Sterrenburg M, Smit J, et al. GnRH antagonists are safer than agonists: an update of a Cochrane review. Hum Reprod Update. 2011;17(4):435.
13. Kolibianakis EM, Albano C, Camus M, Tournaye H, Van Steirteghem AC, Devroey P. Initiation of gonadotropin-releasing hormone antagonist on day 1 as compared to day 6 of stimulation: effect on hormonal levels and follicular development in in vitro fertilization cycles. J Clin Endocrinol Metab. 2003;88(12):5632–7.
14. Kolibianakis EM, Albano C, Kahn J, Camus M, Tournaye H, Van Steirteghem AC, et al. Exposure to high levels of luteinizing hormone and estradiol in the early follicular phase of gonadotropin-releasing hormone antagonist cycles is associated with a reduced chance of pregnancy. Fertil Steril. 2003;79(4):873–80.
15. Huirne JA, van Loenen AC, Schats R, McDonnell J, Hompes PG, Schoemaker J, et al. Dose-finding study of daily GnRH antagonist for the prevention of premature LH surges in IVF/ICSI patients: optimal changes in LH and progesterone for clinical pregnancy. Hum Reprod. 2005;20(2):359–67.
16. Hamdine O, Broekmans FJ, Eijkemans MJ, Lambalk CB, Fauser BC, Laven JS, et al. Early initiation of gonadotropin-releasing hormone antagonist treatment results in a more stable endocrine milieu during the mid- and late-follicular phases: a randomized controlled trial comparing gonadotropin-releasing hormone antagonist initiation on cycle day 2 or 6. Fertil Steril. 2013;100(3):867–74.
17. Abuzeid MI, Mitwally M, Abuzeid YM, Bokhari HA, Ashraf M, Diamond MP. Early initiation of gonadotropin-releasing hormone antagonist in polycystic ovarian syndrome patients undergoing assisted reproduction: randomized controlled trial ISRCTN69937179. J Assist Reprod Genet. 2012;29(11):1193–202.
18. Mokhtar S, Sadeghi MR, Akhondi MM, Zafardoust S, Badenush B, Fatemi F, et al. ART outcomes in GnRH antagonist protocol (flex ible) and long GnRH agonist protocol during early follicular phase in patients with polycystic ovary syndrome: a randomized clinical trial. J Reprod Infertil. 2015;16(3):148–54.
19. Weiss NS, Nahuis M, Bayram N, Mol BW, Van der Veen F, van Wely M. Gonadotrophins for ovulation induction in women with polycystic ovarian syndrome. Cochrane Database Syst Rev. 2015;9:CD010290.
20. Koundouros SN. A comparison study of a novel stimulation protocol and the conventional low dose step-up and step-down regimens in patients with polycystic ovary syndrome undergoing in vitro fertilization. Fertil Steril. 2008;90(3):569–75.
21. Mourad S, Brown J, Farquhar C. Interventions for the prevention of OHSS in ART cycles: an overview of Cochrane reviews. Cochrane Database Syst Rev. 2017;1:CD012103.
22. Pacchiarotti A, Carlomagno G, Antonini G, Pacchiarotti A. Effect of myo-inositol and melatonin versus myo-inositol, in a randomized controlled trial, for improving in vitro fertilization of patients with polycystic ovarian syndrome. Gynecol Endocrinol. 2016;32(1):69–73.
23. Pundir J, Psaroudakis D, Savnur P, Bhide P, Sabatini L, Teede H, et al. Inositol treatment of anovulation in women with polycystic ovary syndrome: a meta-analysis of randomised trials. BJOG. 2018;125(3):299–308.
24. Choi J, Smitz J. Luteinizing hormone and human chorionic gonadotropin: origins of difference. Mol Cell Endocrinol. 2014;383(1-2):203–13.
25. Pellicer A, Albert C, Mercader A, Bonilla-Musoles F, Remohi J, Simon C. The pathogenesis of ovarian hyperstimulation syndrome: in vivo studies investigating the role of interleukin-1beta, interleukin-6, and vascular endothelial growth factor. Fertil Steril. 1999;71(3):482–9.
26. Schmidt DW, Maier DB, Nulsen JC, Benadiva CA. Reducing the dose of human chorionic gonadotropin in high responders does not affect the outcomes of in vitro fertilization. Fertil Steril. 2004;82(4):841–6.
27. Tsoumpou I, Muglu J, Gelbaya TA, Nardo LG. Symposium: update on prediction and management of OHSS. Optimal dose of HCG for final oocyte maturation in IVF cycles: absence of evidence? Reprod Biomed Online. 2009;19(1):52–8.
28. Youssef MA, Abou-Setta AM, Lam WS. Recombinant versus urinary human chorionic gonadotropin for final oocyte maturation triggering in IVF and ICSI cycles. Cochrane Database Syst Rev. 2016;4:CD003719.
29. Babayof R, Margalioth EJ, Huleihel M, Amash A, Zylber-Haran E, Gal M, et al. Serum inhibin A, VEGF and TNFalpha levels after triggering oocyte maturation with GnRH agonist compared with HCG in women with polycystic ovaries undergoing IVF treatment: a prospective randomized trial. Hum Reprod. 2006;21(5):1260–5.
30. Engmann L, Siano L, Schmidt D, Nulsen J, Maier D, Benadiva C. GnRH agonist to induce oocyte maturation during IVF in patients at high risk of OHSS. Reprod Biomed Online. 2006;13(5):639–44.
31. Youssef MA, Van der Veen F, Al-Inany HG, Mochtar MH, Griesinger G, Nagi Mohesen M, et al. Gonadotropin-releasing hormone agonist versus HCG for oocyte triggering in antagonist-assisted reproductive technology. Cochrane Database Syst Rev. 2014;10:CD008046.
32. Griesinger G, Schultz L, Bauer T, Broessner A, Frambach T, Kissler S. Ovarian hyperstimulation syndrome prevention by gonadotropin-releasing hormone agonist triggering of final oocyte maturation in a gonadotropin-releasing hormone antagonist protocol in combination with a "freeze-all" strategy: a prospective multicentric study. Fertil Steril. 2011;95(6):2029–33, 33 e1.
33. Humaidan P, Kol S, Papanikolaou EG, Copenhagen Gn RHATWG. GnRH agonist for triggering of final oocyte maturation: time for a change of practice? Hum Reprod Update. 2011;17(4):510–24.
34. Seyhan A, Ata B, Polat M, Son WY, Yarali H, Dahan MH. Severe early ovarian hyperstimulation syndrome following GnRH agonist trigger with the addition of 1500 IU hCG. Hum Reprod. 2013;28(9):2522–8.
35. Humaidan P, Polyzos NP, Alsbjerg B, Erb K, Mikkelsen AL, Elbaek HO, et al. GnRHa trigger and individualized luteal phase hCG support according to ovarian response to stimulation: two prospective randomized controlled multi-centre studies in IVF patients. Hum Reprod. 2013;28(9):2511–21.
36. Devroey P, Polyzos NP, Blockeel C. An OHSS-free clinic by segmentation of IVF treatment. Hum Reprod. 2011;26(10):2593–7.
37. Krishna D, Dhoble S, Praneesh G, Rathore S, Upadhaya A, Rao K. Gonadotropin-releasing hormone agonist trigger is a better alternative than human chorionic gonadotropin in PCOS undergoing IVF cycles for an OHSS free clinic: a randomized control trial. J Hum Reprod Sci. 2016;9(3):164–72.
38. Das M, Son WY, Buckett W, Tulandi T, Holzer H. In-vitro maturation versus IVF with GnRH antagonist for women with polycystic ovary syndrome: treatment outcome and rates of ovarian hyperstimulation syndrome. Reprod Biomed Online. 2014;29(5):545–51.

39. Durinzi KL, Saniga EM, Lanzendorf SE. The relationship between size and maturation in vitro in the unstimulated human oocyte. Fertil Steril. 1995;63(2):404–6.
40. Russell JB. Immature oocyte retrieval with in-vitro oocyte maturation. Curr Opin Obstet Gynecol. 1999;11(3):289–96.
41. Vitek WS, Witmyer J, Carson SA, Robins JC. Estrogen-suppressed in vitro maturation: a novel approach to in vitro maturation. Fertil Steril. 2013;99(7):1886–90.
42. Shalom-Paz E, Almog B, Wiser A, Levin I, Reinblatt S, Das M, et al. Priming in vitro maturation cycles with gonadotropins: salvage treatment for nonresponding patients. Fertil Steril. 2011;96(2):340–3.
43. Shalom-Paz E, Holzer H, Son W, Levin I, Tan SL, Almog B. PCOS patients can benefit from in vitro maturation (IVM) of oocytes. Eur J Obstet Gynecol Reprod Biol. 2012;165(1):53–6.
44. Lainas TG, Sfontouris IA, Zorzovilis IZ, Petsas GK, Lainas GT, Alexopoulou E, et al. Flexible GnRH antagonist protocol versus GnRH agonist long protocol in patients with polycystic ovary syndrome treated for IVF: a prospective randomised controlled trial (RCT). Hum Reprod. 2010;25(3):683–9.
45. Siristatidis CS, Vrachnis N, Creatsa M, Maheshwari A, Bhattacharya S. In vitro maturation in subfertile women with polycystic ovarian syndrome undergoing assisted reproduction. Cochrane Database Syst Rev. 2013;10:CD006606.
46. Choi MH, Lee SH, Kim HO, Cha SH, Kim JY, Yang KM, et al. Comparison of assisted reproductive technology outcomes in infertile women with polycystic ovary syndrome: in vitro maturation, GnRH agonist, and GnRH antagonist cycles. Clin Exp Reprod Med. 2012;39(4):166–71.
47. Zheng X, Wang L, Zhen X, Lian Y, Liu P, Qiao J. Effect of hCG priming on embryonic development of immature oocytes collected from unstimulated women with polycystic ovarian syndrome. Reprod Biol Endocrinol. 2012;10:40.
48. Reavey J, Vincent K, Child T, Granne IE. Human chorionic gonadotrophin priming for fertility treatment with in vitro maturation. Cochrane Database Syst Rev. 2016;11:CD008720.
49. Gulekli B, Buckett WM, Chian RC, Child TJ, Abdul-Jalil AK, Tan SL. Randomized, controlled trial of priming with 10,000 IU versus 20,000 IU of human chorionic gonadotropin in women with polycystic ovary syndrome who are undergoing in vitro maturation. Fertil Steril. 2004;82(5):1458–9.
50. Wong KM, van Wely M, Mol F, Repping S, Mastenbroek S. Fresh versus frozen embryo transfers in assisted reproduction. Cochrane Database Syst Rev. 2017;3:CD011184.
51. Chen ZJ, Shi Y, Sun Y, Zhang B, Liang X, Cao Y, et al. Fresh versus frozen embryos for infertility in the polycystic ovary syndrome. N Engl J Med. 2016;375(6):523–33.
52. Yarali H, Polat M, Mumusoglu S, Yarali I, Bozdag G. Preparation of endometrium for frozen embryo replacement cycles: a systematic review and meta-analysis. J Assist Reprod Genet. 2016;33(10):1287–304.

29 Laparoscopic Ovarian Drilling in Polycystic Ovary Syndrome

Austin D. Findley and Karen Jessup

Polycystic ovary syndrome (PCOS) is the most common endocrine disorder in reproductive-age women, with an estimated worldwide prevalence of 6–10% [1]. The disorder is characterized by the presence of androgen excess, ovulatory dysfunction, and polycystic ovaries. PCOS is believed to be caused by a complex interaction of genetic traits and environmental factors and is recognized as one of the most common causes of infertility and subfertility in women [2]. Treatment of PCOS-associated infertility consists of medical and surgical options to induce ovulation. The oral ovulation induction agent clomiphene citrate (CC) is considered first-line medical therapy due its efficacy, safety, tolerability, and low cost [3]. For women who are resistant to this treatment, ovulation may be induced with aromatase inhibitors, injectable gonadotropins, or ovarian surgery.

First described by Stein and Leventhal in 1935, bilateral ovarian wedge resection (BOWR) performed via laparotomy was long considered a primary treatment for ovulation induction in women with PCOS and ovulatory dysfunction [4]. BOWR was highly successful at restoring ovulation in women with PCOS. With the development of medical ovulation induction agents, as well as the associated postoperative complications of adhesion formation and diminished ovarian function having a negative impact on fertility, this procedure fell out of favor. In 1984, Gjönnaess first described a laparoscopic surgical approach to restore ovulation in women with PCOS [5]. Laparoscopic ovarian drilling (LOD), also referred to as ovarian diathermy, electrocautery, or electrocoagulation had the promise of restoring ovulation while minimizing ovarian damage and adhesion formation. Additionally, it provided all of the benefits of a minimally invasive procedure over laparotomy. Since its introduction, LOD has proven to be very successful in restoring ovulation in women with PCOS. Typical rates of spontaneous ovulation after LOD have been reported to be around 70–80% [6]. LOD has also proven effective in correcting many of the metabolic changes associated with PCOS, often with long-lasting effects. The introduction of ovarian drilling through operative laparoscopy has allowed surgical treatment of PCOS to remain a second-line option for women who fail to respond to medical ovulation induction and a way to manage the associated endocrine abnormalities in some women. This chapter discusses the role of laparoscopic ovarian drilling for ovulation induction and its effect on metabolic dysfunction in women with PCOS.

29.1 Indications For Surgery

According to the American Society for Reproductive Medicine, laparoscopic ovarian drilling is recommended as a second-line treatment for ovulation induction in women with PCOS who fail to respond to treatment with clomiphene citrate, as more than 75% of women will ovulate with oral therapy [3]. It may also be considered as a primary option for women who are not attempting to conceive in order to manage ovulatory and endocrine dysfunction, in those who are unwilling or unable to use traditional medical therapies, and for patients who find the rates of multiple gestation unacceptable.

29.2 Procedure and Technique

Despite the fact that LOD has been performed for several decades, a standardized approach to the procedure has never been agreed upon. LOD is an outpatient procedure that typically requires three laparoscopic ports. Most commonly, a laparoscopic approach is undertaken where a camera is introduced through an umbilical port and a grasper and monopolar needle electrode are placed through ancillary ports in each lower abdominal quadrant. The ovary is stabilized by grasping it near the hilum, and the monopolar needle

A. D. Findley (✉) · K. Jessup
Department of Obstetrics and Gynecology, Wright-Patterson Medical Center, Wright-Patterson Air Force Base, Dayton, OH, USA
e-mail: austin.findley@us.af.mil

G. N. Allahbadia et al. (eds.), *Textbook of Assisted Reproduction*, https://doi.org/10.1007/978-981-15-2377-9_29

electrode is introduced into the ovarian stroma at multiple sites as the tissue is heated through the activation of electrosurgical energy (Fig. 29.1). Four to ten puncture sites are typically made on one or both ovaries away from the hilum where the blood supply enters the ovary. The goal of the procedure is to cause enough destruction of the ovarian cortex that the metabolic changes seen in women with PCOS are corrected, without inducing damage severe enough to lead to premature ovarian failure.

The exact mechanism of action by which ovarian drilling restores ovulation and improves fertility and endocrine dysfunction is not known. It is believed to result from thermal damage to the androgen producing theca cells in the ovarian stroma. The resultant decrease in LH secretion and reduced androgen production provides an environment within the ovary that is conducive to normal follicular development. The procedure has also been described using carbon dioxide (CO_2), argon, or Nd:YAG lasers, but the use of these instruments is much less common due to the high cost and lack of availability of these instruments.

Multiple studies have tried to address the best practice in regards to the number of holes made in each ovary, the type, amount and time of energy applied, and whether one or both ovaries should be treated. Studies performed to assess the effects of LOD have described anywhere from 4 to 40 puncture sites per ovary. Only one study has directly compared

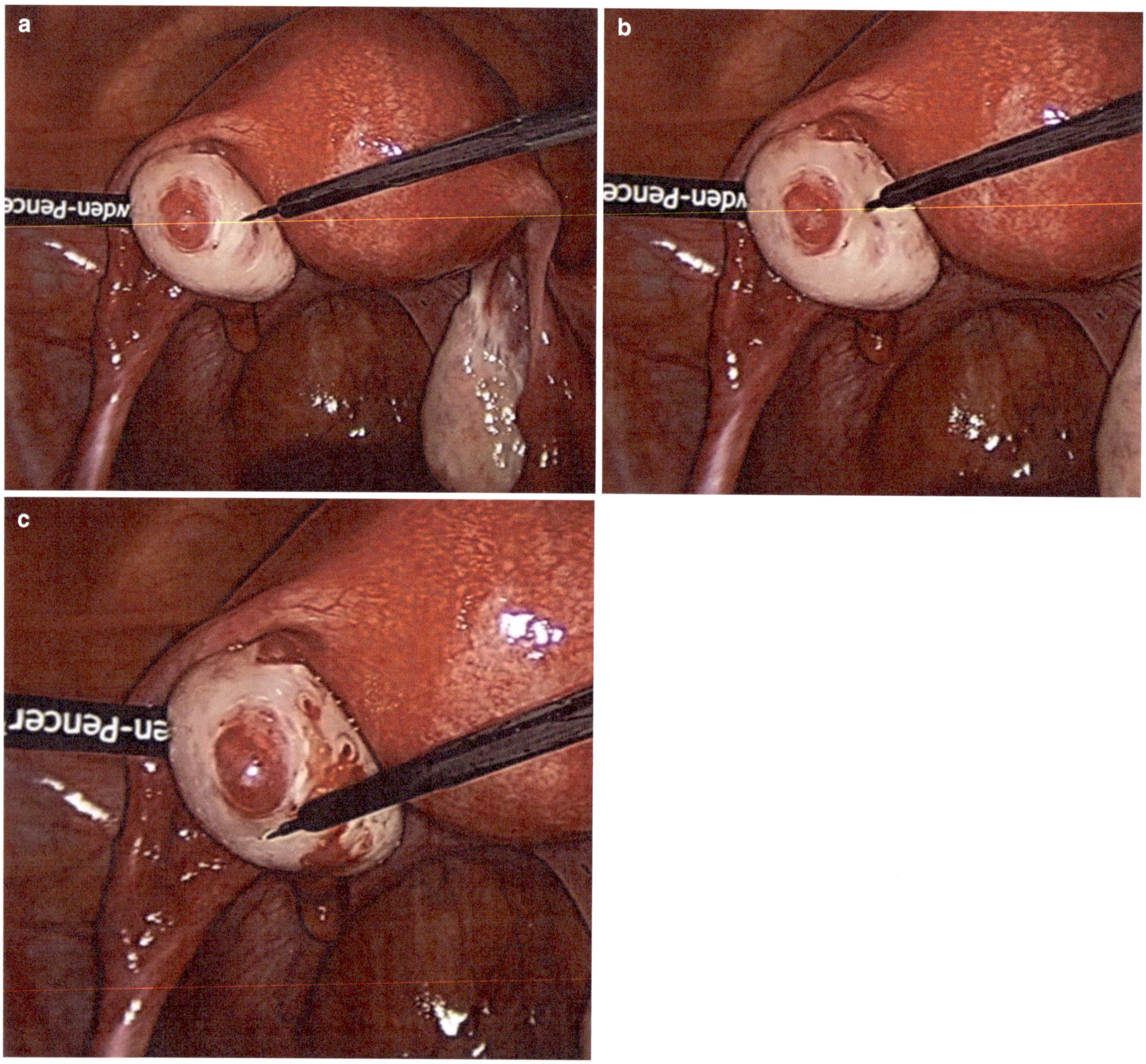

Fig. 29.1 Laparoscopic ovarian drilling with a monopolar needle electrode. (**a**) The ovary is stabilized as a monopolar needle is introduced into the abdomen. (**b**) The monopolar needle is introduced approximately 5–10 mm into the ovarian stroma. (**c**) 4–10 puncture sites are made on each ovary, applying a 4 s burst of 40 W coagulating current

differences in outcomes based on the number of puncture sites [7]. In a 2005 study by Malkawi et al.[7], the authors compared outcomes of LOD in women who received five puncture sites versus ten puncture sites per ovary. The authors found that five punctures on each ovary was equally as effective as ten punctures with respect to resumption of regular menses, ovulation rate, spontaneous and medically assisted conception, multiple gestation, ovarian hyperstimulation, and miscarriage rate. Additionally, performing fewer punctures resulted in equivalent reduction in LH, testosterone, DHEAS, and androstenedione. Although it has been suggested that more puncture sites may lead to more adhesions, a study by Mercorio et al., in which second look laparoscopy was performed after LOD, found no difference in the incidence or severity of adhesions (6 vs. 12 puncture sites) [8].

The amount of energy applied through the monopolar needle electrode is typically 40 W of power. A short burst of cutting current is used to penetrate the capsule of the ovary and the needle tip is advanced 5–10 mm into ovarian cortex. Coagulation current of 40 W is then applied for a total of 4 s at each site. A large systematic review reported no difference in postoperative ovarian reserve when 450–1200 Joules (J = W • s • # puncture sites) was applied to each ovary [9].

In studies examining unilateral vs. bilateral ovarian drilling, there has not been shown to be a difference in live birth rate, pregnancy rate, ovulation rate, or miscarriage rate [10, 11]. Despite this, most studies and descriptions of the procedure perform drilling on both ovaries.

29.3 Outcomes

29.3.1 Pregnancy, Miscarriage, Live Birth, Multiple Pregnancies, Ovarian Hyperstimulation, Cost, and Patient Preferences

Reported pregnancy rates following LOD are widely variable, with observed rates of 13–88% [6]. Higher rates of successful conception are reported when normal anatomy is identified at the time of surgery compared to abnormal surgical findings such as endometriosis (84–87.5% vs. 20–35%) [12, 13]. In a Cochrane systematic review, pooled data showed pregnancy rates of 25–51% following LOD and 30–51% following other medical treatments (OR 0.94, 95% CI 0.78 to 1.14) [10]. In this analysis, there was no difference in pregnancy rates when ovarian drilling was compared to treatment with CC, CC + metformin, CC + tamoxifen, gonadotropins, aromatase inhibitors, or CC + rosiglitazone. LOD did provide benefit when compared to metformin alone (OR 2.47, 95% CI 1.05 to 5.81). Additionally, there was no difference identified in the rate of live birth or miscarriage between groups. Live birth rates ranged from 24 to 44% following LOD and 27 to 62% following medical treatments (OR 0.77, 95% CI 0.59 to 1.01).

Miscarriage rates in women with PCOS are higher than the general public, with an incidence of 30–50% [6, 14]. Several studies have demonstrated a decrease in the miscarriage rate following LOD [15, 16]. However, Farquhar et al. reported no difference in miscarriage rate after LOD compared to medical ovulation induction in their review [10].

When compared to ovulation induction with gonadotropins, LOD results in a significantly lower incidence of multiple pregnancies (OR 0.13, 95% CI 0.03 to 0.52) and ovarian hyperstimulation syndrome (OHSS) (0 vs. 3%). There is no difference in multiple pregnancies or OHSS when LOD was compared to other medical treatments for ovulation induction in the setting of PCOS. When LOD is performed prior to IVF, there were no differences in the pregnancy, miscarriage, live birth, multiple pregnancy, or OHSS rate when compared to IVF alone.

Costs of treatment are significantly lower with LOD compared to ovulation induction with gonadotropins. Additionally, patients tend to prefer LOD to ovulation induction with gonadotropins [17–19].

29.3.2 Ovulation and Endocrine Changes

Ovulatory and endocrine changes after laparoscopic ovarian drilling are well documented. Regular ovulation is reported to occur in 30–90% of women with PCOS who undergo LOD, with a mean of 83% after monopolar diathermy [6, 20]. While LOD does decrease anti-Müllerian hormone and ovarian volume, there is no significant change in antral follicle count [9, 16]. Most studies have demonstrated significant reduction in serum AMH, LH, and androgen levels, while FSH remains relatively unaffected or slightly increased after LOD [6, 14, 21]. Androstenedione, free testosterone, and dehydroepiandrosterone sulfate are decreased and sex hormone binding globulin is not changed [22]. Accordingly, numerous studies have also demonstrated improvement in acne and hirsutism associated with hyperandrogenic PCOS, with the effects often lasting for years. Amer et al. reported that 40% of patients with acne and 25% of patients with hirsutism had noticeable improvement in symptoms 4 to 9 years after laparoscopic ovarian drilling [22]. Mohiuddin et al. reported a decrease in acne from 38 to 14% and no change in hirsutism at 6 to 10 years after LOD [23].

The effects of LOD on serum insulin and glucose levels have been mixed. Tiitinen et al. did not find a significant decrease in serum insulin levels in short-term follow-up after LOD [24]. Api et al. have reported decreased insulin levels but no effect on glucose [21]. Seow et al. found significantly decreased levels of insulin and glucose 3 months after surgery [6].

Table 29.1 Endocrine effects in women with PCOS after LOD

Measurement	Effect
AMH	↓
LH	↓
FSH	↔ or ↑
Antral follicle count	↔
Ovarian volume	↓
Testosterone	↓
Androstenedione	↓
DHEA-S	↓
SHBG	↔
Insulin	↔ or ↓
Lipids	
Total cholesterol	↔ or ↓
LDL	↔ or ↓
HDL	↔ or ↑
Endometrial hyperplasia/cancer	No studies

Very little research exists on the effects of LOD on lipids. In one prospective study of 34 patients, Shokeir et al. reported a significant decrease in total cholesterol, low-density lipoprotein (LDL), and a significant increase in high-density lipoprotein (HDL) [25]. In another small study involving 22 patients with PCOS, Kucuk et al. did not find any significant difference in cholesterol or lipoprotein levels after LOD [26]. Lemieux et al. also failed to find an improvement in insulin and glucose metabolism or changes to serum lipoprotein levels [27].

Although chronic anovulation is a hallmark of PCOS, there are no studies examining a possible reduction in the incidence of endometrial hyperplasia or malignancy as a potential long-term benefit of the procedure. A summary of the endocrine effects is listed in Table 29.1.

29.4 Complications

Other than general complications that may occur during any laparoscopy, the potential for postoperative adhesions and diminished ovarian reserve are the primary concerns that have been raised when examining LOD. Severe adnexal adhesions and premature ovarian failure leading to decreased fertility are the main reasons that bilateral ovarian wedge resection was ultimately abandoned. Although postoperative adhesions of the adnexa are common after laparoscopic ovarian drilling, the severity and effect on fertility appears to be limited.

Postoperative adhesions have been reported in 0 to 100% of women undergoing laparoscopic ovarian drilling during reoperation [20]. In studies where early second-look laparoscopy was performed, adhesions were generally noted to be mild and did not affect pregnancy rates [6, 28]. Additionally, the application of adhesion barriers or early second-look laparoscopy with adhesiolysis does not improve the pregnancy rate following LOD [28–30].

Multiple studies have confirmed a decrease in AMH and ovarian volume after LOD [16]. Amer et al. conducted a meta-analysis on the impact of LOD on AMH and ovarian reserve. In their pooled analysis, they found that AMH was reduced by 2.13 ng/mL after LOD, with the effects lasting for up to 6 months [9]. Although ovarian volume and AMH are significantly reduced for long periods of time after LOD, there is no evidence that suggests this actually results in diminished ovarian reserve or premature ovarian failure. Rather, these changes have been interpreted as a normalization of the abnormal ovarian structure and function that occurs after the procedure [31].

29.5 Alternative and Novel Procedures

In addition to the traditional laparoscopic approach of ovarian drilling with electrosurgery or laser energy, alternative methods of ovarian tissue destruction for the treatment of PCOS have also been described. These include transvaginal hydrolaparoscopy (THL) and high-intensity focused ultrasound (HIFU). Multiple studies have documented the feasibility of ovarian drilling performed via transvaginal hydrolaparoscopy [32–35]. In this procedure, a small incision is made in the posterior vaginal fornix and the pelvis is filled with sterile fluid to elevate the bowel out of the pelvis. A camera allows for visualization of the posterior uterus, ovarian fossa, ovaries, and fallopian tubes. Ovarian drilling can also be achieved through this approach with a bipolar needle electrode. The proposed benefits of this approach include direct access to the adnexa via the posterior cul-de-sac without a need for abdominal incisions. One randomized controlled trial comparing THL to LOD demonstrated shorter operative time (20 vs. 40 min, $p < 0.0001$), equivalent reduction in AMH levels, less pain (1.1 vs. 3.3 VAS scale, $p < 0.0001$), and fewer postoperative adhesions (16% vs. 70%, $p < 0.0001$) in the THL group without any difference in the rate of complications [34, 35].

Another procedure that offers promise in the treatment of PCOS involves the use of noninvasive focused ultrasound therapy. Animal studies examining the use of high-intensity focused ultrasound (HIFU) have demonstrated effectiveness at inducing tissue injury and necrosis within the ovarian stroma without damaging the surface of the ovary [36]. The procedure, similar to MR-guided focused ultrasound for the treatment of uterine fibroids, eliminates the need for surgery altogether and has the potential to prevent the formation of postoperative adhesions associated with ovarian drilling. This procedure has not yet been studied and developed in humans.

29.6 Conclusion

Laparoscopic ovarian drilling is highly effective in restoring ovulation in women with anovulatory PCOS, with the effects often lasting for many years. It remains a viable option for treatment in those who fail to respond to ovulation induction with clomiphene citrate. LOD is just as effective as gonadotropins for achieving pregnancy, but with less risk for multiple pregnancies and OHSS, lower cost, and better acceptability to patients. In addition to the benefits it provides for infertility treatment, it may also result in improvement in the common endocrine abnormalities associated with PCOS. Hirsutism and acne are frequently improved as a result of decreased androgen levels. Results are mixed or lacking as to whether or not LOD may reduce serum insulin and glucose levels, improve lipid profiles, and decrease the long-term risk for endometrial hyperplasia or cancer due to chronic anovulation. While postoperative adhesion formation does occur after LOD, this has generally been noted to be mild and without consequence to fertility. There is no evidence to suggest that standard surgical protocols for ovarian drilling result in premature ovarian failure. Ongoing study of the procedure and novel approaches to restoring ovulation in women with PCOS should continue to be explored.

References

1. Bozdag G, Mumusoglu S, Zengin D, Karabulut E, Yildiz BO. The prevalence and phenotypic features of polycystic ovary syndrome: a systematic review and meta analysis. Hum Reprod. 2016 Dec;31(12):2841–55.
2. Hull MG. Epidemiology of infertility and polycystic ovarian disease: endocrinological and demographic studies. Gynecol Endocrinol. 1987 Sep;1(3):235–45.
3. Thessaloniki ESHRE/ASRM-Sponsored PCOS Consensus Workshop Group. Consensus on infertility treatment related to polycystic ovary syndrome. Fertil Steril. 2008 Mar;89(3):505–22.
4. Stein IF, Leventhal M. Amenorrhea associated with bilateral polycystic ovaries. Am J Obstet Gynecol. 1935;29:181.
5. Gjönnaess H. Polycystic ovarian syndrome treated by ovarian electrocautery through the laparoscope. Fertil Steril. 1984 Jan;41(1):20–5.
6. Seow KM, Juan CC, Hwang JL, Ho LT. Laparoscopic surgery in polycystic ovary syndrome: reproductive and metabolic effects. Semin Reprod Med. 2008 Jan;26(1):101–10.
7. Malkawi HY, Qublan HS. Laparoscopic ovarian drilling in the treatment of polycystic ovary syndrome: how many punctures per ovary are needed to improve the reproductive outcome? J Obstet Gynaecol Res. 2005 Apr;31(2):115–9.
8. Mercorio F, Mercorio A, Di Spiezio SA, Barba GV, Pellicano M, Nappi C. Evaluation of ovarian adhesion formation after laparoscopic ovarian drilling by second-look minilaparoscopy. Fertil Steril. 2008 May;89(5):1229–33.
9. Amer SA, El Shamy TT, James C, Yosef AH, Mohamed AA. The impact of laparoscopic ovarian drilling on AMH & ovarian reserve: a meta-analysis. Reproduction. 2017 Apr 18;154(1):R13–21.
10. Farquhar C, Brown J, Marjoribanks J. Laparoscopic drilling by diathermy or laser for ovulation induction in anovulatory polycystic ovary syndrome. Cochrane Database Syst Rev. 2012 Jun 13;6:CD001122.
11. Zahiri Sorouri Z, Sharami SH, Tahersima Z, Salamat F. Comparison between unilateral and bilateral ovarian drilling in clomiphene citrate resistance polycystic ovary syndrome patients: a randomized clinical trial of efficacy. Int J Fertil Steril. 2015 Apr–Jun;9(1):9–16.
12. Gjønnaess H. Ovarian electrocautery in the treatment of women with polycystic ovary syndrome (PCOS). Factors affecting the results. Acta Obstet Gynecol Scand. 1994 May;73(5):407–12.
13. Armar NA, Lachelin GC. Laparoscopic ovarian diathermy: an effective treatment for anti-oestrogen resistant anovulatory infertility in women with the polycystic ovary syndrome. Br J Obstet Gynaecol. 1993 Feb;100(2):161–4.
14. Flyckt RL, Goldberg JM. Laparoscopic ovarian drilling for clomiphene-resistant polycystic ovary syndrome. Semin Reprod Med. 2011 Mar;29(2):138–46.
15. Colacurci N, Zullo F, De Franciscis P, Mollo A, De Placido G. In vitro fertilization following laparoscopic ovarian diathermy in patients with polycystic ovarian syndrome. Acta Obstet Gynecol Scand. 1997 Jul;76(6):555–8.
16. Amer SA, Banu Z, Li TC, Cooke ID. Long-term follow-up of patients with polycystic ovary syndrome after laparoscopic ovarian drilling: endocrine and ultrasonographic outcomes. Hum Reprod. 2002 Nov;17(11):2851–7.
17. Bayram N, van Wely M, van der Veen F, Bossuyt PM, Nieuwkerk P. Treatment preferences and trade-offs for ovulation induction in clomiphene citrate-resistant patients with polycystic ovary syndrome. Fertil Steril. 2005 Aug;84(2):420–5.
18. Farquhar CM, Williamson K, Gudex G, Johnson NP, Garland J, Sadler L. A randomized controlled trial of laparoscopic ovarian diathermy versus gonadotropin therapy for women with clomiphene citrate-resistant polycystic ovary syndrome. Fertil Steril. 2002 Aug;78(2):404–11.
19. van Wely M, Bayram N, Bossuyt PM, van der Veen F. Laparoscopic electrocautery of the ovaries versus recombinant FSH in clomiphene citrate-resistant polycystic ovary syndrome. Impact on women's health-related quality of life. Hum Reprod. 2004 Oct;19(10):2244–50.
20. Fernandez H, Morin-Surruca M, Torre A, Faivre E, Deffieux X, Gervaise A. Ovarian drilling for surgical treatment of polycystic ovarian syndrome: a comprehensive review. Reprod Biomed Online. 2011 Jun;22(6):556–68.
21. Api M, Görgen H, Cetin A. Laparoscopic ovarian drilling in polycystic ovary syndrome. Eur J Obstet Gynecol Reprod Biol. 2005 Mar 1;119(1):76–81.
22. Amer SA, Gopalan V, Li TC, Ledger WL, Cooke ID. Long term follow-up of patients with polycystic ovarian syndrome after laparoscopic ovarian drilling: clinical outcome. Hum Reprod. 2002 Aug;17(8):2035–42.
23. Mohiuddin S, Bessellink D, Farquhar C. Long-term follow up of women with laparoscopic ovarian diathermy for women with clomiphene-resistant polycystic ovarian syndrome. Aust N Z J Obstet Gynaecol. 2007 Dec;47(6):508–11.
24. Tiitinen A, Tenhunen A, Seppälä M. Ovarian electrocauterization causes LH-regulated but not insulin-regulated endocrine changes. Clin Endocrinol. 1993 Aug;39(2):181–4.
25. Shokeir T, El-Kannishy G. The effects of laparoscopic ovarian drilling on flow mediated dilation in women with PCOS: relationship with insulin resistance and IGF-I. Minerva Ginecol. 2014 Apr;66(2):209–18.
26. Kucuk M, Kilic-Okman T. Hormone profiles and clinical outcome after laparoscopic ovarian drilling in women with polycystic ovary syndrome. Med Sci Monit. 2005 Jan;11(1):CR29–34.
27. Lemieux S, Lewis GF, Ben-Chetrit A, Steiner G, Greenblatt EM. Correction of hyperandrogenemia by laparoscopic ovarian cautery in women with polycystic ovarian syndrome is not accom-

panied by improved insulin sensitivity or lipid-lipoprotein levels. J Clin Endocrinol Metab. 1999 Nov;84(11):4278–82.
28. Greenblatt EM, Casper RF. Adhesion formation after laparoscopic ovarian cautery for polycystic ovarian syndrome: lack of correlation with pregnancy rate. Fertil Steril. 1993 Nov;60(5):766–70.
29. Gürgan T, Kişnişçi H, Yarali H, Develioğlu O, Zeyneloğlu H, Aksu T. Evaluation of adhesion formation after laparoscopic treatment of polycystic ovarian disease. Fertil Steril. 1991 Dec;56(6):1176–8.
30. Saravelos H, Li TC. Post-operative adhesions after laparoscopic electrosurgical treatment for polycystic ovarian syndrome with the application of Interceed to one ovary: a prospective randomized controlled study. Hum Reprod. 1996 May;11(5):992–7.
31. Api M. Is ovarian reserve diminished after laparoscopic ovarian drilling? Gynecol Endocrinol. 2009 Mar;25(3):159–65.
32. Fernandez H, Alby JD, Gervaise A, de Tayrac R, Frydman R. Operative transvaginal hydrolaparoscopy for treatment of polycystic ovary syndrome: a new minimally invasive surgery. Fertil Steril. 2001 Mar;75(3):607–11.
33. Gordts S, Gordts S, Puttemans P, Valkenburg M, Campo R, Brosens I. Transvaginal hydrolaparoscopy in the treatment of polycystic ovary syndrome. Fertil Steril. 2009 Jun;91(6):2520–6.
34. Giampaolino P, Morra I, Tommaselli GA, Di Carlo C, Nappi C, Bifulco G. Post-operative ovarian adhesion formation after ovarian drilling: a randomized study comparing conventional laparoscopy and transvaginal hydrolaparoscopy. Arch Gynecol Obstet. 2016 Oct;294(4):791–6.
35. Giampaolino P, Morra I, Della Corte L, Sparice S, Di Carlo C, Nappi C, et al. Serum anti-Mullerian hormone levels after ovarian drilling for the second-line treatment of polycystic ovary syndrome: a pilot-randomized study comparing laparoscopy and transvaginal hydrolaparoscopy. Gynecol Endocrinol. 2017 Jan;33(1):26–9.
36. Shehata IA, Ballard JR, Casper AJ, Hennings LJ, Cressman E, Ebbini ES. High-intensity focused ultrasound for potential treatment of polycystic ovary syndrome: toward a noninvasive surgery. Fertil Steril. 2014 Feb;101(2):545–51.

30 Care of the Diabetic Woman Undergoing Medically Assisted Reproduction

Hayley Marshall and Kellie Flood-Shaffer

Diabetes mellitus, whether gestational, type 1, or type 2, is associated with a myriad of long-term morbidities, especially as one progresses in age. It is estimated that more than eight million women in the United States have diabetes mellitus prior to pregnancy and that it is observed in up to 1% of all pregnancies [1]. Although gestational diabetes arises with carbohydrate intolerance only during pregnancy, its prevalence varies in direct proportion with type 2 diabetes in a given population or ethnic group, and up to 50% of women with gestational diabetes can proceed to develop type 2 diabetes later in life [2]. With increasing prevalence of diabetes in the general population and advances in biotechnology allowing older women or women with chronic health conditions or complex infertility issues to become pregnant, thought about intentional, specialized preconception and antenatal counseling and care must be undertaken. After reading this chapter, readers will be able to understand the prevalence of obesity and impaired glucose metabolism and the impacts they have on health and assisted reproduction outcomes; explain the current knowledge of pathophysiology behind abnormal glucose metabolism and adverse reproductive outcomes; and recognize recommendations for women with obesity and/or diabetes seeking assisted reproductive techniques. A brief overview of the impact of diabetes on male fertility will also be addressed.

30.1 Pathophysiologic Difference in Diabetic Ovaries

Insulin and insulin-like growth factors are integral in the stimulation of steroidogenesis in the ovary. Diamond et al. studied the effect of diabetes on the process of steroidogenesis by comparing progesterone production in cultured granulosa cells from both diabetic and nondiabetic women, stimulated by hCG or insulin. Progesterone production was noted to increase on day 4 for both diabetic and nondiabetic granulosa cells when stimulated with hCG. When insulin was the stimulus, progesterone production was noted only in the nondiabetic follicles, suggesting that insulin-stimulated progesterone production by granulosa cells in the setting of diabetes is impaired [3]. Impaired progesterone production may then lead to failed pregnancy or early miscarriage.

30.2 Preconception Care for the Subfertile Woman

The maternal and fetal risks associated with diabetes during pregnancy are well documented, including increased maternal risk of hypertension, preeclampsia, and cesarean delivery and increased fetal risks of congenital malformation, large for gestational age, shoulder dystocia, and neonatal hypoglycemia. Children born to women with gestational diabetes have an increased risk for obesity and type 2 diabetes later in life themselves. It seems logical then, especially in the setting of assisted fertility where pregnancies are meticulously mapped out and planned, that diabetes education and management take a top priority for both the patient and physician. In a study by Riskin-Mashiah and Auslander, the quality of preconception and intrapartum care for diabetic women was examined. Three measures were evaluated for the ART group and the spontaneous pregnancy (control) group: folic acid use/prescription fillings 3 months prior to fertility treatment or pregnancy to prevent neural tube defects, evaluation of hemoglobin A1c (HbA1c) levels within 3 months of fertility treatment or pregnancy, and the use of potentially harmful drugs in the first month after fertility treatment or pregnancy (ACE inhibitors, ARBs, and statins) [4]. Surprisingly, there was no statistical difference between the two groups in any of the measures studied. In fact, women in the ART group had a decreased percentage of participants with good diabetic control (as evidenced by an HbA1c of <7 3 months after treatment), with 31.3% in the

H. Marshall · K. Flood-Shaffer (✉)
Department of Obstetrics and Gynecology, John Peter Smith Hospital, Fort Worth, TX, USA
e-mail: kfloodshaf@jpshealth.org

G. N. Allahbadia et al. (eds.), *Textbook of Assisted Reproduction*, https://doi.org/10.1007/978-981-15-2377-9_30

ART group and 40% in the spontaneous pregnancy group. Folic acid use was slightly increased in the ART group (23.9%) versus the spontaneous pregnancy group (20%). In regard to the potentially harmful medications often used to treat co-existing medical conditions, 3 women in the spontaneous pregnancy group filled at least 1 prescription in the month after pregnancy diagnosis, while 12 women in 16 fertility cycles did so in the ART group. This study demonstrates that achieving pregnancy should not be the only goal in diabetic women undergoing ART and that preconception counseling regarding the importance of glycemic control is lacking. As discussed by Tripathi et al., a study originating in the United Kingdom demonstrated the significant improvements preconception counseling had on folic acid use and optimal glycemic control pre- and intrapartum [5]. In diabetic women receiving focused and intentional preconception counseling, 68.4% (as opposed to 31.6% in non-counseled women) took prepregnancy folic acid, and 63.8% (as opposed to 36.3% in non-counseled women) had optimal prepregnancy glycemic control [4]. These studies go to show that specialized attention in the preconception time period is vital for appropriate education and optimizing a woman's health in anticipation of a healthy pregnancy.

30.3 Risk of Diabetes in Art

Many studies have confirmed a baseline increased risk of gestational diabetes with assisted reproductive technologies, perhaps because of the exogenous and exaggerated hormone effects that occur during the induction process, but the underlying cause of infertility must be taken into consideration as well. Polycystic ovarian syndrome (PCOS) is one of the most common endocrinopathies among young women, affecting up to 10% of reproductive-aged females [6, 7]. Anovulation, infertility, hyperandrogenism, hyperinsulinemia, and insulin resistance are all characteristics of this disease process. Elevated insulin levels indirectly increase LH-dependent ovarian androgen biosynthesis and inhibit sex hormone-binding globulin synthesis in the liver, resulting in a hyperandrogenic state [7]. With the relative insulin resistance that exists with PCOS, women with this syndrome produce higher levels of insulin compared to normal. Increased levels of insulin have both a direct effect on the ovaries themselves and cause increased release of other factors such as insulin-like growth factor 1 (IGF-1), which can prevent the growth of ovarian follicles through to ovulation [6]. PCOS is also associated with other conditions such as type 2 diabetes mellitus, gestational diabetes, hypertension, and dyslipidemia. In relation to gestational diabetes in the PCOS patient, Ashrafi et al. reported that the most important and significant predictors for development of GDM in these patients were menstrual irregularity, abnormal lipid profiles, and lack of pregestational metformin consumption [8]. Holte et al. found that women with PCOS who developed GDM had higher serum levels of very low-density lipoproteins and cholesterol than their GDM counterparts who did not have PCOS [9]. Thus, it is reasonable that early screening tests for gestational diabetes in women with PCOS, especially in those with a history of ART treatment, with irregular periods, or with an abnormal lipid profile, be undertaken early in pregnancy to optimize timely management for improved maternal and fetal outcomes. In a study by Levran et al., the incidence of glucose intolerance in women with PCOS who became pregnant after treatment for ovulation was compared to that of healthy women who conceived without intervention. The incidence of abnormal glucose tolerance test results in the treated group was twice that in the normal group [10]. Even more specifically, patients who underwent ovulation induction with HMG had a higher percentage of abnormal test results than those who conceived via other treatment modalities. In one study by Cozzolino et al., a group of women who had gestational diabetes was analyzed to determine the impact of age, body mass index, and mode of conception on the incidence of GDM. In general, this study found that women who conceived through assisted reproductive technology had a significantly higher percentage of women with GDM versus those who conceived spontaneously, 31.1% versus 13.6%, respectively. When separating ART methods, the incidence of GDM was higher in those women undergoing egg donation IVF/ICSI as opposed to homologous IVF/ICSI [11].

Well-known factors that increase the risk of developing gestational diabetes include high prepregnancy body mass index, advanced maternal age, pre-existing hypertension, smoking, parity, multiple gestations, and assisted reproductive technology treatment. ART inherently involves multiple risk factors for gestational diabetes in and of itself, as many ART therapies result in multiple gestations and women undergoing ART are older or have a medical co-morbidity negatively affecting fertility causing them to seek such treatment. In a study by Wang et al., the prevalence of GDM following ART in different cohorts of women was examined. This group found that regardless of method of conception, two conditions were associated with baseline increased risk of gestational diabetes: advanced maternal age and multiple gestation. Within the younger population studied, it was noted that the women undergoing ART had higher odds of developing GDM compared to those who conceived spontaneously. Lastly, within the women undergoing ART, the rate of gestational diabetes was increased in those who were overweight or obese. Although this study did not itself investigate the effects of different ART procedures (single embryo transfer, double embryo transfer, cleavage embryo transfer, blastocyst transfer, or fresh/thawed embryo transfer), there is previously established evidence that certain techniques are associated with increased likelihood of GDM. For example, double embryo transfer inherently increases the risk of multifetal gestation, which is associated with an increased risk of gestational diabetes, and other research has demonstrated that blastocyst transfer, as opposed to cleavage embryo transfer, is also associated with increased risk of GDM [12]. Exact mechanisms of how the ART techniques alter hormones in a manner that increases the risk of gestational diabetes are not completely understood, but there are some theories that exist. Changes in estrogen, progesterone, and insulin-like growth factor during ovarian stimulation are thought to contribute to the increased risk of GDM in ART patients [13]. The etiology of infertility (i.e., PCOS), types of drugs used for ovulation induction and luteal phase support, changes in the hormonal environment after ovulation induction and during early pregnancy, and presence of underlying metabolic and vascular factors exacerbated during ART procedures contribute to the increased risk of gestational diabetes in ART patients [14]. Bals-Pratsch et al. mention how ovulation induction and luteal phase support with hCG during ART may possibly trigger the onset of pathological glucose metabolism and maintain high estrogen levels [15]. In another study by Pieard et al., gestational diabetes was noted to coincide with elevated circulating progesterone levels, and progesterone had an important role in signaling during insulin release. Accordingly, onset of gestational diabetes is often seen in the second trimester of pregnancy as levels of progesterone increase [16]. Ashrafi et al. also found a relationship between progesterone use and development of gestational diabetes in the ART population, as progesterone is used for luteal phase support and preterm labor prevention [14]. In fact, Waters et al. compared the incidence of glucose intolerance during pregnancy in women receiving 17-alpha-hydroxyprogesterone caproate versus those not receiving the injection, and they found that 24% of women receiving the injection developed impaired glucose tolerance versus only 11% of women who did not receive the injection. This effect was also independent of other important risk factors including maternal race, age, body mass index, and parity [17]. Another group, Chen et al., investigated leptin and its relationship between ART and the development of gestational diabetes. Both serum and follicular fluid leptin levels increase during controlled ovarian hyperstimulation. Leptin helps regulate the secretion of sex steroids via the hypothalamic-pituitary-ovarian (HPO) axis as it is involved in energy metabolism throughout the pregnancy, and it can also contribute to the insulin resistance seen with GDM [18]. Increased plasma leptin levels in turn stimulate progesterone secretion from the trophoblast cells. The elevated progesterone levels foster insulin resistance on the molecular level by decreasing glucose transporter-4 in muscle and adipose tissue. Elevated leptin concentrations also affect the aromatization of androstenedione. By inhibiting aromatization, the conversion of androstenedione into estradiol is prevented, resulting in increased androgen levels and thus altered insulin secretion [18].

30.4 Optimizing the Subfertile Woman

Many studies, as will be discussed below, have evaluated metformin for anovulatory infertility in women with PCOS. Obesity and body mass index (BMI) appeared to play a significant role in the efficacy of medication used for fertility treatments. Prior to any medication administration, it is standard recommendation that obese women (BMI >30) undergo lifestyle interventions to enhance weight loss as first-line therapy. After review of multiple studies, it appeared that the pregnancy and live birth rate in obese women was higher for clomiphene versus metformin, but that metformin is a "very suitable" alternative to clomiphene as first-line ovulation induction in non-obese women with PCOS [6]. As Johnson's review article discusses, metformin may carry advantages over clomiphene, such as no known thinning endometrial effect, no known increase in multiple pregnancy rate (which itself increases risk of diabetes during pregnancy), and no concern over long-term adverse effects on the ovary.

There is conflicting data on whether or not the hypersecretion of luteinizing hormone (LH) in PCOS patients is responsible for an increased risk of miscarriage in PCOS patients, as it has also been found that suppression of LH release before conception does not improve the live birth rate [19–21]. The primary outcome in a study by Khattab et al. was miscarriage rate in PCOS patients who did or did not receive metformin. Their data concluded that women who received metformin had a substantially less percentage of miscarriage (11.6%) compared to those who did not (36.3%) [22]. Multiple mechanisms are theorized as to how metformin is beneficial. One suggested mechanism is that by decreasing the serum androgen levels, one decreases the overall risk of early pregnancy loss [23, 24]. Another mechanism involves hyperinsulinemia and insulin resistance. Hyperinsulinemia decreases the expression of glycodelin and insulin-like growth factor binding protein 1 (IGFBP-1) which adversely affects endometrial function and the peri-implantation milieu [25]. Glycodelin is significant in that it may play a role in inhibiting the endometrial immune response to the embryo [26, 27]. IGFBP-1 is critical in that it helps to facilitate the adhesion processes at the maternal-fetal interface [28, 29]. As metformin sensitizes peripheral tissue to insulin, the insulin reduction with its use can increase serum glycodelin and IGFBP-1 and enhance luteal phase uterine vascularity and blood flow in PCOS women [25]. Metformin has been shown to specifically improve endothelial function by improving markers of endothelial activation and coagulation [30–33]. A study by Meenakumari et al. found significant enhancement in luteal phase progesterone concentration in PCOS women who were treated with metformin, which of course helped to decrease early pregnancy loss [34]. Lastly, hyperinsulinemia is also associated with increased levels of plasminogen activator inhibitor-1, which is an independent risk factor for miscarriage in PCOS [35, 36]. Altered glucose metabolism is a well-known feature of PCOS. This altered glucose metabolism has a negative effect on the progesterone synthetic capacity of follicular and long-term cultured granulosa cells. In a study by Maruthini et al., this was alleviated by metformin pretreatment [37].

30.5 Therapies Used in Diabetic and Prediabetic Women Prior to and Postconception

Once pregnancy has been achieved, the next question being studied is whether women who become pregnant following metformin-induced ovulation, or any ART method for that matter, should continue with metformin through early pregnancy, especially in the setting of PCOS. It has been noted that in spontaneously conceiving PCOS women, the frequency of gestational diabetes is approximately 20–30% and that metformin can be safely continued until 6 to 8 weeks of gestation as it does not appear to be associated with any known fetal toxic effect [15]. In a study by Bals-Pratsch et al., an oral glucose tolerance test was performed within 4 weeks after pregnancy was confirmed in a group of ART patients undergoing pre-ART metformin treatment. All of these women continued metformin until a positive heartbeat was seen on sonogram. Overall results showed that 40% of women still proceeded to develop gestational diabetes mellitus and 14% of women had at least some form of impaired glucose tolerance, with the subgroup of pregnant women who suffered from PCOS showing a significantly higher frequency of both [15]. Although the exact amount of time of pre-ART metformin treatment was not distinguished, it is clear from this study that prepregnancy glycemic control is imperative considering such high rates of gestational diabetes and impaired glucose tolerance were seen in ART patients already undergoing glucose optimization therapy. Another group, Ashrafi et al., examined the difference of gestational diabetes incidence among three groups of women: women undergoing ART with PCOS, women undergoing ART without PCOS, and healthy women who neither had PCOS nor underwent ART. This group found that incidence values of gestational diabetes were significantly increased in patients with PCOS and undergoing ART. 44.4% of women with PCOS undergoing ART developed gestational diabetes, while 29.9% of the women without PCOS but undergoing ART and 7.3% of the women without PCOS who conceived spontaneously developed gestational diabetes [8]. This group also found that metformin consumption was associated with a significant reduction in gestational diabetes, a reduction by up to 40%. One of the reasons glycemic control is so important in the early phases of pregnancy, and perhaps why some would want their ART patients (especially women who have pre-existing diabetes) to continue an antidiabetic agent even after a positive pregnancy test is achieved, is that there seems to be a critical time frame for placentation 5–6 days after fertilization [15]. During this time the blastocyst adheres to the endometrium and then proceeds with implantation. It is suggested that implantation and vasculogenesis are affected by altered glucose metabolism, resulting in implantation failure or spontaneous abortion [15].

Ovarian hyperstimulation is a potential life-threatening risk for patients undergoing ART. As many studies mentioned above have demonstrated the potential benefit of metformin for (pre)diabetic and PCOS women, Jacob et al. studied whether or not a course of metformin prior to undergoing ART would reduce the risk of ovarian hyperstimulation syndrome [38]. In general, women with PCOS are the highest risk of ovarian hyperstimulation as they have a more sizable cohort of antral follicles capable of responding to the exogenous hormone administration [39]. Unlike the study by Doldi et al. [40], Jacob et al.'s study did not find any significant reduction in the incidence of moderate-severe OHSS when using metformin as pretreatment for women undergoing ART. Onalan et al. also investigated metformin treatment in patient with PCOS undergoing IVF and found that metformin did not lead to any improvement in IVF/ICSI outcomes among these patients [41].

Ongoing research in China regarding insulin-sensitizing therapies is under evaluation in an effort to reduce altered glucose metabolism in certain patients. A quinolone-derivative alkaloid found in many traditional Chinese medicinal herbs called berberine is currently being investigated and is reported to have comparable insulin-sensitizing capabilities to metformin [7]. Berberine has limited side effects and is currently being used in China for treating intestinal infections and diarrhea. In a study by Wei et al., berberine, when compared to metformin, improved some of the metabolic and hormonal derangement in a group of Chinese women with PCOS [42]. A study by An et al. investigated the effects of berberine, metformin (a 12-week course of administration), and placebo in PCOS women undergoing ART therapies. Berberine and metformin were equivalent on many outcomes (reduction in waist circumference and waist/hip ratio, decreases in total testosterone and free androgens, increases in sex hormone binding globulin, and improvement of glucose metabolism), but a greater reduction in body mass index, total cholesterol, and LDL cholesterol was seen in patients who received the berberine [7]. This study also found significantly higher clinical pregnancy rates in the women who received berberine and metformin and that the live birth rate was highest in those patients taking berberine. The higher rates of clinical pregnancy and live births in the berberine group are partially attributed to berberine's ability to increase energy expenditure and consumption of lipid metabolites, thus resulting in greater weight loss and reduction of BMI. Although the mechanism of action is not completely understood, there have been some studies demonstrating that berberine increased glucose consumption and intake in hepatocytes, adipocytes, and myotubes in a manner independent from, and in the absence of, insulin [43, 44]. Further research has demonstrated berberine's ability to upregulate the expression of the insulin receptor at the transcriptional level by stimulating the insulin receptor promoter via protein kinase C [42, 45]. Unlike metformin, berberine's safety for continued use during pregnancy has not been fully investigated yet, but it appears to have promise for future treatment of preventing or assisting in treatment of the diabetic patient in pregnancy. With the maternal and neonatal morbidities associated with diabetes and increasing patient population with diabetes, more methods of optimizing glucose control are strongly desired and needed.

30.6 Long-Term Complications

Although there is still investigation regarding this topic, there are long-term risks for both the mother and the offspring that were conceived via artificial means, and undergoing IVF is not without taking on potential for significant obstetrical and perinatal morbidity and mortality. Many studies have demonstrated the increased risk of ectopic or heterotopic pregnancies, preterm birth, low birthweight infants, abnormal placentation secondary to supraphysiological levels of E2 [46, 47], gestational diabetes, and preeclampsia [48–51]. However, other studies by Jaques et al. and Thomson et al. have reported increased morbidity in the subfertile population in general who conceived without the use of artificial methods, which points to a possible underlying predisposition of this certain patient population [52, 53]. These groups found that the rates of pregnancy-induced hypertension, perinatal deaths, abnormal placentation, low birthweight infants, cesarean delivery, and preterm labor were all associated with spontaneously conceiving in this group of subfertile women.

Ratson et al. followed a group of women who underwent either IVF or ovulation induction (OI) and studied their risk for long-term ophthalmic complications, such as glaucoma, diabetic retinopathy, macular degeneration, and retinal detachment. This study found that although this group overall did not have a significant increased risk for the aforementioned complications, when the ART group was subdivided between IVF and OI, there was a difference in risk. IVF patients had a significantly higher incidence of retinal detachment, so much so that when controlling for maternal age, obesity, and parity, IVF was noted as an independent risk factor for retinal detachment [54].

Fauser et al. reviewed data from the Sixth Evian Annual Reproduction (EVAR) Workshop group meeting which was held to evaluate the impact of IVF and intracytoplasmic sperm injection on the health of children born via these artificial techniques. Multiple studies that were reviewed at this conference reviewed data which revealed that IVF-conceived children tend to have lower birthweights but higher peripheral fat, blood pressure, and fasting glucose levels than naturally conceived children [55]. The women undergoing ART are often older or perhaps have other medical co-morbidities which increase the chance of selecting gametes that may result in these differences noted in ART conceived children. There have also been previous concerns about genetic imprinting disorders in children born as a result of IVF; however, this compilation of data revealed that the absolute risk of imprinting disorders after assisted reproduction is less than 1% [55]. Hargreave et al. went beyond just looking at the increased glucose levels in ART-conceived children, to looking specifically at the risks of type 1 diabetes mellitus in these children. This study found no association between maternal fertility problems and type 1 diabetes [56]. In the United States, the CDC maintains the National ART Surveillance System, which collects information about treatment outcome. This is difficult, however, as there is a relative infrequency of both ART and the outcomes of interest (birth defects, cancer, developmental disorders) [57].

30.7 Impact of Diabetes on Male Reproduction

Although the main focus of this chapter is on the woman undergoing ART, the male factor is also an important aspect to consider, especially when it is one of the more common reasons for infertility among couples. Diabetes may affect male fertility at multiple levels as a result of its effects on endocrine control of spermatogenesis, spermatogenesis itself, or by impairing penile erection and/or ejaculation [58]. In a study by Agbaje et al., the impact of diabetes on the overall quality of and DNA of sperm was analyzed. The genetic aspect of sperm that was studied, nDNA and mtDNA, is considered molecular biomarkers of fertility potential and genetic integrity [59, 60]. Fertility is noted to decline when sperm DNA fragmentation is elevated [61].

mtDNA deletions are associated with impaired sperm motility and infertility [62] and are subject to much greater oxidative stress than nDNA [63]. In Agbaji's study, semen volume in diabetic men was significantly less; however, no differences were noted in sperm concentration, total sperm output, percentage motility, or percentage normal morphology. Various studies have analyzed semen profiles from diabetic men, all with slight variants on but overall similar results as the study by Agbaje et al. [64–67]. Although this study noted a decreased semen volume from diabetic men, the amount ejaculated still remains within the normal range set by the WHO. As such, this brings up the question on whether or not the standard ranges for current semen analysis should be re-evaluated. Bonde et al. and Saleh et al. have noted that although a man may have an apparently normal semen analysis, he may still be subfertile [68, 69]. Agbaji et al. reported that sperm from diabetic subjects had both a significantly higher mean percentage of fragmented sperm nDNA and higher median number of mtDNA deletions. Damage to sperm DNA is significant because the oocyte has only a limited ability to repair damaged sperm DNA [70, 71] such that fragmentation beyond the oocyte's capacity may result in increased rates of embryonic failure and/or pregnancy loss [72, 73]. Brinkworth, Aitken et al., and Aitken comment on how increased sperm DNA damage has been implicated in the future health of resulting offspring [74–77]. For example, men who smoke have increased levels of oxidative sperm DNA damage [78]; thus their offspring are more likely to suffer from childhood cancers, particularly leukemia and lymphoma [79]. Other etiologies of sperm DNA damage exist, including deficient chromatin packing [80], abortive apoptosis [81], and environmental pollutants and oxidative stress [82] – oxidative stressors such as supraphysiological levels of glucose as seen in diabetic men.

In conclusion, although the amount of research is limited on the diabetic woman undergoing assisted reproductive therapy, it is apparent that special care needs to be taken for these women. Appropriate counseling in the preconception period and early glucose tolerance screening seem to be paramount. Research is actively being conducted in search of screening tools and treatments to better optimize glucose control in these patients to decrease manageable risks. Diabetes affects male fertility factors as well, which is also important to consider when taking care of the couple in the infertility clinic as essentially one patient. Despite the large body of evidence discussed in this chapter, investigation is ongoing with rich opportunity for improved care.

References

1. The American College of Obstetricians and Gynecologists. Pregestational Diabetes Mellitus. 2005. Print.
2. The American College of Obstetricians and Gynecologists. Gestational Diabetes Mellitus. 2013. Print.
3. Diamond M, Lavy G, Polan M. Progesterone production from granulosa cells of individual human follicles derived from diabetic and nondiabetic subjects. Int J Fertil. 1989;34(3):204–8.
4. Riskin-Mashiah S, Auslander R. Quality of medical care in diabetic women undergoing fertility treatment: we should do better! Diabetes Care. 2011;34(10):2164–9.
5. Tripathi A, Rankin J, Aarvold J, Chandler C, Bell R. Preconception counseling in women with diabetes: a population-based study in the north of England. Diabetes Care. 2010;33:586–8.
6. Johnson NP. Metformin use in women with polycystic ovary syndrome. Ann Transl Med. 2014;2(6):56.
7. An Y, Sun Z, Zhang Y, Liu B, Guan Y, Lu M. The use of Berberine for women with polycystic ovary syndrome undergoing IVF treatment. Clin Endocrinol. 2013;80(3):425–31.
8. Ashrafi M, Sheikhan F, Arabipoor A, Hosseini R, Nourbakhsh F, Zolfaghari Z. Gestational diabetes mellitus risk factors in women with polycystic ovary syndrome (PCOS). Eur J Obstet Gynecol Reprod Biol. 2014;181:195–9.
9. Holte J, Gennarelli G, Wide L, Lithell H, Berne C. High prevalence of polycystic ovaries and associated clinical, endocrine, and metabolic features in women with previous gestational diabetes mellitus. J Clin Endocrinol Metabol. 1998;83(4):1143–50.
10. Levran D, Shoham Z, Habib D, Greenwald M, Nebel L, Mashiach S. Glucose tolerance in pregnant women following treatment for sterility. Int J Fertil. 1990;35(3):157–9.
11. Cozzolino M, Serena C, Maggio L, Rambaldi M, Simeone S, Mello G, et al. Analysis of the main risk factors for gestational diabetes diagnosed with International Association of Diabetes and Pregnancy Study Groups (IADPSG) criteria in multiple pregnancies. J Endocrinol Investig. 2017;40(9):937–43.
12. Wang Y, Nikravan R, Smith H, Sullivan E. Higher prevalence of gestational diabetes mellitus following assisted reproduction technology treatment. Hum Reprod. 2013;28(9):2554–61.
13. Maman E, Lunenfeld E, Levy A, Vardi H, Potashnik G. Obstetric outcome of singleton pregnancies conceived by in vitro fertilization and ovulation induction compared with those conceived spontaneously. Fertil Steril. 1998;70(2):240–5.
14. Ashrafi M, Gosili R, Hosseini R, Arabipoor A, Ahmadi J, Chehrazi M. Risk of gestational diabetes mellitus in patients undergoing assisted reproductive techniques. Eur J Obstet Gynecol Reprod Biol. 2014;176:149–52.
15. Bals-Pratsch M, Großer B, Seifert B, Ortmann O, Seifarth C. Early onset and high prevalence of gestational diabetes in PCOS and insulin resistant women before and after assisted reproduction. Exp Clin Endocrinol Diabetes. 2011;119(06):338–42.
16. Pieard F, Wanatabe M, Schoonjans K. Progesterone receptor knockout mice have an improved glucose homeostasis secondary to beta cell proliferation. Proc Natl Acad Sci. 2002;99:16544–5648.
17. Waters T, Schultz B, Mercer B, Catalano P. Effect of 17α-hydroxyprogesterone caproate on glucose intolerance in pregnancy. Obstet Gynecol. 2009;114(1):45–9.
18. Chen R, Fisch B, Ben-Haroush A, Kaplan B, Hod M, Orvieto R. Serum and follicular fluid leptin levels in patients undergoing controlled ovarian hyperstimulation for in vitro cycle. Clin Exp Obstet Gynecol. 2004;31:103–6.
19. Regan L, Owen E, Jacobs H. Hypersecretion of luteinising hormone, infertility, and miscarriage. Lancet. 1990;336:1141–4.
20. Homburg R, Armar N, Eshel A, Adams J, Jacobs H. Influence of serum luteinising hormone concentrations on ovulation, conception, and early pregnancy loss in polycystic ovary syndrome. Br Med J. 1988;297:1024–6.
21. Clifford K, Rai R, Watson H, Franks S, Regan L. Does suppressing luteinising hormone secretion reduce the miscarriage rate? Results of a randomised controlled trial. Br Med J. 1996;312:1508–11.

22. Khattab S, Mohsen I, Foutouh I, Ramadan A, Moaz M, Al-Inany H. Metformin reduces abortion in pregnant women with polycystic ovary syndrome. Gynecol Endocrinol. 2006;22(12):680–4.
23. Okon M. Serum androgen levels in women who have recurrent miscarriages and their correlation with markers of endometrial function. Fertil Steril. 1998;69(4):682–90.
24. Tulppala M, Stenman U, Cacciatore B, Ylikorkala O. Polycystic ovaries and levels of gonadotrophins and androgens in recurrent miscarriage: prospective study in 50 women. BJOG Int J Obstet Gynaecol. 1993;100(4):348–52.
25. Jakubowicz D. Insulin reduction with metformin increases luteal phase serum glycodelin and insulin-like growth factor-binding protein 1 concentrations and enhances uterine vascularity and blood flow in the polycystic ovary syndrome. J Clin Endocrinol Metab. 2001;86(3):1126–33.
26. Bolton A, Clough K, Stoker R, Pockley A, Mowles E, Westwood O, et al. Identification of placental protein 14 as an immunosuppressive factor in human reproduction. Lancet. 1987;329(8533):593–5.
27. Okamoto N, Uchida A, Takakura K, Kariya Y, Kanzaki H, Riittinen L, et al. Suppression by human placental protein 14 of natural killer cell activity. Am J Reprod Immunol. 1991;26(4):137–42.
28. Giudice L, Mark S, Irwin J. Paracrine actions of insulin-like growth factors and IGF binding protein-1 in non-pregnant human endometrium and at the decidual–trophoblast interface. J Reprod Immunol. 1998;39(1–2):133–48.
29. Jones J, Gockerman A, Busby W Jr, Wright G, Clemmons D. Insulin-like growth factor binding protein 1 stimulates cell migration and binds to the alpha5 beta1 integrin by means of is Arg-Gly-Asp sequence. Proc Natl Acad Sci USA. 1993;90:10553–7.
30. Diamanti-Kandarakis E, Alexandraki K, Protogerou A, Piperi C, Papamichael C, Aessopos A, et al. Metformin administration improves endothelial function in women with polycystic ovary syndrome. Eur J Endocrinol. 2005;152(5):749–56.
31. Diamanti-Kandarakis E. Indices of low-grade chronic inflammation in polycystic ovary syndrome and the beneficial effect of metformin. Hum Reprod. 2006;21(6):1426–31.
32. Caballero A, Delgado A, Aguilar-Salinas C, Herrera A, Castillo J, Cabrera T, et al. The differential effects of metformin on markers of endothelial activation and inflammation in subjects with impaired glucose tolerance: a placebo-controlled, randomized clinical trial. J Clin Endocrinol Metabol. 2004;89(8):3943–8.
33. Orio F, Palomba S, Cascella T, De Simone B, Manguso F, Savastano S, et al. Improvement in endothelial structure and function after metformin treatment in young normal-weight women with polycystic ovary syndrome: results of a 6-month study. J Clin Endocrinol Metabol. 2005;90(11):6072–6.
34. Meenakumari K, Agarwal S, Krishna A, Pandey L. Effects of metformin treatment on luteal phase progesterone concentration in polycystic ovary syndrome. Braz J Med Biol Res. 2004;37(11):1637–44.
35. Glueck C, Wang P, Fontaine R, Sieve-Smith L, Tracy T, Moore S. Plasminogen activator inhibitor activity: an independent risk factor for the high miscarriage rate during pregnancy in women with polycystic ovary syndrome. Metabolism. 1999;48(12):1589–95.
36. Gris J, Neveu S, Mares P, Biron C, Hedon B, Schved J. Plasma fibrinolytic activators and their inhibitors in women suffering from early recurrent abortion of unknown etiology. J Lab Clin Med. 1993;122:606–15.
37. Maruthini D, Harris S, Barth J, Balen A, Campbell B, Picton H. The effect of metformin treatment in vivo on acute and long-term energy metabolism and progesterone production in vitro by granulosa cells from women with polycystic ovary syndrome. Hum Reprod. 2014;29(10):2302–16.
38. Jacob S, Brewer C, Tang T, Picton H, Barth J, Balen A. A short course of metformin does not reduce OHSS in a GnRH antagonist cycle for women with PCOS undergoing IVF: a randomised placebo-controlled trial. Hum Reprod. 2016;31(12):2756–64.
39. Ng E, Tang O, Ho P. The significance of the number of antral follicles prior to stimulation in predicting ovarian responses in an IVF programme. Hum Reprod. 2000;15(9):1937–42.
40. Doldi N, Persico P, Di Sebastiano F, Marsiglio E, Ferrari A. Gonadotropin-releasing hormone antagonist and metformin for treatment of polycystic ovary syndrome patients undergoing in vitro fertilization–embryo transfer. Gynecol Endocrinol. 2006;22(5):235–8.
41. Önalan G, Pabuçcu R, Goktolga U, Ceyhan T, Bagis T, Cıncık M. Metformin treatment in patients with polycystic ovary syndrome undergoing in vitro fertilization: a prospective randomized trial. Fertil Steril. 2005;84(3):798–801.
42. Wei W, Zhao H, Wang A, Sui M, Liang K, Deng H, et al. A clinical study on the short-term effect of berberine in comparison to metformin on the metabolic characteristics of women with polycystic ovary syndrome. Eur J Endocrinol. 2011;166(1):99–105.
43. Turner N, Li J, Gosby A, To S, Cheng Z, Miyoshi H, et al. Berberine and its more biologically available derivative, dihydroberberine, inhibit mitochondrial respiratory complex I: a mechanism for the action of berberine to activate AMP-activated protein kinase and improve insulin action. Diabetes. 2008;57(5):1414–8.
44. Zhou L, Yang Y, Wang X, Liu S, Shang W, Yuan G, et al. Berberine stimulates glucose transport through a mechanism distinct from insulin. Metabolism. 2007;56(3):405–12.
45. Zhang H, Wei J, Xue R, Wu J, Zhao W, Wang Z, et al. Berberine lowers blood glucose in type 2 diabetes mellitus patients through increasing insulin receptor expression. Metabolism. 2010;59(2):285–92.
46. Imudia A, Awonuga A, Kaimal A, Wright D, Styer A, Toth T. Elective cryopreservation of all embryos with subsequent cryothaw embryo transfer in patients at risk for ovarian hyperstimulation syndrome reduces the risk of adverse obstetric outcomes: a preliminary study. Fertil Steril. 2013;99(1):168–73.
47. Farhi J, Haroush A, Andrawus N, Pinkas H, Sapir O, Fisch B, et al. High serum oestradiol concentrations in IVF cycles increase the risk of pregnancy complications related to abnormal placentation. Reprod Biomed Online. 2010;21(3):331–7.
48. Jackson R, Gibson K, Wu Y, Croughan M. Perinatal outcomes in singletons following in vitro fertilization: a meta-analysis. Obstet Gynecol. 2004;103(3):551–63.
49. Kallen B, Finnstrom O, Nygren K, Otterblad Olausson P, Wennerholm U. In vitro fertilisation in Sweden: obstetric characteristics, maternal morbidity and mortality. BJOG Int J Obstet Gynaecol. 2005;112(11):1529–35.
50. Zhu L, Zhang Y, Liu Y, Zhang R, Wu Y, Huang Y, et al. Maternal and live-birth outcomes of pregnancies following assisted reproductive technology: a retrospective Cohort study. Sci Rep. 2016;6(1):35151.
51. Qin J, Sheng X, Wu D, Gao S, You Y, Yang T, et al. Worldwide prevalence of adverse pregnancy outcomes among singleton pregnancies after in vitro fertilization/intracytoplasmic sperm injection: a systematic review and meta-analysis. Arch Gynecol Obstet. 2016;295(2):285–301.
52. Jaques A, Amor D, Baker H, Healy D, Ukoumunne O, Breheny S, et al. Adverse obstetric and perinatal outcomes in subfertile women conceiving without assisted reproductive technologies. Fertil Steril. 2010;94(7):2674–9.
53. Thomson F, Shanbhag S, Templeton A, Bhattacharya S. Obstetric outcome in women with subfertility. BJOG Int J Obstet Gynaecol. 2005;112(5):632–7.
54. Ratson R, Sheiner E, Davidson E, Sergienko R, Beharier O, Kessous R. Fertility treatments and the risk for ophthalmic complications: a cohort study with 25-year follow-up. J Matern Fetal Neonatal Med. 2016;29(19):3094–7.

55. Fauser B, Devroey P, Diedrich K, Balaban B, Bonduelle M, Delemarre-van de Waal H, et al. Health outcomes of children born after IVF/ICSI: a review of current expert opinion and literature. Reprod Biomed Online. 2014;28(2):162–82.
56. Hargreave M, Kjaer S, Jørgensen M, Jensen A. Type 1 diabetes risk in children born to women with fertility problems: a cohort study in 1.5 million Danish children. Acta Obstet Gynecol Scand. 2016;95(12):1441–6.
57. Kissin D, Jamieson D, Barfield W. Monitoring health outcomes of assisted reproductive technology. N Engl J Med. 2014;371(1):91–3.
58. Sexton W, Jarow J. Effect of diabetes mellitus upon male reproductive function. Urology. 1997;49(4):508–13.
59. Agbaje I, Rogers D, McVicar C, McClure N, Atkinson A, Mallidis C, et al. Insulin dependant diabetes mellitus: implications for male reproductive function. Hum Reprod. 2007;22(7):1871–7.
60. Trisini A, Singh N, Duty S, Hauser R. Relationship between human semen parameters and deoxyribonucleic acid damage assessed by the neutral comet assay. Fertil Steril. 2004;82(6):1623–32.
61. Evenson DP, Jost LK, Marshall D, et al. Utility of the sperm chromatin structure assay as a diagnostic and prognostic tool in the human fertility clinic. Hum Reprod. 1999;14:1039–49.
62. Lestienne P, Reynier P, Chretien MF, et al. Oligoasthenospermia associated with multiple mitochondrial DNA rearrangements. Mol Hum Reprod. 1997;3(9):811–4.
63. Van Houten B, Woshner V, Santos J. Role of mitochondrial DNA in toxic responses to oxidative stress. DNA Repair. 2006;5(2):145–52.
64. Padrón R, Dambay A, Suárez R, Más J. Semen analyses in adolescent diabetic patients. Acta Diabetol Lat. 1984;21(2):115–21.
65. Garcia-diez L, Corrales Hernandez J, Hernandez-diaz J, Pedraz M, Miralles J. Semen characteristics and diabetes mellitus: significance of insulin in male infertility. Arch Androl. 1991;26(2):119–28.
66. Handelsman DJ, Conway AJ, Boylan LM, et al. Testicular function and glycemic control in diabetic men. A controlled study. Andrologia. 1985;17:488–96.
67. Ali S, Shaikh R, Siddiqi N, Siddiqi P. Semen analysis in insulin-dependent/non-insulin-dependent diabetic men with/without neuropathy. Arch Androl. 1993;30(1):47–54.
68. Bonde J, Ernst E, Jensen T, Hjollund N, Kolstad H, Scheike T, et al. Relation between semen quality and fertility: a population-based study of 430 first-pregnancy planners. Lancet. 1998;352(9135):1172–7.
69. Saleh R, Agarwal A, Nelson D, Nada E, El-Tonsy M, Alvarez J, et al. Increased sperm nuclear DNA damage in normozoospermic infertile men: a prospective study. Fertil Steril. 2002;78(2):313–8.
70. Matsuda Y, Tobari I. Repair capacity of fertilized mouse eggs for X-ray damage induced in sperm and mature oocytes. Mutat Res Fundam Mol Mech Mutagen. 1989;210(1):35–47.
71. Genesca A, Caballin M, Miro R, et al. Repair of human sperm chromosome aberrations in the hamster egg. Hum Genet. 1992;89(2):181–6.
72. Ahmadi A, Ng S. Developmental capacity of damaged spermatozoa. Hum Reprod. 1999;14(9):2279–85.
73. Ahmadi A, Ng S. Fertilizing ability of DNA-damaged spermatozoa. J Exp Zool. 1999;284(6):696–704.
74. Brinkworth M. Paternal transmission of genetic damage: findings in animals and humans. Int J Androl. 2000;23(3):123–35.
75. Aitken R, Baker M, Sawyer D. Oxidative stress in the male germ line and its role in the aetiology of male infertility and genetic disease. Reprod Biomed Online. 2003;7(1):65–70.
76. Aitken R, Ryan AL, Curry BJ, et al. Multiple forms of redox activity in populations of human spermatozoa. Mol Hum Reprod. 2003;9(11):645–61.
77. Aitken R. Founders' lecture. Human spermatozoa: fruits of creation, seeds of doubt. Reprod Fertil Dev. 2004;16(7):655.
78. Fraga C, Motchnik P, Wyrobek A, Rempel D, Ames B. Smoking and low antioxidant levels increase oxidative damage to sperm DNA. Mutat Res Fundam Mol Mech Mutagen. 1996;351(2):199–203.
79. Ji B, Shu X, Zheng W, Ying D, Linet M, Wacholder S, et al. Paternal cigarette smoking and the risk of childhood cancer among offspring of nonsmoking mothers. JNCI J Natl Cancer Inst. 1997;89(3):238–43.
80. Manicardi G, Bianchi P, Pantano S, Azzoni P, Bizzaro D, Bianchi U, et al. Presence of endogenous nicks in DNA of ejaculated human spermatozoa and its relationship to chromomycin A3 accessibility. Biol Reprod. 1995;52(4):864–7.
81. Shen H, Dai J, Chia S-E, et al. Detection of apoptotic alterations in sperm in subfertile patients and their correlations with sperm quality. Hum Reprod. 2002;17(5):1266–73.
82. Aitken J, Fisher H. Reactive oxygen species generation and human spermatozoa: the balance of benefit and risk. BioEssays. 1994;16:259–67.

Vitamin D Deficiency and Medically Assisted Reproduction

31

V. Sarais, E. Giacomini, Alessandra Alteri, and P. Viganò

31.1 Vitamin D Epidemiology, Main Functions, and Metabolism

Vitamin D is a fat-soluble vitamin and a steroid hormone that plays a key role in the regulation of calcium homeostasis and bone health. However, vitamin D system also regulates the expression of several genes (3% of human genome) involved in cell differentiation and cell cycle control and exercising multiple pleiotropic functions on extra-skeletal target tissues, such as immune and cardiovascular system, pancreatic endocrine cells, muscle, and adipose tissue.

Vitamin D is produced in the skin upon exposure to sunshine. Although it is defined as a vitamin, the fact that it can be produced in skin and dietary intake not being required separates it from other vitamins. Vitamin D should be better considered as a prohormone, but not a vitamin. It exists in small amounts in food, being highest in fortified dairy and fish oils. The precursor molecule 7-dehydrocholesterol exists in the skin and is converted to the intermediary pre-vitamin D molecule with exposure to sunlight via a nonenzymatic reaction. Pre-vitamin D slowly isomerizes to vitamin D. The skin must be exposed to UV light of a specific wavelength (280–315 nm) for these reactions to occur. Vitamin D undergoes a two-step activation process to produce the active metabolite 1,25-dihydroxyvitamin D [1,25$(OH)_2$ D].

The tightly regulated activation process involves the synthesis of 25$(OH)_2$D in the liver, followed by the conversion to 1,25$(OH)_2$D by in the kidney. 1,25$(OH)_2$D is the active form that maintains adequate blood levels of calcium and phosphorus (Fig. 31.1).

When the dietary calcium supply is inadequate, 1,25$(OH)_2$D in conjunction with adequate parathyroid hormone (PTH) increases calcium mobilization from the bone into the circulation. 1,25$(OH)_2$D, also together with PTH, reduces urinary calcium excretion by increasing reabsorption of the last 1% of the filtered calcium load from the distal tubule. This is an important quantity since 7 g of calcium is filtered in humans every day. To maintain neutral phosphate balance, the phosphate absorbed in the intestine and mobilized from the bone needs to be excreted, and renal phosphate excretion is increased by endocrine stimuli, such as fibroblast growth factor 23 (FGF23) and PTH [1, 2].

When serum calcium levels are decreased, a calcium-sensing receptor in the parathyroid gland stimulates the synthesis and release of PTH. Upon restoration of calcium levels, calcium-sensing receptor signals suppress PTH production and secretion, and PTH gene transcription is also suppressed by 1,25$(OH)_2$D. 1,25$(OH)_2$D itself and increased PTH levels suppress 1α-hydroxylase activity [3–5].

In nature, the sun is able to provide a radiation of 280–315 nm depending on season and latitude. In Northern populations, there is a high incidence of vitamin D deficiency due to the sunrays not reaching at 280–315 nm to penetrate the skin with enough intensity, during the winter. Vitamin D is acquired from the diet or supplements in the form of cholecalciferol (vitamin D3, animal origin) or ergocalciferol (vitamin D2, plant/fungal origin).

Vitamin D is absorption from the proximal segments of the small intestine is facilitated by bile salt through the formation of micellar solutions [6]. Eighty-eight percent of the vitamin D metabolites in circulation are bound to the vitamin D-binding protein (DBP), while the rest loosely associates with albumin, and less than 0.05% of 25$(OH)_2$D is found in free form [3, 5, 7–9].

DBP polymorphisms with corresponding effects on various diseases have been studied, but conclusive evidence is not available. DBP knockout mice, however, show no impairment of the basic vitamin D functions [10, 11].

V. Sarais (✉) · A. Alteri
Obstetrics and Gynaecology Department, IRCCS San Raffaele Scientific Institute, Milan, Italy
e-mail: sarais.veronica@hsr.it

E. Giacomini · P. Viganò
Division of Genetics and Cell Biology, Reproductive Sciences Laboratory, IRCCS San Raffaele Hospital Institute, Milan, Italy

G. N. Allahbadia et al. (eds.), *Textbook of Assisted Reproduction*, https://doi.org/10.1007/978-981-15-2377-9_31

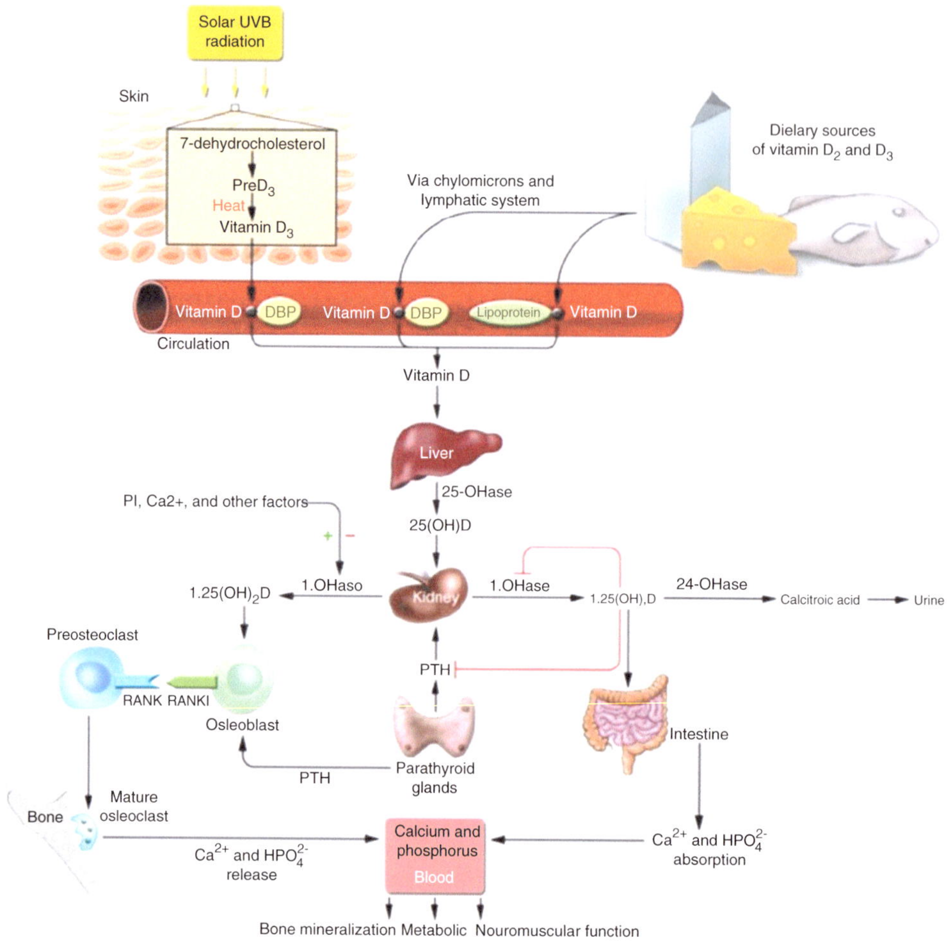

Fig. 31.1 Metabolism of vitamin D. The bio-activation process comprises the synthesis of 25(OH)$_2$D in the liver by 25-hydroxylation, followed by the conversion to 1,25(OH)$_2$D by the 1α-hydroxylase in the kidney under very tightly regulated physiological conditions. (From Querfeld U, Mak RH. Vitamin D deficiency and toxicity in chronic kidney disease: in search of the therapeutic window. Pediatr Nephrol 2010 25(12): 2413–2430, with permission)

Increased 1α-hydroxylase mRNA levels and enzyme activity have been detected in human keratinocytes, in endometrial cells, and in macrophages [12, 13]. The lack of vitamin D receptor (VDR) or 1α-hydroxylase leads to a bone and growth plate phenotype in mice that resembles congenital severe vitamin D deficiency disease in humans. The key target for VDR is the intestine because high calcium intake, or selective VDR rescue in the intestine, restores a normal bone and growth plate phenotype. The VDR is expressed in almost all tissues, and almost all cells respond to 1,25(OH)$_2$D exposure. VDR- or vitamin D-deficient mice shows propensity to autoimmune diseases such as inflammatory bowel disease or type 1 diabetes upon exposure to predisposing factors. VDR is expressed also in endothelium, vascular smooth muscle, and cardiomyocytes [14]. Lifestyle, environmental, and genetic factors can affect vitamin D status. Vitamin D deficiency is widespread in the world affecting developing as well as developed countries [15, 16]. The reasons for this putative increase in vitamin D deficiency are multifactorial including obesity, ethnicity (dark-skinned individuals), latitude, aging, and intestinal malabsorptive syndromes including celiac disease and liver and renal diseases [17].

Reduced sunlight exposure (clothing covering the body, use of sunscreens, reduced time outdoors, sedentary lifestyle, pollution) and reduced intake of vitamin D-rich foods also contribute to Vitamin D deficiency. Melanin-rich, dark skin can absorb UVB rays and reduce sunlight penetration leading to a decreased vitamin D production. In the United States, one third of reproductive-aged women have vitamin D concentrations <20 ng/ml (cut-off of sufficiency). Prevalence of vitamin D deficiency during pregnancy is estimated to range from 8% to 99% depending on the population and cut-offs used [18]. Based on a meta-analysis, pregnant women from Japan, the United States, Canada, Australia/New Zealand, and the United Kingdom have vitamin D intakes below current recommendations [19]. These high figures raise the controversy regarding what is meant by terms such as "requirement."

Potential epigenetic mechanisms underlying some of the beneficial effects of vitamin D in altering the risk of chronic diseases has been suggested [20]. Pereira et al. (2012) have reported that 1,25(OH)$_2$D activation of the VDR induces the transcription of genes that may contribute to epigenetic regulation [21].

31.2 Vitamin D and Pregnancy

Strong evidence supports the crucial role of the vitamin D in the reproductive pathophysiology in nonhuman models. Animal models show that vitamin D deficiency or altered function is associated with reduce liter size or loss of overall fertility together with increased maternal and offspring mortality.

Yoshizawa et al. (1997) have reported that female mice null for VDR have markedly reduced fertility and they are unable to reproduce presumably because of the inadequate uterine development. VDR null mutant mice had normal development and growth until weaning, despite reduced expression of vitamin D target genes. However, the mutants stunted up on weaning had alopecia, hypocalcaemia, and infertility. Bone formation was severely impaired as a typical feature of vitamin D-dependent rickets type II. Unlike humans suffering rickets, most of the VDR null mutant mice died until 15 weeks of age. Uterine hypoplasia and impaired folliculogenesis were observed. The absence of defects as alopecia and uterine hypoplasia in vitamin D deficient animals suggests a critical role for VDR per se in growth, bone formation, and female reproduction [22].

Halloran et al. (1980) studied the effects of vitamin D deficiency on fertility, reproductive capacity in female rats, and fetal and neonatal development were observed. Female weanling rats fed with a vitamin D-replete or vitamin D-deficient diet until maturity were mated with normal males. Although vitamin D-deficient females were fertile, vitamin D deficiency reduced overall fertility by 75%, diminished litter sizes by 30%, and impaired neonatal growth from day 6 to day 15 of lactation. Fetal development adjusted by weight gain and viability appeared normal [23].

It is possible that effects of vitamin D can be substantially different among species. It is also possible that all vitamin D functions on female reproduction are not mediated by VDR. So far the discrepancy between studies in rats and in the VDR null mutant mice remains unexplained and requires further research [24, 25].

Vitamin D plays role in cell signaling, gene regulation, and expression in the placenta [26, 27]. Both the VDR and the 1-α-hydroxylase gene are expressed in the placenta [28, 29]. The presence of 1-α-hydroxylase mRNA was also detected in cultures of human syncytiotrophoblasts from term placentas. High levels of 1-α-hydroxylase expression were found by Evans et al. (2004) in first- and second-trimester placentas, providing strong evidence for an active role of $1,25(OH)_2D$ at the fetal maternal interface after implantation [26].

Serum $1,25(OH)_2D$ levels increase threefold during pregnancy. Vitamin D insufficiency was reported for 46.8% and 56.4% of black and white neonates, respectively [30]. Maternal vitamin D status is the direct determinant of newborn's vitamin D status. Low maternal vitamin D levels affect mother, infant, and developing child. Some observational studies suggest that low maternal vitamin D concentrations could be associated with an increased risk of preeclampsia. Increased risks of low birth weight, gestational diabetes, preterm delivery, abnormal labor, cesarean delivery, and miscarriage are other adverse pregnancy outcomes that have been linked to maternal vitamin D deficiency in some, but not all, studies [31–39].

In the meta-analysis by Aghajafari et al. (2013), a correlation between lower vitamin D level and higher risk of adverse neonatal outcomes and obstetrics complications as gestational diabetes, preeclampsia, and small gestational age babies was found [40].

From a meta-analysis of 24 observational studies, Wei et al. (2013) reported that women with circulating $1,25(OH)_2D$ level less than 20,8 ng/ml in pregnancy experienced an increased risk of preeclampsia [odds ratio (OR) 2.09 (95% confidence intervals 1.50–2.90)], gestational diabetes mellitus (GDM) [OR 1.38 (1.12–1.70)], preterm birth [OR 1.58 (1.08–2.31)], and small for gestational age babies (SGA) [OR 1.52 (1.08–2.15)] [31].

31.3 Vitamin D and Role in Implantation

Rudick et al. (2014) examined the effect of vitamin D on results of egg donation: a model which separates factors that impact implantation (recipient) and factors that influence oocyte and embryo quality (donor and cycle factors), so that the effect of vitamin D on the oocyte and the endometrium can be distinguished. In this retrospective study, each recipient was individually matched with an oocyte donor. The clinical pregnancy rate progressively decreased with the reduction of recipient's vitamin D status. After adjusting for potential confounders, normal levels of vitamin D remained the only factor associated with higher clinical pregnancy rates (78% versus 37%, $p = 0.004$), or with higher live birth rates [41].

The concept that vitamin D can influence IVF outcomes through action on endometrium is supported by biological evidence: the cross talk between the embryo and the endometrium involves indeed the link between vitamin D and its receptor [41]. The activation of expression of the homeobox gene A (HOXA) represents a crucial step for implantation derived from the interaction between vitamin D and its receptor. HOXA genes are an evolutionarily conserved family of transcription factors critical to the control of early embryonic development.

In mammals, the homeobox containing HOXA gene family is essential for normal hematopoietic development.

HOXA10 is expressed in both the embryonic and the adult reproductive tracts, predominantly in the uterus.

HOXA10 gene encodes an evolutionarily conserved transcription factor that is essential to endometrial development and receptivity. HOXA10 expression is apparent in endometrial stroma and glands, where it is regulated by sex steroid hormones and it is significantly upregulated in response to estradiol (E2) in Ishikawa cells [42, 43]. In vitro, vitamin D directly activates HOXA10 expression in a human endometrial stromal cell. Vitamin D, VDR, and HOXA10 function in a common reproductive signaling pathway to effect functional differentiation. Thus, vitamin D upregulates HOXA10 [42].

Vitamin D and HOXA10 similarly effect the phenotype of bone marrow-derived cells as well as endometrial cells. One study suggests that HOXA10 is required for endometrial differentiation and for preparation for implantation in the mouse model. A targeted disruption of the *Hoxa10* gene results in uterine factor infertility in mice [44].

There are also several other immunomodulatory effects that may contribute to implantation through vitamin D action: $1,25(OH)_2D$ reduces decidual natural killer cells, with a consequent decrease of the synthesis of cytokines as colony stimulating factors-2 (CSF2), interleukin-1 (IL-1), interleukin-6 (IL-6), and tumor necrosis factor-α (TNF-α). Vitamin D can interfere with the production of endometrial cytokines in endometrial cells isolated from women with a history of recurrent miscarriage [26].

The effect of vitamin D on the decidua has been studied in greater detail than its effects on trophoblast. Kinetic data are available for decidual 1-α-hydroxylase, showing that the enzyme in this tissue is as efficient as its renal counterpart. The production of $1,25(OH)_2D$ by decidual cells has more in common with macrophages, which are the best characterized extrarenal tissue for 1-α-hydroxylase expression [12, 26].

31.4 Vitamin D and Ovarian Function

Vitamin D and markers of ovarian reserve seem to be associated to some extent. Anti-Müllerian-hormone (AMH) expression and serum levels are altered by environmental factors, including vitamin D levels and body weight. AMH is produced by granulosa cells (GCs) and inhibits primordial to primary follicle transition as well as the rate of the primordial follicle assembly. Vitamin D and AMH seem to be related at both the genetic and serum levels. The active form of vitamin D upregulates AMH production in cultured human prostate cell lines.

In humans, serum AMH levels are correlated with serum $1,25(OH)_2D$ levels in late reproductive-aged women. IVF success varies seasonally in parallel with in AMH levels, being 18% lower in the winter when vitamin D levels are the lowest [45].

The vitamin D receptor has been found in human ovarian cells where vitamin D can stimulate the synthesis of steroid hormones and insulin-like growth factor binding protein receptor (IGFBP-1). Findings from Merhi et al. (2014) indicated that vitamin D might promote the differentiation and development of GCs cells [46]. The authors also showed that $1,25(OH)_2D$ alters AMH sensitivity in GCs obtained from women who underwent oocyte retrieval. In this study, an inverse relationship between follicular fluid $1,25(OH)_2D$ levels and AMHR gene expression was found. Women with insufficient/deficient follicular fluid $1,25(OH)_2D$ had a two-fold increase in AMHR-II expression in GCs. Vitamin D treatment downregulates follicular stimulating hormone receptor (FSHR) and AMH receptor II (AMHR-II) gene expression and increases 3β-hydroxysteroid dehydrogenase expression and progesterone production in GCs. AMHR-II receptor expression indirectly interacts and is positively correlated with FSHR gene expression. How vitamin D affects FSHR is unknown, but it could involve AMH signaling. Possibly vitamin D acts on a common intracellular pathway involved in the regulation of both AMHR-II and FSHR; however, further studies are required [46].

Vitamin D deficiency can be involved in pathological conditions correlated to infertility such as PCOS, insulin resistance, and obesity contributing to the development of impaired glucose clearance and metabolic syndrome, even if this issue is still controversial [47, 48] (Fig. 31.2).

31.5 Vitamin D and Polycystic Ovarian Syndrome

Despite many studies investigating an association of vitamin D and metabolic and endocrine disorders in polycystic ovarian syndrome (PCOS), a conclusive relationship has not been demonstrated [49]. Yet, numerous interventional studies assessed an effect of vitamin D supplementation on PCOS, without success. Some evidence suggest that low vitamin D levels are related to insulin resistance, increased levels of total cholesterol, low-density lipoprotein-cholesterol (LDL-C), glucose, c-reactive protein (CRP), triglycerides, and decreased levels of high-density lipoprotein-cholesterol (HDL-C), and quantitative insulin sensitivity check index (QUICKI) in women affected by PCOS [49].

31.6 Vitamin D and Endometriosis

Endometriosis results from a complex interaction of immunologic, endocrine, genetic, and environmental factors; yet, the etiology is not clearly elucidated. Some evidence suggests that vitamin D might be involved in the pathogenesis of endometriosis through the expression of VDR and

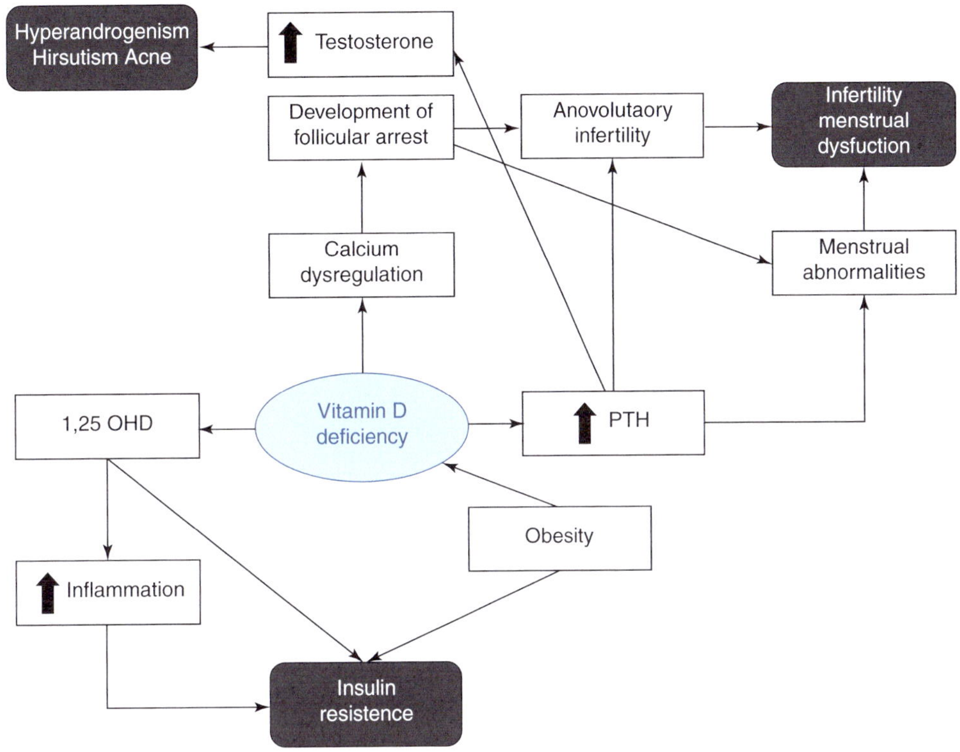

Fig. 31.2 Effect of vitamin D deficiency on ovarian function and menstrual cycle. Low vitamin D levels are related to elevated levels of homeostatic model assessment for insulin resistance (HOMA-IR), total cholesterol, low-density lipoprotein-cholesterol (LDL-C)

1α-hydroxylase in the endometrium, indicating that the endometrium represents an external site for vitamin D production and involvement of vitamin D in the regulation of the immune response. Our group has previously shown that VDR and 1α-hydroxylase are expressed in both eutopic and ectopic endometrium. Their expressions were higher in the endometrium of women with endometriosis compared to the control group [12].

Genetic variation in the VDR could be the link between the vitamin D regulatory network and endometriosis. Vilarino et al. (2011) performed a genetic association study that included 132 women with endometriosis-related infertility, 62 women with idiopathic infertility, and 133 controls to search for a possible association between VDR gene polymorphisms and susceptibility to endometriosis and/or infertility. However, the genotype frequencies of VDR polymorphisms were relatively similar among the groups [50]. A large prospective study reported that predicted plasma levels of $1,25(OH)_2D$ were inversely associated with the risk of endometriosis. Women in the highest quintile of predicted vitamin D concentration had a 24% lower risk of endometriosis than women in the lowest quintile [51]. In contrast, a study from our group including 87 women with endometriosis and 53 controls reported a significant increase in serum levels of $1,25(OH)_2D$ among women with endometriosis (24.9 ± 14.8 ng/ml) compared to the control group (20.4 ± 11.8 ng/ml). The $1,25(OH)_2D$ levels correlated with advanced disease stages [52]. Further studies are required to confirm the possible role of $1,25(OH)_2D$ in endometriosis [52].

31.7 Vitamin D and IVF Outcomes

Studies in women undergoing in vitro fertilization (IVF) suggest an association between vitamin D and IVF success (Table 31.1). However, while the role of vitamin D in human fertility, pregnancy, and neonatal growth has been extensively reviewed, the potential relationship between vitamin D and assisted reproductive technology (ART) outcomes is less scrutinized [53–55].

ART represents an opportunity to draw inferences on vitamin D deficiency in specific aspects of human fertility, allowing individual assessment of the various steps of reproductive process, from sperm function to folliculogenesis and implantation [56, 57].

Our group conducted a cross-sectional study based on the medical records of Caucasian-European female patients who presented to a single academic center for infertility. A total of 1072 women (mean age ± standard deviation 36.3 ± 4.4 years) were included. During the first 5 months of the year, 25(OH) D levels appeared to be completely unaffected by the increased global solar radiation. Then, a rapid increase in 25(OH)D levels could be observed during the month of June with the median value >20 ng/mL, reaching a plateau a few days after the summer solstice.

Median 25(OH)D concentration was <30 ng/mL for 89% of the entire year. 6.5% of patients had $1,25(OH)_2D$ levels ≤10 ng/mL, 40.1% ≤20 ng/mL, and 77.4% ≤30 ng/mL across the year. Global solar radiation was weakly correlated with 25(OH)D levels. A multivariable analysis showed that 25(OH)D levels were inversely associated with BMI [58].

Table 31.1 IVF outcomes in patients with deficient vitamin D levels

Author	Age (mean ± SD)	Cases/controls	CPR	LBR	P/R study
Rudick et al. (2012)	36.7 ± 3.7	109/79	Unchanged	–	R
Polyzos et al. (2014)	30.3 ± 3.8	239/129	Lower	–	R
Paffoni et al. (2014)	37.0 ± 4.3	154/181	Lower	–	P
Franasiak et al. (2015)	35.1 ± 4.0	422/95	Unchanged	–	R
Abadia et al. (2016)	34.9 ± 3.9	30/70	Unchanged	Unchanged	P
Neville et al. (2016)	36.5 ± 3.3	40/24	Unchanged	Unchanged	P
Van der Vijver et al. (2016)	31.2 ± 3.7	127/153	Unchanged	Unchanged	P

CPR clinical pregnancy rate, *LBR* live birth rate, *P* prospective, *R* retrospective

Vitamin D levels were evaluated in follicular fluid (FF) after oocyte retrieval and were observed to be significantly higher in women who achieved a clinical pregnancy with fresh embryo transfer [59].

Controversial results have also been reported about clinical pregnancy outcomes from populations referred to IVF cycles, distinguishing between women with deficiency and normal vitamin D serum levels. Many issues are still unsolved: the possible role of vitamin D on oocyte quality, then if so supplementation may have an impact; however the relevance of ethnicity; different interpretations of levels according to the type of assay used; and the presence of any other molecules apart from $1,25(OH)_2$ D that should be evaluated as they may have a more relevant role [60].

Rudick et al. (2012) in a retrospective cohort study confirmed that vitamin status was related to IVF success in non-Hispanic white women. Pregnancy rate decreased with lower levels of vitamin D. Vitamin D-replete women were four times more likely to achieve a pregnancy than deficient patients. However, among Asian population sufficient levels of vitamin D were not correlated to IVF success but inversely related [60]. Racial differences in the metabolism of vitamin D are reported in many studies. South Asian populations have been reported to have an increased activity of the enzyme responsible for deactivating of $1,25(OH)_2$ D [61]. The positive correlation between maternal vitamin D status and IVF pregnancy rate in non-Hispanic white, but not in Asian women, suggests that this association can be dependent on genetics [60].

Polyzos et al. (2014) reported that women who underwent a single blastocyst transfer, vitamin D deficiency was an independent predictor factor affecting clinical pregnancy rates. They observed significantly lower clinical pregnancy rates in vitamin D-deficient women as compared with vitamin D-insufficient women [41% (98/239) versus 53.3% (49/92), $P = 0.044$] and nonsignificantly lower pregnancy rates compared with vitamin D-replete women [41% (98/239) versus 56.7% (21/37), $P = 0.07$]. Women with vitamin D deficiency were almost 40% less likely to achieve a clinical pregnancy compared with those with serum $1,25(OH)_2D$ levels ≥20 ng/l. Among women undergoing elective single embryo transfer vitamin D deficiency was associated with a 44% lower odds of a clinical pregnancy compared with those with $1,25(OH)_2D$ levels ≥20 ng/ml [62].

Paffoni et al. (2014) prospectively compared IVF outcomes between vitamin D deficient (<20 ng/ml) and vitamin D sufficient (> = 20 ng/ml) women. Ovarian responsiveness, oocyte competence, embryo development, and number of embryos transferred were similar between two groups; however women with sufficient levels of vitamin D had a higher probability of having top quality embryos. Women with vitamin D greater than 20 ng/ml were 2.15 (95% CI 1.23–3.77) more likely to have a clinical pregnancy. The chances of pregnancy were highest for the group with serum levels >30 ng/ml (sufficient level) [63].

Many questions remain unanswered to recommend vitamin D measurement and supplementation to improve fertility [64].

Franasiak et al. (2015) assessed the relationship between serum $1,25(OH)_2D$ levels and implantation and pregnancy rates following an euploid blastocyst embryo transfer. Five hundred twenty-nine cycles with an autologous transfer of one or two euploid blastocysts were analyzed. Pregnancy rates did not differ across strata of vitamin D levels. In women undergoing euploid embryo transfer, vitamin D status was unrelated to pregnancy outcomes. Thus measuring serum $1,25(OH)_2$ D levels did not predict the likelihood of an euploid blastocyst to implant and reach live birth [65].

Possible association between follicular fluid (FF) $1,25(OH)_2D$ levels with number and quality of oocytes was assessed prospectively. While women who achieved a pregnancy had significantly higher follicular fluid vitamin D levels than nonpregnant women both had similar number of oocytes, oocyte quality, number of fertilized oocytes, and serum estradiol levels. A positive correlation was reported between $1,25(OH)_2D$ levels with patient's age and implantation rate. Only a significant difference was found in concentration of follicular fluid $1,25(OH)_2D$ between the two groups as the concentration was higher in the group with a clinical pregnancy [66].

Another prospective cohort study by Neville et al. (2016) did not show any correlation between fertility variables or pregnancy outcomes and male or female vitamin D status [67].

Abadia et al. (2016) examined the association between circulating 1,25$(OH)_2$D concentration and the outcome in women undergoing ART through a prospective cohort study: the serum 1,25$(OH)_2$D concentrations were positively related to fertilization rate, but the observed differences did not translate into improvements in the probability of implantation, clinical pregnancy, or live birth. Each 6 ng/ml increase in serum 1,25$(OH)_2$D was associated with an increase in the odds of fertilization by 19% (OR: 1.19; 95% CI: 1.04, 1.36). Most of the women in this cohort had serum 1,25$(OH)_2$D concentrations between 20 ng/ml and 50 ng/ml [68].

Van de Vijver et al. (2016) investigated whether vitamin D levels effected clinical pregnancy rates following transfer of frozen–thawed embryos, in order to evaluate effects that could only be mediated through the endometrium. Two hundred eighty consecutive women, between 18 and 39 years, underwent frozen embryo transfer (FET) cycles at blastocyst stage. Vitamin D deficiency was defined with a serum level of <20 ng/ml. Clinical pregnancy rates were similar in women with and without vitamin D deficiency. Population included in this study was relatively homogeneous: only one or two good/top quality blastocysts were transferred. However, ethnicity and environmental factors were not assessed. Also, the proportion of SET/DET was significantly higher in the vitamin D deficiency group where there was a lower percentage of top quality embryos [69].

Several meta-analyses have been conducted. However, evidence for a causative effect of 1,25$(OH)_2$D levels on IVF outcomes are still weak, and studies conducted so far rarely satisfy Hill's criteria for causation.

The meta-analysis by Vanni et al. (2014) showed that vitamin D deficiency was highly prevalent among women undergoing controlled ovarian stimulation, ranging from 21% to 31% across studies conducted in Western countries and reaching 75–99% in Iranian studies. Pooled data on 1,25 $(OH)_2$D deficiency from a limited number of studies showed a risk ratio of 0.89 (95% CI 0.53–1.49) and showing a lower but not insignificant likelihood of clinical pregnancy for vitamin D-deficient women compared with vitamin D-sufficient patients [70].

The latest systematic review and meta-analysis [71] on the correlation between vitamin D status and IVF outcomes has included six studies. Four were retrospective, two were prospective studies. The authors concluded that there was not a significant risk of having lower clinical pregnancy rates in the deficient group (RR 0.88, 95% CI 0.69–1.11). However, lower vitamin D status was associated with lower live birth rate (RR 0.76, 95% CI 0.61–0.93).

In conclusion, an association between vitamin D and fertility has been investigated since the 1970s. Yet, almost 50 years later the studies yield conflicting results. As such, there is insufficient evidence to support the routine assessment of vitamin D status in couples undergoing ART. The partly conflicting results of the available studies, potentially explaining the lack of statistical significance for a negative influence of vitamin D deficiency on clinical pregnancy rate, are likely secondary to confounders and insufficient sample size, and further larger studies are required.

References

1. Martin A, Quarles LD. Evidence for FGF23 involvement in a bone-kidney axis regulating bone mineralization and systemic phosphate and vitamin D homeostasis. Adv Exp Med Biol. 2012;728:65–83.
2. Renkema KY, Alexander RT, Bindels RJ, Hoenderop JG. Calcium and phosphate homeostasis: concerted interplay of new regulators. Ann Med. 2008;40(2):82–91.
3. Christakos S, Ajibade DV, Dhawan P, Fechner AJ, Mady LJ. Vitamin D: metabolism. Endocrinol Metab Clin N Am. 2010 Jun;39(2):243–53.
4. De Luca HF. Overview of general physiologic features and functions of vitamin D. Am J Clin Nutr 2004 Dec;80(6 Suppl):1689S–96S. Review.
5. De Luca HF. The development of a bone- and parathyroid-specific analog of vitamin D: 2-methylene-19-Nor-(20S)-1α,25-dihydroxyvitamin D3. Bonekey Rep. 2014 Mar 5;3:514.
6. Lo CW, Paris PW, Clemens TL, Nolan J, Holick MF. Vitamin D absorption in healthy subjects and in patients with intestinal malabsorption syndromes. Am J Clin Nutr. 1985 Oct;42(4):644–9.
7. Bikle DD. The vitamin D receptor: a tumor suppressor in skin. Adv Exp Med Biol 2014;810:282–302. Review.
8. Christakos S, Dhawan P, Porta A, Mady LJ, Seth T. Vitamin D and intestinal calcium absorption. Mol Cell Endocrinol. 2011 Dec 5;347(1–2):25–9.
9. DeLuca HF, Sicinski RR, Tanaka Y, Stern PH, Smith CM. Biological activity of 1,25-dihydroxyvitamin D2 and 24-epi-1,25-dihydroxyvitamin D2. Am J Phys. 1988 Apr;254(4 Pt 1): E402–6.
10. Speeckaert M, Huang G, Delanghe JR, Taes YE. Biological and clinical aspect of the vitamin D binding protein (Gc-globulin) and its polymorphism. Clin Chim Acta. 2006 Oct;372(1–2):33–42.
11. Speeckaert MM, Speeckaert R, van Geel N, Delanghe JR. Vitamin D binding protein: a multifunctional protein of clinical importance. Adv Clin Chem. 2014;63:1–57.
12. Viganò P, Lattuada D, Mangioni S, Ermellino L, Vignali M, Caporizzo E, et al. Cycling and early pregnant endometrium as a site of regulated expression of the vitamin D system. J Mol Endocrinol. 2006 Jun;36(3):415–24.
13. Caprio M, Infante M, Calanchini M, Mammi C, Fabbri A. Vitamin D: not just the bone. Evidence for beneficial pleiotropic extraskeletal effects. Eat Weight Disord. 2016 Aug 23.
14. Merke J, Milde P, Lewicka S, Hügel U, Klaus G, Mangelsdorf DJ, et al. Identification and regulation of 1,25-dihydroxyvitamin D3 receptor activity and biosynthesis of 1,25-dihydroxyvitamin D3. Studies in cultured bovine aortic endothelial cells and human dermal capillaries. J Clin Invest. 1989 Jun;83(6):1903–15.
15. Weisberg P, Scanlon KS, Li R, Cogswell ME. Nutritional rickets among children in the United States: review of cases reported between 1986 and 2003. Am J Clin Nutr. 2004 Dec;80(6 Suppl):1697S–705S.
16. Prentice A. Vitamin D deficiency: a global perspective. Nutr Rev. 2008 Oct;66(10 Suppl 2):S153–64.
17. Uriu-Adams JY, Obican SG, Keen CL. Vitamin D and maternal and child health: overview and implications for dietary requirements. Birth Defects Res C Embryo Today. 2013 Mar;99(1):24–44.

18. Sowell KD, Keen CL, Uriu-Adams JY. Vitamin D and reproduction: from gametes to childhood. Healthcare (Basel). 2015 Nov 9;3(4):1097–120.
19. Blumfield ML, Hure AJ, Macdonald-Wicks L, Smith R, Collins CE. A systematic review and meta-analysis of micronutrient intakes during pregnancy in developed countries. Nutr Rev. 2013 Feb;71(2):118–32.
20. Hossein-nezhad A, Holick MF. Optimize dietary intake of vitamin D: an epigenetic perspective. Curr Opin Clin Nutr Metab Care. 2012 Nov;15(6):567–79.
21. Pereira F, Barbáchano A, Singh PK, Campbell MJ, Muñoz A, Larriba MJ. Vitamin D has wide regulatory effects on histone demethylase genes. Cell Cycle. 2012 Mar 15;11(6):1081–9.
22. Yoshizawa T, Handa Y, Uematsu Y, Takeda S, Sekine K, Yoshihara Y, et al. Mice lacking the vitamin D receptor exhibit impaired bone formation, uterine hypoplasia and growth retardation after weaning. Nat Genet. 1997 Aug;16(4):391–6.
23. Halloran BP, DeLuca HF. Effect of vitamin D deficiency on fertility and reproductive capacity in the female rat. J Nutr. 1980 Aug;110(8):1573–80.
24. Kinuta K, Tanaka H, Moriwake T, Aya K, Kato S, Seino Y. Vitamin D is an important factor in estrogen biosynthesis of both female and male gonads. Endocrinology. 2000 Apr;141(4):1317–24.
25. Johnson LE, DeLuca HF. Vitamin D receptor null mutant mice fed high levels of calcium are fertile. J Nutr. 2001 Jun;131(6):1787–91.
26. Evans KN, Bulmer JN, Kilby MD, Hewison M. Vitamin D and placental-decidual function. J Soc Gynecol Investig 2004 Jul;11(5):263–71. Review.
27. Barrera D, Avila E, Hernández G, Méndez I, González L, Halhali A, et al. Calcitriol affects hCG gene transcription in cultured human syncytiotrophoblasts. Reprod Biol Endocrinol. 2008 Jan 22;6:3.
28. Christakos S, DeLuca HF. Minireview: Vitamin D: is there a role in extraskeletal health? Endocrinology. 2011 Aug;152(8):2930–6.
29. Liu NQ, Hewison M. Vitamin D, the placenta and pregnancy. Arch Biochem Biophys. 2012 Jul 1;523(1):37–47.
30. Bodnar LM, Simhan HN, Powers RW, Frank MP, Cooperstein E, Roberts JM. High prevalence of vitamin D insufficiency in black and white pregnant women residing in the northern United States and their neonates. J Nutr. 2007 Feb;137(2):447–52.
31. Wei SQ, Qi HP, Luo ZC, Fraser WD. Maternal vitamin D status and adverse pregnancy outcomes: a systematic review and meta-analysis. J Matern Fetal Neonatal Med. 2013 Jun;26(9):889–99.
32. Brannon PM, Yetley EA, Bailey RL, Picciano MF. Overview of the conference "Vitamin D and health in the 21st century: an update". Am J Clin Nutr. 2008 Aug;88(2):483S–90S.
33. Bodnar LM, Krohn MA, Simhan HN. Maternal vitamin D deficiency is associated with bacterial vaginosis in the first trimester of pregnancy. J Nutr. 2009 Jun;139(6):1157–61.
34. Dror DK, Allen LH. Vitamin D inadequacy in pregnancy: biology, outcomes, and interventions. Nutr Rev. 2010 Aug;68(8): 465–77.
35. Dror DK. Vitamin D status during pregnancy: maternal, fetal, and postnatal outcomes. Curr Opin Obstet Gynecol. 2011 Dec;23(6):422–6.
36. Hollis BW, Wagner CL. Vitamin D requirements and supplementation during pregnancy. Curr Opin Endocrinol Diabetes Obes. 2011 Dec;18(6):371–5.
37. Lau SL, Gunton JE, Athayde NP, Byth K, Cheung NW. Serum 25-hydroxyvitamin D and glycated haemoglobin levels in women with gestational diabetes mellitus. Med J Aust. 2011 Apr 4;194(7):334–7.
38. Poel YH, Hummel P, Lips P, Stam F, van der Ploeg T, Simsek S. Vitamin D and gestational diabetes: a systematic review and meta-analysis. Eur J Intern Med. 2012 Jul;23(5):465–9.
39. Thorne-Lyman A, Fawzi WW. Vitamin D during pregnancy and maternal, neonatal and infant health outcomes: a systematic review and meta-analysis. Paediatr Perinat Epidemiol. 2012 Jul;26(Suppl 1):75–90.
40. Aghajafari F, Nagulesapillai T, Ronksley PE, Tough SC, O'Beirne M, Rabi DM. Association between maternal serum 25-hydroxyvitamin D level and pregnancy and neonatal outcomes: systematic review and meta-analysis of observational studies. BMJ. 2013 Mar 26;346:f1169.
41. Rudick BJ, Ingles SA, Chung K, Stanczyk FZ, Paulson RJ, Bendikson KA. Influence of vitamin D levels on in vitro fertilization outcomes in donor-recipient cycles. Fertil Steril. 2014 Feb;101(2):447–52.
42. Daftary GS, Taylor HS. Endocrine regulation of HOX genes. Endocr Rev 2006 Jun;27(4):331–55. Review.
43. Taylor HS, Arici A, Olive D, Igarashi P. HOXA10 is expressed in response to sex steroids at the time of implantation in the human endometrium. J Clin Invest. 1998 Apr 1;101(7):1379–84.
44. Satokata I, Benson G, Maas R. Sexually dimorphic sterility phenotypes in Hoxa10-deficient mice. Nature. 1995 Mar 30;374(6521):460–3.
45. Tal R, Seifer DB. Potential mechanisms for racial and ethnic differences in anti-Müllerian hormone and ovarian reserve. Int J Endocrinol 2013;2013:818912. https://doi.org/10.1155/2013/818912. Review.
46. Merhi Z, Doswell A, Krebs K, Cipolla M. Vitamin D alters genes involved in follicular development and steroidogenesis in human cumulus granulosa cells. J Clin Endocrinol Metab. 2014 Jun;99(6):E1137–45.
47. Irani M, Merhi Z. Role of vitamin D in ovarian physiology and its implication in reproduction: a systematic review. Fertil Steril. 2014 Aug;102(2):460–8.
48. Luk J, Torrealday S, Neal Perry G, Pal L. Relevance of vitamin D in reproduction. Hum Reprod. 2012 Oct;27(10):3015–27.
49. He C, Lin Z, Robb SW, Ezeamama AE. Serum vitamin D levels and polycystic ovary syndrome: a systematic review and meta-analysis. Nutrients. 2015 Jun 8;7(6):4555–77.
50. Vilarino FL, Bianco B, Lerner TG, Teles JS, Mafra FA, Christofolini DM, et al. Analysis of vitamin D receptor gene polymorphisms in women with and without endometriosis. Hum Immunol. 2011 Apr;72(4):359–63.
51. Harris HR, Chavarro JE, Malspeis S, Willett WC, Missmer SA. Dairy-food, calcium, magnesium, and vitamin D intake and endometriosis: a prospective cohort study. Am J Epidemiol. 2013 Mar 1;177(5):420–30.
52. Somigliana E, Panina-Bordignon P, Murone S, Di Lucia P, Vercellini P, Vigano P. Vitamin D reserve is higher in women with endometriosis. Hum Reprod. 2007 Aug;22(8):2273–8.
53. Hartwell D, Rødbro P, Jensen SB, Thomsen K, Christiansen C. Vitamin D metabolites-relation to age, menopause and endometriosis. Scand J Clin Lab Invest. 1990 Apr;50(2):115–21.
54. Boyle VT, Thorstensen EB, Mourath D, Jones MB, McCowan LM, Kenny LC, et al. The relationship between 25-hydroxyvitamin D concentration in early pregnancy and pregnancy outcomes in a large, prospective cohort. Br J Nutr. 2016 Oct;116(8):1409–15.
55. Weinert LS, Reichelt AJ, Schmitt LR, Boff R, Oppermann ML, Camargo JL, et al. Vitamin D deficiency increases the risk of adverse neonatal outcomes in gestational diabetes. PLoS One. 2016 Oct 20;11(10):e0164999.
56. Mousa A, Abell S, Scragg R, de Courten B. Vitamin D in reproductive health and pregnancy. Semin Reprod Med. 2016 Mar;34(2):e1–13.
57. Ozkan S, Jindal S, Greenseid K, Shu J, Zeitlian G, Hickmon C, et al. Replete vitamin D stores predict reproductive success following in vitro fertilization. Fertil Steril. 2010 Sep;94(4):1314–9.
58. Anifandis GM, Dafopoulos K, Messini CI, Chalvatzas N, Liakos N, Pournaras S, et al. Prognostic value of follicular fluid 25-OH vitamin D and glucose levels in the IVF outcome. Reprod Biol Endocrinol. 2010 Jul 28;8:91.

59. Pagliardini L, Vigano P, Molgora M, Persico P, Salonia A, Vailati SH, et al. High prevalence of vitamin D deficiency in infertile women referring for assisted reproduction. Nutrients. 2015 Dec 2;7(12):9972–84.
60. Rudick B, Ingles S, Chung K, Stanczyk F, Paulson R, Bendikson K. Characterizing the influence of vitamin D levels on IVF outcomes. Hum Reprod. 2012 Nov;27(11):3321–7.
61. Awumey EM, Mitra DA, Hollis BW, Kumar R, Bell NH. Vitamin D metabolism is altered in Asian Indians in the southern United States: a clinical research center study. J Clin Endocrinol Metab. 1998 Jan;83(1):169–73.
62. Polyzos NP, Anckaert E, Guzman L, Schiettecatte J, Van Landuyt L, Camus M, et al. Vitamin D deficiency and pregnancy rates in women undergoing single embryo, blastocyst stage, transfer (SET) for IVF/ICSI. Hum Reprod. 2014 Sep;29(9):2032–40.
63. Paffoni A, Ferrari S, Viganò P, Pagliardini L, Papaleo E, Candiani M, et al. Vitamin D deficiency and infertility: insights from in vitro fertilization cycles. J Clin Endocrinol Metab. 2014 Nov;99(11):E2372–6.
64. Garcia-Velasco JA, Iglesias C, Fabris A. Vitamin D and in vitro fertilization outcome. Am J Obstet Gynecol. 2015 Mar;212(3):412–3.
65. Franasiak JM, Molinaro TA, Dubell EK, Scott KL, Ruiz AR, Forman EJ, et al. Vitamin D levels do not affect IVF outcomes following the transfer of euploid blastocysts. Am J Obstet Gynecol. 2015 Mar;212(3):315.
66. Farzadi L, Khayatzadeh Bidgoli H, Ghojazadeh M, Bahrami Z, Fattahi A, Latifi Z, et al. Correlation between follicular fluid 25-OH vitamin D and assisted reproductive outcomes. Iran J Reprod Med. 2015 Jun;13(6):361–6.
67. Neville G, Martyn F, Kilbane M, O'Riordan M, Wingfield M, McKenna M, et al. Vitamin D status and fertility outcomes during winter among couples undergoing in vitro fertilization/intracytoplasmic sperm injection. Int J Gynaecol Obstet. 2016 Nov;135(2):172–6.
68. Abadia L, Gaskins AJ, Chiu YH, Williams PL, Keller M, Wright DL, et al. Environment and Reproductive Health Study Team. Serum 25-hydroxyvitamin D concentrations and treatment outcomes of women undergoing assisted reproduction. Am J Clin Nutr. 2016 Sep;104(3):729–35.
69. van de Vijver A, Drakopoulos P, Van Landuyt L, Vaiarelli A, Blockeel C, Santos-Ribeiro S, et al. Vitamin D deficiency and pregnancy rates following frozen-thawed embryo transfer: a prospective cohort study. Hum Reprod. 2016 Aug;31(8):1749–54.
70. Vanni VS, Vigano P, Somigliana E, Papaleo E, Paffoni A, Pagliardini L, et al. Vitamin D and assisted reproduction technologies: current concepts. Reprod Biol Endocrinol. 2014 May 31;12:47.
71. Lv SS, Wang JY, Wang XQ, Wang Y, Xu Y. Serum vitamin D status and in vitro fertilization outcomes: a systematic review and meta-analysis. Arch Gynecol Obstet. 2016 Jun;293(6):1339–45.

Medically Assisted Reproduction and Autoimmunity

32

Keshia Torres-Shafer and Pascal Gagneux

32.1 Chapter Objectives

After reading this chapter the reader will be able to discuss:

1. Common autoimmune diseases and related fertility issues
2. Fertility treatment outcomes including those undergoing assisted reproductive technology
3. Important therapeutic measures to consider in those autoimmune diseases

32.2 Introduction

According to the NIH and American Autoimmune Related Diseases Association (AARDA), autoimmune diseases affect over 50 million people in the United States [1]. There are more than 80 types of autoimmune diseases with overlapping symptoms, making them difficult to diagnose as an individual can be affected with two or more diseases concurrently [2].

Ever since Fleming and others initially discovered adaptive immunity, the term "horror autotoxicus" whereby the immune system attacks its owner has been an important concept [3]. The acquired immune system in vertebrates is an evolution that occurred due to great responsibility placed on misdirected responses [4]. The immune system has a long history of evolutionary trade-offs and albeit complex; it is inherently an "unintelligent design" due to its frequent regulation and dysregulation [5]. Mammalian pregnancy is an immune conundrum, and not surprisingly, dysregulation of normal immune responses including autoimmunity can severely impact reproduction and assisted reproduction technologies [6]. While symptoms may overlap, there are numerous unrelated mechanisms that can contribute to autoimmunity, and the etiology of most autoimmune diseases is unknown. It is clear that environmental effects (infections, parasites, and symbionts, lack of breastfeeding, and excessive hygiene) play important roles in autoimmunity. Genetic factors also play a role as specific genetic variants at important immune loci such as HLA genes have been associated with autoimmune disease. HLA loci are among the most variable loci in the human genome and largely contribute to individual molecular identity [7]. The recent realization that innate and adaptive immune systems can synergize means that polymorphisms at innate immune receptors expressed on antigen presenting cells can also affect risk of autoimmunity [8]. Sex has an important effect on autoimmune disease, which is more prevalent in women than men (up to 75% affect women) as does geographic ancestry [9].

Autoimmunity can lead to a number of conditions including rheumatoid arthritis, systemic lupus erythematosus, celiac disease (sprue), pernicious anemia, vitiligo, scleroderma, psoriasis, inflammatory bowel diseases, Hashimoto's disease, Addison's disease, Graves' disease, reactive arthritis, Sjögren's syndrome, and type 1 diabetes. There are a number of theories regarding the etiology of autoimmune disease including bacterial, viral, medications, chemical irritants, environmental irritants, and multiple underlying genetic components (innate immune receptor polymorphisms and HLA haplotype variation), and many if not all these theories may be valid [10]. As there are many different types of autoimmune diseases, the presenting symptoms vary, but most commonly these include fatigue, fever, and general malaise.

Autoimmune diseases are rarely considered in the infertility work-up, and it is commonly overlooked that these can potentially impair both female and male fertility [11]. This chapter will focus on the impact of common autoimmune

K. Torres-Shafer
Department of Obstetrics & Gynecology, Wright State University Boonshoft School of Medicine, Dayton, OH, USA
e-mail: keshia.torres-shafer@wright.edu

P. Gagneux (✉)
Department of Pathology, University of California San Diego, San Diego, CA, USA
e-mail: pgagneux@ucsd.edu

G. N. Allahbadia et al. (eds.), *Textbook of Assisted Reproduction*, https://doi.org/10.1007/978-981-15-2377-9_32

Table 32.1 Summary of autoimmune diseases and key take home points

Disease	Key points
Premature ovarian failure (POF)	• Autoimmune disorders are associated with POF in 4–30% of cases • Treatment with immunosuppressants has failed to reverse ovarian autoimmunity • DHEA supplementation has been associated with increased pregnancy rates in smaller studies, but there is a need for high quality RCTs • Standard of care remains IVF with donor gametes or embryos
Recurrent implantation failure (RIF)	• Referred to as two or three failed fresh embryo transfers • Small studies have reported benefit with IVIG treatment; however this has not been proven in large quality RCTs • The use of aspirin or enoxaparin in this population is not recommended
Antiphospholipid antibody syndrome (APS)	• Production of autoantibodies against phospholipid-protein complexes • APS is not linked to infertility or poor ART outcome • Patients with APS are not recommended to undergo prophylactic anticoagulant therapy • Patients with APS and RPL are recommended to receive both heparin and aspirin co-therapy during ART and throughout the pregnancy
Rheumatoid diseases	• Women with rheumatoid diseases have same rates of infertility as the general population • Risk of thrombosis is high especially in women with high levels of autoantibodies and nephrotic range proteinuria • Risk of disease flare during ART is low in patients with well-controlled disease • In patients with a history of personal thromboembolic event, proper anticoagulant therapy is required prior to ovulation induction
Autoimmune thyroid disease (AITD)	• Most frequent cause of hypothyroidism in women of reproductive age • Controversy exists on whether there is a link between AITD and infertility • Studies have reported increased pregnancy rates in women treated with levothyroxine during ART • Treatment is not currently recommended for those with subclinical hypothyroidism
Multiple sclerosis (MS)	• MS is an autoimmune degenerative disease • Women with MS undergo menstrual irregularities; however very little literature exists regarding MS and infertility • MS therapies, especially cyclophosphamide, can adversely impact sperm and oocyte quality • MS patients may experience disease exacerbations, but this is not linked to failed IVF rates
Myasthenia gravis (MG)	• MG is a chronic autoimmune disorder which leads to fatigue and progressive muscular weakness • MG is not typically associated with infertility, but it is associated with POF 2% of cases • Course of MG during pregnancy is highly variable. Patients should delay childbirth for 1–2 years after receiving the diagnosis of MG • ART including ovulation induction may lead to disease exacerbation due to increase in estrogen levels
Autoimmune progesterone dermatitis (APD)	• APD is a rare hypersensitivity reaction, which occurs following exposure of progesterone • In infertile patients APD is triggered during ART with administration of exogenous progesterone • Progesterone desensitization is the recommended treatment for patients with APD undergoing ART
Celiac disease (CD)	• CD is a chronic autoimmune disorder which results in intestinal malabsorption and diarrhea • CD can affect women in their reproductive age and is related to delayed menarche, POF, and infertility • Only case reports have noted a benefit with immunomodulatory treatment prior to embryo transfer

diseases on fertility as well as on the outcome of fertility treatments including those undergoing assisted reproductive technology (ART) and for each type will discuss important therapeutic measures to consider (Table 32.1).

32.3 Autoimmunity and Premature Ovarian Failure

Premature ovarian failure (POF) is a syndrome characterized by the cessation of ovarian function before the age of 40 years, in women who present with amenorrhea lasting more than 4 months, and hypoestrogenic hypergonadotropic serum profile (FSH levels >40 mIU/mL with sex steroid deficiency and infertility [10, 12–15]. POF affects 0.3 to 1% of the general population in the United States [16–19]. The majority of POF cases are of unknown etiology but include chromosomal/genetic abnormalities, metabolic/enzymatic factors, metabolic-enzymatic factors, infectious, environmental toxins, autoimmunity, and iatrogenic influences [10, 12].

Autoimmune disorders have been reported to be associated with POF in 4–30% of cases, but the lack of a highly sensitive and specific test precludes an accurate estimate of prevalence, and it is not clear what ovarian antigen may be targeted [10]. The autoimmune involvement has been based on the presence of anti-ovarian antibodies (though there is no current valid serum marker to prove the diagnosis of autoimmune POF), the histological evidence of lymphocytic oophoritis, and the association of other autoimmune disorders which has been reported in up to 10% to 55% of women with POF [20, 21]. These include thyroid (25–60%) [22–24] and adrenal autoimmune diseases (2.5% to 20%) [20, 25, 26] and to a lesser degree including polyglandular syndromes (2%), rheumatoid disease (1%) and SLE, vitiligo, myasthenia gravis, diabetes, and Crohn's disease (<1%) [10, 27]. Cellular infiltration of follicles by macrophages, natural killer cells, T-lymphocytes, plasma cells, and B-lymphocytes represents the characteristic sign of an autoimmune oophoritis [20, 27, 28].

Numerous studies have illustrated that standard treatment outcome for infertility is less effective in the presence of ovarian autoimmunity. However, almost one half of spontaneously affected women have evidence of follicular activity, 25% ovulate after the diagnosis is established, and up 5–10% conceive spontaneously [29, 30]. Cell-mediated and humoral immunity suppression by glucocorticoids or anti-B-cell therapies including the TNF inhibitor Etanercept [31] for reversal of infertility or resumption of ovarian function in selected groups of patients with autoimmune POF has also been recommended in numerous studies [32–38] although, in most instances, treatment with immunosuppressive agents has failed to reverse the course of the ovarian autoimmunity or enhance the ovarian response to gonadotropins [20]. Therapy with dehydroepiandrosterone (DHEA), a precursor of testosterone, androstenedione, and estradiol, promotes activation of the oocytes and inhibits the atretic phenomena. Higher pregnancy rates have been reported following therapy with DHEA supplementation in patients with diminished ovarian function and in women with POF [39, 40], though prospective randomized placebo-controlled studies are required to confirm safety and efficacy.

Other fertility options in POF patients that have been suggested are in vitro maturation of oocyte derived from primordial follicles or stem cells, while IVF (in vitro fertilization) using donor gametes or embryos remains the standard of care in this select group of patients [12].

32.4 Recurrent Implantation Failure (RIF)

The process of implantation in the uterus results from a complex set of events that include highly orchestrated "cross talk" between a euploid blastocyst and a receptive endometrium. These occur through a series of coordinated gene expression, post-translational modifications and hormonal events regulating cell surface molecules, their ligands, and the intracellular signaling resulting from their engagement in both the host uterus and implanting blastocyst [41].

Implantation failure refers to the failure of an embryo(s) to produce detectable amounts of human chorionic gonadotropin (hCG) and/or to reach a stage when an intrauterine gestational sac can be recognized by ultrasonography [42]. Recurrent implantation failure (RIF) refers to the phenomena when the transfer of normal appearing embryos repeatedly fails to lead to the stage of recognizable intrauterine sac. There is no universally accepted definition, and RIF has been defined as either two or three failed fresh IVF transfers or no implantation after the transfer of a total of ten or more cleavage stage embryos or four or more blastocysts [40]. This is in contrast to recurrent IVF failure which has been referred to as the failure to achieve a pregnancy after several IVF attempts attributed to suboptimal embryo quality, advanced maternal age, and uterine factors [43].

The management of infertile couples with failed implantation during IVF is challenging especially in those who are young and good responders and those who generate good quality embryos. Numerous controversial interventions have been tried including assisted hatching, blastocyst transfer, preimplantation genetic screening (PGS), and medical therapies including aspirin, low molecular weight heparin (LMWH), intravenous gamma globulin (IVIG), donor gametes, and gestational surrogacy [44–48].

There is conflicting literature on the value of immunological investigation(s) and treatment in women with RIF. Studies suggest that IVIG may be useful in altering immunological factors including an increased intracellular IgG catabolism, Fc receptor blockade on splenic macrophages and B cells, antibody binding, modulation of cytokine production, and alterations of lymphocyte proliferation [45, 46, 49]. Outcomes in this area are limited. A meta-analysis that included four randomized double-blind trials concluded that given the multiple variables that differ between studies (IVIG scheduling and differing preparations), patient selection, costs, and potential side effects including anaphylaxis, renal insufficiency, and aseptic meningitis syndrome [49], more studies are needed to clarify the role of IVIG-based immune modulation in those with RIF [45].

Similarly, other interventions have been studied such as low-dose aspirin therapy, bed rest, corticosteroids, early scanning in subsequent pregnancies, heparin plus low-dose aspirin therapy, lifestyle adaptation, estrogen therapy, and vitamin supplementation in a meta-analysis including 14 RCTs which failed to demonstrate any of these interventions to be of benefit in women with RIF [50]. A Cochrane review of aspirin and/or enoxaparin therapy also failed to show any benefit in live birth rates. As such, the standard of care currently remains to not treat women with RIF with any anticoagulant therapy. Large high quality RCTs are still needed to elucidate this phenomenon a little further [51].

32.5 Antiphospholipid Antibody Syndrome (APS)

APS is characterized by the production of autoantibodies against phospholipid-protein complexes or plasma proteins (aPL) [52]. Approximately 15 types of antibodies have been described including those directed against cardiolipin, phosphatidylserine (PS), phosphatidylethanolamine (PE), histones, and nucleotides [53], and these have been described as causing issues related to implantation, placentation, and early embryonic vascular compromise [53]. APS is associated with recurrent pregnancy loss (RPL), though the mechanism(s) are incompletely understood. Studies suggest that these antibodies may be involved in the inhibition of cytotrophoblast differentiation and extra-villous cytotrophoblast decidual invasion, as well as inducing syncytiotrophoblast apoptosis [27]. There are also reports of endovascular thrombosis within the microvasculature that supplies the choriodecidual space [52] and abnormal formation of the spiral arterioles [54].

The International Consensus Classification criteria have defined APS if one of the following clinical and laboratory criteria is met which is outlined in Table 32.2. APS is more common in women with a female to male ratio of 5:1 and a reported mean age of diagnosis of 31 years old [55]. There have been retrospective studies done which have suggested a relationship between infertility and APS and similarly between APS and poor ART outcome [55]. Over one dozen existing studies address the relationship between APS and IVF outcome. The majority of these studies showed similar pregnancy and live birth outcomes except for two studies, which showed negative effects of antiphospholipid antibodies on IVF outcomes. A meta-analysis by Bellver et al. failed to show a higher prevalence of APS in infertile women [55]. As such, ASRM does not recommend testing for APS in infertile couples about to undergo IVF as part of the regular work-up [56] as the presence of APS has not been shown to correlate with ART outcomes [55]. However, therapeutic interventions are recommended in the face of recurrent miscarriage and pregnancy complications in the presence of APS [55].

A number of therapeutic approaches have been studied for patients with APS and poor obstetric outcomes including aspirin, unfractionated heparin, low molecular weight heparin (LMWH), corticosteroids, and IVIG. The standard treatment for documented APS and RPL consists of low-dose aspirin (81 mg daily) and twice daily unfractionated heparin. This was found to be superior to treatment with aspirin alone [54, 57]. Heparin is the common name for a poorly defined collection of highly sulfated glycosaminoglycans prepared from porcine intestines. There are documented variations in composition and purity; nonetheless it is the most commonly prescribed drug by weight globally [58]. This medication presumptively works by inhibiting antibodies from binding to the trophoblast and preventing complement activation, thus promoting trophoblastic invasion [59]. Recommendations have included starting heparin 5000–7500 IU twice daily at the time of a positive pregnancy test until delivery and resumed postpartum for 4–6 weeks [59]. Due to its association with thrombocytopenia and osteopenia, platelet counts and partial thromboplastin time should be checked regularly. In addition, additional calcium 1200 mg daily and vitamin D 800–1000 IU daily should be given. Low-dose aspirin should be initiated before conception and discontinued approximately 4 weeks before the expected delivery date. This should be restarted in the postpartum period and continued for life [59].

Table 32.2 Classification criteria for antiphospholipid antibody syndrome [55]

APS diagnostic criteria
– Clinical criteria
– Evidence of vascular thrombosis.
– One or more episodes of arterial or venous thrombosis in any tissue. This must be confirmed by imaging
– History of poor pregnancy outcomes
– One or more unexplained deaths of anatomically normal fetus beyond the tenth week of gestation
– One or more premature births of anatomically normal infant before the 34th week of gestation due to eclampsia, preeclampsia, or clinical signs of placental insufficiency
– Three or more spontaneous abortions before the tenth week of gestation with no other explanation for this outcome
– Laboratory criteria
– Presence of lupus anticoagulants in two different occasions more than 12 weeks apart
– Presence of anti-cardiolipin antibody on two different occasions more than 12 weeks apart
– Presence of anti-beta-2 glycoprotein 1 antibody on two separate occasions more than 12 weeks apart

LMWH enoxaparin 40 mg daily SQ has been compared to unfractionated heparin and reported to have similar efficacy. The use of prednisone has been studied, but results show it does not improve pregnancy rates and may be associated with an increased risk of gestational hypertension and gestational diabetes [54, 60]. In addition, IVIG has been proposed as monotherapy; however, given the costs and lack of level I evidence supporting its efficacy, its use is not recommended [61]. More studies are required to elucidate the benefit of other immunomodulatory agents in patients with RPL/APS.

Given that antiphospholipid antibodies may have a direct embryotoxic effect on preimplantation embryos, it may explain implantation failure after IVF/ET [56, 62]. Women with APS/RPL have demonstrated significant improvement in clinical pregnancy rates when treated with a combination of heparin and aspirin [54], which are believed to positively influence the implantation of the blastocyst including the prevention of thrombosis in the placental vasculature [57]. A meta-analysis of 292 studies by Ziakas et al. concluded that the combination therapy of heparin and aspirin resulted in fewer first trimester losses (OR 0.39, 95% CI 0.24–0.65). As mentioned previously these data hold true in the infertile population with both APS and RPL; however anticoagulation has not been found to be beneficial in women with APS with no RPL.

Current management and guidelines in APS patients undergoing ART may be considered:

- Women with antiphospholipid antibodies and no personal history of thromboembolic events do not require heparin prior to ovum retrieval. Heparin therapy is instead recommended from the time of embryo transfer. Risk of thrombosis is higher during luteal phase [55].

- Women with antiphospholipid antibodies and a personal history of thromboembolic events should be treated with therapeutic doses of heparin for ovarian stimulation. Heparin must be discontinued 12–24 h prior to ovum retrieval and re-started 6–12 h after in order to decrease the risk of bleeding. Low-dose aspirin should also be prescribed but halted 5–7 days prior to oocyte retrieval [55].

In APS patients, ART including ovarian stimulation is a safe process, which has no major health implications as long as appropriate prophylactic anticoagulant therapy is adopted. In terms of risk for thromboembolic events, the risk remains higher in pregnancy than while receiving ART. Data suggest that treatment with aspirin and unfractionated heparin can provide hope to couples suffering from APS/RPL. However, patients with APS without RPL do not appear to benefit from prophylactic anticoagulant therapy.

32.6 Rheumatic Diseases

Rheumatoid arthritis (RA) and systemic lupus erythematosus (SLE) are relatively common, severe disorders. About 1.5 million people or about 0.6 percent of the US adult population have RA. SLE has a reported prevalence of 15–50 cases per 100,000 in Europeans and European Americans and is 3–4 times higher among African Americans, while it is more likely in women between the ages of 13 and 55 years old [63]. RA and SLE represent just two of a larger number of autoimmune disorders, including multiple sclerosis, Crohn's disease, ulcerative colitis, type 1 diabetes, and psoriasis and share defects in immune function and regulation, leading to inflammation that destroys tissues and in the case of SLE can result in a hypercoagulable state and in severe cases can lead to organ failure [64, 65].

Female sex steroid hormones are thought to play an important role in the etiology and pathophysiology of autoimmunity given the preponderance of women affected by chronic immune/inflammatory diseases [66]. Estrogens are known to enhance the humoral immune response through estrogen receptors (ERα) as opposed to ERβ and by their peripheral metabolites [67]. Women are known to have a better response to immunization than men [68]. Anti-ERα antibodies appear to induce cell activation and consequent apoptotic cell death in resting lymphocytes. At the same time, they induce proliferation of anti-CD3-stimulated T-lymphocytes, a mechanism that might contribute to autoreactive T-cell expansion [67]. Several studies support an accelerated aromatase-mediated peripheral metabolic conversion of upstream androgen precursors to estrogen metabolites in peripheral tissues affected by immune/inflammatory reactions [69].

It is unclear in women with rheumatic disease how autoantibodies may be the cause of infertility [70]. However, data do not validate this assumption, though some have asserted that there is a prolonged time to pregnancy compared to women in the general population. In a prospective study of women with RA desiring conception, 42% experienced a greater than 12-month interval until conception [71] and more often appear to require assisted reproduction [72]. While medications (including cyclophosphamide) and serious illness including renal failure may impact pregnancy, primary infertility rates are similar to those in the general population. The Practice Committee of ASRM screening states screening ART candidates for autoantibodies and treating for positive findings is not justified and may cause undue anxiety given the prognostic uncertainty of those findings [72].

In women with SLE who are undergoing infertility therapy, the concern lies in a flare of the disease or thrombosis. The risk of thrombosis remains a significant concern particularly in women with high levels of antiphospholipid antibodies (aPL), nephrotic-range proteinuria, or other conditions that increase thrombotic risk. In those undergoing ovulation induction, thrombosis can result from high supraphysiologic concentrations of estradiol. There is also an associated risk for ovarian hyperstimulation syndrome (OHSS) with results in hemoconcentration which further increases the risk of thrombosis [73]. Data confirms the assertion that thrombosis is usually infrequent [73, 74]. Moreover, the risk has been significantly reduced by using stimulation protocols with gonadotropin-releasing hormone (GnRH) antagonists, oocyte maturation with GnRH agonists, elective cryopreservation, and elective single embryo transfers [75].

The other concern is the risk of disease flare. While studies are retrospective and use different ovarian stimulation protocols in well-controlled disease, the risk for a flare is low particularly when adjuvant therapy is given. However, a flare or exacerbation tends to be greater in active disease [76]. Those with active disease, badly controlled arterial hypertension, pulmonary hypertension, advanced renal disease, severe valvulopathy or heart disease, and major previous thrombotic events are patients in which ART should be discouraged [76]. Fortunately, fertility preservation has made it possible for women who undergo therapy with chemotherapy including cyclophosphamide for lupus nephritis, systemic sclerosis, or vasculitis [77].

Overall, the outcomes of IVF pregnancies in women appear to provide generally optimistic results. Studies in women undergoing IVF have found no association between autoantibody positivity and the number of IVF cycles or fertility success rates, failing to establish an association between rheumatoid diseases and IVF outcome [78–80]. Although this has not been a consistent finding, some retrospective studies have reported a significantly higher miscarriage rate and lower delivery rate in this patient population [79].

In conclusion, ART may be considered for patients with RA including SLE and APS as there does not appear to be an increase in the risk of disease flare or thrombosis as long as disease is well controlled. ART should be avoided in those patients with the complications mentioned above.

Based on existing literature:

- Patients should be in SLE remission for at least 6 months. Those patients with badly controlled hypertension, pulmonary hypertension, advanced renal disease, severe valvulopathy, or heart disease should not undergo ART [64, 72].
- SLE patients can have successful ART outcomes when on proper anticoagulant and immunosuppressive therapy whenever indicated [64, 72].

32.7 Autoimmune Thyroid Disease

Autoimmune thyroid disease (AITD) is by far the most frequent cause of hypothyroidism in women of reproductive age [81]. AITD is characterized by anti-thyroid antibody production including anti-thyroid peroxidase (TPO) or thyroglobulin (TG) resulting from the presence of abnormal or damaged thyroid structure [82]. The prevalence of AITD tends to increase with age with approximately one in five women of childbearing age who have TPO antibodies (Ab) or (TG-Ab) and appears to be more prevalent among infertile women [83, 84].

It has been clearly established that hypothyroidism in pregnancy is associated with miscarriage, placental abruption, neonatal intensive care unit (NICU) admission, and lower intelligence scores [85–87]. Thus, treatment with levothyroxine is recommended in pregnancy in this patient population [88]. It has been reported that a TSH concentration > 2.5 mU/ml may increase the risk of progression to overt hypothyroidism [81]. It has also been advised to treat subclinically hypothyroid in women where thyroid antibodies are detected as well [89].

Controversy remains regarding the significance of AITD and infertility. While no apparent effect has been observed in pregnancy rates [82, 90], some studies have established that even in the absence of overt thyroid dysfunction, AITD is linked with a three- to fivefold increase in the overall miscarriage rate among women with spontaneous pregnancies [91, 92].

With respect to women undergoing ART, where the rapid and robust rise in estradiol concentrations may increase stress on the hypothalamic-pituitary-thyroid axis to maintain a pregnancy, miscarriage rates have also been reported to be increased though this has not been a consistent finding in women with AITD [93–95]. Treatment interventions have included levothyroxine at doses of 1 mg/kg/day, a fixed dose of 50 mcg/day, or titrated doses of levothyroxine [96–98] combined with acetylsalicylic acid, prednisolone, and/or treatment with selenomethionine at 200 mg/day [99, 100]. Studies have reported significantly higher pregnancy rates in those treated with levothyroxine combined with acetylsalicylic acid and prednisolone compared with controls receiving no treatment (RR: 4.14, CI: 1.47–11.66, $P = 0.007$) [98]. In a pooled analysis on miscarriage rates, there was a 52% near significant relative risk reduction in miscarriages (RR: 0.58, CI: 0.32–0.1.06) [98].

In summary, while treatment with levothyroxine is recommended for all women considering pregnancy with clinical hypothyroidism as it lowers the risk for miscarriage and preterm delivery, there is insufficient evidence to recommend treatment for subclinical hypothyroidism. While AITD may identify patients at risk of clinical hypothyroidism and levothyroxine appears to lower the risk for miscarriage and preterm birth in women with thyroid autoimmunity, randomized, placebo controlled trials are warranted.

32.8 Multiple Sclerosis

Multiple sclerosis (MS) is an autoimmune degenerative inflammatory disease that is a result of activation of autoreactive CD4+ T cells, which target proteins of the myelin sheath [101]. Symptoms usually appear between 20 and 40 years of age and are characterized by a female to male ratio of 3:1 [102].

Very little literature exists regarding infertility and ART outcomes, though sexual and endocrine disturbances have been described in MS patients of both genders, leading to lower fertility rates. Disturbances in the hypothalamic-pituitary-gonadal axis affect both female and male MS patients. In women, this may induce menstrual disturbances and subsequent infertility secondary to elevated prolactin, LH, FSH, and total and free testosterone [103, 104]. In men with MS, serum levels for LH, FSH, and testosterone are significantly lower compared to controls and can result in compromised semen parameters including a lower total sperm count, motility, and percent normal morphology [105]. In addition, medical therapy for MS, particularly immunosuppressive therapies (e.g., mitoxantrone, cyclophosphamide), has been shown to adversely impact sperm and oocyte quality [106].

Reports also suggest that fertility does not seem to be impaired in women with MS; however women who undergo ART appear to have an increased risk of MS relapse. In one prospective study of MS patients (n = 16) who had not suffered any relapses or disease activity on MRI in the previous 9 months prior to undergoing ART, 75% of patients experienced exacerbations of their MS symptoms (12 of 16 patients) within 3 months after failed IVF cycles [107]. MRI imaging revealed new or enlarging T2 lesions on MRI [107]. There were no differences in relapse when stratifying for number of ART cycles or pregnancy success [107]. The proposed mechanisms include an interruption of disease modifying medications, stress of undergoing fertility therapy, and a hormonally induced upregulation in pro-inflammatory markers [108]. Further study is required before conclusive recommendations can be given [102].

32.9 Myasthenia Gravis

Myasthenia gravis (MG) is a chronic autoimmune disorder of neuromuscular transmission from production of autoantibodies against the nicotinic acetylcholine receptor, which alters nerve impulses to muscle fibers that lead to fatigue and progressive muscular weakness [109, 110]. While MG commonly affects women in their childbearing years with a reported prevalence of 1 in 5000 [111, 112], it is typically not associated with infertility, though acetylcholine receptor antibodies have been found in 2% of women with POF [111].

Variations in symptoms during menstruation and pregnancy have been reported in women with MG suggesting a functional link between sex steroids and the expression of disease [111, 113]. It has been reported there is an increased expression of estrogen receptors in thymocytes and peripheral blood mononuclear cells in MG patients and with abnormal level of estrogens in MG patients with the development of B-cell hyperplasia and enhanced cytokine production that may exacerbate this autoimmune state [114]. The clinical course of myasthenia gravis may be impacted by the rapid rise in estrogen and progesterone associated with ovulation induction. Other events such as pregnancy, ovarian hyperstimulation syndrome, and hormone fluctuations in the event of failed cycles also have the potential to impact the clinical course of this disease. Nonetheless, very little has been described in the literature surrounding ART and MG making it very challenging to counsel for MG women who request assisted reproduction [111].

Previous studies would suggest that there is no increase in miscarriage rates [113, 115]. While the course of MG during pregnancy has been reported to be highly variable; with exacerbations in 41% of pregnancies (equally distributed in each trimester), remission in 29%, and no change in disease course in 32% [113], while 30% had postpartum exacerbations. In experimentally induced autoimmune MG, conflicting reports exist, where the susceptibility to and the severity of disease by excess estrogen and progesterone administration [116, 117].

One case report by Ricci et al. in a 40-year-old female patient with severe MG who underwent four ART cycles suggested that MG patients should not be excluded IVF. They eloquently reviewed that all MG patients should be properly informed effects both of ovulation induction and assisted reproduction and of pregnancy on the course disease cannot be well estimated. Given that maternal mortality risk is inversely proportionate to the duration of the disease with the highest risk being in the first year, MG patients should delay childbirth for 1–2 years after diagnosis [118]. Particular concerns should be with women who demonstrate hormonal-related exacerbations (during menstruation or pregnancy) of myasthenic symptoms as they may be at higher risk of developing symptom fluctuation with ART. Pre-screening and evaluation with a neurologist, anesthesiologist, and high-risk OB counseling should be performed. Referral to a tertiary infertility medical center where medical emergency services are available should be considered, and MG patients should be monitored closely throughout the assisted reproduction procedure. Selection of appropriate anesthetic technique (general anesthesia) for oocyte retrieval should be considered, and an intensive surveillance in the early postoperative recovery phase should assured. Proper follow-up should be continued both in the case of pregnancy and in the case of unsuccessful procedures. As such, more data regarding MG patients undergoing ovarian stimulation and ART are required to assess the safety of this treatment.

32.10 Autoimmune Progesterone Dermatitis

Autoimmune progesterone dermatitis (APD) is a rare hypersensitivity reaction that has been reported to occur following exposure to endogenous and/or exogenous progesterone during the luteal phase, either prior to or during menses. Symptoms have been reported to vary, ranging from skin lesions including urticaria, eczema, folliculitis, or erythema multiforme to angioedema, folliculitis, vulvovaginal pruritus, and in some severe cases anaphylaxis [119].

The pathogenesis of APD is unknown but is believed to have a Th2 immune mechanism with acute and delayed responses consistent with both type 1 and type 4 hypersensitivity reactions [119]. Treatment consists of topical or systemic corticosteroids as well as medical suppression of endogenous progesterone production. In severe cases in which symptoms are refractory, definitive treatment includes hysterectomy/oophorectomy.

In the infertile patient, APD appears to be triggered with the utilization of exogenous progesterone after oocyte retrieval and embryo transfer [119]. Progesterone desensitization has been reported as an alternative in women with APD with prednisone, 3 days prior to progesterone desensitization and tapered after egg transfer. The desensitization process consists of intravaginal suppositories, with a starting dose of 1 μg and gradually increased to 100 μg. In cases of anaphylactic reaction to progesterone, montelukast, a leukotriene receptor antagonist, has been used as premedication prior to progesterone suppositories. In a small case series, four successfully conceived without any APD exacerbation. Although APD is extremely rare, one should consider the prevalence would continue rise with the increasing utilization of infertility therapy and ART.

32.11 Celiac Disease

Celiac disease (CD) is a chronic autoimmune disease characterized by small intestinal malabsorption and diarrhea, triggered by the ingestion of food products containing gluten [120]. The prevalence of celiac disease has risen in recent decades with reported prevalence of 0.5–1% worldwide which has increased fourfold to fivefold over the past 50 years [121]. Gluten is a protein complex found in wheat, rye, and barley. One of its components, the prolamin gliadin, can be antigenic for certain individuals especially after being deamidated by intestinal transglutaminases. CD predominantly affects the mucosa of the small intestine where the injured small intestinal epithelium impairs digestion and absorption of the nutrients. CD may be classified as asymptomatic, classical, and atypical. Classic cases present with symptoms of malabsorption include diarrhea, steatorrhea, flatulence, and resulting nutritional and vitamin deficiencies. Atypical cases present with extraintestinal manifestations that may include dermatitis herpetiformis, aphthous stomatitis, neurologic dysfunction, osteopathy, and diabetes mellitus. Patients with celiac disease are also at an increased risk of cancer, including a twofold to fourfold increased risk of non-Hodgkin's lymphoma and a more than 30-fold increased risk of small intestinal adenocarcinoma [122].

Celiac disease more often affects women during their reproductive years and has been associated with a wide array of gynecologic disorders including delayed menarche and puberty, polycystic ovarian syndrome, endometriosis amenorrhea, POF, and infertility [123]. Clinical and epidemiological studies reveal that female patients with coeliac disease are at higher risk of spontaneous abortion, low birth weights, and reduced duration of lactation [124]. One study reported that up to 7% tested positive for tissue transglutaminase IgA antibodies in those with RPL and 6% with unexplained infertility and another reported 8% of couples were positive for anti-gliadin antibodies with unexplained infertility [125]. As such, some have suggested that testing women for celiac disease should be considered in those with RPL and/or unexplained infertility.

With respect to therapy, to our knowledge, only case reports have considered treatments including Humira where TNF-alpha is elevated, intravenous intralipids prior to embryo transfer, and low molecular weight heparin, in addition to a gluten-free diet [126, 127].

32.12 Xenosialitis

All cell surfaces are coated by a complex array of glycans. In mammals, the majority of these surface glycans are capped with sialic acids, nine carbon backbone acidic amino sugars. By virtue of their position and high abundance at the outermost cell surface, sialic acids are involved in multiple functions including cellular recognition during development, infection, and immune processes [128]. The role of sialic acids in reproduction is not fully understood, but acquisition of a sialylated glycocalyx is crucial to sperm function [129]. Most recently, it has been shown that sperm sialidases are involved in desialylation during capacitation [130] and that sialic acids of sialyl Lewis X glycans on human egg zona pellucida are essential for sperm binding [131]. Implantation also involves L-selectins on the blastocyst known to interact with sialic acid containing ligands on the endometrium [132, 133]. Highly sialylated glycodelin A is produced by the decidua and engages sialic acid-binding innate immune receptors on trophoblast to suppress trophoblast invasion [134]. The two most common sialic acids in mammals are N-glycolylneuraminic acid (Neu5Gc) and N-acetylneuraminic acid (Neu5Ac) [135]. Most mammals have an abundance of each molecule in different ratios on various cell surfaces. In contrast, humans have lost the ability to convert Neu5Ac to Neu5Gc due to a loss-of-function mutation in the cytidine monophosphate N-acetylneuraminic acid hydroxylase (CMAH) gene encoding the CMAH enzyme [136]. As a result, humans lack glycans capped by endogenous Neu5Gc on their cell surfaces and have an excess of Neu5Ac [137], a difference in hundreds of millions of molecules per cell. Despite the inability to endogenously produce Neu5Gc, dietary intake of red meat and dairy products, the richest sources of Neu5Gc, can result in accumulation and incorporation trace amounts of Neu5Gc into the glycocalyx on human cells [138]. This has been reported in both human tumors such as breast, colon, and skin cancers [139] and normal tissues including secretory epithelium and blood vessels [140]. Moreover, most humans have circulating anti-Neu5Gc antibodies [138, 140] targeting this xenoglycan in serum [138, 141]. Levels of anti-Neu5Gc antibodies vary among different individuals, but it has been suggested that chronic exposure to Neu5Gc and incorporation of this xenoglycan combined with circulating anti-Neu5Gc antibodies can promote chronic inflammatory states contributing to various diseases [128] including some of the diseases associated Hanganutziu-Deicher (HD) antibodies, which are reactive against Neu5Gc [142, 143]. There is also experimental evidence for Neu5Gc acting as a xeno-auto antigen capable of exacerbating an inflammatory reaction within vasculature endothelium [144]. A recent study proved that the dietary xenoglycan Neu5Gc causes increased cancer via systemic inflammation in a mouse model [145]. There is mounting evidence that the dietary bioaccumulation of xenoglycan and production of targeting antibodies might underlie various forms of xenosialitis [146]. A small-scale study carried out on a cohort of infertility patients suggests that the presence of Neu5Gc antigen or anti-Neu5Gc antibodies is present in reproductive tracts of both male and female infertility subjects and may interfere with fertility within the uterine environment [147]. Studies in transgenic mice bearing the same mutation as humans in the sialic acid modifying gene Cmah have shown that dietary incorporation of Neu5Gc can tag sperm for increased attack by uterine leukocytes [135]. Sialic acid-binding innate receptors, so called Siglecs, are expressed in the placenta and the amnion, and this expression is unique to humans. Higher levels of inflammation-related Siglec-6 expression have been associated with preeclampsia [148–150]. Ascending infections of the female reproductive tract such as group B *Streptococcus* and *Neisseria gonorrhoeae* also involve interactions with immune modulatory Siglec receptors expressed in the amnion and sialic acid-binding components of complement such as factor H [151, 152]. It has recently been proposed that the uniquely human sialic acid biology and associated numerous changes in sialic acid sensing Siglec receptors could be contributing to elevated levels of autoimmunity in our species [153]. Further studies are required in order to better understand the role of the Neu5Gc dietary xenoglycan and targeting antibodies in sub or infertile couples.

32.13 Conclusion

Autoimmunity encompasses a large category of diseases with various etiologies that frequently affect women of childbearing age. The pathophysiology and treatment of autoimmune disease(s) is a crucial consideration for the reproductive endocrinology infertility specialist as these can affect women's fertility and fertility treatment outcomes. There is a continued need for further research in this under-appreciated field.

References

1. https://www.aarda.org/autoimmune-information/autoimmune-statistics/
2. Ermann J, Fathman CG. Autoimmune diseases: genes, bugs and failed regulation. Nat Immunol. 2001 Sep;2(9):759–61.
3. Avrameas S. Natural autoantibodies: from "horror autotoxicus" to "gnothi seauton". Immunol Today. 1991 May;12(5):154–9.
4. Hedrick SM. The acquired immune system: a vantage from beneath. Immunity. 2004 Nov;21(5):607–15.
5. McDade TW. Life history theory and the immune system: steps toward a human ecological immunology. Am J Phys Anthropol. 2003;Suppl 37:100–25.
6. Moffett A, Loke YW. The immunological paradox of pregnancy: a reappraisal. Placenta. 2004 Jan;25(1):1–8.
7. Maiers M, Gragert L, Klitz W. High-resolution HLA alleles and haplotypes in the United States population. Hum Immunol. 2007 Sep;68(9):779–88.
8. Hemmer B, Kerschensteiner M, Korn T. Role of the innate and adaptive immune responses in the course of multiple sclerosis. Lancet Neurol. 2015 Apr;14(4):406–19.
9. Cooper GS, Stroehla BC. The epidemiology of autoimmune diseases. Autoimmun Rev. 2003 May;2(3):119–25.
10. Ebrahimi M, Akbari AF. The role of autoimmunity in premature ovarian failure. Iran J Reprod Med. 2015 Aug;13(8):461–72.
11. Carp HJA, Selmi C, Shoenfeld Y. The autoimmune bases of infertility and pregnancy loss. J Autoimmun. 2012 May;38(2–3):J266–74.
12. Goswami D, Conway GS. Premature ovarian failure. Hum Reprod Update. 2005;11:391–410.
13. Laml T, Preyer O, Umek W, Hengstschlager M, Hanzal H. Genetic disorders in premature ovarian failure. Hum Reprod Update. 2002;8:483–91.
14. Schlessinger D, Herrera I, Crisponi I, Mumm S, Percesepe A, Pellegrini M, et al. Genetic and translocations involved in POF. Am J Med Genet. 2002;111:328–33.
15. Matikainen T, Perez GI, Jurisicova A, Pru JK, Schlezinger JJ, Ryu HY, et al. Aromatic hydrocarbon receptor-driven Bax gene expression is required for premature ovarian failure caused by biohazardous environment chemical. Nat Genet. 2001;28:355–60.
16. The Practice Committee of the American Society for Reproductive Medicine. Current evaluation of amenorrhea. Fertil Steril. 2006;86:148–55.
17. Luborsky JL, Meyer P, Sowers MF, Gold EB, Santoro N. Premature menopause in a multi ethnic population study of the menopause transition. Hum Reprod. 2003;18:199–206.
18. Beck-Peccoz P, Persani L. Premature ovarian failure. Orphanet J Rare Dis. 2006;6:1–9.
19. Nolting M, Perez L, Belen M, Martinez Amuchastegui J, Straminsky V, Onetto Claudia C, et al. Importance of detecting transition to the premature ovarian failure. Gynecol Endocrinol. 2008;24:257–8.
20. Lebovic DI, Naz R. Premature ovarian failure: think "autoimmune disorder". Sex Reprod Menopause. 2004;2:230–3.
21. Forges T, Monnier-Barbarino P, Faure GC, Bene MC. Autoimmunity and antigenic targets in ovarian pathology. Hum Reprod Update. 2004;10:163–75.
22. Rees M, Purdie D. Premature menopause. In: Rees M, Purdie D, editors. Management of the menopause: the handbook. London: Royal Society of Medicine Press; 2006. p. 142–9.
23. Poppe K, Glinoer D, Van Steirteghem A, Tournaye H, Devroey P, Schiettecatte J, et al. Thyroid dysfunction and autoimmunity in infertile women. Thyroid. 2002;12:997–1001.
24. Abalovich M, Mitelberg L, Allami C, Gutierrez S, Alcaraz G, Otero P. Subclinical hypothyroidism and thyroid autoimmunity in women with infertility. Gynecol Endocrinol. 2007;23:279–83.
25. Reato G, Morlin L, Chen S, Furmaniak J, Rees SB, Masiero S, et al. Premature ovarian failure in patients with autoimmune Addison, s disease: clinical, genetic, and immunological evaluation. J Clin Endocrinol Metab. 2011;96:1255–61.
26. Bakalov VK, Vanderhoof VH, Bondy CA, Nelson LM. Adrenal antibodies detect asymptomatic auto-immune adrenal insufficiency in young women with spontaneous premature ovarian failure. Hum Reprod. 2002;17:2096–100.

27. Ayesha, Jha V, Goswami D. Premature ovarian failure: an association with autoimmune diseases. J Clin Diagn Res. 2016 Oct;10(10):QC10–2.
28. Bats AS, Barbarino P, Bene MC, Faure GC, Forges T. Local lymphocytic and epithelial activation in a case of autoimmune oophoritis. Fertil Steril. 2008;90:849.
29. Rebar RW, Connolly HV. Clinical features of young women with hypergonadotropic amenorrhea. Fertil Steril. 1990;53:804–10.
30. Nelson LM, Anasti JN, Kimzey LM, Defensor RA, Lipetz KJ, White BJ, et al. Development of luteinized graafian follicles in patients with karyotypically normal spontaneous premature ovarian failure. J Clin Endocrinol Metab. 1994;79:1470–5.
31. Jankowska K. Premature ovarian failure. Prz Menopauzalny. 2017 Jun;16(2):51–6.
32. Corenblum B, Rowe T, Taylor PJ. High dose, short-term glucocorticoids for the treatment of infertility resulting from premature ovarian failure. Fertil Steril. 1993;59:988–91.
33. Wang L, Huang P, Huang X. Analysis of the treatment of 1,020 patients with immunologic infertility. Zhonghua Fu Chan Ke Za Zhi 1999;34: 234–6 (in Chinese).
34. Barbarino-Monnier P, Gobert B, Guillet-May F, Bene MC, Barbarino A, Foliguet B, et al. Ovarian autoimmunity and corticotherapy in an in-vitro-fertilization attempt. Hum Reprod. 1995;10:2006–7.
35. Levesque MC. Translational mini-review series B cell-directed therapies: recent advances in B cell-directed biological therapies for autoimmune disorders. Clin Exp Immunol. 2009;157:198–208.
36. Mamas L, Mamas E. Premature ovarian failure and dehydroepiandrosterone. Fertil Steril. 2009;91:644–6.
37. Barad D, Gleicher N. Increased oocyte production after treatment with dehydroepiandrosterone. Fertil Steril. 2005;84:756.
38. Kalantaridou SN, Braddock DT, Patronas NJ, Nelson LM. Treatment of autoimmune premature ovarian failure. Hum Reprod. 1999;14:1777–82.
39. Barad D, Gleicher N. Effect of dehydroepiandrosterone on oocyte and embryo yields, embryo grade and cell number in IVF. Hum Reprod. 2006;21:2845–9.
40. Barad D, Brill H, Gleicher N. Update on the use of dehydroepiandrosterone supplementation among women with diminished ovarian function. J Assist Reprod Genet. 2007;24:629–34.
41. Dominguez F, Pellicer A, Simón C. Paracrine dialogue in implantation. Mol Cell Endocrinol. 2002;186(2):175–81.
42. Coughlan C, Ledger W, Wang Q, Fenghua L, Demirol A, Gurgan T, et al. Recurrent implantation failure: definition and management. Reprod Biomed Online. 2014;28:14–38.
43. Ferraretti AP, LaMarca A, Fauser BC, Tarlatzis B, Nargund G, Gianaroli L. ESHRE consensus on the definition of 'poor response' to ovarian stimulation for in vitro fertilization: the Bologna criteria. Hum Reprod. 2011;26:1616–24.
44. Blake D, Farquhar C, Johnson N, Proctor M. Cleavage stage versus blastocyst stage embryo transfer in assisted conception. Cochrane Database Syst Rev. 2007;4:CD002118. https://doi.org/10.1002/14651858.CD02118.pub3.
45. Zeyneloglu HB, Onalan G. Remedies for recurrent implantation failure. Semin Reprod Med. 2014;32(4):297–305. https://doi.org/10.1055/s-0034-1375182.
46. American Society Reproductive Medicine. The role of assisted hatching in in vitro fertilization: a review of the literature. Fertil Steril. 2008;90:196–8. https://doi.org/10.1016/j.fertnstert.2008.08.043.
47. Papanikolaou EG, Kolibianakis EM, Tournaye H, Venetis CA, Fatemi H, Tarlatzis B, et al. Live birth rates after transfer of equal number of blastocysts or cleavage-stage embryos in IVF. A systematic review and meta-analysis. Hum Reprod. 2008;23:91–9. https://doi.org/10.1093/humrep/dem339.
48. Petersen CG, Mauri AL, Baruffi RL, Oliveira JB, Massaro FC, Elder K, et al. Implantation failures: success of assisted hatching with quarter-laser zona thinning. Reprod Biomed Online. 2005;10:224–9. https://doi.org/10.1016/S1472-6483(10)60944-3.
49. Li J, Chen Y, Liu C, Hu Y, Li L. Intravenous immunoglobulin treatment for repeated IVF/ICSI failure and unexplained infertility: a systematic review and a meta-analysis. Am J Reprod Immunol. 2013 Dec;70(6):434–47.
50. Duckitt K, Qureshi A. Recurrent miscarriage. BMJ Clin Evid. 2011 Feb;1:2011.
51. Kaandorp S, Di Nisio M, Goddijn M, Middeldorp S. Aspirin or anticoagulants for treating recurrent miscarriage in women without antiphospholipid syndrome. Cochrane Database Syst Rev. 2009 Jan 21;1:CD004734.
52. Ulcova-Gallova Z. Repeated miscarriages in patients with antiphospholipid syndrome and subjected to in vitro fertilization: the importance of preimplantation genetic diagnosis. Lupus. 2012 Jun;21(7):744–6.
53. Lee S-R, Park E-J, Kim S-H, Chae H, Kim C-H, Kang B-M. Influence of antiphospholipid antibodies on pregnancy outcome in women undergoing in vitro fertilization and embryo transfer. Am J Reprod Immunol. 2007 Jan;57(1):34–9.
54. Sher G, Matzner W, Feinman M, Maassarani G, Zouves C, Chong P, et al. The selective use of heparin/aspirin therapy, alone or in combination with intravenous immunoglobulin G, in the management of antiphospholipid antibody-positive women undergoing in vitro fertilization. Am J Reprod Immunol. 1998 Aug;40(2):74–82.
55. Cervera R. Antiphospholipid syndrome. Thromb Res. 2017 Mar;151(Suppl 1):S43–7.
56. Chighizola CB, de Jesus GR. Antiphospholipid antibodies and infertility. Lupus. 2014 Oct;23(12):1232–8.
57. Ziakas PD, Pavlou M, Voulgarelis M. Heparin treatment in antiphospholipid syndrome with recurrent pregnancy loss: a systematic review and meta-analysis. Obstet Gynecol. 2010 Jun;115(6):1256–62.
58. Rosania L. Heparin crisis 2008: a tipping point for increased FDA enforcement in the pharma sector? Food Drug Law J 2010;65(3):489–501, ii.
59. El Hachem H, Crepaux V, May-Panloup P, Descamps P, Legendre G, Bouet P-E. Recurrent pregnancy loss: current perspectives. Int J Women's Health. 2017;9:331–45.
60. Laskin CA, Bombardier C, Hannah ME, Mandel FP, Ritchie JW, Farewell V, et al. Prednisone and aspirin in women with autoantibodies and unexplained recurrent fetal loss. N Engl J Med. 1997 Jul 17;337(3):148–53.
61. Sauer R, Roussev R, Jeyendran RS, Coulam CB. Prevalence of antiphospholipid antibodies among women experiencing unexplained infertility and recurrent implantation failure. Fertil Steril. 2010 May 1;93(7):2441–3.
62. Costa M, Colia D. Treating infertility in autoimmune patients. Rheumatology (Oxford). 2008 Jun;47(Suppl 3):iii38–41.
63. de Macedo JF, de Macedo GC, Campos LA, Baltatu OC. Successful pregnancy following assisted reproduction in woman with systemic lupus erythematosus and hypertension: a case report. Medicine (Baltimore). 2015 Sep;94(37):e1531.
64. Hickman RA, Gordon C. Causes and management of infertility in systemic lupus erythematosus. Rheumatology (Oxford). 2011 Sep;50(9):1551–8.
65. Straub RH, Bijlsma JW, Masi A, Cutolo M. Role of neuroendocrine and neuroimmune mechanisms in chronic inflammatory rheumatic diseases—the 10-year update. Semin Arthritis Rheum. 2013;43(3):392–404.
66. Cutolo M, Brizzolara R, Atzeni F, Capellino S, Straub RH, Puttini PC. The immunomodulatory effects of estrogens: clinical rel-

evance in immune-mediated rheumatic diseases. Ann NY Acad Sci. 2010;1193:36–42.
67. Colasanti T, Maselli A, Conti F, Sanchez M, Alessandri C, Barbati C, et al. Autoantibodies to estrogen receptor α interfere with T lymphocyte homeostasis and are associated with disease activity in systemic lupus erythematosus (SLE). Arthritis Rheum. 2012;64(3):778–87.
68. Klein SL, Flanagan KL. Sex differences in immune responses. Nat Rev Immunol. 2016 Aug 22;16(10):626–38.
69. Capellino S, Straub RH, Cutolo M. Aromatase and regulation of the estrogen-to androgen ratio in synovial tissue inflammation: common pathway in both sexes. Ann NY Acad Sci. 2014;1317:24–31.
70. Brouwer J, Hazes JM, Laven JS, Dolhain R. Fertility in women with rheumatoid arthritis: influence of disease activity and medication. Ann Rheum Dis. 2014;74(10):1836–41.
71. Jawaheer D, Zhu JL, Nohr EA, Olsen J. Time to pregnancy among women with rheumatoid arthritis. Arthritis Rheum. 2011;63:1517–21.
72. Practice Committee of American Society for Reproductive M. Anti-phospholipid antibodies do not affect IVF success. Fertil Steril. 2008;90:S172–3.
73. Bellver J, Pellicer A. Ovarian stimulation for ovulation induction and in vitro fertilization in patients with systemic lupus erythematosus and antiphospholipid syndrome. Fertil Steril. 2009 Dec;92(6):1803–10.
74. Ragab A, Barakat R, Ragheb M, State O, Badawy A. Subfertility treatment in women with systemic lupus erythematosus. J Obstet Gynaecol. 2012;32:569–71.
75. Humaidan P, Polyzos NP, Alsbjerg B, Erb K, Mikkelsen AL, Elbaek HO, et al. GnRHa trigger and individualized luteal phase hCG support according to ovarian response to stimulation: two prospective randomized controlled multi-centre studies in IVF patients. Hum Reprod. 2013;28:2511–21.
76. Guballa N, Sammaritano L, Schwartzman S, Buyon J, Lockshin MD. Ovulation induction and in vitro fertilization in systemic lupus erythematosus and antiphospholipid syndrome. Arthritis Rheum. 2000;43:550–6.
77. von Wolff M, Donnez J, Hovatta O, Keros V, Mataris T, Montag M, et al. Cryopreservation and autotransplantation of human ovarian tissue prior to cytotoxic therapy— a technique in its infancy but already successful in fertility preservation. Eur J Cancer. 2009;45:1547–53.
78. Chilcott IT, Margara R, Cohen H, et al. Pregnancy outcome is not affected by antiphospholipid antibody status in women referred for in vitro fertilization. Fertil Steril. 2000;73:526–30.
79. Sanmarco M, Bardin N, Camoin L, et al. Antigenic profile, prevalence, and clinical significance of antiphospholipid antibodies in women referred for in vitro fertilization. Ann N Y Acad Sci. 2007;1108:457–65.
80. Lee SR, Park EJ, Kim SH, Chae H, Kim CH, Kang BM. Influence of antiphospholipid antibodies on pregnancy outcome in women undergoing in vitro fertilization and embryo transfer. Am J Reprod Immunol. 2007;57:34–9.
81. Vanderpump MP, Tunbridge WM, French JM, Appleton D, Bates D, Clark F, et al. The incidence of thyroid disorders in the community: a twenty year follow-up of the Whickham Survey. Clin Endocrinol. 1995;43:55–68.
82. Poppe K, Glinoer D, Tournaye H, Devroey P, van Steirteghem A, Kaufman L, et al. Assisted reproduction and thyroid autoimmunity: an unfortunate combination? J Clin Endocrinol Metab. 2003 Sep;88(9):4149–52.
83. Zhong Y, Ying Y, Wu H, Zhou C, Xu Y, Wang Q, et al. Relationship between antithyroid antibody and pregnancy outcome following in vitro fertilization and embryo transfer. Int J Med Sci. 2012;9(2):121–5.
84. Reh A, Chaudhry S, Mendelsohn F, Im S, Rolnitzky L, Amarosa A, et al. Effect of autoimmune thyroid disease in older euthyroid infertile woman during the first 35 days of an IVF cycle. Fertil Steril. 2011 Mar 1;95(3):1178–81.
85. Haddow JE, Palomaki GE, Allan WC, Williams JR, Knight GJ, Gagnon J, et al. Maternal thyroid deficiency during pregnancy and subsequent neuropsychological development of the child. N Engl J Med. 1999;341:549–55.
86. Li Y, Shan Z, Teng W, Yu X, Li Y, Fan C, et al. Abnormalities of maternal thyroid function during pregnancy affect neuropsychological development of their children at 25–30 months. Clin Endocrinol. 2010;72:825–9.
87. van den Boogaard E, Vissenberg R, Land JA, van Wely M, van der Post JA, Goddijn M, et al. Significance of (sub)clinical thyroid dysfunction and thyroid autoimmunity before conception and in early pregnancy: a systematic review. Hum Reprod Update. 2011;17:605–19.
88. Abalovich M, Amino N, Barbour LA, Cobin RH, De Groot LJ, Glinoer D, et al. Management of thyroid dysfunction during pregnancy and postpartum: an Endocrine Society Clinical Practice Guideline. J Clin Endocrinol Metab. 2007;92:S1–47.
89. Stagnaro-Green A, Abalovich M, Alexander E, Azizi F, Mestman J, Negro R, et al. Guidelines of the American thyroid association for the diagnosis and management of thyroid disease during pregnancy and postpartum. Thyroid. 2011;21:1081–125.
90. Grassi G, Balsamo A, Ansaldi C, Balbo A, Massobrio M, Benedetto C. Thyroid autoimmunity and infertility. Gynecol Endocrinol. 2001;15:389–96.
91. Prummel MF, Wiersinga WM. Thyroid autoimmunity and miscarriage. Eur J Endocrinol. 2004;150:751–5.
92. Stagnaro-Green A, Glinoer D. Thyroid autoimmunity and the risk of miscarriage. Best Pract Res. 2004;18:167–81.
93. Muller AF, Verhoeff A, Mantel MJ, De Jong FH, Berghout A. Decrease of free thyroxine levels after controlled ovarian hyperstimulation. J Clin Endocrinol Metab. 2000;85:545–8.
94. Poppe K, Glinoer D, Tournaye H, Schiettecatte J, Devroey P, van Steirteghem A, et al. Impact of ovarian hyperstimulation on thyroid function in women with and without thyroid autoimmunity. J Clin Endocrinol Metab. 2004;89:3808–12.
95. Poppe K, Glinoer D, Tournaye H, Schiettecatte J, Haentjens P, Velkeniers B. Thyroid function after assisted reproductive technology in women free of thyroid disease. Fertil Steril. 2005;83:1753–7.
96. Negro R, Mangieri T, Coppola L, Presicce G, Casavola EC, Gismondi R, et al. Levothyroxine treatment in thyroid peroxidase antibody-positive women undergoing assisted reproduction technologies: a prospective study. Hum Reprod. 2005;20:1529–33.
97. Negro R, Formoso G, Mangieri T, Pezzarossa A, Dazzi D, Hassan H. Levothyroxine treatment in euthyroid pregnant women with autoimmune thyroid disease: effects on obstetrical complications. J Clin Endocrinol Metab. 2006;91:2587–91.
98. Revelli A, Casano S, Piane LD, Grassi G, Gennarelli G, Guidetti D, et al. A retrospective study on IVF outcome in euthyroid patients with anti-thyroid antibodies: effects of levothyroxine, acetyl-salicylic acid and prednisolone adjuvant treatments. Reprod Biol Endocrinol. 2009;7:137.
99. Negro R, Greco G, Mangieri T, Pezzarossa A, Dazzi D, Hassan H. The influence of selenium supplementation on postpartum thyroid status in pregnant women with thyroid peroxidase autoantibodies. J Clin Endocrinol Metab. 2007;92:1263–8.
100. Nohr SB, Jorgensen A, Pedersen KM, Laurberg P. Postpartum thyroid dysfunction in pregnant thyroid peroxidase antibody-positive women living in an area with mild to moderate iodine deficiency: is iodine supplementation safe? J Clin Endocrinol Metab. 2000;85:3191–8.

101. Gold SM, Voskuhl RR. Estrogen and testosterone therapies in multiple sclerosis. Prog Brain Res. 2009;175:239–51.
102. Michel L, Foucher Y, Vukusic S, Confavreux C, de Sèze J, Brassat D, et al. Increased risk of multiple sclerosis relapse after in vitro fertilisation. J Neurol Neurosurg Psychiatry. 2012 Aug;83(8):796–802.
103. Haensch CA, Jörg J. Autonomic dysfunction in multiple sclerosis. J Neurol. 2006;253(Suppl 1):I3–9.
104. Grinsted L, Heltberg A, Hagen C, et al. Serum sex hormone and gonadotropin concentrations in premenopausal women with multiple sclerosis. J Intern Med. 1989;226:241–4.
105. Safarinejad MR. Evaluation of endocrine pro le, hypothalamic-pituitary-testis axis and semen quality in multiple sclerosis. J Neuroendocrinol. 2008;20:1368–75.
106. Prévinaire JG, Lecourt G, Soler JM, et al. Sexual disorders in men with multiple sclerosis: evaluation and management. Ann Phys Rehabil Med. 2014;57:329.
107. Correale J, Farez MF, Ysrraelit MC. Increase in multiple sclerosis activity after assisted reproduction technology. Ann Neurol. 2012 Nov;72(5):682–94.
108. Hellwig K, Correale J. Artificial reproductive techniques in multiple sclerosis. Clin Immunol. 2013;149:219–24.
109. Conti-Fine B, Milani M, Kaminski HJ. Myasthenia gravis: past, present, and future. J Clin Invest. 2006;116:2843–54.
110. Vincent A. Unravelling the pathogenesis of myasthenia gravis. Nat Rev Immunol. 2002;2:797–804.
111. Ricci G, De Santis M, Pagnini G, Tamaro LF, Giolo E, Guaschino S. Assisted reproduction treatment in severe myasthenia gravis. Fertil Steril. 2008 Sep;90(3):850.e5–8. https://doi.org/10.1016/j.fertnstert.2007.07.1387.
112. Hoek A, Schoemaker J, Drexhage HA. Premature ovarian failure and ovarian autoimmunity. Endocr Rev. 1997;18:107–34.
113. Plauche WC. Myasthenia gravis in pregnancy: an update. Am J Obstet Gynecol. 1979;135:691–7.
114. Nancy P, Berrih-Aknin S. Diffential estrogen receptor expression in autoimmune myasthenia gravis. Endocrinology. 2005;146:2345–53.
115. Leker RR, Karni A, Abramsky O. Exacerbation of myasthenia gravis during the menstrual period. J Neurol Sci. 1998;156:107–11.
116. Leker RR, Karni A, Brenner T, Weidenfeld J, Abramsky O. Effects of sex hormones on experimental autoimmune myasthenia gravis. Eur J Neurol. 2000;7:203–6.
117. Delpy L, Douin-Echinard V, Garidou L, Bruand C, Saoudi A, Guery JC. Estrogen enhances susceptibility to experimental autoimmune myasthenia gravis by promoting type 1-polarized immune responses. J Immunol. 2005;175:5050–7.
118. Scott JS. Immunological diseases in pregnancy. Prog Allergy. 1977;23:321–66.
119. Prieto-Garcia A, Sloane DE, Gargiulo AR, Feldweg AM, Castells M. Autoimmune progesterone dermatitis: clinical presentation and management with progesterone desensitization for successful in vitro fertilization. Fertil Steril. 2011 Mar 1;95(3):1121.e9–13.
120. Lundin KE, Scott H, Hansen T, et al. Gliadin-specific, HLA-DQ(alpha 1*0501,beta 1*0201) restricted T cells isolated from the small intestinal mucosa of celiac disease patients. J Exp Med. 1993;178:187–96.
121. Rubio-Tapia A, Ludvigsson JF, Brantner TL, et al. The prevalence of celiac disease in the United States. Am J Gastroenterol. 2012;107:1538–44.
122. Ludvigsson JF, Montgomery SM, Ekbom A, et al. Small-intestinal histopathology and mortality risk in celiac disease. JAMA. 2009;302:1171–8.
123. Janet MC, Benjamin L, Jeffrey W, et al. Prevalence of celiac disease in patients with unexplained infertility in the united states: a prospective study. J Reprod Med. 2011;56:199–203.
124. Rostami K, Steegers EA, Wong WY, Braat DD, Steegers-Theunissen RP. Coeliac disease and reproductive disorders: a neglected association. Eur J Obstet Gynecol Reprod Biol. 2001;96:146.
125. Karaca N, Yılmaz R, Aktun LH, Batmaz G, Karaca Ç. Is there any relationship between unrecognized Celiac disease and unexplained infertile couples? Turk J Gastroenterol. 2015;26:484–6.
126. Clark DA. Anti-TNF alpha therapy in immune-mediated subfertility: state of the art. J Reprod Immunol. 2010;85:15–24.
127. Winger EE, Reed JL, Ashoush S, El-Toukhy T, Ahuja S, Taranissi M. Degree of TNF-α/IL-10 cytokine elevation correlates with IVF success rates in women undergoing treatment with Adalimumab (Humira) and IVIG. Am J Reprod Immunol. 2011;65:610–8.
128. Varki A, Schauer R. Sialic acids. In: Varki A, Cummings RD, Esko JD, Freeze HH, Stanley P, Bertozzi CR, et al., editors. Essentials of glycobiology [Internet], 2nd edn. Cold Spring Harbor (NY): Cold Spring Harbor Laboratory Press; 2009 [cited 2017 Dec 21]. Available from http://www.ncbi.nlm.nih.gov/books/NBK1920/
129. Wessel J, Behrens U, Lork E, Watson PG, Schröter M, Mews R. Syntheses and structures of bis(azole)difluorosulfuranes. Inorg Chem. 1999 Oct 18;38(21):4789–94.
130. Ma F, Wu D, Deng L, Secrest P, Zhao J, Varki N, et al. Sialidases on mammalian sperm mediate deciduous sialylation during capacitation. J Biol Chem. 2012 Nov 2;287(45):38073–9.
131. Pang P-C, Chiu PCN, Lee C-L, Chang L-Y, Panico M, Morris HR, et al. Human sperm binding is mediated by the sialyl-Lewis(x) oligosaccharide on the zona pellucida. Science. 2011 Sep 23;333(6050):1761–4.
132. Genbacev OD, Prakobphol A, Foulk RA, Krtolica AR, Ilic D, Singer MS, et al. Trophoblast L-selectin-mediated adhesion at the maternal-fetal interface. Science. 2003 Jan 17;299(5605):405–8.
133. Margarit L, Gonzalez D, Lewis PD, Hopkins L, Davies C, Conlan RS, et al. L-selectin ligands in human endometrium: comparison of fertile and infertile subjects. Hum Reprod. 2009 Nov;24(11):2767–77.
134. Lam KKW, Chiu PCN, Lee C-L, Pang RTK, Leung CON, Koistinen H, et al. Glycodelin-A protein interacts with Siglec-6 protein to suppress trophoblast invasiveness by down-regulating extracellular signal-regulated kinase (ERK)/c-Jun signaling pathway. J Biol Chem. 2011 Oct 28;286(43):37118–27.
135. Ma F, Deng L, Secrest P, Shi L, Zhao J, Gagneux P. A mouse model for dietary xenosialitis: antibodies to xenoglycan can reduce fertility. J Biol Chem. 2016;291(35):18222–31.
136. Chou HH, Takematsu H, Diaz S, Iber J, Nickerson E, Wright KL, et al. A mutation in human CMP-sialic acid hydroxylase occurred after the Homo-Pan divergence. Proc Natl Acad Sci USA. 1998 Sep 29;95(20):11751–6.
137. Chou H-H, Hayakawa T, Diaz S, Krings M, Indriati E, Leakey M, et al. Inactivation of CMP-N-acetylneuraminic acid hydroxylase occurred prior to brain expansion during human evolution. Proc Natl Acad Sci USA. 2002 Sep 3;99(18):11736–41.
138. Tangvoranuntakul P, Gagneux P, Diaz S, Bardor M, Varki N, Varki A, et al. Human uptake and incorporation of an immunogenic nonhuman dietary sialic acid. Proc Natl Acad Sci USA. 2003 Oct 14;100(21):12045–50.
139. Miyake M, Zenita K, Tanaka O, Okada Y, Kannagi R. Stage-specific expression of SSEA-1-related antigens in the developing lung of human embryos and its relation to the distribution of these antigens in lung cancers. Cancer Res. 1988 Dec 15;48(24 Pt 1):7150–8.
140. Padler-Karavani V, Yu H, Cao H, Chokhawala H, Karp F, Varki N, et al. Diversity in specificity, abundance, and composition of anti-Neu5Gc antibodies in normal humans: potential implications for disease. Glycobiology. 2008 Oct;18(10):818–30.
141. Nguyen DH, Tangvoranuntakul P, Varki A. Effects of natural human antibodies against a nonhuman sialic acid that metaboli-

cally incorporates into activated and malignant immune cells. J Immunol. 2005 Jul 1;175(1):228–36.
142. Miwa Y, Kobayashi T, Nagasaka T, Liu D, Yu M, Yokoyama I, et al. Are N-glycolylneuraminic acid (Hanganutziu-Deicher) antigens important in pig-to-human xenotransplantation? Xenotransplantation. 2004 May;11(3):247–53.
143. Varki A. Multiple changes in sialic acid biology during human evolution. Glycoconj J. 2009 Apr;26(3):231–45.
144. Pham T, Gregg CJ, Karp F, Chow R, Padler-Karavani V, Cao H, et al. Evidence for a novel human-specific xeno-auto-antibody response against vascular endothelium. Blood. 2009 Dec 10;114(25):5225–35.
145. Samraj AN, Pearce OMT, Läubli H, Crittenden AN, Bergfeld AK, Banda K, et al. A red meat-derived glycan promotes inflammation and cancer progression. Proc Natl Acad Sci USA. 2015 Jan 13;112(2):542–7.
146. Varki NM, Strobert E, Dick EJ, Benirschke K, Varki A. Biomedical differences between human and nonhuman hominids: potential roles for uniquely human aspects of sialic acid biology. Annu Rev Pathol. 2011;6:365–93.
147. Sroga JM, et al. N-glycolylneuraminic acid (Neu5Gc) xenoglycan (XE) and directed antibodies (ABs) are present in the female reproductive tract. Fertil Steril. 2011;96(3):S68.
148. Winn VD, Gormley M, Paquet AC, Kjaer-Sorensen K, Kramer A, Rumer KK, et al. Severe preeclampsia-related changes in gene expression at the maternal-fetal interface include sialic acid-binding immunoglobulin-like lectin-6 and pappalysin-2. Endocrinology. 2009 Jan;150(1):452–62.
149. Rumer KK, Uyenishi J, Hoffman MC, Fisher BM, Winn VD. Siglec-6 expression is increased in placentas from pregnancies complicated by preterm preeclampsia. Reprod Sci. 2013 Jun;20(6):646–53.
150. Li H, Han L, Yang Z, Huang W, Zhang X, Gu Y, et al. Differential proteomic analysis of syncytiotrophoblast extracellular vesicles from early-onset severe preeclampsia, using 8-Plex iTRAQ labeling coupled with 2D nano LC-MS/MS. Cell Physiol Biochem. 2015;36(3):1116–30.
151. Ali SR, Fong JJ, Carlin AF, Busch TD, Linden R, Angata T, et al. Siglec-5 and Siglec-14 are polymorphic paired receptors that modulate neutrophil and amnion signaling responses to group B Streptococcus. J Exp Med. 2014 Jun 2;211(6):1231–42.
152. Gulati S, Schoenhofen IC, Whitfield DM, Cox AD, Li J, St Michael F, et al. Utilizing CMP-sialic acid analogs to unravel *Neisseria gonorrhoeae* lipooligosaccharide-mediated complement resistance and design novel therapeutics. PLoS Pathog. 2015 Dec;11(12):e1005290.
153. Varki A. Are humans prone to autoimmunity? Implications from evolutionary changes in hominin sialic acid biology. J Autoimmun. 2017 Sep;83:134–42.

33 Immunotherapies and Unexplained Infertility

Tanya L. Glenn and Steven R. Lindheim

33.1 Chapter Objectives

After reading this chapter, the reader will be able to understand the basics of the human immune system, discuss the various theories of changes in the immune system observed in pregnancy, review different therapies used to treat immunologic related infertility and consider the future of immunologic infertility.

33.2 Introduction

Human fertility is a vast, complex, and entirely imperfect system. Overall 20% of clinically recognized pregnancies result in first trimester miscarriage with up to 50% attributed to chromosomal abnormalities [1]. The American Society of Reproductive Medicine (ASRM) defines recurrent pregnancy loss (RPL) as at least two failed clinical pregnancies [2]. By these estimates, 5% of the population have RPL, 1% will experience three or more losses, and up to 50% of these individuals with an unknown etiology [2, 3].

Considering that the human fetus is semi-allogenic, with half of its DNA maternal or "self"; hence half is paternal or "foreign," the maternal immune system inherently should recognize the fetus as "non-self" and attack it. This concept was originally proposed in the 1950s by Sir Philip Medawar when he pioneered the relationship between immunology and fertility [4]. In attempt to downregulate the immune system, steroids and intravenous immune globulin (IVIG) have been used in infertility secondary to immunologic dysfunction, though multiple reports, including a recent Cochrane review, reported this treatment is largely unsuccessful [5–7]. However, there appears to be some type of immune tolerance that is enacted during pregnancy allowing embryos to develop. Understanding this process may give insight to those with infertility secondary to immunologic dysfunction. Thus, the purpose of this chapter is to identify potential mechanisms that cause immunologic dysfunction in pregnancy, review treatments that have been used or studied, and touch upon future directions in infertility. Prior to delving into this vast topic, a basic overview of the immune system is warranted.

T. L. Glenn (✉)
Department of Obstetrics and Gynecology, Wright State University, Dayton, OH, USA
e-mail: tanya.glenn@wright.edu

S. R. Lindheim
Department of Obstetrics and Gynecology, Wright State University, Boonshoft School of Medicine, Dayton, OH, USA

33.3 Immune System Basics

The human immune system is divided into two basic entities: the innate and adaptive system. The innate immune system is our first line of defense and is present prior to any infection (Fig. 33.1). It includes physical barriers and cells such as phagocytes, natural killer cells, and the complement system [8]. The innate immune system uses pattern recognition receptors to identify common ligands that invading organisms display, which induces a cascade of events including the release of cytokines, degradative enzymes, and initiates phagocytosis [8, 9]. We will focus on the natural killer cells (NK), which are antiviral, utilize azurophilic granules to attack intracellular bacteria, and have anti-tumor abilities.

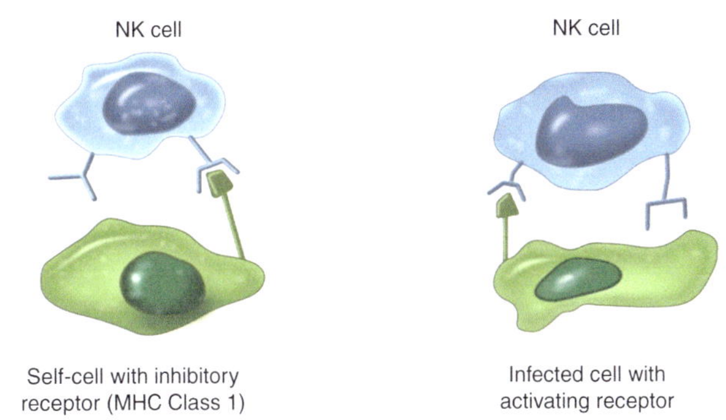

Fig. 33.1 Innate immune system

G. N. Allahbadia et al. (eds.), *Textbook of Assisted Reproduction*, https://doi.org/10.1007/978-981-15-2377-9_33

The NK cells contain both activating and inhibitory receptors on its cell surface, which play a vital role in recognizing "self" antigens, or class I major histocompatibility complex (MHC) molecules [8]. These cell surface molecules are displayed by every nucleated cell in the human body. The two receptors are in balance with each other to destroy cells with the activating receptor, and not those with class 1 MHC ligands. As the embryo contains non-self-ligands, an understanding of how the maternal immune system avoids rejection of the embryo and identifies ways to prevent activation of the maternal immune system is vital [8–10].

The adaptive immune system is more complex and is composed of the humoral and cellular immunity. Humoral immunity deals with extracellular pathogens and toxins by B cells that produce antibodies/immunoglobulins [10]. The cell-mediated immune system plays an important role in intracellular pathogens through T cells [10]. The acquired immune system is triggered after the recognition of antigens that are displayed by toxins or invading organisms. These antigens encounter specific B or T lymphocytes that contain the correct receptor for that antigen and become activated. The B cells become activated by creating antibodies, plasma cells, and memory cells. The T cells are mobilized by creating multiple different forms of T lymphocytes in addition to memory cells. It is these different T lymphocytes that are thought to play a vital role in the immunology of reproduction [8–10].

The T lymphocytes are exposed to specific antigens by antigen presenting cells, such as the dendritic cell or macrophages, which are then activated and create specialized T cells and memory cells [10]. The T helper cells have two subsets, TH1 and TH2. The TH1 cell line produces interferon gamma, IL-2, and TNF- beta, which fight intracellular pathogens, bacteria, inappropriate autoimmunity, and viruses [11]. The TH2 subset produces IL-4, IL-5, IL-10, and IL-13, influencing the humoral immune system and mounting a response against extracellular pathogens, helminth infections, and atopic diseases [11]. The regulatory T cells prevent the immune system for becoming too intense and attacking itself, which is pertinent in reproductive immunology. Failure of this system can lead to autoimmune diseases, such as type 1 diabetes, and may contribute to the destruction of the developing embryo [8–10] (Fig. 33.2).

33.4 History of Immunology and Pregnancy

In the 1940s–1950s, Sir Peter Medawar was one of the first to report on the relationship between the maternal immune system and the fetus. Medawar saw the fetus as semi-allogeneic and created an allograft analogy with three hypotheses concerning the mechanism of maternal tolerance [12]. The first was the physical separation between mom and baby; second was that fetus lacked antigenic properties; and last was that the immune system was inactivated in pregnancy [12].

These ideas have since been rejected. For his first hypothesis, we now know that there is some mixing of maternal and

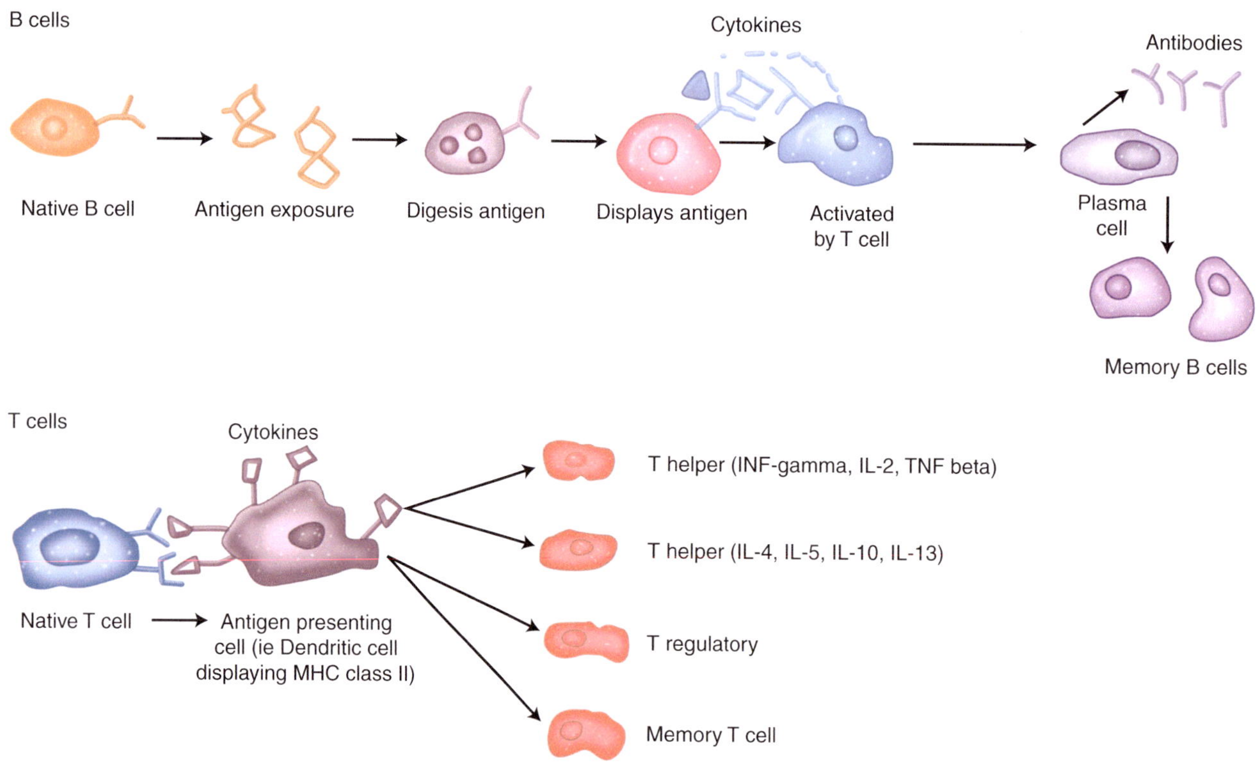

Fig. 33.2 Adaptive immune system

fetal blood throughout pregnancy, which is the basis for cell free DNA testing [9, 13]. The immune system at the placental/decidual interface is also very robust during implantation. Last, the immune system is not arrested during pregnancy; otherwise a rapid progression from HIV to AIDS would be observed [14]. While Medawar's hypotheses have been disproven, he laid the foundation of maternal-fetal tolerance throughout pregnancy, opening the field of reproductive immunology [12].

It was not until 40 years later that Colbert and Main suggested that it was the placenta, not the fetus, that interfaced with the maternal immune system [9]. The human placenta develops from external trophectoderm and is exposed to the immune system through implantation and spiral artery formation.

In the early 1990s, Wegmann proposed the TH1/TH2 hypothesis, in which cytokines produced by TH1 lymphocytes may have an adverse impact on the fetus [15]. However, cytokines produced by TH2 cells, such as granulocyte-macrophage colony-stimulating factor (GM-CSF), IL-3, and CSF-1, are shown to improve differentiation/growth of trophoblasts. They considered pregnancy a state of increased TH2 expression. Mouse studies showed an increase in response of antibodies versus cell-mediated immunity during pregnancy, which they hypothesized was related to the increase in TH2 cell types—that mainly stimulate antibodies—while maternal resistance against intracellular pathogens was less robust [15]. However, there are a large number of pro-inflammatory cytokines and leukocytes that are present during healthy gestations [14]. In addition, the trophoblast does not appear to express the HLA-A/B molecules nor class II molecules, which are required to stimulate lymphocyte activity [16]. It can be postulated that the change in levels of TH1 and TH2 may not be the direct cause of a healthy pregnancy, but rather a reflection of other ongoing events during healthy gestations.

33.5 Cells of Immunologic Interest

33.5.1 T Cells

The CD4 + CD25+ (cell surface ligands) regulatory T cells prevent excessive immune response and may be an essential feature to avoiding embryonic rejection. Treg cells are increased in the decidual tissue, lymph nodes of the uterus, and blood during pregnancy, especially in the first and second trimester [17]. Treg cells act as immunosuppressants by preventing multiplication and production of cytokines by other CD4/8 cells, inhibit NK cells, and certain DC/macrophages [17].

There are multiple mechanisms for the development and maturity of the Treg cells including the control of transcription factor, Foxp3. A loss of function mutation of this transcription factor is associated with the severe auto-immune disease—immune dysregulation, polyendocrinopathy, enteropathy, X-linked syndrome or IPEX [18]. Other mechanisms include specific dendritic cells (DCs) that activate CD4 + TH0 cells into Treg cells. The DCs that activate Treg cells are exposed to transforming growth factor beta (TGF-beta), IL-10, granulocyte-macrophage colony-stimulating factor 4 (GM-CSF-4), and IL-4 during differentiation, which enable them to induce the proper Treg cells [17]. These specific DCs also express Indoleamine 2,3-dioxygenase (IDO), which is vital in the conversion of TH0 to Treg cells and have the capability to downregulate other DCs from activating the TH0. TGF-Beta prevents the pathway to creating T cells that lack the suppressive capacity [17].

The Treg cells can be produced in the periphery or the thymus, and their function in the immune system is dependent on their origin. Peripheral Treg cells (pTreg) are only seen in placental mammals and require an enhancer called conserved noncoding sequence 1 (CNS-1) [19]. Without this enhancer, there is an increase in the activation of effector T cells that precludes correct formation of the placenta [19].

Aluvihare et al. displayed that CD4+/25+ cells were in higher number in pregnant mice, and there was an increase in the Foxp3 mRNA expression within the uterus [20]. This was mainly in first and second trimester and declined in the third trimester and after birth, which has also supported in Guerins' review [17]. Treg cells are also higher during healthy pregnancy versus non-pregnant individuals or in patients with RPL [21]. This suggests that when near term immunosuppressive mechanisms may decline as the body prepares itself to 'reject' the fetus during parturition [22].

Many studies have shown that the elevation of Treg cells needed to be present prior to conception to result in successful implantation. Thus, implying alternative regulatory factors are needed to cause the increase in Treg cells other than the embryo itself. One theory is hormonal fluctuations throughout the menstrual cycle. There is an increase in Treg cells associated with elevations of estrogen in the follicular phase. However, the elevations of estrogen in individuals with RPL do not correlate with an increase in Treg cells, suggesting an underlying mechanism that prevents the beneficial effects estrogen should have [22]. It has also been suggested that the expansion of Treg cells may be due to exposure to paternal antigens and signaling factors released from the trophoblast [9]. Compelling evidence still lacks regarding the mechanism that influences the Treg cell expansion.

33.5.2 Natural Killer Cells

Natural killer cells comprise nearly 40% of the cells within the decidual tissue [9]. These decidual NK cells (dNK) possess different cell surface receptors that are less toxic than the nondiscriminatory cytotoxic role seen by NK cells in the periphery [4, 9]. Decidual NK cells seem to play a vital role in the remodeling required for placentation, implantation, angiogenesis, and spiral arteries [5, 9, 12].

An increase in the cytokines of the inflammatory pathway, IL-6, TNF alpha, IL-12, and CRP, is seen in healthy pregnancies, but there is no systemic infection seen that is anticipated with the elevation of these cytokines. This suggests that a mild inflammatory response may be required for implantation/placental development [23]. However, an exaggerated response with major elevations of IL-18 and interferon gamma may have disastrous consequences: tipping the balance of various interleukins to an inflammatory ratio that causes an abnormal pregnancy [23].

NK cells have also been hailed as one of the primary drivers behind the immune suppression seen in pregnancy versus the T lymphocytes. The placenta displays unique MHC1 molecules including HLA-C, E, and G. Decidual NK cells recognize HLA-C molecules through killer immunoglobulin receptor (KIRs). It has been proposed that without this specific receptor, vascularization does not adequately take place, which can lead to other gestational problems including preeclampsia [12]. The HLA-E and HLA-G receptors are less well known; however HLA-E does play a part in immune recognition, while HLA-G has a defined role in vascularization of the decidua [12]. Both ligands are recognized and activated by specific dNK cells, while T lymphocytes are unable function this way [23]. Studies in mice support the idea that T cells are the primary mediators behind immunosuppression/tolerance in pregnancy [20]. However, human trophoblasts display a specific subset of HLA molecules that are unable to be recognized by T lymphocytes but are recognized by NK cells [12].

It can then be suggested that both dNK cells and T lymphocytes play an influential role in the immune balance required in a health pregnancy. Perhaps neither is the sole requirement for a healthy pregnancy, but rather it is the balance between suppression and activation of T lymphocytes and dNK cells that are required for successful pregnancy.

33.6 Immunologic Concerns

33.6.1 Paternal Alloantigens

Another compelling question is why do the paternal antigens escape detection from the maternal immune system? One simple answer is that they do not. Fetal tissue can be detected in the maternal blood and vice versa. Obviously, there is some crossover, yet most pregnancies are healthy. This returns to the idea of maternal immune system tolerance to paternal alloantigens, perhaps by repeated exposure to semen during intercourse and later trophoblast implantation [17]. Thus, the maternal immune system is slowly primed to accept the semi-allogenic fetus. This has been elegantly displayed by tissue graft experiments, where allogeneic skin grafts with paternal DNA were placed on the pregnant female and were accepted until after the pregnancy [12].

33.6.2 Antiphospholipid Antibody Syndrome

Antiphospholipid syndrome (APAS) is an autoimmune disorder in which normal phospholipids, a portion of all living cell membranes, are attacked by the immune system. During pregnancy, women with APAS that have a history of a thrombotic event are treated with prophylactic heparin and low-dose aspirin [24]. This combination has been reported to improve outcomes, as it prevents the formation of clots within the placental vessels. However, women with implantation failure do not benefit from heparin/aspirin, as their problem lies with the trophoblast's ability to differentiate and develop which is unaffected by anticlotting agents [7].

33.7 Studied Therapies

33.7.1 Large Molecules

33.7.1.1 IVIG

The use of intravenous immunoglobulin (IVIG) for RPL has been controversial and results mixed. Immunoglobulin is the purified plasma from human donors, which contains antibodies and autoantibodies from healthy individuals [3]. There are numerous ways that IVIG can modulate the immune response: by inhibiting autoantibody production, preventing complement activation, increasing Treg cells, and decreasing pro-inflammatory NK cells (Table 33.1) [7].

A meta-analysis by Clark et al., in 2006 reported on three RCTs that supported the use of IVIG prior to conception in patients who had APAS or elevated NK cell activity [25]. Two of the three reported the presence of autoantibodies, one with positive anti-thyroid and the other with positive APA or ANA, and concluded that there was a statistically significant increase in live birth rate in those who were given IVIG, 36% versus 19.3% ($p = 0.012$) [25]. In another systemic review in 2014 on IVIG and elevated NK cells in ART cycles concluded that although the results from IVIG appeared positive, they did not recommend this for standard treatment due to the extreme heterogeneity between study designs, lab standards of elevated NK cell levels, and variable reporting of pregnancy outcomes [5]. This emphasizes the need for adequate studies that are specific to RPL.

Although these meta-analyses do not support IVIG use, they were not performed in individuals with unexplained

Table 33.1 Treatments for immunologic dysfunction in pregnancy

Intervention	Type of study	Author	Year	Outcome	Future research recommendations	ASRM recommendations
Intralipid	Double blind RCT	Dakhly	2016	Increase in ongoing pregnancy/live birth rates with treatment vs placebo (37.5% vs 22.4%; $p = 0.005$)	No meta-analysis	None reported
	RCT	Meng	2016	Individuals with unexplained RPL and elevated NK cells randomized to intralipid vs IVIG. Determined intralipid and IVIG therapy equivalent, with intralipid having less side effects and cost	Few RCTs No Cochrane review	
Leukocyte immunotherapy	Meta-analysis	Cochrane	2012	Individuals with paternal or third party lymphocyte immunization had no increase in live birth rates (OR 1.23; 95% CI 0.89–1.70 and OR 1.39; 95% CI 0.68–2.82)	RCTs specific to RPL	None reported
	Meta-analysis	Borges	2016	Reanalyzed Cochrane data with new RCTs. Live birth rates improved with immunotherapy (OR 1.63; 95% CI 1.13–2.35)		
Cyclosporine	Adaptive clinical trial	Fu	2015	Individuals who failed combination therapy (aspirin, prednisone, heparin, immunotherapy, IVIG) had cyclosporine added, of those who completed the trial 77% had live births ($n = 26$)	No RCTs No meta-analysis No Cochrane review	None reported
Tacrolimus	Prospective cohort	Nakagawa	2014	Individuals received tacrolimus dose (1, 2, 3 mg) pending their elevation in TH1/TH2 levels. Higher pregnancy rates with treatment vs no treatment (64% vs 0%) and higher live birth rates with lower levels of TH1/TH2 (83.3% vs 37.5% vs 40%)	No RCTs No ASRM opinion	None reported
	Prospective cohort	Nakagawa	2017	Elevated TH1/TH2 and RPL, randomized to same treatment as first study. Highest pregnancy/delivery rates with lowest TH1/TH2 (46.3% vs 21.4%, $p < 0.05$), indicating TH1 good predictor for outcome in ART and Tacrolimus can improve outcome	No Cochrane	
Prednisone	Cochrane review	Boomsma	2012	No improvement with prednisone in ART in sub fertile individuals (any etiology)	Limited RCTs with RPL	Advises against use (2012)
	Quasi-RCT	Fawzy	2014	Individuals received prednisone + heparin (not blinded), with 1+ miscarriage and unknown etiology, pregnancy rates >12 weeks higher in treatment arm (38.6% vs 24.6%, $p = 0.016$)		
G-CSF	Systemic review	Borges	2015	2 of 7 RCTs concerned RPL and had improvement in pregnancy/live birth rates, studies heterogenous	No Cochrane review Limited RCTs on RPL in general population (majority in Asian population)	None reported
	Double blind RCT	Barad	2016	Normal IVF patients, G-CSF has no improvement in clinical pregnancy rates		
	Meta-analysis	Xie	2017	Intrauterine perfusion with G-CSF increased implantation and pregnancy rates (RR 2.35; 95% CI1.20–4.60 and RR 2.52; 95% CI 1.39–4.55), in patients undergoing IVF		
	Meta-analysis	Li	2017	Intrauterine perfusion with G-CSF increased implantation and clinical pregnancy rates in individuals undergoing IVF with RPL or thin endometrium in Asian population (RR 1.887; 95% CI 1.256–1.2833 and RR 2.312; 95% CI 1.444–3.701)		

(continued)

Table 33.1 (continued)

Intervention	Type of study	Author	Year	Outcome	Future research recommendations	ASRM recommendations
GM-CSF	RCT	Ziebe	2013	Sub-analysis of individuals with RPL with increase in live birth rates with treatment ($p = 0.02$)	No meta-analysis No Cochrane review No RCT on RPL	None reported
Etanercept	Adaptive clinical trial	Jerzak	2012	Decrease in NK cells with etanercept, and a higher decrease in NK cells in individuals who became pregnant ($p < 0.05$)	No meta-analysis No Cochrane review	None reported
Adalimumab	Prospective cohort	Winger	2009	Increase in live birth rates with adalimumab with IVIG vs no treatment (73% vs 0%, $p < 0.0009$) in individuals with RPL and elevated TH1/TH2	No meta-analysis No Cochrane review	None reported
IVIG	Meta-analysis	Clark	2006	Increase in live birth rates with IVIG in individuals with auto-antibodies (36% vs 19.3%, $p = 0.012$)	Limited RCTs	Advises against use (2006)
	Systemic review	Polanski	2014	Increase in live birth rates with IVIG and elevated NK cells (RR 3.94; 95% CI 2.01–7.69), studies heterogenous and underpowered		

Abbreviations: Randomized control trial (RCT); American Society of Reproductive Medicine (ASRM); Intravenous Immunoglobulin (IVIG); Confidence Interval (CI); Odds Ratio (OR); Recurrent pregnancy loss (RPL); Assisted Reproductive Technology (ART); Granulocyte colony stimulating factor (G-CSF); Granulocyte-Macrophage Colony Stimulating Factor (GM-CSF); Natural Killer Cells (NK Cells); In Vitro Fertilization (IVF)

RPL. A retrospective observational study by Ramos-Medina that included over 400 women with RPL demonstrated a beneficial effect of IVIG [26]. IVIG was only given to individuals who had RPL and expansion of NK or NKT cells (T lymphocytes with properties of NK and T cells). Individuals with IVIG (n = 121) had a live birth rate of 96% versus 30.8% in those without IVIG ($p < 0.0001$) [26]. However, in a small (n = 83) randomized control study in 2016, individuals with secondary RPL were randomized to placebo versus IVIG. No difference was seen in their primary outcome of birth through the first 28 days of life (54.8% vs 50.0%; 95% CI of 0.70–1.74) [27]. Further studies are warranted specific to RPL are pertinent prior to considering the use of IVIG. Currently, the American Society of Reproduction Medicine advises against the use of IVIG for primary RPL, as it has not been proven to benefit the pregnancy and can have significant side effects and cost [28].

33.7.1.2 TNF-Alpha Inhibitors

Tumor necrosing factor alpha inhibitors are a group of biological agents that are designed to suppress the inflammatory response seen in multiple autoimmune diseases. In autoimmune RPL, the root cause may be due to unregulated NK cells, an imbalance in TH1/TH2 lymphocytes, or a combination of these factors. However, due to its intense immune suppression, TNF-alpha inhibitors can lead to the onset of opportunistic infections or activation of latent infections [29]. There are two TNF-alpha inhibitors approved for RPL, adalimumab and etanercept [3].

33.7.1.3 Adalimumab

Winger et al. reported in a prospective cohort study in individuals (n = 76) with levels of TH1/TH2 greater than one standard deviation above the mean, that the monoclonal antibody, adalimumab, would reduce the level of TH1/TH2 and was associated with higher pregnancy rates [30]. There was a statistically significant difference when comparing live birth rates between adalimumab with IVIG (73%) versus no treatment (0%) ($p < 0.0009$) [30]. In addition, they saw a greater number of clinical pregnancies (73%) in those with adalimumab with IVIG versus IVIG alone (52%, $p < 0.05$), although the number of live births was non-significant [30]. Unfortunately, individuals chose their treatment; thus an uneven number were found in each group, introducing bias. In addition, the sample size was small, and the treatment groups were broken down further into four different study groups, dramatically decreasing the power of their results [30]. These encouraging outcomes need to be taken cautiously until RCTs are performed.

33.7.1.4 Etanercept

Etanercept, a TNF-alpha immunoglobulin fusion protein that inactivates TNF-alpha, decreases TH-1 cytokines and was designed for individuals with resistant rheumatoid arthritis [31]. It also downregulates NK cell activation, which may play a role in infertility when NK cells are in elevated or have incorrect functional status [31]. Current literature supports its use in individuals who have a considerable risk of rheumatoid arthritis or have rheumatoid arthritis while pregnant, as pregnancy may increase the severity of symptoms.

Jerzak et al. performed a prospective study utilizing etanercept in individuals with RPL and elevated NK cells ($n = 30$) [31]. Overall, a 57% pregnancy rate was achieved and had a significant decrease in NK cells from baseline. In those who failed to become pregnant, there was no notable change in NK cell levels [31]. Caution should be taken given the small sample size, the primary end point was pregnancy only, and the lack of control group [31]. While promising, there has been no RCT with etanercept and RPL; thus the use of etanercept should be done in research settings only.

33.7.1.5 Granulocyte-Macrophage Colony-Stimulating Factor (GM-CSF)

Colony-stimulating factor (CSF) is a collection of glycoproteins that activate intracellular pathways to stimulate cell proliferation and differentiation required for implantation [32, 33]. Collectively, these factors may effect implantation through its impact on the developing endometrium and upregulates the ability of the dendritic cells to become activated, thus increasing the number of active T cells [17, 33].

Granulocyte-macrophage colony-stimulating factor (GM-CSF) is a specific CSF that helps differentiate and proliferate multiple cell lines including macrophages, neutrophils, and eosinophils [3]. The use of GM-CSF for infertility was studied in a large multicenter randomized control trial ($n = 1332$) comparing embryos cultured in media with and without GM-CSF with a sub-analysis on individuals that have at least one miscarriage [34]. Their secondary analysis had an increase in live birthrates in individuals with one or more miscarriages (28.9% vs 24.1%, OR of 1.35 (95% CI 1.03–1.78)) [34]. Further studies regarding RPL with the use of GM-CSF are warranted.

33.7.1.6 G-CSF

Granulocyte colony-stimulating factor (G-CSF) is a cytokine produced by decidual cells and trophoblastic cells that targets the expansion of neutrophils, increases TH2 expression, activates Tregs cells, and increases dendritic cells [3, 35, 36]. This factor is produced at the placental-endometrial interface, stimulates the endometrium, and may play a significant role in implantation and ovarian function [3, 35]. This role was supported by Ledee et al., where low levels of G-CSF in follicular fluid were a significant negative predictor (97%) of implantation success in women undergoing ICSI or IVF [32]. As G-CSF plays a role in increasing cytokine differentiation and abundance in the endometrium, research has assessed its impact on endometrial thickness and implantation.

Many systemic reviews have covered G-CSF and infertility including a 2017 systematic review/meta-analysis of 11 studies concerning endometrial growth and implantation rate [37]. The conclusion was that intrauterine perfusion with G-CSF increased implantation rates (RR 2.35, 95% CI 1.20–4.60), pregnancy rates (RR = 2.52; 95% CI 1.39–4.55), and endometrial thickness (mean difference 1.79; 95% CI 0.92–2.67; $p < 0.0001$) [37]. However, RPL was not specifically evaluated and a significant variance in the dose and duration was reported [37]. Another meta-analysis of 6 studies with 607 individuals, 3 RCTs, had a subgroup analysis of individuals with RPL and noted an improvement in outcomes (RR 1.8; 95% CI 1.25–1.28) [38]. Both meta-analyses concluded that higher quality RCTs, in a more generalizable population, were required prior to recommending G-CSF as a treatment option.

33.7.2 Small Molecules

33.7.2.1 Prednisone

Prednisone has long been used in patients with inflammatory diseases, severe asthma, and autoimmune disease. Its use was proposed as immunotherapy in patients with RPL thought to have an overactive immune system with elevated NK cells [3].

A 2012 Cochrane Review reported on the use of glucocorticoids in ART cycles (ICSI or IVF) during peri-implantation which included 14 RCTs and 1879 individuals who were sub-fertile with any etiology [38]. Only three studies reported live birth rates, which did not reveal an increase in live birth rates (OR 1.21, 95% CI 0.67–2.19). A subgroup analysis showed an improvement in pregnancy rate in those undergoing IVF vs ICSI (OR 1.50, 95% CI 1.05–2.13) [38]. They concluded that in individuals undergoing ART the use of glucocorticoids should be limited to research only. A quasi-RCT by Fawzy et al., published after the Cochrane review, studied the combination of prednisone and heparin in 334 women with at least one IVF failure utilizing ICSI with no history of hormonal or uterine abnormalities [39]. The study arm was given 20 mg prednisone/day starting at time of ovarian stimulation and continued until the eighth week of pregnancy. Pregnancy rates were significantly higher in the treatment arm (42.8% versus 30.3%, $p = 0.028$), as were ongoing pregnancy rates beyond 12 weeks (38.6% vs 24.6%, $p = 0.016$) [39]. However, the subjects were not blinded, and their primary outcome was not clinically significant.

The mechanism of how prednisone improves fertility in unexplained RPL remains unclear. As such, ASRM has stressed that prednisone is not a benign drug and its use increases pregnancy-related complications including diabetes and hypertension [2]. At present, the ASRM Practice Committee Opinion currently does did not support the use of prednisone in individuals with RPL and APAS [2].

33.7.2.2 Tacrolimus

Tacrolimus is an immunosuppressant that has been mainly used for the prevention of transplant rejection and autoimmune diseases. It specifically blocks multiple regions in the T- lymphocyte pathway by preventing expansion of cytotoxic T cells, blocking IL-2 receptors and mediators of T lymphocytes such as IL2 and INF-gamma [40]. The mechanism of action is along the same lines as other immune modulators: to correct the imbalance between TH1/TH2, with the idea that RPL is caused by an uncontrolled TH1 response.

To our knowledge, there are only two studies on tacrolimus and RPL both by Nakagawa et al. [40, 41]. The first, a prospective cohort study (n = 42) of subjects with unexplained RPL, where baseline levels of TH1/TH2 were assessed by examining the levels of INF-gamma (TH1 marker) and IL-4 (TH2 marker) and then given tacrolimus (1, 2, or 3 mg) prior to embryo transfer based on TH1/TH2 levels. Those that received tacrolimus had a 64% pregnancy rate and 45.7% implantation rate compared to none in the control group. Those with lower TH1/TH2 levels had the highest clinical pregnancy rate (83.3%) and live birth rates (83.3%) compared to the 2 mg group (50.0 and 37.5%) or 3 mg (40.0 and 40.0%) [40]. In a second prospective cohort study (n = 124) of women with elevated TH1/TH2 levels and RPL, the highest ongoing pregnancy/delivery rates were those with the lowest TH1/TH2 level, versus those with the highest TH1/TH2 level (46.3% vs 21.4%, $p < 0.05$) [41]. Their work suggests that an elevated TH1/TH2 may predict reduced ART success and that Tacrolimus improves pregnancy outcomes [41]. We await placebo-controlled RCTs to prove its efficacy and safety.

33.7.2.3 Cyclosporine

Like tacrolimus, cyclosporine has been used to reduce the risk of rejection after organ transplant inhibiting calcium pathways that are essential to the production of T lymphocytes and IL-2 [3]. In addition, it increases IL-4, a TH2-specific cytokines; reduces the production of TH-1-related cytokines, while boosting cytokine expression that assists trophoblasts in implantation, growth, and movement; and prevents trophoblast apoptosis [3].

Limited studies in those with RPL and antiphospholipid antibody (APA) have been performed. Fu assessed subjects (n = 26) with RPL with APA who had failed a combined therapy of prednisone, aspirin, heparin, and IVIG [42]. They used a previous protocol of prednisone 60 mg, aspirin 80 mg, heparin 5000 IU twice daily, and IVIG 400 mg/kg per day, and then added 50 mg of cyclosporine two to three times per day, with the goal of maintaining a stable concentration of cyclosporine between 80 to 150 ng/ml [42]. This was continued throughout pregnancy unless APA became negative, at which time the cyclosporine was gradually decreased and discontinued. Twenty (77%) delivered a live birth, three (11.5%) had stillbirths (13, 22, and 26 weeks), and three (11.5%) were lost to follow-up. Complications noted were gestational hypertension and early delivery. Further work is needed to assess cyclosporine's efficacy and safety [42].

33.7.3 Cell Based

33.7.3.1 Paternal and Third-Party Lymphocyte Immunization

The theory behind the use of lymphocyte immunization is to generate tolerance of the maternal immune system to the semi-allogenic fetus. This has been accomplished using partner or paternal lymphocytes, third party, or donor lymphocytes. Paternal lymphocyte immunization uses lymphocytes with HLA subtypes from the father that are different from the maternal HLA subtypes. This is given in a high dose (100×10^6 or more lymphocytes) to the mother via intradermal or intravenous methods for the largest impact [3]. Third-party lymphocyte immunization differs in that its dose is approximately 10x greater, administered intravenously only, and theoretically provides a more robust response within the maternal immune system as it is a foreign lymphocyte antigen compared to a familiar one from the partner. It is thought that the lymphocyte immunization would "shield" the fetal HLA antigens from the maternal immune system [3]. Multiple studies have been performed; however most have small sample sizes and bias, which make interpreting and applying data difficult.

A Cochrane systematic review attempted to clarify this issue in a review of 20 RCTs on RPL, ≤1 prior live birth, or infertility due to other non-immunologic etiology. They compared lymphocyte immunization, trophoblast membrane infusion, or IVIG [6]. Results demonstrated no increased probability of live births (after 20 weeks) with respect to paternal cell immunization (OR 1.23 with 95% CI of 0.89–1.70) or third-party lymphocyte immunization (OR of 1.39 (95% CI 0.68–2.82) [6]. The conclusion was that none of these interventions should be used for RPL of unknown origin. However, a meta-analysis in 2016 reexamined the Cochrane review and determined that the methods of one of the included studies was inadequate. When this study was eliminated, there was a positive association in the treatment arm (OR 1.63, 95% CI 1.13–2.35) [43]. Some side effects of infection and fever were reported and should not be overlooked.

As with all immunomodulating treatments for RPL, randomized control studies with meticulous patient selection will determine its true efficacy. To date, ASRM has no specific guidelines regarding lymphocyte immunotherapy, thus it should only be undertaken in experimental protocols.

33.7.4 Miscellaneous

33.7.4.1 Intralipid

Intralipids are fat emulsions in intravenous form that suppress NK cells through an ill-defined mechanism. Studies suggest that intralipids may act through a multitude of receptors, suppress macrophages, and stimulate the reticulo-endothelial system. This system removes signals from cells that identify the cells as abnormal, rendering that cell invisible to the immune system [3].

An RCT in women with RPL, unexplained infertility, and elevated NK cells ($n = 296$) using either 2 cc of intralipid (diluted in 250 cc saline) or saline administered at egg retrieval through first trimester showed a significant increase in ongoing pregnancies/live birth rates (37.5% vs 22.4%; $p = 0.05$) [44]. An RCT in 2016 compared IVIG to intralipid through the 12th week of pregnancy [45]. The live birth rates were equivalent in both groups (97.5% vs 98%; $p > 0.05$) [45]. These mixed results suggest further scrutiny is required.

33.8 Future Direction and Conclusions

An ample amount of research has gone into studying immunologic dysfunction of infertility, though conclusive evidence is still lacking. The future of immunologic dysfunction in infertility and RPL has gaps in knowledge that need to be addressed further.

When considering Treg cells, it would be easy to theorize that simply giving women more Treg cells would correct the problem. However, one cannot be sure that Treg cells would be able to be administered in high enough quantities to create a compelling difference, nor that they would not have any antigen switching that may cause a more enhanced immunologic response. Other areas along the pathway to create Treg cells may also serve as targets for intervention. FOXP3, the transcription factor, is vital to the creation of proper Treg cells. FOXP3 is difficult to induce as it is intracellular, but modern technology using viral-induced FOXP3 may help bypass this complication [18]. IDO induction has also been considered via viral or gene therapy, which could then upregulate DCs. In addition, Treg cells can be increased by giving G-CSF, which acts on increasing tolerogenic DCs. Natural Killer cells are also a potential target, yet more knowledge is required to determine the optimal number or percent active, their origin, and the pathway to create dNK cells. Future research with well-designed studies will hopefully uncover the mystery of autoimmunity, ART, and allow for targeted therapy(s) [5].

References

1. Mayo Clinic Staff. Miscarriage. Mayo Clinic [Internet]. 2016 July [cited on 2017 Sept 25]. Available from http://www.mayo-clinic.org/diseases-conditions/pregnancy-loss-miscarriage/home/ovc-20213664.
2. Evaluation and treatment of recurrent pregnancy loss: a committee opinion. American Society of Reproductive Medicine. Fertil Steril [Internet]. 2012 [cited on 2017 Aug 24]. Available from http://www.fertstert.org/article/S0015-0282(12)02242-X/pdf.
3. Abdolmohammadi-Vahid SS, Danzig S, Hamdi K, Jadid-Nicaragua F, Ahmadi M, Yousefi M. Novel immunotherapeutic approaches for treatment of infertility. Biomed Pharmacother [Internet]. 2016. [cited on 2017 Aug 15];84:1449–59. https://doi.org/10.1016/j.biopha.2016.10.062.
4. Colbert GT, Maine EK. Immunology of the maternal-placental interface in normal pregnancy. Semin Perinatol [Internet]. 1991 June [Cited 2017 Aug 01]; 15(3):196–205.
5. Polanski LT, Barbosa MAP, Martins MP, Baumgarten MN, Campbell B, Brosens J, Quenby S, Raine-Fenning N. Interventions to improve reproductive outcomes in women with elevated natural killer cells undergoing assisted reproduction techniques: a systematic review of literature. Hum Reprod [Internet]. 2014 [cited on 2017 Aug 12]; 29(1):65–75. https://doi.org/10.1093/humrep/det414.
6. Wong LF, Porter TF, Scott JR. Immunotherapy for recurrent miscarriage (review). Cochran Library [Internet]. 2014 [cited 2017 Aug 07]. Available from http://www.cochrane.org/CD000112/PREG_immunotherapy-for-recurrent-miscarriage
7. Coulam CB, Acacio B. Does immunotherapy for treatment of reproductive failure enhance live births? Am J Reprod Immunol [Internet]. 2012 Feb 16 [Cited on 12 Aug 2017]; 67(4):296–304. https://doi.org/10.1111/j.1600-0897.2012.01111.x.
8. Kumar V, Abbas A, Fausto N, Aster J. Disease of the immune system. In: Robbins and Cotran pathologic basis of disease. 8th ed. Philadelphia: Saunders Elsevier; 2010. p. 183–257.
9. Creasy RK, Resnik R, Iams JD, Lockwood CJ, Moore TR, Green MF. Immunology of pregnancy. In: Creasy & Resnik's maternal-fetal medicine principle and practice. 7th ed. Philadelphia: Saunders Elsevier; 2014. p. 80–92.
10. Hall JE. Resistance of the body to infection: II. Immunity and allergy. In: Guyton and Hall textbook of medical physiology. 13th ed. Philadelphia: Elsevier; 2016. p. 465–76.
11. Fallon PG, Jolin HE, Smith P, Emson CL, Townsend MJ, Fallon R, Smith P, McKenzie AN. IL-4 induces characteristic Th2 responses even in the combined absence of IL-5, IL-9, and IL-13. Immunity [Internet]. 2002 July [cited on 13 Aug 2017];17(1):7–17.
12. Trowsdale J, Betz AG. Mother's little helpers: mechanisms of maternal-fetal tolerance. Nat Immunol [Internet]. March 2006. [cited 2017 Aug 12];7(3) https://doi.org/10.1038/ni1317.
13. American College of Obstetrics and Gynecology. Cell-Free DNA Screening. ACOG/ SMFM [Internet]. 2015 September [cited 2017 Aug 20]; number 640. Available on https://www.acog.org/Resources-And-Publications/Committee-Opinions/Committee-on-Genetics/Cell-free-DNA-Screening-for-Fetal-Aneuploidy.
14. Sacks G, Sargent S, Redman C. An innate view of human pregnancy. Trends Genet [Internet].1999 March [cited 2017 Aug 08];20(3): 114–118.
15. Wegmann TG, Lin H; Guilbert L, Mosmann TR. Bidirectional cytokine interactions in maternal-fetal relationship: is success in pregnancy a Th2 phenomenon? Immunol Today [Internet]. 1993 [cited 2017 Aug 08];14(7).https://doi.org/10.1016/0167-5699(93)90235-D.
16. Samy E, Setiady YY, Ohno K, Pramoonjago P, Sharp C, Tung KS. The role of physiological self-antigen in the acquisition

and maintenance of regulatory T-cell function. Immunol Rev [Internet]. 2006 [cited on 2017 Aug 12]; 212: 170–184.https://doi.org/10.1111/j.010502896.2006.00404.x.
17. Guerin LR; Prins JR; Robertson SA. Regulatory T-cells and immune tolerance in pregnancy: a new target for infertility treatment? Hum Reprod Update. [Internet]. 2009 Sept-Oct [cited 2017 Aug 01]:15(5);517–535. https://doi.org/10.1093/humupd/dmp004.
18. Gambineri E, Torgerson TR, Ochs HD. Immune dysregulation, polyendocrinopathy, enteropathy, and X-linked inheritance (IPEX), a syndrome of systemic autoimmunity caused by mutations of FOXP3, a critical regulator of T-cell homeostasis. Curr Opin Rheumatol [Internet]. 2003 Jul [cited on 2017 Aug 13];15(4):430–435.
19. Samstein RM, Josefowicz SZ, Arvey A, Treuting PM, Rudensky AY. Extrathymic generation of regulatory T cells in placental mammals mitigates maternal-fetal conflict. Cell [Internet]. 2012 Jul 6 [cited 2017 Aug 07];150(1):29–38. https://doi.org/10.1016/j.cell.2012.05.031.
20. Aluvihare VR, Kallikourdis M, Betz AG. Regulatory T cells mediate maternal tolerance to the fetus. Nat Immunol [Internet]. 2004 March [cited 2017 Aug 07];5(3):266–271. https://doi.org/10.1038/nj1037.
21. Arruvito L, Sanz M, Banham AH, Fainboim L. Expansion of CD4+CD25+ and FOXP3+ regulatory T cells during the follicular phase of the menstrual cycle: implications for human reproduction. J Immunol [Internet]. 2007 Feb 15 [cited on 2017 Aug 12];178(4):2572–2578.
22. Zhao JX, Zeng YY, Liu Y. Fetal alloantigen is responsible the expansion of the CD4+CD25+ regulatory T cell pool during pregnancy. J Reprod Immunol [Internet]. 2007 Aug [cited 2017 Aug 07];75(2):71–81. https://doi.org/10.1016/j.jri.2007.06.052.
23. Sargent IL; Angela M , Borzychowski AM , Redman CWG. NK cells and human pregnancy - an inflammatory view. Trends Immunol [Internet]. 2006 [cited 2017 Aug 08];27(9). https://doi.org/10.1016/j.it.2006.06.009.
24. Antiphospholipid Syndrome. The American College of Obstetricians and Gynecologists [Internet]. 2012 Dec [cited on 2017 Aug 17];132. Available on https://www.acog.org/Resources-And-Publications/Practice-Bulletins/Committee-on-Practice-Bulletins-Obstetrics/Antiphospholipid-Syndrome.
25. Clark DA, Coulam CB, Stricker RB. Is Intravenous immunoglobulins (IVIG) efficacious in early pregnancy failure? A critical review and meta-analysis for patients who fail in vitro fertilization and embryo transfer (IVF). J Assist Reprod Genet [Internet]. 2006 Jan [cited on 2017 Sept 5];23(1). https://doi.org/10.1007/s10815-005-9013-1.
26. Ramos-Medina R, Garcia-Segovia A, Carbone J, Aguaron De La Cruz A, Seyfferth A, Alonso B, Leon JA, Alecsandru D, Melia E, Carrillo de Albornoz E, Ordonez D, Santillan L, Verdu V, Garcia Ruiz De Morales JM, Lopez-Hoyos M, Lopez Larios A, Sampalo A, Carballero P, Ortiz Quintana L, Fernandez-Cruz E, Sanchez-Ramon S. Experience in IVIG therapy for selected women with recurrent reproductive failure and NK cell expansion. Am J Reprod Immunol [Internet]. 2014 [cited on 2017 Aug 13];71:458–466. https://doi.org/10.1111/aji.12217.
27. Christiansen OB, Larsen EC, Egerup E, Lunoee L, Egestad L, Nielsen HS. Intravenous immunoglobulin treatment for secondary recurrent miscarriage: a randomised, double-blind, placebo-controlled trial. BJOG [Internet]. 2015 [cited on 2017 Sept 30];122: 500–508. https://doi.org/10.1111/1471-0528.13192.
28. The Practice Committee Opinion of the American Society of Reproductive Medicine. Intravenous Immunoglobulin (IVIG) and recurrent spontaneous pregnancy loss. Fertil Steril [Internet]. 2006 [cited on 2017 Aug 02];86(4). https://doi.org/10.1016/j.fertstert.2006.08.047.
29. Ali T, Kaitha S, Mahmood S, Ftesi A, Stone J, Bronze M. Clinical use of anti-TNF therapy and increased risk of infections. Drug Healthc Patient Saf [Internet]. 2013 March [cited 2017 Oct 2];5:79–99. https://doi.org/10.2147/DHPS.S28801.
30. Winger EE, Reed JL, Ashoush S, Ahuja S, El-Toukhy T, Taranissi M. Treatment with Adalimumab (Humira) and intravenous immunoglobulin improves pregnancy rates in women undergoing IVF. Am J Reprod Immunol [Internet]. 2009 [cited on 2017 Aug 13];61:113–120. https://doi.org/10.1111/j.1600-0897.2008.00669.x.
31. Jerzak M, Ohams M, Gorski A, Baranowski W. Entanercept immunotherapy in women a history of recurrent reproductive failure. Ginekol Pol [Internet]. 2012 [cited on 2017 Aug 29];83:260–264.
32. Ledee N, Gridelet V, Ravet S, Jouan C, Gaspard O, Wenders F, Thonon F, Hincourt N, Dubois M, Foidart JM, Munaut C, Perrier d'Hauterive S. Impact of follicular G-CSF quantification on subsequent embryo transfer decisions: a proof of concept study. Human Reprod [Internet]. 2013 Feb [cited on 2017 Aug 12];28(2):406–413. https://doi.org/10.1093/humrep/des354.
33. Kumar P, Mahajan S. Preimplantation and postimplantation therapy for the treatment of reproductive failure. J Hum Reprod Sci [Internet]. 2013 Apr-Jun [cited on 2017 Aug 12];6(2):88–92. https://doi.org/10.4103/0974-1208.117165.
34. Ziebe S, Loft A, Povlsen BB, Erb K, Agerholm I, Aasted M, Gabrielsen A, Hnida C, Zobel DP, Munding B, Bendz SH, Robertson SA. A randomized clinical trial to evaluate the effect of granulocyte-macrophage colony-stimulating factor (GM-CSF) in embryo culture medium for in vitro fertilization. Fertil Steril [Internet]. 2013 May 1 [Cited on 2017 Aug 12]; 99(6):1600–1609. https://doi.org/10.1016/j.fertnstert.2012.12.043.
35. Eftekhar M, Hosseinisadat R, Baradaran R, Naghshineh E. Effect of granulocyte colony stimulating factor (G-CSF) on IVF outcomes in infertile women: An RCT. Int J Reprod Biomen (Yazd) [Internet]. 2016 May [cited on 2017 Aug 14];14(5):341–346.
36. Scarpellini F, Sbracia M. Use of granulocyte colony-stimulating factor for the treatment of unexplained recurrent miscarriage: a randomized controlled trial. Hum Reprod [Internet]. 2009 [cited on 2017 Aug 16];24(11):2703–2708. https://doi.org/10.1093/humrep/dep240.
37. Xie Y, Zhang T, Tian Z, Zhang J, Wang W, Zhang H, Zeng Y, Ou J, Yang Y. Efficacy of intrauterine perfusion of granulocyte colony-stimulating factor (G-CSF) for Infertile women with thin endometrium: A systematic review and meta-analysis. Am J Reprod Immunol [Internet]. 2017 April [cited on 2017 Sept 30];78:e12701. https://doi.org/10.1111/aji.12701.
38. Boomsma CM, Keay SD, Macklon NS. Peri-implantation glucocorticoid administration for assisted reproductive technology cycles (review). Cochrane Database System Rev [Internet]. 2012 [cited on 2017 Sept 25];6. Available from www.cochranelibrary.com https://doi.org/10.1002/14651858.CD005996.pub3.
39. Fawzy M, El-Refaeey AAA. Does combined prenisolone and low molecular weight heparin have a role in unexplained implantation failure? Gynecol Endocrinol Reprod Med [Internet]. 2014 [cited on 2017 Aug 24];289:677–680. https://doi.org/10.1007/s00404-013-3020-8.
40. Nakagawa K, Kwak-Kim J, Ota K, Kuroda K, Hisano M, Sugiyama R, Yamaguchi K. Immunosuppression with Tacrolimus improved reproductive outcome of women with repeated implantation failure and elevated peripheral blood Th1/Th2 cell ratios. Am J Reprod Immunol [Internet]. 2014 [cited on 2017 Sept 4];73:353–361. https://doi.org/10.1111/aji.12338.
41. Nakagawa K, Kwak-Kim J, Kuroda K, Sugiyama, R, Yamaguchi K. Immunosuppressive treatment using tacrolimus promotes pregnancy outcome in infertile women with repeated implantation failures. Am J Reprod Immunol [Internet]. 2017 [cited on 2017 Sept 29];78:e12682. https://doi.org/10.1111/aji.12682.

42. Fu, JH. Analysis of the use of cyclosporine A to treat refractory immune recurrent spontaneous abortion. Clin Exp Obstet Gynecol [Internet]. 2015 [cited 2017 Aug 30];42(6):739–742.
43. Borges Cavalcante M, Silva Cost FDA, Barini R, Araujo E Jr. Granulocyte colony-stimulating factor and reproductive medicine: a review. Iran J Reprod Med [Internet]. 2015 Apr [cited on 2017 Sept 29];13(4): 195–202.
44. Dakhly DM, Bayoumi YA, Sharkawy M, Gad Allah SH, Hassan MA, Gouda HM, Hashem AT, Hatem DL, Ahmed MF, El-Khayat W. Intralipid supplementation in women with recurrent spontaneous abortion and elevated levels of natural killer cells. Internal J Gynecol Obstet [Internet]. 2016 [cited on 2017 Sept 4];135:324–327. https://doi.org/10.1016/j.ijgo.2016.06.026.
45. Meng L, Lin J, Chen L, Wang Z, Liu M, Liu Y, Chen X, Zhu L, Chen H, Zhang J. Effectiveness and potential mechanisms of intralipid in treating unexplained recurrent spontaneous abortion. Arch Gynecol Obstet [Internet]. Oct 2015 [cited on 2017 Sept 25];294:29–39. https://doi.org/10.1007/s00404-015-3922-8.

34 Human Leukocyte Antigen (HLA) Typing in Medically Assisted Reproduction

Sana M. Salih, Logan Havemann, and Steven R. Lindheim

34.1 The Immune System in Humans

The immune system plays a central role on human survival and reproduction. The immune response is fine-tuned to prevent over- and under-response to protect against infection and cancer while avoiding autoimmune reaction and accommodating pregnancy. The human body has two main immune mechanisms: innate immunity and adaptive (acquired) immunity. Innate immunity consists of natural immunity such as physical barriers (skin and mucous membranes), normal flora, and nonspecific immune cells (phagocytes and NK cells). Adaptive immunity consists of humoral immune response (production of antibody) and cell-mediated immune response (production of lymphocyte). Adaptive immunity is induced by cell surface proteins known as the human leukocyte antigens (HLAs) that are encoded by the major histocompatibility complex (MHC) genes. The MHC/HLA immune system is responsible for protecting the body against invading microorganisms and foreign proteins, recognition of "self" from "non-self," and removal of damaged tissue and abnormal cells including cancer [1]. HLA-G promotes immune tolerance in pregnancy and plays a critical role in establishing and maintaining normal pregnancy [2]. Perturbations of HLA-G genotypes are associated with infertility and pregnancy complications such as implantation failure and recurrent pregnancy loss. It prompts poor placentation and late pregnancy complications such as pregnancy-induced hypertension, intrauterine growth restriction, and gestational diabetes [3–11]. Recent advances in assisted reproductive technology (ART) allowed the selection of HLA-matching embryos to be used as source of hematopoietic stem cell donors to siblings affected with blood disorders such as Fanconi syndrome and leukemia [12, 13].

S. M. Salih
RMA of Central Pennsylvania at PinnacleHealth, Mechanicsburg, PA, USA

L. Havemann
Wright State University School of Medicine, Dayton, OH, USA

S. R. Lindheim (✉)
Department of Obstetrics and Gynecology, Wright State University, Boonshoft School of Medicine, Dayton, OH, USA
e-mail: steven.lindheim@wright.edu

34.2 HLA Genetic Structure

MHC is a super locus of genes found in all vertebrates that encode a variety of proteins including cell surface markers and antigen-presenting molecules that among several other functions, play an essential role in the immune system. Conventionally, the term human leukocyte antigen (HLA) system is synonymous with human MHC. However, some literature uses the term HLA to refer specifically to the HLA proteins and reserves the term MHC to refer to the region of the genome that encodes for the HLA protein. In this chapter, the terms MHC and HLA will be used interchangeably. The classical human MHC region is located on the short arm of chromosome 6 at position 6p21.3 and spans 3.78 megabases [14–16]. The HLA region has been mapped and includes 224 genes, many of which are not known to be involved in immune function [16]. Recently, the discovery of an additional 23 genes relevant to the MHC outside of the boundaries of the classical MHC led to the use of the term extended MHC region, which spans the classical MHC region and an additional 3.8 megabases [17]. The mapping and understanding of the genes in the classical and extended MHC regions is an area of ongoing research. MCH has a well-established role in regulating immunity. MCG is important for pregnancy maintenance, and it greatly impacts reproduction and social behavior, including mate selection and kin recognition [18–21].

34.3 HLA Organization and Function

One of the most critical functions of the immune system is the ability to discriminate self from non-self, which is accomplished in part by the MHC antigens. The classical

G. N. Allahbadia et al. (eds.), *Textbook of Assisted Reproduction*, https://doi.org/10.1007/978-981-15-2377-9_34

MHC region has been subdivided into three regions: class I, class II, and class III. The extended MHC region also includes extended class I and extended class II regions [17]. Each region contains numerous gene loci which can be classified as protein coding, gene candidate, non-protein coding, and pseudogenes. Of the 253 gene loci in the extended MHC region, only 45 are known to be HLA-like, specifically HLA-class I, MIC, and HLA-class II genes [22].

34.3.1 Class I Region

The class I region includes the genes encoding the six classical and non-classical class I HLA antigens. The three classical class I antigens (HLA-A, HLA-B, and HLA-C) are highly polymorphic and expressed on almost all cells, excluding erythrocytes and trophoblasts [22, 23]. The three non-classical class I antigens (HLA-E, HLA-F, and HLA-G) are distinguished by more limited polymorphisms and restricted tissue expression. The classical class I HLA is responsible for the T-cell-mediated cytotoxicity in response to intracellular foreign proteins. Class I HLA antigens are dimerized membrane-bound proteins that are capable of presenting antigens to the outside. The classical class I HLAs (HLA-A, HLA-B, and HLA-C) present short peptides from inside the cell to CD8 T-cells. In brief, foreign proteins are engulfed by host cells and digested into smaller peptides, which are presented on the surface of cells. The presented peptides are about nine amino acids in length and are produced from proteins that are broken down by proteasomes inside the cell. Peptides derived from foreign (non-self) proteins that are presented on the class I MHC are recognized as foreign antigens by cytotoxic T-cells, and a cascade is initiated that ultimately results in cellular death [22, 23].

34.3.2 Class II Region

The class II region includes the genes encoding the three classical class II HLA antigens (HLA-DP, HLA-DQ, and HLA-DR). These antigens are highly polymorphic and are constitutively expressed on the surface of antigen-presenting cells, specifically immune cells (B-cells, dendritic cells, macrophages, and monocytes) [22, 23]. Research demonstrated that dramatic increases in the expression of the classical class II HLA antigens could occur during immune system activation, and these antigens can be expressed on cell types that generally have little to no expression of the classical class II antigens [24]. The class II region also contains other non-classical class II HLA antigens (HLA-DMA, HLA-DMB, HLA-DMO, HLA-LMP2 and HLA-LMP7, among others), some of which assist in the class I antigen processing and presentation system.

The classical class II HLA antigens consist of two transmembrane chains (alpha and beta), each with two domains. The distal domains on each chain associate non-covalently outside the cell membrane to the peptide-binding groove, where antigens are presented to the T-cells. Class II HLA is mostly responsible for the B-cell-mediated humoral toxicity in response to extracellular foreign proteins [22, 23]. The classical class II HLA (HLA- DP, HLA-DQ, and HLA-DR) present antigens from outside the cell to CD4 T-cells (T-helper cells). In brief, foreign antigen presentation results in the multiplication of CD4 T-cells, which in turn stimulate B-cells to produce antibodies or cell-mediated immune response (cytotoxic T-cells) against a specific foreign antigen [22, 23].

34.3.3 Class III Region

The class III region is found between the class I and II genes and includes the genes encoding for diverse immune responses such as complement components (C2, C4, and factor B), cytokines (TNF, LTA, LTB), and heat shock proteins [25]. Although this region contains no known HLA class I- and class II-like genes, many of the genes expressed in this region mediate immune responses. They have critical roles in various cellular processes such as transcription regulation, housekeeping, biosynthesis, electron transport and hydrolase activity, protein-protein interactions for either intracellular or intercellular interactions, chaperone function, and signaling [22].

34.4 Methods of HLA Typing

Identification of HLA genotyping is complicated by the many sequence and structural variations of the MHC locus in different population. Currently, HLA typing is done using DNA-based typing techniques [26]. DNA-based typing techniques begin with extracting DNA from the leukocytes of a patient's blood. A variety of molecular-based methods are then available to determine which alleles are present, including sequence-specific oligonucleotide probe hybridization (SSOP) [27], sequence-specific primer amplification (SSP) [28], and sequencing-based typing (SBT) [29]. The most commonly used methods are SSOP and SBT, while simpler methods such as PCR-restriction fragment length polymorphism (RFLP) [30] and reference strand-based conformation analysis (RSCA) [31] are no longer used [26].

In SSOP, the extracted DNA undergoes PCR amplification using a set of primers to selectively amplify the desired loci. The amplified section is then probed with various SSOPs designed to bind complement sequences on the PCR product and that have nonradioactive labels. The binding patterns of various SSOPs to an amplified PCR product are pieced together to the identity of the specific allele. Given the complexity and polymorphisms of HLA alleles, a single SSOP probe is rarely able to identify a single allele, and a multitude of various probes must be utilized. In SBT, the extracted DNA also undergoes PCR amplification of desired loci as in SSOP. However, after amplification and isolation of the PCR product, Sanger sequencing is then used to determine the nucleotide sequence of the PCR product to identify the allele.

Both SSOP and SBT methods are very beneficial for clinical and research purposes. However, SSOP gives low-resolution allelic typing results, whereas SBT can give high-resolution results that identify specific polymorphisms. As SBT can sequence both conserved and polymorphic regions of a gene, it thus enables identification of new alleles, which may not be possible with methods such as SSOP that rely on known sequences for identification.

As molecular DNA-based typing techniques remain expensive and time-consuming, a great deal of research has gone into next-generation sequencing (NGS) techniques that offer a combination of clonal amplification with the ability to sequence larger regions of genes, including introns [32]. Additionally, the recent availability of dense genotyping platforms, such as the Immunochip (Illumina SNP chip) [33], has allowed for fine mapping, and genotyping that is a cheaper, faster, and an easier alternative than direct MHC typing and NGS methods [34]. These technologies, although gaining in popularity, are still evolving and carry the promise to further elucidate the role of HLA in reproductive health.

34.5 HLA in Normal Pregnancy

Efficient systems of immunotolerance are required for successful establishment and continuance of pregnancy as mothers and their embryo/fetus are invariably genetically dissimilar. Currently, there is no consensus regarding the exact mechanisms by which the mother host does not reject the "foreign" embryo/fetus, although research has identified multiple overlapping and redundant mechanisms of tolerance. Of relevance are the studies identifying the importance of HLA-G in implantation and pregnancy.

In pregnancy, the uterus and placenta produce several types of soluble immunosuppressive molecules and are populated by several types of leukocytes with immunosuppressing properties [35]. During implantation, the blastocyst invades the mother's decidua resulting in a physical relationship between the maternal and embryo tissues [35]. At this point, cells from the trophectoderm layer of the blastocyst begin to specialize into the villous cytotrophoblasts, syncytiotrophoblasts (cellular layer that forms the barrier between the embryonic/fetal placenta and maternal blood), and extravillous cytotrophoblasts. The latter invade maternal decidua and have a significant role in maintaining maternal blood flow to the placenta from week 10 through parturition [35]. To avoid stimulating rejection of the embryo, these trophoblast cells which are in immediate juxtaposition to maternal blood and immune cells are immune privileged and do not express class Ia HLA-A or HLA-B or class II HLA molecules [35]. On the other hand, trophoblast cells do express class Ib HLA molecules, HLA-E, HLA-F, and HLA-G [8, 35]. The best studied of these three genes is HLA-G which is unique to the trophoblast and has been demonstrated to have diverse functions. Most importantly, it has immunomodulatory properties that may attenuate the maternal immune response at the maternal-fetal interface [35].

The HLA-G molecule is characterized by mRNA alternative splicing that generates seven protein isoforms; four isoforms are membrane-bound (HLA-G1, HLA-G2, HLA-G3, and HLA-G4), whereas three isoforms are soluble (sHLA-G5, sHLA-G6, and sHLA-G7) [36, 37]. According to the IMGT/HLA database, nucleotide variations in HLA-G result in 50 alleles, 16 proteins, and 2 null alleles [15]. Low levels of sHLA-G have been associated with some pregnancy complications, such as recurrent spontaneous miscarriages, pre-eclampsia, and in vitro fertilization (IVF) implantation failure [38, 39]. Multiple genetic and epigenetic factors may modify HLA-G gene expression and protein levels [40]. The soluble HLA-G forms are detectable in the plasma of women, both non-pregnant and pregnant [37]. Most nucleotide polymorphisms of the HLA-G gene do not alter amino acid sequence; however, they may have an impact on transcription and level of mRNA expression. HLA-G gene expression may be modified by specific polymorphisms that are present in the regulatory regions of the gene [41]. Furthermore, the 14-bp insertion/deletion (ins/del) polymorphism in exon 8 also affects the gene expression [42].

Unlike other HLA antigens, the leading role of HLA-G in the embryo/fetal trophoblasts is not the presentation of antigens to leukocytes but instead functions in immunosuppression and tolerance. It has been evidenced that HLA-G is an inhibitory ligand that selectively targets and binds to leukocyte immunoglobulin-like receptors B1 found on uterine lymphocytes, macrophages, and dendritic cells and LILRB2 expressed solely on uterine macrophages and dendritic cells [35]. The result of HLA-G binding to LILRB1/LILRB2 causes interference of the leukocyte activating signals resulting in an immune suppressing effect by (1) inhibiting CD8 T-cell killing; (2) suppressing CD4 T-cell induction and proliferation; (3) negatively impacting natural killer cell killing, migration, proliferation, and cytokine production; (4) regulating cytokine production of maternal mononuclear leukocytes and CD8 T-cells; and (5) modifying dendritic cell activation and maturation [35]. Furthermore, HLA-G interacts with endothelial cells and induces angiogenesis via inducing chemokines and cytokines from uterine natural killer cells (uNK).

Soluble HLA-G is found not only in the plasma of pregnant women but also in the amniotic fluid and supernatant culture media from in vitro-cultured embryos [37]. Studies have demonstrated the sHLA-G influence cytokine production by maternal mononuclear leukocytes and can induce maternal CD8 T-cell death, resulting in an immunosuppressive effect. Several reports suggest that levels of HLA-G may predict reproductive success and that the various polymorphisms of HLA-G may affect the level of sHLA-G in the plasma [35, 43]. Research has associated low expression of sHLA-G in the maternal plasma with HLA-G*01:01:03 and HLA-G*01:05 N alleles, intermediate levels with HLA-G*01:01:08 and HLA-G*01:04b alleles, and high expression levels with HLA-G*01:04:01 and HLA-G*-1:01 g [42, 44]. Reduced sHLA-G protein expression in the maternal plasma is thus linked to HLA-G alleles and had been associated with disruption of the maternal-fetal interface and reproductive failure [38]. Studies have shown that the presence of an HLA-G*0104 or HLA-G*0105 N allele in either partner was significantly associated with an increase in the risk for recurrent miscarriage [45], and fetal allele HLA-G*0106 was associated with increase in the risk for miscarriage and preeclampsia [46, 47].

34.6 HLA and Infertility

The predominance of specific HLA alleles in women seeking fertility and IVF treatment has not been well studied. Costa et al. reported on HLA genotyping in 33 couples undergoing assisted reproduction treatment (cases) and 120 naturally conceiving couples (controls). They demonstrated that the haplotype HLA-G*01:01:01 showed significantly higher frequency in the control group [38]. The promoter region of this haplotype has been described as an "infertility protector," and its coding region has been associated with high serum levels of sHLA-G. Intriguingly, the outcome of this study showed that those with successful outcomes after ART shared the same haplotype (HLA-G*01:01:01) as the control women [38].

34.6.1 HLA and In Vitro Fertilization (IVF)

Recent research into the role of HLA in IVF and intracytoplasmic sperm injection (ICSI) has focused on the association between pregnancy successes and failures with various HLA-G alleles, but no consensus currently exists as to what alleles are "protective" and which alleles render one "susceptible" to having to utilize ART. Much of this has to do with the variability of expression of similar alleles. One study reported that that HLA-G*01:03 was more frequently observed in control couples compared to infertile couples [48], while another study has shown that a very similar allele, HLA-G*01:03:01, was commonly found in couples with implantation failure [38].

Of much focus is a 14 bp insertion/deletion polymorphism in exon 8 of the 3'UTR present in both the HLA-G gene and transcript that has been associated with HLA-gene expression and thus levels of s-HLA-G [49]. HLA-G homozygous for 14 bp deletion allele was associated with the highest mean birth weight and placental weight compared to HLA-G homozygous for 14 bp insertion allele ($P = 0.008$ and $P = 0.009$) [11].

A study by Costa et al. that included 25 ART couples and 94 control couples found that allele HLA-G*01:01:02a with the 14 bp *deletion* was more frequent in the control group and associated with successful pregnancy and adequate levels of sHLA-G (protective), whereas the same allele with the 14 bp *insertion* was more frequent in the case group and associated the need for ART and insufficient levels of sHLA-G (susceptible) [38]. Additionally, stratification of the case group demonstrated that those who underwent ART with failure had a higher frequency of HLA-G*01:01:02a with the 14 bp insertion [38]. Multiple studies and a meta-analysis have demonstrated an association between the 14 bp insertion and decreased sHLA-G levels and increased risk of IVF and recurrent implantation failure, with the risk being greater in those women who are homozygous for the 14 bp insertion [38, 50, 51]. However, the effects of the 14 bp insertion on reproductive processes have shown contradictory results as other authors have found that the 14 bp insertion has no influence on the clinical outcome of patients undergoing ART [52].

A great deal of research has been dedicated to elucidating the role of sHLA-G levels in the culture media on pregnancy success. Multiple studies have focused on the positive association between levels of sHLA-G and implantation success in IVF and ICSI [53]; however, not all studies corroborate these findings [54]. In one study examining the concentration of sHLA-G in the embryo culture media and embryo morphology of 326 embryos from 49 couples undergoing IVF which was associated with pregnancy outcome, all patients who became pregnant had at least one embryo with a culture media sHLA-G concentration ≥2 U/mL, and no patients who had transfers of all embryos with sHLA-G concentration <2 U/mL became pregnant [55]. Findings showed a 65% pregnancy rate with "good grade" embryos (7–8 cells, grade 1–2) with sHLA-G concentration ≥2 U/mL, demonstrating that adequate sHLA-G concentrations are essential, but not sufficient for successful implantation [55]. In contrast, a blinded study examining sHLA-G concentration was performed on 1405 embryo supernatants from 355 patients from three ART centers and found that only in one center was there a significant association between sHLA-G positive embryo supernatants and successful implantation, whereas no association was found in the other centers [54]. The study also determined that the percentage of sHLA-G positive embryo supernatants was significantly higher in those supernatants from IVF than ICSI and that the percentage and concentrations of sHLA-G positive embryo supernatants varied between centers contingent on culture media and ART conditions. A multicenter study of 2364 IVF cycles randomly collected from 29 German ART centers suggested that sHLA-G testing was an independent factor in improving the pregnancy rate from 30 to 40% [56]. A recent meta-analysis of 15 studies over 6170 patients investigating the diagnostic accuracy of sHLA-G concentration in embryo supernatant for predicting pregnancy success concluded that the presence of sHLA-G in the embryo culture medium favored higher pregnancy rate (3.79, 95% CI: 2.69–5.33, $P < 0.00001$). The authors recommended further clinical studies to confirm the beneficial effect [57].

Interestingly, other reproductive organs also secrete HLA-G. sHLA-G was identified in seminal plasma of infertile men [58]. Men with HLA-G del14bp/del14b allele have a higher level and showed a trend toward their female partner becoming pregnant after ART [58]. sHLA-G was also identified in follicular fluids of women undergoing IVF (19/50, 38%) [59]. Further research is needed to determine the clinical application of these measurements.

34.7 HLA and Implantation Failure

The success of IVF is dependent upon implantation of the genetically dissimilar embryo into the maternal endometrium. HLA-G is expressed in the preimplantation embryos which can be secreted by embryonic stem cells [60, 61]. Expression of HLA-G in early embryos is important for the obtainment of pregnancy [8, 62]. The presence of HLA-G-specific transcripts in preimplantation embryos was associated with increased blastocyst cleavage rate and significantly greater number of blastomeres per embryo at 24–48 h after fertilization ($P < 0.001$) [7]. Studies examining the relationship between HLA sharing of partners and adverse pregnancy outcomes have shown mixed findings. Studies from the early 1990s suggested that that genetic similarity, defined as the sharing of more than one HLA loci, may lead to recurrent miscarriages, with a case series demonstrating pregnancy success in couples with HLA similarity and repeated IVF failure after IVIG treatment (ten patients, five pregnant) [63]. Live birth rates were improved after IVIG in a subset of women with repeated IVF failure and elevated circulating natural killer cells (CD56+) (38% and 0%, $P < 0.0001$, 64]. A 2013 systemic review of ten studies showed improved implantation rate, clinical pregnancy rate, and live birth rate in women with repeated IVF/ICSI failure and unexplained infertility; the live birth rate per embryo transferred was nevertheless not impacted [65]. However, a recent study examined the level of HLA dissimilarity between couples with recurrent implantation failure, and those with successful implantation found no association between recurrent implantation failure and the degree of histocompatibility between partners or sharing of a specific HLA antigen ($n = 72$) [66]. Multiple studies corroborating these findings with another study of 25 patients showed that IVIG did not improve the live birth rate in couples with repeated unexplained IVF failure (15% vs.12%, $P = 0.52$) [67]. A 2015 meta-analyses of 41 studies evaluating whether HLA sharing of couples was associated with the occurrence of recurrent miscarriage concluded that although the results demonstrated an association, the studies contained a high degree of bias and results should be interpreted cautiously [68]. More research is needed in this area to elucidate potential associations between HLA sharing, recurrent miscarriages, and the need for ART.

34.8 HLA and Early Pregnancy Loss

Maternal-fetal tolerance and embryo invasion of the uterine lining by the extravillous trophoblast are regulated by uNK [24, 69]. uNK express maternal killer immunoglobulin-like receptors (KIRs) that bind to their ligand, HLA-C and HLA-G, expressed on the extravillous trophoblast [70]. There are multiple KIR receptor isoforms resulting in two KIR receptor haplotypes. KIR A haplotype consists of inhibitory genotypes, whereas KIR B haplotype consists of activating genotypes. The effect of KIR receptor and HLA-C on pregnancy loss in IVF was reported in two studies [71, 72]. Alecsandru et al. studied KIR haplotypes in 1304 IVF cycles in women who received two embryo transfers [71]. Pregnancy loss after IVF was more common in KIR A haplotype carriers when compared to KIR B haplotype carriers (22.8% vs. 11.1%; $P = 0.03$). Similarly, donor egg cycles with two embryo transfers showed a reduction in live birth rate with KIR B haplotype (7.5% vs. 26.4%; $P = 0.006$) [71]. Morin et al. investigated the effect of HLA-C on early pregnancy loss in the context of IVF and uterine natural killer cells (uNK) [72]. The impact of maternal KIR haplotype and embryonic HLA-C genotype on pregnancy outcomes in 668 IVF cycles in which a single euploid embryo was transferred was investigated. Pregnancy loss after IVF was significantly decreased in women with KIR A haplotype compared to KIR B haplotype (16% vs. 27.8%, RR 0.57, 95%; $P < 0.01$). The different effect of KIR haplotype on pregnancy outcome between the two above-mentioned studies may be related to different study design as only euploid embryos were transferred in the later study. Morin et al. also investigated the effect of the blastocyst HLA-C zygosity in relation to KIR haplotype [72]. The pregnancy loss rates were further affected by the embryo's HLA-C genotype status. KIR A patients who received an embryo that was homozygous for the HLA-C genotype (C1/C1) have the least pregnancy loss [72].

34.9 Conclusions

The immunogenetics of the maternal-fetal interface, implantation, pregnancy, and infertility are complex and multifactorial. There is currently no consensus on the roles of different HLA-G alleles in these processes. Currently, findings suggest that variant promoter and coding regions of the different HLA-G alleles are associated with variant levels of gene expression which could be vital to the gestational success of a couple. Certain HLA-G alleles are associated with poor IVF outcome including implantation failure, early pregnancy loss, and poor placentation. Further research is needed into HLA variant alleles to elucidate their effects on gene expression and determine if there is a causal link between variants and infertility and reproductive failure.

References

1. Abrams ET, Miller EM. The roles of the immune system in women's reproduction: evolutionary constraints and life history trade-offs. Am J Phys Anthropol. 2011;146(Suppl 53):134–54.
2. Slukvin II, Lunn DP, Watkins DI, Golos TG. Placental expression of the nonclassical MHC class I molecule Mamu-AG at implantation in the rhesus monkey. Proc Natl Acad Sci U S A. 2000;97:9104–9.
3. Rapacz-Leonard A, Dabrowska M, Janowski T. Major histocompatibility complex I mediates immunological tolerance of the trophoblast during pregnancy and may mediate rejection during parturition. Mediat Inflamm. 2014:579279.
4. Hviid TV, Christiansen OB. Linkage disequilibrium between human leukocyte antigen (HLA) class II and HLA-G--possible implications for human reproduction and autoimmune disease. Hum Immunol. 2005;66:688–99.
5. O'Brien M, McCarthy T, Jenkins D, Paul P, Dausset J, Carosella ED, Moreau P. Altered HLA-G transcription in pre-eclampsia is associated with allele specific inheritance: possible role of the HLA-G gene in susceptibility to the disease. Cell Mol Life Sci. 2001;58:1943–9.
6. Pfeiffer KA, Rebmann V, Passler M, van der Ven K, van der Ven H, Krebs D, Grosse-Wilde H. Soluble HLA levels in early pregnancy after in vitro fertilization. Hum Immunol. 2000;61:559–64.
7. Jurisicova A, Casper RF, MacLusky NJ, Mills GB, Librach CL. HLA-G expression during preimplantation human embryo development. Proc Natl Acad Sci U S A. 1996;93:161–5.
8. Fuzzi B, Rizzo R, Criscuoli L, Noci I, Melchiorri L, Scarselli B, Bencini E, Menicucci A, Baricordi OR. HLA-G expression in early embryos is a fundamental prerequisite for the obtainment of pregnancy. Eur J Immunol. 2002;32:311–5.
9. Emmery J, Hachmon R, Pyo CW, Nelson WC, Geraghty DE, Andersen AM, Melbye M, Hviid TV. Maternal and fetal human leukocyte antigen class Ia and II alleles in severe preeclampsia and eclampsia. Genes Immun. 2016;17:251–60.
10. Martinetti M, Beneventi F, Capittini C, Locatelli E, Simonetta M, Cavagnoli C, De Maggio I, De Silvestri A, Pasi A, Spinillo A. The immunosignature of mother/fetus couples in gestational diabetes mellitus: role of HLA-G 14 bp ins/del and PAPP-A A/C polymorphisms in the uterine inflammatory milieu. Dis Markers. 2017:4254750.
11. Emmery J, Christiansen OB, Nilsson LL, Dahl M, Skovbo P, Moller AM, Steffensen R, Hviid TVF. Associations between fetal HLA-G genotype and birth weight and placental weight in a large cohort of pregnant women—possible implications for HLA diversity. J Reprod Immunol. 2017;120:8–14.
12. Kahraman S, Beyazyurek C, Yesilipek MA, Ozturk G, Ertem M, Anak S, Kansoy S, Aksoylar S, Kuskonmaz B, Oniz H, Slavin S, Karakas Z, et al. Successful haematopoietic stem cell transplantation in 44 children from healthy siblings conceived after preimplantation HLA matching. Reprod Biomed Online. 2014;29:340–51.
13. Tur-Kaspa I, Jeelani R. Clinical guidelines for IVF with PGD for HLA matching. Reprod Biomed Online. 2015;30:115–9.
14. Tripodis N, Mason R, Humphray SJ, Davies AF, Herberg JA, Trowsdale J, Nizetic D, Senger G, Ragoussis J. Physical map of human 6p21.2-6p21.3: region flanking the centromeric end of the major histocompatibility complex. Genome Res. 1998;8:631–43.
15. http://www.ebi.ac.uk/imgt/hla/. IMGT/HLA Database Homepage. 2003.
16. Complete sequence and gene map of a human major histocompatibility complex. The MHC sequencing consortium. Nature. 1999;401:921–3.
17. Dorak MT, Shao W, Machulla HK, Lobashevsky ES, Tang J, Park MH, Kaslow RA. Conserved extended haplotypes of the major histocompatibility complex: further characterization. Genes Immun. 2006;7:450–67.
18. Ziegler A, Kentenich H, Uchanska-Ziegler B. Female choice and the MHC. Trends Immunol. 2005;26:496–502.
19. Beauchamp GK, Yamazaki K, Bard J, Boyse EA. Preweaning experience in the control of mating preferences by genes in the major histocompatibility complex of the mouse. Behav Genet. 1988;18:537–47.
20. Yamazaki K, Beauchamp GK, Shen FW, Bard J, Boyse EA. Discrimination of odortypes determined by the major histocompatibility complex among outbred mice. Proc Natl Acad Sci U S A. 1994;91:3735–8.
21. Manning CJ, Wakeland EK, Potts WK. Communal nesting patterns in mice implicate MHC genes in kin recognition. Nature. 1992;360:581–3.
22. Shiina T, Hosomichi K, Inoko H, Kulski JK. The HLA genomic loci map: expression, interaction, diversity and disease. J Hum Genet. 2009;54:15–39.
23. McCluskey J, Peh CA. The human leucocyte antigens and clinical medicine: an overview. Rev Immunogenet. 1999;1:3–20.
24. Halloran PF, Wadgymar A, Autenried P. The regulation of expression of major histocompatibility complex products. Transplantation. 1986;41:413–20.
25. Gruen JR, Weissman SM. Human MHC class III and IV genes and disease associations. Front Biosci. 2001;6:D960–72.
26. Dunn PP. Human leucocyte antigen typing: techniques and technology, a critical appraisal. Int J Immunogenet. 2011;38:463–73.
27. Cao K, Chopek M, Fernandez-Vina MA. High and intermediate resolution DNA typing systems for class I HLA-A, B, C genes by hybridization with sequence-specific oligonucleotide probes (SSOP). Rev Immunogenet. 1999;1:177–208.
28. Bunce M, O'Neill CM, Barnardo MC, Krausa P, Browning MJ, Morris PJ, Welsh KI. Phototyping: comprehensive DNA typing for HLA-A, B, C, DRB1, DRB3, DRB4, DRB5 & DQB1 by PCR with 144 primer mixes utilizing sequence-specific primers (PCR-SSP). Tissue Antigens. 1995;46:355–67.
29. Dunn PP, Cox ST, Little AM. Sequencing protocols for detection of HLA class I polymorphism. Methods Mol Biol. 2003;210:191–222.

30. Riisom K, Soorensen IJ, Mooller B, Kruse TA, Graugaard B, Lamm LU. HLA-DR typing using restriction fragment length polymorphism (RFLP) with one enzyme and two probes. Tissue Antigens. 1988;31:141–50.
31. Arguello JR, Madrigal JA. HLA typing by reference strand mediated conformation analysis (RSCA). Rev Immunogenet. 1999;1:209–19.
32. Holcomb CL, Hoglund B, Anderson MW, Blake LA, Bohme I, Egholm M, Ferriola D, Gabriel C, Gelber SE, Goodridge D, Hawbecker S, Klein R, et al. A multi-site study using high-resolution HLA genotyping by next generation sequencing. Tissue Antigens. 2011;77:206–17.
33. Cortes A, Brown MA. Promise and pitfalls of the immunochip. Arthritis Res Ther. 2011;13:101.
34. Matzaraki V, Kumar V, Wijmenga C, Zhernakova A. The MHC locus and genetic susceptibility to autoimmune and infectious diseases. Genome Biol. 2017;18:76.
35. Hunt JS, Langat DL. HLA-G: a human pregnancy-related immunomodulator. Curr Opin Pharmacol. 2009;9:462–9.
36. Rizzo R, Melchiorri L, Stignani M, Baricordi OR. HLA-G expression is a fundamental prerequisite to pregnancy. Hum Immunol. 2007;68:244–50.
37. Rizzo R, Andersen AS, Lassen MR, Sorensen HC, Bergholt T, Larsen MH, Melchiorri L, Stignani M, Baricordi OR, Hviid TV. Soluble human leukocyte antigen-G isoforms in maternal plasma in early and late pregnancy. Am J Reprod Immunol. 2009;62:320–38.
38. Costa CH, Gelmini GF, Wowk PF, Mattar SB, Vargas RG, Roxo VM, Schuffner A, Bicalho MG. HLA-G regulatory haplotypes and implantation outcome in couples who underwent assisted reproduction treatment. Hum Immunol. 2012;73:891–7.
39. Hviid TV, Hylenius S, Hoegh AM, Kruse C, Christiansen OB. HLA-G polymorphisms in couples with recurrent spontaneous abortions. Tissue Antigens. 2002;60:122–32.
40. Rebmann V, da Silva NF, Wagner B, Horn PA. HLA-G as a tolerogenic molecule in transplantation and pregnancy. J Immunol Res. 2014;2014:297073.
41. Hviid TV, Rizzo R, Melchiorri L, Stignani M, Baricordi OR. Polymorphism in the 5' upstream regulatory and 3' untranslated regions of the HLA-G gene in relation to soluble HLA-G and IL-10 expression. Hum Immunol. 2006;67:53–62.
42. Rebmann V, van der Ven K, Passler M, Pfeiffer K, Krebs D, Grosse-Wilde H. Association of soluble HLA-G plasma levels with HLA-G alleles. Tissue Antigens. 2001;57:15–21.
43. Morandi F, Rizzo R, Fainardi E, Rouas-Freiss N, Pistoia V. Recent advances in our understanding of HLA-G biology: lessons from a wide spectrum of human diseases. J Immunol Res. 2016;2016:4326495.
44. Hviid TV, Hylenius S, Rorbye C, Nielsen LG. HLA-G allelic variants are associated with differences in the HLA-G mRNA isoform profile and HLA-G mRNA levels. Immunogenetics. 2003;55:63–79.
45. Aldrich CL, Stephenson MD, Karrison T, Odem RR, Branch DW, Scott JR, Schreiber JR, Ober C. HLA-G genotypes and pregnancy outcome in couples with unexplained recurrent miscarriage. Mol Hum Reprod. 2001;7:1167–72.
46. Moreau P, Contu L, Alba F, Lai S, Simoes R, Orru S, Carcassi C, Roger M, Rabreau M, Carosella ED. HLA-G gene polymorphism in human placentas: possible association of G*0106 allele with pre-eclampsia and miscarriage. Biol Reprod. 2008;79:459–67.
47. Tan CY, Ho JF, Chong YS, Loganath A, Chan YH, Ravichandran J, Lee CG, Chong SS. Paternal contribution of HLA-G*0106 significantly increases risk for pre-eclampsia in multigravid pregnancies. Mol Hum Reprod. 2008;14:317–24.
48. Nardi Fda S, Slowik R, Wowk PF, da Silva JS, Gelmini GF, Michelon TF, Neumann J, Bicalho MG. Analysis of HLA-G polymorphisms in couples with implantation failure. Am J Reprod Immunol. 2012;68:507–14.
49. Rousseau P, Le Discorde M, Mouillot G, Marcou C, Carosella ED, Moreau P. The 14 bp deletion-insertion polymorphism in the 3' UT region of the HLA-G gene influences HLA-G mRNA stability. Hum Immunol. 2003;64:1005–10.
50. Fan W, Huang Z, Li S, Xiao Z. The HLA-G 14-bp polymorphism and recurrent implantation failure: a meta-analysis. J Assist Reprod Genet. 2017;34:1559–65.
51. Enghelabifar M, Allafan S, Khayatzadeh J, Shahrokh Abadi K, Hasanzadeh Nazarabadi M, Moradi F, Musavifar N, Jalali M, Mojarrad M. Association of the maternal 14-bp insertion/deletion polymorphism in the histocompatibility leukocyte antigen G gene with recurrent implantation failure. Iran J Reprod Med. 2014;12:641–6.
52. Sipak-Szmigiel O, Cybulski C, Wokolorczyk D, Lubinski J, Kurzawa R, Baczkowski T, Radwan M, Radwan P, Ronin-Walknowska E. HLA-G polymorphism and in vitro fertilization failure in a Polish population. Tissue Antigens. 2009;73:348–52.
53. Sher G, Keskintepe L, Batzofin J, Fisch J, Acacio B, Ahlering P, Ginsburg M. Influence of early ICSI-derived embryo sHLA-G expression on pregnancy and implantation rates: a prospective study. Hum Reprod. 2005;20:1359–63.
54. Tabiasco J, Perrier d'Hauterive S, Thonon F, Parinaud J, Leandri R, Foidart JM, Chaouat G, Munaut C, Lombroso R, Selva J, Bergere M, Hammoud I, et al. Soluble HLA-G in IVF/ICSI embryo culture supernatants does not always predict implantation success: a multicentre study. Reprod Biomed Online. 2009;18:374–81.
55. Roussev RG, Coulam CB. HLA-G and its role in implantation (review). J Assist Reprod Genet. 2007;24:288–95.
56. Rebmann V, Switala M, Eue I, Grosse-Wilde H. Soluble HLA-G is an independent factor for the prediction of pregnancy outcome after ART: a German multi-centre study. Hum Reprod. 2010;25:1691–8.
57. Niu Z, Wang L, Pang RTK, Guo Y, Yeung WSB, Yao Y. A meta-analysis of the impact of human leukocyte antigen-G on the outcomes of IVF/ICSI. Reprod Biomed Online. 2017;34:611–8.
58. Dahl M, Perin TL, Djurisic S, Rasmussen M, Ohlsson J, Buus S, Lindhard A, Hviid TV. Soluble human leukocyte antigen-G in seminal plasma is associated with HLA-G genotype: possible implications for fertility success. Am J Reprod Immunol. 2014;72:89–105.
59. Rizzo R, Fuzzi B, Stignani M, Criscuoli L, Melchiorri L, Dabizzi S, Campioni D, Lanza F, Marzola A, Branconi F, Noci I, Baricordi OR. Soluble HLA-G molecules in follicular fluid: a tool for oocyte selection in IVF? J Reprod Immunol. 2007;74:133–42.
60. Golos TG, Giakoumopoulos M, Gerami-Naini B. Review: trophoblast differentiation from human embryonic stem cells. Placenta. 2013;34(Suppl):S56–61.
61. Verloes A, Van de Velde H, LeMaoult J, Mateizel I, Cauffman G, Horn PA, Carosella ED, Devroey P, De Waele M, Rebmann V, Vercammen M. HLA-G expression in human embryonic stem cells and preimplantation embryos. J Immunol. 2011;186:2663–71.
62. Jurisicova A, Antenos M, Kapasi K, Meriano J, Casper RF. Variability in the expression of trophectodermal markers beta-human chorionic gonadotrophin, human leukocyte antigen-G and pregnancy specific beta-1 glycoprotein by the human blastocyst. Hum Reprod. 1999;14:1852–8.
63. Elram T, Simon A, Israel S, Revel A, Shveiky D, Laufer N. Treatment of recurrent IVF failure and human leukocyte antigen similarity by intravenous immunoglobulin. Reprod Biomed Online. 2005;11:745–9.
64. Coulam CB, Goodman C. Increased pregnancy rates after IVF/ET with intravenous immunoglobulin treatment in women with elevated circulating C56+ cells. Early Pregnancy. 2000;4:90–8.
65. Li J, Chen Y, Liu C, Hu Y, Li L. Intravenous immunoglobulin treatment for repeated IVF/ICSI failure and unexplained infertility: a

systematic review and a meta-analysis. Am J Reprod Immunol. 2013;70:434–47.
66. Lashley LE, van der Westerlaken LA, Haasnoot GW, Drabbels JJ, Spruyt-Gerritse MJ, Scherjon SA, Claas FH. Maternal HLA-C2 and 14 bp insertion in HLA-G is associated with recurrent implantation failure after in vitro fertilization treatment. Tissue Antigens. 2014;84:536–44.
67. Stephenson MD, Fluker MR. Treatment of repeated unexplained in vitro fertilization failure with intravenous immunoglobulin: a randomized, placebo-controlled Canadian trial. Fertil Steril. 2000;74:1108–13.
68. Meuleman T, Lashley LE, Dekkers OM, van Lith JM, Claas FH, Bloemenkamp KW. HLA associations and HLA sharing in recurrent miscarriage: a systematic review and meta-analysis. Hum Immunol. 2015;76:362–73.
69. Nowak I, Wilczynska K, Wilczynski JR, Malinowski A, Radwan P, Radwan M, Kusnierczyk P. KIR, LILRB and their ligands' genes as potential biomarkers in recurrent implantation failure. Arch Immunol Ther Exp. 2017;65:391–9.
70. Moffett A, Colucci F. Uterine NK cells: active regulators at the maternal-fetal interface. J Clin Invest. 2014;124:1872–9.
71. Alecsandru D, Garrido N, Vicario JL, Barrio A, Aparicio P, Requena A, Garcia-Velasco JA. Maternal KIR haplotype influences live birth rate after double embryo transfer in IVF cycles in patients with recurrent miscarriages and implantation failure. Hum Reprod. 2014;29:2637–43.
72. Morin SJ, Treff NR, Tao X, Scott RT 3rd, Franasiak JM, Juneau CR, Maguire M, Scott RT. Combination of uterine natural killer cell immunoglobulin receptor haplotype and trophoblastic HLA-C ligand influences the risk of pregnancy loss: a retrospective cohort analysis of direct embryo genotyping data from euploid transfers. Fertil Steril. 2017;107:677–683 e672.

Bleeding Disorders and ART

35

Veronika Levin, Rachel Booth, and Shahab Minassian

35.1 Physiology of Hemostasis

Hemostasis is a normal physiologic function that is integral to tissue perfusion as well as the appropriate functioning of organs. As such, in the event of inevitable occurrences of vessel injury, they must be resolved quickly. The process is accomplished by a sophisticated balance of clot formation and clot lysis, consisting of an interplay between platelets and the coagulation cascade when functioning correctly [1]. When vessel injury first occurs, it cues von Willebrand factor to bind to subendothelial collagen on one end with platelet receptors at the other end. Following this, platelet adhesion results in the release of numerous mediating factors, all of which contribute to vasoconstriction and platelet activation. Platelet activation is just one component of hemostasis. In the event of a substantial vascular insult, the coagulation cascade must also be involved to form a sufficient fibrin plug, achieving satisfactory hemostasis [1, 2].

Coagulation factors are created by the liver. These initially exist in an inactive state until recruited, at which time they become active through an intricate cascade network. To briefly simplify the coagulation cascade: it involves the intrinsic pathway (factors XII, XI, IX, VIII) and extrinsic pathway (tissue thromboplastin and factor VII), which eventually converge to activate the common pathway (factors X, V, II, and I). This process then allows fibrinogen to convert into fibrin, forming a stabilized clot. Fibrinogen is essential to normal hemostasis as it is a substrate for conversion to fibrin. Fibrin is the support for thrombin generation and platelet aggregation, forming a template for subsequent fibrinolysis and wound healing [1]. When activated, the coagulation cascade is always mitigating hemostasis while also avoiding pathological thrombosis. A prothrombotic state can be a necessary physiologic response to injury; however, equally relevant is how this system is balanced and returns to homeostasis. There are several antithrombotic agents such as protein C and S and antithrombin III, among others that rapidly promote clot lysis. Furthermore, both the platelet system and coagulation cascade must have the appropriate quantity and quality of factors involved in the process to run smoothly, avoiding pathologic states. These pathologic states and inappropriate functioning of elements may ultimately contribute to numerous problems, including failed implantation, and affect assisted reproductive technology (ART) efforts in women desiring pregnancy.

35.2 Assisted Reproductive Technologies (ART)

ART is inclusive of numerous procedures and strategies that target direct manipulation of oocytes [3]. The most common form of ART is in vitro fertilization (IVF), and due to improving technology and updated techniques, the success rates are continuously improving. IVF usually starts with controlled ovarian hyperstimulation by way of exogenous gonadotropins, followed by retrieval of oocytes from the ovaries under transvaginal ultrasound guidance, fertilization in the lab, and ultimately transcervical transfer of embryos into the uterus [3]. The focus of this chapter is on women with thrombophilias and thrombotic disorders undergoing IVF.

V. Levin
Department of Obstetrics and Gynecology, Reading Medical Center, West Reading, PA, USA

R. Booth
Department of Obstetrics & Gynecology, Boonshoft School of Medicine, Wright State University, Dayton, OH, USA
e-mail: rachel.booth@wright.edu

S. Minassian (✉)
Department of Obstetrics and Gynecology, Reading Hospital, West Reading, PA, USA
e-mail: shihab.minassian@towerhealth.org

G. N. Allahbadia et al. (eds.), *Textbook of Assisted Reproduction*, https://doi.org/10.1007/978-981-15-2377-9_35

35.3 Bleeding Disorders

35.3.1 Disorders of Platelets

35.3.1.1 Gestational Thrombocytopenia (GT)

GT can occur commonly during pregnancy and is the most common cause of thrombocytopenia during the third trimester of pregnancy. While the normal platelet count is usually between 150,000 and 450,000/μL, women with GT experience platelet counts drop below the threshold of normal, and this usually is not seen until the third trimester. However, it generally never decreases lower than 70,000/μL. This is important as a progressively decreasing platelet count can be a signal of more serious pathologies and should continue to be monitored. Affected women are asymptomatic and have no history of thrombocytopenia. After delivery, the platelet count is expected to normalize within 3 months. While the pathogenesis of GT remains unclear, it is thought in part to be autoimmune, and the diagnosis does overlap with mild idiopathic thrombocytopenic purpura [4].

35.3.1.2 Idiopathic Thrombocytopenic Purpura (ITP)

ITP is a platelet disorder mediated by platelet antibodies that accelerate platelet destruction and inhibit their production. Specifically, the IgG antibody binds to platelets and renders them susceptible to sequestration and premature damage in the reticuloendothelial system. It is the most common cause of thrombocytopenia during the first two trimesters of pregnancy [4, 5]. ITP is a heterogeneous disorder divided into two discrete entities: acute ITP and chronic ITP. Acute ITP is usually seen in children following a viral illness. The pathophysiology involves the IgG antibody attaching to the viral antigen adsorbed onto the platelet surface, which can result in bleeding from mucous membranes. The disease is self-limiting in the majority of cases, often only requiring observation for treatment. However, if severe bleeding results, oral corticosteroids or intravenous immunoglobulin is used for therapy (typically the treatment modality used for chronic ITP). Chronic ITP has an insidious onset and is most commonly found in adults. It rarely results from a viral illness, and it is not self-limiting as the acute form. Chronic ITP with severe thrombocytopenia and symptoms requires corticosteroids or intravenous immunoglobulin, but if these entities do not help establish hemostasis or improvement in symptoms, then splenectomy may be needed as a last resort [4–6].

35.3.1.3 Thrombotic Thrombocytopenic Purpura (TTP)

TTP is a thrombotic microangiopathy caused by a reduction in von Willebrand factor-cleaving protease, ADAMTS13, activity. This leads to five findings through physical exam and laboratory findings: thrombocytopenia, microangiopathic hemolytic anemia, fever, renal dysfunction, and neurologic signs. The neurologic findings include headache, altered consciousness, seizures, and sensory-motor deficits in most scenarios [7]. The deficiency of ADAMTS13 activity prevents large multimers of circulating von Willebrand factor (vWF) from normal cleavage into normal-sized smaller multimers. This increase in von Willebrand factor causes an imbalance in the cascade that then defaults to inappropriate platelet aggregation and thrombus formation [4]. The condition can either be acquired or familial due to inherited mutations in ADAMTS13, resulting in ADAMTS13 deficiency.

Furthermore, rare cases of drug-induced TTP have been reported after medication exposure to ticlopidine, mitomycin C, cyclosporine, tacrolimus, quinine, and clopidogrel. TTP tends to occur in pregnancy with a mean onset at 23.5 weeks of gestational age; however, it can occur at any point from the first trimester through the postpartum period and usually is present after delivery as well [4]. Treatment of TTP involves plasmapheresis within 24–48 h of diagnosis. While this is the recommended treatment modality, the literature has also shown success rates with fresh frozen plasma infusions and corticosteroids [4, 6].

35.3.1.4 Heparin-Induced Thrombocytopenia (HIT)

HIT is a response to heparin intake and occurs in two distinct types. Type I HIT is not autoimmune in origin and results in no clinical consequences. Type I HIT usually occurs within 2 days of heparin initiation with mild thrombocytopenia, and platelet counts return to normal despite continued heparin exposure. On the other hand, type II HIT usually occurs in individuals who have had more than 4 days of heparin exposure and results due to antibody formation against the heparin-platelet factor 4 complex. This formation causes thrombocytopenia with an average platelet nadir of 60 K and can result in significant thrombosis [6, 8]. Therapy must be initiated immediately for type II HIT, and involves cessation of heparin and institution of a non-heparin anticoagulant (such as argatroban or fondaparinux), while monitoring for bleeding and thrombotic risk. Moreover, Coumadin may serve as an adequate anticoagulant in this situation, but the patient must be anticoagulated with a non-heparin anticoagulant in conjunction while Coumadin is reaching optimal dosing [9].

35.3.2 Inherited Disorders of Platelet Function

35.3.2.1 Bernard-Soulier Syndrome

Bernard-Soulier syndrome is a rare autosomal recessive bleeding disorder, consisting of a combination of platelet dysfunction, thrombocytopenia, and abnormal platelet morphology. The functional platelet defect arises from a mutation in the polypeptides of the glycoprotein (GP) Ib/IX/V complex, which is critical for the initial adhesion of platelets to exposed subendothelium as well as binding of platelets to vWF. Bleeding can be severe and can complicate pregnancy. Affected patients require platelet transfusion for severe bleeding, especially prior to surgery. Antifibrinolytic agents and DDAVP are also useful in some cases [1, 10].

35.3.2.2 Glanzmann's Thrombasthenia

Glanzmann's thrombasthenia is another autosomal recessive disorder of platelets, causing loss or dysfunction of the platelet glycoprotein complex—GP IIb/IIIa. This complex serves as a receptor for adhesion proteins such as fibrinogen and vWF. Without this receptor, platelets cannot aggregate normally to form the initial clot at the site of vessel injury. Onset is usually in the neonatal period and subsequent cutaneous, gastrointestinal bleeding, and menorrhagia can result, requiring platelet transfusions or factor VIIa where possible [1, 10].

35.3.3 Acquired Disorders of Platelet Function

35.3.3.1 Medications

Many medications can affect platelet function. NSAIDs are one of the commonly used medications that affect platelet function. Particularly aspirin, a well-known NSAID, inhibits aggregation of platelets because it irreversibly inhibits cyclooxygenase-1 and cyclooxygenase-2, preventing synthesis of thromboxane A 2 and prostaglandins, which are both essential to platelet aggregation [1]. It is for this reason that aspirin is often held for 5–7 days prior to surgical procedures to avoid the risk of bleeding and hemorrhage. Other medications that can have detrimental effects on platelets include propranolol, lidocaine, penicillin, ampicillin, and amitriptyline as these medications interfere with the platelet membrane. Furthermore, medications such as caffeine, vinblastine, vincristine, and colchicine can also have detrimental effects on platelets as they can inhibit platelet phosphodiesterase, which aids in platelet aggregation [11].

35.3.3.2 Chronic Kidney Disease (CKD)

CKD results in many detrimental effects in the human body which can affect platelet function. Particularly, CKD causes elevations of uremia in the blood in addition to anemia. There is evidence that uremia causes increased production of nitrous oxide (NO) by endothelial cells. The increased NO levels result in increased cyclic GMP levels in the blood, which leads to reductions in thromboxane A2 and ADP levels, impairing platelet aggregation. CKD causes anemia due to decreased production of renal erythropoietin. Normally, red blood cells occupy the center of blood vessels, while platelets are closer to the endothelial surface. This proximity to the surface allows platelets to adhere to the endothelium and form a platelet plug when there is endothelial injury. However, with anemia, the platelets are more dispersed rather than at the surface of the endothelial layer, impairing adherence to the endothelium and thus impairing platelet aggregation and formation of the platelet plug. Anemia also contributes to platelet dysfunction by its effects on ADP and thromboxane release as well as circulating NO and cyclic GMP concentrations [1, 12].

35.3.4 Hemophilias

35.3.4.1 Hemophilia A and B

Hemophilia is an inherited disorder of coagulation. There are two types of x-linked recessive hemophilia: hemophilia A (deficiency of factor VIII) and hemophilia B (deficiency of factor IX, also known as Christmas disease). Both factor VIII (FVIII) and factor IX (FIX) are important elements of the coagulation cascade, thus deficiencies in these elements lead to blood loss. The severity of blood loss depends on the specific factor levels in the serum with clinical severity of bleeding ranging from mild to severe. Severely affected patients can bleed into deep-seated muscles such that the enlarging hematoma can compress adjacent nerves and vasculature [1]. Hemophilia is associated with a prolonged activated partial thromboplastin time (aPTT). Statistically, 50% of male offspring from a female carrier inherit the disorder, whereas 100% of male offspring from an affected mother inherit the disease [4].

Hemophilia A is confirmed by a FVIII assay. Most patients require replacement therapy with FVIII concentrate, depending on the size/severity of the bleed. In patients with mild disease, 1-amino-8-D-arginine vasopressin (DDAVP), given intravenously or by nasal spray, mobilizes FVIII from stores and may avoid the need for concentrate. On the contrary, individuals with hemophilia B require infused FIX. Finally, the other main difference between the two hemophilias is the increased likelihood (~25% of severely affected individuals) of the development of antibodies to FVIII (known as "inhibitors"), leading to hemophilia A [1, 6, 10].

35.3.4.2 Von Willebrand Disease (vWD)

vWD is the most common bleeding disorder caused by mutations in the gene for vWF. vWF is an adhesive glycoprotein secreted by endothelium and megakaryocytes with two major functions: promotion of platelet adhesion to damaged endothelium and platelets and the transport and stabilization of FVIII. Thus, vWD is associated with excessive bleeding due to abnormal platelet function and low FVIII activity. vWD is classified as either type 1 (partial quantitative deficiency of vWF with autosomal dominant inheritance), type 2 (functional defect of the vWF protein separated into four different subtypes; autosomal dominant or recessive inheritance), and type 3 (complete deficiency of vWF with autosomal recessive inheritance). The clinical presentation of vWD is spontaneous bleeding, especially with epistaxis, menorrhagia, gum bleeding, or excessive bleeding following trauma or surgery [1]. vWD usually has a normal prothrombin time (PT), and the activated partial thromboplastin time (aPTT) may be normal or prolonged, depending on the degree of reduction of the FVIII level. Initial screening for vWD consists of three tests: vWF antigen, vWF activity (ristocetin cofactor activity), and FVIII activity. Further specialized assays are needed to determine the type of vWD present as the type of disease dictates the expected treatment/management. Mild bleeding often requires no intervention, but excessive bleeding often requires administration of DDAVP for vWD type 1. DDAVP is less effective for type 2 vWD (and is contraindicated in some subtypes) and has no effect on type 3 vWD. Under these circumstances, appropriate treatment consists of FVIII concentrates with vWF [1, 11, 13].

35.3.4.3 Vitamin K Deficiency

Vitamin K is essential to the clotting cascade as it is the cofactor for γ-glutamyl carboxylation, which is necessary for the activation and functioning of coagulation factors II, VII, IX, and X, as well as proteins C and S. Vitamin K is derived from dietary vegetables and intestinal flora. Vitamin K deficiency occurs in severely malnourished patients, in those with malabsorptive disorders such as celiac disease and tropical sprue, and in newborn babies the first weeks/months of life (babies usually receive a prophylactic 1 mg intramuscular injection of vitamin K injection at birth). Thus, deficiencies in vitamin K will lead to disruption of the coagulation cascade and result in excessive bleeding [1].

35.3.4.4 Plasminogen Activator Inhibitor-1 (PAI-1) Deficiency

Plasminogen activator inhibitor-1 (PAI-1) is an essential protein critical to the down-regulation of the fibrinolytic pathway, resulting in decreased clot breakdown and formation of fibrin degradation products. This deficiency is rare and is inherited as an autosomal recessive disorder that results in excessive clot lysis leading to mild to moderate delayed bleeding. Bleeding, which can be more significant, is expected to be more pronounced after trauma/surgical procedures, paeticvularly involving the oral and urogenital areas. Furthermore, the disorder can also result in increased blood loss during menstruation and pregnancy [6, 10, 14].

35.3.4.5 Rare Bleeding Disorders

The rare bleeding disorders, which comprise about 3–5% of all the inherited bleeding disorders, include the inherited deficiencies of coagulation factors fibrinogen, factor II (FII), factor V (FV), factor VIII (FVIII), factor VII (FVII), factor X (FX), factor XI (FXI), and factor XIII (FXIII). Their clinical manifestations have a wide range of severity, and they are usually transmitted in an autosomal recessive manner. While these bleeding disorders are rare, their prevalence is much higher in countries where consanguineous marriages are relatively common. Due to the rarity of these disorders, limited data are available on the clinical manifestations, diagnosis, and management of affected individuals in general and especially during pregnancy. As such, these individuals should be closely monitored with a multidisciplinary team, including specialized centers and hematologists that can provide more insight into the disease progression and sequelae [13, 15].

Inherited disorders of fibrinogen are divided into quantitative deficiencies (afibrinogenemia and hypofibrinogenemia) and qualitative abnormalities (dysfibrinogenemia). Treatment and sequelae of fibrinogen disorders depend on the type of disorder present. Afibrinogenemia results in blood failing to clot in all coagulation screening tests. While many individuals with inherited disorders of fibrinogen are asymptomatic, the bleeding tendency for afibrinogenemia can be severe with spontaneous hemorrhage and excessive blood loss after surgery. Fibrinogen concentrate is the treatment of choice when fibrinogen replacement is necessary [1, 13].

FII (prothrombin) deficiency is the rarest inherited bleeding disorder with a prevalence of 1:2,000,000 in the general population [13, 14]. Complete deficiency of prothrombin has not been described, suggesting that complete FII deficiency is incompatible with life [14].

FV deficiency is a very rare disorder that often presents with epistaxis and oral cavity bleeding. Severe bleeding is treated with virally inactivated fresh frozen plasma (FFP) as there is no FV concentrate available for repletion. It is also possible to have a combined FV and FVIII deficiency so patients with reduced FV values should also have additional testing to exclude FVIII deficiency [13, 14].

FVII is a vitamin K-dependent glycoprotein, and, through its interaction with tissue factor, it is fundamental to the initiation of coagulation [14]. FVII deficiency is the most common of all the rare inherited coagulation disorders. There is a poor correlation between absolute FVII levels and the risk of bleeding [13, 14]. FVII deficiency has a variable bleeding tendency. A central nervous system hematoma is one of the greatest risks in severe cases and often presents shortly after childbirth. The diagnosis of FVII deficiency is confirmed by FVII assay. Additionally, one must eliminate vitamin K deficiency or other acquired causes of a clotting disorder before the diagnosis of FVII deficiency is made [14]. Recombinant FVII (rFVII) concentrate is available for treatment [1] and is the recommended treatment modality.

Factor X operates its utility as the first enzyme in the common pathway of thrombus formation [14]. Severe (homozygous) FX deficiency has an incidence of 1:1,000,000 in the general population, while the prevalence of heterozygous FX deficiency is about 1:500. While most heterozygotes are typically clinically asymptomatic, some heterozygotes do have a significant bleeding tendency [13, 14]. As mentioned for FVII deficiency, it is important to exclude a vitamin K deficiency or other acquired causes of a clotting disorder before the diagnosis of FX deficiency is made.

FXI deficiency is more common in Ashkenazi Jews. There is a variable relationship between the factor level and bleeding tendency [1]. Bleeding is most commonly provoked by injury or surgery, and women with FXI deficiency have an increased risk of menorrhagia and bleeding in relation to childbirth [14]. Treatment options for severe bleeding include FXI concentrate and recombinant factor VIIa [1]. While all coagulation factors are essential to the coagulation cascade, reports in the literature suggest that FXI is less essential to hemostasis than FVIII and FIX, and, perhaps, other factors may influence the bleeding tendency in FXI deficiency [14].

FXIII deficiency is also very rare, but, should it occur, it can result in severe hemorrhage and poor wound healing. Most affected individuals present early in life with profuse bleeding from the umbilical cord. The most common cause of death is intracranial hemorrhage, which has been reported in 25% of affected patients [16]. There are three subtypes of FXIII deficiency (they vary based on the presence or absence of the subunits A and S), and they all differ in bleeding tendency. FXIII concentrate is available for treatment and is the best replacement therapy. However, if unavailable, FFP and cryoprecipitate can also be used to raise FXIII levels although higher doses are required [14].

35.3.5 Other Causes of Bleeding Disorders

Other causes of bleeding disorders include advanced liver disease, acquired hemophilia (antibodies known as "inhibitors" that block the action of coagulation factors, particularly FVIII), and drug therapy. As mentioned previously, the liver is essential to normal hemostasis as it produces all the factors of the intrinsic and extrinsic coagulation pathway in addition to clearing the body of fibrin degradation products and activated clotting factors. Thus, advanced liver disease can result in numerous hemostatic abnormalities including reduced synthesis of clotting factors, increased consumption of clotting factors (leading to disseminated intravascular coagulopathy), qualitative and quantitative platelet abnormalities, qualitative fibrinogen abnormalities, and accelerated clot lysis leading to excessive blood loss [1]. Acquired hemophilias with antibodies against clotting factors can be associated with other autoimmune disorders such as rheumatoid arthritis (RA), skin disorders, malignancy, drug therapy (especially penicillin), and pregnancy. This too leads to disruption of hemostasis due to excess blood loss [1].

All medications have side effects, and it is essential to individualize the risks and benefits of medications to each patient when determining if that individual should proceed with the chosen therapy. Many different medications can result in the disruption of hemostasis and cause excess blood loss, including NSAIDs (aspirin, ketorolac, etc.), anticoagulants (warfarin, heparin, etc.), antiplatelet agents (clopidogrel, ticlopidine, etc.), and certain antidepressants (paroxetine, fluoxetine, and sertraline) just to name a few. Certain herbal medications and remedies can also result in bleeding, including ginkgo biloba, large amounts of garlic, ginger, ginseng, saw palmetto, and willow bark [1, 10].

35.4 Thrombophilias

Thrombophilia is a predisposition to thrombosis due to enhanced coagulation. Thrombophilia can be either inherited (familial) or acquired. Certain risk factors increase the potential for the presence of thrombophilia. Merely having a history of DVT or PE in a first- or second-degree relative does not warrant a workup for thrombophilia, because this would result in approximately 25% of all patients having a positive family history. Even patients with a strong family history have only a small minority with confirmed inherited thrombophilia [1]. Only individuals with certain risk factors, such as DVT in patients less than 40 years old, arterial thrombosis in patients less than 30 years old, recurrent fetal loss, etc. would require a thrombophilia workup. Initial screening for thrombophilia consists of a blood count and a coagulation screen, while further laboratory testing is dictated by the possible causes of familial or acquired thrombophilia [1].

35.4.1 Inherited Thrombophilias

Familial thrombophilia may be caused by any genetically determined defect of either the coagulation or fibrinolytic systems, which results in accelerated thrombin formation or impaired fibrin dissolution.

35.4.2 Factor V Leiden (FVL)

The most common form of familial thrombophilia is FVL. FVL results in the inherited resistance to the anticoagulant action of activated protein C (APC). This resistance does now allow APC to inactivate the activated cofactors Va and VIIIa by limited proteolysis, resulting in thrombosis. In most cases, resistance to APC is caused by a single point mutation in the factor V gene (factor V Leiden), which results in the mutated form of FVa that is less sensitive than normal FVa to APC-mediated inactivation. FVL has an autosomal dominant mode of inheritance, and the increased risk of venous thrombosis is 4–8-fold in heterozygotes and 50–100-fold in homozygotes. Moreover, the risk of venous thrombosis is highest in patients homozygous for the mutation or in heterozygotes with other risk factors [1].

35.4.3 Prothrombin G20210A

The second most common familial thrombophilia is Prothrombin G20210A. Prothrombin (factor II) is the precursor of thrombin, which is the end-product of the coagulation cascade that converts fibrinogen to fibrin to form a stabilized fibrin clot. The G20210A mutation results from a substitution of adenine (A) for guanine (G) at position 20210 in a non-coding region of the prothrombin gene, resulting in the increased function of prothrombin due to elevated concentrations of prothrombin in plasma. Prothrombin G20210A has an autosomal dominant mode of inheritance, and the risk of thrombosis in heterozygotes is increased approximately 3–4-fold. Just as homozygotes with FVL, homozygotes with Prothrombin G20210A have a larger increased risk for clot compared to heterozygotes. Some individuals have the combined inheritance of both FVL and Prothrombin G20210A, which increases their risk for clot even greater than either mutation alone [1].

35.4.4 Protein C and S Deficiencies

Hereditary deficiency of protein C is an autosomal dominant disorder. Acquired deficiency of protein C can occur in liver disease, DIC, and warfarin treatment. Protein C inactivates procoagulant FVa and FVIIIa, reducing thrombin generation. Familial protein C deficiency results in an increased incidence of venous thromboembolism, ranging from superficial thrombophlebitis to DVT and PE. These events may be either spontaneous or triggered by other factors such as surgery or pregnancy [1]. Protein S is the non-enzymatic cofactor of protein C, and its deficiency will result in inappropriate functioning of protein C. As a result, thrombin generation will not be reduced and the incidence of thrombosis will increase. Hereditary deficiency of protein S has a similar clinical presentation to protein C deficiency. Both proteins C and S undergo vitamin K-dependent gamma-carboxylation and require this for appropriate functioning and clot control [1].

35.4.5 Antithrombin Deficiency

Antithrombin (AT) functions to inhibit thrombin and clotting factors IXa, Xa, XIa, and XIIa. AT deficiency can be inherited in an autosomal dominant manner with variable penetrance, leading to different types of the disorder. Creasy et al. [7] classify the disorders in the following manner: type 1 (reductions in antigen and activity), type 2 (normal levels of antigen but decreased activity), and type 3 (a rare homozygous form with little or no activity). The risk of thrombosis varies between disease subtypes, being greater for an abnormality affecting the reactive (thrombin binding) site as compared to the heparin-binding site. Literature supports that the risk of venous thrombosis is larger in heterozygotes for AT deficiency than for those with APCR, protein C, or protein S deficiency. Thus, although AT deficiency is the least common of the thrombophilias, it is the most thrombogenic [1, 7].

35.4.6 MTHFR Mutation

MTHFR mutation is due to the production of a thermolabile variant of methylenetetrahydrofolate reductase (MTHFR) with reduced enzymatic activity due to a C → T transition at position 677 in the methylenetetrahydrofolate reductase (MTHFR) gene. This mutation results in elevated plasma homocysteine levels. Elevated plasma homocysteine is a risk factor for venous thromboembolism [17] because it induces vascular injury via various mechanisms such as increased smooth muscle cell proliferation, enhanced collagen production, activation of FVIIa and FV, and inhibition of protein C and heparin sulfate to name a few. Although hyperhomocysteinemia was previously reported to be a modest risk factor of venous thromboembolism [18, 19], recent data indicate that elevated homocysteine levels are a weak risk factor of venous thromboembolism [20, 21].

35.4.7 Plasminogen Activator Inhibitor-1 (PAI-1) Mutation

As mentioned previously, PAI-1 is a protein that functions to inhibit tissue plasminogen activator (tPA) and urokinase (uPA), which are the two main activators of plasminogen and fibrinolysis. PAI-1 serves as a balancing mechanism to break down formed clots appropriately, avoiding the risk of VTE. However, the polymorphism that results in a single guanine deletion/insertion polymorphism (4G/5G) in the promoter region of the PAI-1 gene results in disruption of the checks and balances of the coagulation cascade. This results in elevated concentrations of PAI-I in plasma, leading to increased clot formation and buildup without appropriate fibrinolysis [6, 22].

35.4.8 Acquired Thrombophilias

35.4.8.1 Antiphospholipid Syndrome

Antiphospholipid syndrome (APS) is the most common form of acquired thrombophilia [4]. It is an autoimmune disorder that is diagnosed both with clinical findings and laboratory values, needing at least one of both. The initial workup includes identifying any of the antiphospholipid antibodies:

lupus anticoagulant, anticardiolipin antibody, and anti-β2-glycoprotein. APS can be primary, where the patient has no obvious autoimmune disease, or secondary if there is already a diagnosis of systemic lupus erythematosus (SLE) or other rheumatologic diseases. APS results in venous and arterial thrombosis. While the pathogenesis of APS is not clearly understood, studies suggest that the antiphospholipid antibody affects various pathways of coagulation, including protein C, platelets (they interact with phospholipids on the surface of platelets which increases platelet adhesiveness and production of von Willebrand multimers), tissue factor, and impaired fibrinolysis, among others. Moreover, antiphospholipid antibodies inhibit the activity of anticoagulants such as thrombomodulin, protein S, β2-glycoprotein I, and prostacyclin [4].

35.4.8.2 Activated Protein C Resistance (APCR)

As mentioned previously, most cases of APCR are due to inherited FVL mutation. However, there is also a small percentage of cases (<5%) that result in acquired activated protein C resistance not related to FVL. This results from disruptions in the coagulation cascade, creating an imbalance in factors such as protein S deficiency [23], increased antithrombin levels [24], and increased levels of factor VIIIc [25, 26]. Moreover, other ways to acquire APCR are exogenous estrogen use seen in some studies with third-generation oral contraceptives and hormone replacement therapy.

35.4.8.3 Hyperhomocysteinemia

In addition to the inherited MTHFR mutation mentioned above, elevated homocysteine levels can be acquired because of specific vitamin deficiencies. These vitamin deficiencies include deficiencies of folate, vitamin B6, and/or vitamin B12. As mentioned above, recent studies support that elevated homocysteine levels are a weak risk factor for venous thromboembolism [19, 21], and this is likely due to a diet rich in folate due to supplementation in a folate-replete diet of developed nations, including folate supplementation of flour in the United States [7].

35.5 Hemostatic Changes in Pregnancy

Many hemostatic changes occur during pregnancy in preparation for the hemostatic challenge of labor and delivery. In large part, these changes favor a hypercoagulable state to avoid the potential for hemorrhage. Table 35.1. from ACOG practice bulletin #123 [21] summarizes the specific changes in coagulation factors during pregnancy.

Table 35.1 Changes in the normal functioning of the coagulation system during pregnancy

Coagulant factors	Change in pregnancy
Procoagulants	
Fibrinogen	Increased
Factor VII	Increased
Factor VIII	Increased
Factor X	Increased
Von Willebrand factor	Increased
Plasminogen activator inhibitor-1	Increased
Plasminogen activator inhibitor-2	Increased
Factor II	No change
Factor V	No change
Factor IX	No change
Anticoagulants	
Free protein S	Decreased
Protein C	No change
Antithrombin III	No change

Data from Bremme KA. Haemostatic changes in pregnancy. Best Practice & Research Clinical Haematology. 2003;16:153–68 and Medcalf RL, Stasinopoulos SJ. The undecided serpin: the ins and outs of plasminogen activator inhibitor type 2. FEBS J 2005;272:4858–67.

Similar hemostatic responses to pregnancy are seen in women with inherited bleeding disorders, which may lead to normalization of the hemostatic defect in these women. However, this response is variable depending on the type of bleeding disorder present [1]. Moreover, women with factor deficiencies may not achieve the same factor levels during pregnancy compared to women without factor deficiencies. For instance, factor VIII levels increase progressively in carriers of hemophilia A during pregnancy, peaking in the third trimester. Thus, most carriers of hemophilia A have normal FVIII levels at term. On the other hand, FIX levels do not increase significantly during pregnancy; thus, most carriers of hemophilia B with a low baseline level of FXI will continue to have the hemostatic defect at term. This increases the risk for hemorrhage in these affected women. Furthermore, depending on the type of vWD present, levels of FVIII and vWF antigen may change, and thrombocytopenia may develop due to increased production of abnormal intermediate vWF multimers. This may lead to spontaneous platelet aggregation [13]. Thus, it is essential to be aware of the presence of bleeding disorders in women prior to the start of conception, especially for those attempting ART. Patients should be monitored closely to assess the need for specialized treatment/prophylaxis with either factor repletion or anticoagulation as existing bleeding disorders and thrombophilias may or may not be aggravated during pregnancy outside of the normal baseline changes of all factors [1].

35.6 Implantation

Implantation consists of three stages: apposition, adhesion, and invasion. It occurs 5–7 days after fertilization. The implantation of the blastocyst into the endometrium is a complex process of signaling pathways, including specific receptors expressed both on the embryo and the maternal cell's surface [27].

After the shedding of the zona pellucida, the embryo is oriented toward the endometrium, but there is no contact between the endometrium and the embryo. This first step of implantation is called apposition. Following apposition, the adhesion process takes place, which is a time-limited step controlled by cell surface receptor communication between the receptors on the endometrium and the extracellular matrix molecule (ECM) ligands on the embryo. It is during adhesion that the embryo attaches to the endometrial cells [27]. Finally, the last, and most complex step in the implantation process, is invasion of the trophoblast into the endometrium. This process involves the up-regulation and down-regulation of many factors, both on the maternal and embryo side. For instance, the initial invasion of the trophoblast requires the up-regulation of proteases to degrade the ECM. Following this, the extravillous cytotrophoblast (ECT) gains endometrial vessels and breaches their wall, allowing first contact of embryo cells with maternal blood [27]. Hemostasis during vessel invasion is controlled by the up-regulation of tissue factor (TF) and activation of the extrinsic coagulation cascade as well as an increase in plasminogen activator inhibitor (PAI-1). PAI-1 itself regulates cell adhesion and migration.

Most importantly, during implantation, there must exist a specific balance of coagulation, fibrin deposition, and fibrinolysis for normal trophoblast invasion to occur. As fibrin accumulates, it forces the conversion of plasminogen to plasmin and thus stimulates the process of fibrinolysis. Fibrinolysis is essential for modulation of the ECM which itself is mediated by the plasminogen activation system to aid in cell migration through proteolysis to achieve implantation [27].

35.7 Bleeding Disorders and Thrombophilias: Effects on Reproduction and ART

In the literature, many factors have been recognized to affect either the success or failure rate of IVF embryo transfer. Maternal factors affecting this process include age, parity, hormonal levels before stimulation, antral follicle counts, endometrial thickness, and quality of the transformed endometrium. Embryo factors limiting implantation success include embryo grading evaluation and place of embryo transfer in the uterus. Additionally, factors other than the endometrium contribute to the remodeling of the endometrium to appropriately accept the embryo after embryo transfer, including extracellular matrix molecules (ECM molecules), the endothelium, and blood circulation factors [27]. Moreover, factors involved in the coagulation and fibrinolysis cascade have also contributed to the transformation process of the endometrium, affecting the implantation process. As such, studies involving inherited and acquired coagulation disorders in pregnant women, although not many, have been performed to study the effects of these disorders on successful pregnancy outcomes, particularly in the population of women undergoing ART [28].

Multiple studies have shown that inherited thrombophilias increase the risk of recurrent first- and second-trimester pregnancy losses because of placental bed thrombosis [27]. Furthermore, other studies suggest a higher prevalence of inherited thrombophilias in recurrent implantation failure compared with healthy parous women, suggesting that similar mechanisms hampering implantation of embryos and early placentation can occur in women with bleeding disorders undergoing ART [29–32]. On the other hand, other studies in the literature challenge the above-mentioned relationship between poor pregnancy outcomes and thrombophilias, suggesting there is in fact no relationship between the two [27, 29]. For instance, since the development of the intervillous space occurs after 10 weeks of gestation, it is difficult to conclude that implantation failure is solely a result of microthrombosis in decidual vessels [27] attributed to thrombophilias. Additionally, a selective advantage of FVL carriers was first described by Gopel et al. [33] who found a 90% successful implantation rate after first IVF attempt in FVL carriers when compared to only 49% of successful implantation rate in non-carriers [27, 33]. This study not only suggests a positive effect of thrombin deposition during trophoblast invasion but also supports Tan et al.'s study [29] that improved implantation rates is an important genetic advantage for women with the FVL mutation, especially in women attempting ART [29].

Ivanov et al. [27, 34] studied the effects of thrombophilias not only on the success of implantation but also on how thrombophilias influence maternal-embryo receptor interaction and embryo development. In cases of increased thrombin production, such as in women with inherited thrombophilias, decidual cells produce antiangiogenic soluble factors, which inhibit enzymes necessary for ECT invasion. Consequently, this leads to insufficient invasion of ECT into the decidua, resulting in incomplete vascular transformation and underperfused embryonic cells [27].

Underperfused embryonic cells may result in early pregnancy loss, especially in those attempting IVF. In Prothrombin G20210A, there is an increased plasma concentration of prothrombin as well as an increased risk of thrombosis. In FVL, the circulating half-life of FV increases dramatically and thus increases the risk of blood clots. Early recurrent pregnancy losses (<10 weeks of gestational age) were found to be more prevalent in Prothrombin G20210A than FVL. Perhaps this is due to the slightly increased levels of APC at early pregnancy, and maybe this could correlate to an increased IVF failure rate in those with Prothrombin G20210A. Despite these suggestions, the literature provides debatable evidence for increased risk of late and early recurrent pregnancy loss for FVL and Prothrombin G20210A as some studies show no relation between these inherited thrombophilias and implantation failure in IVF attempts [27]. Moreover, while Tan et al. found that poor IVF outcomes are not associated with FVL, prothrombin gene mutation, MTHFR mutations, or APCR mutations, larger sample-sized controlled studies are needed to definitively establish this relationship [29, 32].

Some studies have suggested a link between inherited disorders of platelets and recurrent pregnancy loss development or possible implantation failure. This hypothesis is based on the theory that impaired platelet function results in disturbance of the uteroplacental vascular system. Specifically, increased platelet aggregation may potentially result in a prothrombotic state and increase thrombus formation in the intervillous spaces, resulting in poor fetal outcome [27]. Moreover, platelet dysfunction and polymorphisms may also affect the adhesion process in addition to the endometrium-embryo interaction during implantation. Despite these suggestions, further studies and evidence need to be collected to investigate pregnancy outcomes in women undergoing IVF with inherited disorders of platelets.

Individuals with deficiencies of folic acid or MTHFR mutations result in DNA hypomethylation as well as abnormal biochemical and phenotypic changes in cell development and interaction that may contribute to unsuccessful pregnancies. Furthermore, low MTHFR activity affects methionine metabolism, leading to increased levels of homocysteine in blood plasma. Extreme elevations of serum homocysteine levels have been associated with increased thrombosis due to endothelial injury and coagulation cascade activation. Furthermore, while suggestion exists for the potential impact of MTHFR mutation on early pregnancy loss and implantation failure, this conclusion is still disputed in the literature, and its role in infertility has not been extensively investigated [27]. Moreover, increased supplementation of folic acid during pregnancy can mask the role of MTHFR mutations on IVF failure rates. As such, increased folic acid supplementation should be recommended to those with MTHFR mutations undergoing IVF [27].

As mentioned above, fibrinolysis is necessary for implantation as it modulates the ECM in combination with the plasminogen activation system to aid in cell migration through proteolysis. However, inhibition of fibrinolysis due to PAI-I mutations can result in impaired trophoblast invasion [27]. Specifically, PAI-I mutations inhibit conversion of plasminogen to plasmin, which results in hypofibrinolysis, and thus, impaired implantation due to limited trophoblast invasion into the endometrial tissue.

Inherited bleeding disorders are lifelong conditions that are associated with a broad range of bleeding manifestations, especially in pregnant women. Women with inherited bleeding disorders encounter hemostatic challenges during pregnancy and childbirth. Pregnancy in these women requires individualized management often provided by a multidisciplinary team consisting of an obstetrician, hematologist, and anesthetist. Advanced planning is essential in ensuring an optimal outcome both for mom and child [13].

Von Willebrand disease and hemophilia account for the greatest incidence of inherited bleeding disorders in women. The risks of miscarriage and bleeding during pregnancy are unknown in carriers of hemophilia. Women with vWD have a miscarriage rate of 15%, which is similar to the miscarriage rate of 12–13.5% in the general population [13]. Importantly, the miscarriage and bleeding rate in affected women depends on the type of vWD inherited as mentioned previously. Despite this evidence in the literature and prior studies, our increased knowledge of these disorders suggests that vWD alone does not impair fertility nor does it increase the likelihood of miscarriages [13].

Since FII deficiency is one of the rarest bleeding disorders, other than a few minimal published reports on postpartum hemorrhage, there is no published data on the management or outcomes of pregnancy for this disorder [14]. As such, management of women with this deficiency and desire for ART should be performed in consultation with a hematologist.

Likewise, there is no available data for the management of women with FV or FVII deficiency attempting pregnancy and ART because of their rarity [14].

As mentioned above, FX levels increase during pregnancy. However, in women with severe FX deficiency and a history of adverse outcomes in pregnancy, pregnant women may benefit from aggressive replacement therapy to undergo a successful pregnancy [14]. Importantly, if blood products are administered to maintain FX levels to avoid hemorrhage, thought must always be given to the potential for thrombosis associated with replacement therapy. Thrombosis, as mentioned above, may also be detrimental to the patient and attempted ART. For individuals with severe FX deficiency, prothrombin complex concentrates are the recommended therapy.

Pregnant women with severe FXI deficiency are usually subject to bleeding at the time of birth regardless of route of delivery. In fact, there is no evidence supporting that FXI deficiency affects women in early pregnancy loss that may lead to spontaneous abortion or failed implantation [14]. Although observations of FXI levels in pregnancy are contradictory, any found changes are generally not clinically significant [1].

Some literature has suggested that women with type II FXIII deficiency have inevitable recurrent abortions and that affected men are sterile; however, these studies are not well substantiated [16]. Despite these few reported cases, a policy of universal FXIII replacement starting in childhood may enable more patients to attain reproductive status [16]. Asahina [35] further describes that FXIII deficiency can result in habitual abortions due to decidual bleeding that occurs between 5 and 6 weeks of gestational age [35]. Without appropriate repletion products, spontaneous abortion is inevitable. This is supported by Inbal's work, showing that FXIII has an essential role in placental implantation and the continuation of pregnancy, and up to 50% of severely affected pregnant women will miscarry without appropriate treatment [36]. Maternal fibrinogen and FXIII are essential to the fetus after 4–5 weeks of gestational age as they both are present abundantly in decidual stroma around invasive cytotrophoblasts. When cytotrophoblasts invade the endometrium, it is the maternal fibrinogen and FXIII that is essential for cytotrophoblasts to anchor as adhesive proteins [37].

Minimal small trials have addressed the effects of protein S and protein C deficiency on pregnancy outcomes. Some studies have suggested increased rates of late fetal loss, IUGR, stillbirth, and preeclampsia with either of these deficiencies. However, no firm recommendations for testing have been established because the small sample sizes and lack of research limit the ability to draw specific conclusions. Additionally, if screening for protein S deficiency should occur, it should never be done during pregnancy. This is because protein S levels decrease during pregnancy, thus testing during pregnancy will result in numerous false-positive results [7].

Normal fibrinogen levels are essential in pregnancy to avoid active hemorrhage, risk of thrombosis, and early and recurrent pregnancy loss. Specifically, the importance of fibrinogen in pregnancy has been demonstrated in studies with fibrinogen knockout mice. In these knockout mice, gestation was not maintained to term. Women with fibrinogen deficiencies may conceive and have a normal embryonic implantation if they have adequate fibrinogen levels, especially during 5–8 weeks of gestation, as this is the most common time of pregnancy loss if fibrinogen replacement is not provided [15, 38, 39]. Overall, it has been noted in several studies that fibrinogen plays an essential role in implantation [14]; thus, defective quantity or quality of fibrinogen levels can result in ineffective implantation with ART.

35.8 Preconception Counseling and Evaluation

All individuals planning on attempting IVF require a basic evaluation preceding the start of a cycle outside of having their health and medical comorbidities optimized for attempting pregnancy. Identification of either affected or carrier status should be performed prior to pregnancy for women with a family history of inherited bleeding disorders. This allows for appropriate preconceptual counseling and early pregnancy management. Preconceptual counseling has two main purposes: to provide families with adequate information regarding the genetic implications of their disorders and appropriate management and to allow the implementation of specific plans for pregnancy with therapies if needed [4, 7]. Specifically, in ART, couples can opt for pre-implantation diagnosis (PGD) to test the embryo for their specific genetic condition prior to implantation with IVF. While costly and not always a potential option for patients due to financial reasons, PGD allows patients to avoid implantation of an embryo that will have detrimental effects in the future due to the specific inherited disorder. PGD is different from pre-implantation genetic screening (PGS), which only tests for chromosomal normalcy and not for the presence of a specific genetic disease [3]. This is especially important in carriers of hemophilia due to the severity of the disorder in male offspring and the knowledge of genetic defects in many of the affected families. As mentioned previously, carriers of hemophilia have a 50% chance of having a male fetus that is affected and a 50% chance of having a female fetus who is a carrier of hemophilia [4].

In general, hemostatic coverage is required for women with subnormal factor levels undergoing invasive procedures during pregnancy, or if they experience significant bleeding or hematoma. When prophylaxis or treatment is required, recombinant products should be used if possible to avoid the potential risk of viral transmission with other products [13].

Prenatal testing is a challenge in women with vWD. The specific mutations involved in type 1 and type 3 vWD are not known, while multiple mutations exist in type 2 vWD. While fetal blood vWF levels can be obtained if necessary, inherent risks are associated with this invasive procedure. Affected pregnant women should be informed of these potential risks when counseled about prenatal genetic testing [4]. Genetic counseling should be offered to couples with vWD, especially to couples who are at risk of having severe type III disease newborns [7]. Likewise, the literature supports offering prenatal diagnosis to families affected with Bernard-Soulier syndrome, especially to families who have had previously affected children. Women who have Glanzmann's thrombasthenia and who have been treated with multiple platelet transfusions should undergo evaluation for parental platelet antigen incompatibility and the presence of specific antiplatelet antibodies for fetal antigens prior to conception or attempting ART [7].

All women considering pregnancy should have a thorough medical history evaluation prior to undergoing pregnancy, especially when undergoing ART. All women with SLE should undergo testing for antiphospholipid antibodies prior to conception. Moreover, women who have sustained recurrent spontaneous abortions or a thromboembolic event during a prior pregnancy should also undergo evaluation for APS [4]. False-negative laboratory results may occur, especially during pregnancy due to the increased concentration of clotting factors observed, thus it is very important to evaluate for APS prior to pregnancy if there is high clinical suspicion for this disorder [4]. The necessary lab work needed for testing of APS includes lupus anticoagulant, anticardiolipin antibody, and anti-β2-glycoprotein; furthermore, these labs must be elevated on two occasions at least 12 weeks apart to fulfill lab criteria for APS [7].

A preconception platelet count should always be collected, and it can be helpful in distinguishing between GT and ITP. It is essential to distinguish between the two disorders because there is a small, but significant, risk of neonatal thrombocytopenia in the setting of ITP [4].

As noted above, there is conflicting evidence regarding the relationship between inherited thrombophilias and pregnancy outcomes in the context of ART. Qublan et al. [40] found that thrombophilia has a significant role in IVF-embryo transfer implantation failure, which led to their recommendation of thrombophilia screening (specifically for FVL mutation, prothrombin mutation, MTHFR mutation, deficiencies in proteins S and C, antithrombin III deficiency, or APS) for all women with repeated IVF-embryo transfer failure [40, 41]. On the contrary, Steinvil et al. [42], through a retrospective analysis, found that none of the common thrombophilias tested in women undergoing ART was significantly associated with the number of prior failed ART cycles or with lower fertility. Instead, the authors found that women who had APCR and/or FVL and lupus anticoagulant had significantly higher live birth rates compared to controls and that thrombophilia carrier status was not associated with poorer reproductive outcomes. As such, the data from this large retrospective study confirmed that neither screening for thrombophilia nor anticoagulant treatment is indicated in cases with unexplained reproductive failure in women undergoing ART [28, 42]. On the other hand, Speroff and Fritz [3] recommend that selected screening for the most common thrombophilias (APS, FVL, prothrombin gene mutation) is reasonable for women with unexplained recurrent pregnancy loss with a suspicious loss (after 8 weeks' gestation or detection of embryonic heart activity) or losses that may have been caused by placental insufficiency or thrombosis in prior pregnancies. Finally, although inherited thrombophilias are common, affecting 15% of Western populations, and underlie approximately 50% of VTEs in pregnancy, VTE complicates only 0.1% of pregnancies [43]. Thus, the rarity of VTE during pregnancy and postpartum, and the high prevalence of inherited thrombophilias, makes universal screening of pregnant patients for thrombophilia cost-ineffective [43], which can be extrapolated to women attempting pregnancy with ART. The American Society for Reproductive Medicine, in its Practice Bulletin, does not currently support testing for inherited thrombophilias in cases of recurrent pregnancy loss [44].

35.9 Ovarian Hyperstimulation Syndrome (OHSS) and Bleeding Disorders and Thrombophilias

OHSS results from excess exogenous gonadotropins that may occur in women undergoing ART [3]. On rare occasions, OHSS can occur in women who undergo ovulation induction with clomiphene-induced cycles. While the exact pathophysiology of OHSS is unknown, it is iatrogenic and has a broad pathophysiologic spectrum, ranging from mild to severe disease. The etiology is likely due to increased capillary permeability, leading to leakage of fluid from the vascular compartment, with third space fluid accumulation and intravascular dehydration. Furthermore, it is a massive transudation of protein-rich fluid that causes an imbalance in hydrostatic pressures and shifts fluid significantly. Vascular endothelial growth factor (VEGF) is thought to contribute to this and shifting fluid out of the vascular spaces resulting in excess peritoneal fluid.

Although the disease is often self-limited and resolves spontaneously after a few days, it may persist for longer and appear to be more aggressive in conception cycles [3]. The most severe form of OHSS includes massive ovarian enlargement, severe abdominal pain, ascites, pleural effusion, hemoconcentration, oliguria, electrolyte imbalances, and hypercoagulability, which can result in a life-threatening derangement in hemostasis. In fact, the incidence of moderate OHSS in women undergoing ART is 2–4% and severe OHSS is 0.1–0.5% [44]. Risk factors for OHSS include young age (<35 years), low body weight, PCOS, higher doses of gonadotropins, previous hyperstimulation, and HCG luteal supplementation [3, 44]. Severe OHSS requires hospitalization, careful monitoring, and aggressive treatment to repair fluid shifts, electrolyte imbalances, hemoconcentration, and thrombosis prophylaxis.

The major complication of OHSS is arterial and venous thrombosis that can occur in any anatomical site. The risk of thrombosis increases during OHSS with increased estradiol levels, dehydration, and thrombophilia [44]. Some studies support an increased risk of thromboembolism in women with a known thrombophilia undergoing ART. Mor and Schenker suggest that women desiring ART and undergoing ovarian stimulation should undergo thrombophilia screening to identify those at higher risk for thrombotic events [44]. On the contrary, Anderson et al. conclude [45] that the risk of thrombosis in women undergoing ovarian hyperstimulation is low (~0.1% per treatment cycle); thus, thrombophilia testing is not routinely recommended for women undergoing ovarian stimulation. This is supported by the American College of Chest Physicians (ACCP) who recommends against the use of routine thrombosis prophylaxis in women undergoing ART [46]. Furthermore, Mor and Schenker [44] support an absolute indication for anticoagulation prophylaxis in women who develop OHSS and have thrombophilia. Likewise, the ACCP recommends thrombosis prophylaxis only in the population of women undergoing ART who develop ovarian hyperstimulation syndrome (OHSS), recommending thrombosis prophylaxis with prophylactic LMWH for 3 months post-resolution of clinical OHSS [46]. Finally, Ata and Urman [28] also recommend prophylactic heparin or LMWH treatment for women with severe OHSS.

35.10 Management of Bleeding Disorders and Thrombophilias for ART

The concern for women undergoing ART is the potential for bleeding during or after egg retrieval. As mentioned before, the severity of the bleeding depends on the type of vWD. For example, about 75% of women with moderate to severe vWD experience significant peripartum bleeding with an overall 20% risk of postpartum hemorrhage in women with vWD [4]. The risk of peripartum bleeding for these patients is related to the levels of vWF/Ag, FVIIIc, and vWF/RCo. In general, therapy is administered either in the setting of a spontaneous bleeding event or in a prophylactic context for the high-risk individual. Mainstays of therapy include DDAVP, a synthetic analog of vasopressin, and vWF-FVIII concentrates. DDAVP rapidly and transiently increases levels of FVIII and vWF. It is administered by continuous intravenous infusion over 30 min in an acute bleeding event, or it can be given subcutaneously or inhaled nasally for prophylaxis [47]. Like all medications, DDAVP does have side effects and can result in fluid retention and hyponatremia. Furthermore, DDAVP has uncertain utility in the management of women with type 2 and type 3 vWD; thus, vWF-FVIII concentrate is indicated for these patients. Cryoprecipitate can be used emergently if vWF-FVIII concentrates are unavailable. While antifibrinolytic therapy plays a role in the management of individuals with vWD, it is avoided during pregnancy and lactation because of its potential teratogenicity and effects on newborns [4]. Multidisciplinary care by an experienced obstetrician, hematologist, and anesthesiologist should be provided for women with vWD. FVIIIc and vWF/RCo levels, partial thromboplastin time (PTT), type and crossmatch, and a complete blood count are obtained at the time of hospital admission or any invasive procedure. Women with vWD should be monitored for bleeding at the time of egg retrieval, with blood cell products and DDAVP available for use as needed. While there are no clear recommendations suggesting testing or treatment for women with vWD, perhaps this should be considered and discussed with a hematologist prior to the start of ART, especially with any planned potentially invasive procedures such as egg retrieval.

Women with hemophilia require complex management in association with hematology and anesthesia consultation. Factor levels and optimization of the patient's bleeding disorder should be considered when planning for ART, in addition to discussing management with the hematologist regarding blood product infusions or further testing.

As mentioned above, management of many factor deficiencies is not fully known due to the rarity of these deficiencies. As such, when encountering women with these rare deficiencies, it is best to discuss management with a hematologist. Bolton et al., [14] suggest that pregnant women with FV levels <1 U/dL should undergo administration of FFP to avoid bleeding. The FFP should be administered once the patient is in labor, prior to surgery, or any invasive procedure. Perhaps this can be extrapolated to the egg retrieval process as this invasive procedure on occasion may result in excess bleeding if the inadvertent puncture of vasculature occurs. Additionally, with product administration, close monitoring of FV levels is essential to maintain minimum hemostatic FV levels. On the other hand, patients with a partial deficiency of FV and no prior history of bleeding during invasive procedures could be managed expectantly [14]. As such, perhaps affected women with adequate FV levels and no history of bleeding can be managed expectantly during egg retrieval rather than receiving unnecessary blood products. Furthermore, the literature suggests that FVII and FVIIa levels maintained between 100 and 150 U/dL result in no bleeding problems. Thus, perhaps these ranges of FVII can accommodate an uneventful egg retrieval and normal implantation in women undergoing IVF.

For a patient with FXI deficiency and without a history of bleeding, prophylaxis is not necessary, but FFP should be available if needed. Conversations with the anesthesiologist should occur prior to any plans of egg retrieval to counsel the patient on need of lab collection or expectations for blood products on the day of egg retrieval. For instance, if consideration for regional block anesthesia is made, it is usually administered with FFP prior to the procedure and with documentation of normalization of the PTT [4]. Furthermore, in patients with FXI deficiency and a bleeding history, FFP should be administered before delivery, as well as 2–3 days later, to reduce the risk of delayed hemorrhage [4]. A similar management plan could be considered in the ART patient.

As discussed above, FXIII and fibrinogen are both essential for appropriate implantation. Moreover, in patients with FXIII deficiency, the occurrence of spontaneous recurrent abortions and uterine bleeding is elevated; thus, these individuals need regular infusions of FFP or FXIII concentrate to maintain their pregnancy [4]. Thus, administration of FXIII should be administered by 5 weeks of gestational age to prevent miscarriage. Adequate fibrinogen levels are essential during 5–8 weeks of gestation, as this is the most common time of pregnancy loss if fibrinogen replacement is not provided [15, 38, 39]. Maintaining the fibrinogen trough level above 0.6 g/L, and, if possible, over 1.0 g/L, is recommended [39]. Perhaps this can be extrapolated to women undergoing ART who may also require infusions prior to egg retrieval and embryo transfer.

Yoni et al. [48] state that arterial thrombotic complications usually occur 10.5 days after embryo transfer (ET), while venous thrombotic complications typically occur 40 days after ET. Furthermore, in women undergoing ART, the risk for a thrombotic event is approximately ten times higher compared to women who are not undergoing ART. This increased risk may be attributed to an increased level of estradiol in addition to other factors, as well as the key finding that both the coagulation and fibrinolysis systems are activated during IVF, especially in the presence of OHSS [49]. As mentioned from the above discussions, the influence of thrombophilic factors on pregnancy outcome after ART is linked to the modification of the endometrium adhesion properties and the effect on the ability of trophoblastic invasion [27]. Despite these links, it is difficult to assess each individual bleeding disorder on IVF failure risk and poor pregnancy outcome, because a variety of factors other than these bleeding disorders can contribute to pregnancy failure in ART. However, because thrombogenic factors can modify the implantation process, it is essential to establish the type, dose, and effective treatment needed if warranted that will aid in the imbalance of hemostatic proteins and time of implantation to improve pregnancy outcomes after ART [27]. What is important to remember is that every patient with thrombophilia during pregnancy needs to be assessed on a case-by-case basis as every patient's treatment plan is individualized based on their personal and family history. Asymptomatic women who harbor thrombophilic conditions, but have never experienced clinical manifestations, do not require anticoagulation therapy during pregnancy or ART [4]. Prophylactic anticoagulation treatment for carriers of low-risk mutations with any personal or family history of VTE is not indicated. There have been varied results in clinical trials using anticoagulation in the setting of recurrent miscarriage; however, in the large, multicenter, randomized, placebo-controlled study examining the use of aspirin or aspirin plus heparin in women with unexplained miscarriage, there was no improvement in the live birth rate compared with placebo [4, 48].

On the contrary, some clinicians prescribe antithrombotic drugs in infertile women after ART, especially in the presence of previous implantation failures and positive testing for thrombophilia, not due to proven efficacy, but for suspected biologic plausibility of having a successful outcome with better control of hemostasis [34]. Grandone et al. [50] investigated this approach and its impact on improved live births for women with and without thrombophilias. Grandone et al. found that in a general population of infertile couples, thrombophilic women do not have a lower chance of good pregnancy outcomes, consistent with prior research [50, 51]. In support of other studies, Grandone et al. found that the use of aspirin in general infertile women is not justified to improve pregnancy outcome, either in the presence or in the absence of thrombophilia [50, 52]. On the other hand, the study supports the potential benefit of LMWH in improving the number of live births, independently of the presence of thrombophilia [50]. Ivanov et al. [34] support the beneficial role of heparin on embryo implantation as it not only helps to prevent thrombosis but also aids in interactions with several adhesion molecules, growth factors, cytokines, and enzymes such as matrix metalloproteinases, which are all essential in the success of implantation [53]. While some studies and clinicians support the use of anti-thrombolytic therapy in women attempting ART with thrombophilias, the literature confirms that universal thrombophilia screening is not useful in infertile couples or prior failed IVF cycles to discriminate women with a worse pregnancy prognosis [50]. The ACCP has specific recommendations for antithrombotic prophylaxis with LMWH in pregnant women with thrombophilias, depending on the thrombophilia type, personal history of VTE, and family history of VTE, which are somewhat consistent with the American College of Obstetricians and Gynecologists [21] recommendations. Both governing bodies recommend anticoagulation for high-risk thrombophilias, including homozygous FVL or Prothrombin G20210A mutation [34, 54]. ACOG extends high-risk thrombophilias to include antithrombin deficiency and double heterozygous for Prothrombin G20210A mutation and FVL [7, 54]. These recommendations are further supported by Ata and Urman [28] who disagree with routine testing or treatment for congenital or acquired thrombophilia in the setting of ART or in couples with implantation failure. Furthermore, they suggest that a careful personal and family history along with a risk assessment for VTE should be obtained in every woman undergoing controlled ovarian stimulation with ART, such that if these assessments are positive, only then would testing for thrombophilia be warranted. Again, while heparin may have potential implantation enhancing effects, if it should be administered to increase success rates of ART, it needs to be investigated in further large-scale randomized trials, especially because prior studies were methodologically limited and inadequate [7, 28].

Several studies that examined the association between the prothrombin gene mutation and ART failure [28, 31, 40, 55] showed an overall non-significant association (OR, 1.48; 95% CI, 0.71–3.06), and the risk of ART failure was similar between heterozygotes and homozygotes compared with normal controls. Likewise, several other studies evaluated the association between MTHFR mutation and ART outcome, and there was no association between MTHFR carrier status and ART outcomes [28], and both homozygotes and heterozygotes performed similarly. Overall, neither prothrombin gene mutation nor MTHFR mutation increases the risk of failure in ART; thus, no specific testing or management for women attempting ART is required [28, 56].

Because antiphospholipid antibodies exert prothrombotic effects on the body via various mechanisms, the risk of thrombosis is significantly increased during pregnancy in patients with APS. Additionally, antiphospholipid antibodies decrease levels of annexin V, a potent vascular endothelial anticoagulant produced by placental trophoblasts. As such, pregnant women with APS not only may develop thrombotic events but also may experience spontaneous abortions, preeclampsia, HELLP syndrome, as well as IUGR [4, 7]. Women with APS who have sustained prior thrombotic events should receive therapeutic anticoagulation during pregnancy with aspirin and heparin, while those with antiphospholipid antibodies but no manifestations of the clinical syndrome should receive prophylactic anticoagulation during pregnancy [4, 7].

Since PAI-I plays a crucial role in fibrinolysis regulation and thus implantation, early diagnosis of hypofibrinolytic disorders in pregnancy is essential. Most importantly, if hypofibrinolysis is identified early, the initiation of LMWH therapy may avoid the complications of pregnancy in coagulation disorders and perhaps aid in successful implantation and pregnancy rates for women undergoing ART. Furthermore, studies have shown that metformin is also a potential management option for women with PAI-I mutations as it aids in reducing PAI-I levels, decreasing hypofibrinolysis and increasing appropriate implantation [27, 57]. As mentioned before, it would be best to discuss optimal patient management for these women undergoing ART with a hematologist.

Given the potential role of platelet dysfunction on implantation failure, studies have suggested that perhaps a prophylactic anti-aggregate therapy to prevent poor pregnancy outcome can be considered in this patient population [27, 58]. This anti-aggregate therapy would need to be individualized and discussed with a hematologist as this is not a firm or supported recommendation for the standard of care.

In severe ITP, maternal antiplatelet IgG can cross the placenta and cause thrombocytopenia in fetuses. Treatment options for ART patients with ITP are generally similar to those for patients with ITP except for the use of teratogenic supplements such as danazol, cyclophosphamide, and vinca alkaloids. Platelet transfusions are reserved for life-threatening bleeding because the lives of transfused platelets are short-lived in ITP. Glucocorticoids are considered first-line treatment, and prednisone is usually initiated at 1 mg/kg based on the patient's baseline weight. Potential side effects of prednisone should be discussed with the patient prior to the start of therapy and include weight gain, bone loss, hypertension, and gestational diabetes. IVIG is another treatment modality that can aid in a rapid increase in platelet count. It is particularly used to help increase platelet counts a few days before delivery or other invasive procedures. IVIG is administered at a dose of 2 g/kg over 2 days; however, it is important to realize that the improvement in platelet count is transient [4]. Although no clear evidence or studies have investigated the use of IVIG for patients with ITP undergoing ART, perhaps IVIG can be considered prior to egg retrieval for those with severe disease or those with a history of prior ITP. Prior to pursuing treatment, this should be discussed with a hematologist to investigate whether this is truly needed and could potentially improve patient outcomes for ART.

Treatment of TTP involves emergent plasmapheresis within 24–48 h of diagnosis. Long-term sequelae of TTP in surviving patients include chronic renal failure, hypertension, and recurrence of TTP. While infusion of FFP is an alternative to plasmapheresis for TTP treatment, plasmapheresis is the preferred treatment modality. Finally, corticosteroids have also been used successfully in the treatment of pregnancy-associated TTP [4]. TTP should be treated prior to the start of ART, and prior TTP should be documented in the patient's history to plan for future potential predicaments once already starting IVF cycles.

Women who desire ART should undergo an extensive history collection to screen for any potential medical comorbidities or medications that can predispose them to inadequacies of hemostasis as this can potentially affect their success with ART. Some medications may need to be held during invasive procedures, such as aspirin or LMWH, while others may need to be adjusted to avoid teratogenicity to the offspring. This discussion with patients is essential, because every woman will have an individualized treatment plan based on her history. There may be some teratogenic medications that need to be continued during pregnancy and attempted conception, such as warfarin for women with mechanical heart valves; thus, discussion of medications is essential. Finally, herbal medications also need to be discussed as some of these medicines may need to be avoided during ART and invasive procedures to prevent increased risk for bleeding.

35.11 Conclusions

Hemostasis is essential and plays an important role in reproduction, conception, and final delivery. Pregnancy favors a thrombogenic state to overcome and compensate for the potential bleeding that can occur during the time of delivery. However, overcompensation of the thrombogenic state can alter normal reproductive processes, and result in poor outcomes for women attempting pregnancy, especially those undergoing ART. This chapter was aimed to portray a comprehensive review of existing bleeding disorders and thrombophilias and how they may affect women attempting pregnancy, focusing on women undergoing ART in the form of IVF. While available data exists to define the etiology and consequences of bleeding disorders and thrombophilias, there are still many questions that remain unanswered. This is not only due to the lack of knowledge for certain disorders but also due to the lack of adequate, powered, randomized controlled trials that can delineate a clear recommendation on the effect of bleeding or thrombophilia disorders on pregnancy and ART, as well as the potential benefit of antithrombotic agents for women with a history of thrombophilia undergoing ART. Overall, there is no clear clinical evidence or support of routine screening for thrombophilia in all women undergoing ART or in those who have had multiple IVF implantation failures, nor are there distinct guidelines to provide thromboprophylaxis to women with thrombophilias undergoing ART. It is only women with a thrombophilia who develop the complication of OHSS that thromboprophylaxis during ART is recommended. Finally, individuals with bleeding disorders should be managed based on their distinct bleeding disorder and the knowledge that is available on their specific bleeding disorder.

As such, it is our role as physicians to counsel our patients to the best of our ability with the most updated guidelines and studies and to individualize our patient care based on the patient's relative family and personal history in addition to her desires. Moreover, it is essential to work with a multidisciplinary team to manage patients with bleeding and thrombophilia disorders to provide optimal care and avoid potential complications that could be anticipated by experts. The multidisciplinary team may consist of an obstetrician, hematologist, anesthesiologist, and in some cases maternal-fetal medicine specialist.

References

1. Howard MR, Hamilton PJ, Britton R. Haematology: an illustrated colour text. Fourth ed. Edinburgh: Elsevier. Accessed via Clinical Key; 2013.
2. Pettker CM, Lockwood CJ. Chap. 45, Thromboembolic disorders in pregnancy. In: Obstetrics: normal and problem pregnancies. 7th ed. Philadelphia, PA: Elsevier; 2017. p. 965–80.
3. Fritz MA, Speroff L. Recurrent early pregnancy loss. In: Clinical gynecologic endocrinology and infertility. 8th ed. Philadelphia, PA: Lippincott Williams & Wilkins; 2011.
4. Cromwell C, Paidas M. Chap. 151: Hematologic changes in pregnancy. In: Hematology: basic principles and practice, Thrombophilia and pregnancy. 7th ed. Philadelphia, PA: Elsevier; 2018. p. 2203–2214.e5.
5. McCrae KR. Thrombocytopenia in pregnancy: differential diagnosis, pathogenesis, and management. Blood Rev. 2003;17:7.
6. International RBDD Registry, the Indiana Hemophilia & Thrombosis Center, and the Rare Coagulation Disorders Subcommittee of the National Hemophilia Foundation. 2014. Rare Coagulation Disorders Resource Room. Retrieved from http://www.rarecoagulationdisorders.org/.
7. Creasy RK, Resnik R, Iams JD, Lockwood CJ, Moore TR, Greene MF. Coagulation disorders in pregnancy. In: Creasy & Resnik's maternal-fetal medicine principles and practice. Seventh ed. Philadelphia, PA: Elsevier Saunders; 2014.
8. Greinacher A. Heparin-induced thrombocytopenia. J Thromb Haemost. 2009;1:9–12. https://doi.org/10.1111/j.1538-7836.2009.03385.x.
9. Linkins LA, Dans AL, Moores LK, et al. Treatment and prevention of heparin-induced thrombocytopenia: antithrombotic therapy and prevention of thrombosis, ninth ed.: American College of Chest Physicians Evidence-Based Clinical Practice Guidelines. Chest. 2012;141(2):e495S–530S. https://doi.org/10.1378/chest.11-2303.141:e495S.
10. Schulman S. Bleeding disorders, World Federation of Hemophilia. 2010. Accessed via https://www.wfh.org/en/page.aspx?pid=639
11. Baz R, Mekhail T. Disorders of platelet function and number. Lyndhurst, OH: The Cleveland Clinic Foundation; 2009.. Retrieved from http://www.clevelandclinicmeded.com/medicalpubs/diseasemanagement/hematology-oncology/disorders-platelet-function/
12. Hedges SJ, Dehoney SB, Hooper JS, et al. Evidence-based treatment recommendations for uremic bleeding. Nat Clin Pract Nephrol. 2007;3(3):138–53.
13. Chi C, Kadir RA. Inherited bleeding disorders in pregnancy. Best Pract Res Clin Obstet Gynecol. 2012;26(1):103–17.
14. Bolton-Maggs PH, Perry DJ, Chalmers EA, et al. The rare coagulation disorders–review with guidelines for management from the United Kingdom haemophilia centre doctors' organisation. Haemophilia. 2004;10(5):593–628. https://doi.org/10.1111/j.1365-2516.2004.00944.x.
15. Huq FY, Kadir RA. Management of pregnancy, labor and delivery in women with inherited bleeding disorders. Haemophilia. 2011;17:20–30. https://doi.org/10.1111/j.1365-2516.2011.02561.x.
16. Burrows RF, Ray JG, Burrows EA. Bleeding risk and reproductive capacity among patients with factor XIII deficiency: a case presentation and review of the literature. Obstet Gynecol Surv. 2000;55(2):103–8.
17. den Heijer M, Koster T, Blom HJ, et al. Hyperhomocysteinemia as a risk factor for deep-vein thrombosis. N Engl J Med. 1996;334:759–62.
18. den Heijer M, Rosendaal FR, Blom HJ, Gerrits WB, Bos GM. Hyperhomocysteinemia and venous thrombosis: a meta-analysis. Thromb Haemost. 1998;80:874–7.
19. Eichinger S. Homocysteine, vitamin B6 and the risk of recurrent venous thromboembolism. Pathophysiol Haemost Thromb. 2003;33:342–4.
20. den Heijer M, Lewington S, Clarke R. Homocysteine, MTHFR and risk of venous thrombosis: a meta-analysis of published epidemiological studies. J Thromb Haemost. 2005;3:292–9.
21. The American College of Obstetricians and Gynecologists. Practice bulletin #123: Thromboembolism in pregnancy. In ACOG. 2011. Retrieved from https://www.acog.org/Clinical-Guidance-and-Publications/Practice-

Bulletins/Committee-on-Practice-Bulletins-Obstetrics/Thromboembolism-in-Pregnancy
22. Goodman C, Hur J, Goodman CS, Jeyendran RS, Coulam C. Are polymorphisms in the ACE and PAI-1 genes associated with recurrent spontaneous miscarriages? Am J Reprod Immunol. 2009;62(6):365–70. https://doi.org/10.1111/j.1600-0897.2009.00744.x.
23. De Ronde H, Bertina RM. Laboratory diagnosis of APC-resistance: a critical evaluation of the test and the development of diagnostic criteria. Thromb Haemost. 1994;72:880–6.
24. Freyburger G, Javorschi S, Labrouche S, Bernard P. Proposal for objective evaluation of the performance of various functional APC-resistance tests in genotyped patients. Thromb Haemost. 1997;78:1360–5.
25. Koster T, Rosendaal FR, De Ronde H, Briet E, Vandenbroucke JP, Bertina RM. Venous thrombosis due to poor anticoagulant response to activated protein C: Leiden Thrombophilia Study. Lancet. 1993;342:1503–6.
26. Kraaijenhagen RA, In'T Anker PS, Koopman MMW, Reitsma PH, Prins MHH, Van Den Ende A, Buller HR. High plasma concentration of factor VIIIc is a major risk factor for venous thromboembolism. Thromb Haemost. 2000;83:5–9.
27. Ivanov P, Tsvyatkovska T, Konova E, Komsa-Penkova R. Inherited thrombophilia and IVF failure: the impact of coagulation disorders on implantation process. Am J Reprod Immunol. 2012;68(3):189–98. https://doi.org/10.1111/j.1600-0897.2012.01156.x.
28. Ata B, Urman B. Thrombophilia and assisted reproduction technology-any detrimental impact or unnecessary overuse? J Assist Reprod Genet. 2016;33(10):1305–10.
29. Tan X, Yu Z, Sao J, Chen L, Shen Y, Ding J, Shi W. Association between in vitro fertilization outcomes and inherited thrombophilias: a meta-analysis. J Assist Reprod Genet. 2016;33(8):1093–8. https://doi.org/10.1007/s10815-016-0726-0.
30. Bellver J, Soares SR, Álvarez C, Muñoz E, Ramírez A, Rubio C, et al. The role of thrombophilia and thyroid autoimmunity in unexplained infertility, implantation failure and recurrent spontaneous abortion. Hum Reprod. 2008;23:278–84.
31. Vaquero E, Lazzarin N, Caserta D, Valensise H, Baldi M, Moscarini M, et al. Diagnostic evaluation of women experiencing repeated in vitro fertilization failure. Eur J Obstet Gynecol Reprod Biol. 2006;125:79–84.
32. Di Nisio M, Rutjes AW, Ferrante N, Tiboni GM, Cuccurullo F, Porreca E. Thrombophilia and outcomes of assisted reproduction technologies: a systematic review and meta-analysis. Blood. 2011;118(10):2670–8. https://doi.org/10.1182/blood-2011-03-340216.
33. Göpel W, Ludwig M, Junge AK, Kohlmann T, Diedrich K, Möller J. Selection pressure for the factor-V-Leiden mutation and embryo implantation. Lancet. 2001;358:1238–9.
34. Ivanov P, Tomov SI, Tsvyatkovska T, Konova E, Komsa-Penkova R. Thrombophilia in assisted reproductive technology — Place and needs of thromboprophylaxis. In: Ivanov P, editor. Pregnancy thrombophilia - the unsuspected risk. Croatia: InTech; 2013. https://doi.org/10.5772/56793.. Available from: https://www.intechopen.com/books/pregnancy-thrombophilia-the-unsuspected-risk/thrombophilia-in-assisted-reproductive-technology-place-and-needs-of-thromboprophylaxis.
35. Asahina T, Kobayashi T, Takeuchi K, Kanayama N. Congenital blood coagulation factor XIII deficiency and successful deliveries: a review of the literature. Obstet Gynecol Surv. 2007;62(4):255–60.
36. Inbal A, Muszbek L. Coagulation factor deficiencies and pregnancy loss. Semin Thromb Hemost. 2003;29(2):171–4. https://doi.org/10.1055/s-2003-38,832.
37. Asahina T, Kobayashi T, Okada Y, et al. Studies on the role of adhesive proteins in maintaining pregnancy. Horm Res. 1998;50(2):37.
38. Grech H, Majumdar G, Lawrie AS, Savidge GF. Pregnancy in congenital afibrinogenaemia: report of a successful case and review of the literature. Br J Haematol. 1991;78(4):571–2. https://doi.org/10.1111/j.1365-2141.1991.tb04491.x.
39. de Moerloose P, Casini A, Neerman-Arbez M. Congenital fibrinogen disorders: an update. Semin Thromb Hemost. 2013;39(6):585–95. https://doi.org/10.1055/s-0033-1,349,222.
40. Qublan HS, Eid SS, Ababneh HA, Amarin ZO, Smadi AZ, Al-Khafaji FF, Khader YS. Acquired and inherited thrombophilia: implication in recurrent IVF and embryo transfer failure. Hum Reprod. 2006;21(10):2694–8.
41. Fatemi HM, Popovic-Todorovic B. Implantation in assisted reproduction: a look at endometrial receptivity. Reprod BioMed Online. 2013;27(5):530–8.
42. Steinvil A, Raz R, Berliner S, Steinberg DM, Zeltser D, Levran D, et al. Association of common thrombophilias and antiphospholipid antibodies with success rate of in vitro fertilisation. Thromb Haemost. 2012;108(6):1192–7. https://doi.org/10.1160/TH12-06-0381.
43. Mark PE. Venous thromboembolism in pregnancy. Clin Chest Med. 2010;31(4):731–40.
44. Practice Committee of the American Society for Reproductive Medicine. Evaluation and treatment of recurrent pregnancy loss: a committee opinion. Fertil Steril. 2012;98(5):1103–11.
45. Mor YS, Schenker JG. Ovarian hyperstimulation syndrome and thrombotic events. Am J Reprod Immunol. 2014;72(6):541–8. https://doi.org/10.1111/aji.12310.
46. Anderson JA, Hogg KE, Weitz JI. Chap. 140, Hypercoagulable states. In: Hematology: basic principles and practice. Seventh ed. Philadelphia, PA: Elsevier; 2018. p. 2076–87.. Retrieved from https://www.clinicalkey.com/#!/content/book/3-s2.0-B9780323357623001402?scrollTo=%23hl0000517.
47. Bates SM, Greer IA, Middeldorp S, Veenstra DL, Prabulos AM, Vandvik PO. American College of Chest Physicians. VTE, thrombophilia, antithrombotic therapy, and pregnancy: antithrombotic therapy and prevention of thrombosis, ninth ed.: American College of Chest Physicians Evidence-Based Clinical Practice Guidelines. Chest. 2012;141(2):e691S–736S.
48. Yoni C, Tulandi T, Almog B, Zohav E, Deutsch V, Many A, Amit A, Cohen A. Prolonged activation of the coagulation system during in vitro fertilization cycles. Eur J Obstet Gynecol Reprod Biol. 2017;216:111–5.
49. Lipe BC, Dumas MA, Ornstein DL. Von Willebrand disease in pregnancy. Hematology/Oncology Clin N Am. 2011;25(2):335–58.
50. Kaandorp SP, Goddijn M, van der Post JA, et al. Aspirin plus heparin or aspirin alone in women with recurrent miscarriage. N Engl J Med. 2010;362:1586.
51. Grandone E, Villani M, Tiscia GL, Dentali F, Colaizzo D, Cappucci F, Chinni E, Ageno W, Margaglione M. Clinical pregnancies and live births in women approaching ART: A follow-up analysis of 157 women after thrombophilia screening. Thromb Res. 2014;133(2):168–72.
52. Ricci G, Bogatti P, Fischer-Tamaro L, Giolo E, Luppi S, Montico M, et al. Factor V Leiden and prothrombin gene G20210A mutation and in vitro fertilization: prospective cohort study. Hum Reprod. 2011;26:3068–77.
53. Dentali F, Ageno W, Rezoagli E, Rancan E, Squizzato A, Middeldorp S, et al. Low-dose aspirin for in vitro fertilization or intracytoplasmic sperm injection: a systematic review and a meta-analysis of the literature. J Thromb Haemost. 2012;10:2075–85.
54. Nelson SM, Greer IA. The potential role of heparin in assisted conception. Hum Reprod Update. 2008;14:623–45.
55. The American College of Obstetricians and Gynecologists. Practice Bulletin #138: Inherited thrombophilias in pregnancy. In ACOG. 2013. Retrieved from https://www.acog.org/Clinical-Guidance-and-Publications/Practice-Bulletins/Committee-on-Practice-Bulletins-Obstetrics/Inherited-Thrombophilias-in-Pregnancy

56. Grandone E, Colaizzo D, Lo Bue A, Cappucci F, Cittadini E, Margaglione M. Clinical relevance of inherited thrombophilia in implantation failure: who needs to be screened? Haematologica. 2003;88(12):35.
57. Simur A, Ozdemir S, Acar H, Colakoğlu MC, Görkemli H, Balci O, Nergis S. Repeated in vitro fertilization failure and its relation with thrombophilia. Gynecol Obstet Investig. 2009;67(2):109–12. https://doi.org/10.1159/000165776.
58. Velazquez EM, Mendoza SG, Wang P, Glueck CJ. Metformin therapy is associated with decreased plasminogen activator inhibitor-1, lipoprotein (a), and immunoreactive insulin levels in patients with polycystic ovary syndrome. Metabolism. 1997;46:454–7.

36 Medically Assisted Reproduction in Organ Transplant Recipients

Megan C. Smith and Steven R. Lindheim

36.1 Background

Over a century of trial and error in organ transplantation gives insight to the modern approach to the procedure. In 1902, experimental surgeon Emerich Ullmann demonstrated the feasibility of renal transplantation and vascular grafting by transplanting a functional kidney into a canine model [1]. Ullmann's description of the challenges of maintaining allograft perfusion and avoiding host rejection was corroborated by several researchers over the next several decades, citing similar obstacles until 1954, when the first successful human renal transplant was reported where the organ donor was the identical twin of the recipient [2]. The success of this pioneering procedure was attributed to immunological similarity of the donor to the recipient, evading the pervasive concern of organ rejection. Refinements in transplant technique were soon applied to successful liver and heart transplants in the 1960s [3]. Today, transplantation medicine has progressed so that even "non-essential" transplants are possible, as demonstrated by the first successful transplantation of a uterus with full child-bearing capacity in 2013 [4] (Fig. 36.1).

Given the progress of transplantation medicine, it is not surprising that patients of child-bearing age and younger are undergoing allograft transplantation. With advances in vascular anastomosis, infection control, and immunosuppression, post-organ transplant pregnancies have, with proper clinical management, had excellent outcomes since the 1950s [5]. Despite the positive prognosis of post-operative pregnancies, clinicians still consider these gestations to be high-risk. Thus, aggressive pre-, peri-, and post-natal care of both mother and fetus is crucial.

Additional challenges include persistent post-operative infertility. In these patients, assisted reproductive technology (ART) may be considered. ART can enhance reproductive success in the post-transplant population. Management of these patients must emphasize the maintenance of allograft function and optimization of maternal health throughout treatment.

This chapter will introduce several issues including the most pressing challenges in modern organ transplantation, and how the anticipation and management of these risks are altered in the pregnant transplant recipient; immunosuppressive therapy and its impact on post-operative fertility with the patient's future reproductive goals in mind; fetal and maternal complications of post-transplant gestations demonstrating the necessity of careful patient monitoring; the modern prospect of uterine transplantation as well as possibilities for future innovations in the field of transplantation medicine; and, finally, special considerations of ART in organ transplant recipients will be reviewed.

36.2 Fertility and Immunosuppressants

Modern organ transplantation has the capacity to prolong survival with excellent results in patients with end-stage organ disease. This is especially important in young women of child-bearing age with hopes of maintaining post-operative fertility. Heavy immunosuppression is necessary to prevent graft rejection in these patients, but the use of immunosuppressive agents requires knowledgeable administration to avoid infertility in both male and female patients.

A study of immunosuppressive agents on male fertility demonstrated that cyclosporine and sirolimus, agents commonly used in post-transplant immunosuppression, have concerning effects on the male reproductive system (Table 36.1). Both agents were found to severely impair spermatogenesis and derail the hypothalamic-pituitary-gonadal axis by decreasing serum levels of testosterone. Tacrolimus, however, only mildly inhibited spermatogenesis and produced no histological evidence of testicular injury [6]. If the injurious nature of immunosuppressive agents

M. C. Smith · S. R. Lindheim (✉)
Department of Obstetrics and Gynecology, Wright State University, Boonshoft School of Medicine, Dayton, OH, USA
e-mail: steven.lindheim@wright.edu

G. N. Allahbadia et al. (eds.), *Textbook of Assisted Reproduction*, https://doi.org/10.1007/978-981-15-2377-9_36

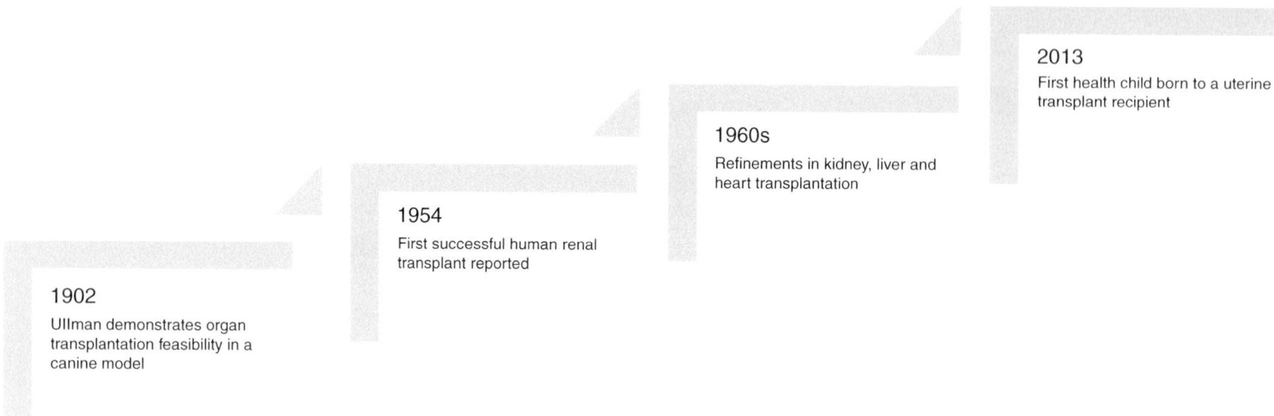

Fig. 36.1 Timeline of significant achievements in transplantation medicine

Table 36.1 Impact of immunosuppressive agents on male fertility

Drug	Effect	Overall impact on fertility
Cyclosporine	Impair spermatogenesis and decrease testosterone (T) levels	Negative
Sirolimus	Impair spermatogenesis and decrease T levels	Negative
Tacrolimus	Mild, reversible inhibition of spermatogenesis	Neutral

demonstrated in animal models is applicable to human reproductive function, clinical evidence suggests that these harmful effects are reversible. Overall fertility rates in post-transplant males remain similar to those of the general population, supporting the finding that gonadal dysfunction caused by post-transplant medication resolves within 6 months of transplant [7, 8].

Female transplant patients show similar recovery of reproductive function, though registry data on the subject of successful post-transplant pregnancies is limited [9]. Physiologically, the immune response encourages pregnancy by enhancing endometrial reception of the embryo and promoting deep placentation [10]. Thus, it follows that the immunosuppression necessary for successful organ transplant may negatively impact fertility rates and pregnancy outcomes in these patients. Though many post-transplant pregnancies are successful and without complication, studies have found an increased incidence of premature delivery, low birth weight, and stillbirth in transplant patients [11]. Fetal outcomes are discussed below.

36.3 Counseling Transplant Recipients

Patients receiving immunosuppressive therapy should be counseled regarding these possible impacts of post-transplant treatment on fertility, pregnancy, and outcomes for future offspring. In addition, transplant patients of reproductive age should be pre-operatively counseled on contraception and pregnancy options after receiving the organ graft.

36.3.1 Contraception

Oral contraceptive use must be tailored to the individual patient's post-transplant reproductive desires and risks. The estrogen component may increase levels of angiotensinogen, the substrate for renin activity [12]. Increased enzymatic activity secondary to substrate availability enhances the activity of the renin-angiotensin-aldosterone system, causing hypertension. This potential exacerbation of hypertension is an important consideration in the post-organ transplant population. On the other hand, progestin-only oral contraceptives are associated with less serious adverse side effects and may be considered safer than estrogen/progestin formulations [13]. However, progestin-only oral contraceptives are notably less effective than combined oral contraceptives and carry a higher risk of irregular bleeding [13]. These qualities of oral contraceptives should be considered in the context of desired reproductive outcomes post-transplant, expense to the patient, and thorough and individualized risk-benefit analysis [14].

There is mixed evidence regarding the post-transplant use of intrauterine devices (IUDs). Earlier studies raised concerns about a potential negative effect of immunosuppression on IUD efficacy and increased risk of infection with post-transplant IUD usage [15]. Evidence within the last decade suggests, however, that the T-cell-inhibiting mechanism of most immunosuppressants used in organ transplantation does not affect the mechanism of IUDs, which rely on macrophage function [16]. Furthermore, evidence demonstrates no increased risk of infection in immunosuppressed IUD users when compared to immunocompetent patients

[17]. Thus, IUDs may be considered an alternative method of contraception for patients with a contraindication to estrogen or progestin use.

36.3.2 Post-transplant Delay Period Before Attempting Conception

When approaching post-transplant fertility in organ transplant patients, it is vital to review the dysfunction of fertility caused by underlying pre-transplant conditions. This dysfunction is most apparent and well-studied in patients with end-stage renal disease (ESRD).

Patients with ESRD are subject to a plethora of medical complications, including infertility and sexual dysfunction. ESRD patients often undergo regular dialysis in an effort to mitigate the negative impact of their renal condition. Dialysis-dependent patients have imbalances in gonadotropin production and a resultant elevation of luteinizing hormone (LH). In women, the cyclic LH surge does not occur, leading to anovulation [18]. In men, spermatogenesis is impaired by the hormonal dysfunction, impacting sperm quality and quantity [18]. In addition to hormonal imbalance, vascular calcification is also highly prevalent in patients with chronic kidney disease (CKD), leading to pelvic vascular insufficiency and further impairing sexual function [19]. Neurological complications are common comorbidities in patients with CKD, potentially manifesting as autonomic neuropathy. Inadequate sympathetic and parasympathetic stimulation during intercourse may lead to impotence, another confounding factor for renal-impaired patients attempting to conceive [20].

Even if medical complications of organ failure do not directly contribute to infertility, the psychological impact of severe illness may lead to decreased libido in potential renal and non-renal transplant patients, limiting reproductive desire and capacity. Despite the prevalence of fertility concerns in end-stage renal disease, fertility is commonly restored following a successful organ transplant. However, patients should be counseled regarding the unique fertility challenges presented by his or her post-transplant condition.

If conception is desired post-transplant, the clinician and patient should discuss the length of time the patient should wait before attempting conception. McKay and members of the Consensus Conference on Reproductive Issues and Transplantation in 2005 recommend attempting conception as early as 1 year post-transplant in patients with adequately functioning grafts, low risk for infection, and no teratogenic medications [14]. In other circumstances, including acute graft rejection and serum creatinine above 1.5 mg/dL, patience beyond 1 year post-transplant should be considered prior to attempting conception [14].

36.4 Management of Pregnancy in Solid-Organ Transplant Recipients

In organ transplantation, proper risk management is crucial to the patient's long-term health and quality of life. Rejection, infection, and maintenance of adequate graft function are the most pressing concerns in any organ transplant recipient. Female transplant patients of reproductive age carry the additional risk of potential teratogenic effects of immunosuppressant medications. Pregnancy should be managed cautiously in these patients.

36.4.1 Maternal Considerations

Pregnancies in organ transplant recipients should be considered high risk, with special attention paid to treatment goals relevant to the gestation. The key issues include rapid resolution of hypertensive complications and maintenance of transplant function [14].

36.4.1.1 Hypertension

One of the most commonly encountered complications of solid-organ transplantation is hypertension, with a prevalence of 70–90% in the transplant population [21]. Though hypertension is common among all solid-organ transplant recipients, special attention should be paid to the management of elevated blood pressure in renal transplant recipients, as many hypertensive mechanisms depend on renal function. A high incidence of hypertension has been reported in female pregnant renal transplant patients, carrying a six-fold higher risk of progression to preeclampsia when compared to the general pregnant population [22].

The mechanism of this condition in the early post-transplant period is related to intravascular volume expansion in the face of persistent systemic vascular resistance (Fig. 36.2). Peripheral renin concentration is elevated during the early post-transplant period in kidney recipients by an uncertain mechanism that may be related to autonomic denervation of the allograft, resulting in increased sodium and fluid retention [23]. In an acute condition, the vasculature responds to this increased intravascular blood volume by lowering peripheral resistance, in order to preserve a normalized blood pressure at the expense of cardiac output. However, in chronic states of elevated intravascular blood volume, such as the post-transplant period, vascular tone increases, resulting in elevated arterial blood pressure [24]. This mechanism attempts to return cardiac output to normal and preserve cardiac function in the long term but presents an ongoing challenge with hypertension in the renal transplant patient.

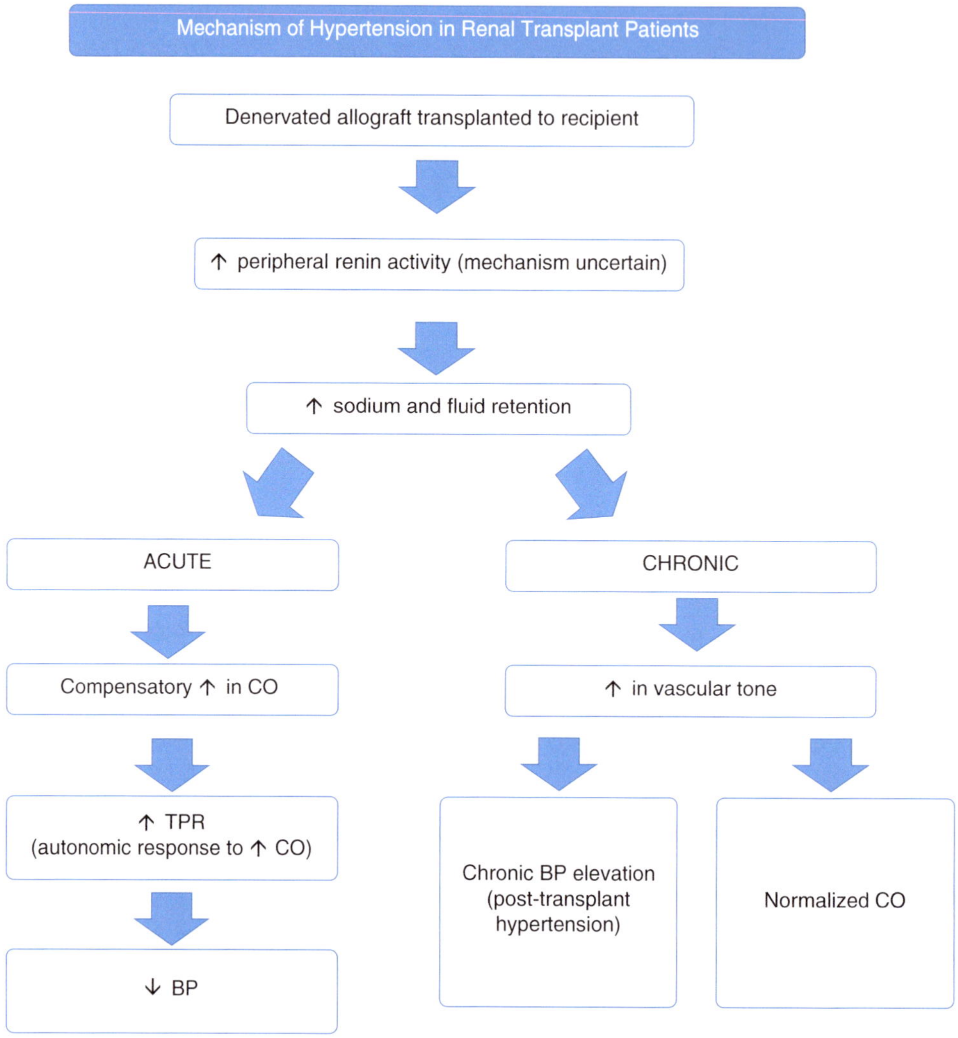

Fig. 36.2 Mechanism of hypertension in renal transplantation. *CO* cardiac output, *TPR* total peripheral resistance, *BP* blood pressure

36.4.1.2 Maintenance of Graft Function

In nonpregnant renal transplant patients, serial serum creatinine levels may be compared in order to monitor graft function [25]. However, pregnancy induces a physiological hyperfiltration in the kidneys, whether the organ is endogenous or transplanted, thereby reducing the accuracy of serum creatinine as an indicator of transplant function [9, 26]. Ultrasound-guided renal biopsy is a safe alternative in detecting rejection at the histological level, if suspected in the context of unexplained reduction of allograft function [14]. Mass spectrometry (MS) urine analysis has emerged as a noninvasive means of diagnosing acute renal transplant rejection and may be useful in detecting functional decline in the allograft before histological damage is evident on biopsy [27]. MS testing allows for early detection of matrix degradation products, indicative of acute rejection, in the urine.

36.4.1.3 Infection

Transplant patients have a remarkably high incidence of post-operative infection, leading to morbidity and potential mortality in many patients despite advances in transplantation medicine. Though immunosuppression is necessary to prevent graft rejection, these agents carry an increased risk of infection due to an underactive immune response. Infections occur at a rate of 45 per 100 patients, with cytomegalovirus (CMV) as the most common identifiable causative organism [28]. Other common pathogens infecting transplant recipients are listed in Table 36.2.

Table 36.2 Common specific pathogens in post-transplantation infections. (In descending order of frequency by type)

Type	Pathogen
Virus	Cytomegalovirus (CMV)
	Varicella-zoster virus (VZV)
	Herpes simplex virus (HSV)
	Hepatitis C virus (HCV)
	Hepatitis B virus (HBV)
Bacteria	*Mycobacterium tuberculosis*
Fungus	*Candida albicans*
	Pneumocystis jiroveci

CMV has been identified in 6–8% of renal transplant patients [28, 29]. CMV infection is of particular concern in pregnant transplant recipients and is a member of a group of infections known as TORCH. TORCH organisms, including *Toxoplasma gondii*, *Rubella virus*, *Cytomegalovirus*, herpes simplex virus, and "Other", are transmissible in utero and are known to cause spontaneous abortions and serious congenital malformations, including limb hypoplasia, microcephaly, and cleft lip/palate [30]. "Other" represents a growing list of organisms with similar attributes, including *Treponema pallidum* (the causative agent of syphilis), varicella-zoster virus, and parvovirus B19 [30].

The impact of CMV infection in transplant patients is compounded in pregnancy. In immunocompetent patients, CMV causes a mild infection resembling mononucleosis or is completely asymptomatic. Nearly 50–100% of normal adults carry CMV antibodies indicating previous exposure [31]; however, a key determinant in the virulence of CMV is the host's immune status [31]. In immunocompromised individuals, including transplant recipients, CMV causes a disseminated infection resulting in pneumonitis and colitis [31]. These findings may progress to acute respiratory distress and extensive gastrointestinal ulceration [31]. CMV transmitted to the fetus can result in devastating consequences including intracranial calcifications, intrauterine growth retardation, and liver dysfunction, all of which can result in fetal and neonatal morbidity [31]. Infants who survive may be afflicted with permanent sensorineural hearing loss and other neurological deficits [31].

It is crucial to initiate surveillance for CMV and other potential infections throughout the post-transplant period. Serology, while useful in establishing the pre-transplant CMV status of both donor and recipient, cannot detect active infection [32]. Molecular methods, specifically polymerase chain reaction (PCR), are more sensitive and accurate than other diagnostic methods in detecting and quantifying CMV infection [32]. CMV prophylaxis may be initiated, especially in CMV-naïve recipients receiving allografts from CMV-positive donors [32]. The majority of adults and potential donors have been exposed, creating a difficult treatment situation in these patients. Pre-operative determination of CMV status by serology of both the donor and patient allows proactive management of potential infection.

36.4.2 Fetal and Neonatal Considerations

If the transplant patient is pregnant during immunosuppression, the fetus will unavoidably be exposed to these medications. The maternal-fetal circulation is not equipped to sequester immunosuppressive agents within the maternal blood. All medications used for immunosuppression have been known to cross into placental and fetal circulation during pregnancy [9]. Methotrexate, mycophenolate mofetil, and leflunomide are decidedly teratogenic and should be avoided in pregnancy [33]. However, research suggests that hydroxychloroquine, corticosteroids, azathioprine, and sulfasalazine may be less disruptive to fetal development when used as immunosuppressive agents in transplant recipients [33].

There has been some concern among the medical community that immunosuppression during pregnancy may lead to congenital anomalies. Though pregnancies in immunosuppressed patients demonstrate a higher incidence of adverse gestational outcomes including low birth weight and premature delivery, evidence does not suggest that immunosuppression inherently leads to birth defects [34, 35]. The specific teratogenic medications discussed above, however, do carry a developmental risk to the fetus.

Though most immunosuppression regimens have not been shown to cause adverse outcomes in children of transplant patients, this population does demonstrate a high incidence of fetal complications. The incidence of preterm birth (52–53%), low birth weight (42–46%), and intrauterine growth restriction (30–50%) are elevated in renal allograft recipients, especially in those with poorly managed maternal hypertension and serum creatinine level over 17 mg/dL [22]. In the absence of maternal risk factors including hypertension, impaired allograft function, and proteinuria, there does not appear to be a higher risk of miscarriage [22]. On the other hand, in the presence of any of these risk factors, a miscarriage rate of 11–26% has been reported, approximately twofold higher than that of the general population [22].

36.5 Pregnancy in Uterine Transplant Patients

36.5.1 Historical Perspective

Pregnancy in solid-organ transplant patients is well-studied, but the notion of transplanting a functional uterus, capable of carrying a pregnancy, has become a burgeoning area of interest for researchers. For decades, there has been no successful treatment available that would allow women with an absent or otherwise dysfunctional uterus to carry a child to term, and many women have settled for using a gestational surrogate. Infertility has shown strong associations with clinical depression, anxiety, and a reduced quality of life [36, 37]. Restoring the capability of child-bearing to patients with absolute uterine factor infertility (AUFI) is a life-changing possibility for women, one that today's patients show a keen interest in pursuing [38]. Uterine transplant is an emerging treatment option for AUFI, which may also be attributed to congenital malformations of the uterus, severe intrauterine adhesions, or prior hysterectomy [4, 39].

The possibility of genital transplantation began to be explored in 1896, when an Austrian gynecological team experimented with ovarian autotransplantation in rabbits [40]. After the turn of the century, researchers began to study the possibility of uterine transplantation, though published research from this time period is scarce. With the rise of in vitro fertilization during the late 1970s, the majority of infertile couples were able to conceive, deferring interest in the field of uterine transplantation until the 1990s. Animal models including rodents and primates were studied, soon followed by the experimental clinical stage of the procedure in humans [41].

The first report of a human uterus transplantation was published in 2002 by a Saudi Arabian team [41, 42]. Performed on 26-year-old patient who lost her uterus at age 20 due to post-partum hemorrhage, the procedure was ultimately unsuccessful. The patient suffered acute vascular thrombosis months after the transplant, and the donor uterus was removed. However, histopathological study showed no signs of transplant rejection, an encouraging observation in the face of the procedure's failure.

Clinical interest in the procedure has more recently been spurred with the birth of the first healthy child 1 year after a uterine transplant in Sweden in 2013. The transplant patient was diagnosed with congenital absence of the uterus, one of many causes of absolute uterine factor infertility [4]. An intense triple immunosuppression regimen and swift resolution of three mild rejection episodes were vital to the success of the Swedish operation. Results of this procedure are promising for the future of elective uterine transplants, though the nature of the procedure poses unique medical risks that must continue to be addressed [43]. As highlighted by the concentrated efforts of the transplant team in Sweden, immunosuppression and meticulous follow-up are essential components of future procedures. To date, 11 cases of uterine transplantation have been reported worldwide. Seven of these cases resulted in pregnancy, three of which achieved live births [41].

Following Sweden's successful uterine transplant, the procedure was then attempted in the United States in 2016. The operation appeared successful until the donor uterus was emergently removed 2 weeks following the procedure, after a fungal infection compromised the integrity of the graft's vascular flow [44]. These cases illustrate three critical components of a successful uterine transplant: maintenance of adequate blood flow, aggressive immunosuppression, and scrupulous infection control.

36.5.2 Ethical Considerations

Unlike other organs, including the kidneys, liver, and heart, the uterus is regarded as "non-vital," presenting ethical concerns of clinical legitimacy when approaching the procedure. In this context, an argument in favor of non-vital transplantation is the rising prevalence and clinical acceptance of these procedures [45]. Penile and testicular transplantations have been performed, as well as hand and face transplantations [46, 47]. These body parts are not necessary for survival, but the psychological and functional benefits of transplantation justify the procedure, as can be argued for uterine transplantations.

The ethical concern of potential harm outweighing the benefits of elective uterine transplantation must also be considered. From a technical aspect, the surgical procedure and management of uterine transplantation is similar to that of vital organ transplants, implying no increased risk to the uterus recipient or the potential fetus. Some immunosuppressive agents necessary for rejection control have demonstrated teratogenic effects, as discussed above, but the flexibility of regimens allow clinicians to evade this risk.

Lefkowitz et al. considered the ethical issues surround this procedure in 2011, creating the Montreal Criteria for the Ethical Feasibility of Uterine Transplantation [45] (Table 36.3). Considering that the procedure is medically safe for the pregnant patient and her fetus, and assuming that uterine transplantation will lead to a viable pregnancy, the criteria below are proposed for the recipient, donor, and healthcare team [45]. It has been proposed that all ethical criteria must be met before proceeding with uterine transplantation.

36.5.3 Future of Uterine Transplantation

Clinical forays into uterine transplantation procedure may soon be made less treacherous by the development of "unrejectable" bioengineered organs. Whole organ engineering is a promising means of evading the common challenges of immunosuppression and rejection in transplantation. A technique known as decellularization has been employed, stripping donor organs down to scaffolds of extracellular matrix material. The scaffold, free of any donor cells (and thus, potential donor antigens), may then be seeded with stem cells derived from the desired organ [48]. Originally developed in hopes of improving solid-organ transplant technology, decellularization/recellularization techniques show promise for achieving a viable bioengineered uterus or regeneration of a partially excised uterus, without the risk of organ rejection [49].

36.6 Assisted Reproductive Technology in Organ Transplant Recipients

Though fertility is re-established in many organ transplant recipients, especially those well within their child-bearing years, many may struggle with infertility that may be caused

Table 36.3 Montreal Criteria for the Ethical Feasibility of Uterine Transplantation

The recipient…	…is a genetic female of reproductive age with no medical contraindications to transplantation
	…has documented congenital or acquired UFI which has failed all current gold standard and conservative therapy
	…has a personal or legal contraindication to surrogacy and adoption measures or seeks the UTx solely as a measure to experience gestation, with an understanding the limitations provided by the UTx in this respect
	…has not had her decision to undergo UTx deemed as irrational by expert psychological evaluation, and has no psychological comorbidity that interferes with diagnostic workup of treatment
	…does not exhibit frank unsuitability for motherhood
	… is likely to take antirejection medication and follow up with the treating team in a responsible manner
	…is responsible enough to consent, informed enough to make a responsible decision
The donor…	…is a female of reproductive age with no medical contraindications to donation
	…has repeatedly attested to her conclusion of parity or has signed an advanced directive for postmortem organ donation
	…has no history of uterine damage or disease
	…is responsible enough to consent, informed enough to make a responsible decision, and not under coercion
The health care team…	…is part of an institution that meets Moore's third criterion[a] as it pertains to institutional stability
	…has provided adequate informed consent to both parties regarding risks, potential sequelae, and chances of success and failure
	…has no conflict of interest independently or with either party
	…has the duty to preserve anonymity if the donor or recipient do not explicitly waive this right

[a]Moore and Kinne defined field strength, laboratory background, and institutional stability as key components for ethical analysis of surgical innovation. Reprinted with permission from Elsevier

UTx uterine transplantation

From Lefkowitz A, Edwards M, Balayla J. Ethical considerations in the era of the uterine transplant: an update of the Montreal criteria for the ethical feasibility of uterine transplantation. Fertil Steril. 2013;100 [4]:924–26, with permission

by a separate reproductive abnormality or from graft dysfunction.

In those with fertility issues secondary to impaired graft function, the underlying dysfunction should be treated and controlled before attempting conception. Postponing conception for at least a year after achieving adequate graft function has been recommended, as discussed above [14]. Graft function is particularly relevant in renal transplant patients, as impaired reproductive function is a known comorbidity in patients with renal insufficiency [50]. Overall, though data is limited on infertility rates in other solid-organ transplant patients, renal allograft recipients appear to demonstrate similar fecundity when compared to the general population [50]. This suggests that the same standard diagnostic and treatment approach used in the typical infertility patient should be used in these patients, with the added caution of allograft monitoring throughout the treatment [41].

36.6.1 In Vitro Fertilization

Indications for in vitro fertilization (IVF) in transplant patients are similar to that of general population including tubal disease and male factor infertility. IVF is a first-line treatment for infertility due to its safety, efficacy, and minimal invasiveness [51]. Overall, discussions on IVF in transplant patients are few, though even greater caution must be entertained in this patient population. While data is lacking on response to gonadotropins, implantation, and pregnancy rates, risks including ovarian hyperstimulation syndrome and multiple gestations have the potential for even greater consequences in this patient population.

Reports that exist focus primarily on renal transplant patients, with the first reported IVF pregnancy was in 1995, thus establishing the efficacy of this procedure in the transplant population [52]. Several case reports since have demonstrated that IVF pregnancies have no direct impact on graft function and that pregnancy in these patients does not increase renal morbidity [52–54]. However, some cases suggest that ART may indirectly contribute to graft dysfunction. It has been hypothesized that medically enlarged ovaries caused by ART may lead to compression of the graft and secondary renal obstruction, reversible by symptomatic treatment [55].

36.6.2 Alternative Approaches to ART

A number of options used to minimize IVF complications in the general population should be considered and applied to this patient population. These include minimal stimulation protocols, elective single embryo transfer, elective cryopreservation, and subsequent embryo transfer.

36.6.2.1 Minimal Stimulation Protocols

Minimal stimulation (MS) protocols aim to produce a fewer number of high-quality oocytes for IVF, rather than simply producing a greater quantity of oocytes, as in conventional controlled ovarian stimulation. The pregnancy rate and number of retrieved oocytes in patients receiving MS IVF has been reported to be similar to that in conventional IVF patients, and in addition MS offers several benefits [56, 57].

MS using SERM or gonadotropin triggers carries a lower risk of OHSS, in contrast to traditional ovarian stimulation protocols where supraphysiologic estradiol levels and multiple follicular recruitment are often seen [56]. These are the main factors leading to an increased risk of OHSS and resultant fluid shift from the vasculature to the interstitial space causing ascites, hemoconcentration, and a hypercoagulable state [58]. This is crucial to avoid particularly in those with renal transplants.

36.6.2.2 GnRH-Agonist Triggers

Another consideration is the use of GnRH-agonist (GnRH-a) to induce oocyte maturation (trigger) with GnRH-antagonist (GnRH-ant) protocols to minimize OHSS risk, instead of using human chorionic gonadotropins (hCG). Data suggests that levels of key hormones implicated in the pathogenesis of OHSS (vascular endothelial growth factor, tumor necrosis factor α, and estradiol) are significantly lower in patients receiving GnRH-a trigger when compared to hCG trigger. The suggested mechanism for this finding is the shorter half-life of GnRH-a, which stimulates LH release for 24 h [59]. This is a relatively narrow duration of action when compared to hCG trigger, which sustain gonadotropin production for more than a week [59]. Meta-analysis suggests that GnRH-a triggers are significantly safer than hCG trigger [60]. Several studies have reported that the use of a GnRH-a trigger significantly reduces the risk of OHSS to 0–2%, a striking decrease compared to the 5–31% incidence of OHSS with hCG triggers [60–62].

GnRH-a trigger during GnRH-ant regimens may either be given as an independent 0.1 mg dose of triptorelin (a synthetic GnRH-a analogue) or concomitantly with a 1500 IU bolus of hCG (dual-trigger) 34–37 h prior to oocyte retrieval [63]. Alternatively, a 0.15 mg bolus of leuprolide acetate (Lupron) or a 300 μg intranasal dose of nafarelin acetate (Synarel) may be administered to stimulate final oocyte maturation [64, 65]. Overall, while the use of a GnRH-a trigger minimizes the risk of OHSS, its benefits must be balanced against its less desirable pregnancy outcomes. The odds of pregnancy are significantly less with GnRH-a than with hCG (OR 0.75, 95% CI 0.59–0.96) [57]. This strategy is currently recommended for use only in patients who intend to have their oocytes cryopreserved for later use [57]. GnRH-a triggers may have wider application beyond cryopreservation, but further research is needed with respect to pregnancy outcomes.

36.6.2.3 Elective Cryopreservation

With improved cryopreservation techniques with vitrification, pregnancy outcomes have been reported to be comparable to fresh embryo transfers (ETs) [66, 67]. Elective cryopreservation and subsequent frozen thaw cycles also provides the benefit of avoiding OHSS by allowing the supraphysiologic estradiol to normalize from ovulation induction and oocyte retrieval [68]. A combination of GnRH-a trigger with elective cryopreservation appears to essentially eliminate the risk of OHSS in patients undergoing this approach and should be considered in the transplant population [69].

36.6.2.4 Elective Single Embryo Transfer

Elective single embryo transfer (eSET) has been demonstrated to result in similar pregnancy outcomes when compared to multiple embryo transfer (MET), while avoiding the risk of multifetal gestation [70]. As such, the American Society for Reproductive Medicine (ASRM) currently recommends eSET when the prognosis for implantation is good, in patients under age 35 with several high-quality embryos available for transfer [71].

The pregnant transplant patient is already at a six-fold increased risk of preeclampsia (discussed above) and multiple pregnancy itself confers a further threefold risk of developing this condition, taxing the renal system well beyond normal limits [72]. In the transplant patient, particularly the renal transplant patient, preeclampsia can have catastrophic implications. While no data exists on implantation and pregnancy rates, following ASRM's recommendations of eSET would be a prudent approach and should be strongly considered [71].

36.7 Conclusion

The organ transplant population presents a unique set of challenges when considering post-operative pregnancy. The immunosuppressive therapy necessary to combat allograft rejection presents potential reproductive concerns. The majority of transplant patients regain pre-operative fertility levels within 6 months post-procedure. However, additional risks appear during pregnancy. The allograft encounters an increased workload in the face of pregnancy, potentially complicating maternal health throughout gestation. Pregnant transplant recipients also carry an increased risk of adverse fetal outcomes, including fetal growth restriction and preterm birth. With careful consideration of these factors, as well as the concerns of hypertension, infection, and rejection in transplant patients, birth outcomes can be excellent. For patients with uterine factor infertility, uterine transplant is a viable prospect. Properly managed organ transplantation has the potential to save and prolong lives, affording patients the full experience of life, including family planning and childbirth.

References

1. Nagy J. A note on the early history of renal transplantation: Emerich (Imre) Ullmann. Am J Nephrol. 1999;19:346–9.
2. Murray JE, Merrill JP, Harrison JH. Renal homotransplantations in identical twins. Surg Forum. 1955;6:432–6.
3. Barker CF, Markmann JF. Historical overview of transplantation. Cold Spring Harb Perspect Med. 2013;3(4):a014977.

4. Brännström M, Johanneson L, Bokström H, Kvarnström N, Mölne J, Dahm-Kähler P, et al. Livebirth after uterus transplantation. Lancet. 2015;385:607–16.
5. Coscia LA, Constantinescu S, Moritz MJ, Frank AM, Ramirez CA, Doria C, et al. Report from the National Transplant Pregnancy Registry (NTPR): outcomes of pregnancy after transplantation [abstract]. Clin Transpl. 2008:89–105.
6. Chen Y, Zhang Z, Lin Y, Lin H, Li M, Nie P, et al. Long-term impact of immunosuppression at therapeutic doses on male reproductive system in unilateral nephrectomized rats: a comparative study. Biomed Res Int. 2013;2013:690382.
7. Akbari F, Alavi M, Esteghamati A, Mehrsai A, Djaladat H, Zohrevand R, et al. Effect of renal transplantation on sperm quality and sex hormone levels. BJU Int. 2003;92(3):281–3.
8. Saha MT, Saha HH, Niskanen LK, Salmela KT, Pasternack AI. Time course of serum prolactin and sex hormones following successful renal transplantation. Nephron. 2002;92:735–7.
9. McKay DB, Josephson MA. Pregnancy after kidney transplantation. Clin J Am Soc Nephrol. 2008;3(Suppl 2):S117–25.
10. Robertson SA, Jin M, Yu D, Moldenhauer LM, Davies MJ, Hull ML, Norman RJ. Corticosteroid therapy in assisted reproduction – immune suppression is a faulty premise. Hum Reprod. 2016;31(10):2164–73.
11. Stratta P, Canavese C, Giacchino F, Mesiano P, Quaglia M, Rossetti M. Pregnancy in kidney transplantation: satisfactory outcomes and harsh realities. J Nephrol. 2003;16(6):792–806.
12. Kang AK, Duncan JA, Cattran DC, Floras JS, Lai V, Scholey JW, et al. Effect of oral contraceptives on the renin angiotensin system and renal function. Am J Physiol Regul Integr Comp Physiol. 2001;280(3):R807–13.
13. Chrousos GP. The gonadal hormones and inhibitors. In: Katzung BG, Trevor AJ, editors. Basic and clinical pharmacology. New Delhi: McGraw-Hill; 2015. p. 708–12.
14. McKay DB, Josephson MA. Reproduction and transplantation: report on the AST consensus conference on reproductive issues and transplantation. Am J Transplant. 2005;5:1592–9.
15. Zerner J, Doil KL, Drewry J, Leeber DA. Intrauterine contraceptive device failures in renal transplant patients [abstract]. J Reprod Med. 1981;26(2):99–102.
16. Perry R, et al. Medical interactions with contraceptives. In: Allen RH, Cwiak CA, editors. Contraception for the medically challenging patient. New York: Springer; 2014. p. 356.
17. Browne H, Manipalviratn S, Armstrong A. Using an intrauterine device in immunocompromised women. Obstet Gynecol. 2008;112(3):667–9.
18. Schmidt RJ, Holley JL. Fertility and contraception in end-stage renal disease [abstract]. Adv Ren Replace Ther. 1998;5(1):38–44.
19. Gorriz JL, Molina P, Cerveron MJ, Vila R, Bover J, Nieto J, et al. Vascular calcification in patients with non-dialysis CKD over 3 years. Clin J Am Soc Nephrol. 2015;10(4):654–66.
20. Arnold R, Issar T, Krishnan AV, Pussell BA. Neurological complications in chronic kidney disease. JRSM Cardiovasc Dis. 2016;5:2048004016677687.
21. Zbroch E, Malyszko J, Mysliwiec M, Przybylowski P, Durlik M. Hypertension in solid organ transplant recipients [abstract]. Ann Transplant. 2012;17(1):100–7.
22. Shah S, Verma P. Overview of pregnancy in renal transplant patients. Int J Nephrol. 2016;2016:1.
23. Kornerup HJ. The patterns of peripheral plasma renin concentration in the early post-transplant period. Scand J Urol Nephrol. 1979;13(2):185–9.
24. MacAllister RJ, Vallance P. Systemic vascular adaptation to increases in blood volume: the role of the blood-vessel wall. Nephrol Dial Transplant. 1996;11:231–40.
25. Josephson MA. Monitoring and managing graft health in the kidney transplant recipient. Clin J Am Soc Nephrol. 2011;6(7):1774–80.
26. Helal I, Fick-Brosnahan GM, Reed-Gitomer B, Schreir RW. Glomerular hyperfiltration: definitions, mechanisms and clinical implications [abstract]. Nat Rev Nephrol. 2012;8(5):293–300.
27. Zapf A, Gwinner W, Karch A, Metzger J, Haller H, Koch A. Non-invasive diagnosis of acute rejection in renal transplant patients using mass spectrometry of urine samples – a multicenter phase 3 diagnostic accuracy study. BMC Nephrol. 2015;16:153.
28. Snyder JJ, Israni AK, Peng Y, Zhang L, Simon TA, Kasiske BL. Rates of first infection following kidney transplant in the United States. Kidney Int. 2009;75(3):317–26.
29. Karutha S, Blumberg EA. Common infections in kidney transplant recipients. Clin J Am Soc Nephrol. 2012;7:2058. https://doi.org/10.2215/CJN.04410512.
30. Yadav RK, Maity S, Saha S. A review on TORCH: groups of congenital infections during pregnancy. J Sci Innovative Res. 2014;3(2):258–64.
31. McAdam AJ, Milner DA, Sharpe AH. Infectious disease. In: Kumar V, Abbas AK, Aster JC, editors. Robbins and Coltran pathologic basic of disease. 9th ed. Philadelphia, PA: Elsevier; 2015. p. 359–60.
32. Azevedo LS, Pierrotti LC, Abdala E, Costa SF, Strabelli TM, Campos SV, et al. Cytomegalovirus infection in transplant recipients. Clinics (Sao Paulo). 2015;70(7):515–23.
33. Leroy C, Rigot J, Leroy M, Decanter C, Mapiphan KL, Parent AS, et al. Immunosuppressive drugs and fertility. Orphanet J Rare Dis. 2015;10:136. https://doi.org/10.1186/s13023-015-0332-8.
34. Cooper WO, Cheetman TC, Li D, Stein CM, Callahan ST, Morgan TM. Brief report: risk of adverse fetal outcomes associated with immunosuppressive medications for chronic immune-mediated diseases in pregnancy. Arthritis Rheum. 2014;66(2):440–50.
35. Motta M, Tincani A, Meroni PL, Cimaz R. Follow-up of children exposed antenatally to immunosuppressive drugs. Rheum. 2008;47(3)
36. Sut HK, Kaplan B. Quality of life in women with infertility via the FertiQol and the hospital anxiety and depression scales [abstract]. Nurs Health Sci. 2015 Mar;17(1):84–9.
37. Ramezanzadeh F, Aghssa MM, Abedinia N, Zayeri F, Khanafshar N, Shariat M, Jafarabadi M. A survey of relationship between anxiety, depression and duration of fertility. BMC Womens Health. 2004 Nov 6;4:9.
38. Saso S, Clark A, Bracewell-Milnes T, Saso A, Al-Memar M, Thum M, et al. Psychological issues associated with absolute uterine factor infertility and attitudes of patients toward uterine transplantation. Prog Transplant. 2016;26(1):28–39.
39. Saravelos SH, Cocksedge KA, Li TC. Prevalence and diagnosis of congenital uterine anomalies in women with reproductive failure: a critical appraisal. Hum Reprod Update. 2008;14:415–29.
40. Knauer E. An attempt at ovary transplantation in rabbits. Zentralblatt für Gynäkologie. 1896;20:524–8.. Germanica
41. Johanneson L, Järvholm S. Uterus transplantation: current progress and future prospects. Int J Women's Health. 2016;8:43–51.
42. Fageeh W, Raffa H, Jabbad H, Marzouki A. Transplantation of the human uterus. Int J Gynaecol Obstet. 2002;76(3):245–51.
43. Farrell RM, Falcone T. Uterine transplant: new medical and ethical considerations. Lancet. 2015 Feb 14;385(9968):581–2.
44. Common infection caused first U.S. transplant to fail, hospital says. University of Utah Health Library. 2016 Apr 8. Retrieved from http://healthcare.utah.edu/healthlibrary/related/doc.php?type=6&id=709834.
45. Lefkowitz A, Edwards M, Balayla J. Ethical considerations in the era of the uterine transplant: an update of the Montreal criteria for the ethical feasibility of uterine transplantation. Fertil Steril. 2013;100(4):924–6.
46. Donati-Bourne J, Roberts HW, Rajjoub Y, Coleman RA. A review of transplantation practice of the urologic organs: is it only achievable for the kidney? Rev Urol. 2015;17(2):69–77.

47. Gander B, Brown CS, Vasilic D, Furr A, Banis JC Jr, Cunningham M, et al. Composite tissue allotransplantation of the hand and face: a new frontier in transplant and reconstructive surgery. Transpl Int. 2006;19(11):868–80.
48. Scarritt ME, Pashos NC, Bunnell BA. A review of cellularization strategies for tissue engineering of whole organs. Front Bioeng Biotechnol. 2015 Mar 30;3:43.
49. Miyazaki K, Maruyama T. Partial regeneration and reconstruction of the rat uterus through recellularization of a decellularized uterine matrix. Biomaterials. 2014 Oct;35(31):8791–800.
50. Ghazizadeh S, Lessan-Pezeshki M, Khatami MR, Mahdavi-Mazdeh M, Abbasi MR, Azmandian J, et al. Infertility among kidney transplant recipients. Saudi J Kidney Dis Transpl. 2007;18(1):79–82.
51. Huang LN, Tan J, Hitkari J, Dahan MH. Should IVF be used a first-line treatment or as a last resort? A debate presented at the 2013 Canadian Fertility and Andrology Society meeting. Reprod Biomed Online. 2015;30(2):128–36.
52. Lockwood GM, Ledger WL, Barlow DH. Successful pregnancy outcome in a renal transplant patient following in-vitro fertilization. Hum Reprod. 1995;10(6):1528–30.
53. Tamaki M, Ami M, Kimata N, Tsutsui T, Watanabe Y, Saito T, et al. Successful singleton pregnancy outcome resulting from in vitro fertilization after renal transplantation. Transplantation. 2003;75(7):1082–3.
54. Nouri K, Bader Y, Helmy S, Ott J, Jirecek S, Tempfer CB. Live birth after in vitro fertilization and single embryo transfer in a kidney transplant patient: a case report and review of the literature. J Assist Reprod Genet. 2011;28(4):351–3.
55. Khalaf Y, Elkington N, Anderson H, Taylor A, Braude P. Ovarian hyperstimulation syndrome and its effect on renal function in a renal transplant patient undergoing IVF treatment: case report. Hum Reprod. 2000;15(6):1275–7.
56. Zhang JJ, Merhi Z, Yang M, Bodri D, Chavez-Badiola A, Repping S, et al. Minimal stimulation IVF vs conventional IVF: a randomized controlled trial. Am J Obstet Gynecol. 2016;214(1):96.e1–8.
57. Youssef MAF, Abdelmoty HI, Ahmed MAS, Elmohamady M. GnRH agonist for final oocyte maturation in GnRH antagonist co-treated IVF/ICSI treatment cycles: systematic review and meta-analysis. J Adv Res. 2015;6(3):341–9.
58. Kumar P, Sait SF, Sharma A, Kumar M. Ovarian hyperstimulation syndrome. J Hum Reprod Sci. 2011;4(2):70–5.
59. Babayof R, Margalioth EJ, Huleihel M, Amash A, Zylber-Haran E, Gal M, et al. Serum inhibin A, VEGF, and TNFalpha levels after triggering oocyte maturation with GnRH agonist compared with HCG in women with polycystic ovaries undergoing IVF treatment: a prospective randomized trial. Hum Reprod. 2006;21(5):1260–5.
60. Youssef MA, Van der Veen F, Al-Inany HG, Mochtar MH, Griesinger G, Nagi Mohesen M, et al. Gonadotropin-releasing hormone agonist versus HCG for oocyte triggering in antagonist-assisted reproductive technology. Cochrane Database Syst Rev. 2014;10:CD008046.
61. Engmann L, DiLuigi A, Schmidt A, Nulsen J, Maier D, Benadiva C. The use of gonadotropin-releasing hormone (GnRH) agonist to induce oocyte maturation after cotreatment with GnRH antagonist in high-risk patients undergoing in vitro fertilization prevents the risk of ovarian hyperstimulation syndrome: a prospective randomized controlled study. Fertil Steril. 2008;89(1):84–91.
62. Acevedo B, Gomez-Palomares JL, Ricciarelli E, Hernández ER. Triggering ovulation with gonadotropin-releasing hormone agonists does not compromise embryo implantation rates. Fertil Steril. 2006;86(6):1682–7.
63. Oliveira JB, Baruffi R, Petersen CG, Mauri AL, Cavagna M, Franco JG. Administration of single-dose GnRH agonist in the luteal phase in ICSI cycles: a meta-analysis. Reprod Bio Endocrinol. 2010;8:107.
64. Zhang J, Chang L, Sone Y, Silber S. Minimal ovarian stimulation (mini-IVF) for IVF utilizing vitrification and cryopreserved embryo transfer. Reprod Biomed. 2010;21(4):485–95.
65. Sismanoglu A, Tekin HI, Erden HF, Ciray NH, Ulug U, Bahceci M. Ovulation triggering with GnRH agonist vs hCG in the same egg donor population undergoing donor oocyte cycles with GnRH antagonist: a prospective randomized cross-over trial. J Assist Reprod Genet. 2009;26(5):251–6.
66. Maheshwari A, Raja EA, Bhattacharya S. Obstetric and perinatal outcomes after either fresh or thawed frozen embryo transfer: an analysis of 112,432 singleton pregnancies recorded in the human fertilisation and embryology authority anonymized dataset. Fertil Steril. 2016;106(7):1703–8.
67. Pereira N, Petrini AC, Lekovich JP, Schattman GL, Rosenwaks Z. Comparison of perinatal outcomes following fresh and frozen-thawed blastocyst transfer. Int J Gynaecol Obstet. 2016;135(1):96–100.
68. Roque M, Lattes K, Serra S, Solà I, Geber S, Carreras R, et al. Fresh embryo transfer versus frozen embryo transfer in in vitro fertilization cycles: a systematic review and meta-analysis. Fertil Steril. 2013;99(1):156–62.
69. Griesinger G, von Otte S, Schroer A, Ludwig AK, Diedrich S, et al. Elective cryopreservation of all pronuclear oocytes after GnRH agonist triggering of final oocyte maturation in patients at risk of developing OHSS: a prospective, observational proof-of-concept study. Hum Reprod. 2007;22(5):1348–52.
70. Thurin A, Hausken J, Hillensjö T, Jablonowska B, Pinborg A, Strandell A, et al. Elective single-embryo transfers versus double-embryo transfer in in vitro fertilization. N Engl J Med. 2004;351:2392–402.
71. Practice Committee of the Society for Assisted Reproductive Technology and Practice Committee of the American Society for Reproductive Medicine. Elective single-embryo transfer. Fertil Steril. 2012;97(4):835–42.
72. Duckitt K, Harrington D. Risk factors for pre-eclampsia at antenatal booking: systematic review of controlled studies. BMJ. 2005;330:565. https://doi.org/10.1136/bmj.38380.674340.E0.

Ovarian Hyperstimulation Syndrome

37

Sule Yildiz and Baris Ata

Ovarian hyperstimulation syndrome (OHSS) is characterized by increased capillary permeability causing fluid shift into the third space. OHSS can present with ascites, pleural effusion, hypovolemia, hemoconcentration, and hypercoagulability. Thromboembolism is the most serious complication, which potentially can lead to death. As such, OHSS is the most serious complication of infertility treatments.

37.1 Pathophysiology of Ovarian Hyperstimulation Syndrome

Ovarian hyperstimulation syndrome occurs most often following ovarian stimulation with gonadotropin for assisted reproductive technology (ART). It is very rarely reported in spontaneously conceived pregnancies. Overactivating FSH receptor gene mutations cause predisposition to OHSS [1, 2]. Very high levels of endogenous hCG can also trigger OHSS in a molar pregnancy [3–7].

The hallmark of OHSS is increased capillary permeability leading to ascites and pleural effusion. Vascular endothelial growth factor (VEGF) is the major molecule responsible for increased vascular permeability [8–11]. There are three VEGF receptors: VEGF receptor-1 (VEGFR-1), VEGFR-2, and VEGFR-3 [12, 13]. VEGFR-1 and VEGFR-2 are expressed by endothelial cells. VEGF receptors are also expressed on the granulosa cells of the follicles [14–16]. Moreover, endothelial cells produce a soluble form of VEGFR-1 (sVEGRFR-1), that is indeed an antagonist; since on it binds free VEGF and prevents the latter from binding and stimulating membrane bound receptors [17, 18].

VEGFR-2 activation increases mitogenic activity in endothelial cells and results in a rapid increase in vascular permeability [19]. Moreover, VEGF causes fenestration of the endothelial barrier in small vessels [20, 21].

VEGF is produced in granulosa cells during folliculogenesis. Human chorionic gonadotropin (hCG) augments VEGF expression following gonadotropin stimulation [22–25]. In the presence of multifollicular development, hCG multiplies the already increased VEGF expression in ovarian follicles.

Ovarian renin-angiotensin system (RAS) overactivation can be an intermediate step between hCG exposure and VEGF over-expression. Ovarian RAS is dependent on gonadotropins and probably plays a role in the selection and development of a dominant follicle and in ovulation [26, 27]. HCG administration increases plasma concentration of prorenin, the primary molecule of RAS pathway [28]. Prorenin is converted to angiotensin also in the ovary [29]. Angiotensin 2 is a strong stimulator of VEGF expression, and VEGF expression can be suppressed by the administration of angiotensin receptor blockers [30–37].

37.2 Risk Factors for Ovarian Hyperstimulation Syndrome

Effective prevention requires identification of women at risk for OHSS. The number of luteinized granulosa cells determines both the incidence and the severity of the syndrome; the increased VEGF production by these cells is the main cause of OHSS [38]. Obviously multiple follicular growth brings about the risk. Risk factors can be grouped as primary and secondary risk factors. *Primary risk factors* are endogenous factors regardless of the risks superimposed by controlled ovarian stimulation (COS) protocol, while *secondary risk factors* appear during the COS cycle.

S. Yildiz
Department of Obstetrics and Gynecology, Koc University Hospital, Istanbul, Turkey

B. Ata (✉)
Division of Reproductive Endocrinology and Infertility, Department of Obstetrics and Gynecology, Koç University School of Medicine , Istanbul, Turkey

Department of Obstetrics, Gynecology and Reproductive Sciences, Yale University School of Medicine, New Haven, CT, USA
e-mail: barisata@ku.edu.tr

G. N. Allahbadia et al. (eds.), *Textbook of Assisted Reproduction*, https://doi.org/10.1007/978-981-15-2377-9_37

37.2.1 Primary Risk Factors

Young age, low body weight, polycystic ovarian syndrome (PCOS), and previous history of OHSS are primary risk factors [39, 40]. However, the absence of these factors is not 100% reassuring. Fatal cases of OHSS have also been reported in women older than 40 years [41–43]. The relationship between body mass index (BMI) and risk of OHSS is equivocal. The administration of standard gonadotropin dosage disregarding the BMI might have led to administration of relatively higher amount of gonadotropin to lean women [39]. On the other hand, many women with PCOS have high BMI. Accordingly, BMI alone should not be considered as a risk factor. Women developing OHSS in the absence of other primary risk factors had sixfold higher anti-Müllerian Hormone (AMH) levels as compared to those without OHSS [44]. AMH was found to be a better predictor of OHSS as compared with age and BMI, with a sensitivity of 90.5% and a specificity of 81.3% for a cutoff value set at 3.36 ng/ml [45].

Clear-cut threshold levels do not exist for any of these primary risk factors to allow precise identification of women who will develop OHSS. Furthermore, absence of these primary risk factors does not provide reassurance. Hence the risk of OHSS should always be considered at the beginning of a treatment cycle.

37.2.2 Secondary Risk Factors

Serum estradiol (E2) levels during a stimulation cycle, the rate of E2 increase, follicle number and size, and number of collected retrieved have been assessed as secondary risk factors for OHSS. E2 molecule itself does not have a direct vasoactive effect, and high E2 levels alone do not cause OHSS in the absence of HCG [21, 46, 47]. Serum E2 levels merely represent granulosa cell activity in the context of OHSS.

Serum E2 levels largely overlap between women with and without OHSS, yielding only a modest predictive value [42, 48–50]. Women with partial 17,20 desmolase deficiency can develop OHSS with low E2 levels [51].

The relationship between the number of growing follicles and the risk of OHSS has been evaluated in several studies [41, 52–54]. Although the two are strongly correlated, there is not a precise cutoff denoting significantly increased risk of OHSS. Further, follicle count and size show high variation in the presence of multifollicular growth [48]. Follicle count per se does not improve sensitivity, specificity, and positive or negative predictive values [45].

Identification of primary and secondary risk factors is useful for risk assessment during COS even in the absence of well-defined threshold levels. However, their interpretation varies considerably among clinics and physicians [38].

37.3 Prevention of OHSS

OHSS develops due to excessive VEGF production from a high number of luteinized granulosa cells. Exogenous hCG administration, endogenous luteinizing hormone, or endogenous hCG of a developing pregnancy can all cause and sustain excessive luteinization. Exogenous hCG injection or very rarely endogenous LH triggered by a single bolus of GnRH agonist injection is responsible for the development of *early OHSS* (within the first 8 days of oocyte collection), while hCG of pregnancy for *late OHSS* (8 days after oocyte collection). In addition to the categorization according to the time of onset, OHSS is also categorized according to the symptomatology and laboratory findings. Mild OHSS is characterized by abdominal distention, bilateral ovarian enlargement, and nausea with normal biochemistry. Vomiting and diarrhea can occur. Mild OHSS is usually self-limiting and does not require intervention other than close monitoring. However, occurrence of pregnancy can lead to progression of the condition. Moderate OHSS is characterized by ultrasound evidence of ascites and increased hematocrit over 41%, white blood cell count (WBC) above 10,000/μL, and hypoproteinemia, in addition to the symptoms of mild OHSS. Abdominal distention and other symptoms are more prominent in moderate OHSS. Features of severe OHSS include, in addition to the findings of moderate OHSS, massive ascites with clinical findings, hydrothorax and dyspnea, hypotension, oliguria, and hepatic dysfunction. Laboratory findings of severe OHSS are hematocrit >45%, WBC > 15,000/μ, and creatinine levels between 1 and 1.5 mg/dl. Critical OHSS is the most severe form and can become life-threatening. Symptoms and findings of critical OHSS include tense ascites, hypoxemia, pericardial effusion, renal failure with oliguria/anuria, thromboembolic phenomena, and adult respiratory distress syndrome. Laboratory findings of critical OHSS are hematocrit >55% and creatinine level >1.5 mg/dl [55].

Two factors are critical for the development of OHSS: (1) increased number of growing follicles and (2) prolonged luteinizing stimulus to granulosa cells. Preventive measures must address these two factors. *Primary measures* aim to limit the number of developing follicles and *secondary measures* to decrease the number of luteinized cells.

Identification of high-risk women, implementing appropriate pre-stimulation measures, and choosing the optimal stimulation protocol with regard to choice of suppressing agent and gonadotropin dosage are primary preventive strategies.

Metformin co-administration in PCOS women undergoing IVF treatment decreased the incidence of OHSS [56–58]. All randomized trials consistently demonstrated a benefit regardless of the duration and dose of metformin (1000–2550 mg daily). Metformin did not affect the number of oocytes and the maximum estradiol levels [56]. The effect of metformin on the incidence of OHSS seems to be mediated by declined insulin levels decreasing VEGF production. Indeed, insulin stimulates VEGF production and secretion in vascular endothelial cells [59].

Lower gonadotropin doses would be associated with fewer growing follicles and decreased risk of OHSS. In women who over-responded to 150–225 IU, lower cycle cancellation rates were reported when the starting rFSH dose was decreased to 75 IU/day [60]. Lower dose cycles had similar clinical outcome, while the number of collected oocytes and the peak E2 levels were significantly decreased, and no OHSS was observed. Using lower gonadotropin doses may be considered despite lack of high-quality evidence.

The incidence of OHSS with human menopausal gonadotropins or recombinant gonadotropins is comparable in ART cycles [61–63]. However, studies excluded women with PCOS who are at the highest risk to develop OHSS [64].

The use of GnRH antagonists for pituitary suppression is associated with fewer follicles and lower incidence of OHSS [65, 66]. Moreover, pituitary suppression with GnRH antagonist allows using GnRHa rather than hCG for final oocyte maturation as a secondary preventive measure. The use of GnRH antagonists is a better choice for women at risk of OHSS. GnRH agonist trigger will be discussed in detail below.

Immature oocytes collection in an unstimulated cycle followed by in vitro maturation (IVM) is a treatment option for women polycystic ovaries. OHSS does not occur after IVM. However, pregnancy rate of IVM is lower than that of conventional IVF. Another alternative can be limited ovarian stimulation, i.e., gonadotropin administration until the leading follicle reaches 12 mm, followed by IVF [67, 68]. Forty percent clinical pregnancy rate without any severe OHSS has been reported in 20 women who had had a history of severe OHSS in previous stimulated cycles.

37.3.1 Secondary Preventive Measures

Secondary preventive strategies are measures that can be taken in women who already developed cohort of multiple follicles.

An effective secondary measure to prevent OHSS is withholding hCG injection and cancelling the treatment. OHSS can still occur following a spontaneous LH surge and achievement of a pregnancy, albeit rarely [69]. Today, widespread use of GnRH antagonists for pituitary suppression enables the use of GnRH agonist triggering and cryopreservation of all embryos without a fresh transfer as the best option. The GnRH agonist trigger provides rapid luteolysis and would be better than merely cancelling the cycle without any trigger at all.

Urinary hCG (uhCG) at the traditional dose of 10,000 IU provides an augmented and prolonged luteinizing stimulus as compared to spontaneous LH surge of a natural cycle. The half-lives of uhCG and LH are approximately 33 h and 1 h, respectively. Recombinant human LH (rLH), recombinant hCG, and finally GnRH analogues are tried as alternatives to uhCG. Recombinant LH (rLH) adequately induces oocyte maturation with a lower incidence of moderate OHSS, but not of severe OHSS [70–72]. In addition to its ineffectiveness to prevent severe OHSS, rLH preparations in the market lack the required dose for this purpose, and rLH triggering is not an option in practice.

Reducing the hCG dosage has been suggested as a means of secondary prevention [40, 73]. However, we are not aware of any RCTs to support this approach. A meta-analysis comparing the efficacy and safety of recombinant and uhCG has reported similar rate of OHSS [72].

The pituitary gland retains its sensitivity to GnRH agonist in GnRH antagonist cycles. Thus, GnRH agonist maintains its capability to induce an endogenous LH surge. Following the GnRHa trigger, LH peaks around 4 h after administration and rapidly returns to its baseline value in about 20 h. In contrast, it takes LH 14 h to reach the peak, followed by a 14-h-long plateau before returning to baseline after 48 h in a natural cycle [74, 75]. Combined with the short half-life of LH, the short LH peak decreases the luteinizing stimulus on the granulosa cells, limiting the production of VEGF. While decreased luteinization diminishes the risk of OHSS, it also impacts on pregnancy and live birth rates following a fresh embryo transfer. The addition of smaller dosages of hCG to rescue the luteal phase was suggested to maintain clinical outcome while almost eliminating OHSS [74, 76, 77]. However, even the small 1500 IU hCG can cause early severe OHSS [78]. Severe OHSS cases have been reported following even GnRH agonist trigger alone, without any hCG [79, 80].

37.3.1.1 Coasting

"Coasting" refers to stopping gonadotropin injections and deferring hCG injection until serum E2 levels decline. The purpose is to allow apoptosis of granulosa cells in smaller FSH-dependent follicles by withholding FSH stimulation, thus decreasing VEGF production in response to HCG. Indeed, Garcia-Velasco et al. prospectively showed that coasting induces apoptosis in granulosa cells from follicles of all sizes [81]. However, a trend toward decreased implantation and pregnancy rates with increased duration of coasting is consistently observed [81–84]. With the availability of GnRH agonist triggering, coasting is seldom used nowadays, yet it may be considered an option perhaps in GnRH agonist cycles, where the agent for ovulation trigger has to be hCG.

37.3.1.2 Dopamine Agonists

Dopamine decreases vascular permeability through decreasing VEGFR-2 phosphorylation [85–87]. Accordingly, dopamine agonist cabergoline (Cb2) significantly reduces VEGFR-2-dependent vascular permeability without a luteolytic effect.

In clinical trials, the incidence of moderate and severe OHSS was significantly reduced with Cb2 administration, without an adverse effect on ovarian functions, implantation, and pregnancy rates [88–90]. Cabergoline is easy to use, safe, and effective in the prevention of OHSS. The proposed dose is 0.5 mg/day orally starting from the day of ovulation trigger or oocyte collection.

37.3.1.3 Renin Angiotensin System Blockage

The use angiotensin converting enzyme (ACE) inhibitors in high-risk patients has been evaluated [91, 92]. Due to its teratogenicity, it could be used only in cycles that do not involve embryo transfer, such as oocyte donors or when all embryos are to be cryopreserved. While one study reported no cases of OHSS in four women, another study reported a 20% incidence of severe OHSS with a similar protocol in ten women [91, 92].

37.3.1.4 Administration of Macromolecules

Albumin and hydroxyethyl starch (HES) solutions decrease fluid leakage by increasing intravascular oncotic pressure. Albumin is also expected to bind and inactivate the circulating vasoactive molecules.

In contrast to a Cochrane report in 2002, more recent large RCTs showed that albumin infusion does not prevent severe OHSS [93–95]. Prophylactic albumin administration is not only ineffective, but it might even be hampering pregnancy outcome as well. Albumin may bind and inactivate molecules necessary for successful embryo implantation. Lower clinical and ongoing pregnancy rates were observed in the albumin-treated group as compared to the placebo group [94].

HES is another macromolecule, and unlike albumin it does not bind other molecules. The larger molecular weight of HES allows it to stay in the intravascular space for a longer period than albumin to maintain oncotic pressure. One RCT reported that infusion of 500 ml 6% HES solution at the time of oocyte collection was more effective than both albumin and placebo [96]. Other studies support this observation [97, 98]. However, the use of HES is debatable since the European Medicines Agency's Pharmacovigilance Risk Assessment Committee recommended withdrawal of HES solutions from the market [99].

37.3.1.5 GnRH Antagonists

GnRH antagonist injections during the luteal phase decrease endogenous LH stimulation of corpora lutea and accelerate luteolysis [100]. Even though this has not been assessed as a preventive strategy, administration of GnRH antagonists for a couple of days can be considered in GnRH agonist triggered cycles if the risk of OHSS is deemed to be high.

37.3.1.6 Decreasing the Number of Transferred Embryos and Embryo Cryopreservation

Since the endogenous hCG leads to late onset of OHSS, embryo transfer should be postponed in a high-risk cycle. Some experts have suggested that multiple pregnancies are also associated with a higher risk of OHSS because of higher HCG levels [101–103]. However the mere presence of hCG seems sufficient to induce OHSS [103]. Clearly, avoiding pregnancy can decrease late-onset OHSS. As of 2019, with the high success rate of embryo vitrification, and studies demonstrating already decreased live birth rates following fresh embryo transfer in women with excessive ovarian response, total embryo cryopreservation is the best compromise in women at high risk [104].

37.3.1.7 Avoiding HCG as a Luteal Support Agent

Use of HCG for luteal phase support has been shown to be associated with significantly higher incidence of OHSS [105]. Hence, luteal phase support with hCG should be avoided in women at risk.

Importantly, the abovementioned strategies to prevent OHSS have different modes of action and can be successfully used together especially when fresh embryo transfer is forfeited [106]. We suggest the following combination for women who are at high risk of OHSS:

- Plan stimulation with a GnRH antagonist followed by GnRH agonist trigger.
- Avoid hCG for trigger and luteal support.
- Plan to freeze all embryos without a fresh embryo transfer.
- Administer Cb2 at a dose of 0.5 mg/day for 7 days starting from the day of trigger or oocyte retrieval.
- Restart GnRH daily GnRH antagonist injections for 5 days following oocyte retrieval.

Such combination is shown to accelerate luteolysis as evidenced by earlier start of menses, to be associated with smaller ovarian volume.

37.4 Management of OHSS

Even though OHSS is a self-limiting condition, thromboembolism and pulmonary edema can lead to death. Today, renal failure is rare, and hepatic failure is not a major risk in the absence of preexisting liver damage. Most cases can be managed in an ambulatory setting.

- On admission vital signs and the respiratory rate should be recorded. The woman should be evaluated for ascites and hydrothorax. Complete blood count, renal and liver function tests including albumin, and coagulation tests are the initial laboratory tests to establish the diagnosis and guide the management.
- Circulating volume must be maintained. Intravenous fluid administration is required for hospitalized patients. Care must be taken to avoid rapid and massive hydration since acute respiratory distress syndrome can occur following massive hydration [107]. Administration of fluid in the presence of endothelial barrier damages contributes to the loss in a short time [108].
- Although albumin administration has been advocated to maintain oncotic pressure and replace the fluid deficit, it remains in the circulation for less than 36 h and moves to the interstitium, contributing to extravasation of the remaining intravascular fluid [108]. RCTs reported decreased requirement for paracentesis, shorter hospital stay, and faster recovery from hemoconcentration with administration of other macromolecule solutions as compared with albumin [109–111]. Dextran is preferable over albumin.
- Decision about the timing of paracentesis and the amount of fluid to be drained depends on clinical judgment. Absolute indications for paracentesis are dyspnea due to ascites, oliguria due to compression of urinary system due to ascites, and severe abdominal distention. Paracentesis acutely decreases intra-abdominal pressure, hence increases venous return, cardiac output, and renal blood flow without adversely affecting uterine circulation [112, 113]. Abdominal or transvaginal paracentesis yields similar results. Due to the concern of protein loss, gradual aspiration has been recommended [114]. Yet, drainage of large amounts, even without albumin replacement has been done without any adverse events [115, 116]. Draining large amounts once paracentesis is done decreases the number of procedures until resolution of the condition.
- Hospitalization is seldom necessary. Moderate/severe OHSS can be reasonably managed on an outpatient basis with paracentesis, hydration, and anticoagulation [116, 117].
- Restarting GnRH antagonist injections can accelerate resolution [100, 118, 119].
- While anticoagulant therapy is generally reserved for patients with thrombophilias, thromboembolic phenomenon, immobility, or obesity, women with severe OHSS can benefit from prophylactic anticoagulant therapy. Once started, anticoagulation should be continued for a minimum of 4–6 weeks after resolution of clinical OHSS or throughout the first trimester.
- Thoracocentesis and pericardiocentesis may be necessary when respiration is impaired or in the presence of cardiac tamponade. Such cases may require monitoring in an intensive care unit [92].
- Diuretics can lead to further hemoconcentration and have resulted in arterial thrombosis, renal failure, and death [43]. They must be avoided.

References

1. Smits G, Olatunbosun O, Delbaere A, Pierson R, Vassart G, Costagliola S. Ovarian hyperstimulation syndrome due to a mutation in the follicle-stimulating hormone receptor. N Engl J Med. 2003;349:760–6.
2. Vasseur C, Rodien P, Beau I, Desroches A, Gerard C, de Poncheville L, Chaplot S, Savagner F, Croue A, Mathieu E, Lahlou N, Descamps P, Misrahi M. A chorionic gonadotropin-sensitive mutation in the follicle-stimulating hormone receptor as a cause of familial gestational spontaneous ovarian hyperstimulation syndrome. N Engl J Med. 2003;349:753–9.
3. Arora R, Merhi ZO, Khulpateea N, Roth D, Minkoff H. Ovarian hyperstimulation syndrome after a molar pregnancy evacuation. Fertil Steril. 2008;90:1197 e5–7.
4. Ludwig M, Gembruch U, Bauer O, Diedrich K. Ovarian hyperstimulation syndrome (OHSS) in a spontaneous pregnancy with fetal and placental triploidy: information about the general pathophysiology of OHSS. Hum Reprod. 1998;13:2082–7.
5. Nappi RG, Di Naro E, D'Aries AP, Nappi L. Natural pregnancy in hypothyroid woman complicated by spontaneous ovarian hyperstimulation syndrome. Am J Obstet Gynecol. 1998;178:610–1.
6. Check JH, Choe JK, Nazari A. Hyperreactio luteinalis despite the absence of a corpus luteum and suppressed serum follicle stimulating concentrations in a triplet pregnancy. Hum Reprod. 2000;15:1043–5.
7. Suzuki S. Comparison between spontaneous ovarian hyperstimulation syndrome and hyperreactio luteinalis. Arch Gynecol Obstet. 2004;269:227–9.
8. McClure N, Healy DL, Rogers PA, Sullivan J, Beaton L, Haning RV Jr, Connolly DT, Robertson DM. Vascular endothelial growth factor as capillary permeability agent in ovarian hyperstimulation syndrome. Lancet. 1994;344:235–6.
9. Goldsman MP, Pedram A, Dominguez CE, Ciuffardi I, Levin E, Asch RH. Increased capillary permeability induced by human follicular fluid: a hypothesis for an ovarian origin of the hyperstimulation syndrome. Fertil Steril. 1995;63:268–72.
10. Soares SR, Gomez R, Simon C, Garcia-Velasco JA, Pellicer A. Targeting the vascular endothelial growth factor system to prevent ovarian hyperstimulation syndrome. Hum Reprod Update. 2008;14:321–33.
11. Albert C, Garrido N, Mercader A, Rao CV, Remohi J, Simon C, Pellicer A. The role of endothelial cells in the pathogenesis of ovarian hyperstimulation syndrome. Mol Hum Reprod. 2002;8:409–18.
12. Waltenberger J, Claesson-Welsh L, Siegbahn A, Shibuya M, Heldin CH. Different signal transduction properties of KDR and Flt1, two receptors for vascular endothelial growth factor. J Biol Chem. 1994;269:26988–95.
13. Pajusola K, Aprelikova O, Korhonen J, Kaipainen A, Pertovaara L, Alitalo R, Alitalo K. FLT4 receptor tyrosine kinase contains

seven immunoglobulin-like loops and is expressed in multiple human tissues and cell lines. Cancer Res. 1992;52:5738–43.
14. Tammela T, Enholm B, Alitalo K, Paavonen K. The biology of vascular endothelial growth factors. Cardiovasc Res. 2005;65:550–63.
15. Gomez R, Simon C, Remohi J, Pellicer A. Administration of moderate and high doses of gonadotropins to female rats increases ovarian vascular endothelial growth factor (VEGF) and VEGF receptor-2 expression that is associated to vascular hyperpermeability. Biol Reprod. 2003;68:2164–71.
16. Gomez R, Gonzalez M, Simon C, Remohi J, Pellicer A. Tyroxine hydroxylase (TH) down regulation in hyperstimulated ovaries reveals the dopamine agonist bromocriptine (Br2) as an effective and specific method to block increased vascular permeability (VP) in OHSS. Fertil Steril. 2003;80:43–4.
17. Hornig C, Barleon B, Ahmad S, Vuorela P, Ahmed A, Weich HA. Release and complex formation of soluble VEGFR-1 from endothelial cells and biological fluids. Lab Investig. 2000;80:443–54.
18. He Y, Smith SK, Day KA, Clark DE, Licence DR, Charnock-Jones DS. Alternative splicing of vascular endothelial growth factor (VEGF)-R1 (FLT-1) pre-mRNA is important for the regulation of VEGF activity. Mol Endocrinol. 1999;13:537–45.
19. Wang D, Donner DB, Warren RS. Homeostatic modulation of cell surface KDR and Flt1 expression and expression of the vascular endothelial cell growth factor (VEGF) receptor mRNAs by VEGF. J Biol Chem. 2000;275:15905–11.
20. Roberts WG, Palade GE. Neovasculature induced by vascular endothelial growth factor is fenestrated. Cancer Res. 1997;57:765–72.
21. Villasante A, Pacheco A, Ruiz A, Pellicer A, Garcia-Velasco JA. Vascular endothelial cadherin regulates vascular permeability: implications for ovarian hyperstimulation syndrome. J Clin Endocrinol Metab. 2007;92:314–21.
22. Wang TH, Horng SG, Chang CL, Wu HM, Tsai YJ, Wang HS, Soong YK. Human chorionic gonadotropin-induced ovarian hyperstimulation syndrome is associated with up-regulation of vascular endothelial growth factor. J Clin Endocrinol Metab. 2002;87:3300–8.
23. Pellicer A, Albert C, Mercader A, Bonilla-Musoles F, Remohi J, Simon C. The pathogenesis of ovarian hyperstimulation syndrome: in vivo studies investigating the role of interleukin-1beta, interleukin-6, and vascular endothelial growth factor. Fertil Steril. 1999;71:482–9.
24. Yamamoto S, Konishi I, Tsuruta Y, Nanbu K, Mandai M, Kuroda H, Matsushita K, Hamid AA, Yura Y, Mori T. Expression of vascular endothelial growth factor (VEGF) during folliculogenesis and corpus luteum formation in the human ovary. Gynecol Endocrinol. 1997;11:371–81.
25. Kamat BR, Brown LF, Manseau EJ, Senger DR, Dvorak HF. Expression of vascular permeability factor/vascular endothelial growth factor by human granulosa and theca lutein cells. Role in corpus luteum development. Am J Pathol. 1995;146:157–65.
26. Itskovitz J, Sealey JE. Ovarian prorenin-renin-angiotensin system. Obstet Gynecol Surv. 1987;42:545–51.
27. Lightman A, Tarlatzis BC, Rzasa PJ, Culler MD, Caride VJ, Negro-Vilar AF, Lennard D, DeCherney AH, Naftolin F. The ovarian renin-angiotensin system: renin-like activity and angiotensin II/III immunoreactivity in gonadotropin-stimulated and unstimulated human follicular fluid. Am J Obstet Gynecol. 1987;156:808–16.
28. Glorioso N, Atlas SA, Laragh JH, Jewelewicz R, Sealey JE. Prorenin in high concentrations in human ovarian follicular fluid. Science. 1986;233:1422–4.
29. Morris RS, Paulson RJ. Ovarian derived prorenin-angiotensin cascade in human reproduction. Fertil Steril. 1994;62:1105–14.
30. Huang W, Wu YL, Zhong J, Jiang FX, Tian XL, Yu LF. Angiotensin II type 1 receptor antagonist suppress angiogenesis and growth of gastric cancer xenografts. Dig Dis Sci. 2008;53:1206–10.
31. Shi RZ, Wang JC, Huang SH, Wang XJ, Li QP. Angiotensin II induces vascular endothelial growth factor synthesis in mesenchymal stem cells. Exp Cell Res. 2009;315:10–5.
32. Anandanadesan R, Gong Q, Chipitsyna G, Witkiewicz A, Yeo CJ, Arafat HA. Angiotensin II induces vascular endothelial growth factor in pancreatic cancer cells through an angiotensin II type 1 receptor and ERK1/2 signaling. J Gastrointest Surg. 2008;12:57–66.
33. Sataranatarajan K, Lee MJ, Mariappan MM, Feliers D. PKCdelta regulates the stimulation of vascular endothelial factor mRNA translation by angiotensin II through hnRNP K. Cell Signal. 2008;20:969–77.
34. Walter A, Etienne-Selloum N, Sarr M, Kane MO, Beretz A, Schini-Kerth VB. Angiotensin II induces the vascular expression of VEGF and MMP-2 in vivo: preventive effect of red wine polyphenols. J Vasc Res. 2008;45:386–94.
35. Herr D, Rodewald M, Fraser HM, Hack G, Konrad R, Kreienberg R, Wulff C. Regulation of endothelial proliferation by the renin-angiotensin system in human umbilical vein endothelial cells. Reproduction. 2008;136:125–30.
36. Ohnuma Y, Toda M, Fujita M, Hosono K, Suzuki T, Ogawa Y, Amano H, Kitasato H, Hayakawa K, Majima M. Blockade of an angiotensin type I receptor enhances effects of radiation on tumor growth and tumor-associated angiogenesis by reducing vascular endothelial growth factor expression. Biomed Pharmacother. 2009;63(2):136–45.
37. Fukumoto M, Takai S, Ishizaki E, Sugiyama T, Oku H, Jin D, Sakaguchi M, Sakonjo H, Ikeda T, Miyazaki M. Involvement of angiotensin II-dependent vascular endothelial growth factor gene expression via NADPH oxidase in the retina in a type 2 diabetic rat model. Curr Eye Res. 2008;33:885–91.
38. Delvigne A, Rozenberg S. Preventive attitude of physicians to avoid OHSS in IVF patients. Hum Reprod. 2001;16:2491–5.
39. van Dop P. Epidemiology and primary risk factors for ovarian hyperstimulation syndrome. In: Gerris J, Delvigne A, Olivennes F, editors. Ovarian hyperstimulation syndrome. Oxon: Informa Healthcare; 2006. p. 7–11.
40. Practice Committee of American Society for Reproductive Medicine. Ovarian hyperstimulation syndrome. Fertil Steril. 2008;90:S188–93.
41. Enskog A, Henriksson M, Unander M, Nilsson L, Brannstrom M. Prospective study of the clinical and laboratory parameters of patients in whom ovarian hyperstimulation syndrome developed during controlled ovarian hyperstimulation for in vitro fertilization. Fertil Steril. 1999;71:808–14.
42. Delvigne A, Demoulin A, Smitz J, Donnez J, Koninckx P, Dhont M, Englert Y, Delbeke L, Darcis L, Gordts S, et al. The ovarian hyperstimulation syndrome in in-vitro fertilization: a Belgian multicentric study. I. Clinical and biological features. Hum Reprod. 1993;8:1353–60.
43. Braat D, Bernardus R, Gerris J. Anonymous reports of lethal cases of ovarian hyperstimulation syndrome. In: Gerris J, Delvigne A, Olivennes F, editors. Ovarian hyperstimulation syndrome. Oxon: Informa Healthcare; 2006. p. 59–70.
44. Nakhuda GS, Chu MC, Wang JG, Sauer MV, Lobo RA. Elevated serum Mullerian-inhibiting substance may be a marker for ovarian hyperstimulation syndrome in normal women undergoing in vitro fertilization. Fertil Steril. 2006;85:1541–3.
45. Lee TH, Liu CH, Huang CC, Wu YL, Shih YT, Ho HN, Yang YS, Lee MS. Serum anti-Mullerian hormone and estradiol levels as predictors of ovarian hyperstimulation syndrome in assisted reproduction technology cycles. Hum Reprod. 2008;23:160–7.

46. Delvigne A, Rozenberg S. Systematic review of data concerning etiopathology of ovarian hyperstimulation syndrome. Int J Fertil Womens Med. 2002;47:211–26.
47. Aboulghar MA, Mansour RT. Ovarian hyperstimulation syndrome: classifications and critical analysis of preventive measures. Hum Reprod Update. 2003;9:275–89.
48. Asch RH, Li HP, Balmaceda JP, Weckstein LN, Stone SC. Severe ovarian hyperstimulation syndrome in assisted reproductive technology: definition of high risk groups. Hum Reprod. 1991;6:1395–9.
49. Morris RS, Paulson RJ, Sauer MV, Lobo RA. Predictive value of serum oestradiol concentrations and oocyte number in severe ovarian hyperstimulation syndrome. Hum Reprod. 1995;10: 811–4.
50. Mathur RS, Akande AV, Keay SD, Hunt LP, Jenkins JM. Distinction between early and late ovarian hyperstimulation syndrome. Fertil Steril. 2000;73:901–7.
51. Pellicer A, Miro F, Sampaio M, Gomez E, Bonilla-Musoles FM. In vitro fertilization as a diagnostic and therapeutic tool in a patient with partial 17,20-desmolase deficiency. Fertil Steril. 1991;55:970–5.
52. Blankstein J, Shalev J, Saadon T, Kukia EE, Rabinovici J, Pariente C, Lunenfeld B, Serr DM, Mashiach S. Ovarian hyperstimulation syndrome: prediction by number and size of preovulatory ovarian follicles. Fertil Steril. 1987;47:597–602.
53. Tal J, Paz B, Samberg I, Lazarov N, Sharf M. Ultrasonographic and clinical correlates of menotropin versus sequential clomiphene citrate: menotropin therapy for induction of ovulation. Fertil Steril. 1985;44:342–9.
54. MacDougall MJ, Tan SL, Balen A, Jacobs HS. A controlled study comparing patients with and without polycystic ovaries undergoing in-vitro fertilization. Hum Reprod. 1993;8:233–7.
55. Navot D, Bergh PA, Laufer N. Ovarian hyperstimulation syndrome in novel reproductive technologies: prevention and treatment. Fertil Steril. 1992;58:249–61.
56. Costello MF, Chapman M, Conway U. A systematic review and meta-analysis of randomized controlled trials on metformin co-administration during gonadotropin ovulation induction or IVF in women with polycystic ovary syndrome. Hum Reprod. 2006;21:1387–99.
57. Moll E, van der Veen F, van Wely M. The role of metformin in polycystic ovary syndrome: a systematic review. Hum Reprod Update. 2007;13:527–37.
58. Mourad S, Brown J, Farquhar C. Interventions for the prevention of OHSS in ART cycles: an overview of Cochrane reviews. Cochrane Database Syst Rev. 2017 Jan 23;1:CD012103.
59. Doronzo G, Russo I, Mattiello L, Anfossi G, Bosia A, Trovati M. Insulin activates vascular endothelial growth factor in vascular smooth muscle cells: influence of nitric oxide and of insulin resistance. Eur J Clin Investig. 2004;34:664–73.
60. Marci R, Senn A, Dessole S, Chanson A, Loumaye E, De Grandi P, Germond M. A low-dose stimulation protocol using highly purified follicle-stimulating hormone can lead to high pregnancy rates in in vitro fertilization patients with polycystic ovaries who are at risk of a high ovarian response to gonadotropins. Fertil Steril. 2001;75:1131–5.
61. Daya S. Updated meta-analysis of recombinant follicle-stimulating hormone (FSH) versus urinary FSH for ovarian stimulation in assisted reproduction. Fertil Steril. 2002;77:711–4.
62. Van Wely M, Westergaard LG, Bossuyt PM, Van der Veen F. Human menopausal gonadotropin versus recombinant follicle stimulation hormone for ovarian stimulation in assisted reproductive cycles. Cochrane Database Syst Rev. 2003:CD003973.
63. Coomarasamy A, Afnan M, Cheema D, van der Veen F, Bossuyt PM, van Wely M. Urinary hMG versus recombinant FSH for controlled ovarian hyperstimulation following an agonist long down-regulation protocol in IVF or ICSI treatment: a systematic review and meta-analysis. Hum Reprod. 2008;23:310–5.
64. Tan SL, Child TJ, Cheung AP, Fluker MR, Yuzpe A, Casper R, Leung P, Cadesky K, Davis VJ. A randomized, double-blind, multicenter study comparing a starting dose of 100 IU or 200 IU of recombinant follicle stimulating hormone (Puregon) in women undergoing controlled ovarian hyperstimulation for IVF treatment. J Assist Reprod Genet. 2005;22:81–8.
65. Al-Inany HG, Abou-Setta AM, Aboulghar M. Gonadotrophin-releasing hormone antagonists for assisted conception. Cochrane Database Syst Rev. 2006;3:CD001750.
66. Lambalk CB, Banga FR, Huirne JA, Toftager M, Pinborg A, Homburg R, van der Veen F, van Wely M. GnRH antagonist versus long agonist protocols in IVF: a systematic review and meta-analysis accounting for patient type. Hum Reprod Update. 2017;23:560–79.
67. El-Sheikh MM, Hussein M, Sheikh AA, Fouad S, El-Sheikh R, Al-Hasani S. Limited ovarian stimulation results in the recovery of mature oocytes in polycystic ovarian disease patients: a preliminary report. Eur J Obstet Gynecol Reprod Biol. 1999;83:81–3.
68. El-Sheikh MM, Hussein M, Fouad S, El-Sheikh R, Bauer O, Al-Hasani S. Limited ovarian stimulation (LOS), prevents the recurrence of severe forms of ovarian hyperstimulation syndrome in polycystic ovarian disease. Eur J Obstet Gynecol Reprod Biol. 2001;94:245–9.
69. Lipitz S, Ben-Rafael Z, Bider D, Shalev J, Mashiach S. Quintuplet pregnancy and third degree ovarian hyperstimulation despite withholding human chorionic gonadotropin. Hum Reprod. 1991;6:1478–9.
70. The European Recombinant LH Study Group. Human recombinant luteinizing hormone is as effective as, but safer than, urinary human chorionic gonadotropin in inducing final follicular maturation and ovulation in in vitro fertilization procedures: results of a multicenter double-blind study. J Clin Endocrinol Metab. 2001;86:2607–18.
71. Manau D, Fabregues F, Arroyo V, Jimenez W, Vanrell JA, Balasch J. Hemodynamic changes induced by urinary human chorionic gonadotropin and recombinant luteinizing hormone used for inducing final follicular maturation and luteinization. Fertil Steril. 2002;78:1261–7.
72. Al-Inany H, Aboulghar MA, Mansour RT, Proctor M. Recombinant versus urinary gonadotropins for triggering ovulation in assisted conception. Hum Reprod. 2005;20:2061–73.
73. Delvigne A. Secondary prevention of threatening ovarian hyperstimulation syndrome. In: Gerris J, Delvigne A, Olivennes F, editors. Ovarian hyperstimulation syndrome. Oxon: Informa Healthcare; 2006. p. 217–38.
74. Humaidan P, Kol S, Papanikolaou EG. GnRH agonist for triggering of final oocyte maturation: time for a change of practice? Hum Reprod Update. 2011;17:510–24.
75. Atkinson P, Koch J, Susic D, Ledger WL. GnRH agonist triggers and their use in assisted reproductive technology: the past, the present and the future. Womens Health (Lond). 2014;10:267–76.
76. Humaidan P. Luteal phase rescue in high-risk OHSS patients by GnRHa triggering in combination with low-dose HCG: a pilot study. Reprod Biomed Online. 2009;18:630–4.
77. Humaidan P, Ejdrup Bredkjaer H, Westergaard LG, Yding Andersen C. 1500 IU human chorionic gonadotropin administered at oocyte retrieval rescues the luteal phase when gonadotropin-releasing hormone agonist is used for ovulation induction: a prospective, randomized, controlled study. Fertil Steril. 2010;93: 847–54.
78. Seyhan A, Ata B, Polat M, Son WY, Yarali H, Dahan MH. Severe early ovarian hyperstimulation syndrome following GnRH agonist trigger with the addition of 1500 IU hCG. Hum Reprod. 2013;28:2522.

79. Fatemi HM, Popovic-Todorovic B, Humaidan P, Kol S, Banker M, Devroey P, Garcia-Velasco JA. Severe ovarian hyperstimulation syndrome after gonadotropin-releasing hormone (GnRH) agonist trigger and "freeze-all" approach in GnRH antagonist protocol. Fertil Steril. 2014;101:1008–11.
80. Gurbuz AS, Gode F, Ozcimen N, Isik AZ. Gonadotropin-releasing hormone agonist trigger and freeze-all strategy does not prevent severe ovarian hyperstimulation syndrome: a report of three cases. Reprod Biomed Online. 2014;29:541–4.
81. Garcia-Velasco JA, Zuniga A, Pacheco A, Gomez R, Simon C, Remohi J, Pellicer A. Coasting acts through downregulation of VEGF gene expression and protein secretion. Hum Reprod. 2004;19:1530–8.
82. Mansour R, Aboulghar M, Serour G, Amin Y, Abou-Setta AM. Criteria of a successful coasting protocol for the prevention of severe ovarian hyperstimulation syndrome. Hum Reprod. 2005;20:3167–72.
83. Ulug U, Bahceci M, Erden HF, Shalev E, Ben-Shlomo I. The significance of coasting duration during ovarian stimulation for conception in assisted fertilization cycles. Hum Reprod. 2002;17:310–3.
84. Isaza V, Garcia-Velasco JA, Aragones M, Remohi J, Simon C, Pellicer A. Oocyte and embryo quality after coasting: the experience from oocyte donation. Hum Reprod. 2002;17:1777–82.
85. Basu S, Nagy JA, Pal S, Vasile E, Eckelhoefer IA, Bliss VS, Manseau EJ, Dasgupta PS, Dvorak HF, Mukhopadhyay D. The neurotransmitter dopamine inhibits angiogenesis induced by vascular permeability factor/vascular endothelial growth factor. Nat Med. 2001;7:569–74.
86. Sarkar C, Chakroborty D, Mitra RB, Banerjee S, Dasgupta PS, Basu S. Dopamine in vivo inhibits VEGF-induced phosphorylation of VEGFR-2, MAPK, and focal adhesion kinase in endothelial cells. Am J Physiol Heart Circ Physiol. 2004;287:H1554–60.
87. Quinn TP, Peters KG, De Vries C, Ferrara N, Williams LT. Fetal liver kinase 1 is a receptor for vascular endothelial growth factor and is selectively expressed in vascular endothelium. Proc Natl Acad Sci U S A. 1993;90:7533–7.
88. Alvarez C, Marti-Bonmati L, Novella-Maestre E, Sanz R, Gomez R, Fernandez-Sanchez M, Simon C, Pellicer A. Dopamine agonist cabergoline reduces hemoconcentration and ascites in hyperstimulated women undergoing assisted reproduction. J Clin Endocrinol Metab. 2007;92:2931–7.
89. Alvarez C, Alonso-Muriel I, Garcia G, Crespo J, Bellver J, Simon C, Pellicer A. Implantation is apparently unaffected by the dopamine agonist Cabergoline when administered to prevent ovarian hyperstimulation syndrome in women undergoing assisted reproduction treatment: a pilot study. Hum Reprod. 2007;22:3210–4.
90. Carizza C, Abdelmassih V, Abdelmassih S, Ravizzini P, Salgueiro L, Salgueiro PT, Jine LT, Nagy P, Abdelmassih R. Cabergoline reduces the early onset of ovarian hyperstimulation syndrome: a prospective randomized study. Reprod Biomed Online. 2008;17:751–5.
91. Ando H, Furugori K, Shibata D, Harata T, Murata Y, Mizutani S. Dual renin-angiotensin blockade therapy in patients at high risk of early ovarian hyperstimulation syndrome receiving IVF and elective embryo cryopreservation: a case series. Hum Reprod. 2003;18:1219–22.
92. Ata B, Yakin K, Alatas C, Urman B. Dual renin-angiotensin blockage and total embryo cryopreservation is not a risk-free strategy in patients at high risk for ovarian hyperstimulation syndrome. Fertil Steril. 2008;90:531–6.
93. Aboulghar M, Evers JH, Al-Inany H. Intravenous albumin for preventing severe ovarian hyperstimulation syndrome: a Cochrane review. Hum Reprod. 2002;17:3027–32.
94. Bellver J, Munoz EA, Ballesteros A, Soares SR, Bosch E, Simon C, Pellicer A, Remohi J. Intravenous albumin does not prevent moderate-severe ovarian hyperstimulation syndrome in high-risk IVF patients: a randomized controlled study. Hum Reprod. 2003;18:2283–8.
95. Isikoglu M, Berkkanoglu M, Senturk Z, Ozgur K. Human albumin does not prevent ovarian hyperstimulation syndrome in assisted reproductive technology program: a prospective randomized placebo-controlled double blind study. Fertil Steril. 2007;88:982–5.
96. Gokmen O, Ugur M, Ekin M, Keles G, Turan C, Oral H. Intravenous albumin versus hydroxyethyl starch for the prevention of ovarian hyperstimulation in an in-vitro fertilization programme: a prospective randomized placebo controlled study. Eur J Obstet Gynecol Reprod Biol. 2001;96:187–92.
97. Graf MA, Fischer R, Naether OG, Baukloh V, Tafel J, Nuckel M. Reduced incidence of ovarian hyperstimulation syndrome by prophylactic infusion of hydroxyaethyl starch solution in an in-vitro fertilization programme. Hum Reprod. 1997;12:2599–602.
98. Konig E, Bussen S, Sutterlin M, Steck T. Prophylactic intravenous hydroxyethyl starch solution prevents moderate-severe ovarian hyperstimulation in in-vitro fertilization patients: a prospective, randomized, double-blind and placebo-controlled study. Hum Reprod. 1998;13:2421–4.
99. Pharmacovigilance Risk Assessment Committee of European Medicines Association. 2018. Available from: https://www.ema.europa.eu/en/news/prac-recommends-suspending-hydroxyethyl-starch-solutions-infusion-market.
100. Lainas GT, Kolibianakis EM, Sfontouris IA, Zorzovilis IZ, Petsas GK, Lainas TG, Tarlatzis BC. Serum vascular endothelial growth factor levels following luteal gonadotropin-releasing hormone antagonist administration in women with severe early ovarian hyperstimulation syndrome. BJOG. 2014;121:848–55.
101. Lyons CA, Wheeler CA, Frishman GN, Hackett RJ, Seifer DB, Haning RV Jr. Early and late presentation of the ovarian hyperstimulation syndrome: two distinct entities with different risk factors. Hum Reprod. 1994;9:792–9.
102. Papanikolaou EG, Tournaye H, Verpoest W, Camus M, Vernaeve V, Van Steirteghem A, Devroey P. Early and late ovarian hyperstimulation syndrome: early pregnancy outcome and profile. Hum Reprod. 2005;20:636–41.
103. De Neubourg D, Mangelschots K, Van Royen E, Vercruyssen M, Gerris J. Singleton pregnancies are as affected by ovarian hyperstimulation syndrome as twin pregnancies. Fertil Steril. 2004;82:1691–3.
104. Chen ZJ, Shi Y, Sun Y, Zhang B, Liang X, Cao Y, Yang J, Liu J, Wei D, Weng N, Tian L, Hao C, Yang D, Zhou F, Shi J, Xu Y, Li J, Yan J, Qin Y, Zhao H, Zhang H, Legro RS. Fresh versus frozen embryos for infertility in the polycystic ovary syndrome. N Engl J Med. 2016;375:523–33.
105. Daya S, Gunby JL. Luteal phase support in assisted reproduction cycles. Cochrane Database Syst Rev. 2008:CD004830.
106. Dahan MH, Tannus S, Seyhan A, Tan SL, Ata B. Combined modalities for the prevention of ovarian hyperstimulation syndrome following an excessive response to stimulation. Gynecol Endocrinol. 2018;34:252–5.
107. Abramov Y, Elchalal U, Schenker JG. Pulmonary manifestations of severe ovarian hyperstimulation syndrome: a multicenter study. Fertil Steril. 1999;71:645–51.
108. Rackow EC, Falk JL, Fein IA, Siegel JS, Packman MI, Haupt MT, Kaufman BS, Putnam D. Fluid resuscitation in circulatory shock: a comparison of the cardiorespiratory effects of albumin, hetastarch, and saline solutions in patients with hypovolemic and septic shock. Crit Care Med. 1983;11:839–50.
109. Abramov Y, Fatum M, Abrahamov D, Schenker JG. Hydroxyethyl starch versus human albumin for the treatment of severe ovarian hyperstimulation syndrome: a preliminary report. Fertil Steril. 2001;75:1228–30.

110. Gamzu R, Almog B, Levin Y, Avni A, Lessing JB, Baram A. Efficacy of hydroxyethyl starch and Haemaccel for the treatment of severe ovarian hyperstimulation syndrome. Fertil Steril. 2002;77:1302–3.
111. Endo T, Kitajima Y, Hayashi T, Fujii M, Hata H, Azumaguchi A. Low-molecular-weight dextran infusion is more effective for the treatment of hemoconcentration due to severe ovarian hyperstimulation syndrome than human albumin infusion. Fertil Steril. 2004;82:1449–51.
112. Levin I, Almog B, Avni A, Baram A, Lessing JB, Gamzu R. Effect of paracentesis of ascitic fluids on urinary output and blood indices in patients with severe ovarian hyperstimulation syndrome. Fertil Steril. 2002;77:986–8.
113. Chen CD, Yang JH, Chao KH, Chen SU, Ho HN, Yang YS. Effects of repeated abdominal paracentesis on uterine and intraovarian haemodynamics and pregnancy outcome in severe ovarian hyperstimulation syndrome. Hum Reprod. 1998;13:2077–81.
114. Ron-El R, Friedler S, Schachter M, Raziel R. Clinical management, ascites management and obstetrical outcome in patients with ovarian hyperstimulation syndrome. In: Gerris J, Delvigne A, Olivennes F, editors. Ovarian hyperstimulation syndrome. Oxon: Informa Healthcare; 2006. p. 149–58.
115. Ozgun MT, Batukan C, Oner G, Uludag S, Aygen EM, Sahin Y. Removal of ascites up to 7.5 liters on one occasion and 45 liters in total may be safe in patients with severe ovarian hyperstimulation syndrome. Gynecol Endocrinol. 2008;24:656–8.
116. Smith LP, Hacker MR, Alper MM. Patients with severe ovarian hyperstimulation syndrome can be managed safely with aggressive outpatient transvaginal paracentesis. Fertil Steril. 2009;92(6):1953–9.
117. Csokmay JM, Yauger BJ, Henne MB, Armstrong AY, Queenan JT, Segars JH. Cost analysis model of outpatient management of ovarian hyperstimulation syndrome with paracentesis: "tap early and often" versus hospitalization. Fertil Steril. 2010;93:167–73.
118. Lainas TG, Sfontouris IA, Zorzovilis IZ, Petsas GK, Lainas GT, Kolibianakis EM. Management of severe early ovarian hyperstimulation syndrome by re-initiation of GnRH antagonist. Reprod Biomed Online. 2007;15:408–12.
119. Lainas GT, Kolibianakis EM, Sfontouris IA, Zorzovilis IZ, Petsas GK, Lainas TG, Tarlatzis BC. Pregnancy and neonatal outcomes following luteal GnRH antagonist administration in patients with severe early OHSS. Hum Reprod. 2013;28:1929–42.

38 Same-Sex Couples and Single Women Undergoing Medically Assisted Reproduction

Ilana B. Ressler

While a "traditional" nuclear family has been defined as a heterosexual married couple and their biologically conceived children, this model is far from universally true. There are an increasing number of unmarried heterosexual couples, divorced individuals, same-sex married and unmarried couples, and single individuals who have or desire to have children. Along with the changing landscape of social family structures, assisted reproductive technology (ART) or medically assisted reproduction (MAR) continues to evolve, offering an increasing number of family building options and techniques. This chapter will examine the different methods available for same-sex couples and single women to have children and the matters pertaining to these specific populations.

38.1 Background

While the majority of births in the USA are to heterosexual married couples, there are increasing numbers of children born to single or unmarried persons. A recent publication of the 2015 National Vital Statistics reports that there were over 1.6 million births (40.3% of all births) to unmarried women [1]. This accompanies a societal shift of both acceptance regarding out-of-wedlock births and attitudes toward the lesbian, gay, bisexual, or transgender (LGBT) community.

It has been estimated that 5.2–9.5 million adults in the USA identify as LGBT, which is 2–4% of the adult population [2]. It has also been estimated that up to six million US children and adults have an LGBT parent, but only about 200,000 children are being raised in a same-sex couple household [3]. There is little population data regarding the birth circumstances of those children in same-sex households (e.g., whether the children were born to a previous heterosexual couple versus into a same-sex couple household).

I. B. Ressler (✉)
Department of Reproductive Endocrinology, Reproductive Medicine Associates of Connecticut, Norwalk, CT, USA

The increasing trend of those forming families outside of the heterosexual couple structure is due to several factors, not only the greater acceptance of these family units but improved ART technology and options and changing legalities regarding adoption and marriage [4, 5]. When looking to create families, single women and same-sex couples have hurdles that heterosexual couples do not face. They must decide first if they wish to have a biologic link to the child(ren). If not, adoption may be pursued, which may present a separate set of obstacles. If a biologic link is desired, ART involving third-party reproduction must be employed. We will now focus on the ART options and surrounding issues for each of these specific populations.

38.2 Single Women

The fertility treatment available to single women is intrauterine insemination or IVF with donor sperm. Some claim that the first attempt at artificial insemination was done by Henry IV, King of Castile, whose nickname was "the Impotent." He was married in 1455 to Princess Juana and 6 years later had a daughter. It was assumed that he was impotent, and the idea of artificial insemination was introduced [6]. In 1784, scientist Lazzaro Spallanzani reported the first artificial insemination in a dog, which resulted in the birth of three puppies [7, 8]. The first documented human artificial insemination was in the 1770s by John Hunter, "the founder of scientific surgery" [6]. The use of artificial insemination increased in the 1800s in several countries, including the USA, Russia, England, and Denmark. This led to the growth of its use first in animals and later in humans in the 1940s. In 1953, Dr. Jerome Sherman introduced a technique of preserving human sperm with glycerol, slow cooling, and storage with solid carbon dioxide. This resulted in the first human pregnancy with frozen sperm in 1953 and finally to the commercialization of sperm banks in the 1970s [6].

Historically, therapeutic donor insemination (TDI) was used primarily by heterosexual couples with male factor

G. N. Allahbadia et al. (eds.), *Textbook of Assisted Reproduction*, https://doi.org/10.1007/978-981-15-2377-9_38

infertility. A study examining the use of TDI by physicians in 1979 compared to a decade later reported that in 1979, 9.5% of physicians using TDI had performed this on unmarried women; this statistic rose to 35% in 1990 [9]. While professional society guidelines for sperm donation include several indications for the use of TDI, they do not specify single women or same-sex female couples. The guidelines do, however, include "females without male partners" [10]. This could include single heterosexual women, single lesbians, or lesbian couples.

There is large oversight of specific aspects of gamete donation. In the USA, there are professional society guidelines regarding screening and testing potential donors, as well as Food and Drug Administration (FDA) guidelines [10–13]. Evaluation of the female recipient should include a thorough medical and reproductive history, a complete physical examination, standard preconception counseling and screening, psychological consultation, evaluation of ovulation, and evaluation for tubal and uterine abnormalities [10].

When selecting a sperm donor, the patient has a choice of selecting an anonymous or known donor. In either case, the following apply: In general, a donor in good health with no known genetic problems and with known established paternity is ideal. The screening process for sperm donors includes semen analysis, psychological evaluation, genetic screening for commonly inherited genetic diseases, medical history, physical exam, and laboratory testing (including infectious diseases, blood type, and Rh). After the sperm is cryopreserved, it should be quarantined for 6 months and the infectious disease testing repeated. Practices utilizing sperm from commercial sperm banks must ensure that the sperm bank is in compliance with legal requirements, both local and federal.

When selecting a sperm donor, the patient should consider what characteristics are important to her. These may include physical characteristics, race, ethnicity, and religious and educational background. If the recipient is Rh negative or CMV negative, consideration of these factors should be made as well.

One study compared single heterosexual and lesbian women and lesbian couples who utilized TDI [14]. This study found that heterosexual women started TDI treatment at an older age as compared to lesbian women. Common factors affecting the timing of when they initiated treatment were job security, the sense of time running out, having worked out concerns regarding parenting, and sufficient social support. Other studies have reported that among those utilizing TDI, single heterosexual and lesbian women were similar to married women demographically, in regard to concerns surrounding TDI and in regard to TDI outcome [15, 16].

In general, single women should not be considered as "infertile" or "subfertile," unless their pre-treatment fertility workup indicates otherwise. While one of the biggest predictors of success with intrauterine insemination with donor sperm is the age of the woman [17, 18], other considerations include use of ovarian stimulation with oral agents or injectable gonadotropins, timing of insemination, and frequency of insemination. Intrauterine insemination has a higher success rate per cycle than intracervical insemination [19, 20]. In a study of single and lesbian women utilizing TDI, the overall pregnancy rate for women <35 years old was 18.5%, 11.9% if 35–40 years old, and 5.4% if >40 years old. The cumulative pregnancy rate after 8 cycles was 86% for those <35 years old, 51% for those 35–40, and 32% if >40 years old. There were no differences in pregnancy rates when correcting for age in relation to the stimulation regimen (natural cycle, clomiphene citrate versus gonadotropins) [17]. Others have shown higher pregnancy rates in those being treated with gonadotropins [21].

38.3 Same-Sex Female Couples

Access to ART is limited or unavailable to lesbian couples in many countries. In some instances, access is as a single woman, not a couple [22]. In 1985, a survey reported that only 0.7% of patients requesting TDI were lesbian couples [23]; a more recent study reports that the majority of those utilizing TDI at their center are lesbian couples [24].

There is more than one option for conception for lesbian couples. This includes one partner providing the oocytes and carrying the pregnancy (with use of TDI or IVF), and sometimes the other partner will do the same in a subsequent pregnancy. If both partners wish to be involved biologically in the same pregnancy, the oocytes from one woman can be retrieved, fertilized with donor sperm, and the embryo(s) transferred to the other's uterus. This process has several names, including reception of oocytes from partner (ROPA), reciprocal IVF, shared maternity, shared conception, shared parenthood, or intrapartner oocyte donation [22, 25, 26].

Studies have investigated the decision-making process regarding which of the partners will conceive and carry the child [27–30]. Reasons include a desire to experience pregnancy and childbirth, the importance of a genetic connection, age, and employment situation. While theoretically possible for both partners to carry, evidence suggests that the minority of lesbian couples desire this approach [24, 29, 30].

When considering their reproductive options, lesbian couples will have a medical consult with a reproductive endocrinologist to review both partners' histories and discuss treatment options as above. A discussion regarding anonymous versus known sperm donation will take place. Preconception testing is similar to a heterosexual woman, including blood type and Rh with antibody status, infectious disease screening (HIV, hepatitis B and C, syphilis, gonorrhea, chlamydia), immunity status to rubella and varicella, cytomegalovirus antibody status, and recent PAP smear results. Pre-conception genetic carrier screening is typically offered. Additional tests include ovarian reserve testing (day 3 follicle stimulating hormone (FSH) with estradiol, anti-Müllerian hormone (AMH), antral follicle count), thyroid function, and prolactin. In addition to the medical consultation, it is recommended that the clinician encourage psychological counseling for sperm donor recipients [10].

When selecting donor sperm for TDI, IVF, or reciprocal IVF, lesbian couples must decide whether to use a known or anonymous sperm donor. One study found that 59% of the women wanted an anonymous donor, primarily to avoid interference from a third party [27]. A different small study found that the majority of women wanted a known donor because they felt their children have the right to know their genetic origin and form relationships with the donors [31]; others are worried that their children might have psychological or identity problems later in life if they did not know their paternity [32]. Importantly, no differences have been seen in the psychological well-being of adolescents with known versus anonymous donors [30, 32].

Evidence suggests that couples have a higher chance of success with achieving a live birth if both partners are willing to go through treatment. A recent study showed that when both partners attempted conception, 88.9% achieved a live birth, compared to 68% when only one partner attempted. Those who were successful with TDI took an average of 3 cycles, and those with IVF took a mean of 6 TDI and 1.7 IVF cycles [24]. A comparison of heterosexual and lesbian women utilizing donor sperm (both TDI and IVF) showed no differences in live birth outcome in relation to sexual orientation [33]. Lesbian couples should be counseled that despite not having a diagnosis of "infertility," it often takes several treatment cycles to be successful and their best chances of success may be if both partners are willing to try. As with all patients, age is one of the biggest predictors of success.

38.4 Same-Sex Male Couples

Studies have shown that gay men decide to become fathers for the same reasons as heterosexual men. These reasons include the desire to nurture children, achieving a sense of immortality, the sense of family that children provide, and constancy of children in their lives [34]. Gay men, however, must decide how they will achieve parenthood. Choices include adoption, providing foster care, and ART with use of oocyte donation and surrogacy. Having a genetic link to the child and allowing for more control over the process are two of the most common reasons why men choose to utilize ART [4, 35].

While many gay men choose adoption as their method for achieving parenthood, an increasing number now choose ART. A strong motivating factor for the latter is having a biological tie to the child. Barriers remain, however, for gay men utilizing ART. One of the most common barriers is cost, as the price can be upward of $100,000 dollars to pay for the process; this includes fees for donor and surrogacy agencies, compensation for the donor and gestational surrogate, fertility treatment fees, medications, and legal fees. For many this becomes cost prohibitive. Some countries do not allow egg donation or gestational surrogacy. Those living in areas with such restrictions may choose to travel and have the treatments elsewhere, which is termed "reproductive tourism" or "cross border reproductive care." Reasons for reproductive tourism include legal purposes and better access to treatment and quality of care [36]. In the USA, laws regarding surrogacy vary by state.

Gay men using ART must select both an oocyte donor and gestational surrogate. There are two types of surrogacy, traditional genetic surrogacy and gestational surrogacy. Traditional surrogacy involves inseminating a woman with the sperm of the intended parent and carrying the pregnancy of a fetus who is genetically related to her. Gestational surrogacy involves utilizing IVF with oocytes from a donor, sperm from the intended parent(s), and creating embryos that are then transferred to a different woman's uterus than the source of the oocytes. Therefore, the surrogate has no genetic connection to the child. The first successful case of surrogacy was reported in 1985 [37]. Its use has increased in recent years from 1.0% of ART cycles in 1999 to 2.5% in 2013, and traditional surrogacy is seldom used [38].

The medical screening and assessment of a gay man is the same as for a heterosexual man utilizing donor oocytes and a surrogate. When a surrogate is involved, the man providing the sperm is considered a "directed donor." FDA donor eligibility must be determined for him, but if deemed to be "ineligible," use of the sperm is not prohibited [39]. If results are positive for one of the FDA-mandated infectious diseases, the tissue must be labeled as such; the physician must evaluate and discuss this with all parties involved, and they may choose to proceed with use of that sperm [10].

A semen analysis should be done on any sperm source under consideration. A gay couple may choose to inseminate the oocytes with one partner's sperm or to split the donor oocytes so that half are inseminated with each partner's sperm. When deciding the sperm source, factors that are considered include the following: the intended parents' ages (one may be older, and they choose to use his first), one may already have a child and feel the other should have the opportunity, one may be considered to have "better genes," and one may feel more strongly about having a biological connection [40]. One study showed that 76% of couples chose to have sperm from both partners inseminate the donor oocytes [41].

When selecting an oocyte donor, intended parents have the option of choosing an anonymous donor or someone with whom they may contact (a known donor or an open-identity donor). Many utilize a donor agency to assist with the donor selection. As with the use of a donor sperm, oocyte donors must go through a rigorous screening process regulated by the FDA. An optimal donor is in good health, has no known genetic problems, and has proven fertility. Donors must be of legal age and ideally 21–34 years old. The evaluation process includes psychological evaluation and screening, ovarian reserve testing, genetic screening for commonly inherited genetic diseases, medical history, physical exam, and laboratory testing (including infectious diseases and ovarian reserve markers) [10]. FDA blood work must be performed within 7 days of sperm collection and within 30 days of oocyte retrieval.

Contracts must be in place prior to starting the stimulation cycle. It is recommended that donors undergo a maximum of six stimulation cycles during their lifetime [42]. The stimulation of an oocyte donor is similar to that of any woman undergoing IVF treatment. Oocyte donors generally have excellent ovarian reserve and are at increased risk for ovarian hyperstimulation syndrome. Monetary compensation to the donor reflects the time and physical and emotional elements that are associated with the donation. Travel costs must sometimes be taken under consideration as well. More recently, the utilization of cryopreserved donor oocytes has increased. This is due to the increasing availability of cryopreserved oocytes since the "experimental" label was lifted from cryopreserving oocytes in 2013 [43]. Donor oocyte banks are now available as donor sperm banks have been for years.

There are several considerations when selecting a surrogate. They should be of legal age and ideally between the ages of 21 and 45 years. It is optimal if they have had at least one prior full-term, uncomplicated pregnancy, but no more than five prior vaginal deliveries or three prior cesarean sections. All potential surrogates and their partners should undergo psychosocial evaluation and counseling by a mental health professional. It is important that the surrogate have a supportive family and/or social network and not feel coerced into the surrogacy arrangement [44]. The majority of surrogates report that they are motivated by altruism and a desire to help a family have a child [35]. In addition, their compensation is a large motivating factor [45]. Some intended parents may have family or friends who are willing to be a surrogate, but most utilize surrogacy agencies to help select one.

There are multiple components to the screening and testing of potential surrogates. A medical professional must thoroughly review their medical history, particularly their pregnancy history. They should be cleared medically to undergo pregnancy. While the FDA does not require screening of surrogates for possible transmissible infectious diseases, ASRM does recommend testing for all surrogates and their partners within 30 days of embryo transfer. It is important to carefully review the risks of the ART procedures and pregnancy and obtain informed consent. Surrogates should have independent legal counsel, and legal contracts must be in place prior to initiating treatment [44].

There are limited studies regarding relationships between gay men and their surrogates. The relationships tend to extend beyond the time of the pregnancy and are overall positive [40, 46]. Many surrogates go on to meet the children and other family members [46]. Gay men utilizing ART to create their families must decide when and how to disclose the details of this process to their children, including use of donor oocytes, a surrogate, and which father has a biological tie to the child. Most disclose this information in an age-appropriate manner and discuss more details as the child ages [46].

38.5 Legal Considerations

Massachusetts was the first state to legalize same-sex marriage in 2004. The US Supreme Court declared that the provision of the federal Defense of Marriage Act that limited federal recognition of marriage to heterosexual couples was unconstitutional in 2013 [47]. In June 2015, the US Supreme Court ruled that same-sex marriage is legal [48].

Legal barriers still exist for gay men wishing to adopt or utilize ART. Adoption by gay parents was prohibited in certain states until recently. In March 2016, a federal judge overturned the last same-sex adoption ban in the USA (in Mississippi), making it legal in all 50 states [49].

All patients utilizing third-party reproduction must have a legal contract. Each party involved should have their own independent legal counsel. Depending on what state (or country) the men come from, and where the surrogate delivers, they may not be able to have both partners' names on the birth certificate. Patients must be clear on the laws of their home state, the home state of the surrogate, and the state where the surrogate delivers, as there are states in which compensated surrogacy contracts are prohibited.

38.6 Ethical Considerations

The debate over the use of artificial insemination began in the USA in 1909 and in Europe in the 1940s. The Catholic Church objected to its use altogether. The main arguments against artificial insemination were that it was a form of adultery that looked past the religious importance of intercourse and encouraged masturbation, which is viewed by the Catholic Church as a vice [6]. Despite these views, the donor sperm bank industry grew. Still today, many countries do not allow the use of donor sperm insemination for single women or lesbian couples. A study in 1984 regarding single women and the use of TDI reports that while it may be permissible in select cases of single women, the physician has the right to refuse treatment [50]. More recent professional society guidelines state that there is no ethical basis to deny reproductive services to unmarried, gay, or lesbian people [51]. All requests for fertility treatment should be treated equally, regardless of marital status or sexual orientation.

One concern with sperm donation is that a man may donate his sperm too many times, which may lead to unknown sexually intimate relationships or marriage between biological siblings. There are no national or international registries that track how many times a man has donated his sperm nor how many children have resulted. While the American Society of Reproductive Medicine recommends a limit to six cycles of oocyte donation for an individual, there is no current method of tracking or proving how many cycles have previously been done [42]. Due to this lack of accurate record keeping, there are no reliable statistics regarding how many children are conceived via donor sperm insemination annually.

Concerns have been raised regarding the offspring of single or lesbian or gay couples, arguing that the best environment is a married, heterosexual family. Some opponents claim that a mother is necessary to provide a more caring and nurturing environment and that lesbian women are less maternal than heterosexual women. Other opponents have said that children of gay and lesbian parents will be socially isolated and have gender identity and sexual orientation difficulties and that the children are at greater risk for pedophilia or sexual abuse [52–55]. There is no scientific data, however, to support any of these claims. The American Psychological Association task force reviewed the data and concluded that parenting effectiveness is not related to the sexual orientation of the parents; lesbian and gay parents are equally likely to provide healthy, supportive environments for their children [56]. Studies of personal and sexual identity development have found few differences between children of lesbian and heterosexual parents [57–60]. Overall, research shows little difference between the development, adjustment, and well-being of children of lesbian and gay parents and heterosexual parents. The ASRM Ethics Committee therefore concludes that there is no ethical basis for which to deny reproductive services to single, lesbian, or gay people [51].

38.7 Conclusion

The landscape of building families and the paths to parenthood is continually changing. The scientific technology and tools with which to build families also continue to rapidly evolve. While the medical building blocks of creating families with ART may not differ in regard to marital status or sexual orientation, there are several other factors to consider when treating patients, including the psychological and legal components. It takes a well-informed team approach to provide the best care and address all considerations.

References

1. Martin JA, Hamilton BE, Osterman MJ, Driscoll AK, Mathews TJ. Births: final data for 2015. Natl Vital Stat Rep. 2017;66(1):1–69.
2. Gates GJ. LGBT demographics: comparisons among population-based surveys (Los Angeles, CA: Williams Institute, UCLA School of Law). 2014. [cited 2017 May 18]. Available from: http://williamsinsitute.law.ucla.edu/wp-content/uploads/lgbt-demogs-sep-2014.pdf.
3. Gates GJ. Marriage and family: LGBT individuals and same-sex couples. 2015. [cited 2017 May 18]. Available from: https://www.princeton.edu/futureofchildren/publications/docs/MarriageandFamily.pdf.
4. Goldberg AE. Lesbian and gay parents and their children: research on the family life cycle. Washington, DC: American Psychological Association; 2010.
5. Stacey J. In the name of the family: rethinking family values in the postmodern age. Boston, MA: Beacon Press; 1996.
6. Ombelet W, Van Robays J. Artificial insemination history: hurdles and milestones. Facts Views Vis Obgyn. 2015;7(2):137–43.
7. Belonoschkin B. The science of reproduction and its traditions. Int J Fertil. 1956;1:215–24.
8. Zorgniotti AW. The spermatozoa count – a short history. Urology. 1975;5:672–3.
9. Shapiro S, Saphire DG, Stone WH. Changes in American A.I.D. practice during the past decade. Int J Fertil. 1990;35(5):284–91.
10. The Practice Committee of the American Society for Reproductive Medicine and the Practice Committee of the Society for Assisted Reproductive Technology. Recommendations for gamete and embryo donation: a committee opinion. Fertil Steril. 2013;99(1):47–62.
11. U.S. Food & Drug Administration. Tissue and tissue products. [cited 2017 May 26]. Available from: https://www.fda.gov/BiologicsBloodVaccines/TissueTissueProducts/default.htm
12. U.S. Food & Drug Administration. Tissue and tissue products. [cited 2017 May 26]. Available from: https://www.fda.gov/BiologicsBloodVaccines/default.htm
13. U.S. Food & Drug Administration. Tissue & tissue products. [cited 2017 May 26]. Available from: https://www.fda.gov/BiologicsBloodVaccines/GuidanceComplianceRegulatoryInformation/ActsRulesRegulations/TissueProposedFinalRules/default.htm
14. Leiblum SR, Palmer MG, Spector IP. Non-traditional mothers: single heterosexual/lesbian women and lesbian couples electing motherhood via donor insemination. J Psychosom Obstet Gynaecol. 1995;1:11–20.
15. Wendland CL, Byrn F, Hill C. Donor insemination: a comparison of lesbian couples, heterosexual couples and single women. Fertil Steril. 1996;65(4):764–70.
16. Ferrara I, Balet R, Grudzinskas JG. Intrauterine donor insemination in single women and lesbian couples: a comparative study of pregnancy rates. Hum Reprod. 2000;15(3):621–5.
17. Ferrara I, Balet R, Grudzinskas JG. Intrauterine insemination with frozen donor sperm. Pregnancy outcome in relation to age and ovarian stimulation regime. Hum Reprod. 2002;17(9):2320–4.
18. Kang BM, Wu TC. Effect of age on intrauterine insemination with frozen donor sperm. Obstet Gynecol. 1996;88(1):93–8.

19. Wainer R, Merlet F, Ducot B, Bailly M, Tribalat S, Lombroso R. Prospective randomized comparison of intrauterine and intracervical insemination with donor sperm. Hum Reprod. 1995;10:2919–22.
20. Guzick D, Carson SM, Coutifaris C, Overstreet J, Factor-Litvak P, Steinkampf MP, et al. Efficacy of superovulation and intrauterine insemination in the treatment of infertility. N Engl J Med. 1999;340:177–83.
21. Matorras R, Diaz T, Corcostegui B, Ramón O, Pijoan JI, Rodriguez-Escudero FJ. Ovarian stimulation in intrauterine insemination with donor sperm: a randomized study comparing clomiphene citrate in fixed protocol versus highly purified urinary FSH. Hum Reprod. 2002;17(8):2107–11.
22. Marina S, Marina D, Marina F, Fosas N, Galiana N, Jové I. Sharing motherhood: biological lesbian co-mothers, a new IVF indication. Hum Reprod. 2010;25(4):938–41.
23. U.S. Congress, Office of Technology Assessment. Artificial insemination: practice in the United States: summary of a 1987 survey – background paper, OTA-13P-BA-48. Washington, DC: U.S. Government Printing Office; 1988.
24. Carpinello OJ, Jacob MC, Nulsen J, Benadiva C. Utilization of fertility treatment and reproductive choices by lesbian couples. Fertil Steril. 2016;106(7):1709–13.
25. Woodward BJ, Norton WJ. Lesbian intra-partner oocyte donation: a possible shake-up in the Garden of Eden? Hum Fertil (Camb). 2006;9:217–22.
26. Marshall LA, Lynn JM. "Shared maternity": gay marriage calls for new language. LGBT Health. 2015;2:367.
27. Goldberg AE. The transition to parenthood for lesbian couples. J GLBT Fam Stud. 2006;2:13–42.
28. Chabot JM, Ames BD. "It wasn't let's get pregnant and go do it": decision-making in lesbian couples planning motherhood via donor insemination. Fam Relat. 2004;53:348–56.
29. Baetens P, Camus M, Devroey P. Counseling lesbian couples: request for donor insemination on social grounds. Reprod Biomed Online. 2003;6:75–83.
30. Bos HM, van Balen F, van den Boom DC. Planned lesbian families: their desire and motivation to have a child. Hum Reprod. 2003;18:2216–24.
31. Touroni E, Coyle A. Decision-making in planned lesbian parenting: an interpretative phenomenological analysis. J Commun Appl Soc Psychol. 2002;12:194–209.
32. Gartrell N, Hamilton J, Banks A, Mosbacher D, Reed N, Sparks CH, et al. The national lesbian family study: 1. Interviews with prospective mothers. Am J Orthopsychiatry. 1996;66:272–81.
33. Nordqvist S, Sydsjö G, Lampic C, Åkerud H, Elenis E, Skoog SA. Sexual orientation of women does not affect outcome of fertility treatment with donated sperm. Hum Reprod. 2014;29(4):704–11.
34. Bigner JJ, Jacobsen BR. Parenting behaviors of homosexual and heterosexual fathers. J Homosex. 1989;18:173–86.
35. Lev AI. Gay dads: choosing surrogacy. Lesbian Gay Psychol Rev. 2006;7:73–7.
36. Shenfield F, de Mouzon J, Pennings G, Ferraretti AP, Nyboe Andersen A, de Wert G, et al. Cross border reproductive care in six European countries. Hum Reprod. 2010;25(6):1361–8.
37. Utian WH, Sheean L, Goldfarb JM, Kiwi R. Successful pregnancy after in vitro fertilization and embryo transfer from an infertile woman to a surrogate. N Engl J Med. 1985;313:1351–2.
38. Perkins KM, Boulet SL, Jamieson DJ, Kissin DM. Trends and outcomes of gestational surrogacy in the United States. Fertil Steril. 2016;106:435–42.
39. U.S. Food & Drug Administration. [cited 2017 July 13] Available from: https://www.fda.gov/downloads/biologicsbloodvaccines/guidancecomplianceregulatoryinformation/guidances/tissue/ucm091345.pdf
40. Greenfeld D, Seli E. Gay men choosing parenthood through assisted reproduction: medical and psychological considerations. Fertil Steril. 2011;95:225–9.
41. Grover SA, Shmorgun Z, Moskovtsev S, Baratz A, Librach CL. Assisted reproduction in a cohort of same-sex male couples and single men. Reprod Biomed Online. 2013;27(2):217–21.
42. Practice Committee of the American Society for Reproductive Medicine and Practice Committee of the Society for Assisted Reproductive Technology. Repetitive oocyte donation: a committee opinion. Fertil Steril. 2014;102(4):964–6.
43. Practice Committee of the American Society for Reproductive Medicine. Mature oocyte cryopreservation: a guideline. Fertil Steril. 2013;99:37–43.
44. Practice Committee of the American Society for Reproductive Medicine. Recommendations for practices utilizing gestational carriers: a committee opinion. Fertil Steril. 2017;107(2):e3–10.
45. Dillaway HE. Mothers for others: a race, class, and gender analysis of surrogacy. Int J Sociol Fam. 2008;34:301–26.
46. Blake L, Carone N, Slutsky J, Raffanello E, Ehrnhardt AA, Golombok S. Gay father surrogacy families: relationships with surrogates and egg donors and parental disclosure of children's origins. Fertil Steril. 2016;106(6):1503–9.
47. Windsor v. United States 570 US 12. 2013.
48. U.S. Supreme Court. Obergefell v. Hodges, no. 14–556. (June 26, 2015).
49. Campaign for Southern Equality, et al. v. Mississippi Department of Human Services, et al. (March 31, 2016).
50. Strong C, Schinfeld JS. The single woman and artificial insemination by donor. J Reprod Med. 1984;29(5):293–9.
51. The Ethics Committee of the American Society for Reproductive Medicine. Access to fertility treatment by gays, lesbians, and unmarried persons: a committee opinion. Fertil Steril. 2013;100:1524–7.
52. Dunstan GR. Ethical aspects of donor insemination. J Med Ethics. 1975;1:42–4.
53. Fletcher JC. Artificial insemination in lesbians: ethical considerations. Arch Intern Med. 1985;145:419–20.
54. Cairney J, Boyle M, Offord DR, Racine Y. Stress, social support and depression in single and married mothers. Soc Psychiatry Psychiatr Epidemiol. 2003;38:442–9.
55. Avison WR. Single motherhood and mental health: implications for primary prevention. Can Med Assoc J. 1997;156:661–3.
56. American Psychological Association. Sexual orientation, parents, and children. 2004. [cited 2017 July 28]. Available from: http://www.apa.org/about/policy/parenting.aspx
57. Patterson CJ. Family relationships of lesbians and gay men. J Marriage Fam. 2000;62:1052–69.
58. Patterson CJ. Lesbian and gay parents and their children: summary of research findings. In: Lesbian and gay parenting: a resource for psychologists. Washington, DC: American Psychological Association; 2004.
59. Perrin EC, The Committee on Psychosocial Aspects of Child and Family Health. Technical Report: Coparent or second-parent adoption by same-sex parents. Pediatrics. 2002;109:341–4.
60. Tasker F. Children in lesbian-led families – a review. Clin Child Psychol Psychiatry. 1999;4:153–66.

Treating Transgender People

39

Kelly Tilleman, Chloë De Roo, Sylvie Lierman, and Petra De Sutter

39.1 The Desire to Parent

A child wish is as present in transgender individuals as it is in cisgender individuals. Evidence from patient surveys shows that 40–50% of transgender individuals wish to have children [1–3]. Many years ago, there was still a debate as to whether trans-persons would be "good parents." This debate, similar to the discussion on the parenting skills of homosexual couples, is now clearly in the past. Although there are not that many studies, especially on the long-term health of children in trans-families, it seems that transgenderism does not impact on the psychosexual or gender identity development of children raised in families having a trans-parent [4–6]. The younger the children were at the time of their parent's transitioning, the better the relationship was with the transitioning parent [7].

In cases where the transitioning of the parent occurred before the birth of the child, it is important to discuss the transgender identity of the parent early in childhood, rather than later in life. If this does not take place in the closeness and safety of the family, it is possible that the gender transition of the parent could be told to the child by another person who is not the parent. This should be avoided, as such a scenario may be devastating for the child [8].

It has been shown that transgender people with children have better mental health and vitality scores than transgender individuals without children [9]. Additionally, having children has even been identified as a suicide protective factor among trans-adults [10].

As eloquently stated by T'Sjoen et al. [6], it is no longer a question of whether transgenders need to be assisted in this desire to parent, but how. Gender confirming treatments imply an effect on the capability to reproduce. Cross-sex hormone therapy almost always has a reversible effect on the spermatogenesis or oocyte maturation, accepting that it can result in permanent loss of fertility [11, 12]. Surgical interventions, including the removal of the gonads, will obviously lead to sterility.

The type of medically assisted reproduction (MAR) offered to transgender people seeking to fulfill the desire to parent depends on many factors. For example, do they wish to conceive a genetically-related child, what is the gender of their partner (if they have one), what is the timing of the MAR in relation to the gender-affirming treatment, and what is the local legislation on access to MAR for them? As a general rule, any form of MAR is best carried out before cross-hormone treatment or at least after periodic cessation of the treatment, since this most probably gives the transgender patients the best MAR outcome chances.

39.2 Medical-Assisted Reproduction in Trans-persons

The seventh version of the World Professional Association for Transgender Health (WPATH) Standards of Care recommends that fertility options should be discussed with patients prior to starting any ART or medical intervention [13]. Furthermore, the impact of each MAR option on fertility should be addressed, including fertility preservation options to offer the possibility of genetically related children. This chapter follows on from a recent review of De Roo et al. [14] and provides information on the effects of therapy on fertility, fertility preservation options, success rates, and how transgender people can use their cryopreserved gametes in the future.

39.3 Fertility Preservation for Transgender Women

Fertility preservation options for transgender women comprise of the cryopreservation of sperm collected through ejaculation or direct testicular surgery/extraction or the

K. Tilleman (✉) · C. De Roo · S. Lierman · P. De Sutter
Department of Reproductive Medicine, Ghent University Hospital, Ghent, Belgium
e-mail: Kelly.Tilleman@UZGent.be

G. N. Allahbadia et al. (eds.), *Textbook of Assisted Reproduction*, https://doi.org/10.1007/978-981-15-2377-9_39

Table 39.1 Fertility preservation options in transgender women

Technique	Description	Considerations	Future use
Sperm cryopreservation	Cryopreservation of ejaculated sperm through masturbation or vibratory stimulation	– Established technique – Masturbation – Post pubertal	*Male partner* Need of a donor oocyte and surrogate mother *Female partner* IUI or IVF/ICSI, depending on sperm quality followed by embryo transfer in partner
Surgical sperm extraction	Percutaneous aspiration of sperm from the testis or epididymis	– Established technique – No masturbation – Surgical procedure – Post pubertal	*Male partner* Need of a donor oocyte and surrogate mother *Female partner* IVF/ICSI treatment followed by embryo transfer in partner
Testicular tissue cryopreservation	Surgical biopsy of testicular tissue	– Experimental – Prepubertal or post pubertal – Possible at moment of genital reconstructive surgery	*Male partner* In vitro maturation and need of a donor oocyte and surrogate mother (not possible at this stage) *Female partner* In vitro maturation and IVF/ICSI followed by embryo transfer in partner (not possible at this stage)

Reprinted from De Roo C. et al. 2016 [14] with permission

freezing of immature testicular tissue. An overview of fertility preservation options in transgender women is provided in Table 39.1. For each option, it should be clearly indicated if this treatment is established, innovative, or experimental. Furthermore, the future use of cryopreserved gametes should be discussed in relation to the gender of the partner.

39.3.1 Sperm Cryopreservation

Sperm obtained through masturbation or vibratory stimulation can be preserved for future use by freezing. Transgender women can find it challenging to masturbate for the purpose of producing a semen sample for cryopreservation. The storage of cryopreserved semen may remind transgender women of their (male) past and could make a transgender woman feel as if she is not a true woman, as cisgender females do not have sperm banked [3, 15–18]. The sperm quality will decide what type of MAR will be most effective in the future.

39.3.2 Surgical Sperm Extraction

This technique requires a needle puncture of the testes in order to extract or aspirate the sperm. This is a standard method in ART. Although this has been presented as an option for transgender women for whom masturbation is extremely difficult, it is important to take into account that this still is a surgical procedure [19].

39.3.3 Testicular Tissue Cryopreservation

Testicular tissue cryopreservation involves surgical biopsy of testicular tissue. This option overcomes the need for masturbation and is also possible in prepubertal boys [19]. It is also a surgical procedure that can be combined with genital reconstructive surgery, accepting that this option is experimental.

When it comes to thawing the tissue, an in vitro maturation procedure would be necessary in order to obtain mature sperm. At the moment, this is not possible as the process is still being optimized in a basic research setting. However, tissue transplantation could also be an option, followed by ART. Transplantation, although technically possible, can restore the male endocrine environment, but this is not desired by transgender women.

39.4 Fertility Preservation for Transgender Men

For transgender men, fertility preservation options include the cryopreservation of embryos, oocytes, or ovarian tissue (the theoretical options are presented and summarized in Table 39.2).

39.4.1 Oocyte Cryopreservation

Human oocyte cryopreservation (often called "egg freezing") requires the trans-man to have hormonal stimulation, the retrieval of the oocyte(s), and subsequent cryopreservation, mostly via the process of vitrification.

The hormonal stimulation includes frequent vaginal ultrasound monitoring. A transvaginal surgical procedure is then performed for the oocyte aspiration [3, 19, 20]. A recent qualitative study by Armaund et al. [20] clearly indicated that the vaginal examinations, and additionally the physiological changes associated with the discontinuation of testos-

Table 39.2 Fertility preservation options in transgender men

Technique	Description	Considerations	Future use
Embryo cryopreservation	Controlled ovarian stimulation for oocyte retrieval and fertilization to obtain embryos for cryopreservation (to freeze)	– Established method – Controlled ovarian stimulation – Vaginal procedure – Post pubertal – Partner or donor sperm	*Male partner* Use of partner's sperm prior to cryopreservation, need of a surrogate mother *Female partner* Fertilization by donor sperm prior to cryopreservation, implantation into the partner's uterus
Oocyte cryopreservation	Controlled ovarian stimulation to obtain oocytes for cryopreservation	– Innovative method – Controlled ovarian stimulation – Vaginal procedure – Post pubertal – No partner required	*Male partner* Use of partner's sperm, need of a recipient uterus (surrogate mother) *Female partner* Fertilization by donor sperm, implantation into the partner's uterus
Ovarian tissue cryopreservation	Surgical excision of ovarian tissue for cryopreservation	– Experimental – Prepubertal or post pubertal – No controlled ovarian stimulation – Possible at moment of genital reconstructive surgery – No partner required	*Male partner* In vitro maturation and use of partner's sperm, need of a recipient uterus (surrogate mother) (not possible at this stage) *Female partner* In vitro maturation, fertilization by donor sperm, implantation into the partner's uterus (not possible at this stage)

Reprinted from De Roo C. et al. 2016 [14] with permission

terone and hormonal stimulation, can trigger gender incongruence and dysphoria. Therefore, this issue should be carefully considered prior to embarking on any treatment.

However, provided oocytes are successfully retrieved and cryopreserved, each oocyte can then be used in the future, via warming, fertilization, and subsequent transfer into a uterus as an embryo. It should be noted that cryopreservation of oocytes does not require fertilization to take place on the day of collection, so there is no need for sperm at this stage.

39.4.2 Embryo Cryopreservation

Embryo cryopreservation is the process of preserving embryos, and this is a good option for post-pubertal transgender men with a male partner. It gives the possibility for such couples to have genetically related offspring. Alternatively, donor sperm can also be used to create embryos. This fertility preservation method requires an ovarian stimulation accompanied with the same psychological and emotional stress in transgender women as described above.

39.4.3 Ovarian Tissue Cryopreservation

Ovarian tissue cryopreservation requires a surgical removal of the ovary. However, there is no need for the patient to undergo ovarian stimulation using hormones as per the techniques previously described. Since cross-sex hormone treatment does not impact the number of primordial follicles in the ovary, the removal of the organ could be performed at the time of genital reconstructive surgery [21].

However, it should be stressed that this technique is presently considered highly experimental, since the future use of this tissue for the patient is doubtful. When (and if) the cryopreserved ovarian tissue is warmed for use, it could theoretically either be transplanted, or the follicles could be matured in the IVF laboratory. The transplantation of the ovarian tissue will most likely cause side effects, by restoring female hormone activity in the trans person. Natural conception is theoretically possible in cases where the oviduct and the uterus are still in situ. Furthermore, exogenous hormonal stimulation of the transplanted ovarian tissue could be tried to obtain mature oocytes for IVF or ICSI.

In the future, it may be possible to mature the follicles from the warmed ovarian tissue in the IVF laboratory, thus negating the need for transplantation. This technique, called in vitro maturation (IVM) of follicles, would prevent the transgender men experiencing the recovery of female hormone activity that would be associated with tissue transplantation. However, safe IVM of these immature follicles in the laboratory is not yet possible. IVM is still highly experimental and, at the moment, only available in basic scientific settings, such as research laboratories. For further reading on this topic, please see Ladanyi et al. [22], who have provided a concise overview of the advances in the field of ovarian cryopreservation and future possibilities for research.

39.5 Transgender Gestation

In the USA, unlike in many European countries, hysterectomy with oophorectomy is not necessary for legal gender reassignment [6]. In Sweden, the requirement of sterilization for gender reassignment legalization was ruled unconstitutional in 2013, while in Belgium, new legislation was put in place in 2018, where a change in gender can be executed solely based on an administrative procedure without the necessity for treatment, diagnosis, or surgery [23]. These changes clearly affect clinical practice [24].

When transgender men decide to keep their ovaries and uterus, they have the option to possibly regain fertility after discontinuing androgen therapy. Transgender men can become pregnant, regardless of prior testosterone use [25]. This also emphasizes the need for specialized obstetric care, addressing the needs of pregnant transgender men.

Being pregnant and giving birth is still not possible for transgender women. The Swedish research unit of Prof Brännström performed a series of uterine transplants and reported the first live birth in 2014 [26]. This could open the possibility for assisted gestation for transgender women [12]. There are, however, medical concerns regarding uterine transplantation if introduced to transgender people [6, 16]. A difficult surgical procedure would be needed in order to change the anatomy of the male pelvis with the intention to perform a successful uterus transplantation. Immunosuppressive therapy would also be necessary and is possibly contraindicated during a pregnancy [6]. However, this in itself would not be any different from a uterine transplantation in a cisgender female patient.

39.6 Trans-centered Reproductive Care

There are many possibilities to aid trans-persons in their desire to parent. However, it is clear from the literature that although technically possible, the specific patient population undergoing these treatments needs special and specific care. Trans-persons experience physical discomfort, emotional stress, and significant gender dysphoria while undergoing MAR [20, 27, 28]. Additionally, "misgendering" can take place via medical staff in communications [27], such as using the wrong pronouns when talking to the patients [20] and the constant use of gender-specific words like "egg," "vagina," and "ovaries" [20].

A gender-neutral environment should be provided, where medical staff are up-to-date on the unique primary care needs for trans-persons. Easy changes to existing clinical practices may be necessary to create the right environment. These could include:

1. A section on patient forms for gender identity as male, female, transgender, or gender-neutral, such as those produced by the Human Fertilization and Embryology Authority (HFEA) in the UK
2. Offering restrooms that are unisex
3. Taking care of gender-neutral communications
4. Being aware of the distress trans-persons experience and creating a trusting patient relationship [20, 28]

Specific training for staff working in fertility clinics is therefore necessary, in order to address all aspects when trans-persons seek MAR. Only by doing this can clinics provide the optimal trans-centered reproductive care.

References

1. Tornello SL, Bos H. Parenting intentions among transgender individuals. LGTB Health. 2017;4(2):115–20.
2. Wierkcx K, Van Caeneghem E, Pennings G, Elaut E, Dedecker D, Van de Peer F, et al. Reproductive wish in transsexual men. Hum Reprod. 2012;27(2):483–7.
3. De Sutter P, Kira K, Verschoor A, Hotimsky A. The desire to have children and the preservation of fertility in transsexual women: a survey. Int J Transgenderism. 2002;6(3):215–21.
4. Green R. Sexual identity of thirty-seven children raised by homosexual or transsexual parents. Am J Psychiatry. 1978;135:692–7.
5. Green R. Transsexuals children. Int J Transgenderism. 1998;2(4).
6. T'Sjoen G, Van Caeneghem E, Wierckx K. Transgenderism and reproduction. Curr Opin Endocrinol Diabetes Obes. 2013;20(6):575–9.
7. White T, Ettner R. Disclosure, risks and protective factors for children whose parents are undergoing a gender transition. J Gay Lesb Psychother. 2004;8(1–2):129–45.
8. Chiland C, Clouet AM, Golse B, Guinot M, Wolf J. A new type of family: transmen as fathers thanks to donor sperm insemination. A 12-year follow-up exploratory study of their children. Neuropsychiatrie de l'enfance et de l'adolescence. 2013;61(6):365–70.
9. Wierckx K. Clinical effects of cross-sex hormone therapy in adult trans persons (chapter 4). Ghent: Ghent University, Faculty of Medicine and Health Sciences; 2014.. http://hdl.handle.net/1854/LU-8535726
10. Moody C, Smith NG. Suicide protective factors among trans adults. Arch Sex Behav. 2013;42(5):739–52.
11. Wallace SA, Blough KL, Kondapalli LA. Fertility preservation in the transgender patient: expanding oncofertility care beyond caner. Gynecol Endocrinol. 2014;30(12):868–71.
12. Murphy TF. The ethics of fertility preservation in transgender body modifications. J Bioeth Inq. 2012;9(3):311–6.
13. Coleman E, Bockting W, Botzer M, Cohen-Kettenis P, DeCuypere G, Feldman J, et al. Standards of care for the health of transsexual, transgender, and gender-nonconforming people, version 7. Int J Transgenderism. 2012;13(4):165–232.
14. De Roo C, Tilleman K, T'Sjoen G, De Sutter P. Fertility options for transgender people. Int Rev Psychiatry. 2016;28(1):112–29.
15. Payer AF, Meyer WJ, Walker PA. The ultrastructural response of human Leydig cells to exogenous estrogens. Andrologia. 1979;11(6):423–36.

16. Hamada A, Kingsberg S, Wierckx K, T'Sjoen G, De Sutter P, Knudson G, Agarwal A. Semen characteristics of transwomen referred for sperm banking before sex transition: a case series. Andrologia. 2014;47(7):832–8.
17. Lübbert H, Leo-Rossberg I, Hammerstein J. Effects of ethinyl estradiol on semen quality and various hormonal parameters in a eugonadal male. Fertility Sterility. 1992;58(3):603–8.
18. Wierckx K, Stuyver I, Weyers S, Hamada A, Agarwal A, De Sutter P, T'Sjoen G. Sperm freezing in transsexual women. Arch Sex Behav. 2012;41(5):1069–71.
19. Wallace SA, Blough KL, Kondapalli LA. Fertility preservation in the transgender patient: expanding oncofertility care beyond cancer. Gynecol Endocrinol. 2014;30:868–71.
20. Armaund G, Dhejne C, Olofsson JI, Rodriguez-Wallberg KA. Transgender men' experiences of fertility preservation: a qualitative study. Hum Reprod. 2017;32(2):383–90.
21. Van Den Broecke R, Van der Elst J, Liu J, Hovatta O, Dhont M. The female-to-male transsexual patient: a source of human ovarian cortical tissue for experimental research. Hum Reprod. 2001;16(1):145–7.
22. Ladanyi C, Mor A, Christianson MS, Dhillon N, Segars JH. Recent advances in the field of ovarian tissue cryopreservations and opportunities for research. J Assist Reprod Genet. 2017;34:709–22.
23. Wet 25 juni 2017 – Wet tot hervorming van regelingen inzake transgender wat de vermelding van een aanpassing van de registratie van het geslacht in de akten van de burgerlijke stand en de gevolgen hiervan betreft. http://www.ejustice.just.fgov.be/eli/wet/2017/06/25/2017012964/justel
24. Rodriguez-Wallberg KA, Dhejne C, Stefenson M, Degerblad M, Olofsson JI. Preserving eggs for men's fertility. A pilot experience with fertility preservation for female-to-male transsexuals in Sweden. Fertil Steril. 2014;102(3 Suppl):e160–1.
25. Light AD, Obedin-Maliver J, Sevelius JM, Kernis JL. Transgender men who experienced pregnancy after female-to-male gender transitioning. Obstet Gynecol. 2014;124(6):1120–7.
26. Brännström M, Johannesson L, Bokström H, Kvarnström N, Mölne N, Dahm-Kähler P, et al. Live birth after uterus transplantation. Lancet. 2015;385(9968):607–16.
27. Chen D, Simons L, Johnson EK, Lockart BA, Finlayson C. Fertility preservation for transgender adolescents. J Adolesc Health. 2017;61:120–3.
28. Selix NW, Rowniak S. Provision of patient-centered transgender care. J Midwifery Woman's Health. 2016;61(6):744–51.

Transvaginal Sonography-Guided Management of Ectopic Pregnancies

40

Luwam Ghidei and Gary N. Frishman

While most ectopic pregnancies implant in the fallopian tube, 10% of extrauterine pregnancies occur outside of the fallopian tube posing an even greater potential to cause significant morbidity and mortality [1]. These non-tubal or complex ectopic pregnancies, such as cesarean scar, cervical, interstitial, ovarian, and heterotopic pregnancies, may be associated with a delayed presentation and diagnosis and thereby a higher risk of emergent surgery, life-threatening hemorrhage and hysterectomy. Fortunately, due to advances in ultrasound technology and clarifications in the criteria for diagnosing ectopic pregnancies, these pregnancies are detected earlier, allowing for timely and less invasive treatment measures. Local injection of ectopic pregnancies with chemotherapeutic agents in place of, or as an adjuvant to, systemic medical or surgical therapy is becoming established as a safe and effective treatment option in appropriately selected patients [2].

Local injection of non-tubal or complex ectopic pregnancies offers many advantages over traditional treatment protocols. By performing the procedure using ultrasound guidance, the provider can immediately confirm cessation of fetal cardiac activity if present. The successful resolution of non-tubal and heterotopic ectopic pregnancies with fetal cardiac activity by local injection alone or after systemic methotrexate failure has been well established [3, 4]. The addition of local injection to systemic methotrexate therapy may improve conservative management success rates in patients with prognostic factors for systemic methotrexate therapy failure, such as cervical pregnancies with gestational age >9 weeks, B-hCG levels >10,000 mIU/mL, crown-rump length >10 mm, and presence of fetal cardiac activity [5, 6].

Conservative management using transvaginal-guided local injection is an attractive alternative that minimizes morbidity compared to surgical management of cervical and cesarean scar pregnancies, which are associated with a significant risk of hemorrhage and rupture [7]. Successful conservative management also potentially preserves fertility as it is associated with a lower risk of hysterectomy than surgical management [8, 9]. Furthermore, monotherapy with local injection chemotherapy to the pregnancy may limit toxicities associated with systemically administered methotrexate. In the event of a heterotopic pregnancy, treatment with local injection allows for the preservation of the intrauterine pregnancy, an outcome that is not possible with systemic methotrexate therapy. There are several case reports of heterotopic pregnancies managed successfully with local injection of methotrexate or potassium chloride and subsequent preterm and term deliveries of the intrauterine gestation [10–12]. Potassium chloride may be theoretically safer with heterotopic pregnancies given the potential absorption of methotrexate by the intrauterine pregnancy. The goals of this chapter are to review patient selection criteria for local treatment, injection techniques, agents used to perform local injection, and treatment outcomes.

40.1 Patient Selection Criteria

40.1.1 Diagnosis

Non-tubal ectopic and heterotopic pregnancies can be diagnosed early in gestation using transvaginal ultrasound (TVUS) and highly sensitive quantitative B-hCG assays. Table 40.1 outlines ultrasound findings suggestive of non-tubal ectopic and heterotopic pregnancies. In hemodynamically stable patients with inconclusive ultrasound findings but a high index of suspicion for ectopic pregnancy exists, further imaging with repeat ultrasound, three-dimensional ultrasound, or magnetic resonance imaging (MRI) may help clarify the diagnosis [13]. Of

L. Ghidei
Department of Obstetrics and Gynecology, Women & Infants Hospital, Alpert Medical School of Brown University, Providence, RI, USA

G. N. Frishman (✉)
Division of Reproductive Endocrinology and Infertility, Department of Obstetrics and Gynecology, Women & Infants Hospital, Alpert Medical School of Brown University, Providence, RI, USA
e-mail: gary.fishman@brown.edu

G. N. Allahbadia et al. (eds.), *Textbook of Assisted Reproduction*, https://doi.org/10.1007/978-981-15-2377-9_40

Table 40.1 Ultrasound criteria suggestive of non-tubal ectopic and heterotopic pregnancies

Type of ectopic pregnancy	Incidence	Ultrasound criteria
Cervical pregnancy [14]	0.01%	1. Empty uterus 2. Barrel-shaped cervix 3. Gestational sac below the level of the internal os 4. Absence of the "sliding sign"[a] 5. Blood flow around the gestational sac using color Doppler
Interstitial pregnancy [15]	0.02–0.04%	1. Empty uterus 2. Eccentrically located gestational sac greater than 1 cm from the endometrial stripe with a continuous rim of myometrium measuring less than 5–8 mm 3. Interstitial line—echogenic line that runs from the endometrial cavity to the cornual region, abutting the interstitial mass or gestational sac
Caesarean scar pregnancy [14]	0.1–0.45%	1. Empty uterus 2. Gestational sac located anteriorly at the level of the internal os covering the visible or presumed site of the previous lower uterine segment caesarean section scar 3. Evidence of functional trophoblastic/placental circulation on Doppler examination 4. Absence of the "sliding sign"[a]
Heterotopic pregnancy [14]	0.03%	1. Intrauterine pregnancy 2. Tubal or non-tubal ectopic pregnancy
Ovarian pregnancy	0.015–0.03%	

[a]Sliding sign: when pressure is applied to the cervix using the probe, the gestational sac slides against the endocervical canal in a miscarriage, but does not in an implanted cervical pregnancy

note, color Doppler should only be used on the uterus when the possibility of a viable intrauterine pregnancy has been ruled out.

40.1.2 Criteria for Local Treatment

When a non-tubal ectopic or heterotopic pregnancy is diagnosed, local treatment should be considered. Contraindications for local treatment mimic those for systemic methotrexate and include ruptured ectopic pregnancy, hemodynamic instability, inability or unwillingness to follow up closely, and contraindications to the agents used for local treatment [2]. In addition, experienced surgeons and equipment are essential. Unstable patients and/or those with ruptured ectopic pregnancies should undergo immediate surgical treatment. Similar to systemic therapy, with local treatment, candidates must be reliable to follow up for the necessary blood tests, ultrasounds, and evaluations to monitor treatment and be able to seek immediate medical attention if symptoms of rupture develop. Of note, B-hCG may downtrend over a course of months following local injection and expectations; follow-up after treatment should be managed accordingly [16]. Surgical therapy is preferred for patients who cannot comply with the prolonged monitoring required after local treatment. Contraindications to the agents themselves should be considered when evaluating candidates for local treatment. Absolute contraindications to methotrexate include breastfeeding, immunodeficiency, sensitivity to methotrexate, active pulmonary disease, peptic ulcer disease, and hepatic, renal, or hematologic dysfunction [3]. In patients with contraindications to methotrexate, potassium chloride and hyperosmolar glucose are alternative agents that can be used for local injection and, as noted above, may be theoretically better in a heterotopic pregnancy. Contraindications to potassium chloride are rare. No maternal complications were reported in the largest series of 239 potassium chloride injections. Isolated cases reveal one maternal cardiac arrest and maternal toxicity if the needle is misdirected to the maternal pelvis and uterus.

There are several types of patients who may significantly benefit from conservative management of non-tubal or complex ectopic pregnancies. Conservative treatment with local therapy should strongly be considered for patients with ectopic pregnancies who desire future fertility. In a systematic review that included 90 cervical ectopic pregnancies treated conservatively, only 4 cases (4.4%) required hysterectomy. This represents a significant reduction from historical accounts that reached nearly a 100% hysterectomy rate after treatment of cervical ectopic pregnancies [17, 18]. Tubal patency was preserved in 91.7% of patients with interstitial pregnancies managed with local injection, and 67% of patients conceived within 1 year of treatment in one case series [19]. Uneventful subsequent pregnancies and deliveries have also been reported in case series of patients with cervical and cesarean scar pregnancies successfully managed with local injection [8, 20]. Another patient population who may substantially benefit from local injection therapy are those patients who are at an increased risk for failure of systemic methotrexate therapy who have prognostic factors for systemic methotrexate therapy failure such as fetal cardiac activity [5]. As noted above, the immediate successful cessation of fetal cardiac activity by local injection of non-tubal ectopic pregnancies alone, or in conjunction with systemic methotrexate or after systemic methotrexate failure, represents a significant advantage of this treatment option compared to systemic treatment alone [3, 4]. Local injection should also be considered in cervical pregnancies with B-hCG levels >10,000 mIU/mL, CRL > 10 mm, or >9 weeks gestational age [6].

Lastly, patients with a heterotopic pregnancy who desire to preserve the intrauterine pregnancy should be offered local injection. As noted earlier, viable deliveries of the intrauterine pregnancies have occurred after this technique [10–12].

40.2 Local Injection Procedures

40.2.1 Approach

Non-tubal and complex ectopic pregnancies may be treated with local injection of cytotoxic agents via a variety of different approaches, including laparoscopic, ultrasonographic, and hysteroscopic guidance [21, 22]. The ultrasonographic approach affords immediate evidence regarding a key endpoint of treatment (i.e., cessation of fetal cardiac activity) while still being able to assess for potential intraoperative complications such as rupture of the ectopic. The route of ultrasound guidance is typically transvaginal, although transabdominal ultrasound-guided approaches have also been reported as a safe alternative [23]. Framarino et al. published a series of 14 cases involving interstitial ectopic pregnancies successfully treated with transabdominal ultrasound-guided injection of methotrexate (25 mg) without complications [24].

40.2.2 Procedure

Ideally, practitioners new to this technique should perform local injection under transvaginal ultrasound guidance in the operating room given the risk of hemorrhage. This procedure is usually performed under sedation, although it has been performed using local anesthesia consisting of 1% lidocaine or no anesthesia (although this latter treatment was with a tubal ectopic) [25] (Fig. 40.1).

For the surgery, the patient is placed in dorsal lithotomy position before being prepped and draped in the usual sterile fashion. A draped transvaginal ultrasound probe is used to assess baseline free pelvic fluid and to visualize the ectopic pregnancy, which may be facilitated via reverse Trendelenburg positioning. The endocavitary needle guide attached to the probe allows for the introduction of a needle directly into the gestational sac in a predictable path. A typical 17-gauge IVF needle works well. Fluid within the gestational sac may be aspirated in an attempt to disrupt the gestation, calculate the volume of fluid to be injected safely, and minimize the distension and risk of rupture of the ectopic with instillation of the embryocide [26]. A double-lumen IVF needle may be especially suited to this procedure as it allows for pre-loading the treatment solution all the way to the needle tip avoiding the injection of air while permitting the withdrawal of fluid within the gestational sac via the second lumen. Slow injection of the agent, under ultrasound guidance, is performed to evaluate for leakage or signs of impending rupture. If fetal cardiac activity is present, intracardiac or intrathoracic injection of solution may be used, and cessation of fetal cardiac activity should be observed. In addition, mechanical disruption of the ectopic with passes of the needle within the sac may be performed. Evaluation for post-procedural bleeding is performed again in reverse Trendelenburg position. Color Doppler flow ultrasound is used at the beginning of the case to assess surrounding vascularity and evaluate the fetal heart activity. This is especially useful since bubbles introduced during the treatment may make traditional ultrasound confirmation of cessation of fetal heart activity difficult at the end

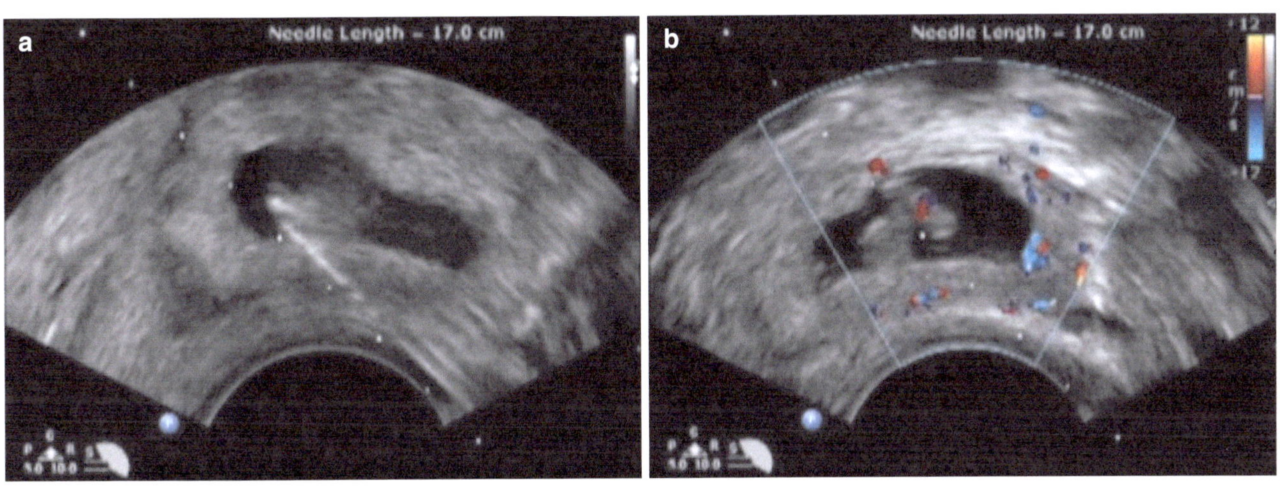

Fig. 40.1 (**a**) Transvaginal ultrasound of a cesarean scar pregnancy with fetal cardiac activity. (**b**) Introduction of a 17-gauge needle into the gestational sac with ultrasound guidance. The fluid was aspirated, and the cesarean scar pregnancy was mechanically disrupted and injected with potassium chloride with cessation of fetal cardiac activity noted

of the procedure. The path chosen for the needle depends on the location of the ectopic and the associated structures and vascularity. Although prospective data is lacking (except for a heterotopic pregnancy), consideration should be given for treating interstitial ectopic pregnancies by attempting to pass the needle medially to laterally to enter the ectopic via the uterine side rather than the potentially thinner aspects of the sac. For example, with an interstitial ectopic, the needle is guided through the uterus into the ectopic taking care to avoid the uterine artery. This also allows any bleeding to take place within the uterus (potentially tamponading it in addition to being able to identify the bleeding) rather than into the pelvis.

40.2.3 Monitoring

Patients should be monitored closely for signs of impending hemorrhage or rupture during and following local injection therapy. Once patients have demonstrated stability following the immediate postoperative period, they can be discharged on the day of the surgery and followed on an outpatient basis provided they are able to return with symptoms of rupture or hemorrhage. Postoperative counseling should also include recommending pelvic rest similar to any significant pelvic surgery.

Non-tubal ectopic pregnancies can be followed with serial B-hCG levels alone, and ultrasounds may be of limited value in the routine protocol. The serial B-hCG levels can be drawn at intervals recommended for the single-dose methotrexate protocol to monitor for response [27]. However, serial B-hCG levels may not be useful in the case of heterotopic pregnancies if the intrauterine pregnancy is undisturbed. In addition, the provider should keep in mind that B-hCG levels may initially rise before starting to decline. If utilizing ultrasounds, it is important to counsel the patient that the ectopic site may persist for 2–3 months. As such, one should not routinely intervene in a stable patient with declining B-hCG levels and a persistent mass. One report documented persistence of a mass by ultrasound in the third trimester at the site of a heterotopic cesarean scar pregnancy after it was managed by local injection [12]. If local injection is combined with systemic multidose methotrexate, serial B-hCG levels, complete blood counts, and liver and renal function tests should be assessed at intervals recommended for the multidose protocol and leucovorin given to minimize the side effects of systemic methotrexate [27]. Although a single dose of systemic methotrexate may be given, we do not typically administer multidose methotrexate in patients in whom local injection has been performed.

40.3 Agents

40.3.1 Selection of Agent

The most commonly used embryotoxic agents used during local injection for non-tubal ectopic and heterotopic pregnancies include methotrexate, potassium chloride, and hyperosmolar glucose. Methotrexate appears to be the most efficacious choice based on the few studies to date. One prospective, randomized, double-blind study compared the efficacy of local injection of methotrexate and hyperosmolar glucose for the treatment of intact tubal ectopic pregnancies. The study found methotrexate to be superior to hyperosmolar glucose [28]. Although there have been no trials comparing local injection of agents for non-tubal or complex ectopic pregnancies, one case series reviewed the outcomes of tubal, cornual, and cervical ectopic pregnancies treated by either methotrexate or potassium chloride. Both agents successfully led to cessation of cardiac activity when locally injected, and there was no difference in the time for resolution following treatment [29]. However, treatment with potassium chloride necessitated systemic methotrexate in 70% of cases. These cases were more likely to undergo complications, suggesting that MTX may be the preferred embryocide for cases at risk for treatment failure. Still, reports have demonstrated a 93–100% success rate using either agent [5, 30]. Therefore, selection of an agent for local injection should be individualized based on patient characteristics and surgeon preference. There are also no trials comparing local injection with an agent to a placebo or needle disruption of the gestational sac alone. It remains unclear whether it is the embryotoxic agent or the act of mechanically disrupting the sac which contributes more to resolving the ectopic, but it is our opinion that the two distinct treatment methods (injection of agent and disruption of sac) both contribute to a successful outcome. The technique of injection is the same for all agents.

40.3.2 Methotrexate

Methotrexate is a folic acid antagonist, which inhibits DNA synthesis and cell proliferation. Local injection of methotrexate may result in a higher dose and prolonged exposure at the site of the ectopic pregnancy while minimizing systemic side effects. In comparing serum levels between local and intramuscular methotrexate for treatment of tubal ectopic pregnancies, conflicting results have been reported, and it has not been confirmed that local administration is associated with lower serum methotrexate levels [31]. No pharmacokinetic studies have been performed in non-tubal ectopic or heterotopic pregnancies managed with local injection of methotrexate. Local injection of methotrexate should not be substituted for systemic methotrexate in patients with absolute contraindications to methotrexate therapy. In the case of cesarean scar ectopic pregnancies, local injection may be more effective than systemic treatment alone due to presence of fibrotic tissue in the scar, which limits access of medication [1]. Local methotrexate alone is successful in resolving ectopic pregnancies with cardiac activity, but may still be combined with other local agents or systemic methotrexate therapy [32]. There have been no trials comparing the dosing regimens. Reported local injection doses of methotrexate have ranged from 25 to 75 mg in 1–2 cm^3 volume, 1 mg/kg, 100 mg single dose, and unadjusted dose of 12.5 mg for non-tubal or complex ectopic pregnancies [11, 22, 33–35]. We use a 50 mg per cc dosing regimen replacing a volume slightly less than the gestational sac fluid aspirated. An alternative method describes injecting 25 mg methotrexate into the area of the embryo and an additional 25 mg into the area of the placenta [35].

As noted earlier, methotrexate administered via local injection may be associated with slower resolution of B-hCG levels. After treatment with local injection, B-hCG may take anywhere from 21 to 177 days to decline to an undetectable value [16, 26, 36]. Two case series of 27 patients illustrated the postoperative course through B-hCG resolution patterns and the associated ultrasound findings. B-hCG tended to increase within the few days after local injection, although no additional treatment was needed. Similarly, both the gestational sac volume and vascularization increased after local methotrexate chemotherapy combined with systemic treatment. Local methotrexate injection combined with systemic methotrexate therapy led to a 100% success rate but required a long follow-up [16, 36].

40.3.3 Potassium Chloride

Potassium chloride, a cardiotoxic agent, may be selected for local injection when fetal cardiac activity is present in a non-tubal ectopic pregnancy or when treating a heterotopic pregnancy given its avoidance of systemic toxicity to the intrauterine gestation [37]. In addition, potassium chloride can be utilized in patients with contraindications to methotrexate who are still eligible for local therapy. Reported doses of potassium chloride include 1–3 mL of 2 mEq/mL potassium chloride solution [11].

A series of 27 non-tubal ectopic pregnancies including 18 cervical pregnancies, 2 cesarean scar pregnancies, 4 cornual pregnancies, and 3 heterotopic pregnancies treated with ultrasound-guided local potassium chloride reported a 93% success rate. Notably, one cesarean scar pregnancy presented with heavy bleeding and was therefore managed with dilation and evacuation rather than KCL. HCG levels were undetectable within 4 months [5].

40.3.4 Hyperosmolar Glucose

Hyperosmolar glucose creates an osmotic effect resulting in the dehydration and necrosis of trophoblastic tissue. Hyperosmolar glucose has been employed in heterotopic pregnancies with no toxicity to the intrauterine pregnancy noted and, similar to potassium chloride, is an alternative agent to methotrexate in patients with contraindications. Reported doses include 5 mL of 20–50% hyperosmolar glucose [21, 38].

40.3.5 Combination Approach

Combining agents such as potassium chloride and methotrexate for local injection or combining local injection with systemic methotrexate has been reported, and the decision may be based upon the initial B-hCG level, fetal cardiac activity, rate of decline following treatment, and/or clinical judgment. Additional systemic methotrexate injection may be needed if B-hCG levels are more than 20,000 mIU/mL at diagnosis [39]. Combination local and systemic methotrexate may reduce time interval for B-hCG to become negative. A report of a cervical pregnancy treated with the combination of local potassium chloride and systemic methotrexate demonstrated a gradual decline in B-HCG levels in addition to a slowly collapsing gestational sac when observed on serial ultrasounds. The patient, who was followed weekly, had B-HCG values that measured <10 IU/L on the 56th day after methotrexate administration [40].

Successful combination treatment with local KCL injection followed by local MTX injection has been reported and is recommended for advanced pregnancies [41]. Local KCL followed by systemic MTX after perceived treatment failure has been reported to yield successful outcomes; however, it may be associated with significant risks and warrants careful patient selection and counseling. Monteagudo et al. reported a series of 14 non-tubal ectopic pregnancies [29]. Seven of the ten pregnancies treated with potassium chloride subsequently received intramuscular methotrexate. Of these, four patients experienced complications including loss of intrauterine pregnancy, hemorrhage necessitating uterine artery embolization, thrombocytopenia, and ruptured embryonic sac. Notably, all four of the above cases had B-hCG titers greater than 29,000, suggesting the complications may be attributable to the characteristics of the case rather than the treatment protocol [29].

40.4 Outcomes

Experience with local treatment for non-tubal ectopic and heterotopic pregnancy is limited to case reports and case series. There are no prospective randomized trials comparing local treatment to medical management or surgical management. When evaluating published outcomes, one must also consider the impact of publication bias.

40.4.1 Cervical Pregnancy

The prevalence of cervical ectopic pregnancies is 0.01% in the general population and IVF pregnancies [42]. Several recent reports suggest intra-amniotic management of cervical ectopic pregnancies is an effective treatment method. A series of 38 women received transvaginal-guided local methotrexate or potassium chloride for cervical pregnancies [8]. Fetal cardiac activity was present in 22 cases. Three patients experienced significant bleeding at the time of local injection, which was successfully managed with conservative measures (intracervical tamponade with a Foley catheter and systemic methotrexate). Two advanced pregnancies (11 and 12 weeks' gestational age) required additional systemic methotrexate for non-declining B-hCG levels after local treatment. No adverse effects of methotrexate were reported. After a mean 4.5 years of follow-up, 18 of 21 women who desired pregnancy delivered, with 1 preterm delivery reported. None of the patients experienced recurrent cervical pregnancies. While this large case series suggests that local treatment for cervical pregnancy, including those which are greater than 10 weeks of gestation and therefore considered advanced, is a safe and effective option for women who desire future fertility, data informing the risk of failed treatment, hemorrhage, and hysterectomy are limited [43]. Junior et al. reported the outcomes of a series of eight patients with cervical ectopic pregnancies with fetal heart activity. B-hCG levels ranged from 3000 to 71,000 mUI/mL. All eight cases were successfully treated with local methotrexate and potassium chloride therapy. Of note, B-hCG levels became undetectable by 12 weeks, and the pregnancies visually regressed by 14 weeks post-injection [44].

40.4.2 Cesarean Scar Pregnancy

The first case of cesarean section scar ectopic pregnancy was described in 1978 by Larsen and Solomon. The incidence of cesarean scar ectopic pregnancies is unknown but continues to rise. Estimated rates range from 1/800 to 1/2216 pregnancies. The incidence will likely continue to rise given modern obstetric practice, in which cesarean deliveries account for 32.2% of all US birth delivery methods [45]. The cesarean scar ectopic pregnancy tends to have a more aggressive behavior with a risk of uterine rupture and bleeding in the first and second trimesters of pregnancy [1]. A case of a cesarean section scar ectopic with B-HCG 18,000 was reported and treated with an aggressive regimen consisting of local methotrexate 1 mg/kg and then IM methotrexate every 2 days for two doses with 0.1 mg/kg folinic acid. After immediate treatment, methotrexate was given weekly until absence of Doppler flow on ultrasound. B-HCG trended from 18,000 to negative in 58 days. On note, the gestational sac was still evident on ultrasound for 2 months after methotrexate therapy. Because of the theoretical obstruction of systemic therapy from fibrotic tissue in cesarean scar ectopic pregnancies, local treatment may be more efficacious. Indeed, local treatment with methotrexate can reduce the time interval for B-hCG to become negative [1]. In a review of 751 cases of cesarean scar ectopic pregnancies that underwent treatment using various methods, complications occurred in 44.1% of cases. Treatment using systemic methotrexate, dilation and curettage, and uterine artery embolization carried the highest rate of complications (62.1%, 61.9%, and 46.9%, respectively) ranging from persistent ectopic pregnancy to acute bleeding due to uterine rupture [36]. Notably, treatment via local injection with methotrexate or potassium chloride achieved the lowest rates of complications of all treatment modalities (9.6%).

Jukovic et al. reported on a case series of seven patients with cesarean scar pregnancies that were managed with local methotrexate, local potassium chloride, or a combination of local methotrexate and potassium chloride [46]. Successful treatment was reported in five of the seven patients with resolution of B-hCG in 6–10 weeks. Two patients experienced heavy bleeding that required blood transfusions and surgical management. One patient had a heterotopic cesarean scar pregnancy that was managed with local injection of potassium chloride alone, and the intrauterine pregnancy progressed to 31 weeks, when hemorrhage originating from the prior cesarean scar necessitated emergent cesarean delivery.

After local injection therapy, similar to other non-tubal ectopic pregnancies, cervical scar ectopics may take weeks to months to resolve. Timor-Tritsch et al. reported a series of 26 cervical scar ectopic pregnancies treated with a regimen of 25 mg MTX injected in the embryo, 25 mg MTX injected in the placental area, and 25 mg systemic MTX administered system. The mean time to resolution was 88.6 days with an initial increase of the serum B-hCG, the sac volume, and its vascularity before their slow resolution. The reasons for the initial increase of the serum B-hCG are unclear but suggested to be related to the release of stored hCG during the initial necrosis of trophoblastic cells. Interestingly, vascularity index (VI) may play a role in monitoring and predicting significant complications. In three patients who suffered from acute bleeding warranting hysterectomy, the VI was significantly higher when compared to the 23 patients who did not have their uteri removed (63.1% vs. 17.8%) [36]. The VI also tends to increase immediately after treatment along with B-hCG and gestational sac volume.

40.4.3 Interstitial Pregnancy

Interstitial pregnancies occur at a prevalence of 0.02–0.04% [47]. In a case series of ten patients with interstitial pregnancies managed with local injection of methotrexate, a success rate of 100% was reported [30]. Tubal patency and subsequent healthy pregnancies have been reported after local injection for interstitial pregnancies, but the risk of recurrence or risk of uterine rupture during subsequent pregnancies remains uncertain [19].

40.4.4 Heterotopic Pregnancy

The incidence of heterotopic pregnancies was historically estimated as 1 in 30,000 deliveries, but more recent data suggests a much higher incidence of 0.03% [48]. An analysis of US assisted reproductive technology (ART) registries demonstrated an incidence of 0.15% among patients receiving ART [49]. Although rare, more concurrent intrauterine and cervical pregnancies are being diagnosed due to the advent and success of assisted reproduction technology. A review of case reports of cervical heterotopic pregnancies managed with local potassium chloride injection reported successful resolution of the cervical pregnancy, but miscarriage of the intrauterine pregnancy, maternal hemorrhage, and preterm delivery were seen [50]. Methotrexate may be successfully used for treatment of cervical heterotopic pregnancy; however, it may not be the first choice when there is a desire to preserve the intrauterine pregnancy. There are successful cases of using local injection therapy with methotrexate for cervical heterotopic pregnancies [51, 52]. One case demonstrated the use of combined local injection therapy with methotrexate and potassium chloride, whereas the other used local injection with methotrexate alone. There are several cases reports of heterotopic pregnancies managed successfully with local injection of methotrexate or potassium chloride and subsequent preterm and term deliveries of the intrauterine pregnancies [10–12].

40.4.5 Ovarian Pregnancy

Ovarian pregnancies are extremely rare occurring in 0.015–0.03% of all pregnancies [53]. Although ovarian ectopic pregnancies may be mistaken for corpus luteum cysts and/or misdiagnosed at the time of surgery, transvaginal-guided aspiration and injection have proven to be successful in the event of an early diagnosis of ovarian ectopic pregnancy. A case report that used a total dose of 50 mg of methotrexate directly into the ectopic followed by disruption of the corpus luteum cyst reported B-hCG levels declined appropriately until undetectable by 8 weeks. The patient subsequently conceived an intrauterine pregnancy and delivered a healthy child. The original four Spiegelberg clinical criteria for the diagnosis of ovarian ectopic pregnancy are outdated because they require surgical intervention for evaluation. Guidelines should be reformed to incorporate new and effective treatment regimens such as ultrasound-guided local management of ovarian ectopic pregnancies [54].

40.5 Conclusions

With early diagnosis of non-tubal ectopic and heterotopic pregnancies, transvaginal ultrasound-guided local treatment alone or as an adjuvant to systemic medical management may be an option for advanced pregnancies in compliant patients and especially those who desire future fertility. Transabdominal ultrasound-guided local injection therapy may be a feasible alternative for patients in whom transvaginal ultrasound-guided therapy is difficult or not feasible based on leiomyomas, elevated BMI, pelvic adhesions, or long distances between the ectopic pregnancy and the vaginal fornices precluding safe intra-amniotic entry [24]. Local injection of agents such as methotrexate, potassium chloride, and hyperosmolar glucose can be safely accomplished with ultrasound guidance and appropriate post-treatment monitoring. Case reports and series suggest high success rates and subsequent fertility after local treatment, although complications such as hemorrhage and need for emergent surgical management still exist as with systemic treatment protocols. It is reasonable to image the uterus via sonohysterography, hysterosalpingography, or hysteroscopy several months after the disappearance resolution to reassess the uterine cavity and facilitate counseling of the patient. Multicenter prospective randomized trials are needed to clearly identify appropriate candidates, compare local treatment to medical and surgical management, and optimize the procedure of local injection.

References

1. Leite JF, et al. Local management with methotrexate of cesarean scar ectopic pregnancy with live embryo guided by transvaginal ultrasound: a case report. Rev Assoc Med Bras. 2016;62(2):184–5.
2. Raughley MJ, Frishman GN. Local treatment of ectopic pregnancy. Semin Reprod Med. 2007;25(2):99–115.
3. Cerveira I, et al. Cervical ectopic pregnancy successfully treated with local methotrexate injection. Fertil Steril. 2008;90(5):2005.e7–10.

4. Moon HS, et al. Use of Tuohy needle for intraamniotic methotrexate injection through the cervical canal in a cervical pregnancy after failure of systemic methotrexate treatment. Am J Obstet Gynecol. 2010;202(5):e4–6.
5. Doubilet PM, et al. Sonographically guided minimally invasive treatment of unusual ectopic pregnancies. J Ultrasound Med. 2004;23(3):359–70.
6. Hung TH, et al. Prognostic factors for an unsatisfactory primary methotrexate treatment of cervical pregnancy: a quantitative review. Hum Reprod. 1998;13(9):2636–42.
7. Hwang JH, et al. Classification and management of cervical ectopic pregnancies: experience at a single institution. J Reprod Med. 2010;55(11–12):469–76.
8. Jeng CJ, Ko ML, Shen J. Transvaginal ultrasound-guided treatment of cervical pregnancy. Obstet Gynecol. 2007;109(5):1076–82.
9. Rotas MA, Haberman S, Levgur M. Cesarean scar ectopic pregnancies: etiology, diagnosis, and management. Obstet Gynecol. 2006;107(6):1373–81.
10. Perez JA, et al. Local medical treatment of interstitial pregnancy after in-vitro fertilization and embryo transfer (IVF-ET): two case reports. Hum Reprod. 1993;8(4):631–4.
11. Verma U, Goharkhay N. Conservative management of cervical ectopic pregnancy. Fertil Steril. 2009;91(3):671–4.
12. Wang CN, et al. Successful management of heterotopic cesarean scar pregnancy combined with intrauterine pregnancy after in vitro fertilization-embryo transfer. Fertil Steril. 2007;88(3):706.e13-6.
13. Bourdel N, et al. Interstitial pregnancy. Ultrasonographic diagnosis and contribution of MRI. A case report. Gynecol Obstetrique Fertilite. 2007;35(2):121–4.
14. Kirk E, Bourne T. Diagnosis of ectopic pregnancy with ultrasound. Best Pract Res Clin Obstet Gynaecol. 2009;23(4):501–8. https://doi.org/10.1016/j.bpobgyn.2008.12.010.
15. Timor-Tritsch IE, Monteagudo A, Matera C, Veit CR. Sonographic evolution of cornual pregnancies treated without surgery. Obstet Gynecol. 1992;79(6):1044–9.
16. Yamaguchi M, et al. Transvaginal methotrexate injection for the treatment of cesarean scar pregnancy: efficacy and subsequent fecundity. J Minim Invasive Surg. 2014;21(5):877–83.
17. Kirk E, et al. The conservative management of cervical ectopic pregnancies. Ultrasound Obstet Gynecol. 2006;27(4):430–7.
18. Kamoi S. Fertility-preserving surgery for cervical ectopic pregnancy, from past to present. In: Ectopic pregnancy – modern diagnosis and management, Chapter 14. 2011. pp. 220–8.
19. Benifla JL, et al. Alternative to surgery of treatment of unruptured interstitial pregnancy: 15 cases of medical treatment. Eur J Obstet Gynecol Reprod Biol. 1996;70(2):151–6.
20. de Vaate AJ, et al. Therapeutic options of caesarean scar pregnancy: case series and literature review. J Clin Ultrasound. 2010;38(2):75–84.
21. Goldenberg M, et al. Treatment of interstitial pregnancy with methotrexate via hysteroscopy. Fertil Steril. 1992;58(6):1234–6.
22. Lin YS, et al. Successful rescue of an early interstitial pregnancy after failed systemic methotrexate treatment: a case report. J Reprod Med. 2007;52(4):332–4.
23. Hartung J, Meckies J. Management of a case of uterine scar pregnancy by transabdominal potassium chloride injection. Ultrasound Obstet Gynecol. 2003;21(1):94–5.
24. Framarino M, et al. Transabdominal ultrasound-guided injection of methotrexate in the treatment of ectopic interstitial pregnancies. J Clin Ultrasound. 2014;42(9):522–6.
25. Darai E, et al. Transvaginal intratubal methotrexate treatment of ectopic pregnancy. Report of 100 cases. Hum Reprod. 1996;11(2):420–4.
26. Brasic N, et al. Conservative management of cesarean scar pregnancy with sonographically guided transvaginal methotrexate injection. J Ultrasound Med. 2013;32(6):1061–3.
27. Medicine, The Practice Committee of the American Society of Reproductive. Medical treatment of ectopic pregnancy. Fertil Steril. 2006;86(4):S96–S102.
28. Sadan O, et al. 'Methotrexate versus hyperosomolar glucose in the treatment of extrauterine pregnancy'. Arch Gynecol Obstet. 2001;265(2):82–4.
29. Monteagudo A, et al. Non-surgical management of live ectopic pregnancy with ultrasound-guided local injection: a case series. Ultrasound Obstet Gynecol. 2005;25(3). Version of Record online: 25 Feb 2005.
30. Hafner T, et al. The effectiveness of non-surgical management of early interstitial pregnancy: a report of ten cases and review of the literature. Ultrasound Obstet Gynecol. 1999;13(2):131–6.
31. Fernandez H, et al. Treatment of unruptured tubal pregnancy with methotrexate: pharmacokinetic analysis of local versus intramuscular administration. Fertil Steril. 1994;62(5):943–7.
32. Tulandi T, et al. Treatment of ectopic pregnancy by transvaginal intratubal methotrexate administration. Obstet Gynecol. 1991;77(4):627–30.
33. Fernandez H, et al. Methotrexate treatment of ectopic pregnancy: 100 cases treated by primary transvaginal injection under sonographic control. Fertil Steril. 1993;59(4):773–7.
34. Sagiv R, et al. Three conservative approaches to treatment of interstitial pregnancy. J Am Assoc Gynecol Laparosc. 2001;8(1):154–8.
35. Timor-Tritsch IE, et al. Successful management of viable cervical pregnancy by local injection of methotrexate guided by transvaginal ultrasonography. Am J Obstet Gynecol. 1994;170(3):737–9.
36. Timor-Tritsch IE, et al. The diagnosis, treatment, and follow-up of cesarean scar pregnancy. Am J Obstet Gynecol. 2012;207(1).
37. Evans MI, Britt DW. Fetal reduction. Semin Perinatol. 2005;29(5):321–9.
38. Allison JL, et al. Hyperosmolar glucose injection for the treatment of heterotopic ovarian pregnancy. Obstet Gynecol. 2012;120(2 Pt 2):449–52. https://doi.org/10.1097/AOG.0b013e31824f6379.
39. Seow KM, Wang PH, Huang LW, et al. Transvaginal sono-guided aspiration of gestational sac concurrent with a local methotrexate injection for the treatment of unruptured cesarean scar pregnancy. Arch Gynecol Obstet. 2013;288(2):361–6.
40. Petousis S, et al. Conservative management of cervical pregnancy with intramuscular administration of methotrexate and KCl injection: case report and review of the literature. World J Clin Cases. 2015;3(1):81–4.
41. Yazici G, et al. Treatment of a cervical viable pregnancy with a single intraamniotic methotrexate injection: a case report. Arch Gynecol Obstet. 2004;270(1):61–3.
42. Vela G, et al. Cervical pregnancy: the importance of early diagnosis and treatment. J Minim Invasive Gynecol. 2007;14(4):481.
43. Mitra AG, Harris-Owens M. Conservative medical management of advanced cervical ectopic pregnancies. [Review]. Obstet Gynecol Surv. 2000;55(6):385–9.
44. Junior JE, Musiello RB, Araujo Junior E, et al. Conservative management of cervical pregnancy with embryonic heart activity by ultrasound-guided local injection. an eight case series. J Matern Fetal Neonatal Med. 2014;27(13):1378–81.
45. Hamilton BE, Martin JA, Osterman MJK, et al. Births: final data for 2014. National vital statistics reports, vol. 64(12). Hyattsville, MD: National Center for Health Statistics; 2015.
46. Jurkovic D, et al. First-trimester diagnosis and management of pregnancies implanted into the lower uterine segment Cesarean section scar. Ultrasound Obstet Gynecol. 2003;21(3):220–7.

47. Damario MA, Rock JA. Ectopic pregnancy. In: Rock JA, Jones III HW, editors. Te Linde's operative gynecology. 9th ed. Philadelphia, PA: Lippincott Williams & Wilkins; 2003. p. 507–36.. ISBN 0-7817-2859-2.
48. Tal J, Haddad S, Gordon N, et al. Heterotopic pregnancy after ovulation induction and assisted reproductive technologies: a literature review from 1971 to 1993. Fertil Steril. 1996;66(1):1–12.
49. Clayton HB. A comparison of heterotopic and intrauterine-only pregnancy outcomes after assisted reproductive technologies in the United States from 1999 to 2002. Fertil Steril. 2007;87(2):303–9.
50. Faschingbauer F, et al. Treatment of heterotopic cervical pregnancies. Fertil Steril. 2010;2010.
51. Deka D, Bahadur A, Singh A, et al. Successful management of heterotopic pregnancy after fetal reduction using potassium chloride and methotrexate. J Hum Reprod Sci. 2012;5(1):57–60.
52. Sijanovic S, Vidosavljevic D, Sijanovic I. Methotrexate in local treatment of cervical heterotopic pregnancy with successful perinatal outcome: case report. J Obstet Bynaecol Res. 2011;37(9):1241–5.
53. Gaudoin MR, et al. Is the incidence of ovarian ectopic pregnancy increasing? J Obstet Gynecol Reprod Biol. 1996;70(2):141.
54. Huber WJ, Frishman G. In: Tulandi T, editor. Ectopic pregnancy: a clinical casebook. New York: Springer; 2014.

Part IV

Improving Outcomes in Medically Assisted Reproduction

Multiple Pregnancies as a Complication of Medically Assisted Reproduction

41

John Wu, David Prokai, and Orhan Bukulmez

Multiple gestations have long been a subject of interest to the medical community. In 1895, Polish pathologist Dyonizy Hellin established a formula for calculating the rate of multiples in the general population: he estimated twinning in 1 in 89 pregnancies; triplets 1 in 89^2, or 7921; and quadruplets 1 in 89^3, or 704,969. To this day, these calculations provide a reasonable approximation of naturally occurring multiple pregnancy rates [1]. However, current worldwide rates of multiple gestations significantly outpace Hellin's law. Why? The introduction of fertility treatments has caused an explosion of multiple gestations, especially in higher-order multiples (triplets or greater). Recent estimates show that 36% of twin births and 77% of high-order births result from fertility treatments.

Multifetal pregnancies can result from in vitro fertilization (IVF) or medically assisted reproduction (MAR), as well as non-IVF fertility treatments such as ovulation induction and superovulation. In 2011, IVF was responsible for 17% of twins and 32% of higher-order pregnancies in the United States [2]. The proportion of twin pregnancies due to IVF has been steadily increasing, while the proportion of higher-order multiples is decreasing (Fig. 41.1). Among women who had live births after IVF with fresh non-donor embryos in 2015, the rates of singleton, twin, and higher-order multiples were 77.2%, 22.1%, and 0.6%, respectively (Fig. 41.2) [3]. It is important to note that superovulation with both clomiphene citrate and/or injectable gonadotropins often combined with intrauterine insemination now accounts for a majority of the burden of higher-order multiple gestations and the attendant risks (2). For the purposes of this chapter, discussion will be focused on multiple gestations following IVF.

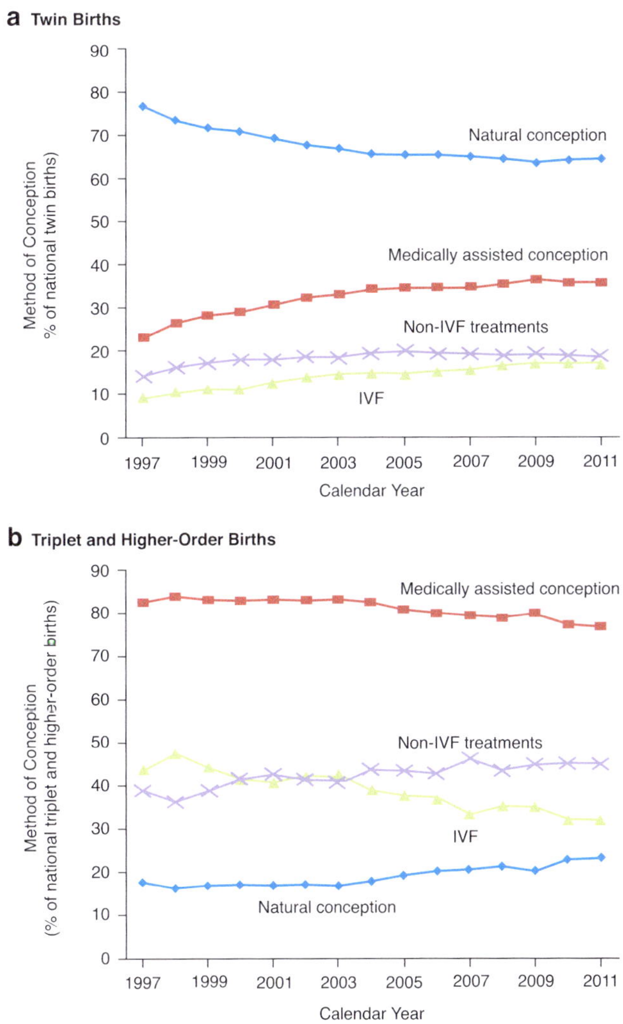

Fig. 41.1 Multiple births, according to method of conception, 1997–2011. (From Kulkarni AD, Jamieson DJ, Jones HW, Kissin DM, Gallo MF, Macaluso M, et al. Fertility Treatments and Multiple Births in the United States. Centers Dis Control Prev N Engl J Med. 2013;23369(5):2218–25, with permission)

J. Wu · D. Prokai · O. Bukulmez (✉)
Division of Reproductive Endocrinology and Infertility, Department of Obstetrics and Gynecology, University of Texas Southwestern Medical Center, Dallas, TX, USA
e-mail: orhan.bukulmez@utsouthwestern.edu

G. N. Allahbadia et al. (eds.), *Textbook of Assisted Reproduction*, https://doi.org/10.1007/978-981-15-2377-9_41

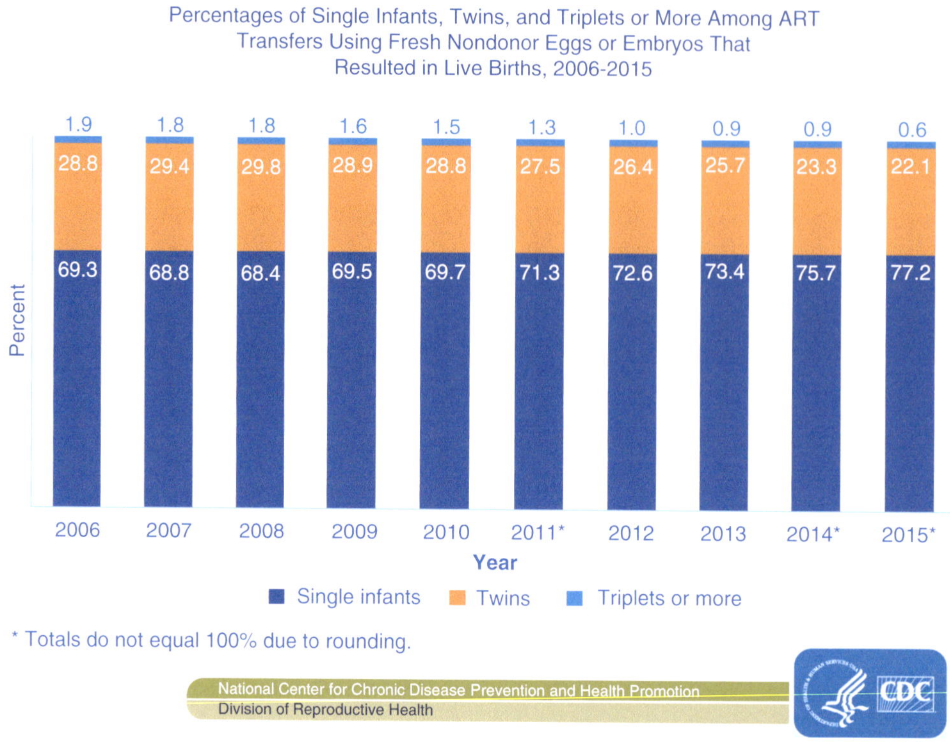

Fig. 41.2 The annual live birth rates of singleton, twin, and higher-order multiples with fresh non-donor eggs or embryos over a period of 10 years. US Department of Health and Human Services, Centers for Disease Control and Prevention. Figures from the 2015 Assisted Reproductive Technology National Summary Report. (From https://www.cdc.gov/art/pdf/2015-national-summary-slides/art_2015_graphs_and_charts.pdf)

41.1 Monozygotic Twinning in Art

The strongest driver of multiple births as a result of IVF is the number of embryos transferred. There is a smaller but still significant contribution from monozygotic twinning. Monozygotic twinning occurs in approximately 1.6–5.6% of single-embryo transfers, above the natural monozygotic rate of approximately 0.4% [4–10]. Risk factors for monozygotic twinning are controversial. It is generally accepted that younger oocytes and good quality embryos are more likely to result in monozygotic twinning [11, 12]. Two meta-analyses reported a two to threefold increased risk with blastocyst transfer in comparison to cleavage stage transfer [13, 14]. However, recent studies have failed to redemonstrate this increased risk. These contradictory results may be a reflection of advancements in embryo culture systems and improvements in laboratory technique over time [7, 8]. Although the debate is not settled, in 2013, the American Society of Reproductive Medicine Practice (ASRM) Committee recommended that patients should be counseled that there may be a small increased risk of monozygotic twinning with blastocyst stage embryo transfer [15].

41.1.1 Vanishing Twins

Approximately 10–15% of singleton pregnancies after IVF, began as twin gestations in early pregnancy. Although these pregnancies ultimately resulted in singleton live births, studies show that there is an increased risk for low birth weight <2500 g, very low birth weight <1500 g, and preterm birth in singleton survivors of vanishing twin pregnancies as compared to pure single gestations. These risks increase with spontaneous reductions that occurred after 8 weeks of gestation [16].

41.2 Complications of Multiple Gestation Pregnancies

Where many patients struggling with infertility may consider multiple gestation a desirable outcome [17, 18], there are many complications secondary to multiple gestation pregnancies that must be taken seriously.

41.2.1 Maternal Complications

Many complications seen in singleton pregnancies are exacerbated by multiple gestations, including but not limited to hyperemesis, hypertension, increased rates of cesarean delivery, and postpartum depression [19–21].

41.2.1.1 Hyperemesis

Nausea and vomiting in the first trimester occur in the majority of pregnancies. Although the exact mechanism is unclear, it is widely believed that elevated levels of human chorionic gonadotropins (hCG) are the culprit. In conditions in which hCG is very elevated, such as molar pregnancies and multiple gestation, there is increased incidence of severe symptoms including *hyperemesis gravidarum*, which is characterized by intractable nausea and vomiting leading to weight loss and/or electrolyte disturbances. Symptoms can significantly reduce a woman's quality of life and may be so severe as to require hospitalization [22].

41.2.1.2 Hypertensive Disorders

Women with multifetal pregnancies are at increased risk for hypertensive disorders. Singleton pregnancies have 6.5% baseline risk for hypertensive disease. This risk multiplies with increasing fetal number: 12.7% for twins and 20.0% for triplets and beyond. Similar trends are seen for the most severe pregnancy-related hypertensive conditions with a baseline of 0.5% for singletons, 1.6% in twins, and 3.1% in higher-order pregnancies [23].

Preeclampsia, a syndrome in pregnancy characterized by hypertension and proteinuria, is increased in multiple gestation with a relative risk of 2.6 [19]. Severe maternal sequelae of preeclampsia can include kidney and liver dysfunction, coagulopathy, cerebral edema, seizure, and stroke. Pregnancies complicated by preeclampsia also lead to fetal morbidity and mortality, with even higher risk for multifetal gestations, especially related to increased preterm delivery before 35 weeks of gestation (34.5% twins vs. 6.3% in singletons) and placental abruption (4.7% twins vs. 0.7% singletons) [19].

41.2.1.3 Cesarean Delivery

Worldwide, 18.6% of all births occur by cesarean delivery. Cesarean delivery rates range from 6.0% to 27.2%, with increased rates seen in developed countries [24]. Although cesarean delivery can be an effective life-saving measure for both the fetus and the mother, it is a major surgery with maternal and perinatal risks. Potential complications of cesarean delivery include endometritis, wound complications, hemorrhage, injury to other organs, and thrombotic events (Table 41.1).

Currently, the estimated rate of cesarean delivery for twin births is 44% [25]. It has been previously argued that planned cesarean delivery for all twin pregnancies may reduce the risk of neonatal morbidity for the second twin. However, more recent literature supports selection of delivery route based on fetal presentation and amnionicity, as studies on planned cesarean delivery show limited neonatal benefit with known maternal risks. The Twin Birth Study randomly assigned patients with twin pregnancy with the first twin in cephalic presentation to planned cesarean versus planned vaginal delivery regardless of the presentation of the second twin. The study found no significant difference in fetal or neonatal death or severe neonatal morbidity (2.2 vs. 1.9%), and follow-up at 2 years of age showed both groups had similar rates of death or developmental delay [25]. Despite evidence supporting the increased role for vaginal delivery in some twin gestations, cesarean rates remain high. Change may be limited by a lack of training in vaginal breech extractions for many obstetricians. The optimal route of delivery for women with higher-order multifetal gestations is unknown, but the rates of cesarean delivery are much increased in comparison to singleton pregnancies. Higher-order multiples also have a high incidence of abnormal presentation at time of delivery.

Table 41.1 Complications of primary cesarean delivery

Complications	Rate (%)
Endometritis	6
Wound complications	1–2
Hemorrhage requiring blood transfusion	2–4
Surgical injury	0.2–0.5

From Hammad IA, Chauhan SP, Magann EF, Abuhamad AZ. Peripartum complications with cesarean delivery: a review of Maternal-Fetal Medicine Units Network publications. J Matern Fetal Neonatal Med [Internet]. 2014 Mar 11 [cited 2017 Nov 14];27(5):463–74, with permission. Available from: http://www.tandfonline.com/doi/full/10.3109/14767058.2013.818970

41.2.1.4 Postpartum Depression

In a prospective study of 207 women who conceived after IVF, mothers of multiples were found to be at threefold increased risk for clinically significant postnatal depression as determined by the Edinburgh postnatal depression scale. These women are more likely to feel tired, feel down, or stressed and even question parenthood [21]. One of the possible etiologies for postpartum depression is a mismatch between expectations and the reality of motherhood. This can be amplified for IVF patients who invest so much emotionally and financially even prior to conception [26].

Postpartum depression not only affects the psychological state of the mother; it can impair other life areas such as decreased duration of breastfeeding, impaired bonding with the infant, care of the infant and other children, and relationship with her partner [27, 28].

41.2.1.5 Maternal Death

Maternal mortality is the ultimate and most tragic maternal complication, although fortunately it is rare in developed countries. There is minimal data on maternal death specifically related to multiple pregnancy. However, in developing countries such as Malawi (with a multiple pregnancy rate of 2.2%), multiple gestation contributed to 11.5% of maternal deaths in the population studied [29].

41.2.2 Neonatal Risks

Multiple pregnancy infants are at higher risk of adverse outcomes compared to singletons, with risk increasing with plurality.

Table 41.2 Gestational age and birth weight characteristics, by plurality: United States, 2015

	All births	Singletons	Twins	Triplets	Quadruplets	Quintuplets and higher-order multiples[a]
Number[a]	3,978,497	3,841,219	133,155	3871	228	24
Percent very preterm[b]	1.59	1.23	10.70	37.12	81.14	95.83
Percent preterm[c]	9.63	7.82	59.11	98.63	98.25	100.00
Percent very low birth weight[d]	1.40	1.08	9.56	36.35	79.09	100.00
Percent low birth weight[e]	8.07	6.34	55.41	95.65	98.64	100.00

Adapted from Martin JA, Hamilton BE, Osterman MJKS, Driscoll AK, Mathews TJ. National Vital Statistics Reports, Volume 66, Number 1, January 5, 2017. 2015 [cited 2017 Nov 15]; 66(1). Available from: https://www.cdc.gov/nchs/data/nvsr/nvsr66/nvsr66_01.pdf

[a]Quintuplets, sextuplets, and higher-order multiple births are not differentiated in the national data set

[b]Under 32 completed weeks of gestation

[c]Under 37 completed weeks of gestation

[d]Less than 1500 g

[e]Less than 2500 g

41.2.2.1 Preterm Delivery

The most common fetal complication of multiple gestation is spontaneous preterm delivery, which is associated with increased perinatal morbidity and mortality and may result in long-term morbidity [30]. More than half of twins and more than 90% of triplets are born either preterm (<37 weeks) or low birth weight (<2500 g) (Table 41.2) [31]. There is additional evidence that preterm birth resulting from multiple gestations correlates with an increased risk for death and significant morbidity compared to similarly preterm singletons [30].

Short-term complications of preterm delivery include hypothermia, respiratory abnormalities, cardiovascular abnormalities, intraventricular hemorrhage, glucose abnormalities, necrotizing enterocolitis, infection, and retinopathy of prematurity [32].

One of the most significant long-term complications of preterm delivery is cerebral palsy, a permanent neurological disorder affecting motor skills and potentially affecting thinking, learning, and communication. The incidence of cerebral palsy in at least one child is approximately 1.5%, 8.0%, and 42.9% in twin, triplet, and quadruplet pregnancies, respectively, in comparison to 0.2% in singleton pregnancies [33].

41.2.2.2 Intrauterine Growth Restriction

Impaired fetal growth in multiple gestations is directly proportional to plurality. This is thought to arise from the inability of the placenta to meet the nutritional needs of multiple fetuses [34].

Low birth weight is correlated with preterm delivery, hypoglycemia, asphyxia, impaired thermoregulation, polycythemia, impaired immune function, and ultimately increased mortality [35]. Long-term effects seen in singleton children who were growth restricted in utero include obesity, metabolic dysfunction, diabetes, and cardiovascular and renal disorders. Specific evidence in twin pregnancies is lacking and confounded by high incidence of preterm delivery [36].

41.2.2.3 Infant Mortality

For multiple births, the infant mortality rate is five times the rate of singleton births (25.84 vs. 5.25 per 1000 live births). Infant mortality rates increase with increasing plurality, with mortality rates for triplets and quadruplets being 12 and 26 times the rate for singleton births, respectively. In the United States, multiple pregnancy accounted for 3% of all births but accounted for 15% of all infant deaths [31].

41.2.3 Costs

41.2.3.1 Financial Implications of Neonatal and Infant Morbidity

Based on numerous cost analyses, the cost of caring for infants from a twin pregnancy is approximately three times that of a singleton pregnancy during the perinatal period [37]. Much of increased costs are due to birth admission with increased utilization of neonatal intensive care units (NICU). Estimates for NICU admissions are 25% for all twins, 75% for triplets, and 100% for all quadruplets [38]. In a recent study conducted by a large university hospital in Canada, 17% of all NICU admissions were infants from multiple gestations after ART [39]. Hospital costs from birth to age 5 remain 3.3-fold higher for IVF multiples in comparison to IVF singletons [40]. The costs of caring for these infants are extended in event of long-term conditions such as cerebral palsy. The Centers for Disease Control and Prevention (CDC) estimates that the average cost per person with cerebral palsy is $921,000 [41]. Overall, the estimated cost of caring for preterm infants resulting from ART in the United States is $1 billion annually, which approximates the total cost of ART treatment itself [38].

41.2.3.2 Financial Implications for Maternal Morbidity

The antenatal and obstetric costs for multiple pregnancy also must be accounted for. Multiple gestation pregnancies are inherently high risk, thus requiring more frequent visits to the obstetrician, increased number of procedures such as ultrasounds, and likely care from perinatologists in event of complications such as gestational diabetes or hypertension. Furthermore, obstetric costs are increased due to increased rates of cesarean delivery. In a large multihospital study conducted in Great Britain, multiple pregnancy doubled the cost of antenatal and obstetric care in comparison to normal singleton pregnancies [42].

41.3 Prevention of Multiple Gestation Pregnancies

Primary prevention of multiple pregnancies is most directly addressed by limiting the number of embryos transferred. As iatrogenic multiple pregnancies are a result of the decision-making between patients and clinicians, careful education must be aimed at both parties.

41.3.1 Society Transfer Guidelines

As previously described, the use of ART has contributed significantly to the incidence of twins and higher-order multiples. Recognizing the increased rate of complications as well as the increased cost to the health system, many countries have enacted strict laws that place limits on the stimulation protocols and the number of embryos transferred to limit the incidence of multiple gestations. In the United States, the American Society for Reproductive Medicine (ASRM) and the Society for Assisted Reproductive Technology (SART) published guidelines to restrict the number of embryos transferred as a means of decreasing the incidence of multiple gestations [43]. Using the age of the patient, stage of the embryo, and preimplantation genetic screening for aneuploidy (PGS) if performed, the upper limit of embryos recommended to be transferred is shown in Table 41.3. In addition to guidelines, careful and thorough discussion with the patient regarding the number of embryos to transfer is required. A strong patient-clinician relationship is needed to support these complex discussions.

Table 41.3 American Society for Reproductive Medicine (ASRM) recommendations for the limit of the number of embryos to transfer

Factors	Age (years)			
Embryo classification	<35	35–37	38–40	41–42
Cleavage stage embryos				
Euploid	1	1	1	1
Other favorable	1	1	≤3	≤4
All others	≤2	≤3	≤4	≤5
Blastocysts				
Euploid	1	1	1	1
Other favorable	1	1	≤2	≤3
All others	≤2	≤2	≤3	≤3

Adapted from Penzias A, Bendikson K, Butts S, Coutifaris C, Fossum G, Falcone T, et al. Guidance on the limits to the number of embryos to transfer: a committee opinion. Fertil. Steril. 2017;107:901–3, with permission

Other favorable = Any one of the following criteria—fresh cycle, expectation of one or more high-quality embryos available for cryopreservation or previous live birth after an IVF cycle; FET cycle, available vitrified day 5 or day 6 blastocysts, euploid embryos first FET cycle, or previous live birth after an IVF cycle

41.3.2 Elective Single-Embryo Transfer

Recent studies demonstrate the effect of increasing elective single-embryo transfer (eSET) rates. In the United States, one study demonstrated that increasing the eSET rate from 9.6 to 22.5% over a period of 3 years only decreased the twin rate in women under age 35 slightly, from 32.4 to 28.3% [44]. Nordic countries like Sweden and Finland, as well as Belgium, have achieved less than 10% multiple birth by more robust use of eSET. The rate of eSET in Sweden was reported to reach 69.9% [45].

Elective single-embryo transfer has not been embraced globally for many reasons, including prognostic factors like female age, reproductive treatment history, embryo grade, as well as economic issues including public funding, national legislation, and accessibility of effective embryo cryopreservation [45]. One cost-effectiveness study also failed to show superiority of eSET as compared to double-embryo transfer (DET), and the authors concluded that the choice should be decided by the financial coverage for ART, the prognostic factors, and the preference of patients [46].

In fact, randomized controlled trials comparing eSET with DET demonstrated that the rate of live birth is decreased with eSET unless it is combined with a highly successful frozen-thawed embryo transfer program [47, 48]. A meta-analysis suggested that eSET of cleavage stage embryos decreases the likelihood of live birth by 38% and multiple birth by 94%. However, increasing the number of both fresh and frozen eSET attempts results in cumulative live birth rate (LBR) comparable to that of DET [49]. Hence the cumulative LBR with eSET is comparable to DET only when a single-embryo transfer following a failed eSET is included [50].

An analysis of United Kingdom's Human Fertilization and Embryology Authority data recommended that transfer of three or more embryos at any age should be avoided, and eSET versus DET decision can be based on factors including female age [51]. Government-sponsored eSET programs in some countries like Canada reduced the total number of IVF offspring by up to one-third but did drop twin rates profoundly [52].

Currently, eSET is offered for good prognosis patients like those younger than 35 years of age. One retrospective cohort study from Finland suggested acceptable outcomes for eSET at cleavage stage in women aged 40–44 years if combined with subsequent frozen-thawed embryo transfer cycles [53]; however the feasibility of an eSET approach to the advanced reproductive age population remains controversial [52]. High-quality evidence to definitively direct patient selection for eSET or DET is not yet available.

The use of morphology, PGS with comprehensive chromosomal analysis, and new techniques such as mitochondrial DNA content [54] can also be employed as means of selecting the "best" single embryo to transfer in order to increase the likelihood of a successful pregnancy and live birth.

Forman et al. conducted an important randomized trial comparing ongoing pregnancy rate and risk of multiple gestation between transfer of a single, PGS-tested euploid blastocyst stage embryo and transfer of two untested blastocysts. Overall, they showed similar ongoing pregnancy rates (60.7% vs. 65.1%, respectively) and a significantly decreased risk of multiple gestation from 53.4% to 0%. This meant that patients with single euploid blastocyst transfer were nearly twice as likely to have an ongoing singleton pregnancy (60.7% vs. 33.7%; RR, 1.8; 95% CI, 1.3–2.5) [55]. The findings of this paper and others [56] demonstrated the efficacy and non-inferiority of elective single-embryo transfer with PGS in appropriately selected patients.

Guidelines for eSET currently include preimplantation aneuploidy screening (43), although PGS for embryo selection has its own controversies [57]. Newer technology measuring mitochondrial DNA content is also controversial; one recent study failed to show any correlation between mitochondrial DNA content and blastocyst ploidy, age, and viability [58].

Another approach to minimizing the number of embryos transferred while maintaining successful pregnancy outcomes is the use of mild or minimal stimulation IVF [59]. One randomized controlled trial demonstrated that while a conventional stimulation protocol produced twice as many embryos as a mild stimulation protocol, the total number of euploid embryos produced (tested at cleavage stage with 10 chromosome analysis) was no greater [60]. Conventional stimulation, focused on maximizing oocyte yield, may therefore result in a pool containing a mix of euploid and aneuploid embryos. If mild stimulation produces a higher-quality pool for embryo selection, then embryo biopsy (and PGS, with its attendant limitations) may not be required to ensure quality prior to transfer.

Overall, the approach to preventing multiple pregnancies after IVF has evolved over time. Limiting the number of embryos transferred has resulted in a decrease especially in high-order multiple pregnancies. This trend accelerated after the publication of a landmark paper in 1998 showing that, in good prognosis patients, DET resulted in comparable pregnancy rates but greatly reduced high-order multiples when compared to the transfer of three or more embryos [61]. In 1999, eSET was proposed to additionally reduce twin gestations [62]. Nowadays, research and discussion are focused on refining eSET protocols to optimize outcomes as described above. It will be important to continue studying the outcomes of ART as new protocols are identified and refined, in order to establish the safest and most effective clinical practices as well as direct patient counseling for complex decision-making including eSET.

41.3.3 Barriers to eSET

Despite strong evidence in favor of eSET, both patients and clinicians may still be reluctant to embrace this approach for a number of reasons.

Many patients continue to request multiple-embryo transfer. Patient factors including the duration of infertility, desire to limit the number of IVF cycles, income, and level of knowledge regarding risks of multiples may contribute to this decision [63–65]. In one survey of 449 infertile women, 1 out of 5 patients cited twins as the outcome they most desire. In these patients, researchers showed a significant underestimation of the risks and complications related to multiple gestations [64]. Interestingly, favorable media portrayals of multiple gestations may contribute to the desire for multiple pregnancy [66]. In the United States, the high out-of-pocket cost associated with IVF affects patients' decision-making. Multiple single-embryo transfer cycles incur more cost to the patient than a single multiple-embryo transfer. Patients may view a twin or triplet pregnancy as the fastest and least expensive way to achieve an "instant family." Importantly, the costs of a high-risk pregnancy and delivery are not as visible.

Physician and clinical factors may play a role as well. A desire to boost clinic success rates may motivate a physician to transfer more embryos to achieve more favorable pregnancy statistics. Finally, as discussed, even with perfect adherence to eSET guidelines, the possibility of multiple gestations exists via the monozygotic splitting of a single transferred embryo [5].

41.4 Prevention of the Complications from Multiple Pregnancies

Primary prevention of multiple gestations with the use of careful ovarian stimulation protocols and a carefully chosen embryo strategy, including comprehensive patient counseling, is the preferred means to limiting the incidence of multiple pregnancies. However, when twins and especially higher-order multiples do occur, patients and providers are often placed in a difficult position to decide on the best management options.

41.4.1 Multifetal Pregnancy Reduction (MFPR)

In the 1980s, fetal reduction techniques were developed to decrease morbidity and mortality associated with multifetal pregnancies. The first case reports in Europe [67] and the United States [68] described surgical techniques to achieve the desired reduction to singleton or twin. Various methods have been described, but the most common technique involves the use of transabdominal imaging followed by intrathoracic injection of potassium chloride (KCl) to achieve cardiac asystole [69]. Classically, the fetus chosen to be reduced is based on technical factors, chiefly accessibility to the intended intervention. With the advent of advancing ultrasound techniques as well as prenatal genetic diagnosis, now reduction techniques are often combined with chorionic villus sampling (CVS) and nuchal translucency measurements in an effort to reasonably exclude the chance of reducing a healthy fetus in favor of a fetus with genetic or anatomical abnormalities [70].

41.4.1.1 Pregnancy Outcomes Following MFPR

Since the publications of the earliest case reports of MFPR, successive publications have shown improved pregnancy outcomes when the total fetal count is reduced.

When MFPR was introduced, the procedure was offered to pregnancies with quadruplets or more. Technical safety was established in a multicenter report showing low fetal loss rates (16% pregnancy loss rate through 24 completed weeks of gestation) and lower proportions of preterm deliveries relative to control groups [71]. A series of papers demonstrated that there was a consistent improvement in pregnancy outcomes, with the largest benefit seen in the highest-order pregnancies [72].

With clear benefits seen in quadruplet and higher pregnancies, investigators began to expand the use of MFPR to triplet pregnancies. Yaron et al. looked at the outcomes of unreduced triplets as opposed to triplets reduced to twins and found substantially improved rates of miscarriage (25% for expectantly managed triplets and 6.2% for triplets reduced to twins) and significantly later gestational age at delivery (32.9 ± 4.7 weeks for expectantly managed triplets and 35.8 ± 3.9 weeks for triplets reduced to twins). Mean birth weights were also significantly higher in the triplet to twin group [73]. Another study showed a reduction in pregnancy loss from 15.41% to 4.76% by reducing from triplets to twins, as well as decreased incidence of low birth weight from 28% to 11% [74].

Additional ethical questions remain regarding the limits of MFPR and to whom it should be offered. Some have posited that offering MFPR is ethically permissible in twin pregnancies regardless of mode of conception, as there is data to suggest improvement in outcomes when the pregnancy is reduced to a singleton [75].

41.4.1.2 Emotional Burden

Couples undergoing infertility treatments are faced with many decisions that provoke significant anxiety. Following the initial joy of a positive pregnancy test, multiple gestations force parents to confront dilemmas they may have never considered before. Couples who opt for MFPR are faced with a unique set of emotional and psychological stressors that can have long-lasting impacts.

The long-term emotional impact of MFPR was first looked at by a group in France [76]. Couples who underwent pregnancy reduction were followed for a total of 2 years after reduction. In the first year following MFPR, the reduction group reported higher rates of depressive symptoms related to their decision to reduce. At the 2-year mark, all but two women no longer had negative feelings toward their decision to reduce and actually had less anxiety and depression when compared to parents with triplets. Regardless of this evidence, each patient and family will have a unique emotional experience. Broaching the subject of reduction requires considerable sensitivity, regardless of the patient's treatment phase.

41.5 Conclusion

Efforts at educating clinicians, patients, and the public can pay huge dividends toward reducing the number of ART-related multiple births and the associated risks. A culture shift is needed in terms of redefining the meaning of a successful outcome in assisted reproduction. Societal guidelines and carefully selected clinic performance metrics need to place greater emphasis on reducing multiples. Comprehensive patient education, in conjunction with interdisciplinary education for perinatologists and general obstetricians, is needed to fully realize the goal of improving maternal and fetal outcomes.

References

1. Fellman J, Eriksson AW. On the History of Hellin's Law. Twin Res Hum Genet. 2009;12:183–190. http://www.journals.cambridge.org/abstract_S1832427400009774. Accessed 6 Nov 2017.
2. Kulkarni AD, Adashi EY, Jamieson DJ, Crawford SB, Sunderam S, Kissin DM. Affordability of fertility treatments and multiple births in the United States. Paediatr Perinat Epidemiol. 2017;31:438–48.
3. Centers for Disease Control, and Prevention AS for R, Medicine S for ART. 2015 Assisted Reproductive Technology National Summary Report. 2017;1–80. https://www.cdc.gov/art/pdf/2015-report/ART-2015-National-Summary-Report.pdf%0Ahttp://www.

cdc.gov/art/ART2011/PDFs/ART_2011_National_Summary_Report.pdf%5Cnpapers2://publication/uuid/94DB174F-EBB0-409F-9B77-49937BA934E3%0Ahttp://www.cdc.gov/art/nas/. Accessed 6 Nov 2017.
4. Knopman JM, Krey LC, Oh C, Lee J, McCaffrey C, Noyes N. What makes them split? Identifying risk factors that lead to monozygotic twins after in vitro fertilization. Fertil Steril. 2014;102:82–9. http://www.ncbi.nlm.nih.gov/pubmed/24794318. Accessed 14 Nov 2017.
5. Milki AA, Jun SH, Hinckley MD, Behr B, Giudice LC, Westphal LM. Incidence of monozygotic twinning with blastocyst transfer compared to cleavage-stage transfer. https://ac.els-cdn.com/S0015028202047544/1-s2.0-S0015028202047544-main.pdf?_tid=bf771c14-c959-11e7-94f3-00000aacb35d&acdnat=1510677477_ea72c204e892f3470fc70d7e31731cb9. Accessed 14 Nov 2017.
6. Sharara FI, Abdo G. Incidence of monozygotic twins in blastocyst and cleavage stage assisted reproductive technology cycles. Fertil Steril. 2010;93:642–5. https://ac.els-cdn.com/S0015028208048243/1-s2.0-S0015028208048243-main.pdf?_tid=267823b8-c95a-11e7-b5c5-00000aab0f01&acdnat=1510677650_49a33481159fdc6031f27852c02365a9. Accessed 14 Nov 2017.
7. Papanikolaou EG, Fatemi H, Venetis C, Donoso P, Kolibianakis E, Tournaye H, et al. Monozygotic twinning is not increased after single blastocyst transfer compared with single cleavage-stage embryo transfer. Fertil Steril. 93:592–7. https://ac.els-cdn.com/S0015028208047730/1-s2.0-S0015028208047730-main.pdf?_tid=2f4d6250-c95a-11e7-a406-00000aab0f27&acdnat=1510677665_725ae5c859a497390cb588d9d34b32e0. Accessed 14 Nov 2017.
8. Moayeri SE, Behr B, Lathi RB, Westphal LM, Milki AA. Risk of monozygotic twinning with blastocyst transfer decreases over time: an 8-year experience. https://ac.els-cdn.com/S0015028206044487/1-s2.0-S0015028206044487-main.pdf?_tid=43b37d06-c95a-11e7-9c5a-00000aab0f02&acdnat=1510677698_0a40b0025bc95ae4cbe6b8e26bcd4e67. Accessed 14 Nov 2017.
9. Sermon K, Capalbo A, Cohen J, Coonen E, DeRycke M, DeVos A, et al. The why, the how and the when of PGS 2.0: current practices and expert opinions of fertility specialists, molecular biologists, and embryologists. Mol Hum Reprod. 2016;22:545–7. http://www.ncbi.nlm.nih.gov/pubmed/27256483. Accessed 27 Sept 2016.
10. Blastocyst transfer is not associated with increased rates of monozygotic twins when controlling for embryo cohort quality. Fertil Steril. 2015;103:95–100. http://www.sciencedirect.com/science/article/pii/S0015028214022638?via%3Dihub#bib1. Accessed 14 Nov 2017.
11. Sheiner E, Har-Vardi I, Potashnik G. The potential association between blastocyst transfer and monozygotic twinning. Fertil Steril. 2001;75:217–8. http://www.ncbi.nlm.nih.gov/pubmed/11163843. Accessed 14 Nov 2017.
12. Tarlatzis BC, Qublan HS, Sanopoulou T, Zepiridis L, Grimbizis G, Bontis J. Increase in the monozygotic twinning rate after intracytoplasmic sperm injection and blastocyst stage embryo transfer. Fertil Steril. 2002;77:196–198. http://www.ncbi.nlm.nih.gov/pubmed/11779618. Accessed 14 Nov 2017.
13. Chang HJ, Lee JR, Jee BC, Suh CS, Kim SH. Impact of blastocyst transfer on offspring sex ratio and the monozygotic twinning rate: a systematic review and meta-analysis. Fertil Steril. 2009;91:2381–2390. http://www.ncbi.nlm.nih.gov/pubmed/18718582. Accessed 14 Nov 2017.
14. Vitthala S, Gelbaya TA, Brison DR, Fitzgerald CT, Nardo LG. The risk of monozygotic twins after assisted reproductive technology: a systematic review and meta-analysis. Hum Reprod Update 2009;15:45–55. http://www.ncbi.nlm.nih.gov/pubmed/18927071. Accessed 14 Nov 2017.
15. Blastocyst culture and transfer in clinical-assisted reproduction: a committee opinion. Fertil Steril. 2013;99:667–672. http://www.sciencedirect.com/science/article/pii/S0015028213001295?via%3Dihub#bib14. Accessed 14 Nov 2017.
16. Pinborg A, Loft A, Schmidt L, Andersen AN. Attitudes of IVF/ICSI-twin mothers towards twins and single embryo transfer. Hum Reprod. 2003;18:621–7. http://www.ncbi.nlm.nih.gov/pubmed/12615836. Accessed 6 Nov 2017.
17. Child TJ, Henderson AM, Tan SL. The desire for multiple pregnancy in male and female infertility patients. Hum Reprod. 2004;19:558–561. https://academic.oup.com/humrep/article-lookup/doi/10.1093/humrep/deh097. Accessed 6 Nov 2017.
18. Chiu W, Chamley L. Clinical associations and mechanisms of action of antisperm antibodies. Fertil Steril. 2004;82:529–535. https://ac.els-cdn.com/S001502820303067X/1-s2.0-S001502820303067X-main.pdf?_tid=9ab979c8-c335-11e7-98b0-00000aab0f01&acdnat=1510002247_b8f57b6472f2786f09c00813a9f3cc9d. Accessed 6 Nov 2017.
19. Sibai BM, Hauth J, Caritis S, Lindheimer MD, MacPherson C, Klebanoff M, et al. Hypertensive disorders in twin versus singleton gestations. National Institute of Child Health and Human Development Network of Maternal-Fetal Medicine Units. Am J Obstet Gynecol. 2000;182:938–42. http://www.ncbi.nlm.nih.gov/pubmed/10764477. Accessed 14 Nov 2017.
20. Conde-Agudelo A, Belizán JM, Lindmark G. Maternal morbidity and mortality associated with multiple gestations. Obstet Gynecol. 2000;95:899–904. http://www.ncbi.nlm.nih.gov/pubmed/10831988. Accessed 14 Nov 2017.
21. Sheard C, Cox S, Oates M, Ndukwe G, Glazebrook C. Impact of a multiple, IVF birth on post-partum mental health: a composite analysis. Hum Reprod. 2007;22:2058–65.. http://www.ncbi.nlm.nih.gov/pubmed/17545565. Accessed 14 Nov 2017
22. Attard CL, Kohli MA, Coleman S, Bradley C, Hux M, Atanackovic G, et al. The burden of illness of severe nausea and vomiting of pregnancy in the United States. Am J Obstet Gynecol. 2002;186:S220–7. http://www.ncbi.nlm.nih.gov/pubmed/12011890. Accessed 16 Nov 2017.
23. Day MC, Barton JR, O'Brien JM, Istwan NB, Sibai BM. The effect of fetal number on the development of hypertensive conditions of pregnancy. Obstet Gynecol. 2005;106:927–31. http://www.ncbi.nlm.nih.gov/pubmed/16260508. Accessed 14 Nov 2017.
24. Betrán AP, Ye J, Moller A-B, Zhang J, Gülmezoglu AM, Torloni MR. The increasing trend in caesarean section rates: global, regional and national estimates: 1990–2014. PLoS One. 2016;11:e0148343. http://www.ncbi.nlm.nih.gov/pubmed/26849801. Accessed 14 Nov 2017.
25. Barrett JFR, Hannah ME, Hutton EK, Willan AR, Allen AC, Armson BA, et al. A randomized trial of planned cesarean or vaginal delivery for twin pregnancy. N Engl J Med. 2013;369:1295–305. http://www.ncbi.nlm.nih.gov/pubmed/24088091. Accessed 14 Nov 2017.
26. Klock SC. Psychological adjustment to twins after infertility. Best Pract Res Clin Obstet Gynaecol. 2004;18:645–56. http://www.ncbi.nlm.nih.gov/pubmed/15279823. Accessed 14 Nov 2017.
27. Stein A, Pearson RM, Goodman SH, Rapa E, Rahman A, McCallum M, et al. Effects of perinatal mental disorders on the fetus and child. Lancet (London) 2014;384:1800–19. http://www.ncbi.nlm.nih.gov/pubmed/25455250. Accessed 14 Nov 2017.
28. Dias CC, Figueiredo B. Breastfeeding and depression: a systematic review of the literature. J Affect Disord. 2014;171:142–54. https://ac.els-cdn.com/S016503271400576X/1-s2.0-S016503271400576X-main.pdf?_tid=4f820f8a-c97d-11e7-9343-00000aacb35e&acdnat=1510692751_08a209ab96a213b2369dec3902420738. Accessed 14 Nov 2017.
29. Mcdermott JM, Steketee R, Wirima J. Mortality associated with multiple gestation in Malawi. Int J Epidemiol. 1995;24:413–9. http://www.ncbi.nlm.nih.gov/pubmed/7635604. Accessed 14 Nov 2017.
30. Bodeau-Livinec F, Zeitlin J, Blondel B, Arnaud C, Fresson J, Burguet A, et al. Do very preterm twins and singletons differ in their neurodevelopment at 5 years of age? Arch Dis Child Fetal Neonatal

Ed. 2013;98:F480–7. http://fn.bmj.com/lookup/doi/10.1136/archdischild-2013-303737. Accessed 15 Nov 2017.
31. Martin JA, Hamilton BE, Osterman MJKS, Driscoll AK, Mathews TJ. National vital statistics reports. 2015;66(1). https://www.cdc.gov/nchs/data/nvsr/nvsr66/nvsr66_01.pdf. Accessed 15 Nov 2017.
32. Stoll BJ, Hansen NI, Bell EF, Shankaran S, Laptook AR, Walsh MC, et al. Neonatal outcomes of extremely preterm infants from the NICHD Neonatal Research Network. Pediatrics. 2010;126:443–56. http://pediatrics.aappublications.org/cgi/doi/10.1542/peds.2009-2959. Accessed 15 Nov 2017.
33. Yokoyama Y, Shimizu T, Hayakawa K. Prevalence of cerebral palsy in twins, triplets and quadruplets. Int J Epidemiol. 1995;24:943–8. http://www.ncbi.nlm.nih.gov/pubmed/8557451. Accessed 16 Nov 2017.
34. Bleker OP, Wolf H, Oosting J. The placental cause of fetal growth retardation in twin gestations. Acta Genet medicae Gemellol Twin Res. 1995;44:103–6. https://www.cambridge.org/core/product/identifier/S0001566000001768/type/journal_article. Accessed 16 Nov 2017.
35. Liu J, Wang X-F, Wang Y, Wang H-W, Liu Y. The incidence rate, high-risk factors, and short- and long-term adverse outcomes of fetal growth restriction: a report from Mainland China. Medicine (Baltimore). 2014;93:e210. http://www.ncbi.nlm.nih.gov/pubmed/25501078. Accessed 16 Nov 2017.
36. Muhlhausler BS, Hancock SN, Bloomfield FH, Harding R. Are twins growth restricted? Pediatr Res. 2011;70:117–22. http://www.nature.com/doifinder/10.1203/PDR.0b013e31821f6cfd. Accessed 16 Nov 2017.
37. Chambers GM, Chapman MG, Grayson N, Shanahan M, Sullivan EA. Babies born after ART treatment cost more than non-ART babies: a cost analysis of inpatient birth-admission costs of singleton and multiple gestation pregnancies. Hum Reprod. 2007;22:3108–15. https://academic.oup.com/humrep/article-lookup/doi/10.1093/humrep/dem311. Accessed 15 Nov 2017.
38. Bromer JG, Ata B, Seli M, Lockwood C, Seli E. Preterm deliveries that result from multiple pregnancies associated with assisted reproductive technologies in the USA: a cost analysis. Curr Opin Obstet Gynecol. 2011;23:168–73. http://content.wkhealth.com/linkback/openurl?sid=WKPTLP:landingpage&an=00001703-201106000-00005. Accessed 15 Nov 2017.
39. Janvier A, Spelke B, Barrington KJ. The epidemic of multiple gestations and neonatal intensive care unit use: the cost of irresponsibility. 2011.. https://ac.els-cdn.com/S0022347611001806/1-s2.0-S0022347611001806-main.pdf?_tid=b03fba54-caed-11e7-b45b-00000aab0f02&acdnat=1510850976_8be722374e0a4bba69c614b4949e7a53. Accessed 16 Nov 2017.
40. Van Heesch MMJ, Evers JLH, Van Der Hoeven MAHBM, Dumoulin JCM, Van Beijsterveldt CEM, Bonsel GJ, et al. Hospital costs during the first 5 years of life for multiples compared with singletons born after IVF or ICSI. Hum Reprod. 2015;30:1481–90. http://www.ncbi.nlm.nih.gov/pubmed/25840426. Accessed 15 Nov 2017.
41. Centers for Disease Control and Prevention (CDC). Economic costs associated with mental retardation, cerebral palsy, hearing loss, and vision impairment–United States, 2003. MMWR Morb Mortal Wkly Rep. 2004;53:57–9. http://www.ncbi.nlm.nih.gov/pubmed/14749614. Accessed 16 Nov 2017.
42. Mistry H, Dowie R, Young T, Gardiner H. Costs of NHS maternity care for women with multiple pregnancy compared with high-risk and low-risk singleton pregnancy. BJOG Int J Obstet Gynaecol. 2007;114:1104–12. http://doi.wiley.com/10.1111/j.1471-0528.2007.01458.x. Accessed 16 Nov 2017.
43. Penzias A, Bendikson K, Butts S, Coutifaris C, Fossum G, Falcone T, et al. Guidance on the limits to the number of embryos to transfer: a committee opinion. Fertil Steril. 2017;107:901–3.
44. Department of Health U, Services Centers for Disease Control H. 2013 Assisted reproductive technology fertility clinic success rates report. 2013.. https://www.cdc.gov/art/pdf/2013-report/art-2013-fertility-clinic-report.pdf. Accessed 27 Dec 2017.
45. Harbottle S, Hughes C, Cutting R, Roberts S, Brison D, Association Of Clinical Embryologists & The (ACE) British Fertility Society (BFS). Elective single embryo transfer: an update to UK Best Practice Guidelines. Hum Fertil. 2015;18:165–83. http://www.ncbi.nlm.nih.gov/pubmed/26391438. Accessed 27 Dec 2017.
46. Hernandez Torres E, Navarro-Espigares JL, Clavero A, López-Regalado M, Camacho-Ballesta JA, Onieva-García M, et al. Economic evaluation of elective single-embryo transfer with subsequent single frozen embryo transfer in an in vitro fertilization/intracytoplasmic sperm injection program. Fertil Steril. 2015;103:699–706. http://linkinghub.elsevier.com/retrieve/pii/S0015028214025151. Accessed 27 Dec 2017.
47. Lukassen HGM, Braat D, Wetzels AMM, Zielhuis GA, Adang EMM, Scheenjes E, et al. Two cycles with single embryo transfer versus one cycle with double embryo transfer: a randomized controlled trial. Hum Reprod. 2005;20:702–8. http://www.ncbi.nlm.nih.gov/pubmed/15618254. Accessed 27 Dec 2017.
48. van Montfoort APA, Fiddelers AAA, Janssen JM, Derhaag JG, Dirksen CD, Dunselman GAJ, et al. In unselected patients, elective single embryo transfer prevents all multiples, but results in significantly lower pregnancy rates compared with double embryo transfer: a randomized controlled trial. Hum Reprod. 2006;21:338–43. http://www.ncbi.nlm.nih.gov/pubmed/16253973. Accessed 27 Dec 2017.
49. Gelbaya TA, Tsoumpou I, Nardo LG. The likelihood of live birth and multiple birth after single versus double embryo transfer at the cleavage stage: a systematic review and meta-analysis. Fertil Steril. 2010;94:936–45. http://www.ncbi.nlm.nih.gov/pubmed/19446809. Accessed 27 Dec 2017.
50. Pandian Z, Marjoribanks J, Ozturk O, Serour G, Bhattacharya S. Number of embryos for transfer following in vitro fertilisation or intra-cytoplasmic sperm injection. In: Pandian Z, editor. Cochrane Database Syst. Rev. Chichester: Wiley; 2013. p. CD003416. http://www.ncbi.nlm.nih.gov/pubmed/23897513. Accessed 27 Dec 2017.
51. Lawlor DA, Nelson SM. Effect of age on decisions about the numbers of embryos to transfer in assisted conception: a prospective study. Lancet. 2012;379:521–7. http://www.ncbi.nlm.nih.gov/pubmed/22243709. Accessed 27 Dec 2017.
52. Gleicher N. The irrational attraction of elective single-embryo transfer (eSET). Hum Reprod. 2013;28:294–7. https://academic.oup.com/humrep/article-lookup/doi/10.1093/humrep/des401. Accessed 27 Dec 2017.
53. Niinimaki M, Suikkari A-M, Makinen S, Soderstrom-Anttila V, Martikainen H. Elective single-embryo transfer in women aged 40–44 years. Hum Reprod. 2013;28:331–5. http://www.ncbi.nlm.nih.gov/pubmed/23175499. Accessed 27 Dec 2017.
54. Wells D. Mitochondrial DNA quantity as a biomarker for blastocyst implantation potential. Fertil Steril. 2017;108:742–7.
55. Forman EJ, Hong KH, Ferry KM, Tao X, Taylor D, Levy B, et al. In vitro fertilization with single euploid blastocyst transfer: a randomized controlled trial. Fertil Steril. 2013;100:100–107.e1.
56. Mancuso AC, Boulet SL, Duran E, Munch E, Kissin DM, Van Voorhis BJ. Elective single embryo transfer in women less than age 38 years reduces multiple birth rates, but not live birth rates, in United States fertility clinics. Fertil Steril. 2016;106:1107–14.
57. Paulson RJ. Preimplantation genetic screening: what is the clinical efficiency? Fertil Steril. 2017;108:228–30. http://www.ncbi.nlm.nih.gov/pubmed/28697911. Accessed 27 Dec 2017.
58. Victor AR, Brake AJ, Tyndall JC, Griffin DK, Zouves CG, Barnes FL, et al. Accurate quantitation of mitochondrial DNA reveals uniform levels in human blastocysts irrespective of ploidy, age, or implantation potential. Fertil Steril. 2017;107:34–42.e3. http://link-

inghub.elsevier.com/retrieve/pii/S0015028216628480. Accessed 27 Dec 2017.
59. Nargund G, Datta AK, Fauser BCJM. Mild stimulation for in vitro fertilization. Fertil Steril. 2017;108:558–67. http://www.ncbi.nlm.nih.gov/pubmed/28965549. Accessed 27 Dec 2017.
60. Baart EB, Martini E, Eijkemans MJ, Van Opstal D, Beckers NGM, Verhoeff A, et al. Milder ovarian stimulation for in-vitro fertilization reduces aneuploidy in the human preimplantation embryo: a randomized controlled trial. Hum Reprod. 2007;22:980–8. http://www.ncbi.nlm.nih.gov/pubmed/17204525. Accessed 27 Dec 2017.
61. Templeton A, Morris JK. Reducing the risk of multiple births by transfer of two embryos after in vitro fertilization. N Engl J Med. 1998;339:573–7. http://www.ncbi.nlm.nih.gov/pubmed/9718375. Accessed 27 Dec 2017.
62. Vilska S, Tiitinen A, Hydén-Granskog C, Hovatta O. Elective transfer of one embryo results in an acceptable pregnancy rate and eliminates the risk of multiple birth. Hum Reprod. 1999;14:2392–5. http://www.ncbi.nlm.nih.gov/pubmed/10469718. Accessed 27 Dec 2017.
63. Newton CR, McBride J, Feyles V, Tekpetey F, Power S. Factors affecting patients' attitudes toward single- and multiple-embryo transfer. Fertil Steril. 2007;87:269–78.
64. Ryan GL, Zhang SH, Dokras A, Syrop CH, Van Voorhis BJ. The desire of infertile patients for multiple births. Fertil Steril. 2004;81:500–4.
65. Ismail L, Mittal M, Kalu E. IVF twins: buy one get one free? J Fam Plan Reprod Heal Care. 2012;38:252–7.
66. Letterie GS. Multiple births: does the news media influence public perceptions? Hum Reprod. 2004;19:2680–1.
67. Dumez Y, Oury JF. Method for first trimester selective abortion in multiple pregnancy. Contrib Gynecol Obstet. 1986;15:50–3. http://www.ncbi.nlm.nih.gov/pubmed/3743080. Accessed 17 Dec 2017.
68. Evans MI, Fletcher JC, Zador IE, Newton BW, Quigg MH, Struyk CD. Selective first-trimester termination in octuplet and quadruplet pregnancies: clinical and ethical issues. Obstet Gynecol. 1988;71:289–96. http://www.ncbi.nlm.nih.gov/pubmed/3347412. Accessed 17 Dec 2017.
69. Antsaklis A, Anastasakis E. Selective reduction in twins and multiple pregnancies. J Perinat Med. 2011;39:15–21. https://www.degruyter.com/view/j/jpme.2011.39.issue-1/jpm.2010.114/jpm.2010.114.xml. Accessed 17 Dec 2017.
70. Rosner M, Pergament E, Andriole S, Gebb J, Dar P, Evans MI. Detection of genetic abnormalities by using CVS and FISH prior to fetal reduction in sonographically normal appearing fetuses. Prenat Diagn. 2013;1–5.
71. Evans MI, Dommergues M, Wapner RJ, Lynch L, Dumez Y, Goldberg JD, et al. Efficacy of transabdominal multifetal pregnancy reduction: collaborative experience among the world's largest centers. Obstet Gynecol. 1993;82:61–6.
72. Evans MI, Andriole S, Britt DW. Fetal reduction: 25 years' experience. Fetal Diagn Ther. 2014;35:69–82.
73. Yaron Y, Bryant-Greenwood PK, Dave N, Moldenhauer JS, Kramer RL, Johnson MP, et al. Multifetal pregnancy reductions of triplets to twins: comparison with nonreduced triplets and twins. Am J Obstet Gynecol. 1999;180:1268–71.
74. Antsaklis A, Souka AP, Daskalakis G, Papantoniou N, Koutra P, Kavalakis Y, et al. Embryo reduction versus expectant management in triplet pregnancies. J Matern Neonatal Med. 2004;16:219–22.
75. Evans MI, Kaufman MI, Urban AJ, Britt DW, Fletcher JC. Fetal reduction from twins to a singleton. Obstet Gynecol. 2004;104:102–9.
76. Garel M, Stark C, Blondel B, Lefebvre G, Vauthier-Brouzes D, Zorn JR. Psychological reactions after multifetal pregnancy reduction: a 2-year follow-up study. Hum Reprod. 1997;12:617–22.

Multiple Birth Minimisation Strategies

42

V. Peddie, Rachel Cutting, and Jane Denton

Since the birth of Louise Brown in 1978, advances in assisted reproductive technology (ART) have resulted in excess of 5 million births worldwide [1, 2]. However, this has not been without risk: 0.9% and 1.4% of all births in England and Wales in the early 1980s and late 1990s being multiples [3] with the rest of Europe reporting a similar trend [4]. Triplets and higher-order multiples experienced a similar rise, with Kulkarni and colleagues [5] estimating a total of 36% of twin births and 77% of triplet and higher-order births resulting from ART in the United States (US).

Twin and triplet pregnancies are concomitant with increased obstetric and neonatal morbidity and mortality, usually related to preterm delivery [3]. Complications include gestational diabetes, hypertension and pre-eclampsia, preterm delivery, intrauterine growth restriction, congenital abnormality and cerebral palsy. Inevitably these complications lead to increased healthcare costs, not only in the short term (neonatal care) but in the health and development needs of children [6]. In 2011, the European Society for Human Reproduction and Embryology (ESHRE) published data from 32 European countries on ART, which highlighted the risk of extremely preterm birth rate (gestational weeks 20–27) as 0.8% for a singleton delivery, increasing to 2.6% for twins and 7.4% for triplets. The same trend was noted for very preterm (28–32 weeks), from 2.5 to 11.0% and 37.4%, and for preterm (33–36 weeks), from 8.7 to 39.3 and 43.9%, respectively [7].

The original version of this chapter was revised. The correction to this chapter can be found at https://doi.org/10.1007/978-981-15-2377-9_93

V. Peddie
Division of Applied Health Sciences, Department of Obstetrics and Gynaecology, School of Medicine and Dentistry, University of Aberdeen, Aberdeen Maternity Hospital, Aberdeen, Scotland

R. Cutting
Human Fertilization and Embryology Authority, 10 Spring Gardens, London, UK

J. Denton (✉)
Queen Charlotte's & Chelsea Hospital, Imperial College Health Care NHS Trust, London, UK
e-mail: jane.denton1@nhs.net

It is now widely accepted that these risks to both mother and child are unacceptable. Although there has been a range in uptake of elective single embryo transfer (eSET), varying from 2.8% in the USA to 69.4% in Sweden [8], there is now pressure from both professional society and regulatory bodies for IVF clinics to act responsibly and implement multiple birth minimization strategies.

This chapter aims to review the historical aspect of the number of embryos to transfer the current global variation in adoption of eSET policies and common strategies which have been implemented to ensure eSET does not compromise the chance of patients achieving live births.

42.1 Worldwide Picture

In 1993, Sweden provided the catalyst for a worldwide shift in embryo transfer policy, with a voluntary reduction in the number of embryos transferred in IVF cycles from three to two. This resulted in almost complete eradication of higher-order multiple pregnancy (triplets or more), with the overall pregnancy and delivery rates unaffected at around 1:3 per embryo transfer [9]. However, the twinning rate remained relatively stable at 1:4 per delivery [10] which promoted a multicentre trial to compare the outcome of one fresh embryo (transfer), and if no pregnancy occurred, the addition of a frozen embryo compared to a double fresh embryo transfer [11]. The study concluded there was no difference in the chance of achieving a pregnancy and Swedish legislation quickly ensued to specify that only one embryo could be replaced in the majority of cases.

Interest was sustained, and in 2004, Pinborg and colleagues published results from a retrospective study on the outcome of 8602 children born as a result of ART, concluding that the outcome of twins was considerably poorer than singleton deliveries, thus drawing the attention of clinicians to elective single-embryo transfer (eSET) [12]. The same year, European countries such as Belgium published data to show that from a health economic perspective, the transfer of

G. N. Allahbadia et al. (eds.), *Textbook of Assisted Reproduction*, https://doi.org/10.1007/978-981-15-2377-9_42

a single top-quality embryo in women <38 years of age was equally as effective, with the added benefit of being cost-effective from a health economic perspective [13].

In March 2004, the fertility sector in the UK witnessed an amendment in Human Fertilization and Embryology Authority [14] policy with the maximum number of embryos to be replaced (in women <40 years) reduced to two. However, this transition significantly reduced triplet, but not twin pregnancy rates.

To address this issue, the HFEA commissioned an expert group in 2005, who published the report 'One Child at a Time: Reducing Multiple births after IVF' [15]. This led to the best outcome from IVF being expressed not simply as a live birth but as a healthy term infant of normal weight.

This inevitably led to consideration of eSET in good prognosis patients and the development of policies specifically addressing multiple births. The UK formed a 'One at a Time' multidisciplinary stakeholder group, consisting of representatives of professional organisations involved in aspects of fertility care, in collaboration with colleagues facilitating obstetric and paediatric care. As a result, a consensus statement and directives were issued by the HFEA in 2007, requiring all licenced centres to have a clear and concise multiple birth minimisation strategy (MBMS) in place by 2009. This movement was endorsed by the British Fertility Society (BFS) [16] and the Association of Clinical Embryologists (ACE) [17].

The HFEA set a national threshold for a multiple pregnancy rate (MPR) of 10% to be achieved by a stepwise progression, by setting an annual maximum MPR target that would reduce each year: from 24% in 2009 to 15% in 2011 [18]. To support the UK sector in this cultural change, the 'One at a Time' Editorial Board agreed guiding principles and focussed on themes prioritised by the expert group [15] in reviewing the literature, national data and health and psychosocial outcomes of twins born as a consequence of fertility treatment.

The group worked to endorse eSET by developing tools to improve clinical practice, including written and web-based information for patients and healthcare professionals. In addition, the HFEA facilitated a number of workshops for clinic staff to share experiences and best practice of ET polices, audit and multiple pregnancy rates.

The policy has resulted in a significant decrease in multiple births (from 1:4 IVF live births in 2008; 1:6 in 2013 to 1:7 in 2015), whilst maintaining stable success rates (Fig. 42.1). Such a positive step is testament to the fertility sector auditing and reviewing their strategies and making use of the data available to them [19].

By 2010, Turkey had also introduced legislation for eSET in women aged 35 years and under, in both first and second cycles [20]. Equally, central funding in Canada enabled the rollout of eSET legislation across the Atlantic, its aim being eSET in every treatment cycle, irrespective of age or history, which resulted in an impressive reduction in the MPR from 25.6% to 3.7% [21].

In the USA, Kulkarni and colleagues [4] reported a 1.9 factor increase in twin deliveries from 1971 to 2009 and 6.7 factor increase in triplet and higher-order births from 1971 to 1998. However, the latter decreased by 29% from 1998 to 2011. This decline in number of triplet and higher-order multiples coincided with a 70% reduction in the transfer of three or more embryos during IVF programmes.

Nevertheless, more than a third of all treatments in the USA resulted in triplet and higher-order births. In 2012, the Practice Committee won the backing of the American

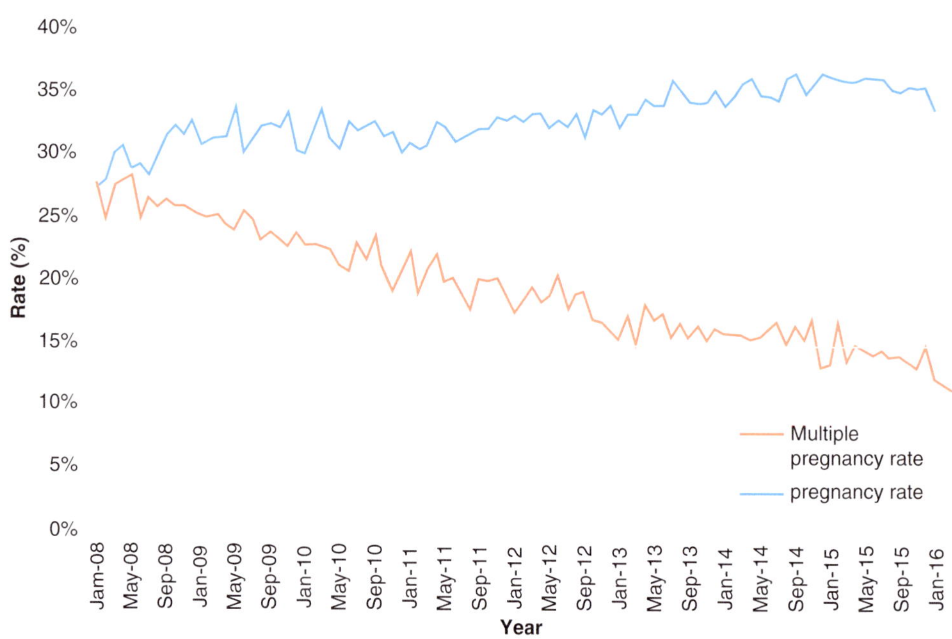

Fig. 42.1 HFEA (UK) data reflecting the continued downward trend in multiple pregnancy whilst maintaining pregnancy rates. (From Human Fertilization & Embryology Authority (2015) Improving outcomes for fertility patients: multiple births. http://www.hfea.gov.uk/docs/Multiple_Births_Report_2015.pdf)

Society for Reproductive Medicine (ASRM) with the adoption of eSET for all good prognosis patients [22].

42.2 Influence of Funding and Insurance on eSET

In 2003, Belgium introduced a policy to support funding for up to six cycles of IVF treatment for all couples, provided the female was less than 43 years old. The Belgian government recognised that this would reduce perinatal costs associated with multiple pregnancies if eSET was actively encouraged. This policy subsequently led to a dramatic increase in the use of eSET [23]. Other countries such as Australia—where there is generous public funding—have seen this aspect positively influencing voluntary uptake of eSET [24] and a subsequent successful MPR reduction.

It is important to recognise the contribution that increased state-funding affords. However, this is not the case for all countries. For example, state-funding via the National Health Service (NHS) remains low in the UK, where there is disparate commissioning of IVF services. Some areas of the UK have full NHS funding for IVF treatment, with patients are more willing to accept eSET; conversely, other areas have restricted NHS funding, e.g. for only one NHS-funded cycle, with patients more reluctant to accept eSER, especially if the cost of cryopreservation is not included.

For self-funding patients with only two good quality embryos available on day of transfer, the decision regarding eSET is not always morally and ethically determined, irrespective of prognosis [25]. As a result, and irrespective of multidisciplinary engagement with the eSET policy, healthcare professionals may find themselves 'empathising' with a rationale that supports the request for double-embryo transfer (DET). Nevertheless, where ambiguity and uncertainty exist, it is imperative that healthcare professionals consider the obstetric and general medical history.

42.3 Influence of Technological Advances on eSET: Embryo Selection in a MBMS

Embryo quality is one of the most influential factors in the prediction of IVF treatment success [13], and until very recently, focus has been solely on static morphological assessment. Embryo quality is primarily based on the number of blastomeres, evenness of cell division, and degree of fragmentation, although oocyte quality can also be considered [26]. In the UK, a MBMS algorithm scheme was proposed over a decade ago, based on the number of top quality embryos available [17]. Whilst external quality assurance schemes have tried to drive consistency, grading of embryo morphology is notoriously subjective. The challenge, therefore, to select the most viable embryo has intensified with the introduction of eSET. This has contributed towards development of two technologies: an increase in blastocyst transfer and development of technologies such as time-lapse imaging (TLI) and preimplantation genetic testing for aneuploidy (PGT-A, formerly called preimplantation genetic screening [PGS]).

42.3.1 Blastocyst Culture

Scientists in Australia were one of the first to explore the potential for blastocyst transfer in 1998, with Gardner and colleagues comparing day 3 implantation rates with embryos cultured to day 5 in serum-free medium [27]. They concluded that transfer of blastocysts in IVF would result in sustainable pregnancy rates, whilst reducing the number of embryos transferred, thereby minimising the risk of multiple pregnancy (Fig. 42.2). Furthermore, inconsistent and unreliable day 2–3 embryo selection invariably led to development of blastocyst culture programmes with promising pregnancy rates, where patients had a number of top quality embryos available [28].

The development of sequential media to meet the metabolic requirements of the human embryo further encouraged the use of blastocyst culture, with reports of an increase in implantation rates [29], possibly because the timing of transfer more closely reflected that of normal conception and improved embryo selection [30].

A Cochrane review [30] concluded that it was questionable whether the stage of embryo replaced impacted on live birth rates. Whilst blastocyst transfer was recognised as beneficial and able to improve live birth rates, the low quality of the evidence led to the conclusion that further well-designed randomised controlled trials (RCTs) are required, specifically relating to eSET.

National overview

	Trend	Oct13-Sep14	Oct14-Sep15	Oct15-Sep16
Multiple pregnancy rate		16%	15%	14%
Multiple birth rate		14%	14%	–
Pregnancy rate		35%	36%	35%
eSET		29%	31%	36%
Blastocyst		54%	61%	65%

Fig. 42.2 HFEA (UK) data reflecting the National overview from Oct 2013 to Feb 2016. (Human Fertilization & Embryology Authority (2015) Improving outcomes for fertility patients: multiple births. http://www.hfea.gov.uk/docs/Multiple_Births_Report_2015.pdf)

Whilst we have witnessed increased interest in blastocyst culture, it does have practical drawbacks; the technique is more labour-intensive and requires specialist incubators (low oxygen tension) and, thus, increases overall cost.

There have also been compromises in the context of number of embryos cryopreserved [31] and the potential for gene expression modification (epigenetics) with the adoption of blastocyst culture strategies. Epigenetics refers to modifications of gene expression (active versus inactive genes) that can alter phenotypic characteristics. According to De Ryke et al. [32], there are at least two critical periods in which epigenetic reprogramming occurs, one during the process of gametogenesis and the other throughout the preimplantation embryonic stage. Recent changes in ET timing and prolonged culture may interrupt methyltransferase activity and gene expressions. Whilst many successful eSET programmes recommend extended culture, further research should be conducted to evaluate the safety.

42.3.2 Time-Lapse Imaging

Although TLI was used as early as 1929 to visualise preimplantation development of rabbit embryos [33], its use remained predominantly experimental. However, in 1997, a report was published showing the value of serial imaging in assessing pronuclear formation and polar body extrusion in human embryos [34]. These findings, together with the drive to learn more about preimplantation embryo development, founded the interest in using continual monitoring of embryos for non-invasive assessment. TLI has rapidly advanced with great interest, and no doubt in response to worldwide pressure towards implementation of a MBMS. TLI allows the investigation of the morphology and developmental kinetics (collectively termed morphokinetics) without disturbing the culture environment [35], especially if a single-step culture medium is used [36].

One of the first TLI studies of human preimplantation embryos showed that synchrony in the appearance of nuclei after the first cleavage correlated with pregnancy rates ($P < 0.05$) [35]. Another Danish group concluded that high-quality blastocysts could be predicted within the first 48 h of culture, although this did not correlate with pregnancy rates [36].

Since then, further research to develop algorithms to aid embryo selection has been undertaken with many studies showing promising results [37, 38]. Negative predictors, which lead to embryos having lower implantation potential, include direct cleavage from one to three cells, uneven blastomeres at the two-cell stage and multinucleation at the four-cell stage [39]. However, a recent critical appraisal of the literature concluded that the current evidence fails to support routine use of the TLI; therefore patients should not be subject to a surcharge for application of this 'add-on' [40]. Furthermore, a Cochrane review stated that there is insufficient evidence of differences in live birth, miscarriage, stillbirth or clinical pregnancy to promote use of TLI over conventional incubation and that further studies are required to further elucidate the perceived benefits [41].

42.3.3 Preimplantation Genetic Testing for Aneuploidy

It is well established that embryonic aneuploidy is prevalent in IVF cycles and that these fatal genetic flaws are responsible for implantation failure and early miscarriage following ET of a morphologically good quality embryo. This prevalence increases with female age: the estimated aneuploidy rate increases from 25% for oocytes from women under 35 years to in excess of 75% for women over 40 years [42].

Chromosomal analysis can be used to help select euploid embryos for ET, which, in theory, should improve implantation rates, decrease miscarriage rates and reduce time to achieve a successful pregnancy. Innovative methods allow for comprehensive chromosomal screening—such as microarray comparative genomic hybridisation (a-CGH)—which utilises a whole genome amplification technique prior to labelling the DNA with a fluorescent dye and applying it to a microarray. Used alongside trophectoderm biopsy, this technique is increasingly being used clinically, although the results from well-designed multicentre RCTs are eagerly awaited. Published trials have reported initial benefits with statistically significant higher delivery rates being achieved after PGT-A [43]. Furthermore, a systematic review suggested that PGT-A improved embryo selection methods and could decrease multiple pregnancy rates in good prognosis patients [44].

42.3.4 Assessment of Embryo Metabolism

Although not routinely implemented in clinical practice, a promising area that may in the future be used to improve minimisation strategies is assessment of embryo metabolism. Embryo viability can be measured by analysing the components in culture media, which are either taken up or released by the human embryo [45]. Further research is required to determine whether metabolomics, oxygen consumption or amino acid turnover will provide us with a definitive model to select viable embryos.

42.4 Cryopreservation

Cryopreservation of supernumerary good quality embryos is a fundamental adjunct to IVF cycles. Successful implementation of eSET is therefore strongly dependent on successful cryopreservation programmes, since there is no evidence of a significant difference in the cumulative live birth rate from a single cycle of DET compared to cumulative cycles of eSET (e.g. one fresh eSET cycle followed by one frozen eSET cycle) [46].

More recently, there has been a shift towards vitrification with the more traditional slow-freeze methods becoming less common practice. Current evidence appears to favour vitrification in yielding more consistent results with extended culture embryos and metaphase II oocytes [47]. Loutradi and colleagues [48] conducted a systematic review and meta-analysis and similarly concluded that vitrification of blastocysts was superior to slow-freezing methods; nevertheless, some argue that slow freezing still has a place.

Regardless of the cryopreservation technique used, both rely on morphological selection beforehand, as restricting cryopreservation to good quality embryos may lead to better recovery after thawing/warming [22]. Further RCTs, using the same criteria for post-thaw/warm survival and defined outcome points, are required before one method can be recommended over another.

In addition, studies that assess the safety and efficacy of vitrification and its application of high concentration of cryoprotectants are also required. However, improvements and confidence in vitrification programmes appear to have positively influenced the uptake of eSET and as a result should be assimilated with minimisation strategies.

42.5 Reinvigorating MBMS in the UK

In the UK, the HFEA continues to work with the fertility sector via their online tool 'Cumulative Sum Analysis (CUSUM)' to monitor multiple clinical pregnancy rates in real time. Since 2012, IVF clinics have been able to access CUSUM directly through the HFEA online 'clinic portal'. CUSUM plots have an upper threshold, which, if breached, suggests that where clinic's multiple clinical pregnancy rates continue at the same rate or upward trend, they are unlikely to meet the annual target. However, if clinics engage in monthly key performance indicator (KPI) meetings, they can involve the multidisciplinary team in reviewing their MBMS and make a case for positive change.

The HFEA continues to gather evidence via patient surveys, engagement with clinics, and further field-based data analysis. This helps to drive the HFEA's proactive engagement with NHS Commissioners to discuss equitable funding to further support the uptake of eSET.

42.6 Conclusion

This chapter has described the worldwide collaborative efforts to reduce the public health issue of iatrogenic multiple births. Where one or more good quality blastocysts are available on day 5, there is overwhelming evidence that eSET should be implemented.

eSET success is dependent on accurate embryo assessment and selection methods together with a good cumulative pregnancy rate, which is heavily dependent on effective cryopreservation programmes. New technologies such as TLI and PGT-A may further help quantify embryo health, viability and potential. Many clinics are already integrated these within an MBMS, to attempt to further optimise the chance of pregnancy with eSET.

Whilst IVF outcomes and patient satisfaction can be measured in numerical form, there is no substitute for engaging the patients in what many would perceive as the most significant part of the treatment programme. Multidisciplinary involvement is therefore crucial for informed consent to occur. Within the UK, IVF clinics have the autonomy to develop and implement individualised MBMS. However, these must be harmonised with an active audit programme to allow for continual review and subsequent improvement in response to both pregnancy and multiple pregnancy rates.

Since the inception of the HFEA's MBMS in 2009, the views of the fertility sector have shifted in response to its successful implementation. Accepting and respecting professional roles (and boundaries), together with confidence in multidisciplinary involvement, have been key to the successful application of the eSET policy. The way in which the information and data is presented, coupled with acceptance and belief in the regulatory functions, will ensure maintenance of effective eSET programmes and, most importantly, improve the obstetric outcome for mother and baby.

References

1. Bionews. Five million births from IVF. 2013. www.bionews.org.uk/page_354987.asp. Accessed 25 Apr 2017.
2. Kamel RM. Assisted Reproductive Technology after the Birth of Louise Brown. J Reprod Infertil. 2013;14(3):96–109.
3. Smith L, Manktelow BN, Draper ES, Boyle EM, Johnson SJ, Filed DJ. Trends in the incidence and mortality of multiple births by socioeconomic deprivation and maternal age in England: population-based cohort study. BMJ Open. 2014;4:e004514. https://doi.org/10.1136/bmjopen-2013-004514.
4. Blondel B, Macfarlane A, Gissler M, et al. Preterm birth and multiple pregnancy in European countries participating in the PERISTAT project. BJOG. 2006;113:528–3.
5. Kulkarni AD, Jamieson DJ, Jones HW, Kissin DM, Gallo MF, Macaluso M, Adashi EY. N Engl J Med. 2013;369:2218–25. https://doi.org/10.1056/NEJMoa1301467

6. Chambers GM, Hoang VP, Lee E, Hansen M, Sullivan EA, Bower C, Chapman M. Hospital costs of multiple-birth and singleton-birth children during the first 5 years of life and the role of assisted reproductive technology. JAMA Paediat. 2014;168(11):1045–53. https://doi.org/10.1001/jamapediatrics.2014.1357.
7. De Mouzon J, Goossens V, Bhattacharya S, Castilla JA, Ferraretti AP, Korsak V, Kupka M, Nygren KG, Nyboe Andersen A. European IVF-monitoring (EIM) Consortium, for the European Society of Human Reproduction and Embryology (ESHRE). Assisted reproductive technology in Europe, 2006: results generated from European registers by ESHRE. Hum Reprod. 2010;25(8):1851–62.
8. Maheshwari A, Griffiths S, Bhattacharya S. Global variations in the uptake of single embryo transfer. 2011;17(1):107–20.
9. National Board of Health and Welfare. Official Statistics of Sweden. 2004. http://www.sos.se
10. Bergh C. Single embryo transfer: a mini-review. Hum Reprod. 2005;20(2):323–7.
11. Thurin A, Hausken J, Hillensjo T, Jablanowska B, Pinborg A, Strandell A, Bergh C. Elective single-embryo transfer versus double-embryo transfer in in-vitro fertilization. N Engl J Med. 2004;351:2392–402.
12. Pinborg A, Loft A, Nyboe-Anderson A. Neonatal outcome in a Danish cohort of 8602 children born after in-vitro fertilization or intracytoplasmic sperm injection: the role of twin pregnancy. Acta Obstet Gynaecol Scand. 2004;83(11):1071–8.
13. Gerris JM. Single embryo transfer and IVF/ICSI outcome: a balanced appraisal. Hum Reprod Update. 2005;11(2):105–21.
14. Human Fertilisation & Embryology Authority. Code of practice. 6th ed. 2003. http://www.hfea.gov.uk/docs/Code_of_Practice_Sixth_Edition.pdf. P83: 8.17-20.
15. Braude P. One child at a time: reducing multiple births after IVF. HFEA. 2006;5
16. Hamilton M. Multiple births in the United Kingdom: a consensus statement. Hum Fertil. 2009;10(2):71–4.
17. Cutting R, Morroll D, Roberts SA, Pickering S, Rutherford A. Elective single embryo transfer: guidelines for practice, British fertility society and association of clinical embryologists. Hum Fertil. 2008;11(3):131–46.
18. Human Fertilisation & Embryology Authority. Multiple births from fertility treatment in the UK: a consensus statement. 2011. http://www.hfea.gov.uk/docs/2011-05_Multiple_Births_Consensus_Statement_-_FINAL.pdf
19. Human Fertilisation & Embryology Authority. Improving outcomes for fertility patients: multiple births. 2015. http://www.hfea.gov.uk/docs/Multiple_Births_Report_2015.pdf
20. Kultursay N, Yalaz M, Ozge Koroglu A, MAR Neonatal Study Group. Neonatal outcome following new assisted reproductive technology regulations in Turkey – a nationwide multicenter point prevalence study. J Matern Fetal Neonatal Med. 2015;28(2)
21. Bissonnette F, Phillips SJ, Gunby J, Holzer H, Mahutte N, St-Michel P, Kadoch IJ. Working to eliminate multi-pregnancies: a success story in Quebec. Reprod BioMed Online. 2011;23:500–4.
22. Alpha Scientists in Reproductive Medicine, ESHRE Special Interest Group in Reproductive Medicine. The alpha consensus meeting on cryopreservation key performance indicators and benchmarks: proceedings of an expert meeting. RBM Online. 2012;25:146–67.
23. Ombelet W, De Sutter P, Van der Elst J, Martens G. Multiple gestation and infertility treatment: registration, reflection and reaction – the Belgian project. Hum Reprod Update. 2005;11:3–14.
24. Umstad MP, Hale L, Wang YA, Sullivan EA. Multiple deliveries: the reduced impact of in vitro fertilisation in Australia. Aust N Z J Obstet Gynaecol. 2013;53(2)
25. Chambers GM, Ledger W. The economic implications of multiple pregnancy following ART. Semin Fetal Neonatal Med. 2014;19(4):254–61. https://doi.org/10.1016/j.siny.2014.04.004.. Epub 2014 Jun 3
26. Serhal PF, Ranieri DM, Knins A, Marchant S, Davies M, Khadum IM. Oocyte morphology predicts outcome of intracytoplasmic sperm injection. Hum Reprod. 1998;13:1267–70.
27. Gardner DK, Vella P, Lane M, Wagley L, Schlenker T, Schoolcraft WB. Culture and transfer of human blastocysts increases implantation rates and reduces the need for multiple embryo transfers. Fertil Steril. 1998;69(1):84–8.
28. Blake DA, Farquhar CM, Johnson N, Proctor M. Cleavage stage versus blastocyst stage embryo transfer in assisted conception. Cochrane Database Syst Rev. 2007:CD002118.
29. Gardner DK. Blastocyst culture: toward single embryo transfer. Hum Fertil. 2000;3(4):229–37.
30. Glujovsky D, Farquhar C, Quinteiro Retamar AM, Sedo CR, Blake D. Cleavage stage versus blastocyst stage embryo transfer in assisted reproductive technology. Cochrane Database Syst Rev. 2016;30(6):CD002118.
31. Pavone ME, Innes J, Hirshfeld-Cytron J, Kazer R, Zhang J. Comparing thaw survival, implantation and live birth rates from cryopreserved zygotes, embryos and blastocysts. J Hum Reprod Sci. 2011;4(1):23–8.
32. De Rycke M, Liebaers I, Van Steirteghem A. Epigenetic risks related to assisted reproductive technologies risk analysis and epigenetic inheritance. Hum Reprod. 2002;17(10):2487–94.
33. Lewis WH, Gregory PW. Cinematographs of living developing rabbit eggs. Science. 1929;69:226–9.
34. Payne D, Flaherty SP, Barry MF, Matthews CD. Preliminary observations on polar body extrusion and pronuclear formation in human oocytes using time-lapse video cinematography. Hum Reprod. 1997;12:532–41.
35. Lemmen JG, Agerholm I, Ziebe S. RBM Online. 2008;17(3):385–91.
36. Summers M, Biggers JD. Chemically defined media and culture of mammalian preimplantation embryos: historical perspective and current issues. Hum Reprod Update. 2003;9:557–82.
37. Wong CC, Loewke KE, Bossert NL, Behr B, De Jonge CJ, Baer TM, Reijo Pera RA. Non-invasive imaging of human embryos before embryonic genome activation predicts development to the blastocyst stage. Nat Biotechnol. 2010;28:1115–21.
38. Meseguer M, Herrero J, Tejera A, Hilligsoe JM, Ramsing NB, Remohi J. The use of morphokinetics as a predictor of embryo implantation. Hum Reprod. 2011;26:2658–71.
39. Rubio I, Kuhlmann R, Agerholm I, Kirk J, Herrero J, Escriba MJ, Bellver J, Meseguer M. Limited implantation success of direct cleaved human zygotes: a time lapse study. Fertil Steril. 2012;98(6):1458–63.
40. Racowsky C, Kovacs P, Martins WP. A critical appraisal of time-lapse imaging for embryo selection: where are we and where do we need to go? J Assist Reprod Genet. 2015;32(7):1025–30.
41. Armstrong S, Arroll N, Cree LM, Jordan V, Farquhar C. Time-lapse systems for embryo incubation and assessment in assisted reproduction. Cochrane Database Syst Rev. 2015;27(2):CD011320.
42. Fragouli E, Alfarawati S, Goodall NN, Sánchez-García JF, Colls P, Wells D. The cytogenetics of polar bodies: insights into female meiosis and the diagnosis of aneuploidy. Mol Hum Reprod. 2011;17(5):286–95.
43. Scott RT, Upham KM, Forman EJ, Hong KH, Scott KL, Taylor D, Tao X, Treff NR. Blastocyst biopsy with comprehensive chromosome screening and fresh embryo transfer significantly increases in vitro fertilization implantation and delivery rates: a randomized controlled trial. Fertil Steril. 2013;100(3):697–703.

44. Dahdouh EM, Balayla J, García-Velasco JA. Comprehensive chromosome screening improves embryo selection: a meta-analysis. Fertil Steril. 2015;104(6):1503–12.
45. Leese HJ, Guerif F, Allgar V, Brison DR, Lundin K, Sturmey RG. Biological optimization, the Goldilocks principle, and how much is lagom in the preimplantation embryo. Mol Reprod Dev. 2016;83(9):748–54.
46. Pandian Z, Marjoribanks J, Ozturk O, Serour G, Bhattacharya S. Number of embryos for transfer following in vitro fertilisation or intra-cytoplasmic sperm injection. 2013;29(7):CD003416.
47. Edgar DH, Gook DA. A critical appraisal of cryopreservation (slow cooling versus vitrification) of human oocytes and embryos. Hum Reprod Update. 2012;0:1–19.
48. Loutradi K, Kolibianakis E, Venetis C, Evangelos E, Pados G, Bontis I, Tarlatzis B. Cryopreservation of human embryos by vitrification or slow freezing: a systematic review and meta analysis. Fertil Steril. 2008;90(1):186–93.

Multifetal Reduction Following Medically Assisted Reproduction

43

Neil Seligman and Stephanie C. Laniewski

43.1 Background

The ideal goal of assisted reproductive technology is to facilitate the conception and birth of a healthy child; the unintended consequence of efforts to meet this objective has been the dramatic rise in multiple gestations [1]. The incidence of higher-order multiples steadily increased in the United States between 1980 and 1998, rising from 37.0 to 193.5 per 100,000 births [2]. In part, the increasing numbers of twin, triplet, and higher-order multiples can be attributed to both ovulation induction and in vitro fertilization with multiple-embryo transfer [1–5]. In 2012, 44% of infants resulting from assisted reproductive technology were part of a multiple birth, whereas only 3% originated from naturally conceived multiple gestations [3].

The increased risk for both perinatal and postnatal complications in multiple gestations has been well established [4–7]. Table 43.1 shows the fetal risks with the percentage of risk increasing proportionately with the number of fetuses present. The trend toward delayed childbearing has resulted in a disproportionate number of older women utilizing assisted reproductive technology [6], a cohort that is more apt to have pre-existing medical conditions. The physiological changes of pregnancy can exacerbate maternal disease, the effects of which can be further exaggerated by a multiple gestation [7]. Maternal cardiovascular disease is a major cause of both morbidity and mortality during pregnancy; women over the age of 35 years are 2–4 times more likely to have prepregnancy chronic hypertension [8]. The rate of preeclampsia is essentially doubled in women who are over the age of 40 years. Multiple gestations further magnify these risks, as well as the risk for gestational diabetes, anemia, thrombocytopenia, hyperemesis gravidarum, placenta previa, and postpartum hemorrhage. Women carrying multiples may experience earlier disease onset and faster progression. Higher-order multiples almost always necessitate cesarean delivery, which carries its own inherent risks [4–8].

Higher-order multiples also confer greater economic and psychosocial burdens [1, 4, 5–7]. The cost of prenatal care is increased in multiple gestations due to the need for more intensive fetal monitoring, more frequent prenatal appointments, a higher risk for pregnancy-related complications (gestational diabetes, etc.), and a greater chance for hospitalization and in-patient monitoring [9]. Premature and low birth weight infants are typically cared for in the neonatal intensive care unit rather than the newborn nursery, resulting in longer hospitalization, increased surveillance, and a higher incidence of procedures and interventions [9, 10]. Beyond the delivery and initial hospitalization, parents of multiples have the ongoing costs of caring for multiple children of the same age. Diapers, clothing, and childcare (or lost wages if a parent stops working to care for their multiples) can impose significant economic strain [9, 10]. Exclusively breastfeeding higher-order multiples is rarely an achievable goal, thus adding the financial burden of providing infant formula and bottles. The greater psychosocial burden of higher-order multiples cannot be overlooked; studies have shown higher rates of parental depression, anxiety, marital discord and/or divorce, child abuse, and maladaptive behavior in older siblings [7, 11, 12].

43.2 Terminology and Rationale

Multifetal pregnancy reduction (MFPR) is a procedure, the intent of which is to reach a "safer" number of fetuses, to decrease the risk for adverse outcome associated with higher-order multiples [4, 6, 7, 13, 14]. Multifetal pregnancy reduction cannot eliminate risk altogether, nor can it guarantee the desired outcome of a healthy term infant [15]. As such, it should be presented to patients as a means of risk mitigation, rather than one of risk prevention.

N. Seligman (✉) · S. C. Laniewski
Division of Maternal-Fetal Medicine, Department of Obstetrics and Gynecology, University of Rochester Medical Center, Rochester, NY, USA
e-mail: Neil_Seligman@URMC.Rochester.edu

G. N. Allahbadia et al. (eds.), *Textbook of Assisted Reproduction*, https://doi.org/10.1007/978-981-15-2377-9_43

Table 43.1 Fetal risks of multiple pregnancies increase proportionally to the number of fetuses

Risk (%)	Singleton	Twin	Triplet	Quadruplet	Quintuplet+
Preterm birth (all)	7.74	58.71	98.35	97.97	100
Preterm birth <32 weeks	1.23	10.58	39.27	71.95	100
Average gestational age at delivery (weeks) (Stone—higher-order multiples)	40	35.3	31.9	29.5	<30
Low birth weight	6.24	55.26	95.14	97.53	100
Very low birth weight	1.07	9.56	36.96	65.43	90.91
Risk per 1000					
Early mortality (20 weeks gestation—age 1 year)	5.24	24.37	61.08	137.04	Not available
Cerebral palsy	2.3	12.6	44.8	NA	NA

Conversely, selective termination (ST) is performed when fetal anomalies have been detected in at least one fetus (but not all) of a multiple gestation. The goal of selective termination is twofold: to terminate the anomalous fetus and to allow continuation of the pregnancy for the unaffected fetus, with the anticipated outcome being a healthy live birth [4, 13, 14].

43.3 Ethical Issues

Multifetal reduction represents a conflict between "the value for human life, reduction of harm, prevention of suffering, or benefit of health" [16]. Although the increased risk of complications in multiple gestations is well established, debate remains about whether contemporary outcomes warrant reduction. Advancements in care have improved the outcome of triplets. For example, the risk of delivering an extremely low birth weight baby is greatly increased with triplets, but there is still a 90% chance of delivering infants weighing >1000 g, for which survival is almost certain in a modern neonatal intensive care unit [17]. Furthermore, plurality itself does not significantly influence short-term outcome, that is, infants of similar birth weight have similar outcomes [17, 18]. This argument notwithstanding, the goal of assisted reproduction techniques should be to achieve a singleton pregnancy [19].

From a legal perspective, it is unclear whether MFPR should be, or is, considered a form of abortion. Laws vary from state to state, but in general, where abortion is legal, MFPR is legal. The terms "abortion" and "termination" refer to removal of an embryo or fetus and placenta from the uterus to end a pregnancy. Many experts argue that MFPR is not really "termination of pregnancy" and distinct ethical features and justifications distinguish the two procedures. Multifetal reduction is a procedure to secure a healthier pregnancy outcome; by reducing one or more fetuses, those remaining may be more likely to do better [19]. In this instance, fetal death is an indirect consequence of the therapy which is a necessary, but not necessarily desirable, result [20, 21]. As an analogy, think of the life boat full of people while others still in the water are about to drown. Letting some people perish is possibly justified because too many passengers will cause the vessel to sink, with all lives lost [22]. In other words, some sacrifices are, every so often, necessary and legitimate when the interest of the many precedes those of the few (aka the reduced fetuses) [14].

In addition to the distinctions between MFPR and abortion, opinions on fetal reduction do not follow the traditional "pro-life/prochoice dichotomy" [16]. Up to one-third of couples with multiple pregnancies refuse MFPR for moral, religious, and ethical reasons that parallel arguments against abortion [23]. But, some individuals who oppose abortion justify MFPR either to improve the life and well-being of the remaining fetus(es) or because of lifestyle preferences [16]. Viewing "health" as a simply biological concept would preclude the desire to raise a child with financial security or adequate attention and emotional support [24].

Most providers see the decision to undergo reduction as that of the patient's, and the same arguments that justify abortion also justify fetal reduction. Principle among these is respect for autonomy, which is the foundation for informed consent, acknowledges a woman's right to hold views and make choices based on her personal values and beliefs [4]. Whether a woman's autonomy to determine a state of pregnancy should extend to determination of the number of fetuses she is pregnant with remains controversial [25]. For now, so long as abortion remains controversial, MFPR will remain controversial as well.

From both a procedural and ethical perspective, MFPR and ST are very similar. Possibly the biggest distinction is that while the reduced fetus(es) are presumably normal in MFPR, in ST the reduced fetus is abnormal [14]. The notion of overlapping risks, lifestyle framework, the nature and acceptability of disability, and patient autonomy arguably apply to both procedures [26].

43.4 Professional Society Recommendations

Though many professional societies have statement about the need for strategies to minimize the risk of multifetal pregnancies, few offer statements about MFPR. The American College of Obstetricians and Gynecologists (ACOG) and International Federation of Gynecology and

Obstetrics (FIGO) state that women should be provided nondirective counseling about the risks of multifetal pregnancy and the possible benefits of MFPR in the setting of higher-order multiple (typically triplets or more) conceived either spontaneously or with assisted reproductive technology [4, 5, 19]. Studies have shown that patients pursuing assisted reproductive technology may view a twin or triplet gestation as a positive outcome; this may be influenced by many factors, including the amount of time spent trying to conceive, the financial aspects of assisted reproductive technology, parental age, and desire for a large family [1, 6, 9, 10, 27]. The perinatal risks of multiple gestations are often not well understood and may be largely underestimated by patients who have not been appropriately counseled [1, 14].

43.5 Counseling

Informed consent is more than a single conversation, and it is the responsibility of the rendering provider to make sure that all information is adequately conveyed to patients in a way that is both understandable and meaningful [4, 28–31]. While multifetal pregnancy reduction should by no means be viewed as a bulwark for assisted reproductive technology, patients must be accurately counseled of its availability, both before and, when necessary, after conception occurs. Nondirective counseling is essential when discussing topics such as reproductive planning, prenatal diagnostic testing, and feticide [29–31]. Regardless of personal convictions, there is a professional responsibility to convey information that is complete and accurate, while respecting patient autonomy [4, 29–31]. For both providers offering multifetal reduction as well as providers who may directly or indirectly facilitate such a referral, information should be provided to patients, in as many iterations as is necessary, to allow them to make their own best decision for their personal circumstances. Not only does this mean an accurate depiction of the risks, benefits, and limitations of multifetal pregnancy reduction but a similar explanation of any alternative, including expectant management of higher-order multiples. Likewise, it is paramount that patients know that they will receive support for their decision without fear of provider coercion or disapproval [4, 29–31]. When MFPR is discordant with a physician's value system, he/she should provide a referral to an experienced physician [4].

43.6 Genetic Testing

An increasing number of tests are available to women during pregnancy to assess the health of the fetus; the information provided by these tests focuses primarily on karyotypic abnormalities. Non-invasive screening, which assays maternal serum analytes or cell-free fetal DNA, provides an estimation of risk for fetal aneuploidy without posing any risk of fetal injury or loss. However, the sensitivity and specificity of screening tests are decreased in twin gestations; currently, neither maternal serum screening nor cell-free fetal DNA screening can be performed in higher-order multiples [7, 15]. This is problematic in that multifetal gestations are inherently at greater risk for aneuploidy (Table 43.2). While the risk for a chromosome abnormality in any one fetus is the same as that of a singleton, the risk is additive in multifetal gestations, thereby conveying a higher overall risk [4, 5–7, 15, 32]. In the absence of other identifiable risk factors, a maternal age of 35 years at the time of delivery has historically been the turning point for which invasive prenatal testing is offered as part of routine prenatal care [27]. With each additional fetus, the threshold for the age at which a woman should be considered "high-risk" is lowered.

Table 43.2 Risk of aneuploidy by maternal age and fetal number

Maternal age	Singleton (1/x)	Twin	Triplet	Quadruplet
24	670	335	223	**168**
26	625	313	208	**156**
28	560	280	**187**	140
30	465	233	155	116
32	350	**175**	117	88
34	230	115	77	58
35	**180**	90	60	45
36	135	68	45	34

If the goal of multifetal reduction is to curtail the risk of adverse pregnancy outcome, testing for fetal chromosome abnormalities—which inherently increase the risk for spontaneous loss, stillbirth, and neonatal death—should be considered [4, 5–7]. Early sonographic findings such as lagging fetal growth, increased nuchal translucency, absent nasal bone, or non-physiologic ventral wall herniation are all indicative of a potential fetal anomaly [7, 15, 27, 32]. As such, there would be little perceived benefit to obtaining a karyotype for an abnormal-appearing fetus. However, not all aneuploid fetuses will present with visible markers [15], and it is therefore prudent to initiate a conversation with the patient about prenatal diagnostic testing prior to multifetal reduction. This counseling should focus on the risks, benefits, and limitations of both electing and declining invasive prenatal testing [6, 32].

Chorionic villus sampling is technically more challenging in a multiple gestation; when being performed prior to fetal reduction, it is cardinal that every effort be made to minimize the risk of sampling error (e.g., unintentional sampling of the same placement more than once). Accurate mapping of each fetus and its placenta is crucial, and the respective locations should be well documented for future reference [5–7, 27, 32]. Samples should be obtained for fetuses that are not slated for reduction to confirm a normal karyotype. Whether one additional fetus should be sampled depends upon multiple factors such as index of suspicion for aneuploidy, potential risk of the additional procedure, and the technical feasibility of obtaining the extra sample [27]. Another discussion point is the type of results desired before proceeding with a planned reduction. A full karyotype will rule out any numerical or large structural rearrangements; however, results are not available for 7–10 days. Fluorescent in situ hybridization (FISH) allows for more immediate information, with results available in as little as 24 h; however, FISH is less comprehensive than a full karyotype. Direct FISH screens for common aneuploidies (Trisomy 13, 18, 21, and sex chromosome aneuploidies), which account for approximately 70% of aneuploidies present at the time of chorionic villus sampling [6, 15, 27, 32]. The provider and patient should therefore have a conversation about goals of testing, including the relative acceptability of postponing fetal reduction in anticipation of a full karyotype versus lessening the interval between chorionic villus sampling and fetal reduction by proceeding with more limited test results because of the ongoing risk of loss of unreduced multiples [16].

43.7 Outcomes

Multiple studies have demonstrated improvement in pregnancy outcome with MFPR [33–35]. In a meta-analysis of 2240 triplets reduced to twins compared to 604 triplets managed conservatively, fetal loss <24 weeks was 5.1% vs. 11.5% (OR 0.45 95% CI 0.3–0.6), delivery <28 weeks was 2.9% vs. 8.4% (OR 0.35 95% CI 0.2–0.6), delivery <32 weeks was 10.1% vs. 20.3% (0.5 95% CI 0.4–0.7), and perinatal mortality was 26.6/1000 vs. 92/1000 (OR 0.3 95% CI 0.2–0.7) [36]. The benefits can be loosely summarized as "one month, one pound." That is, for each fetus reduced, the benefit is approximately 1 month longer gestation and 1 pound greater birth weight. Pregnancies reduced to twins have an outcome similar to pregnancies starting as twins [37].

Factors most closely linked to pregnancy outcome following fetal reduction are:

- Starting number
- Ending number
- Gestational age
- Operator/center experience

43.7.1 Starting and Ending Number

Fetal loss rates and prematurity vary with both the starting and ending number (Table 43.3) [32]. The loss rate is the lowest when twins are reduced to singletons; remains stable when the starting number is three, four, or five fetuses; and increases substantially when the starting number is greater than five or the finishing number is three or more [32]. The pregnancy loss rate when starting with sextuplets exceeds 20% [35].

Table 43.3 Loss rates by starting and ending number

Starting number of fetuses	Loss rate if ending as twins	Loss rate if ending as singleton
≥5	12.1%	Na
4	5.8%	4.0%
3	4.5%	6.1%
2	Na	2.1%

From Stone, J., Ferrara, L., Kamrath, J., Getrajdman, J., Berkowitz, R., Moshier, E., Eddleman, K., 2008. Contemporary outcomes with the latest 1000 cases of multifetal pregnancy reduction (MPR). Am. J. Obstet. Gynecol. 199, e1–e4, with permission

43.7.2 Gestational Age

Most fetal reductions are performed between 10 and 13 weeks for reasons outlined below. For procedures performed within this time frame, there is no significant difference in loss rates [35]. Whether procedures performed at later gestational ages are associated with higher rates of loss is not entirely clear [38, 39] and the data is confounded by indication since procedures performed at later gestational ages tend to be for discordant anomalies or genetic conditions. In a group of women undergoing ST, the loss rate was 5.4% for procedures between 9 and 12 weeks versus 8.7%, 6.8%, and 9.1% for procedures carried out between 13–18, 19–24, and over 25 weeks, respectively, but the difference was not statistically significant [39].

43.7.3 Operator Experience

In 1988, Berkowitz et al. published the first reports using a transabdominal technique in which three of nine women lost the entire pregnancy (33%) [40]. Subsequently, Berkowitz and colleagues published their results with another 200 consecutive cases in which the rate of loss was 9.5% and decreased to 8% as their experience increased to 400 cases [41, 42]. This group has now performed >2000 cases with a loss rate of 4.7% in the last 1000 procedures performed from 1999 to 2006 [32]. The reduction in loss rate with experience was also seen in another large, multicenter study of 3513 women in which the losses decreased from 13.2% before 1990 to 9.4% from 1991 to 1994 and to 6.4% from 1995 to 1998 [35]. The overall loss rate was 9.6% which is higher than reported by Berkowitz's group (5.4% in 1000 consecutive cases from 1986 to 1999) [34]. The difference is attributed to all of the procedures being performed at a single center and only using a transabdominal technique. Improvements in loss rates over time have also been explained by improvements in ART leading to smaller proportion of higher-order multiples, better ultrasound visualization, and use of CVS which lowers the risk of leaving behind an abnormal fetus [36].

All said, compared to the spontaneous background loss rate, the incremental added risk of the procedure is <1% [43].

43.7.4 Selective Termination

Outcomes following ST are generally good with loss rates that are similar to those seen in MFPR (4.0% and 7.5% in the two largest series) [27, 39]. The effect of starting and ending number is similar to that seen in MFPR; however, the biggest risk of loss occurs when more than one fetus is reduced. Median gestational age at delivery after ST is 36–37 weeks. While gestational age does not appear to be a significant factor in the loss rate, ST should be performed as soon as possible once the decision is made [39].

43.8 Technique

The critical steps in planning a MFPR can be outlined as follows: (1) counseling, (2) "mapping" ultrasound, (3) CVS (optional), (4) reduction, and (5) follow-up. At the first encounter (optimally at 9–10 weeks), the patient is scheduled for consultation and a mapping ultrasound. The mapping scan serves several purposes:

- Confirm pregnancy number and viability of all fetuses.
- Confirm dating and assess growth.
- Confirm chorionicity (rule out monochorionicity) and document location of the placenta and associated fetus/sac.
- Evaluate for gross anomalies (e.g., thickened nuchal translucency).

Labs (complete blood count, type and screen, HIV, and hepatitis C) should be obtained prior to the visit. When there are known concerns about fetal growth, an ultrasound before the consult is preferred to ensure the viability of all the fetuses.

Most women who opt for chorionic villus sampling (CVS) are scheduled for a follow-up visit (typically 10–11 weeks). Separating the consult/mapping and CVS visits serves two major purposes. First, it maintains a neutral and bias-free counseling environment, and second, it aids in scheduling. Trying to accomplish everything in a single visit can put tremendous pressure on resources because of the time needed. Additionally, many women are undecided about MFPR, decline after counseling, or have abnormal ultrasound findings like spontaneous co-twin demise, discordant growth, or major anomalies. Factors which are considered when selecting fetuses for reduction include:

- Location
  - Distance from the cervix
  - Accessibility of the placenta for sampling
  - Feasibility of reduction without disrupting an adjacent fetus
- Growth
- Gross anomalies

All factors being equal, we sample the fetuses closest to the cervix. Sampling is limited to two fetuses in a single visit and no more than two passes per placenta (if needed to ensure adequate sample size).

Reduction is scheduled as soon as possible once the patient has opted to proceed; for women who elected sampling, scheduling should coincide with the availability of cytogenetic test results (typically 13 weeks). A follow-up ultrasound is performed to evaluate for interval changes and correlate fetal labeling/location with the previous ultrasounds. When choosing the fetuses for reduction, the same factors used in selecting fetuses for placental sampling are considered with the addition of cytogenetic testing results (if any). Again, all things being equal, we reduce the fetus/es farthest from cervix. When possible, the fetus closest to the cervix is avoided because of the theoretical risk of infection and to reduce fluid leakage.

Reduction is performed transabdominally under sterile conditions as an outpatient procedure. The abdomen is prepped with betadine or chlorhexidine, and a sterile cover is placed over the ultrasound probe. A 22-gauge amniocentesis needle is inserted into the fetal thorax, ideally intracardiac, under real-time ultrasound guidance. Once placement is confirmed visually, 0.5–2.0 cc of 2 mEq/mL potassium chloride (KCl) is injected, and the fetus is observed for cessation of cardiac activity for 60–120 s before removal of the needle. Additional fetuses are reduced following the same technique either through the same puncture site or, more often, through a second needle insertion. Reduction of five or more fetuses is separated into two appointments a week apart. Other techniques, including transvaginal or transcervical aspiration, have been described but have higher loss rates.

An ultrasound is repeated in 30–60 min to confirm absence of fetal heart motion in the reduced fetus and viability of the remaining fetus/es. If reactivation of the fetal heart rate was to occur, the procedure should be repeated. Neither prophylactic antibiotics nor local analgesia is used; however, a small prescription of benzodiazepines (typically Ativan) to be used immediately before the procedure and in the immediate post-procedure period is offered for anxiety.

Selective termination is very similar though some key elements are different. In general, ST is most commonly performed in twins. The procedure is typically performed at a later gestational age for anomalies and/or aneuploidy diagnosed often at the time of a routine anatomy ultrasound. Amniocentesis is performed rather than CVS when cytogenetic testing is required and can be done as a separate procedure or immediately prior to injection of KCl. A larger gauge needle (typically 20-gauge) and larger volume of KCl (typically 1–5 cc) are used. More attention is paid to intracardiac placement of the needle.

43.9 Post-Procedure Care and Follow-Up

Patients are counseled to observe for leakage of fluid, vaginal bleeding, abdominal pain, and fever. Some leakage of amniotic fluid, or even a large "gush," from the sac of the reduced fetus, is not uncommon and typically occurs within the first few days [43]. We perform a follow-up ultrasound for reassurance though even when imaging confirms oligo- or anhydramnios this fluid loss does not appear to increase the risk of loss. A short course of antibiotics, such as azithromycin, is sometimes given. Some cramping immediately following the procedure is common and can be treated with acetaminophen. Pain unrelieved with acetaminophen, heavy vaginal bleeding, or any fever requires evaluation.

A follow-up ultrasound is scheduled 1 week after reduction to confirm cessation of fetal cardiac activity. In most series, intracardiac KCl has a 0% first dose failure rate [44]. We counsel our patients that return of cardiac activity is possible but very unlikely. In the unlikely event that there is return of cardiac activity, a repeat procedure is strongly advised. After this, the referring provider is advised to follow growth every 4 weeks in the third trimester. The reduced fetuses will be visible for several weeks after the procedure until the tissue is resorbed. By the time of delivery, it is often difficult to identify any tissue from the reduced fetuses. In ST, the larger fetus does not resorb; however over time the tissue will compact, and the amniotic fluid will disappear. The reduced fetus is delivered along with the placenta and is not often identifiable to the patient. Although it is typical to send the fetal remains and placenta to pathology, the degree of maceration limits the utility of this evaluation.

43.10 Special Issues

43.10.1 Reduction to Singleton

An increasing proportion of women are reducing to a singleton [6, 45]. From 2000 to 2007, Stone and colleagues observed a threefold increase in the number of patients reducing to a singleton compared to the period from 1986 to 1999 (11.8% vs. 31.8%). Yet reduction to singleton is still somewhat controversial because depending on perspective, it is less likely to improve outcome. Reduction of triplets to a singleton, compared to twins, is associated with a higher rate of term deliveries and higher birth weight [45–47]. Similar findings were noted by Haas et al. using transvaginal fetal aspiration at 6–8 weeks [48]. However, a higher rate of early fetal loss <24 weeks with a lower finishing number (typically 1–2% higher) may not justify increases in gestational age and birth weight that are of marginal clinical significance. For example, the mean gestational age at delivery of triplets reduced to twins compared to singletons was 35.2 vs. 37.7 weeks, arguably an acceptable either way outcome for many parents [32]. Nonetheless, this is a complex discussion which should also take into account reductions in severely preterm birth and maternal complications like gestational hypertension/preeclampsia and gestational diabetes [46, 48].

Another consideration is that a woman's individual circumstance may justify reduction to a singleton irrespective of the difference in outcome noted in these studies. Reduction to singleton may reduce the risk of preterm birth in women whose history places them at marked risk [5]. For example, in a woman with a history of mid-trimester loss secondary to cervical insufficiency, twins will not only further increase already high risk of recurrent preterm birth but also limit the options for intervention. Reduction to a singleton may also be justifiable to reduce the physiologic stress in women with medical comorbidities like heart disease [4]. Other, less tangible factors include economic and psychosocial factors as well as preference [4].

A related issue is reduction of a twin pregnancy to singleton which has also become increasingly common [47]. The same obstetrical, medical, and psychosocial rationale can be used to justify reduction of twins, but patients and providers are less comfortable with this scenario [49]. Age appears to be a factor in choosing to reduce twins. There is conflicting evidence as to whether obstetrical outcomes are improved with reduction of twins to a singleton. Some authors have reported no change in outcome [50], while others have shown lower prematurity rates but no reduction in early preterm birth or birth weight <5th percentile [51–53]. Regarding the results of a study by Haas and colleagues, Drugan et al. stated "considering a 5% risk of pregnancy loss following fetal reduction, two pregnancies will be lost because of fetal reduction for each case of (not necessarily fatal) RDS prevented" [47].

In our view, while elective termination of pregnancy is legal, women should have the option to reduce higher-order multiples to a singleton. Reduction of twins to a singleton is not routinely discussed in our practice unless warranted by historical factors or requested by the patient. Paraphrasing from Dr. Evan, in a pluralistic society where the emphasis is on curbing a state's interference with the choice of abortion, how could it be wrong to respect a couple's right to noninterference in the freedom to choose to have one infant rather than two [6].

43.10.2 Monochorionic

Multiples with a monochorionic pair have become more common rising from 2.1% of patients undergoing reduction during the period from 1986 to 1999 to 5.7% in the decade following, largely as a result of assisted reproductive technology [45]. These multiples are at increased risk of adverse outcomes largely because of the unique complications which result from placental vascular communication, namely, twin-twin transfusion syndrome and selective intrauterine growth restriction. Demise of one twin in a monochorionic pair has serious implications for the surviving twin including neurologic injury or death (30–50%) [36]. To give perspective, the risk of a monochorionic pair in a multiple pregnancy is equivalent to that of an additional fetus (i.e., the outcome of dichorionic triamniotic triplets is equivalent to that of quadrachorionic quadruplets).

Most experts agree that, as long as the other fetus(es) appears healthy, reduction of the monochorionic pair provides the best outcome. The report by Myers et al. was one of the first to suggest that, in higher-order multiples, reduction of the monochorionic pair improves pregnancy outcome [54]. A second report published around the same time showed higher rates of immediate complications in 12 pregnancies in which a monochorionic pair was reduced; however, the complications were rupture of the reduced sac and all had favorable outcomes [55]. Several other studies have shown similar improvements in pregnancy outcome largely attributable to a reduction in preterm birth at the expense of a higher miscarriage rate and lower rate of survival of at least one fetus [56–58]. Morlando and colleagues modeled the results of a systematic review in a hypothetical cohort of 1000 dichorionic triamniotic triplets. Preterm birth <32 weeks was 5.5% following reduction of the monochorionic pair compared to 33.3% and 17.6% in unreduced triplets and reduction of the fetus with a separate placenta, respectively [57]. Selective termination in monochorionic twins requires cord coagulation, cord ablation, radiofrequency ablation, or microwave ablation, procedures which carry much higher risk and are performed in a limited number of centers.

References

1. Practice Committee of the American Society for Reproductive Medicine. Multiple gestation associated with infertility therapy: an American Society for Reproductive Medicine Practice Committee opinion. Fertil Steril. 2012;97(4):825–34.
2. MacDorman MF, Gregory ECW. National Vital Statistics Reports. 2015;64(8).
3. Sunderam S, Kissin DM, Crawford S, Folger SG, Jamieson DJ, Warner L, Barfield WD. Assisted reproductive technology surveillance–United States, 2013. MMWR Surveill Summ. 2015;64(11):1–25.
4. American College of Obstetricians and Gynecologists. ACOG Committee opinion no. 553: multifetal pregnancy reduction. Obstet Gynecol. 2013;121(2 Pt 1):405.
5. American College of Obstetricians and Gynecologists. Perinatal risks associated with assisted reproductive technology. ACOG Committee Opinion No. 671. Obstet Gynecol. 2016;128(3):e61–8.
6. Evans MI, Andriole S, Britt DW. Fetal reduction: 25 years' experience. Fetal Diagn Ther. 2014;35(2):69–82.
7. Stone J, Kohari KS. Higher-order multiples. Clin Obstet Gynecol. 2015;58(3):668–75.
8. Norwitz ER, Edusa V, Park JS. Maternal physiology and complications of multiple pregnancy. Semin Perinatol. 2005;29(5):338–48.
9. Chambers GM, Ledger W. The economic implications of multiple pregnancy following ART. Semin Fetal Neonat Med. 2014;19(4):254–61.
10. Miller VL, Ransom SB, Shalhouba A, Sokol RJ, Evans MI. Multifetal pregnancy reduction: perinatal and fiscal outcomes. Am J Obstet Gynecol. 2000;182(6):1575–80.
11. Bryan E. The impact of multiple preterm births on the family. BJOG Int J Obstet Gynaecol. 2003;110(s20):24–8.
12. Leonard LG. Depression and anxiety disorders during multiple pregnancy and parenthood. J Obstet Gynecol Neonat Nurs. 1998;27(3):329–37.
13. Stone J, Berkowitz RL. Multifetal pregnancy reduction and selective termination. Semin Perinatol. 1995;19(5):363–74.
14. Legendre CM, Moutel G, Drouin R, Favre R, Bouffard C. Differences between selective termination of pregnancy and fetal reduction in multiple pregnancy: a narrative review. Reprod BioMed Online. 2013;26(6):542–54.
15. Rosner M, Pergament E, Andriole S, Gebb J, Dar PE, Evans MI. Detection of genetic abnormalities by using CVS and FISH prior to fetal reduction in sonographically normal appearing fetuses. Prenat Diagn. 2013;33(10):940–4.
16. Evans MI, Britt DW. Multifetal pregnancy reduction: evolution of the ethical arguments. Semin Reprod Med. 2010;28:295–302.
17. Blickstein I. Who is afraid of triplet pregnancies? www.comtecmed.com/cogi/cogi5/abstracts/Blickstein_triplets.doc
18. Shinwell ES, Blickstein I, Lusky A, Reichman B. Excess risk of mortality in very low birthweight triplets: a national, population based study. Arch Dis Child Fetal Neonat Ed. 2003;88(1):F36–40.
19. Serour GI. Ethical recommendations on multiple pregnancy and multifetal reduction. Int J Gynecol Obstet. 2006;92(3):331–2.
20. Pinchuk S. A difficult choice in a different voice: multiple births, selective reduction and abortion. Duke J Gender Law Policy. 2000;7:29.
21. Daar JF. Selective reduction of multiple pregnancy: lifeboat ethics in the womb. Univ Calif Davis Law Rev. 1992;25(4):773–843.
22. Berkowitz RL. Ethical issues involving multifetal pregnancies. The Mount Sinai J Med (New York). 1998;65(3):185–90.
23. Davis C, Douglas H. Selective reduction of fetuses in multiple pregnancies and the law in Australia. J Law Med. 2014;22:155–73.
24. McClimans L. Elective twin reductions: evidence and ethics. Bioethics. 2009;24(6):295–303.
25. Rorty MV, Pinkerton JV. Elective fetal reduction: the ultimate elective surgery. J Contemp Health Law Policy. 1996;13:53.
26. Wale J. Selective termination of pregnancy and fetal reduction in multiple pregnancy: terminology, blurred lines and ethical discourse. https://doi.org/10.13140/RG.2.1.5099.7368
27. Eddleman KA, Stone JL, Lynch L, Berkowitz RL. Chorionic villus sampling before multifetal pregnancy reduction. Am J Obstet Gynecol. 2000;183(5):1078–81.

28. Effect of advanced age on fertility and pregnancy in women. https://www.uptodate.com/contents/effect-of-advanced-age-on-fertility-and-pregnancy-in-women?source=search_result&%3Bsearch=maternal+age&%3BselectedTitle=1~150
29. Cheong MA, Tay CS. Application of legal principles and medical ethics: multifetal pregnancy and fetal reduction. Singap Med J. 2014;55(6):298.
30. Chervenak FA, McCullough LB. An ethically justified practical approach to offering, recommending, performing, and referring for induced abortion and feticide. Am J Obstet Gynecol. 2009;201(6):560–e1.
31. Seller MJ. Ethical aspects of genetic counselling. J Med Ethics. 1982;8(4):185–8.
32. Ferrara L, Gandhi M, Litton C, McClung EC, Jandl K, Moshier E, Eddleman K, Stone J. Chorionic villus sampling and the risk of adverse outcome in patients undergoing multifetal pregnancy reduction. Am J Obstet Gynecol. 2008;199(4):408–e1.
33. Stone J, Ferrara L, Kamrath J, Getrajdman J, Berkowitz R, Moshier E, Eddleman K. Contemporary outcomes with the latest 1000 cases of multifetal pregnancy reduction (MPR). Am J Obstet Gynecol. 2008;199:e1–4.
34. Stone J, Eddleman K, Lynch L, Berkowitz RL. A single center experience with 1000 consecutive cases of multifetal pregnancy reduction. Am J Obstet Gynecol. 2002;187(5):1163–7.
35. Evans MI, Berkowitz RL, Wapner RJ, Carpenter RJ, Goldberg JD, Ayoub MA, Horenstein J, Dommergues M, Brambati B, Nicolaides KH, Holzgreve W. Improvement in outcomes of multifetal pregnancy reduction with increased experience. Am J Obstet Gynecol. 2001;184(2):97–103.
36. Wimalasundera RC. Selective reduction and termination of multiple pregnancies. Semin Fetal Neonat Med. 2010;15(6):327–35.
37. Antsaklis A, Anastasakis E. Selective reduction in twins and multiple pregnancies. J Perinat Med. 2011;39(1):15–21.
38. Evans MI, Dommergues M, Wapner RJ, Lynch L, Dumez Y, Goldberg JD, Zador IE, Nicolaides KH, Johnson MP, Golbus MS, Boulot P. Efficacy of transabdominal multifetal pregnancy reduction: collaborative experience among the world's largest centers. Obstet Gynecol. 1993;82(1):61–6.
39. Evans MI, Goldberg JD, Horenstein J, Wapner RJ, Ayoub MA, Stone J, Lipitz S, Achiron R, Holzgreve W, Brambati B, Johnson A. Selective termination for structural, chromosomal, and Mendelian anomalies: international experience. Am J Obstet Gynecol. 1999;181(4):893–7.
40. Berkowitz RL, Lynch L, Chitkara U, Wilkins IA, Mehalek KE, Alvarez E. Selective reduction of multifetal pregnancies in the first trimester. N Engl J Med. 1988;318(16):1043–7.
41. Berkowitz RL, Lynch L, Lapinski R, Bergh P. First-trimester transabdominal multifetal pregnancy reduction: a report of two hundred completed cases. Am J Obstet Gynecol. 1993;169(1):17–21.
42. Berkowitz RL, Lynch L, Stone J, Alvarez M. The current status of multifetal pregnancy reduction. Am J Obstet Gynecol. 1996;174(4):1265–72.
43. Obican S, Brock C, Berkowitz R, Wapner RJ. Multifetal pregnancy reduction. Clin Obstet Gynecol. 2015;58(3):574–84.
44. Diedrich J, Drey E. Induction of fetal demise before abortion. Contraception. 2010;81(6):462–73.
45. Stone J, Belogolovkin V, Matho A, Berkowitz RL, Moshier E, Eddleman K. Evolving trends in 2000 cases of multifetal pregnancy reduction: a single-center experience. Am J Obstet Gynecol. 2007;197(4):394–e1.
46. Kuhn-Beck F, Moutel G, Weingertner AS, Kohler M, Hornecker F, Hunsinger MC, Kohler A, Mager C, Neumann M, Nisand I, Favre R. Fetal reduction of triplet pregnancy: one or two? Prenat Diagn. 2012;32:122–6.
47. Drugan A, Weissman A. Multi-fetal pregnancy reduction (MFPR) to twins or singleton–medical justification and ethical slippery slope. J Perinat Med. 2016.
48. Haas J, Hourvitz A, Dor J, Yinon Y, Elizur S, Mazaki-Tovi S, Barzilay E, Shulman A. Pregnancy outcome of early multifetal pregnancy reduction: triplets to twins versus triplets to singletons. Reprod BioMed Online. 2014;29(6):717–21.
49. Klitzman RL. Reducing the number of fetuses in a pregnancy: providers' and patients' views of challenges. Hum Reprod. 2016;31(11):2570–6.
50. Hasson J, Shapira A, Many A, Jaffa A, Har-Toov J. Reduction of twin pregnancy to singleton: does it improve pregnancy outcome? J Matern Fetal Neonat Med. 2011;24:1362–6.
51. Haas J, Sasson AM, Barzilai E, Mazaki Tovi S, Orvieto R, Weisz B, et al. Perinatal outcome after fetal reduction from twin to singleton: to reduce or not to reduce? Fertil Steril. 2015;103:428–32.
52. Gupta S, Fox NS, Feinberg J, Klauser CK, Rebarber A. Outcomes in twin pregnancies reduced to singleton pregnancies compared with ongoing twin.
53. Evans MI, Kaufman MI, Urban AJ, Britt DW, Fletcher JC. Fetal reduction from twins to a singleton: a reasonable consideration? Obstet Gynecol. 2004;104(1):102–9.
54. Myers V, Cramer D, Rychlek K, Finney T, Weiner S. OC9. 06: Reduction of the monochorionic pair in multifetal pregnancies improves outcome. Ultrasound Obstet Gynecol. 2005;26(4):324.
55. Athanasiadis AP, Zafrakas M, Tarlatzis BC, Vaitsi V, Mikos T, Bontis J. Multifetal pregnancy reduction in pregnancies with a monochorionic component. Fertil Steril. 2005;83(2):474–6.
56. Chaveeva P, Kosinski P, Puglia D, Poon LC, Nicolaides KH. Trichorionic and dichorionic triplet pregnancies at 10–14 weeks: outcome after embryo reduction compared to expectant management. Fetal Diagn Ther. 2013;34:199–205.
57. Morlando M, Ferrara L, D'antonio F, Lawin-O'Brien A, Sankaran S, Pasupathy D, Khalil A, Papageorghiou A, Kyle P, Lees C, Thilaganathan B. Dichorionic triplet pregnancies: risk of miscarriage and severe preterm delivery with fetal reduction versus expectant management. Outcomes of a cohort study and systematic review. BJOG Int J Obstet Gynaecol. 2015;122(8):1053–60.
58. Skiadas CC, Missmer SA, Benson CB, Acker D, Racowsky C. Impact of selective reduction of the monochorionic pair in in vitro fertilization triplet pregnancies on gestational length. Fertil Steril. 2010;94(7):2930–1.

44 Perinatal Outcome of Medically Assisted Reproduction Pregnancies

Galia Oron and Benjamin Fisch

Currently more than 1.6% of all infants born in the United States are conceived by medically assisted reproduction (MAR) [1]. The most recent report of the European Society of Human Reproduction and Embryology found that the percentage of infants born after ART varied from 0.2% to 6.1% of the total national birth cohort in 2013 [2]. That same year, an estimated five million babies worldwide were born using MAR [3], and by the time you read this chapter, the number will have increased substantially.

MAR is associated with an increased risk of adverse maternal and perinatal outcomes, including pregnancy-induced hypertension, gestational diabetes, placenta previa and placental abruption, cesarean section, preterm delivery (PDT), and low birth weight (LBW). In the past, most of these complications were attributed to the increased prevalence of multiple gestations associated with ART treatment. However, systematic reviews and meta-analyses since the mid-2000s have revealed that MAR-conceived singletons are also at higher risk of adverse perinatal outcomes than spontaneously conceived singletons, [4–10] even after controlling for maternal risk factors such as age, parity, smoking, duration of infertility, and preexisting diseases [11–13]. This finding is important as these maternal risk factors, in addition to obesity, alcohol use, and previous pregnancy loss, are themselves strong predictors of adverse obstetric outcomes [14].

The perinatal safety of MAR is of growing concern given its increasing use and potential long-term health effects that may arise later in life in the offspring [15, 16].

Definitions

- Low birth weight, <2500 g; very low birth weight, <1500 g
- Preterm delivery, <37 weeks of gestation; very preterm delivery, >32 weeks of gestation
- Perinatal mortality, still birth from 20 weeks of gestation, or neonatal deaths at 0–27 completed days after birth

G. Oron (✉) · B. Fisch
IVF and Infertility Unite, Beilinson Hospital, Petah Tikva, Israel

44.1 Perinatal Outcomes of ART

44.1.1 Perinatal Outcomes in Singletons

The most recent national surveillance reports prepared by the Centers for Disease Control and Prevention (CDC) for 2013 reported LBW rates of 29.1% for MAR-conceived infants compared to 8.0% for general population of infants in the United States [1]. Additionally, 33.6% of all ART-conceived singletons were born preterm and 6.1%, very preterm. The corresponding rates in the general population were 11.4% and 1.9%. Overall, MAR-conceived infants accounted for approximately 5.8% of all LBW infants and 5.1% of all very low birth weight (VLBW) infants and approximately 4.6% of all preterm infants and 6.1% of all very preterm infants.

These data are in line with the results of systematic reviews and meta-analyses published in the early 2000s which showed that singletons conceived by MAR were at increased risk of LBW, VLBW, PTD, and very preterm delivery (VPTD) in both matched and non-matched studies [14–19]. These studies were the first to rebut the traditional notion that the relatively poor perinatal outcome of ART newborns was due to the higher frequency of multiple pregnancies associated with the new technology. Although by the time of their publication the absolute risk for LBW had decreased from the more than twofold increased risk in the 1990s, it was still considerably higher than that in the general population, even after adjusting for maternal age, parity, and ethnicity. Proposed explanations for the decline included advances in MAR procedures, technical improvements in ultrasound-guided embryo transfer, and changes in obstetric practices leading to closer monitoring and intervention [20].

In 2012, a meta-analysis of 30 cohort studies (20 matched and 10 unmatched) comparing MAR-conceived and spontaneously conceived singletons observed that in the 19 studies (total 28,352 ART singletons) in which the rate of LBW was reported, the relative risk (RR) of LBW in the MAR group was 1.65 (95% CI 1.56–1.75), with an absolute increased risk of 3% compared to spontaneous conception. In the 14

G. N. Allahbadia et al. (eds.), *Textbook of Assisted Reproduction*, https://doi.org/10.1007/978-981-15-2377-9_44

studies in which the rate of VLBW was reported (total 27,105 MAR singletons), the RR of VLBW in the MAR group was 1.93 (95% CI 1.72–2.17), with an absolute increased risk of 1%. In the 22 studies reporting PTD (total 27,819 ART singletons), the RR was 1.54 (95% CI 1.47–1.62) and the absolute risk, 3%, and in the 11 studies reporting VPTD (total 24,170 ART singletons), the RR was 1.68 (95% CI 1.48–1.91).

The most recent meta-analysis conducted to date included 50 cohort studies with a total of 161,370 MAR-conceived singletons and 2,280,241 spontaneously conceived singletons. The RRs of LBW and VLBW in the MAR group were 1.6 (95% CI 1.49–1.75) and 2.2 (95% CI 1.84–2.43), respectively, and of PTD and VPTD, 1.71 (95% CI 1.59–1.83) and 2.12 (95% CI 1.73–2.59), respectively. The risk of perinatal death was 64% higher in the ART singletons than the controls (RR 1.64, 95% CI 1.41–1.90). MAR was also associated with significantly higher risks of maternal and obstetric complications: 30%, pregnancy-induced hypertension; 31%, gestational diabetes; 27% placenta previa; 83%, placental abruption; and 58%, cesarean section. The risks persisted even when the data analysis was restricted to studies using matched controls or adjusting for such confounders as maternal age, parity, smoking, preexisting medical conditions, and socioeconomic and demographic parameters [21, 22].

44.1.2 Perinatal Outcomes in Twins

According to the CDC MAR surveillance report, in 2013, 41.1% of all MAR pregnancies ended in multiple-birth deliveries compared with 3.5% in the general population [1]. The MAR-conceived twins were approximately 4.5 times more likely to be born before term and 6 times more likely to be born with LBW compared to MAR-conceived singletons. Consequently, there has been a widespread trend to transfer only single embryos, leading to a 22.6% decline in the percentage of MAR-conceived multiple-birth infants in the United States, from 53.1% in 2000 to 41.1% in 2013 [1].

In 2010 a Swedish national cohort study of dizygotic born in 1982–2007, 1545 MAR-conceived and 8675 spontaneously conceived, reported an increased risk of VPTD in the ART group, even after adjusting for maternal age, parity, and smoking [23]. These findings were in line with a another meta-analysis published in the same year that included a total of 4385 ART-conceived twins and 11,793 spontaneously conceived twins wherein the ART group showed a greater likelihood of premature birth and LBW after adjusting for maternal confounding factors [24]. In 2016, a meta-analysis of 15 cohort studies including 6420 ART-conceived and 13,650 spontaneously conceived dichorionic twins concluded that ART twins were at increased risk of preterm birth (RR 1.13, 95% CI 1.00–1.29; $p = 0.05$), very preterm birth (RR 1.39, 95% CI 1.07–1.82; $p = 0.01$), and LBW (RR 1.11, 95% CI 1.00–1.23; $p = 0.05$), with no statistically significant between-group difference in VLBW and perinatal mortality. However, the number of participants in each outcome analysis varied according to the number of studies reporting that outcome such that substantial heterogeneity was observed across the studies [25].

Nevertheless some studies show comparable perinatal risks of MAR multiples. A Danish national cohort study of twins born between 1995 and 2000, including 3438 conceived by ART and 10,362 conceived spontaneously, found that after stratification for maternal age and parity, there was no between-group difference in the risk of LBW, PTD, or perinatal mortality. When the study population was restricted to dizygotic twins, including 1650 ART-conceived and 3546 spontaneously conceived, the ART group had a significantly lower mean birth weight and gestational age, but these differences disappeared after the analysis was adjusted for maternal age and parity [26]. Also in 2016, a Dutch study evaluated the outcome of 6694 dizygotic twins: 470 after ovulation induction, 511 after controlled ovarian stimulation and intrauterine insemination (COH-IUI), 2437 after in vitro fertilization (IVF), and 3276 after natural conception (controls). Similar rates of LBW and prematurity were noted in the COH-IUI and IVF groups compared to controls [27].

44.1.3 Perinatal Outcomes of Fresh Versus Frozen Embryo Transfers

The practice of cryopreservation of supernumerary embryos is increasing worldwide in the wake of the cumulative, generally reassuring data in recent years in terms of achieving pregnancy, live birth rate, and obstetric and perinatal outcomes with frozen embryo transfer. However, in the absence of randomized controlled trials comparing the obstetric and perinatal outcomes of singletons born of fresh or frozen-thawed embryos, the available data so far are derived from large cohort studies and meta-analyses of observational studies.

Large registry studies from Denmark [26], Finland [28], and Sweden [29] reported a better outcome for singletons born after frozen-thawed rather than fresh embryo transfer even after adjusting for confounding variables known to have an effect on pregnancy outcome. In all three studies, infants in the frozen-thawed embryo group had a lower rate of LBW and, in some cases, a decreased risk of PTD. Perinatal mortality was comparable between the groups in the Danish and Finnish studies, whereas the Swedish study reported higher rates in the frozen-thawed embryo group.

Others compared perinatal outcome between singleton infants born after ART with frozen-thawed or fresh embryo transfer and spontaneously conceived singletons, but the results were mixed. A large retrospective Nordic population-based cohort study of singletons born in the late 1990s to 2007 found that those born after frozen-thawed embryo transfer ($n = 6647$) had a lower rate of LBW (aOR 0.81 95% CI 0.71–0.91) and PTD (aOR 0.84, 95% CI 0.76–0.92) than those born after fresh embryo transfer ($n = 42{,}242$) but a higher rate of perinatal mortality (aOR 1.49, 95% CI 1.07–2.07). Compared to the spontaneous conception ($n = 288{,}542$), the frozen embryo transfer group had higher rates of LBW, PTD, VLBW, and VPTD, after adjusting for maternal age, parity, offspring sex, and year of birth. The authors also reported a significant increase in the rate of cesarean section in the frozen embryo transfer group (26.3% vs. 22.6% in the fresh embryo transfer group and 15.4% in the spontaneous conception group; $p < 0.001$) [30]. These findings were corroborated by other meta-analyses which showed an association of singleton frozen-thawed pregnancies with LBW and PTD [31, 32]. In the study of Maheshwari et al. [31], the absolute risk reduction was 3% for LBW (RR 0.69, 95% CI 0.62–0.76) and 2% for PTD (RR 0.84, 95% CI 0.78–0.9), and the RR of perinatal mortality was 0.68 (95% CI 0.48–0.96). Analyses restricted to matched cohort, good-quality studies yielded a persistent risk reduction with the transfer of frozen-thawed embryos. In their meta-analysis including 32,349 frozen embryo transfer cycles and 94,472 fresh embryo transfer cycles, Zhao et al. [32] noted a decreased risk of LWB and PDT in the singletons born after fresh embryo transfer. There was no significant difference from controls in perinatal mortality.

It should be noted that all the findings described above were derived from meta-analyses of different studies with heterogeneous populations using different methods of cryopreservation (slow freezing or vitrification at the cleavage and/or the blastocyst stage), which may have affected the reported outcome.

Wennerholm et al. [30] also reported a higher birth weight of singletons following frozen embryo transfer compared with fresh embryo transfer and spontaneous conception and an increased risk of being born large for gestational age (LGA) (5.8% vs. 4% and 3.9%, respectively) and macrosomic (>4000 g) (5.7% vs. 2.8% and 3.4%, respectively). These risks were supported in a cohort study of 550 children with a sibling combination of first child fresh embryo transfer/second child frozen embryo transfer (group 1) and 116 children with a sibling combination of first child frozen embryo transfer/second child fresh embryo transfer (group 2), with adjustment for birth order. Taking into account that second children are generally heavier than first-born children, the authors found a higher risk of LGA for the first sibling combination, although it was still significantly increased for the second sibling combination [33]. The reason for the higher birth weight in singletons born after frozen embryo transfer is still unclear. One possible mechanism is compromise of the intrauterine environment by COH in fresh cycles, with better placentation and overgrowth in frozen cycles. However, this does not explain the higher risk of LGA in singletons born after frozen embryo transfer than in naturally conceived singletons. Another possible mechanism involves fetal growth-related epigenetic modifications of the human embryo during cryopreservation and thawing.

A recent study based on data provided by the Human Fertilization and Embryology Authority (HFEA) included 112,432 singletons born in 1991–2011 in the United Kingdom: 95,911 after fresh embryo transfer and 16,521 after frozen embryo transfer. The frozen embryo transfer group had a decreased risk for LBW (RR 0.73, 95% CI 0.66–0.80) and VLBW (RR 0.78, 95% CI 0.63–0.96) and an increased risk of high birth weight (>4 kg) (RR 1.64, 95% CI 1.53–1.76), with no between-group difference in the risk of preterm and very preterm deliveries. This study had the advantages of access to one of the largest national datasets available in addition to the possibility to adjust for important confounding factors of maternal age and parity and cause and duration of infertility [34].

44.2 Causes of Adverse Outcomes

There is an ongoing debate as to whether adverse perinatal outcomes of MAR pregnancies are related to the technology or to the infertility itself. There is an inherent problem in studies comparing MAR-conceived with spontaneously conceived singletons because of the a priori condition of the mothers: subfertile with underlying reproductive abnormalities or healthy and fertile and drawn from the general population. Accordingly, singletons born to women with at least 1 year of involuntary childlessness were found to be at increased obstetric and perinatal risks compared to singletons born to fertile women, after adjusting for age and parity [35, 36].

In a further attempt to isolate the effects of these factors, several groups from different countries used a sibship study design. The cohorts consisted of consecutive singleton sibling pairs in which one sibling was MAR-conceived and the other, spontaneously conceived, However, the results were conflicting. In the study from Norway including 2546 sibling pairs, perinatal outcome was similar in the MAR and spontaneous conception groups, and the authors conclude that the increased perinatal risk of MAR babies was related to factors that led to the mothers' infertility [37]. A larger, more recent, study from Holland analyzed 272,551 sibling pairs using both inter-sibling and sibship analyses, taking mode of conception, maternal characteristics, and birth order into account. The results showed that maternal characteristics, including subfertility, were associated with an increased risk of perinatal mortality, LBW, and PTD [38]. By contrast, however, a Danish sibship study of 13,692 singleton sibling pairs demonstrated an increased perinatal risk in the MAR babies than in the spontaneously conceived babies. Although the risk in the MAR group showed a trend toward a decrease, the difference from controls was significant and persistent. These findings indicated that treatment factors may be at least partially liable for the adverse outcome associated with MAR [39].

Using another approach, several studies compared singletons born after different fertility treatments, namely, ovulation induction, intrauterine insemination, and in vitro fertilization; spontaneously conceived singletons served as controls. They found an increased risk associated with fertility treatment regardless of the type of treatment used, indicating that the technology itself was apparently not exclusively responsible for adverse outcome [12, 40]. The authors suggested that ovarian stimulation may lead to the production of several corpora lutea of varying function or adversely affect the growing follicle and developing oocyte. Alternatively, ovarian stimulation may be associated with an increased excretion of insulin-like growth factor binding protein (IGFBP)-1, which is linked to fetal growth restriction and placental structural abnormalities [41].

To date the largest prospective study of this issue was conducted in China in 2016. A total of 5639 singleton babies were included: 1260 born after IVF, 1899 born after non-ART treatments to subfertile women, and 2480 naturally conceived babies of fertile women. The analyses were adjusted for important confounding factors. Compared to the spontaneously conceived group, the babies born to subfertile mothers were at increased risk of LBW and PTD. However, the ART-conceived babies were at highest risk of all the groups, with an aOR of 1.75 for LBW (95% CI 1.12–2.92) and aOR of 1.26 for PTD (95% CI 1.01–1.53) [13].

44.3 Attempts to Reduce the Adverse Perinatal Outcome of MAR Singletons

44.3.1 Single-Embryo Transfer

To avoid multiple pregnancies in MAR and their accompanying adverse effects, researchers are attempting to transfer only single embryos in MAR cycles. This has been made possible with recent improvements in culture conditions and cryopreservation and the establishment of morphologic criteria defining the highest quality embryos with the best chance of implantation. Greater emphasis has also been placed on patient education for better implementation of this practice worldwide.

In regular stimulated IVF cycles, it is often possible to select the embryo of highest quality among the high-quality embryos available. This procedure is termed elective single-embryo transfer (e-SET). Randomized controlled studies of cleavage-stage embryos have shown that fresh e-SET yields comparable pregnancy rates to the transfer of two embryos simultaneously, with a significant reduction in the rate of multiple gestations and adverse perinatal and obstetric outcomes. Similar findings were noted for blastocyst-stage embryos. Birth rates were not significantly compromised when either cleavage-stage or blastocyst-stage embryos were used. [42]. Others reported that singletons born after elective SET had a substantially reduced risk of PTD (RR 0.37, 95% CI 0.25–0.55) and LBW (RR 0.25, 95% CI 0.15–0.45) than singletons born after double-embryo transfer. Compared to spontaneously conceived singletons, they had a barely detectable increased risk of PTD, placenta previa, and gestational diabetes [43].

Promising findings for SET have also been reported in terms of perinatal mortality relative to double-embryo transfer (DET). A large population study from Australia and New Zealand including more than 50,000 singleton births noted a 53% higher perinatal mortality rate in the DET group than the SET group (aRR 1.53, 95% CI 1.29–1.8) [44]. Furthermore, the transfer of a single embryo, whether elective or not, almost completely eliminated the vanishing twin phenomenon (birth of a singleton after the co-twin disappeared), which has been associated with an increased likelihood of LBW and PTD compared to IVF pregnancies that were originally singletons [45]. It is still unknown if the increased adverse outcome of IVF singletons with a vanished co-twin is due to the absorption of necrotic fetoplacental tissue by the remaining twin, followed by the release of cytokines and prostaglandins, or to impaired utero-fetal interaction leading to the fetal demise of one twin [45, 46]. Nevertheless, it should be borne in mind that monozygotic twinning can still occur with the transfer of a single embryo [47] and that twins born after DET have half the risk of perinatal mortality than monozygotic twins born after SET (aRR 0.48, 95% CI 0.32–0.72) [44].

The most recent large population study of SET included more than 140,000 live births in Japan between 2007 and 2012. The results showed that the use of SET has substantially reduced perinatal morbidity, including PTD and LBW, and perinatal mortality [48].

44.3.2 Day of Embryo Transfer: Blastocyst Versus Cleavage

Culturing cleavage-stage embryos (day 2–3) to the blastocyst stage (day 5–6) enables the clinician to select the highest-quality embryos for transfer based on the morphological score. Furthermore, women who undergo blastocyst-stage embryo transfer constitute a selective cohort with distinct characteristics and a good prognosis. They are possibly younger with a higher ovarian response to treatment than women who undergo cleavage-stage embryo transfer. Nevertheless, there is still a risk of cancelled embryo transfer due to unsuccessful culturing. Extending embryo time in culture conditions beyond genomic activation could have genetic and epigenetic effects on trophoectodermic cells, triggering differences in implantation and placentation and leading to adverse perinatal outcomes [49–52]. Although the current literature suggests that transferring a fresh single blastocyst embryo yields higher rates of clinical pregnancy and live birth than transferring a cleavage-state embryo [53, 54], the quality of the evidence is moderate to low, and large randomized controlled studies are still needed to draw a definitive conclusion [55].

A large population-based Swedish registry study compared the perinatal outcome of singletons born after blastocyst-stage transfer (n = 4819), cleavage-stage transfer (n = 25,747), or spontaneous conception (n = 1,196,394) between 2002 and 2013. The blastocyst-transfer group was found to be at increased risk of perinatal mortality (aOR 1.16, 95% CI 1.14–2.29) compared to the cleavage-embryo group and at increased risk of PTD compared to the spontaneous-conception group (aOR 1.17, 95% CI, 1.05–1.31). They also had an increased risk of placenta previa and placental abruption. There was a lower rate of LBW and a higher rate of macrosmic (>4500 g) infants despite lower rates of gestational diabetes in the blastocyst group [56].

Systematic reviews and meta-analyses report an increased risk of PTD and VPTD with extended culture [57–59]. However, these findings referred to singletons resulting from the transfer of more than one embryo, with no way to account for the vanishing twin phenomenon which is known to affect perinatal outcome. Some of the studies that adjusted for the vanishing twin phenomenon and possible maternal confounders reported an increased risk of PTD and VPTD with extended embryo culture (aOR 1.39, 95% CI 1.29–1.50 and aOR 1.35, 95% CI 1.13–1.61) [60] whereas others found comparable perinatal outcomes, including LBW and PTD, to cleavage-stage transfer [61]. The latter studies were in agreement with a large recent population study from Australia and New Zealand including more than 40,000 singleton deliveries which yielded similar rates of PTD and LBW in the two groups [62]. Studies analyzing singletons born after SET of a cleavage or a blastocyst embryo also found no between-group differences [63] even when the groups were matched for maternal confounders and embryo quality [64].

The largest study to date evaluated the outcome of 277,042 singletons from single-embryo transfers of fresh and frozen-thawed cleavage- and blastocyst-stage embryos in Japan between 2008 and 2010. Frozen transfer was associated with a significantly reduced risk of PTD and LBW but a higher incidence of placenta accrete. There was no significant association between blastocyst transfer and maternal risk [65].

Studies evaluating perinatal outcome after fresh and vitrified-thawed blastocyst embryo transfers show comparable findings, although vitrification was associated with an overall higher birth weight [66] even when restricted to e-SETs [67] similar to findings reported for cleavage-stage embryo transfers.

44.3.3 Type of Culture Medium

Not only extended time under culture conditions but also the type of culture medium has an effect on the perinatal outcome. Genes responsible for cell cycle and DNA replication have been shown to favor certain types of media over others [68]. Furthermore, the source of the proteins found in embryo culture was found to be an independent factor affecting birth weight [69].

However, the effect of the type of culture medium on birth weight is controversial. A study from Holland was the first to report an association of lower mean singleton birth weight with in vitro embryo culture in Cook medium as opposed to Vitrolife medium, regardless of whether the embryos were fresh or frozen-thawed [70, 71]. Others reported a higher rate of LBW among singletons conceived after embryo culture in Medicult ISMI medium compared to Medicult Universal or Vitrolife GI medium [72, 73]. By contrast, numerous studies failed to find significant differences in the mean singleton birth weight by type of culture medium used (G1.3/Global/G1.5, HTF/Sage, G5tm/Global/Quinn Advantage, Medicult/Cook/Vitrolife, and Cook/Medicult) [74–78]. Most recently, no significant differences in mean singleton birth weight were observed between Medicult- and Vitrolife-cultured embryos after controlling for potential confounders and adjusting for culture duration [79]. A review summarizing the current literature concluded that although extreme differences in birth weight have been observed in animal studies, the relationship between certain types of culture medium and birth weight in humans is less clear-cut. Of the 11 relevant studies published to date, 5 reported a significant relationship [80].

44.3.4 Embryo Quality

Embryo quality, defined by strict morphological parameters, is a major predictor of the success of ART. The association of cleavage-stage embryo quality with implantation rate and pregnancy outcome is well established [81–83]. There are numerous reports of an association between blastocyst morphology and rates of implantation, clinical pregnancy, and live birth. Which of the three main morphologic characteristics of blastocysts, namely, blastocyst expansion and hatching [84, 85], appearance of the trophectoderm cells [86, 87], or appearance of the inner cell mass (ICM) [88], is the strongest predictor of implantation and live birth remains unclear.

The first study to evaluate the possible association of embryo quality with perinatal complications was performed on singletons born after fresh cleavage- or blastocyst-stage SET to ensure that the baby delivered was from the embryo that was morphologically graded. Good-quality single-embryo transfers were compared with poor-quality SETs. The good-quality embryo transfers were associated with higher clinical pregnancy rate, but there was no significant between-group difference in maternal or neonatal adverse outcomes after adjusting for important confounders [89]. A more recent study from Japan also found comparable perinatal outcomes for good-quality and poor-quality cleavage-stage embryos, but it included both fresh and frozen embryo transfer and did not adjust for potential confounders [90]. There is strong need for additional large randomized controlled studies to corroborate the absence of short- and long-term adverse consequences to the offspring with the use of poor-quality as opposed to good-quality embryos.

44.3.5 Minimal Ovarian Stimulation

It is unclear if the response to ovarian stimulation affects the obstetric outcomes of IVF treatment. A recent study based on data provided by the Human Fertilization and Embryology Act (HFEA) included 591,003 fresh IVF cycles, of which 584,835 were stimulated and 6168 were unstimulated, resulting in 98,667 singleton live births. After adjusting for potential confounders, no significant difference was found between the stimulated and unstimulated cycles in the risk of preterm birth (aOR 1.43, 95% CI 0.91–2.26) and LBW (aOR 1.58, 95% CI 0.96–2.58) [91]. When the same group analyzed the role of ovarian response using a large national database of 402,185 stimulated fresh IVF cycles resulting in 65,868 singleton live births, they found a significantly higher risk of adverse outcomes in women with an excessive response (≥20 oocytes) than in women with a normal response (10–15 oocytes) (preterm birth: aOR 1.15, 95% CI 1.03–1.28; LBW: aOR 1.17, 95% CI 1.05–1.30). There was no increased risk in the women with a suboptimal (4–9 oocytes) or poor response (<3 oocytes). This study, however, was limited by a failure to adjust for confounding factors and the inclusion of women with more than one cycle in the dataset such that the true sample size was unknown. Furthermore, the high-responder group had a high prevalence of women with polycystic ovary syndrome, which is known to be associated with preterm birth and LBW [92]. Therefore, further studies are needed to determine if the increased risk is attributable to the underlying diagnosis or to treatment-associated parameters such as the high estradiol level during embryo implantation.

44.4 Conclusions

Singletons conceived by ART are at increased risk of adverse maternal and perinatal outcomes compared to spontaneously conceived singletons. Although the underlying infertility is probably at least partly responsible, the technology plays an important role as well. Great effort has been exerted to improve perinatal outcome, including the use of single-embryo transfer, avoiding hyperstimulated cycles with vastly elevated E2 levels, employing different culture conditions, and freezing all embryos. While all of these methods are promising, none are without risk themselves.

References

1. Sunderam S, Kissin DM, Crawford SB, Folger SG, Jamieson DJ, Warner L, Barfield WD. Assisted reproductive technology surveillance – United States, 2013. Centers for Disease Control and Prevention (CDC). MMWR Surveill Summ. 2015;64:1–25.
2. Calhaz-Jorge C, de Geyter C, Kupka MS, de Mouzon J, Erb K, Mocanu E, et al. Assisted reproductive technology in Europe, 2012: results generated from European registers by ESHRE. Hum Reprod. 2016;3:1638–52.
3. Kissin DM, Jamieson DJ, Barfield WD. Monitoring health outcomes of assisted reproductive technology. N Engl J Med. 2014;371:91–3.
4. Jackson RA, Gibson KA, Wu YW, Croughan MS. Perinatal outcomes in singletons in vitro fertilization: a meta-analysis. Obstet Gynecol. 2004;103:551–3.
5. Romundstad LB, Romundstad PR, Sunde A, von Düring V, Skjaerven R, Vatten LJ. Increased risk of placenta previa in pregnancies following IVF/ICSI; a comparison of ART and non-ART pregnancies in the same mother. Hum Reprod. 2006;21:2353–8.
6. Reddy UM, Wapner RJ, Rebar RW, Tasca RJ. Infertility, assisted reproductive technology, and adverse pregnancy outcomes: executive summary of a National Institute of Child Health and Human Development workshop. Obstet Gynecol. 2007;109:967–77.
7. McDonald SD, Han Z, Mulla S, Murphy KE, Beyene J, Ohlsson A, Knowledge Synthesis Group. Preterm birth and low birth weight among in vitro fertilization singletons: a systematic review and meta-analyses. Eur J Obstet Gynecol Reprod Biol. 2009;146:138–48.
8. Cooper AR, O'Neill KE, Allsworth JE, Jungheim ES, Odibo AO, Gray DL, et al. Smaller fetal size in singletons after infertility therapies: the influence of technology and the underlying infertility. Fertil Steril. 2011;96:1100–6.
9. Pandey S, Shetty A, Hamilton M, Bhattacharya S, Maheshwari A. Obstetric and perinatal outcomes in singleton pregnancies resulting from IVF/ICSI: a systematic review and meta-analysis. Hum Reprod Update. 2012;18:485–503.
10. Pinborg A, Wennerholm UB, Romundstad LB, Loft A, Aittomaki K, Soderstrom-Anttila V, et al. Why do singletons conceived after assisted reproduction technology have adverse perinatal outcome? Systematic review and meta-analysis. Hum Reprod Update. 2013;19:87–104.
11. Sazonova A, Källen K, Thurin-Kjellberg A, Wennerholm UB, Bergh C. Obstetric outcome after in vitro fertilization with single or double embryo transfer. Hum Reprod. 2011;26:442–50.
12. Hayashi M, Nakai A, Satoh S, Matsuda Y. Adverse obstetric and perinatal outcomes of singleton pregnancies may be related to maternal factors associated with infertility rather than the type

of assisted reproductive technology procedure used. Fertil Steril. 2012;98:922–8.
13. Qin J, Sheng X, Wu D, Gao S, You Y, Yang T, Wang H. Adverse obstetric outcomes associated with in vitro fertilization in singleton pregnancies: a prospective cohort study. Reprod Sci. 2016. [Epub ahead of print].
14. Sazonova A, Källen K, Thurin-Kjellberg A, Wennerholm UB, Bergh C. Factors affecting obstetric outcome of singletons born after IVF. Hum Reprod. 2011;26:2878–86.
15. Barker DJ. The origins of the developmental origins theory. J Intern Med. 2007;261:412–7.
16. Calkins K, Devaskar SU. Fetal origins of adult disease. Curr Probl Pediatr Adolesc Health Care. 2011;41:158–76.
17. Helmerhorst FM, Perquin DA, Donker D, Keirse MJ. Perinatal outcome of singletons and twins after assisted conception: a systematic review of controlled studies. BMJ. 2004;328:261–5.
18. Jackson RA, Gibson KA, Wu YW, Croughan MS. Perinatal outcomes in singletons following in vitro fertilization: a meta-analysis. Obstet Gynecol. 2004;103:551–63.
19. McGovern PG, Llorens AJ, Skurnick JH, Weiss G, Goldsmith LT. Increased risk of preterm birth in singleton pregnancies resulting from in vitro fertilization-embryo transfer or gamete intrafallopian transfer: a meta-analysis. Fertil Steril. 2004;82:1514–20.
20. Schieve LA, Ferre C, Peterson HB, Macaluso M, Reynolds MA, Wright VC. Perinatal outcome among singleton infants conceived through assisted reproductive technology in the United States. Obstet Gynecol. 2004;103:1144–53.
21. Qin J, Liu X, Sheng X, Wang H, Gao S. Assisted reproductive technology and the risk of pregnancy-related complications and adverse pregnancy outcomes in singleton pregnancies: a meta-analysis of cohort studies. Fertil Steril. 2016;105:73–85.e1–6.
22. Pinborg A, Loft A, Rasmussen S, Schmidt L, Langhoff-Roos J, Greisen G, Andersen AN. Neonatal outcome in a Danish national cohort of 3438 IVF/ICSI and 10,362 non-IVF/ICSI twins born between 1995 and 2000. Hum Reprod. 2004;19:435–41.
23. Kallen B, Finnström O, Lindam A, Nilsson E, Nygren KG, Olausson PO. Selected neonatal outcomes in dizygotic twins after IVF versus non-IVF pregnancies. BJOG. 2010;11:676–82.
24. McDonald SD, Han Z, Mulla S, Ohlsson A, Beyene J, Murphy KE, Knowledge Synthesis Group. Preterm birth and low birth weight among in vitro fertilization twins: a systematic review and meta-analyses. Eur J Obstet Gynecol Reprod Biol. 2010;148:105–13.
25. Qin JB, Wang H, Sheng X, Xie Q, Gao S. Assisted reproductive technology and risk of adverse obstetric outcomes in dichorionic twin pregnancies: a systematic review and meta-analysis. Fertil Steril. 2016;105:1180–92.
26. Pinborg A, Loft A, Aaris Henningsen AK, Rasmussen S, Andersen AN. Infant outcome of 957 singletons born after frozen embryo replacement: the Danish National Cohort Study 1995–2006. Fertil Steril. 2010;94:1320–7.
27. Bensdorp AJ, Hukkelhoven CW, van der Veen F, Mol BW, Lambalk CB, van Wely M. Dizygotic twin pregnancies after medically assisted reproduction and after natural conception: maternal and perinatal outcomes. Fertil Steril. 2016;106:371–7.e2.
28. Pelkonen S, Koivunen R, Gissler M, Nuojua-Huttunen S, Suikkari AM, Hydén-Granskog C, et al. Perinatal outcome of children born after frozen and fresh embryo transfer: the Finnish cohort study 1995-2006. Hum Reprod. 2010;25:914–23.
29. Sazonova A, Källen K, Thurin-Kjellberg A, Wennerholm UB, Bergh C. Obstetric outcome in singletons after in vitro fertilization with cryopreserved/thawed embryos. Hum Reprod. 2012;27:1343–50.
30. Wennerholm UB, Henningsen AK, Romundstad LB, Bergh C, Pinborg A, Skjaerven R, et al. Perinatal outcomes of children born after frozen-thawed embryo transfer: a Nordic cohort study from the CoNARTaS group. Hum Reprod. 2013;28: 2545–53.
31. Maheshwari A, Pandey S, Shetty A, Hamilton M, Bhattacharya S. Obstetric and perinatal outcomes in singleton pregnancies resulting from the transfer of frozen thawed versus fresh embryos generated through in vitro fertilization treatment: a systematic review and meta-analysis. Fertil Steril. 2012;98:368–77.
32. Zhao J, Xu B, Zhang Q, Li YP. Which one has a better obstetric and perinatal outcome in singleton pregnancy, IVF/ICSI or FET? A systematic review and meta-analysis. Reprod Biol Endocrinol. 2016;14:51–7.
33. Pinborg A, Henningsen AA, Loft A, Malchau SS, Forman J, Andersen AN. Large baby syndrome in singletons born after frozen embryo transfer (FET): is it due to maternal factors or the cryotechnique? Hum Reprod. 2014;29:618–27.
34. Maheshwari A, Raja EA, Bhattacharya S. Obstetric and perinatal outcomes after either fresh or thawed frozen embryo transfer: an analysis of 112,432 singleton pregnancies recorded in the Human Fertilisation and Embryology Authority anonymized dataset. Fertil Steril. 2016;106:1703–8.
35. Ghazi HA, Spielberger C, Källén B. Delivery outcome after infertility–a registry study. Fertil Steril. 1991;55:726–32.
36. Thomson F, Shanbhag S, Templeton A, Bhattacharva S. Obstetric outcome in women with subfertility. BJOG. 2005;112:632–7.
37. Romundstad LB, Romundstad PR, Sunde A, von Düring V, Skjaerven R, Gunnell D, Vatten LJ. Effects of technology or maternal factors on perinatal outcome after assisted fertilisation: a population-based cohort study. Lancet. 2008;372:737–43.
38. Seggers J, Pontesilli M, Ravelli AC, Painter RC, Hadders-Algra M, Heineman MJ, et al. Effects of in vitro fertilization and maternal characteristics on perinatal outcomes: a population-based study using siblings. Fertil Steril. 2016;105:590–8.e2.
39. Henningsen AK, Pinborg A, Lidegaard Ø, Vestergaard C, Forman JL, Andersen AN. Perinatal outcome of singleton siblings born after assisted reproductive technology and spontaneous conception: Danish national sibling-cohort study. Fertil Steril. 2011;95:959–63.
40. Olivennes F, Rufat P, Andre B, Pourade A, Quiros MC, Frydman R. The increased risk of complication observed in singleton pregnancies resulting from in-vitro fertilization (IVF) does not seem to be related to the IVF method itself. Hum Reprod. 1993;8:1297–300.
41. Johnson MR, Irvine R, Hills F, Bolton VN, Abbas AA, Brooks AA, et al. Superovulation, IGFBP-1 and birth weight. Eur J Obstet Gynecol Reprod Biol. 1995;59:193–5.
42. Steinberg ML, Boulet S, Kissin D, Warner L, Jamieson DJ. Elective single embryo transfer trends and predictors of a good perinatal outcome–United States, 1999 to 2010. Fertil Steril. 2013;99:1937–43.
43. Grady R, Alavi N, Vale R, Khandwala M, McDonald SD. Elective single embryo transfer and perinatal outcomes: a systematic review and meta-analysis. Fertil Steril. 2012;97:324–31.
44. Sullivan EA, Wang YA, Hayward I, Chambers GM, Illingworth P, McBain J, Norman RJ. Single embryo transfer reduces the risk of perinatal mortality, a population study. Hum Reprod. 2012;27:3609–15.
45. Zhou L, Gao X, Wu Y, Zhang Z. Analysis of pregnancy outcomes for survivors of the vanishing twin syndrome after in vitro fertilization and embryo transfer. Eur J Obstet Gynecol Reprod Biol. 2016;203:35–9.
46. Márton V, Zádori J, Kozinszky Z, Keresztúri A. Prevalences and pregnancy outcome of vanishing twin pregnancies achieved by in vitro fertilization versus natural conception. Fertil Steril. 2016;106:1399–406.
47. Vitthala S, Gelbaya TA, Brison DR, Fitzgerald CT, Nardo LG. The risk of monozygotic twins after assisted reproductive technology: a systematic review and meta-analysis. Hum Reprod Update. 2009;15:45–55.
48. Takeshima K, Jwa SC, Saito H, Nakaza A, Kuwahara A, Ishihara O, et al. Impact of single embryo transfer policy on perinatal outcomes in fresh and frozen cycles-analysis of the Japanese Assisted

Reproduction Technology registry between 2007 and 2012. Fertil Steril. 2016;105:337–46.e3.
49. Rizos D, Lonergan P, Boland MP, Arroyo-García R, Pintado B, de la Fuente J, Gutiérrez-Adán A. Analysis of differential messenger RNA expression between bovine blastocysts produced in different culture systems: implications for blastocyst quality. Biol Reprod. 2002;66:589–95.
50. Rizos D, Ward F, Duffy P, Boland MP, Lonergan P. Consequences of bovine oocyte maturation, fertilization or early embryo development in vitro versus in vivo: implications for blastocyst yield and blastocyst quality. Mol Reprod Dev. 2002;61:234–48.
51. Turan N, Katari S, Gerson LF, Chalian R, Foster MW, Gaughan JP, et al. Inter- and intra-individual variation in allele-specific DNA methylation and gene expression in children conceived using assisted reproductive technology. PLoS Genet. 2010;6:e1001033.
52. Nelissen EC, van Montfoort AP, Dumoulin JC, Evers JL. Epigenetics and the placenta. Hum Reprod Update. 2011;17:397–417.
53. Papanikolaou EG, Camus M, Kolibianakis EM, Van Landuyt L, Van Steirteghem A, Devroey P. In vitro fertilization with single blastocyst-stage versus single cleavage-stage embryos. N Engl J Med. 2006;354:1139–46.
54. Papanikolaou EG, Kolibianakis EM, Tournaye H, Venetis CA, Fatemi H, Tarlatzis B, Devroey P. Live birth rates after transfer of equal number of blastocysts or cleavage-stage embryos in IVF. A systematic review and meta-analysis. Hum Reprod. 2008;23(1):91–9.
55. Glujovsky D, Farquhar C, Quinteiro Retamar AM, Alvarez Sedo CR, Blake D. Cleavage stage versus blastocyst stage embryo transfer in assisted reproductive technology. Cochrane Database Syst Rev. 2016;6:CD002118.
56. Ginström Ernstad E, Bergh C, Khatibi A, Källén KB, Westlander G, Nilsson S, Wennerholm UB. Neonatal and maternal outcome after blastocyst transfer: a population-based registry study. Am J Obstet Gynecol. 2016;214:378.e1–10.
57. Maheshwari A, Kalampokas T, Davidson J, Bhattacharya S. Obstetric and perinatal outcomes in singleton pregnancies resulting from the transfer of blastocyst-stage versus cleavage-stage embryos generated through in vitro fertilization treatment: a systematic review and meta-analysis. Fertil Steril. 2013;100:1615–21.e1–10.
58. Martins WP, Nastri CO, Rienzi L, van der Poel SZ, Gracia CR, Racowsky C. Obstetrical and perinatal outcomes following blastocyst transfer compared to cleavage transfer: a systematic review and meta-analysis. Hum Reprod. 2016;31:2561–9.
59. Dar S, Librach CL, Gunby J, Bissonnette F, Cowan L. Increased risk of preterm birth in singleton pregnancies after blastocyst versus day 3 embryo transfer: Canadian ART register (CARTER) analysis. Hum Reprod. 2013;28:924–8.
60. Kalra SK, Ratcliffe SJ, Barnhart KT, Coutifaris C. Extended embryo culture and an increased risk of preterm delivery. Obstet Gynecol. 2012;12:69–75.
61. Fernando D, Halliday JL, Breheny S, Healy DL. Outcomes of singleton births after blastocyst versus nonblastocyst transfer in assisted reproductive technology. Fertil Steril. 2012;97:579–84.
62. Chambers GM, Chughtai AA, Farquhar CM, Wang YA. Risk of preterm birth after blastocyst embryo transfer: a large population study using contemporary registry data from Australia and New Zealand. Fertil Steril. 2015;104:997–1003.
63. Oron G, Sokal-Arnon T, Son WY, Demirtas E, Buckett W, Zeadna A, et al. Extended embryo culture is not associated with increased adverse obstetric or perinatal outcome. Am J Obstet Gynecol. 2014;211:165.e1–7.
64. Oron G, Nayot D, Son WY, Holzer H, Buckett W, Tulandi T. Obstetric and perinatal outcome from single cleavage transfer and single blastocyst transfer: a matched case-control study. Gynecol Endocrinol. 2015;31:469–72.
65. Ishihara O, Araki R, Kuwahara A, Itakura A, Saito H, Adamson GD. Impact of frozen-thawed single-blastocyst transfer on maternal and neonatal outcome: an analysis of 277,042 single-embryo transfer cycles from 2008 to 2010 in Japan. Fertil Steril. 2014;101:128–33.
66. Wikland M, Hardarson T, Hillensjö T, Westin C, Westlander G, Wood M, Wennerholm UB. Obstetric outcomes after transfer of vitrified blastocysts. Hum Reprod. 2010;25:1699–707.
67. Roy TK, Bradley CK, Bowman MC, McArthur SJ. Single-embryo transfer of vitrified-warmed blastocysts yields equivalent live-birth rates and improved neonatal outcomes compared with fresh transfers. Fertil Steril. 2014;101:1294–301.
68. Kleijkers SH, Eijssen LM, Coonen E, Derhaag JG, Mantikou E, Jonker MJ, et al. Differences in gene expression profiles between human preimplantation embryos cultured in two different IVF culture media. Hum Reprod. 2015;30:2303–11.
69. Zhu J, Li M, Chen L, Liu P, Qiao J. The protein source in embryo culture media influences birthweight: a comparative study between G1 v5 and G1-PLUS v5. Hum Reprod. 2014;29:1387–92.
70. Dumoulin JC, Land JA, Van Montfoort AP, Nelissen EC, Coonen E, Derhaag JG, et al. Effect of in vitro culture of human embryos on birthweight of newborns. Hum Reprod. 2010;25:605–12.
71. Nelissen EC, Van Montfoort AP, Coonen E, Derhaag JG, Geraedts JP, et al. Further evidence that culture media affect perinatal outcome: findings after transfer of fresh and cryopreserved embryos. Hum Reprod. 2012;27:1966–76.
72. Eskild A, Monkerud L, Tanbo T. Birthweight and placental weight; do changes in culture media used for IVF matter? Comparisons with spontaneous pregnancies in the corresponding time periods. Hum Reprod. 2013;28:3207–14.
73. Hassani F, Eftekhari-Yazdi P, Karimian L, Valojerdi MR, Maovaghar B, Fazel M, et al. The effects of ISM1 medium on embryo quality and outcomes of IVF/ICSI cycles. Int J Fertil Steril. 2013;7:108–15.
74. Eaton JL, Lieberman ES, Stearns C, Chinchilla M, Racowsky C. Embryo culture media and neonatal birthweight following IVF. Hum Reprod. 2012;27:375–9.
75. Vergouw CG, Kostelijk EH, Doejaaren E, Hompes PG, Lambalk CB, Schats R. The influence of the type of embryo culture medium on neonatal birthweight after single embryo transfer in IVF. Hum Reprod. 2012;27:2619–26.
76. Carrasco B, Boada M, Rodriguez I, Coroleu B, Barri PN, Veiga A. Does culture medium influence offspring birth weight? Fertil Steril. 2013;100:1283–8.
77. Lin S, Li M, Lian Y, Chen L, Liu P. No effect of embryo culture media on birthweight and length of newborns. Hum Reprod. 2013;28:1762–7.
78. Lemmen JG, Pinborg A, Rasmussen S, Ziebe S. Birthweight distribution in ART singletons resulting from embryo culture in two different culture media compared with the national population. Hum Reprod. 2014;29:2326–32.
79. De Vos A, Janssens R, Van de Velde H, Haentjens P, Bonduelle M, Tournaye H, Verheyen G. The type of culture medium and the duration of in vitro culture do not influence birthweight of ART singletons. Hum Reprod. 2015;30:20–7.
80. Zandstra H, Van Montfoort AP, Dumoulin JC. Does the type of culture medium used influence birthweight of children born after IVF? Hum Reprod. 2015;30:530–42.
81. Giorgetti C, Terriou P, Auquier P, Hans E, Spach JL, Salzmann J, Roulier R. Embryo score to predict implantation after in vitro fertilization: based on 957 single embryo transfers. Hum Reprod. 1995;10:2427–31.
82. Ziebe S, Petersen K, Lindenberg S, Andersen AG, Gabrielsen A, Andersen AN. Embryo morphology or cleavage stage: how to select the best embryos for transfer after in-vitro fertilization. Hum Reprod. 1997;12:1545–9.

83. Van Royen E, Mangelschots K, De Neubourg D, Valkenburg M, Van de Meerssche M, Ryckaert G, et al. Characterization of a top quality embryo, a step towards single-embryo transfer. Hum Reprod. 1999;14:2345–9.
84. Balaban B, Urman B, Sertac A, Alatas C, Aksoy S, Mercan R. Blastocyst quality affects the success of blastocyst-stage embryo transfer. Fertil Steril. 2000;74:282–7.
85. Van den Abbeel E, Balaban B, Ziebe S, Lundin K, Cuesta MJ, Klein BM, et al. Association between blastocyst morphology and outcome of single-blastocyst transfer. Reprod Biomed Online. 2013;27:353–61.
86. Ahlstrom A, Westin C, Reismer E, Wikland M, Hardarson T. Trophectoderm morphology: an important parameter for predicting live birth after single blastocyst transfer. Hum Reprod. 2011;26:3289–96.
87. Hill MJ, Richter KS, Heitmann RJ, Graham JR, Tucker MJ, DeCherney AH, et al. Trophectoderm grade predicts outcomes of single-blastocyst transfers. Fertil Steril. 2013;99: 1283–9.
88. Richter KS, Harris DC, Daneshmand ST, Shapiro BS. Quantitative grading of a human blastocyst: optimal inner cell mass size and shape. Fertil Steril. 2001;76:1157–67.
89. Oron G, Son WY, Buckett W, Tulandi T, Holzer H. The association between embryo quality and perinatal outcome of singletons born after single embryo transfers: a pilot study. Hum Reprod. 2014;29:1444–51.
90. Nakagawa K, Ojiro Y, Nishi Y, Sugiyama R, Motoyama H, Sugiyama R. Perinatal outcomes of patients who achieved pregnancy with a morphologically poor embryo via assisted reproductive technology. Arch Gynecol Obstet. 2016;293:183–8.
91. Sunkara SK, LaMarca A, Polyzos NP, Seed PT, Khalaf Y. Live birth and perinatal outcomes following stimulated and unstimulated IVF: analysis of over two decades of a nationwide data. Hum Reprod. 2016;31:2261–7.
92. Sunkara SK, La Marca A, Seed PT, Khalaf Y. Increased risk of preterm birth and low birthweight with very high number of oocytes following IVF: an analysis of 65 868 singleton live birth outcomes. Hum Reprod. 2015;30:1473–80.

45 Effect of Conception Using Assisted Reproduction Technologies (ARTs) on Infant Health and Development

Virender Verma and Priya Soni

45.1 Background and Introduction

A detailed expatiation of what artificial reproduction technologies (ARTs) are and what are their various methods, their indication, and pros and cons have already been described in preceding chapters of this book. The first test tube baby was born in 1978 [1], and after that about 7 million children have been born so far by assisted reproduction techniques, and 2–3% of deliveries in developed countries are ART conceptions [2]! The number is significant enough to warrant a detailed analysis of the problems (if any) which might be associated with these babies.

The artificial reproduction technology procedures are way different than the natural way of conceiving, and it clearly associated with pumping of hormones and other drugs to the mother, also artificial reproduction technology is often tried in relatively older females, all these factors result in mental, physical and social stress which might have some effects over the fetal and newborn health. Further, more the perinatal events, viz., multiple pregnancies, premature labor, small for gestation babies, etc., might add into the increased risk of morbidity.

There is an array of published literature on growth and well-being of ART-conceived babies, and this chapter will look into major evidence available so far and find out "Are children conceived through artificial reproduction technologies at more risk of developing health issues in comparison to normally conceived babies?"

V. Verma (✉)
Ruban's Ratan Hospital for Women and Children, Patna, India

P. Soni
Emergency Medicine, Ruban Memorial Hospital, Patna, India

45.2 Pregnancies Conceived by Artificial Reproduction Technologies and Perinatal Outcomes

45.2.1 Immediate Neonatal Outcomes

Babies born after ART conception are considered to be at increased likelihood of being low birth weight, preterm and/or premature labor/delivery, in utero growth retardation (IUGR), morbidity and neonatal intensive care unit (NICU) admission [3]. This can be because of multiple embryo implantations resulting to multiple pregnancies. Almost one quarter to half of artificial reproduction technology-conceived deliveries are multiple deliveries [4]. Single embryo transfer (SET) is a relatively newer technique which is associated with lower likelihood of multiple gestation [5] and thus has potential to provide better outcomes in terms of lower rates of premature labor and hence lesser low birth weight babies (LBW) [6].

There are studies which eliminated confounding factor (i.e., multiple pregnancy) by considering only singleton deliveries, and it was found that the likelihood of adverse events (preterm delivery, low birth weight, neonatal intensive care unit admission rates and hospital stay, etc.) was still high [7, 8]. One meta-analysis concluded that in artificial reproduction technology-conceived singleton pregnancies, there was almost double chances of adverse perinatal events, viz., death, low birth weight delivery, and/or premature birth; substantially increased risk of delivery a small for gestation baby; and almost 30–40% increment in risk of birth of a baby with congenital malformation [9]. Henningsen et al., in a large cohort of 13,692 singleton children born after artificial reproduction technology conception, concluded that an artificial reproduction technology baby was approximately 65 g lighter and there were 40% more chances of delivering a low birth weight baby and 30% increased likelihood of premature delivery [7]. Furthermore, artificial reproduction technologies are mostly a treatment option for subfertility and/or any other etiology when normal conception is not possible; thus,

G. N. Allahbadia et al. (eds.), *Textbook of Assisted Reproduction*, https://doi.org/10.1007/978-981-15-2377-9_45

the baseline problem might change the course of perinatal events [10]. A Norwegian study concluded that perinatal morbidity and mortality were significantly higher in ART-conceived babies, but when the perinatal adverse events were compared with previous pregnancies in the same couple, the differences became non-significant [11]. Hayashi et al., in their retrospective study (which was published in 2012), compared the perinatal events in singleton deliveries conceived after ART methods (viz., intrauterine stimulation, ovulation stimulation, in vitro fertilization) with who were conceived through ovulation stimulation, intrauterine insemination (IUI), in vitro fertilization (IVF) and normal conception, and it was found that adverse events were similar regardless of the type of artificial reproduction technology used [10].

The mortality and morbidity statistics in ART-assisted twin pregnancies is inconclusive because many articles advocate that ART-assisted twin pregnancies have increased perinatal adverse outcomes, viz., increased chances of low birth weight babies, premature deliveries, and neonatal intensive care unit admissions when compared with twin deliveries conceived naturally [12, 13]. On the contrary few studies differ in outcomes [9, 14].

Therefore, generally speaking, the newborn is at increased risk of morbidity and mortality if the conception was assisted by artificial reproduction technologies. One of the etiological contributors could be subfertility.

45.3 Congenital Malformation

There are several articles which conclude that babies born after artificial reproduction technology-assisted conception have increased chances of having congenital malformations [9, 15–17]. Wen et al., in their meta-analysis consisting of 1,24,468 children born by different artificial reproduction technologies (like in vitro fertilization (IVF)/intracytoplasmic sperm injection, etc.), estimated a pooled-risk equal to 1.37 [CI 95% (1.26–1.48)], but when individual ART methods, (i.e., in vitro fertilization and intracytoplasmic sperm injection) were compared in subgroup analysis, the risk difference was insignificant. The risk of congenital malformation was maximum in the nervous system (more than double the risk as compared to natural conception), followed by the renal and genitourinary system, gastrointestinal system, and cardiovascular system [17]. On the other hand, a large Chinese study showed no significant difference in incidence of congenital malformation as compared to normal population [18].

As alluded earlier, subfertility is a confounding factor for congenital defects [19]; therefore, it could be an independent risk factor for causation of birth defects in the offspring. Hence it is unfair to blame the ART conception as a sole reason for congenital malformations unless we have enough evidence. It was shown by Davies et al. that infertility is an independent contributor to birth defects irrespective of mode of conception [16]. Bonduelle et al. compared birth defects in 5-year-old children born after in vitro fertilization (IVF) versus intracytoplasmic sperm injection (ICSI) and found that the birth defects were clearly more frequent ICSI-assisted conceptions [20]. An Australian study also found similar results [16]. However, many later articles found insignificant difference in congenital malformations on comparing children born as a result of ICSI technology with in vitro fertilization (IVF)-conceived children [17, 21].

At present we can state that more research is warranted to firmly conclude about the real etiological causes of birth defect in ART-conceived offspring whether it is a mode of conception, subfertility, or any other dependent/independent factor.

45.4 Long-Term Health Outcome in ART-Conceived Offspring

45.4.1 Growth and Gonadal Development

A myriad of studies supports the notion that the growth is similar in ART-conceived children when compared to naturally conceived children [20, 22, 23]. On the contrary, a few studies also say that ART-conceived children have more height [24]. It is hypothesized that increased quantity of insulin-like growth factors I and insulin-like growth factor binding protein is responsible for increased growth in these children [25].

The sexual organ development is an important concern in this subgroup of population because artificial reproduction is a modality for subfertile/infertile parents, and it has always been a point of concern that the children born out of ART conception have normal sexual development. There are studies to confirm that sexual development is normal in ART-conceived children [26–29].

The size of penis and testes volume was found to be normal in boys in the age group of 8–14 years. This study also found normal level of anti-Mullerian hormone (AMH) [26]. Belva et al. found salivary testosterone and inhibin B were within normal range [28]. A research on the pubertal girls (born by intracytoplasmic sperm injection) found insignificant difference in gonadal development, pubic hair growth, and menarche, but the development of breasts was lagging in these girls [29].

45.5 Physical Health

Most of the published articles about physical well-being support the fact that there is hardly any difference in pattern of childhood illnesses of children conceived through ARTs as compared to those conceived naturally. Beydoun et al. found insignificant difference in chronic diseases pattern of ART conceived in young adults (18–26 years) when compared with population in general [30].

However, there are studies which disagree with above findings [20, 31, 32]. Bonduelle et al. found that likelihood of illness, seeking medical advice, hospital admission, or surgery was significantly higher in the children born after ART-assisted conception [20]. Ludwig et al. found that the risk of urogenital surgery in boys who were conceived after intracytoplasmic sperm injection was higher because of an increased incidence of undescended testis/testes [32].

45.6 Cardiovascular System

Some reports say that there is an increased incidence of hypertension and glucose intolerance in adolescents born after some or other ART-assisted conceptions [33]. Moreover, Scherrer et al. concluded that the children conceived through ART who look apparently health might have systemic or pulmonary vascular dysfunction [34]. Furthermore, Wikstrand et al. found aberrations in retinal vascularization in those 5-year-old children who were born after conception through intracytoplasmic sperm injection [35].

All of the above evidences are enough to conclude that a long-term follow-up is advocated for all the children born after conception assisted by artificial reproduction technologies.

45.7 Nervous System and Neurodevelopment

A number of studies found that children born after ART-assisted conception more often suffer neuro-sequelae, viz., cerebral palsy [36, 37]. Even though multiple pregnancies and preterm labor are considered to be responsible for this primarily [36, 38, 39], a positive correlation was seen in singletons also [40].

Nevertheless, most of the studies in ART-conceived kids (born at term) found insignificant differences in neurodevelopment when compared to those conceived naturally [31, 41–43].

As of now if we remove the confounding factors like multiple pregnancy and prematurity, the neurodevelopment of children born after ART-assisted conception is at par with children conceived naturally; however, long-term follow-up and further studies are advocated.

45.8 Psychosocial Development and Pervasive Thought Disorders

Wagenaar et al. studied social, emotional, and behavioral parameters in 9–18-year-old children who were born after ART-assisted conception by assessment through parent and teachers. In artificial reproduction technology-conceived children, externalizing behaviors were less pronounced, but depressive and withdrawal behavior was more common [44].

Leunens et al. found no significant difference in motor as well as cognitive development in children of 8–10 year age group conceived through artificial reproduction technologies when compared to normal conception group [45]. In a Chinese study, children (4–6 year age) born after intracytoplasmic sperm injection and in vitro fertilization (IVF) were compared, and no difference was found in social, psychological, and emotional parameters [46]. However, autism spectrum disorder (ASD) was found more prevalent in the intracytoplasmic sperm injection group [47].

45.9 Risk for Cancer

This is one of the most controversial issues because a few published studies showed there are increased chances of some particular cancers in children born after artificial reproduction technologies.

One study initially found an elevated risk of retinoblastoma in children conceived via ART [48], but later on the analysis of the extended data confirmed no correlation was there [49].

In conclusion, the cancer risk in children born after conception assisted by artificial reproduction technologies is difficult to assess because of the rarity of the disease, yet larger case-control and follow-up studies are recommended to find any association if exists.

45.10 Epigenetic Abnormalities

Epigenetics means modifications in gene functions by external means (viz., DNA methylation and histone modification) without changing the sequence of the genes. Genomic imprinting refers to process of silencing of one of the two allyls which results in expression of only one allyl (maternal or paternal), and it is a normal phenomenon and its aberrations can cause diseases [50].

Coming on to epigenetics in children born after ART-assisted conception, Laprise reported that some rare genetic disorders, viz., Beckwith-Wiedemann syndrome (BWS), Angelman syndrome (AS), and retinoblastoma, were more common in this subgroup of population [51]. On the other hand, insignificant correlation between Beckwith-Wiedemann syndrome, Angelman syndrome, retinoblastoma, and Prader-Willi syndrome has been reported by most of other researchers. Furthermore, the disorders are exceedingly uncommon and an exact risk estimation is very difficult.

Some epigenetic changes might result into adult onset disorders: Katari et al. found altered methylation of CpG sites (which may influence gene expression) in cord blood and placental samples of babies born after ART conception; many of these genes have association with metabolic disorders, viz., obesity and diabetes [52].

On the brighter side, most of the recent publications showed no significant correlation between ART-assisted conception and occurrence of epigenetic abnormalities in offspring [53].

Finally, the minor difference in epigenetic disorder between ART conceived and naturally conceived is difficult to explain unless more robust studies and extensive follow-up is conducted.

45.11 Conclusions

In conclusion, it can be stated that largely the children born after artificial reproduction technologies are healthy if we remove the confounding factors like problems arise because of perinatal events (e.g., prematurity). The issues which should be planned more assiduously are aggressive prenatal and perinatal management. The delivery should be attempted in a center which is well equipped with level 3 or level 4 neonatal intensive care unit and adept neonatal team. These children should be screened for metabolic disorders, congenital defects, and epigenetic disorders in case of slightest suspicion.

Nevertheless, it is still to be investigated whether it is the ART procedure itself or the underlying subfertility which is the cause of these issues. At this point of time the first batch of IVF babies are adults and many have their own healthy progeny now.

References

1. Dow K. 'The men who made the breakthrough': how the British press represented Patrick Steptoe and Robert Edwards in 1978. Reprod Biomed Soc Online. 2017;4:59–67.
2. Berntsen S, Söderström-Anttila V, Wennerholm UB, Laivuori H, Loft A, Oldereid NB, et al. The health of children conceived by ART: 'the chicken or the egg?'. Hum Reprod Update. 2019;25(2):137–58.
3. Schieve LA, Meikle SF, Ferre C, Peterson HB, Jeng G, Wilcox LS. Low and very low birth weight in infants conceived with use of assisted reproductive technology. N Engl J Med. 2002;346(10):731–7.
4. de Mouzon J, Goossens V, Bhattacharya S, Castilla JA, Ferraretti AP, Korsak V, et al. Assisted reproductive technology in Europe, 2006: results generated from European registers by ESHRE. Hum Reprod. 2010;25(8):1851–62.
5. Källén B, Finnström O, Lindam A, Nilsson E, Nygren KG, Otterblad OP. Trends in delivery and neonatal outcome after in vitro fertilization in Sweden: data for 25 years. Hum Reprod. 2010;25(4):1026–34.
6. Kjellberg AT, Carlsson P, Bergh C. Randomized single versus double embryo transfer: obstetric and paediatric outcome and a cost-effectiveness analysis. Hum Reprod. 2006;21(1):210–6.
7. Henningsen AK, Pinborg A, Lidegaard Ø, Vestergaard C, Forman JL, Andersen AN. Perinatal outcome of singleton siblings born after assisted reproductive technology and spontaneous conception: Danish national sibling-cohort study. Fertil Steril. 2011;95(3):959–63.
8. Sazonova A, Källen K, Thurin-Kjellberg A, Wennerholm UB, Bergh C. Obstetric outcome after in vitro fertilization with single or double embryo transfer. Hum Reprod. 2011;26(2):442–50.
9. Bower C, Hansen M. Assisted reproductive technologies and birth outcomes: overview of recent systematic reviews. Reprod Fertil Dev. 2005;17(3):329–33.
10. Hayashi M, Nakai A, Satoh S, Matsuda Y. Adverse obstetric and perinatal outcomes of singleton pregnancies may be related to maternal factors associated with infertility rather than the type of assisted reproductive technology procedure used. Fertil Steril. 2012;98(4):922–8.
11. Romundstad LB, Romundstad PR, Sunde A, von Düring V, Skjaerven R, Gunnell D, et al. Effects of technology or maternal factors on perinatal outcome after assisted fertilisation: a population-based cohort study. Lancet. 2008;372(9640):737–43.
12. Hansen M, Colvin L, Petterson B, Kurinczuk JJ, de Klerk N, Bower C. Twins born following assisted reproductive technology: perinatal outcome and admission to hospital. Hum Reprod. 2009;24(9):2321–31.
13. Kanat-Pektas M, Kunt C, Gungor T, Mollamahmutoglu L. Perinatal and first year outcomes of spontaneous versus assisted twins: a single center experience. Arch Gynecol Obstet. 2008;278(2):143–7.
14. Boulet SL, Schieve LA, Nannini A, Ferre C, Devine O, Cohen B, et al. Perinatal outcomes of twin births conceived using assisted reproduction technology: a population-based study. Hum Reprod. 2008;23(8):1941–8.
15. Mozafari Kermani R, Nedaeifard L, Nateghi MR, Shahzadeh Fazeli A, Ahmadi E, Osia MA, et al. Congenital anomalies in infants conceived by assisted reproductive techniques. Arch Iran Med. 2012;15(4):228–31.
16. Davies MJ, Moore VM, Willson KJ, Van Essen P, Priest K, Scott H, et al. Reproductive technologies and the risk of birth defects. N Engl J Med. 2012;366(19):1803–13.
17. Wen J, Jiang J, Ding C, Dai J, Liu Y, Xia Y, et al. Birth defects in children conceived by in vitro fertilization and intracytoplasmic sperm injection: a meta-analysis. Fertil Steril. 2012;97(6):1331–7.e1-4.
18. Yan J, Huang G, Sun Y, Zhao X, Chen S, Zou S, et al. Birth defects after assisted reproductive technologies in China: analysis of 15,405 offspring in seven centers (2004 to 2008). Fertil Steril. 2011;95(1):458–60.
19. Zhu JL, Basso O, Obel C, Bille C, Olsen J. Infertility, infertility treatment, and congenital malformations: Danish national birth cohort. BMJ. 2006;333(7570):679.
20. Bonduelle M, Wennerholm UB, Loft A, Tarlatzis BC, Peters C, Henriet S, et al. A multi-centre cohort study of the physical health of 5-year-old children conceived after intracytoplasmic sperm injection, in vitro fertilization and natural conception. Hum Reprod. 2005;20(2):413–9.
21. Tararbit K, Houyel L, Bonnet D, De Vigan C, Lelong N, Goffinet F, et al. Risk of congenital heart defects associated with assisted reproductive technologies: a population-based evaluation. Eur Heart J. 2011;32(4):500–8.
22. Lee SH, Lee MY, Chiang TL, Lee MS, Lee MC. Child growth from birth to 18 months old born after assisted reproductive technology–results of a national birth cohort study. Int J Nurs Stud. 2010;47(9):1159–66.

23. Woldringh GH, Hendriks JC, van Klingeren J, van Buuren S, Kollée LA, Zielhuis GA, et al. Weight of in vitro fertilization and intracytoplasmic sperm injection singletons in early childhood. Fertil Steril. 2011;95(8):2775–7.
24. Makhoul IR, Tamir A, Bader D, Rotschild A, Weintraub Z, Yurman S, et al. In vitro fertilisation and use of ovulation enhancers may both influence childhood height in very low birthweight infants. Arch Dis Child Fetal Neonatal Ed. 2009;94(5):F355–9.
25. Miles HL, Hofman PL, Peek J, Harris M, Wilson D, Robinson EM, et al. In vitro fertilization improves childhood growth and metabolism. J Clin Endocrinol Metab. 2007;92(9):3441–5.
26. De Schepper J, Belva F, Schiettecatte J, Anckaert E, Tournaye H, Bonduelle M. Testicular growth and tubular function in prepubertal boys conceived by intracytoplasmic sperm injection. Horm Res. 2009;71(6):359–63.
27. Belva F, Bonduelle M, Painter RC, Schiettecatte J, Devroey P, De Schepper J. Serum inhibin B concentrations in pubertal boys conceived by ICSI: first results. Hum Reprod. 2010;25(11):2811–4.
28. Belva F, Bonduelle M, Schiettecatte J, Tournaye H, Painter RC, Devroey P, et al. Salivary testosterone concentrations in pubertal ICSI boys compared with spontaneously conceived boys. Hum Reprod. 2011;26(2):438–41.
29. Belva F, Roelants M, Painter R, Bonduelle M, Devroey P, De Schepper J. Pubertal development in ICSI children. Hum Reprod. 2012;27(4):1156–61.
30. Beydoun HA, Sicignano N, Beydoun MA, Matson DO, Bocca S, Stadtmauer L, et al. A cross-sectional evaluation of the first cohort of young adults conceived by in vitro fertilization in the United States. Fertil Steril. 2010;94(6):2043–9.
31. Källén B, Finnström O, Nygren KG, Olausson PO. In vitro fertilization in Sweden: child morbidity including cancer risk. Fertil Steril. 2005;84(3):605–10.
32. Ludwig AK, Katalinic A, Thyen U, Sutcliffe AG, Diedrich K, Ludwig M. Physical health at 5.5 years of age of term-born singletons after intracytoplasmic sperm injection: results of a prospective, controlled, single-blinded study. Fertil Steril. 2009;91(1):115–24.
33. Ceelen M, van Weissenbruch MM, Vermeiden JP, van Leeuwen FE, Delemarre-van de Waal HA. Cardiometabolic differences in children born after in vitro fertilization: follow-up study. J Clin Endocrinol Metab. 2008;93(5):1682–8.
34. Scherrer U, Rimoldi SF, Rexhaj E, Stuber T, Duplain H, Garcin S, et al. Systemic and pulmonary vascular dysfunction in children conceived by assisted reproductive technologies. Circulation. 2012;125(15):1890–6.
35. Wikstrand MH, Niklasson A, Strömland K, Hellström A. Abnormal vessel morphology in boys born after intracytoplasmic sperm injection. Acta Paediatr. 2008;97(11):1512–7.
36. Källén AJ, Finnström OO, Lindam AP, Nilsson EM, Nygren KG, Olausson PM. Cerebral palsy in children born after in vitro fertilization. Is the risk decreasing? Eur J Paediatr Neurol. 2010;14(6):526–30.
37. Zhu JL, Hvidtjørn D, Basso O, Obel C, Thorsen P, Uldall P, et al. Parental infertility and cerebral palsy in children. Hum Reprod. 2010;25(12):3142–5.
38. Hvidtjørn D, Grove J, Schendel D, Svaerke C, Schieve LA, Uldall P, et al. Multiplicity and early gestational age contribute to an increased risk of cerebral palsy from assisted conception: a population-based cohort study. Hum Reprod. 2010;25(8):2115–23.
39. Saunders NR, Hellmann J, Farine D. Cerebral palsy and assisted conception. J Obstet Gynaecol Can. 2011;33(10):1038–43.
40. Strömberg B, Dahlquist G, Ericson A, Finnström O, Köster M, Stjernqvist K. Neurological sequelae in children born after in-vitro fertilisation: a population-based study. Lancet. 2002;359(9305):461–5.
41. Carson C, Kurinczuk JJ, Sacker A, Kelly Y, Klemetti R, Redshaw M, et al. Cognitive development following ART: effect of choice of comparison group, confounding and mediating factors. Hum Reprod. 2010;25(1):244–52.
42. Mains L, Zimmerman M, Blaine J, Stegmann B, Sparks A, Ansley T, et al. Achievement test performance in children conceived by IVF. Hum Reprod. 2010;25(10):2605–11.
43. Tsai CC, Huang FJ, Wang LJ, Lin YJ, Kung FT, Hsieh CH, et al. Clinical outcomes and development of children born after intracytoplasmic sperm injection (ICSI) using extracted testicular sperm or ejaculated extreme severe oligo-astheno-teratozoospermia sperm: a comparative study. Fertil Steril. 2011;96(3):567–71.
44. Wagenaar K, van Weissenbruch MM, Knol DL, Cohen-Kettenis PT, Delemarre-van de Waal HA, Huisman J. Behavior and socio-emotional functioning in 9-18-year-old children born after in vitro fertilization. Fertil Steril. 2009;92(6):1907–14.
45. Leunens L, Celestin-Westreich S, Bonduelle M, Liebaers I, Ponjaert-Kristoffersen I. Cognitive and motor development of 8-year-old children born after ICSI compared to spontaneously conceived children. Hum Reprod. 2006;21(11):2922–9.
46. Xing LF, Qian YL, Chen LT, Zhang FH, Xu XF, Qu F, et al. Is there a difference in cognitive development between preschool singletons and twins born after intracytoplasmic sperm injection or in vitro fertilization? J Zhejiang Univ Sci B. 2014;15(1):51–7.
47. Knoester M, Helmerhorst FM, van der Westerlaken LA, Walther FJ, Veen S. (L-art-FUP) LARTF-uP. Matched follow-up study of 5 8-year-old ICSI singletons: child behaviour, parenting stress and child (health-related) quality of life. Hum Reprod. 2007;22(12):3098–107.
48. Moll AC, Imhof SM, Cruysberg JR, Schouten-van Meeteren AY, Boers M, van Leeuwen FE. Incidence of retinoblastoma in children born after in-vitro fertilisation. Lancet. 2003;361(9354):309–10.
49. Marees T, Dommering CJ, Imhof SM, Kors WA, Ringens PJ, van Leeuwen FE, et al. Incidence of retinoblastoma in Dutch children conceived by IVF: an expanded study. Hum Reprod. 2009;24(12):3220–4.
50. Koerner MV, Barlow DP. Genomic imprinting-an epigenetic gene-regulatory model. Curr Opin Genet Dev. 2010;20(2):164–70.
51. Laprise SL. Implications of epigenetics and genomic imprinting in assisted reproductive technologies. Mol Reprod Dev. 2009;76(11):1006–18.
52. Katari S, Turan N, Bibikova M, Erinle O, Chalian R, Foster M, et al. DNA methylation and gene expression differences in children conceived in vitro or in vivo. Hum Mol Genet. 2009;18(20):3769–78.
53. Rancourt RC, Harris HR, Michels KB. Methylation levels at imprinting control regions are not altered with ovulation induction or in vitro fertilization in a birth cohort. Hum Reprod. 2012;27(7):2208–16.

Effectiveness and Safety of Freeze-All Strategy with Regard to Medically Assisted Reproduction and Perinatal Outcomes

46

Engin Turkgeldi, Sule Yildiz, Bulent Urman, and Baris Ata

Despite differences in patient management and variations in practice, the final aim of all medically assisted reproduction (MAR) cycles is pregnancy culminating in a healthy singleton baby, ideally in the shortest time and at a reasonable cost. Such an approach would also minimize the psychological and financial stress on the couple.

The two main components of successful implantation are an embryo endowed with the potential to implant and a receptive endometrium. While implantation failure and miscarriages are mostly attributed to aneuploid embryos, about 35% of euploid embryos also fail to implant, suggesting a significant role of endometrial receptivity in achieving pregnancy [1].

More oocytes equate to higher pregnancy rate in MAR [2, 3]; however, supraphysiological levels of sex steroids during ovarian stimulation (OS) to achieve this goal may impair endometrial receptivity and result in lower birth rates [4]. The effect may be due to different gene expression patterns, differences in endometrial morphology, and/or hormonal advancement of the endometrium rendering it less receptive to the embryo. Endometrial gene expression and endometrial morphology were shown to be different in stimulated vs. non-stimulated cycles [5]. Elevation of serum progesterone levels during the follicular phase which appears to be a relatively common phenomenon shifts the implantation window that may affect MAR success [4]. Moreover, medications used during MAR may affect endometrial receptivity. For instance, triggering ovulation with human chorionic gonadotropin (hCG) may result in downregulation of luteinizing hormone receptors in the endometrium due to extended exposure to hCG, possibly decreasing the positive effect of the hCG secreted by the blastocyst during implantation [6].

Besides the suggested detrimental effect of OS on endometrial receptivity and implantation, some observational studies imply that the rates of preterm delivery and low birth weight (LBW) are higher in pregnancies resulting from the transfer of fresh embryos [7].

It is against this background, and with the support of highly effective cryopreservation techniques such as vitrification, some experts have proposed that bypassing the aforementioned detrimental effects of ovarian stimulation by freezing all embryos and performing elective frozen-thawed embryo transfer (eFET) increases implantation rates, and this approach should be the standard in ART practice [8].

In this chapter, our aim was to examine the current evidence on the effect of eFET from the ART and maternal/perinatal outcome perspectives and determine if there is any benefit in applying a universal freeze-all strategy.

46.1 A Review of Randomized Controlled Trials of Fresh and Elective Frozen-Thawed Embryo Transfers

The studies on which universal freeze-all strategy is based are mostly laboratory-based and do not report live birth rates, the ultimate endpoint in MAR. This raises doubt about the applicability of this approach for two reasons: in vitro findings do not always translate into clinical results, and even if they do, it is not known whether eFET will overcome the suggested problems with OS. Currently, the ideal method to test this hypothesis is performing randomized control trials (RCTs) comparing the effectiveness of fresh transfers with eFET. Up to date, seven RCTs have tested this hypothesis.

Assuming that ovarian stimulation and multiple follicular growth impair endometrial receptivity, this effect would be

E. Turkgeldi · S. Yildiz
Department of Obstetrics and Gynecology, Koc University Hospital, Istanbul, Turkey

B. Urman
Department of Obstetrics and Gynecology, Koc University Faculty of Medicine, Istanbul, Turkey

B. Ata (✉)
Division of Reproductive Endocrinology and Infertility, Department of Obstetrics and Gynecology, Koç University School of Medicine, Istanbul, Turkey

Department of Obstetrics, Gynecology and Reproductive Sciences, Yale University School of Medicine, New Haven, CT, USA
e-mail: barisata@ku.edu.tr

G. N. Allahbadia et al. (eds.), *Textbook of Assisted Reproduction*, https://doi.org/10.1007/978-981-15-2377-9_46

expected to be more apparent in patients with a high ovarian response, as seen in a dose-response pattern [9]. Of the seven RCTs performed to date, six include high responders, that is, patients with an average estradiol level >3000 pg/ml on the trigger day or a mean number of 12 or more oocytes collected. We will review these studies starting from the one with the highest response.

In a short communication that did not evolve into an original article, Shapiro et al. reported performing an RCT specifically in women with an antral follicle count of at least 16, who are expected to be high responders [10]. One-hundred and twenty-two patients were randomized into fresh or frozen embryo transfer. Fresh transfers were done on day 5, while other embryos were cryopreserved using slow-freezing method at the two-pronuclear stage and cultured to blastocyst stage after thawing. Peak serum estradiol levels were 5427 vs. 5263 pg/ml, and mean number of oocytes that were retrieved were 20.9 vs. 19.3 in the frozen and fresh transfer groups, respectively. Ongoing pregnancy rates were 77.6% in the frozen transfer group and 65.4% in the fresh transfer group ($p = 0.19$). The authors performed an arbitrary regression analysis controlling for embryo quality and reported statistically significant higher clinical pregnancy rates in the frozen embryo transfer group. Clearly, embryo quality might have been affected by the freezing and thawing process and should be regarded as a factor related to the intervention tested. Thus, an analysis adjusting for embryo quality is not suitable. An intention to treat (ITT) analysis shows similar ongoing pregnancy rates in frozen and fresh embryo transfer groups, 38/60 (63.3%) vs. 34/62 (54.9%), respectively ($p = 0.63$) [11].

Chen et al. recruited 1508 infertile women with polycystic ovary syndrome (PCOS) undergoing their first IVF cycle and randomized them to fresh or frozen embryo transfer at the cleavage stage [12]. As can be expected from the study population, the patients responded excessively reaching an average serum estradiol level of 4288 vs. 4141 pg/ml on the trigger day and an average of 14.4 vs. 14.2 oocytes collected in frozen and fresh embryo groups, respectively. While biochemical (66% vs. 64.6%, $p = 0.57$), clinical (58.7% vs. 56.2%, $p = 0.32$), and ongoing (52.7% vs. 48.8%, $p = 0.13$) pregnancies were similar, live birth rates were significantly higher in the frozen embryo transfer group (49.3% vs. 42%, rate ratio = 1.17, 95% confidence interval CI of 1.05–1.31, $p = 0.004$). This translates to a number needed to treat of 14, meaning that one extra live birth would be achieved for every 14 frozen embryo transfer performed instead of fresh embryo transfer.

Coates et al. undertook a study that compared live birth rates between fresh and elective frozen euploid blastocyst transfers [13]. While the primary objective of the study was to investigate the optimal strategy for transferring embryos following preimplantation genetic screening (PGS), the study provides valuable information about the outcomes of fresh and frozen embryo transfer cycles. One-hundred and seventy-nine patients undergoing PGS were randomized into freeze-all or sixth day fresh embryo transfer groups. The mean serum estradiol levels were not reported in the article; however, median number of oocytes collected were 14 and 17 in fresh and eFET groups, respectively, implying a high ovarian response. Implantation rates were similar in fresh and eFET groups (67.4% vs. 76%, $p = 0.19$); however as the pregnancies progressed, outcomes became significantly more favorable in the eFET group, with ongoing clinical pregnancy rates reported as 40.9% vs. 62.6% ($p < 0.01$) and live birth rates as 39.8% vs. 61.5% ($p < 0.01$), in fresh and eFET groups, respectively. Yet, it is important to note that the results were presented according to an intention-to-treat analysis. Due to technical and logistics problems in availability of PGS results, a number of patients originally randomized to the fresh transfer group were moved to eFET group. The objective of the study was to develop a strategy for the clinical management, justifying an intention-to-treat analysis; however, a per-protocol analysis serves the current review better since we are interested in whether endometrium provides a more favorable environment for embryos in a stimulated or a non-stimulated cycle. Per-protocol analysis yielded similar rates for implantation (67% vs. 78%, $p = 0.23$), ongoing pregnancy (61% vs. 78%, $p = 0.1$), and live birth (59% vs. 70%, $p = 0.3$) in fresh and eFET cycles, respectively.

Shapiro et al. performed an RCT on women with 8–15 AFC undergoing their first IVF cycles who were expected to be normo-responders [14]. Originally, a sample size of 411 was aimed at, however, the study was prematurely halted after an interim analysis following the 100th blastocyst transfer. By that time, 137 patients were randomized into fresh and frozen transfer groups, with 50 and 53 blastocysts transferred, respectively. The mean serum estradiol level on the trigger day was 3418 pg/ml vs. 3076 pg/ml; and mean number of oocytes collected were 14.1 vs. 12.9 in the fresh and frozen transfer groups, respectively. It is interesting that the study defines itself to be dealing with normo-responders whereas these values imply a high ovarian response. Authors reported clinical pregnancy rate per transfer of 54.7% vs. 84% ($p = 0.0013$) and ongoing pregnancy rate per transfer at 10th gestational week of 50.9% vs. 78% ($p = 0.0072$) in fresh and frozen transfer groups, respectively. However, it is interesting that these values are not derived from an intention-to-treat analysis. As the study question is to discover if fresh or frozen transfer policy will yield a better clinical outcome, an intention-to-treat analysis would have provided results that could be generalized and applied to the clinical setting. In fact, an intention-to-treat analysis of the study data reveals similar ongoing pregnancy rates in both groups, 27/67 (40.3%) vs. 39/70 (55.7%) $p = 0.11$, in fresh and frozen transfer groups, respectively. Another drawback of the Shapiro trials is cryopreservation of embryos at the two-pronuclear stage using the slow-freezing technique. Current validity of their data is questionable since almost all clinics worldwide prefer vitrification at the cleavage or blastocyst stages.

Chronologically, the first trial to compare the outcomes of fresh and frozen transfer cycles was by Afflatoonian et al. in 2010 [15]. Three-hundred and seventy-four patients with serum estradiol levels greater than 3000 pg/ml or 15 oocytes collected were included in the study. Significant difference was reported with implantation rates of 17.5% vs. 24.7% and ongoing pregnancy rates of 27.8% vs. 39% in fresh and frozen embryo transfer groups, respectively. However, we will neither analyze this study in detail nor take it into consideration in our review since it was retracted by the American Society of Reproductive Medicine Publications Committee due to serious methodological problems [16].

A recent RCT by Shi et al. investigated the outcomes of fresh and frozen embryo transfers in 2157 ovulatory women [17]. Participants were aged between 20 and 35 years, had regular menstrual cycles, and were undergoing their first in vitro fertilization cycle. Mean estradiol levels were 3110 pg/ml in the fresh embryo transfer group and 3188 in the frozen embryo transfer group, with mean number of oocytes retrieved 12.3 and 12.5, respectively. Live birth rates (LBR) were similar between the fresh and eFET groups (48.7% and 50.2%, respectively; relative risk, 0.97; 95% confidence interval [CI], 0.89–1.06; $p = 0.50$). Likewise, implantation, clinical pregnancy, overall pregnancy loss, and ongoing pregnancy rates were similar in the two groups. It is noteworthy that risk of second-trimester pregnancy loss was significantly lower in the eFET group. However, this was a post hoc analysis. Even though the risk of moderate–severe ovarian hyperstimulation syndrome was significantly lower in the eFET group, the general incidence of this complication was low (0.6% vs. 2.0%; relative risk, 0.32; 95% CI, 0.14–0.74; $p = 0.005$). A high withdrawal rate (15.3% and 18.8%, in the fresh and eFET groups, respectively, $p = 0.03$) was a study limitation.

Another recently published RCT by Vuong et al. included infertile women without PCOS [18]. Seven hundred eighty-two women were randomly assigned to fresh or eFET of cleavage stage embryos. A maximum of two embryos were transferred in both groups. The primary outcome was ongoing pregnancy after the first embryo transfer. The mean serum estradiol level on trigger day was 2029 pg/ml and 2019 pg/ml in the fresh and frozen transfer groups, respectively. Ongoing pregnancy rate was 36.3% and 34.5% in the fresh and eFET groups (RR, 1.05; 95% CI, 0.87–1.27; $p = 0.65$). Live birth rates after the first transfer were 33.8% and 31.5%, respectively (RR = 1.07; 95% CI, 0.88–1.31). Implantation and clinical pregnancy were similar in both groups. The incidence of ectopic pregnancy, miscarriage, multiple pregnancy, OHSS in the primary cycle, or pregnancy complications were not significantly different. Live birth rate after the first cycle and the ongoing pregnancy rates at 12 months were similar between the groups. Singleton birth weight was the only significant difference in perinatal outcomes to the benefit of frozen embryo group. In summary, frozen embryo transfer resulted in a rate of live birth that was similar to that of fresh-embryo transfer. The risk of moderate or severe ovarian hyperstimulation syndrome was lower with frozen embryo transfer. A summary of the aforementioned RCTs can be found in Table 46.1.

In conclusion, it has been hypothesized that the uterine environment of a fresh embryo transfer cycle may be less affected in ovulatory women with a normal ovarian response due to lower estradiol levels when compared with PCOS or those with a high ovarian response. However, one study aside, all were dealing with high responders. Furthermore, even in this setting, clinical outcomes did not consistently favor frozen embryo transfers. Chen et al. showed a significant benefit for frozen embryo transfer, but it should be recognized that PCOS comprise a very specific group of patients and due to their increased risk for OHSS, they would be best served with a freeze all policy. Still, it is noteworthy that although not significant, a trend for improved clinical outcome was observed in patients with a high ovarian response. However, as demonstrated above, such a benefit or trend dwindles and finally ceases to exist as ovarian response reduces from high to normal. Moreover, freeze-all strategy increases time to reach pregnancy, costs, and possible risks by delaying the treatment and subjecting the embryo to additional procedures. Finally, based on the current evidence, offering a universal freeze-all strategy seems to be an overgeneralization of data from a specific group, and changing the clinical practice dramatically for all patients undergoing IVF based on this is a leap too big to take.

46.2 A Review of Studies on the Effect of Frozen Embryo Transfer on Perinatal Outcomes

Early studies comparing perinatal outcomes of fresh and frozen ART cycles have shown differences in the incidences of preterm birth (PTB), fetal weight, and preeclampsia [19, 20]. It is difficult to pinpoint the effect of a single factor such as fresh or frozen embryo transfer, since ART includes a number of variables that interact with each other, parental factors, medications used, fertilization method, culture media, and transfer stage to name a few. It should also be noted that most studies on the subject are observational, with few randomized controlled trials. The relatively low incidence of some

Table 46.1 Randomized controlled trials of fresh vs. elective frozen embryo transfer

	Shapiro et al. [10]		Shapiro et al. [14]		Chen et al. [12]		Coates et al. [13]		Vuong et al. [18]		Shi et al. [17]	
	Fresh	Frozen	Fresh	Frozen	Fresh	Frozen	Fresh	Frozen	Fresh	Frozen	Fresh	Frozen
Number randomized	67	70	62	60	762	746	46	82	391	391	1080	1077
Mean serum estradiol level on day of trigger in pg/ml (SD)	3418 (1501)	3076 (1438)	5263 (2832)	5427 (3037)	4141 (2159)	4288 (2210)	N/A	N/A	2029 ± 1616	2019 ± 1470	3110 ± 1525	3188 ± 1558
Embryo cryopreservation stage	N/A	2 PN oocyte	N/A	2 PN oocyte	N/A	Cleavage	N/A	Blastocyst	N/A	Cleavage	N/A	Cleavage
Embryo transfer stage	Blastocyst	Blastocyst	Blastocyst	Blastocyst	Cleavage	Cleavage	Euploid blastocyst	Euploid blastocyst	Cleavage	Cleavage	Cleavage	Cleavage
Live birth rate (%)	60/129 (46.5)	74/130 (56.9)			320/762 (42)	368/746 (49.3)	27/46 (71.2)	60/82 (73.2)	123/391 (31.5)	132/391 (33.8)	542/1080 (50.2)	525/1080 (48.7)

adverse perinatal outcomes renders it difficult to assess them in the RCT setting [21]. Supraphysiological hormone levels in a stimulated cycle is one of the suspected factors leading to adverse perinatal outcomes following fresh embryo transfer.

The risk of SGA delivery is thought to be increased in ART pregnancies, but results are controversial. Recently, a record linkage study compared 5536 spontaneous singleton pregnancies with 6470 singleton ART pregnancies, and after adjusting for maternal age, ethnicity, marital status, maternal education, smoking status, prenatal care, parity, gestational hypertension, and sex of the infant, they showed no statistically significant difference between the two groups regarding (OR = 1.1, 95% CI 0.96–1.27) [22]. On the other hand, preterm delivery and low birth weight (LBW) risks were higher in ART pregnancies (aOR 1.23, 95% CI: 1.08–1.41 and aOR 1.26, 95% CI: 1.08–1.47, respectively) [22]. An observational study of all ART cycles in the United Kingdom between 1991 and 2008 included 65,868 singleton deliveries from 402,185 cycles, and after adjusting for treatment period, female age, indication for ART, type of infertility (primary or secondary), number of embryos transferred, and pregnancies initiated as singletons or multiples, women from whom 20 or more oocytes were collected were at higher risk for LBW and PTB compared to women from whom 10–15 oocytes were retrieved [23]. Pregnancies followed by frozen transfer IVF cycles were less likely to be complicated by SGA, LBW, and PTB compared with children born after fresh embryo transfers in this large Nordic cohort study [19]. Moreover, the rates of LGA and birthweight >4500 g were significantly increased for singletons conceived from cryopreservation cycles compared with singletons conceived from fresh cycles [24]

Kalra et al. compared 38,626 and 18,166 pregnancies following the transfer of fresh and frozen embryos, respectively. In singletons, preterm delivery rates did not show any difference. However, the odds of overall LBW following fresh embryo transfer were significantly higher (AOR 1.35, 95% CI 1.20–1.51) [25]. Recently, Weinerman et al. compared perinatal outcomes following transfer of fresh and vitrified blastocysts in a transgenic mouse model [26]. Embryo transfer in a superovulated cycle resulted in smaller term fetuses regardless of the transferred blastocysts being fresh or frozen. This suggests that fetal growth disorders can be a consequence of altered placental vasculogenesis and blood flow caused by the superovulated environment. These findings suggest that supraphysiological hormone levels can have a detrimental effect on endometrial function, leading to LBW and SGA.

Although observational studies showed small yet significant differences regarding fetal weight between fresh and frozen cycles, the difference was not that prominent in RCTs. Results from the RCTs are contradictory with the observational data. Three of the four RCTs reporting birthweight did not indicate a significant difference between fresh and frozen embryo transfers, whereas one RCT reported significantly lower birthweight and higher incidence of low birth weight with fresh embryo transfer [12, 18, 27].

It should be noted that the vast majority of the data from observational studies and RCTs are cleavage stage embryo transfer cycles. It is questionable whether observations on cleavage stage transfers are applicable to blastocyst transfers, a practice that is increasingly becoming more common. A population-based registry study examining 4819 singletons born after blastocyst transfer; 25,747 after cleavage stage transfer; and 1,196,394 spontaneous conceptions found that the risk of SGA was significantly lower with blastocyst transfers compared to cleavage stage transfers (AOR 0.71, 95% CI: 0.56–0.88) or spontaneous conceptions (AOR 0.70, 95% CI: 0.57–0.87) [28]. Recently, a systematic review and meta-analysis assessed perinatal outcomes of singleton pregnancies followed by blastocyst vs. cleavage stage embryo transfers. Primary outcomes were preterm birth before 37 weeks and low birth weight (<2500 g). They reported significantly higher rates of preterm birth <37 weeks after blastocyst transfer in fresh cycles (RR 1.15, 95% CI, 1.05–1.25; $p = 0.002$). Also, they found fewer SGA deliveries after blastocyst transfer in fresh cycles. However, after blastocyst transfers in frozen cycles, LGA births were observed more than cleavage transfers. In fresh cycles, no differences were observed for LGA in both groups [29].

In addition to PTB, LBW, or SGA, other pregnancy-related complications such as ectopic pregnancy, hypertensive disorders, perinatal mortality, and placenta anomalies can occur at different rates following fresh or frozen transfer. These are discussed below.

Registry-based studies and a few RCTs consistently reported an increased risk of preeclampsia following frozen embryo transfer. Preeclampsia rate was found to increase threefold after eFET in Chen et al.'s study (rate ratio 3.12, 95% CI: 1.26–7.73, $p = 0.009$) [12]. CoNARTaS group and registry-based studies from Sweden and Japan reported similar results [20, 24, 30]. The odds of hypertensive disorders were increased 2.63-fold (1.73–3.99) after eFET in the Nordic registry. Likewise, risk of preeclampsia was significantly higher following eFET in Swedish (aOR: 1.32, 95% CI: 1.07–1.63) and Japanese (aOR: 1.58, 95% CI: 1.35–1.86) registries [20]. In a recently published retrospective study including 15,937 births from ART, 9417 singletons and 6520 twin pregnancies compared preeclampsia risk between fresh and frozen transfer in both singleton and twin pregnancies as well pregnancies from autologous and donor eggs. They categorize preeclampsia in groups as preeclampsia without severe features, preeclampsia with severe features, preeclampsia with preterm delivery, and chronic hypertension with superimposed preeclampsia. The results showed increased preeclampsia risk after cryopreserved-warmed ET than after fresh transfer in all groups in singleton pregnancies. Preeclampsia rates in singleton pregnancies conceived with donor eggs were similar between the cryopreserved transfer and fresh transfer groups (10.78% vs. 12.13%, respectively, $p = 0.56$). However, pregnancies from donor egg transfers showed 2.69-fold higher preeclampsia rates than pregnancies from autologous eggs. The underlying mechanism is suggested as different HLA-C pattern originating from the donor egg. In twin pregnancies from autologous eggs, preeclampsia with severe features and preeclampsia with preterm delivery were also more frequent after cryopreserved–warmed transfers than fresh ETs (9.26% vs. 5.70%, $p < 0.01$, and 14.81% vs. 11.74%, $p = 0.04$, respectively) [31]. However, findings from most recent RCTs by Shi et al. [17] and Vuong et al. [18] involving normo-ovulatory women are contradictory with the abovementioned data. Both studies reported no significant difference regarding preeclampsia between fresh and frozen transfers (rate ratio 1.36, 95% CI: 0.77–2.42 and rate ratio 2, 95% CI: 0.18–21.97), respectively.

A number of studies showed that cleavage stage and fresh embryo transfers pose higher risk for ectopic pregnancy compared to blastocyst and frozen embryo transfers, respectively [32–35].

In a recently published retrospective study based on the results of 69,756 in vitro fertilization–embryo transfer cycles including 45,960 (65.9%) fresh and 23,796 (34.1%) frozen–thawed embryo transfer cycles, a lower rate of ectopic pregnancy per clinical pregnancy after frozen-thawed embryo transfer pregnancies was observed, compared with fresh embryo transfers (odds ratio = 0.31; 95% confidence interval = 0.24–0.39) [36].

Overall incidence of ectopic pregnancy is reported to be about 1.5% in these studies. The absolute difference between fresh and frozen embryo transfers ranges between 0.5 and 1.4%, in favor of frozen embryo transfers. However, the three recent RCTs comparing fresh and frozen embryo transfers that report ectopic pregnancy rates report similar rates in the two groups [12, 17, 18]. Moreover, two studies, one of which examines the 153,115 ART pregnancies in the United Kingdom registry, found similar rates for ectopic pregnancy after fresh and frozen transfer [37, 38]. Data are conflicting about ectopic pregnancy rates between fresh and frozen cycles. ART indications such as tubal pathologies, transfer technique, number of embryos transferred in each cycle, and the method of endometrial preparation should be considered prior to a causal inference of the embryo status can be concluded [39].

In Chen et al.'s RCT, the fact that there were two stillbirth and five neonatal deaths in the eFET group and none in the fresh embryo transfer group is disturbing. The p value comparing neonatal deaths was 0.06, just short of statistical significance. Similarly, increased risk for perinatal death after eFET was shown in a registry-based study (aOR 1.9, 95% CI: 1.03–3.54) [24]. A recent meta-analysis reported conflicting results [21]. On the contrary, Vuong et al. reported three stillbirths all of which occurred in the fresh embryo group versus none in the frozen transfer group [18]. As stillbirth and perinatal mortality are grave outcomes, even a minor increase is worrisome and can solely be a strong argument against eFET. It is relieving to observe that recent findings are comforting.

Placenta accreta is a rare complication of pregnancy with potentially severe consequences. Several studies investigated placenta-associated complications regarding frozen or fresh embryo transfers. Ishiara et al. reported an association between advanced maternal age and increased odds of both placenta previa (AOR 1.05 [95% CI 1.02–1.08]) and PIH which is also categorized as a placenta-associated complication (AOR 1.07 [95% CI 1.06–1.09]). A remarkable finding of this study was significantly higher odds of both placenta accreta (AOR 3.16 [95% CI 1.71–6.23]) and PIH (AOR 1.58 [95% CI 1.35–1.86]) following FET [20].

Since the analyses were not controlled for known risk factors, these observations do not comprise proof of a causal relationship between FET and placenta accreta. However, in a case control study, with the aim to investigate an association between placenta accreta and frozen embryo transfer, 50 women with placenta accreta were matched with 150 women without accreta for age and prior cesarean section status; the aOR was 3.2 (95% CI: 1.14–9.02) with fresh embryo transfer as the referent [20, 40]. The suggested mechanism regarding association between FET and placenta accreta was low serum estradiol levels in FET cycles. In a murine model, it was shown that low doses of estradiol permit trophoblast ingrowth by maintaining uterus in a prolonged receptive state. In addition, the endometrium is supposed to be thinner causing exuberant trophoblastic growth [40, 41].

To sum up, although some evidence suggests that frozen embryo transfer may be associated with better outcomes for PTB, LBW, SGA, and ectopic pregnancy, the data are far from conclusive. Furthermore, there is some evidence suggesting that frozen embryo transfer may be associated with an increased risk of hypertensive disorders, stillbirth, perinatal mortality, and placental anomalies.

46.3 Conclusion

The hypothesis that the supraphysiological sex hormone levels may have a detrimental effect on ART outcomes and a universal freeze-all strategy could overcome this effect appears to be less plausible with the recent high-quality studies. According to the current evidence, normal and poor responders do not seem to benefit from eFET. On the other hand, FET can be regarded as a medically indicated intervention for hyperresponders since fresh ET should already be avoided in order to prevent ovarian hyperstimulation syndrome in these patients. Hence, deferring fresh ET in favor of eFET should be based on ovarian response, rather than a universal strategy for all ART cycles.

Likewise, the available evidence on the effects of frozen embryo transfer on maternal and perinatal outcomes is conflicting and not robust enough to prefer one method of transfer over the other.

References

1. Scott RT Jr, Ferry K, Su J, Tao X, Scott K, Treff NR. Comprehensive chromosome screening is highly predictive of the reproductive potential of human embryos: a prospective, blinded, nonselection study. Fertil Steril. 2012;97(4):870–5.
2. Ata B, Kaplan B, Danzer H, et al. Array CGH analysis shows that aneuploidy is not related to the number of embryos generated. Reprod BioMed Online. 2012;24(6):614–20.
3. Sunkara SK, Rittenberg V, Raine-Fenning N, Bhattacharya S, Zamora J, Coomarasamy A. Association between the number of eggs and live birth in IVF treatment: an analysis of 400 135 treatment cycles. Hum Reprod (Oxford). 2011;26(7):1768–74.
4. Venetis CA, Kolibianakis EM, Bosdou JK, Tarlatzis BC. Progesterone elevation and probability of pregnancy after IVF: a systematic review and meta-analysis of over 60 000 cycles. Hum Reprod Update. 2013;19(5):433–57.
5. Horcajadas JA, Riesewijk A, Polman J, et al. Effect of controlled ovarian hyperstimulation in IVF on endometrial gene expression profiles. Mol Hum Reprod. 2005;11(3):195–205.
6. Evans J, Salamonsen LA. Too much of a good thing? Experimental evidence suggests prolonged exposure to hCG is detrimental to endometrial receptivity. Hum Reprod (Oxford). 2013;28(6):1610–9.
7. Turkgeldi E, Yagmur H, Seyhan A, Urman B, Ata B. Short and long term outcomes of children conceived with assisted reproductive technology. Eur J Obstet Gynecol Reprod Biol. 2016;207:129–36.
8. Evans J, Hannan NJ, Edgell TA, et al. Fresh versus frozen embryo transfer: backing clinical decisions with scientific and clinical evidence. Hum Reprod Update. 2014;20(6):808–21.
9. Hill AB. The environment and disease: association or causation? Proc R Soc Med. 1965;58:295–300.
10. Shapiro BS, Daneshmand ST, Garner FC, Aguirre M, Hudson C, Thomas S. Evidence of impaired endometrial receptivity after ovarian stimulation for in vitro fertilization: a prospective randomized trial comparing fresh and frozen-thawed embryo transfers in high responders. Fertil Steril. 2011;96(2):516–8.
11. Ata B, Seli E. A universal freeze all strategy: why it is not warranted. Curr Opin Obstet Gynecol. 2017;29(3):136–45.
12. Chen ZJ, Shi Y, Sun Y, et al. Fresh versus frozen embryos for infertility in the polycystic ovary syndrome. N Engl J Med. 2016;375(6):523–33.
13. Coates A, Kung A, Mounts E, et al. Optimal euploid embryo transfer strategy, fresh versus frozen, after preimplantation genetic screening with next generation sequencing: a randomized controlled trial. Fertil Steril. 2017;107(3):723–730.e723.
14. Shapiro BS, Daneshmand ST, Garner FC, Aguirre M, Hudson C, Thomas S. Evidence of impaired endometrial receptivity after ovarian stimulation for in vitro fertilization: a prospective randomized trial comparing fresh and frozen-thawed embryo transfer in normal responders. Fertil Steril. 2011;96(2):344–8.
15. Aflatoonian A, Oskouian H, Ahmadi S, Oskouian L. Retracted Article: Can fresh embryo transfers be replaced by cryopreserved-thawed embryo transfers in assisted reproductive cycles? A randomized controlled trial. J Assist Reprod Genet. 2010;27(7):357–63.
16. Retraction note to: Can fresh embryo transfers be replaced by cryopreserved-thawed embryo transfers in assisted reproductive cycles? A randomized controlled trial. J Assist Reprod Genet. 2013;30(9):1245.
17. Shi Y, Sun Y, Hao C, et al. Transfer of fresh versus frozen embryos in ovulatory women. N Engl J Med. 2018;378(2):126–36.
18. Vuong LN, Dang VQ, Ho TM, et al. IVF transfer of fresh or frozen embryos in women without polycystic ovaries. N Engl J Med. 2018;378(2):137–47.
19. Wennerholm UB, Henningsen AK, Romundstad LB, et al. Perinatal outcomes of children born after frozen-thawed embryo transfer: a Nordic cohort study from the CoNARTaS group. Hum Reprod (Oxford). 2013;28(9):2545–53.
20. Ishihara O, Araki R, Kuwahara A, Itakura A, Saito H, Adamson GD. Impact of frozen-thawed single-blastocyst transfer on maternal and neonatal outcome: an analysis of 277,042 single-embryo transfer cycles from 2008 to 2010 in Japan. Fertil Steril. 2014;101(1):128–33.
21. Zhao J, Xu B, Zhang Q, Li YP. Which one has a better obstetric and perinatal outcome in singleton pregnancy, IVF/ICSI or FET?: a systematic review and meta-analysis. Reprod Biol Endocrinol. 2016;14(1):51.
22. Declercq E, Luke B, Belanoff C, et al. Perinatal outcomes associated with assisted reproductive technology: the Massachusetts Outcomes Study of Assisted Reproductive Technologies (MOSART). Fertil Steril. 2015;103(4):888–95.
23. Sunkara SK, La Marca A, Seed PT, Khalaf Y. Increased risk of preterm birth and low birthweight with very high number of oocytes following IVF: an analysis of 65 868 singleton live birth outcomes. Hum Reprod (Oxford). 2015;30(6):1473–80.
24. Sazonova A, Kallen K, Thurin-Kjellberg A, Wennerholm UB, Bergh C. Obstetric outcome in singletons after in vitro fertilization with cryopreserved/thawed embryos. Hum Reprod (Oxford). 2012;27(5):1343–50.
25. Kalra SK, Ratcliffe SJ, Coutifaris C, Molinaro T, Barnhart KT. Ovarian stimulation and low birth weight in newborns conceived through in vitro fertilization. Obstet Gynecol. 2011;118(4):863–71.
26. Weinerman R, Ord T, Bartolomei MS, Coutifaris C, Mainigi M. The superovulated environment, independent of embryo vitrification, results in low birthweight in a mouse model. Biol Reprod. 2017;97(1):133–42.
27. Shapiro BS, Daneshmand ST, Bedient CE, Garner FC. Comparison of birth weights in patients randomly assigned to fresh or frozen-thawed embryo transfer. Fertil Steril. 2016;106(2):317–21.
28. Ginstrom Ernstad E, Bergh C, Khatibi A, et al. Neonatal and maternal outcome after blastocyst transfer: a population-based registry study. Am J Obstet Gynecol. 2016;214(3):378.e1–10.
29. Alviggi C, Conforti A, Carbone IF, Borrelli R, de Placido G, Guerriero S. Influence of cryopreservation on perinatal outcome after blastocyst- vs cleavage-stage embryo transfer: systematic review and meta-analysis. Ultrasound Obstet Gynecol. 2018;51(1):54–63.
30. Opdahl S, Henningsen AA, Tiitinen A, et al. Risk of hypertensive disorders in pregnancies following assisted reproductive technology: a cohort study from the CoNARTaS group. Hum Reprod (Oxford). 2015;30(7):1724–31.
31. Sites CK, Wilson D, Barsky M, et al. Embryo cryopreservation and preeclampsia risk. Fertil Steril. 2017;108(5):784–90.
32. Huang B, Hu D, Qian K, et al. Is frozen embryo transfer cycle associated with a significantly lower incidence of ectopic pregnancy? An analysis of more than 30,000 cycles. Fertil Steril. 2014;102(5):1345–9.

33. Fang C, Huang R, Wei LN, Jia L. Frozen-thawed day 5 blastocyst transfer is associated with a lower risk of ectopic pregnancy than day 3 transfer and fresh transfer. Fertil Steril. 2015;103(3):655–661.e653.
34. Londra L, Moreau C, Strobino D, Garcia J, Zacur H, Zhao Y. Ectopic pregnancy after in vitro fertilization: differences between fresh and frozen-thawed cycles. Fertil Steril. 2015;104(1):110–8.
35. Li Z, Sullivan EA, Chapman M, Farquhar C, Wang YA. Risk of ectopic pregnancy lowest with transfer of single frozen blastocyst. Hum Reprod (Oxford). 2015;30(9):2048–54.
36. Zhang X, Ma C, Wu Z, et al. Frozen-thawed embryo transfer cycles have a lower incidence of ectopic pregnancy compared with fresh embryo transfer cycles. Reprod Sci (Thousand Oaks). 2017:1933719117746759.
37. Aflatoonian A, Karimzadeh Maybodi MA, Aflatoonian N, et al. Perinatal outcome in fresh versus frozen embryo transfer in ART cycles. Int J Reprod Biomed (Yazd, Iran). 2016;14(3):167–72.
38. Santos-Ribeiro S, Tournaye H, Polyzos NP. Trends in ectopic pregnancy rates following assisted reproductive technologies in the UK: a 12-year nationwide analysis including 160 000 pregnancies. Hum Reprod (Oxford). 2016;31(2):393–402.
39. Ishihara O, Kuwahara A, Saitoh H. Frozen-thawed blastocyst transfer reduces ectopic pregnancy risk: an analysis of single embryo transfer cycles in Japan. Fertil Steril. 2011;95(6):1966–9.
40. Kaser DJ, Melamed A, Bormann CL, et al. Cryopreserved embryo transfer is an independent risk factor for placenta accreta. Fertil Steril. 2015;103(5):1176–1184.e1172.
41. Ma WG, Song H, Das SK, Paria BC, Dey SK. Estrogen is a critical determinant that specifies the duration of the window of uterine receptivity for implantation. Proc Natl Acad Sci U S A. 2003;100(5):2963–8.

47 Outcome of Vitrified-Thawed Embryo Transfer in the GnRH Agonist Versus Antagonist Protocols

Mete Isikoglu

47.1 Rationale

Considerable proportion of the adverse treatment outcome in assisted reproductive techniques (ART) is the result of multiple pregnancies, including twins. Thus, one of the main challenges is to avoid multiple pregnancies without significantly lowering the overall pregnancy rates. This can be done if the best embryo can be selected for transfer and if the freezing and thawing techniques can be improved.

Since the mid-1980s, cryopreservation and storage of in vitro-derived cleavage stage embryos have been employed. The first successful pregnancy via frozen embryo transfer (FET) was reported in 1983 in Australia [1] followed by the first live birth following embryo cryopreservation in 1984 in the Netherlands [2]. The major advantages of frozen embryo transfer are increased cumulative pregnancy rate after oocyte pickup, decreased multiple birth rate, decreased cost, and prevention of ovarian hyperstimulation syndrome (OHSS) and related complications [3]. The economic costs of multiple births are much higher compared with singleton births. The mean medical cost of delivering a singleton baby was estimated to be $9329, whereas a set of twins costs $20,318, and triplets costs $153,335 [4].

Conventional slow-freezing protocols have been extensively used for cryopreservation of human embryos. These procedures are based on low cryoprotectant concentrations and a slow cooling rate. Vitrification (i.e., a glass-like state) is an increasingly popular method, based on an ultra-rapid method of cryopreservation, the aim of which is to overcome the damages due to cryopreservation including chilling injury, intracellular ice formation, and fracture damages. The principle of dehydration also applies in vitrification, but concepts such as hydraulic permeability play a less significant role. To achieve vitrification within a cell, both a reduction in water content and a highly viscous cytoplasm are necessary. This is facilitated by exposure to high concentrations of permeating and non-permeating cryoprotectants which result in extreme shrinkage together with rapid cooling rates. In order to minimize the impact of the hyper-osmotic conditions, the exposure time is reduced followed by loading on to microtools. Further improvements, such as artificial collapse of the blastocoel and use of minute volume holding devices (e.g., electron microscopic grid and Cryoloop), have greatly improved the survival rates of vitrified blastocysts.

The first successful pregnancy following transfer of vitrified blastocyst was reported in 2000 followed 1 year later by the first report of live delivery via vitrified blastocyst.

In their critical review of the published literature, Edgar et al. reported that available evidence suggests that vitrification is the current method of choice when cryopreserving metaphase II oocytes. Early cleavage stage embryos can be cryopreserved with equal success using slow cooling and vitrification. Successful blastocyst cryopreservation may be more consistently achieved with vitrification, but optimal slow cooling can produce similar results [5].

The effect of many factors on the outcome of FET has been the subject of the studies so far including controlled ovarian hyperstimulation (COH) protocol, freezing protocol, the selection of embryos for freezing and transfer, and endometrial preparation before embryo transfer, as well as the age of women undergoing FET.

Interestingly, in the existing literature, comparison of the outcome of vitrified-thawed embryos generated from gonadotrophin releasing hormone (GnRH) agonist and antagonist protocols has not been rigorously evaluated so far. In a scarce number of studies, the issue is mentioned among other stimulation parameters.

This chapter will discuss the effect of the type of the GnRH analog used in a COH program on the outcome of vitrified/thawed cycles.

M. Isikoglu (✉)
Gelecek The Center For Human Reproduction, Antalya, Turkey

G. N. Allahbadia et al. (eds.), *Textbook of Assisted Reproduction*, https://doi.org/10.1007/978-981-15-2377-9_47

47.2 Introduction

The ultimate goal of assisted reproductive techniques is to get the woman pregnant with a singleton pregnancy. Elective single embryo transfer and cryopreservation of the excess embryos with a good cryopreservation program may results in acceptable pregnancy rates with a low risk for multiples. Besides, cryopreservation may provide safety for patients with a high risk of OHSS. Furthermore, for patients whose endometrium is not favorable, cryopreservation of the entire cohort of embryos and FET may provide better implantation rates.

Based on the data generated from European registers by ESHRE, IVF practitioners have a tendency to transfer lesser number of embryos over the last decade (Fig. 47.1).

According to the same database, in 2009 the proportion of FET cycles to "fresh" cycles was 28.0% (26% in 2008), but in some countries the proportion was much higher: 43% in Switzerland, 32% in Sweden, and 40% in Finland [6].

In the United States, the contribution of frozen-thawed embryo transfers to the number of total live births has been increasing continuously for the last 15 years (Fig. 47.2a, b).

Because vitrification appears to be an efficient and safe method for preservation, the prevalence of vitrification increased worldwide in the last decade. Factors related to the outcome of frozen/thawed embryo transfers are COH protocol, freezing protocol, selection of embryos for freezing and transfer, pregnancy in the fresh IVF/ICSI cycle from where the frozen embryos originated, female age at embryo freezing, the age of women undergoing FET, embryo quality before freezing, thawed embryos resume cleaving, cryopreservation-associated damage, progesterone supplementation, hormonal substitution, antral follicle count, basal serum FSH level, endometrial thickness, mean number of embryos transferred, mean number of good-quality embryos, reason for freezing, damaged blastomere, and observed compaction [7–9].

47.3 Clinical Discussion

In their retrospective analysis, Ashrafi et al. investigated the impact of the clinical and embryological factors on the pregnancy outcome of frozen-thawed embryo transfer. Evaluation of 247 cycles in which slow-freezing technique was used revealed that the pregnancy outcome was better and implantation rate was higher in women who were stimulated with the GnRH long agonist protocol in their fresh cycles than those stimulated with the antagonist protocol [7]. Contradictory results were reported by some other researchers: Seelig et al. found that pregnancy rates were similar independent of whether they resulted from the long-protocol cycles with hMG (15.4%) and recFSH (13.1%) or from the antagonist protocol cycles with hMG (25.0%) and recFSH (17.5%) [10]. In parallel to these findings, Eldar-Geva et al. found similar outcome for cryopreserved embryo transfer following GnRH-antagonist/GnRH-agonist, GnRH-antagonist/HCG, or long protocol ovarian stimulation [11].

Shi et al. retrospectively analyzed 2313 vitrified-thawed embryo transfer cycles regarding 22 clinical variables. Blastocyst transfers were excluded. The pregnancy rates were higher in long agonist protocol (51.6%) compared to short protocol (33.7%) and other protocols (35.5%) [12]. In

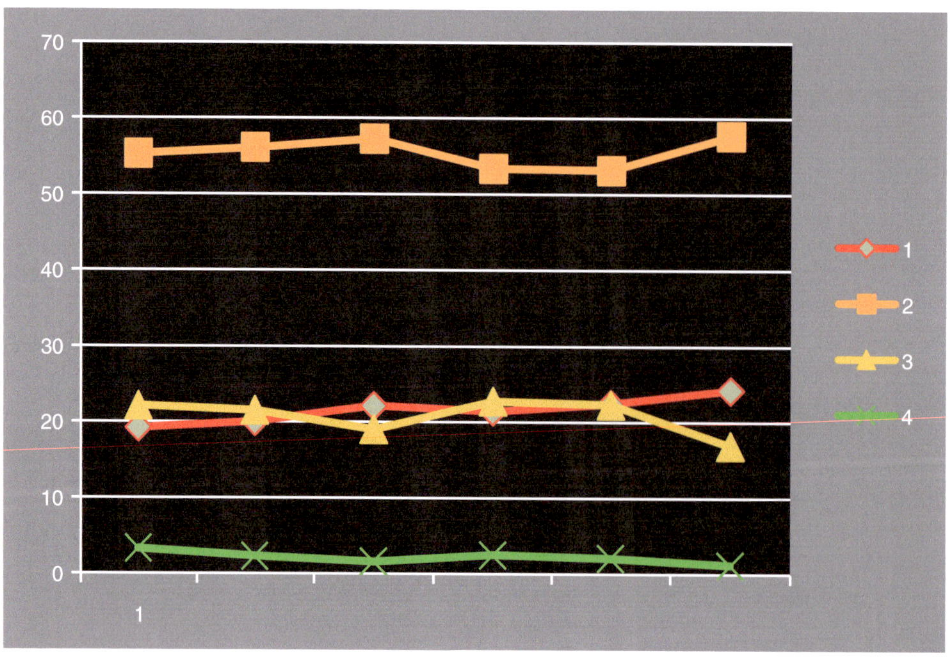

Fig. 47.1 Percentages of number of embryos transferred per fresh cycle in European countries between 2004 and 2011

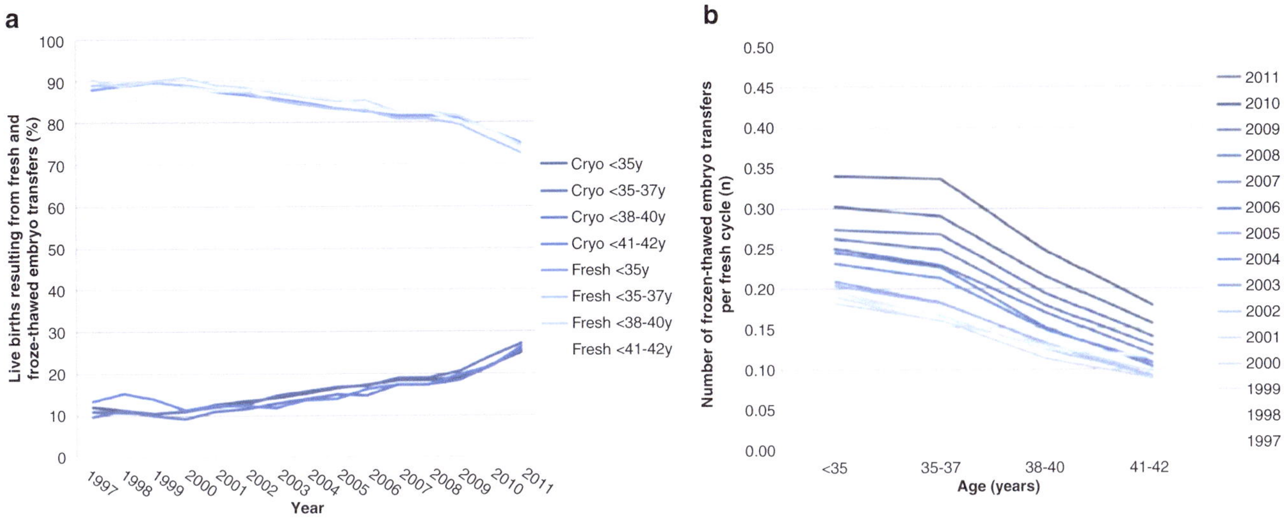

Fig. 47.2 (**a**) The contribution of fresh and frozen-thawed embryo transfers to the number of total live births after ART per age group from 1997 to 2011 in the United States. (**b**) The number of frozen-thawed embryo transfers per the number of fresh cycles per year from 1997 to 2011 in the United States (adapted from CDC 2013)

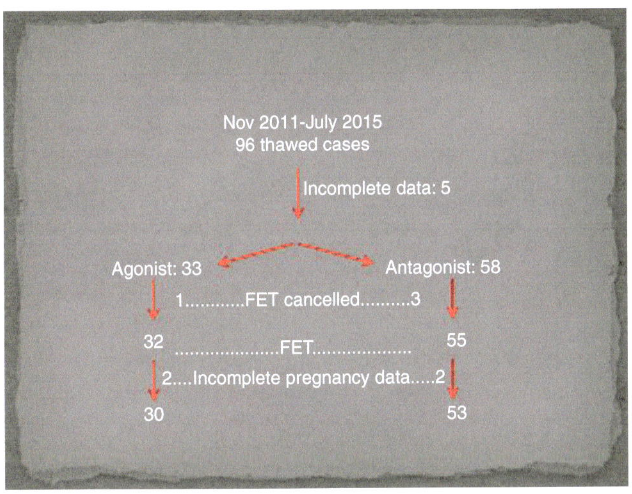

Fig. 47.3 Flowchart of the retrospective descriptive analysis of the vitrified-thawed embryo transfers

another retrospective study, Ahlström et al. evaluated several variables for the prediction of live birth in frozen-thawed single blastocyst transfer cycles. Live birth rates after agonist and antagonist cycles were 39.2% and 38.8%, respectively ($p = 0.98$) [13].

We retrospectively analyzed our own data pertaining to the period between November 2011 and July 2015 on vitrification/thawing cycles (Fig. 47.3). In all agonist and antagonist cycles, final triggering was performed by recombinant human chorionic gonadotrophin.

Of the 91 cryopreservation cases, 48 were vitrified at cleavage stage (on day 2 or day 3), while 43 were vitrified at blastocyst stage.

Table 47.1 Demographic and general characteristics of both groups

	Agonist	Antagonist	*p*
# Patients	33	58	NA
Age	31.7 ± 5.1	31.7 ± 5.2	0.97
Husband's age	35.6 ± 4.5	36.1 ± 6.6	0.68
BMI	24.4 ± 4.0	23.3 ± 4.0	0.24
Previous IVF attempts	3 (9%)	6 (10%)	0.52

During the mentioned time period, all FETs were performed in hormonally supplemented cycles. For the preparation of the endometrium, hormone replacement with 2 mg/day estradiol valerate was started from day 1 of the cycle and gradually increased to 6 mg/day, and 90 mg intravaginal progesterone was commenced 2 days before FET. Endometrial thickness was assessed by transvaginal ultrasound.

Age of the patients, husbands' ages, BMIs, and the number of previous IVF attempts were similar in both groups (Table 47.1).

The etiology of the patients is depicted in Table 47.2. The percentage of tubal factor infertility was much higher in agonist group. There is not a conceivable explanation except coincidence for this finding. Higher number of patients would be helpful to exclude the effect of chance.

The stimulation parameters for the fresh cycles did not show any statistically significant difference (Table 47.3).

Pre-freeze parameters are shown in Tables 47.4 and 47.5.

Post-thaw parameters, pregnancy rates, and implantation rates for cleavage phase transfers (Table 47.6) and blastocyst transfers did not show any statistically significant difference (Table 47.7).

The percentage of subgroups with immediate FET and FET after post-thaw extended culture were found to be

Table 47.2 Etiologic classification in both groups

	Agonist	Antagonist	*p*
Male factor	11 (33%)	14 (24%)	0.35
Endometriosis	1 (3%)	1 (1.7%)	1
Tubal factor	9 (27%)	2 (3.4%)	0.001
Unexplained	3 (9.1%)	11 (19%)	0.20
Ovulatory	5 (15%)	14 (24%)	0.31
Combined	1 (3%)	2 (3%)	1

Table 47.3 COH variables of the groups

	Agonist	Antagonist	*p*
Duration of COH	9.8 ± 1.5	9.5 ± 1.5	0.27
GN used	1977 ± 586	1925 ± 579	0.68
Peak E2 value	2225± 1205	2244 ± 2443	0.97
# Antral follicles	14.65 ± 5.9	13.38 ± 7.8	0.47

Table 47.4 Pre-freeze parameters for day 2–3 freezing

	Agonist	Antagonist	*p*
	13	35	NA
# MII oocytes	12.3 ± 6.7	12.1 ± 6.2	0.93
Fertilization rate	93%	89%	0.49
Use of testicular sperm	1/13	2/35	1

Table 47.5 Pre-freeze parameters for day 5 freezing

	Agonist	Antagonist	*p*
	20	23	NA
# MII oocytes	18.75 ± 7.5	17.22 ± 6.6	0.48
Fertilization rate	93%	88%	0.46
Use of testicular sperm	1/20	0/23	0.46

Table 47.6 Post-thaw parameters, pregnancy rates, and implantation rates for cleavage phase embryo transfers

	Agonist	Antagonist	*p*
	13	35	NA
# Embryos frozen	3.75 ± 2.7	4.75 ± 3.7	0.49
Survival rate %	89.9 ± 24.9	83.9 ± 24.6	0.56
Partial degeneration %	10.13 ± 24.9	16.13 ± 24.6	0.56
# Embryos transferred	2.38 ± 0.92	2.33 ± 0.70	0.89
Pregnancy rate%	42.9	26.1	0.64
Implantation rate%	19.0 ± 25.8	6.6 ± 15.7	0.12

Table 47.7 Post-thaw parameters, pregnancy rates, and implantation rates for blastocyst transfers

	Agonist	Antagonist	*p*
	20	23	NA
# Embryos frozen	5.63 ± 2.8	5.19 ± 2.6	0.55
Survival rate %	86.3 ± 22.7	85.2 ± 21.8	0.86
# Embryos transferred	2.5 ± 0.8	2.32 ± 0.7	0.48
Pregnancy rate %	33.3	34.5	0.93
Implantation rate %	14.0 ± 0.2	13.0 ± 0.3	0.87

Table 47.8 Percentage of immediate FET and FET after post-thaw culture for day 2–3 frozen embryos

	Agonist	Antagonist	*p*
Immediate FET	9 (70%)	26 (74%)	1
FET after follow-up	4 (30%)	9 (26%)	0.72

Table 47.9 Percentage of immediate FET and FET after post-thaw culture for day 5 frozen embryos

	Agonist	Antagonist	*p*
Immediate FET	18 (90%)	22 (96%)	0.32
FET after follow-up	2 (10%)	1 (4%)	0.59

similar for the agonist and antagonist groups (Tables 47.8 and 47.9).

47.4 Recent Advances and Conclusion

FET has been successfully performed worldwide and provides further opportunities for patients to achieve pregnancy in addition to fresh embryo transfers. However consensus is still lacking on the best practice for embryo cryopreservation. Even though several variables of patients' profiles, controlled ovarian stimulation, embryo morphokinetics, and freezing-thawing techniques were rigorously investigated; the effect of the type of GnRH analog on the outcome of vitrified-thawed embryo transfers has not been the major concern of the studies so far. Our study is the first one focusing directly on the effect of the type of the GnRH analog on the outcome of the vitrified-thawed embryo transfer. It also is unique since it compares the outcome of both cleavage stage embryos as well as blastocysts. In the present data, post-thaw embryo parameters and pregnancy outcome were very similar in vitrified-thawed embryo transfers in agonist and antagonist cycles. Thus, the potential for frozen-thawed embryos to implant and develop following transfer seems to be independent of the GnRH analog. This issue still needs high-quality prospective randomized trials for stronger evidence.

References

1. Trounson A, Mohr L. Human pregnancy following cryopreservation, thawing and transfer of an eight-cell embryo. Nature. 1983;305(5936):707–9.
2. Zeilmaker GH, Alberda AT, van Gent I, Rijkmans CM, Drogendijk AC. Two pregnancies following transfer of intact frozen-thawed embryos. Fertil Steril. 1984;42(2):293–6.
3. Tiitinen A, Halttunen M, Härkki P, Vuoristo P, Hyden-Granskog C. Elective single embryo transfer: the value of cryopreservation. Hum Reprod. 2001;16(6):1140–4.

4. Hidlebaugh DA, Thompson IE, Berger MJ. Cost of assisted reproductive technologies for a health maintenance organization. J Reprod Med. 1997;42:570–4.
5. Edgar DH, Gook DA. A critical appraisal of cryopreservation (slow cooling versus vitrification) of human oocytes and embryos. Hum Reprod Update. 2012;18(5):536–54. https://doi.org/10.1093/humupd/dms016. Epub 2012 Apr 25.
6. Kupka MS, Ferraretti AP, de Mouzon J, Erb K, D'Hooghe T, Castilla JA, Calhaz-Jorge C, De Geyter C, Goossens V, European IVF-Monitoring Consortium, for the European Society of Human Reproduction and Embryology. Assisted reproductive technology in Europe, 2010: results generated from European registers by ESHRE. Hum Reprod. 2014;29(10):2099–113. https://doi.org/10.1093/humrep/deu175. Epub 2014 Jul 27.
7. Ashrafi M, Jahangiri N, Hassani F, Akhoond MR, Madani T. The factors affecting the outcome of frozen-thawed embryo transfer cycle. Taiwan J Obstet Gynecol. 2011;50(2):159–64. https://doi.org/10.1016/j.tjog.2011.01.037.
8. Sun Y, Feng Y, Zhang A, Lu X, Niu Z, Gu R. Frozen–thawed embryo transfer cycles in China: clinical outcomes of two and three multicellular embryos transfers. J Assist Reprod Genet. 2012;29:417–21.
9. Balaban B, Urman B, Ata B, Isiklar A, Larman MG, Hamilton R, Gardner DK. (2008). A randomized controlled study of human day 3 embryo cryopreservation by slow freezing or vitrification: vitrification is associated with higher survival, metabolism and blastocyst formation. Hum Reprod. 2008;23:1976–82.
10. Seelig AS, Al-Hasani S, Katalinic A, Schöpper B, Sturm R, Diedrich K, Ludwig M. Comparison of cryopreservation outcome with gonadotropin-releasing hormone agonists or antagonists in the collecting cycle. Fertil Steril. 2002;77(3):472–5.
11. Eldar-Geva T, Zylber-Haran E, Babayof R, Halevy-Shalem T, Ben-Chetrit A, Tsafrir A, Varshaver I, Brooks B, Margalioth EJ. Similar outcome for cryopreserved embryo transfer following GnRH-antagonist/GnRH-agonist, GnRH-antagonist/HCG or long protocol ovarian stimulation. Reprod Biomed Online. 2007;14(2):148–54.
12. Shi W, Zhang S, Zhao W, Xia X, Wang M, Wang H, Bai H, Shi J. Factors related to clinical pregnancy after vitrified-warmed embryo transfer: a retrospective and multivariate logistic regression analysis of 2313 transfer cycles. Hum Reprod. 2013;28(7):1768–75. https://doi.org/10.1093/humrep/det094. Epub 2013 Apr 18.
13. Ahlström A, Westin C, Wikland M, Hardarson T. Prediction of live birth in frozen-thawed single blastocyst transfer cycles by pre-freeze and post-thaw morphology. Hum Reprod. 2013;28(5):1199–209. https://doi.org/10.1093/humrep/det054. Epub 2013 Mar 10.

48 Blastocyst Transfer For Everyone?

J. Preston Parry and John S. Rushing

One of the hardest questions in medicine is "What does it mean to do right by our patients?" When it comes to deciding whether patients should have only blastocyst transfers, this is not as clear cut as it would seem. At first glance, transferring only blastocysts makes sense if wishing to maximize fecundity while following current standards for the number of embryos to transfer [1]. Though a case can be made for this approach resulting in the best outcomes, what may be right for the patient may not always be the approach that leads to the highest fecundity per transfer. Several factors such as patient autonomy, lab capabilities, and cost-effectiveness may result in circumstances where a cleavage-stage transfer may be reasonable. Patients are heterogeneous in their diagnoses and desires, so a one-size-fits-all approach is difficult to justify, even if one size will fit most. By reviewing core considerations for blastocyst relative to cleavage-stage transfer, it is easier for clinicians to delineate their personal balance between the ideal and the real, which helps their patients find this balance as well.

The primary objectives for this chapter are to assess transferring only blastocysts relative to cleavage-stage embryos, explore the underlying evidence, and then address considerations that may favor cleavage-stage over cavitating-stage transfer.

48.1 The Case for Blastocyst Transfer for Everyone

When combined, three considerations suggest that most, if not all, patients should have blastocyst-stage transfer preferred to cleavage stage. These are:

1. Current standards for the number of embryos to transfer typically recommend transferring a similar number of cleavage- and blastocyst-stage embryos.
2. For the same number of embryos, blastocyst transfer results in a higher pregnancy rate per transfer than cleavage stage.
3. Relative to extended culture, transfer of poor-quality cleavage-stage embryos does not increase the likelihood of a live birth, even if waiting until a cavitating stage would increase the risk of having no embryos to transfer.

Taken in combination, if extended culture allows embryos to demonstrate their true viability, when only one embryo (or two) should be transferred regardless of stage, it makes sense to choose one that has declared itself to have a better prognosis.

48.2 How Many Embryos Should Be Transferred?

The American Society for Reproductive Medicine (ASRM) and the Society for Assisted Reproductive Technology (SART) have been leaders in trying to reduce the "multiple birth epidemic." Popular awareness for this issue dates back to *Life Magazine* in their August 25, 1965, issue describing Pergonal as "the fantastic drug that creates quintuplets." Though this article predates IVF, for the USA in the 1980s when IVF started to become more available, a meaningful gap started to develop between observed and age-adjusted rates of twin as well as triplet and higher-order births [2]. Between 1971 and 2001, twin births increased almost twofold and triplet and higher-order births increased more than sevenfold.

Advances in technology have been important in allowing fewer embryos to be transferred for comparable or even higher rates of success. However, public pressure as well as guidance from ASRM, SART, and other organizations has also helped in stemming the tide of multiple gestation. As a

J. P. Parry (✉) · J. S. Rushing
Department of Obstetrics and Gynecology, University of Mississippi Medical Center, Jackson, MS, USA

G. N. Allahbadia et al. (eds.), *Textbook of Assisted Reproduction*, https://doi.org/10.1007/978-981-15-2377-9_48

result, between 1998 and 2011, transfer of three or more embryos during an IVF cycle declined from 79% to 24% [2]. As a result, the proportion of twins associated with IVF appears to be plateauing, and the proportion of triplet and higher-order births from IVF has declined by 33% over a 13-year period from 48% to 32%.

To make further progress in reducing multiple gestations, ASRM and SART Practice Committees issued in 2017 even more stringent guidelines for the number of embryos to transfer (Table 48.1) [1]. With these guidelines, all women with euploid embryos should have single-embryo transfer, regardless of whether it is cleavage stage or blastocyst. Similarly, if euploidy is unknown but the patient has a favorable prognosis, all women up to age 37 should have single-embryo transfer, regardless of whether it is cleavage stage or blastocyst. Moreover, if the woman is under the age of 35 and does not have known euploidy or favorable prognosis, she should only receive one to two embryos, regardless of whether they are cleavage stage or blastocyst. Outside of these circumstances, the guidelines start to allow for greater flexibility with increasing advanced maternal age, which makes sense because of higher rates of aneuploidy. However, based on the national statistics for age distributions for IVF, one would expect at least half to two thirds of women undergoing IVF with their own eggs to have the same number of embryos recommended for transfer, regardless of whether they are cleavage stage or blastocysts. Therefore, if patients are wanting to maximize pregnancy rates and are constrained in the quantity to transfer, then selecting the best quality embryos optimizes per cycle fecundity.

Table 48.1 Recommendations for the limit to the number of embryos to transfer

	Age (years)			
Prognosis	<35	35–37	38–40	41–42
Cleavage-stage embryos[a]				
Euploid	1	1	1	1
Other favorable[b]	1	1	≤3	≤4
All others	≤2	≤3	≤4	≤5
Blastocysts[a]				
Euploid	1	1	1	1
Other favorable[b]	1	1	≤2	≤3
All others	≤2	≤2	≤3	≤3

From Guidelines for limits on how many embryos should be transferred. (Reproduced with permission from the Practice Committee of the American Society for Reproductive Medicine and the Practice Committee of the Society for Assisted Reproductive Technology. Guidance on the limits to the number of embryos to transfer: a committee opinion. Fertil Steril. 2017;107(4): p. 901–3, with permission

[a]See text for more complete explanations

[b]Other favorable-Any ONE of these criteria: Fresh cycle: expectation of one or more high-quality embryos available for cryopreservation, or previous live birth after an IVF cycle; FET cycle: availability of vitrified day 5 or day 6 blastocysts, euploid embryos, first FET cycle, or previous live birth after an IVF cycle

Please note: Justification for transferring additional embryos beyond recommended limits should be clearly documented in the patient's medical record. ASRM

Limits on number of embryos to transfer. Fertil Steril. 2017

48.3 Does Blastocyst Transfer Result in a Higher Pregnancy Rate than Cleavage-Stage Transfer?

Embryology can be humbling. Suboptimal-appearing early-stage embryos can progress into healthy-appearing blastocysts. High-grade embryos can be aneuploid. Even a few hours can sometimes result in an "ugly duckling" turning in to a "swan," where embryos selected for transfer in the morning may change by the afternoon. Multiple factors contribute to this and preimplantation genetic screening will be an important step for further understanding embryonic viability, as well as potentially technologies such as metabolomics and time-lapse embryo monitoring.

One of the critical underlying factors may relate to the influence of paternal DNA on embryonic development. Though maternal genes drive the first two embryonic cell divisions [3], poor-quality sperm have progressively more negative effects throughout the rest of embryonic development [4, 5]. As a result, though marked damage may be readily apparent, the longer an embryo develops past the cleavage stage, the greater the chance for identifying DNA-associated defects, particularly for sperm-associated problems, which may be why cleavage-stage morphology is limited in predicting blastocyst quality [6]. Additionally, even if a single viable embryo is present, there may be an advantage to transferring at a cavitating stage relative to a cleavage stage, as uterine contractility seems to decrease as time progresses from hCG administration [7]. Also, the hyperestrogenic environment may be more disadvantageous to early-stage embryos as a result of less than ideal conditions for growth [8].

Regardless of mechanism, multiple publications have shown the theoretical benefits of blastocyst transfer to result in higher pregnancy rates relative to cleavage stage after controlling for the number of embryos transferred [9–11]. A 2016 Cochrane review showed an odds ratio of 1.48 (95% CI 1.20–1.82) from blastocyst transfer relative to cleavage-stage transfer (Fig. 48.1) [12]. These findings were pooled from 13 studies with a total of 1630 participants (couples or women using donor sperm). Clinical pregnancy rates (OR 1.3, 95% CI 1.14–1.47) and cumulative pregnancy rates with vitrification (OR 2.44, 95% CI 1.17–5.12) also favor blastocyst transfer. (Cumulative pregnancy rates were higher for cleavage stage than blastocyst transfers when looking at four older studies using slow freeze protocols, but freezing technology and extended culture were less advanced at the time of those studies as a potential source of bias.) Also of note, because

Study of Subgroup	Day 5/6 Events	Day 5/6 Total	Day 2/3 Events	Day 2/3 Total	Weight	Odds Ratio M-H, Fixed, 95% CI
Brugnon 2010	22	55	21	52	8.8%	0.98 [0.45, 2.13]
Devreker 2000	3	11	1	12	0.5%	4.13 [0.36, 47.30]
Elgindy 2011	52	100	35	100	11.4%	2.01 [1.14, 3.55]
Emiliani 2003	33	82	41	89	16.0%	0.79 [0.43, 1,45]
Fernandez-Shaw 2015	25	60	11	60	4.4%	3.18 [1.39, 7.31]
Frattarelli 2003	15	29	8	28	2.7%	2.68 [0.89, 8.02]
Levitas 2004	3	23	3	31	1.5%	1.40 [0.26, 7.66]
Levron 2002	8	46	15	44	8.6%	0.41 [0.15, 1.09]
Livingstone 2002	14	30	11	29	4.1%	1.43 [0.51, 4.04]
Papanikolaou 2005	38	80	23	84	8.0%	2.40 [1.25, 4.60]
Papanikolaou 2006	56	175	38	176	17.5%	1.71 [1.06, 2.76]
Rienzi 2002	24	50	24	48	8.7%	0.92 [0.42, 2.04]
Van der Auwera 2002	24	70	17	66	7.8%	1.50 [0.72, 3.15]
Total (95% CI)		**811**		**819**	**100.0%**	**1.48 [1.20, 1.82]**
Total events	317		248			

Heterogeneity: Chi^2 = 21.83, df = 12 (P = 0.04); I^2 = 45%
Test for overall effect: Z = 3.68 (P = 0.0002)

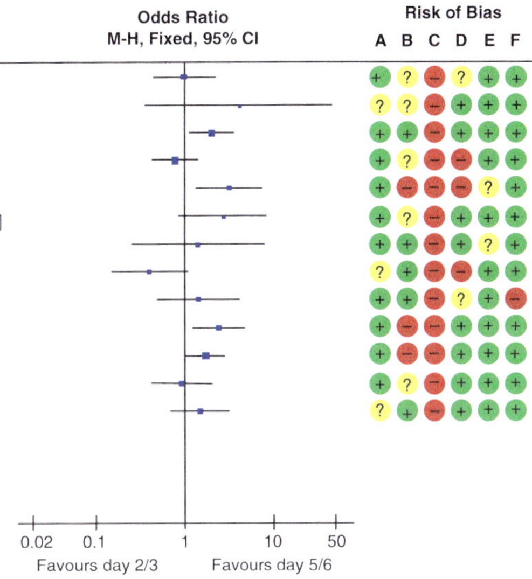

Risk of bias legend
(A) Random sequence generation (selection bias)
(B) Allocation concealment (selection blas)
(C) Blinding (performance bias and detection bias)
(D) Incompleted outcome data (attrition bias)
(E) Selective reporting (reporting bias)
(F) Other biase

Fig. 48.1 Forest plot comparing live birth rates for blastocyst vs. cleavage-stage transfer. (From Glujovsky D, Farquhar C, Quinteiro Retamar A, Alvarez Sedo C, Blake D. Cleavage stage versus blastocyst embryo transfer in assisted reproductive technology. The Cochrane Library. 2016; 6(Jan 1), with permission)

clinicians tend to transfer more cleavage stage than blastocyst-stage embryos, subgroup analysis where only equal numbers of embryos were transferred still showed a persistent advantage to blastocyst transfer. Though the data did not show a statistically significant increase in twin (OR 1.05, 95% CI 0.83–1.33) or high-order multiple gestation (OR 0.45, 95% CI 0.18–1.15), there was a trend toward the latter increasing with cleavage-stage transfer. Also of note, surprisingly there was a slight trend toward a higher likelihood of miscarriage with blastocyst transfer (OR 1.15, 95% CI 0.88–1.50), though this also was not statistically significant. Finally, the Cochrane analysis did not see a difference in cumulative pregnancy rates between cleavage- and blastocyst-stage transfers, but this conclusion (or lack thereof) came from very-low-quality evidence.

48.4 Are Poor-Quality Cleavage-Stage Embryos More Likely to Survive in Utero than in Culture Until the Blastocyst Stage?

If patients have favorable prognosis and are planning to freeze all embryos with subsequent transfer, doing this at the blastocyst stage seems to result in higher pregnancy rates than freeze all at the cleavage stage [13]. Part of this difference relates to embryo selection. However, even when selecting good-quality embryos, blastocysts seem to have a slightly higher survival rate with vitrification than cleavage-stage embryos [14], so if there are embryos in excess of those that would be transferred, many will culture embryos until they are cavitating. Accordingly, decisions for blastocyst transfer are easier if extended culture is intended anyway.

If extended culture for transfer and freezing indications is probable in good prognosis patients, then the decision for cleavage-stage transfer may apply more to poor prognosis patients with fewer embryos of lower quality. Though day 3 of culture is a snapshot in time and some embryos can make a remarkable recovery, many poor-quality cleavage-stage embryos do not progress to the blastocyst stage. This is consistent with the Cochrane findings that culturing to the blastocyst stage increases the probability that there are no embryos to transfer (OR 2.5, 95% CI 1.76–3.55, day 2–3 3.6%, day 5–6 8.5%) [12]. However, the lack of embryos to transfer does not necessarily mean that pregnancy outcomes were changed. If focusing on patients with poor-quality cleavage-stage embryos, limited data suggests that continuing culture to blastocyst stage doesn't hurt and may help. According to one prospective case study using historic controls for comparable poor-quality embryos, transferring at cleavage stage resulted in a 27.2% pregnancy rate per transfer, which increased to a net pregnancy rate of 33.5% if embryos were cultured to the blastocyst stage before transfer (even after accounting for 7.6% of patients having no blastocysts to transfer) [15]. The higher pregnancy rate with blastocyst transfer for similar poor-quality embryos was not statistically significant nor was the lower rate of miscarriage (cleavage stage 20.4% vs. blastocyst 13.2%) nor the lower rate of multiple gestation (cleavage stage 13.6% vs. blastocyst 9.4%). However, a mean of 5.2 embryos were transferred in the cleavage stage relative to a mean of 2.4 embryos in the blastocyst stage. More research needs to be performed specifically comparing immediate transfer to extended culture for patients with poor-quality cleavage-stage embryos; however, the trend does not show cleavage-stage transfer to be advantageous, and it may even be disadvantageous. Moreover, if ASRM/SART guidelines for a patient would recommend a similar number of cleavage-stage and blastocyst embryos for transfer, yet more than doubling the number of cleavage-stage embryos transferred does not increase fecundity; the case for blastocyst transfer in poor prognosis patients becomes even stronger.

48.5 The Case Against Blastocyst Transfer for Everyone

48.5.1 Patient Autonomy

A central principle of medical ethics is patient autonomy. Predating both the Nuremberg Code and the Tuskegee syphilis study, the landmark 1914 New York case *Schloendorff v. Society of New York Hospital* ruled that medical intervention without consent could be considered battery [16]. Clinicians caring for hypertension, diabetes, and cancer frequently find their patients have different preferences relative to their own, and the balance of autonomy with beneficence and nonmaleficence can be difficult. Procreative therapy is rife with patients using complementary and alternative medicines, and this is accepted by clinicians even when these can be associated with up to 30% lower pregnancy and live birth rates [17]. Many patients will choose blastocyst transfer when presented with data that it overall results in higher live birth rates per fresh transfer and that cleavage-stage transfer even with poor-quality embryos does not seem to improve pregnancy outcomes. However, not all patients will make such choices any more than they will all agree on ICSI, assisted hatching, or complementary and alternative medicines. Though autonomy does not give patients the right to force clinicians into dangerous or unethical practice, it does give patients the right to choose less effective therapies if on a scale comparable to other accepted treatment alternatives. Informing and respecting our patients is central to great care, even when their choices may not mirror our own, including when it comes to cleavage stage relative to blastocyst transfer.

48.5.2 Laboratory Technology

Though advances in embryology have led to "extended culture" becoming relatively standard, not all practices in the world use extended culture. This is comparable to the persistence of ZIFT and GIFT after culture to cleavage stage became more successful. With favorable outcomes being associated with blastocyst transfer, as well as programs able to offer extended culture likely having a level of technology contributing to higher fecundity, ideally patients should be steered to programs that can offer the best chance of pregnancy. However, access to fertility care can be limited, where geographic and other barriers may hinder patients from receiving the full range of therapies [18]. Accordingly, all practices that offer IVF should strive to be able to culture embryos to the blastocyst stage effectively, even if rare exceptions may exist.

48.5.3 Cost-Effectiveness

No economic analyses have been performed comparing cleavage-stage and blastocyst transfer. However, the cumulative live birth rates for cleavage-stage and blastocyst transfer are not statistically different, even though it favors blastocyst transfer when using vitrification for embryo freezing [12]. (Of note, the literature is underpowered statistically on this issue, and because this metric tends to bias towards the null, a better measure with future research may be the total cumulative number of live births per fresh cycle.) Extended culture adds to the cost of an IVF cycle, but there is also a cost to freezing embryos at cleavage stage as well as the potential for multiple additional transfer-associated costs for an offsetting cumulative pregnancy rate. It has also been argued the costs of repeating IVF should be accounted for if there is a higher likelihood of having no embryos to transfer with extended culture [19], but this likely applies primarily to poor prognosis patients, who may be at greater risk for needing repeat IVF with either approach [15]. Also, in addition to live birth rates, miscarriage rates, culture, and freezing costs, cost-effectiveness modeling should consider neonatal outcomes. With blastocyst transfer there seems to be a higher rate of preterm birth (22–31%), but a lower rate of small for gestational age (12–23%), but this data comes from observational studies [19]. Finally, costs need to distinguish those directly to the patient relative to those to society, and these will depend on whether patients have insurance coverage for IVF and other factors.

48.6 Conclusions

It is hard to determine best practice when better-quality studies are needed. There is sufficient heterogeneity and doubt in published research such that cases can be made for both cleavage-stage and blastocyst transfer. Many patients facing difficult medical choices redirect questions to their physician and ask "What would you do for your family?" The question is more easily answered if stratified by prognosis. If in good prognosis patients the likelihood of having no embryos to transfer is low, and similar numbers of cleavage- and blastocyst-stage embryos are to be transferred according to ASRM and SART guidelines, but blastocysts have a higher implantation rate, choosing blastocyst transfer will likely shorten the time to pregnancy. If in poor prognosis patients "compassionate transfer" at the cleavage stage does not improve outcomes and may even worsen them, the belief that "at least I had a chance" may be a counterproductive illusion. Accordingly, blastocyst transfer should be preferred for most patients, though not all, particularly in the context of respecting patient autonomy. Further research such as cost-effectiveness data could change such a perspective. However, given the increasing trend toward preimplantation genetic screening, where cleavage-stage biopsy is less accurate and more harmful to the embryo than blastocyst biopsy [20], the future may lead to blastocyst transfer for everyone.

References

1. Practice Committee of the American Society for Reproductive Medicine and the Practice Committee of the Society for Assisted Reproductive Technology. Guidance on the limits to the number of embryos to transfer: a committee opinion. Fertil Steril. 2017;107(4):901–3.
2. Kulkarni A, Jamieson D, Jones H Jr, Kissin D, Gallo M, Macaluso M, et al. Fertility treatments and multiple births in the United States. N Engl J Med. 2013;369(23):2218–25.
3. Braude P, Bolton V, Moore S. Human gene expression first occurs between the four and eight cell stages of preimplantation development. Nature. 1988;332(6163):459–61.
4. Dar S, Grover S, Moskovtsev S, Swanson S, Baratz A, Librach C. In vitro fertilization intracytoplastmic sperm injection outcome in patietns with a markedly high DNA fragmentation index (>50%). Fertil Steril. 2013;100(1):75–80.
5. Simon L, Murphy K, Shamsi M, Liu L, Emery B, Aston K, et al. Paternal influence of sperm DNA integrity on early embryonic development. Hum Reprod. 2014;29(11):2402–12.
6. Graham J, Han T, Porter R, Levy M, Stillman R, Tucker M. Day 3 morphology is a poor predictor of blastocyst quality in extended culture. Fertil Steril. 2000;74(3):495–7.
7. Fanchin R, Ayoubi J, Righini C, Olivennes F, Schönauer L, Frydman R. Uterine contractility decreases at the time of blastocyst transfers. Hum Reprod. 2001;16(6):1115–9.
8. Valbuena D, Martin J, de Pablo J, Remohi J, Pellicer A, Simon C. Increasing levels of estradiol are deleterious to embryonic implantation because they affect the embryo. Fertil Steril. 2001;76(5):962–8.
9. Marek D, Langley M, Gardner D, Confer N, Doody K, Doody K. Introduction of blastocyst culture and transfer for all patients in an in vitro fertilization program. Fertil Steril. 1999;72(6):1035–40.
10. Gardner D, Lane M, Stevens J, Schlenker T, Schoolcraft W. Blastocyst score affects implantation and pregnancy outcome: towards a single blastocyst transfer. Fertil Steril. 2000;73(6):1155–8.
11. Papanikolaou E, Camus M, Kolibianakis E, Van Landuyt L, Van Steirteghem A, Devroey P. In vitro fertilization with single blastocyst stage versus single cleavage stage embryos. N Eng J Med. 2006;354(11):39–46.
12. Glujovsky D, Farquhar C, Quinteiro Retamar A, Alvarez Sedo C, Blake D. Cleavage stage versus blastocyst embryo transfer in assisted reproductive technology. Cochrane Lib. 2016;6.
13. Chen H, Lv J, Wu X, Xiao Y, Xi H, Zhu C, et al. Blastocyst-stage versus cleavage stage embryo transfer in the first frozen cycles of OHSS-risk patients who deferred from fresh embryo transfer. Gynecol Endocrinol. 2015;31(9):698–701.
14. Cobo A, de los Santos M, Castello D, Gamiz P, Campos P, Remohi J. Outcomes of vitrified early cleavage-stage and blastocyst-stage embryos in a cryopreservation program: evaluation of 3,150 warming cycles. Fertil Steril. 2012;98(5):1138–46.
15. Balaban B, Urman B, Alatas C, Mercan R, Aksoy S, Isiklar A. Blastocyst-stage transfer of poor-quality cleavage stage embryos results in higher implantation rates. Fertil Steril. 2001;75(3):514–8.
16. Madeira J, Coyne K, Jaeger A, Parry J, Lindheim S. Inform and consent: more than just "sign here". Fertil Steril. 2017;108(1):40–1.
17. Boivin J, Schmidt L. Use of complementary and alternative medicines associated with a 30% lower ongoing pregnancy/live birth rate during 12 months of fertility treatment. Hum Reprod. 2009;24(7):1626–31.
18. Adashi E, Dean L. Access to and use of infertility services in the United States: framing the challenges. Fertil Steril. 2016;105(5):1113–8.
19. Glujovsky D, Farquhar C. Cleavage-stage or blastocyst transfer: what are the benefits and harms? Fertil Steril. 2016;106(2):244–50.
20. Scott R, Upham K, Forman E, Zhao T, Treff N. Cleavage-stage biopsy significantly impairs human embryonic implantation potential while blastocyst biopsy does not: a randomized and paired clinical trial. Fertil Steril. 2013;100(3):624–30.

49 Endometrial Receptivity Testing

Jacqueline Y. Maher, Rebecca A. Garbose, and Mindy S. Christianson

Chapter Objectives

After reading this chapter, the reader will be able to:

1. Understand the regulation of endometrial receptivity by ovarian hormone production and the implanting blastocyst.
2. Explain the current knowledge of endometrial receptivity testing, including biomarkers for endometrial receptivity.
3. Describe diagnostic modalities utilized to determine optimal endometrial receptivity and improve pregnancy rates, which include endometrial histology, biochemical markers, and the endometrial receptivity array.

49.1 Introduction

The act of an embryo implanting into the uterus is the culmination of three major actions, which include development, synchronization, and signaling between the developing blastocyst and endometrium. The uterine lining and the embryo communicate in a complex manner with orchestrated genetic and hormonal interaction [1]. In order for successful ongoing pregnancy to occur, precise coordination of these events is critical. Endometrial receptivity is defined as the ability of the uterine lining to permit an embryo to attach, implant into the myometrium, and develop a placenta and ultimately result in a successful pregnancy. While the implantation process is complex and multifactorial, interaction between a viable embryo and an endometrial receptivity is paramount. Accurate testing to diagnose endometrial receptivity over the years has been challenging. Many researchers have studied and developed endometrial histology, biomarkers, and noninvasive ultrasound markers to detect defects in endometrial receptivity [2].

Despite advances in assisted reproduction technology (ART) over the past 40 years, overall implantation and pregnancy rates have remained relatively low. This suboptimal implantation rate occurs despite optimized embryo factors such as preimplantation genetic screening to confirm euploid embryos are transferred, demonstrating that success of in vitro fertilization and embryo transfer (IVF-ET) cycles relies not only on a viable embryo but also on uterine receptivity [3]. Unsuccessful embryo transfers of high-quality euploid embryos are generally assessed to be due to a failure at the level of endometrial receptivity [4].

In recent years, investigators have started to reveal the complexities of uterine receptivity, in both human and animal models [1]. However, specifics of the concerted relationships between the endometrium and embryo remain unclear, mostly because an in vitro model to study implantation does not exist and there are ethical obstacles involved in early embryo research [5]. In this chapter, we will provide an overview of endometrial receptivity and its relationship with ovarian hormone production and the implanting blastocyst with special focus on the window of implantation. We will also highlight diagnostic modalities utilized to diagnose ideal endometrial receptivity and optimize pregnancy rates. Key areas reviewed include endometrial histology, biochemical markers, and the endometrial receptivity array (ERA).

49.2 The "Window of Implantation"

Specific molecular, genetic, and hormonal factors guide endometrial development and receptivity, allowing for a blastocyst to implant only under optimal conditions with precise timing [1, 6]. Implantation has a specific timeline that begins at the start of progesterone exposure, transitioning the endometrium from a pre-receptive phase to a receptive phase

J. Y. Maher (✉) · R. A. Garbose · M. S. Christianson
Division of Reproductive Endocrinology and Infertility, Department of Gynecology and Obstetrics, Johns Hopkins University School of Medicine, Baltimore, MD, USA
e-mail: jyano3@jhmi.edu

G. N. Allahbadia et al. (eds.), *Textbook of Assisted Reproduction*, https://doi.org/10.1007/978-981-15-2377-9_49

called the window of implantation (WOI). The receptive time frame is then followed quickly by a nonreceptive or refractory phase [1]. In pre-receptive phase, blastocysts can survive in the endometrial cavity until the receptive state begins. When window of implantation ends and the endometrium transforms to the nonreceptive phase, embryo survival in the uterine cavity is no longer possible [1].

In a typical 28-day natural cycle, the WOI begins on day 19 or 20 and remains open for 4 to 5 days when serum progesterone levels peak [2, 7]. The term implantation failure may refer to two different situations: (1) no detectable β-hCG level or (2) a detectable β-hCG level, but no visible gestational sac seen on transvaginal ultrasound, also known as a biochemical pregnancy [8]. The WOI is tightly controlled by ovarian hormonal regulation and cross talk between the uterus and early embryo impacting various implantation factors.

49.3 Ovarian Hormonal Regulation of the Endometrial Development and Receptivity

The endometrium is morphologically divided into the functionalis and basalis layers. The functionalis is thickened and sloughed due to actions of ovarian hormones, while the basalis, located near the myometrium, remains during the menstrual cycle [9]. The functionalis layer is comprised of two primary cellular areas: (1) a single layer of epithelial cells on the surface and overlaying the epithelial glands and (2) the stroma, which consists of extracellular matrix, fibroblasts, blood vessels, and immune cells [10]. The endometrial cycle is divided into three phases: proliferative, secretory, and menstrual phases, which interact with the ovarian, follicular, and luteal phases (Fig. 49.1). During the proliferative phase, ovarian estradiol causes stromal cell and glandular prolifera-

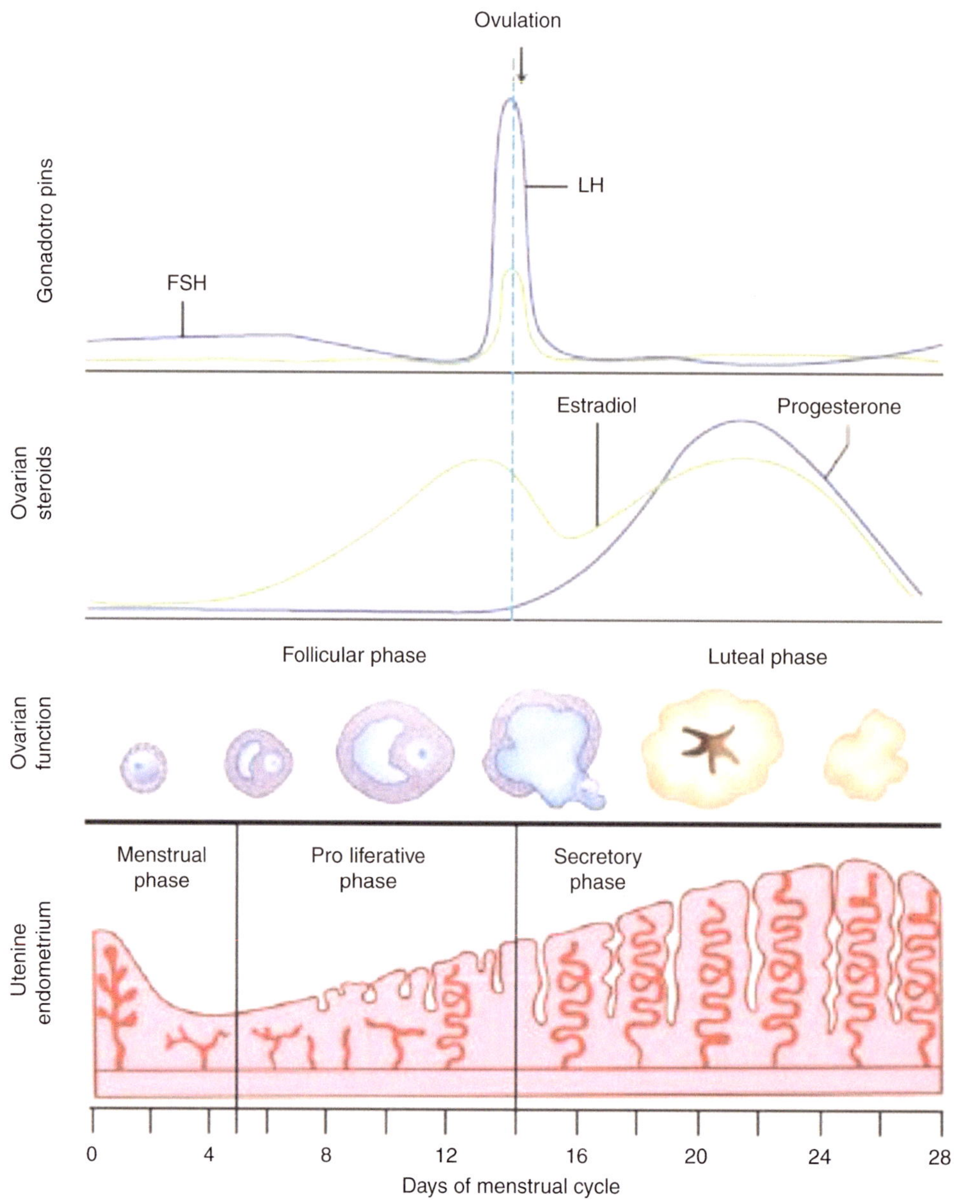

Fig. 49.1 The menstrual cycle (From Emans SJ, Laufer MR, Goldstein DP. The Physiology of Puberty. Pediatric and Adolescent Gynecology. 5th ed. Lippincott Williams & Wilkins; 2005)

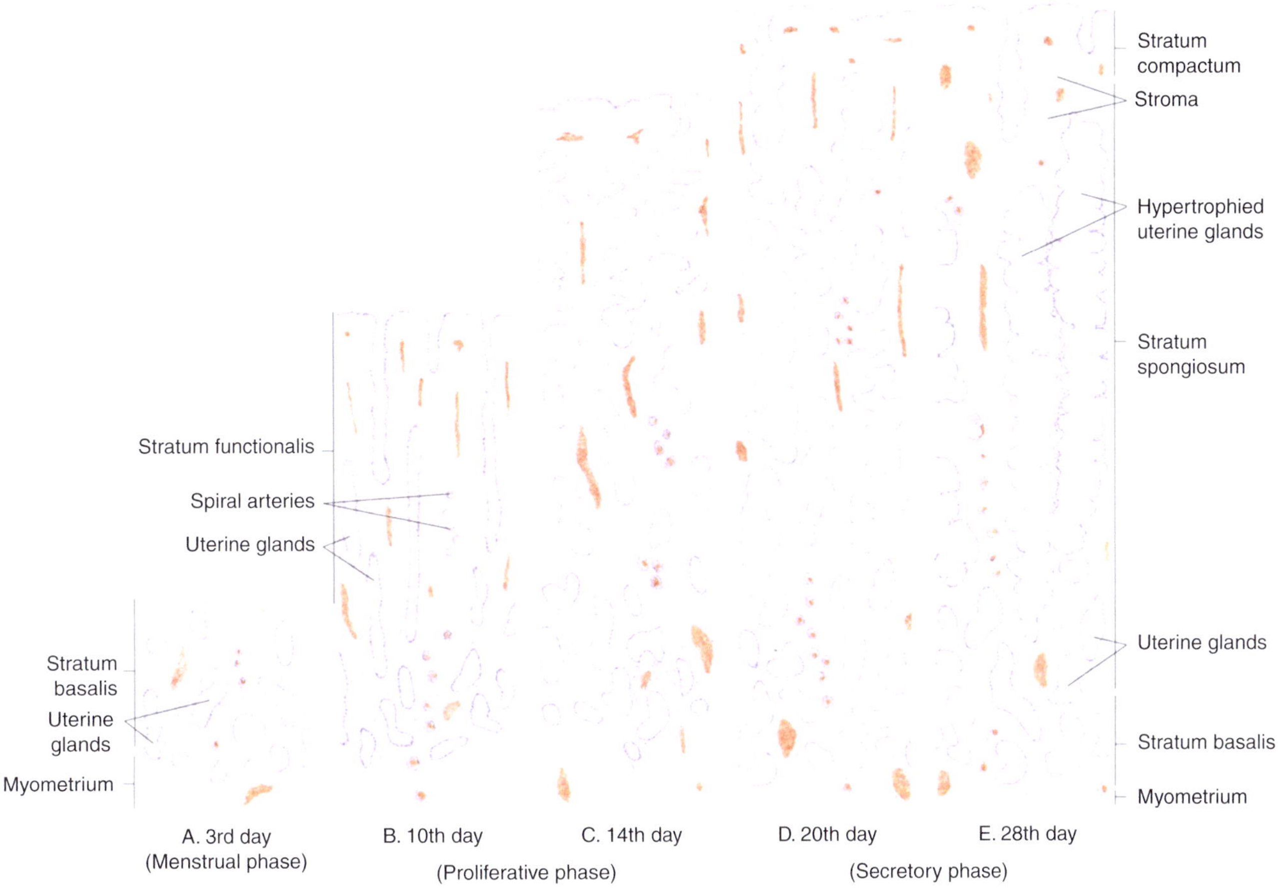

Fig. 49.2 Menstrual cycle: structural modification of endometrium (From Zhang S-X. An Atlas of Histology. New York: Springer; 1999, with permission)

tion and elongation of the spiral arteries. After ovulation, during the secretory phase, progesterone produced by the corpus luteum changes the endometrium to a receptive phenotype essential for implantation (Figs. 49.2 and 49.3).

Ovarian production of estradiol and progesterone is a critical factor for regulating and activating the endometrium for implantation. While progesterone has long been known to play a pivotal role for both implantation and pregnancy maintenance, the role of ovarian estrogen production on implantation is less elucidated and species specific [11]. Prior studies have demonstrated that estrogen is necessary for proliferation of the endometrial lining and for it to be primed for implantation. This development may also play a role in blastocyst activation and continued growth, therefore being essential for effective implantation [6, 12].

49.3.1 Estrogen Priming of the Endometrium

Estrogen, specifically estradiol, induces endometrial proliferation during the follicular phase of the menstrual cycle. Aside from proliferation, estradiol endometrial priming promotes molecular changes necessary for implantation [13]. Notably, estrogen upregulates activity of both estrogen receptors (ER) and progesterone receptors (PR) within the endometrium [14]. Two distinct isoforms of the estrogen receptor (ER), ERα and ERβ, regulate the estrogen's impact on the endometrial lining. ERα is most abundant in the endometrium and has its greatest activity during the follicular phase, with activity declining after ovulation. ERβ, localized within the glandular epithelium and vascular epithelium, also has decreased activity after ovulation due to progesterone-induced downregulation of both ER isoforms [13].

In cases of exogenous estradiol administration, such as programmed FET cycles or donor egg embryo recipient cycles, estradiol doses similar to serum levels during a natural cycle induce ER and PR activity within the endometrium. To achieve proper endometrial priming, duration of estradiol exposure must exceed a certain level. However, once this time length is exceeded, length of time of estrogen treatment has a broad temporal window until initiation of progesterone supplementation. Navot et al. examined the flexibility of length of estrogen treatment in donor-recipient cycles and reported that adequate estrogen treatment could range from

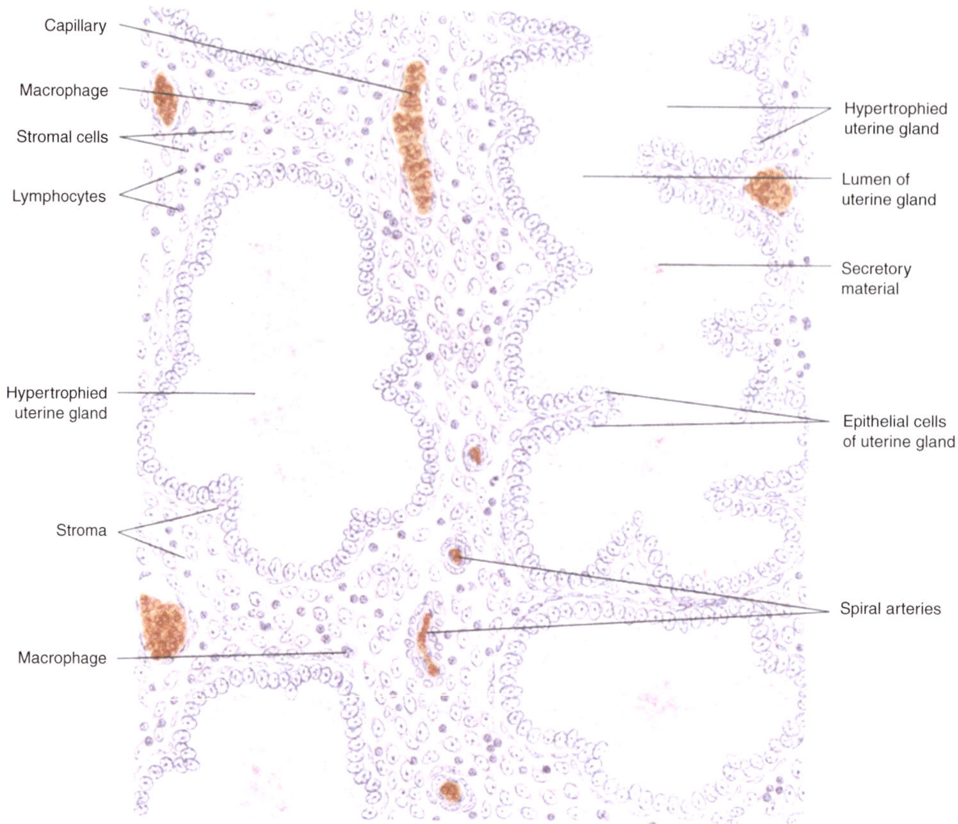

Fig. 49.3 Endometrium: secretory phase (From Zhang S-X. An Atlas of histology. New York: Springer; 1999, with permission)

5 days to 6 weeks without negatively impacting pregnancy rates [15]. Alternative researchers have demonstrated that prolonged estrogen exposure does not decrease rate of successful pregnancy outcomes after up to 14 weeks of estrogen treatment [16–18]. However, since abnormal uterine bleeding often commences after 9 weeks of estrogen therapy, it is recommended to discontinue plans for an embryo transfer after 9 weeks to optimize outcomes [16].

49.3.2 Progesterone Regulation of the Implantation Window

After ovulation, the secretory phase is characterized by complex actions that result in defined endometrial histologic changes [19]. Progesterone receptor (PR) isoforms, PR-A and PR-B, allow progesterone to antagonize estrogen activity. Progesterone downregulates ER and epithelial PR, while stromal PR concentration is consistent [6]. In rodent models, gene mutations in PR-A cause infertility, while treatment with RU-486, a progesterone antagonist, can postpone the endometrial receptivity window [1]. One critical aspect of the WOI, however, is that endometrial receptivity is irreversible and cannot be lengthened in duration or reversed [20, 21]. Entry into the nonreceptive phase ultimately results in lack of embryo survival and has a negative impact on implantation [1, 7].

Progesterone treatment results in a defined window of receptivity that lasts for only 24 to 48 h [22]. In early studies, Navot et al. reported pregnancy rates of 40% when cleavage stage embryos were transferred between days 17 and 19 (day 15 defined as the first day of progesterone administration), while no pregnancies occurred if ET occurred on day 16 or ≥20 days [7]. While this suggests an optimal embryo transfer time between 3 and 5 days post-progesterone exposure, defining the optimal WOI remains controversial [23, 24].

49.4 Uterine-Embryonic Cross Talk

Successful implantation requires a complex sequence of interaction and signaling between the endometrium and blastocyst, with the specific steps of apposition, adhesion, and penetration. While apposition is the initial contact of trophoblastic tissue to the luminal epithelium of the endometrium, blastocyst adhesion requires an increase in stromal vascular permeability [25, 26]. The final stage, penetration, involves trophoblastic invasion through the luminal epithelium into the stroma, connecting to maternal blood supply and commencing endometrial decidualization [1, 26].

In order for the chain of events described above to occur, communication must occur between the endometrium and embryo. Several genes have been identified as playing a role in endometrial receptivity. For example, *HOX* genes, specifically *HOXA10* and *HOXA11*, have demonstrated increased expression in the secretory phases, correlating with increased estradiol and progesterone levels. After implantation and in early pregnancy, the decidua demonstrates high levels of HOXA10 and HOXA11 mRNA [27, 28]. The HOX genes also regulate expression of other genes that impact implantation including pinopodes, integrins, and IGFBP-1 [29–32].

Numerous cytokines and growth factors are associated with receptivity and implantation, including leukemia inhibitory factor (LIF), a member of the interleukin 6 family of proteins, heparin-binding epidermal growth factor (HB-EGF), integrins, mucin 1 (MUC1), Wnt signaling, and β-catenin proteins [33–35]. Endometrial LIF secretion is regulated by prokinextin1 (PROK1) in the secretory phase of the menstrual cycle. In the rodent model, LIF-null mothers experience implantation failure. While LIF-null blastocyst embryos transferred into a wild-type pseudopregnant uterus implant normally [36], embryo demise occurs subsequently, suggesting maternal LIF is critical for both implantation and embryo development [37]. In humans, LIF's role in implantation remains unclear. Integrins are also associated with embryo-endometrium communication [35, 38]. Expression of the integrin $\alpha v\beta 3$ is upregulated by *HOX* genes during the WOI [38–40] and demonstrates decreased levels in conditions that negatively impact fertility such as endometriosis [39, 41], though other studies have not corroborated these findings [41, 42]. Another potential mediator of implantation includes MUC1, which is downregulated by the blastocyst in the uterine epithelium. Although its specific role remains unknown, MUC1 is increased during the follicular phase of the menstrual cycle [43] and remains increased for the first half of the luteal phase [44].

Wnt proteins, a large group of cysteine-rich molecules, play a role in blastocyst activation [45] and also induce LIF expression in the endometrium [1, 5]. Uterine Wnt signaling has been stimulated at the time of embryo attachment before implantation occurs and is necessary to promote the activated blastocyst's attachment to the endometrium [46]. Blocking the Wnt/β-catenin signaling pathway results in decreased implantation as demonstrated by smaller litter sizes in the mouse model [11, 45, 46].

49.5 Endometrial Biopsy, Histology, and Biomarkers

49.5.1 Endometrial Dating

Noyes et al. [47] first reported histological changes in the endometrium over the menstrual cycle and published a sentinel paper establishing criteria for dating the endometrium by endometrial biopsy and subsequent histology [47]. Their findings were identified as sentinel findings in gynecologic practice to evaluate luteal function and diagnose luteal phase deficiency for many years. More recently, however, the Reproductive Medicine Network examined the utility of endometrial biopsy in the fertility evaluation. In a multicenter study of fertile and infertile women (n = 847), the objective was to examine if there was a difference in endometrial histologic dating between the two groups [48]. After detection of a urinary luteinizing hormone surge, subjects were randomized to biopsy in the luteal phase. When the research team compared biopsies from fertility and infertile women in the luteal phase, they found that the percentage of endometrial biopsies that had delayed maturation of the endometrium were not significantly different. The findings of this study led to the clinical finding that histological dating of the endometrium should not be used in routine fertility evaluation [48, 49].

Another application of endometrial histology is in the evaluation of luteal phase defect (LPD), which is when an abnormal corpus luteum results in decreased progesterone production, hindering the receptivity of the endometrium for implantation. The premise is that if not enough progesterone is produced to support a functional secretory endometrium, then an embryo would not be able to implant and grow. Additionally, one could theoretically observe endometrial histology to evaluate the secretory endometrium. In the late 1940s, Dr. Georgeanna Seegar Jones pioneered this idea by looking at basal body temperatures, pregnanediol levels, and endometrial biopsy specimens based on the Noyes criteria to identify LPD [50]. As more sensitive serum assays were developed, Jones corroborated these findings reporting that those with LPD diagnosed by tissue biopsy had a significant decreased in serum progesterone levels during the luteal phase of the menstrual cycle [51]. Smitz et al. [52] reported that administering either progesterone in oil (50 mg daily) or intravaginal micronized progesterone could correct a LPDs in women [52]. Progesterone and HCG have both been used with similar efficacy for luteal phase support in stimulated IVF cycles [53, 54]. Today, however, there are no consensus definitions, tests, or treatment for LPD. Additionally, a 2015 committee opinion from the American Society for Reproductive Medicine concluded that "although progesterone is important for the process of implantation and early embryonic development, LPD as an independent entity causing infertility has not been proven" [55].

49.5.2 Pinopodes

Pinopodes, also called uterodomes, are progesterone-dependent organelles that project from the endometrium from days 20 to 21 of the natural menstrual cycle [56, 57] (Fig. 49.4). While the precise mechanism of action of pinopodes is unknown, they are thought to be necessary for blastocyst adhesion and considered a biomarker for endometrial receptivity. Pinopodes typically appear after 6 to 8 days of progesterone exposure; expression occurs for approximately 48 h within the human endometrium, with fully developed pinopodes existing for little as 1 day [56, 58]. The utility of

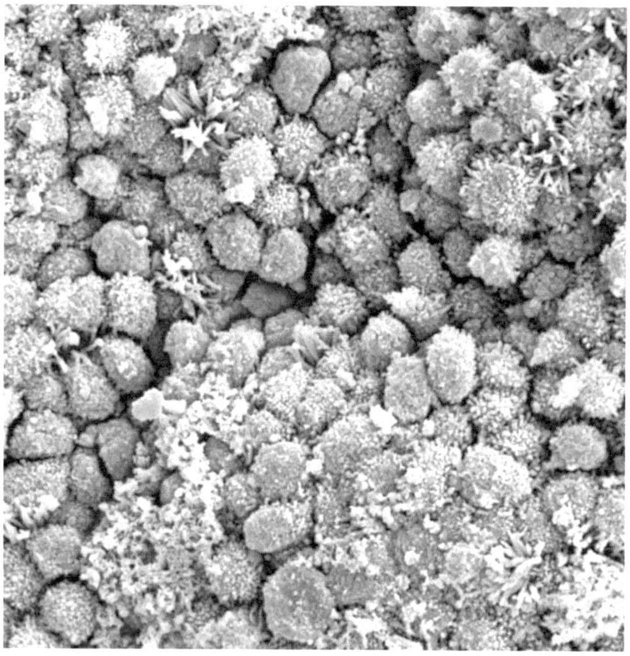

Fig. 49.4 Electron microscopy. Pinopode formation. Endometrial sample obtained on cycle day LH +7 (From Gemzell-Danielsson K, Bygdeman M. Effects of Progestogens on Endometrial Maturation in the Implantation Phase. In: Croxatto HB, Schürmann R, Fuhrmann U, Schellschmidt I, editors. New Mechanisms for Tissue-Selective Estrogen-Free Contraception; Berlin, Heidelberg Springer; 2005. p. 119-38, with permission)

pinopodes to elucidate the window of receptivity is based on the assumptions that pinopodes last for a short <48 h period and can be used to predict endometrial receptivity.

In 1995, Nikas et al. used biopsy to examine pinopodes as an indicator for endometrial receptivity in 14 women undergoing artificial cycles for IVF. Based on the variance of the timing of the fully developed pinopodes and the brief window of maturity, they were hopeful that pinopodes could be used as a tool to determine the ideal timing of implantation for an individual [56]. The same group also found that controlled ovarian hyperstimulation (COH) did not impact pinopode formation in terms of quality and lifespan, but that pinopodes formed 1–2 days earlier in COH cycles compared to natural cycles [59]. However, more recent human studies by Ordi et al. [60] and Quinn et al. [61] have found that infertile women regularly exhibit pinopode formation, calling into question the utility of pinopodes as a marker of the window of implantation in a clinical setting [60, 61].

Overall, endometrial biopsy and histology and evaluation of endometrial pinopodes are techniques used less frequently in current clinical practice.

49.6 Biochemical Receptivity Biomarkers

During the secretory phase of the menstrual cycle, the endometrium undergoes biochemical changes to prepare for implantation. The histologic and molecular properties of the receptive secretory endometrium are a source of investigation to identify markers critical for implantation and altered in infertility. Abnormalities in these biomarkers could be due to intrinsic abnormalities in the individual, inadequate hormonal stimulation, or systemic disorders causing altered function of the endometrium [62]. A summary of the candidate biomarkers evaluated in the literature are detailed in Table 49.1. Although these biomarkers offer hope in the evaluation of endometrial receptivity, lack of accuracy, predictability, and the need for invasive technique are some of the ongoing limitations, and more research is needed in this direction. Innovations in the future to improve endometrial receptivity include endometrial stem cell and gene therapy [76].

49.7 Endometrial Receptivity Array (ERA)

Molecular influences as well as endometrial gene expression play a key role in endometrial receptivity and implantation [77]. The endometrial receptivity assay (ERA) test, developed over the last decade, is a microarray analysis of tissue obtained by endometrial biopsy [78]. The ERA test can determine a specific transcriptomic signature and identify the receptive endometrium in both natural and artificially stimulated cycles [79, 80]. The ERA test compares the genetic profile of a test sample with biopsies from control patients taken 7 days after an LH surge (LH +7) in a natural cycle or 5 days after progesterone administration (P + 5) and after estrogen priming in an artificial endometrial preparation cycle. The test is a customized array that contains 238 genes that are differentially expressed and coupled to a computational predictor. The bioinformatic predictor creates a gene signature by selecting genes whose expression was consistent among different models of endometrial receptivity [81, 82]. The ERA determines if the endometrium is receptive or not and calculates a personalized WOI to optimize the timing of embryo transfer [82].

The test classifies an endometrial sample as "receptive" when the endometrium is suitable for blastocyst implantation or "nonreceptive" when implantation is not favorable. The "nonreceptive" ERA is then sub-classified as "pre-receptive" or "post-receptive" and assigned an exact endometrial status at time of biopsy [81]. With ERA testing, some patients have a delayed WOI, while others may have an advanced WOI. Another subset of patients have an unusually short window of receptivity. The test has been shown to be accurate and reproducible with a specificity of 0.89 and sensitivity of 0.99 for endometrial dating and a specificity of 0.16 and a sensitivity of 0.99 for the pathological classification [81, 83]. These observations suggest that ERA is a superior test over histological dating and has value as a diagnostic tool.

In a pilot study of 17 patients with RIF, clinical pregnancy rates increased from 19% to 60% in patients who had ERA testing and subsequent personalized embryo transfer [84]. In a prospective multicenter trial, women with RIF (n = 85) were compared to controls (n = 25) with no previous IVF

Table 49.1 Summary of endometrial receptivity biomarkers

Biomarker(s)	Function	Author/study	Research and conclusion
PGR-beta, PAEP, CXCL14	• PGR-B: Uterine receptivity and implantation • PAEP and CXCL14: Upregulation of mRNA transcripts during mid-secretory phase	Leach et al. 2012 [62]	• Hypothesized proteins are regulated during the secretory phase, and expression patterns are altered in infertile women • Endometrial biopsies taken during the secretory phase of infertile patients • Decreased PGR-B and increased in PAEP and CXCL14, suggesting that the implantation interval could be closing early • Possible diagnostic marker or therapeutic target
Beta-3, alpha-1, alpha-4 human endometrial integrins	• Integrins: receptor proteins that bind cells to the extracellular matrix to direct growth and function of the epithelium • 9 different integrin subunits on different types of endometrial cells	Lessey et al. 2011 [2]	• Receptive epithelium in a healthy patient may differ from an infertile patient as discordant luteal phase biopsies (≥ 3 days "out of phase") • Infertile patients exhibited delayed epithelial β3 immunostaining • Regulation of integrins at key phases of the menstrual cycle or disruption of integrin expression may decrease uterine receptivity • Regulation of integrins expression may be of therapeutic value
Calcitonin	• Peptide hormone involved in calcium homeostasis • Transiently induced by progesterone in the glandular epithelium of rat models at the time of implantation	Kumar et al. [63]	• Impaired implantation of rat embryos when administered calcitonin antisense oligodeoxynucleotides to attenuate calcitonin • Decreased expression of calcitonin in endometrium during the mid-secretory phase • Progesterone's regulatory role in endometrial calcitonin expression • Progesterone-induced expression of calcitonin in the secretory endometrium temporally coincides with the putative WOI
Leukemia inhibitory factor (LIF)	• IL-6 family cytokine • Crucial role in implantation in mice, since LIF-deficient mice are totally infertile	Aghajanova et al. [64]	• Prior conflicting results regarding decreased expression of LIF in patients with recurrent SABs or infertility • Identified a correlation between the spatial and temporal expression of pinopodes and LIF in human endometrium during the WOI
		Mikołajczyk et al. [65]	• Studied spatial and temporal expression of pinopodes and LIF in endometrial tissue of infertile patients and patients with recurrent SABs vs. fertile controls • Results suggest that decreased LIF was not necessarily associated with infertility or recurrent spontaneous abortions
HoxA10	• Homeobox-containing transcription factor responsible for proper uterine development • Cyclical endometrial expression with peak during WOI • Regulated in response to estrogen and progesterone	Zanatta et al. [66]	• Found women with endometriosis do not demonstrate the expected mid-luteal rise of HOXA10 expression • Concluded that HoxA10 expression could partially explain the infertility in endometriosis patients
Mucin-1 (MUC-1)	• Glycoprotein believed to provide lubrication and protection against bacterial and proteolytic attacks to the endometrium • Expression of cell adhesion molecules and important in blastocyst implantation	Bastu et al. [67]	• Hypothesized that relatively low levels of MUC-1 are necessary successful implantation • Evaluated endometrial and blood samples from women with RIF and control women • Blood and tissue measurements of MUC-1 were significantly lower in women with RIF than in fertile women during the WOI
Stathmin I	• Cytoskeleton-related protein • Regulator of microtubule dynamics during cell-cycle progression • Specifically regulated at the embryo implantation site	Dominguez et al. [68]	• Hypothesized implication of stroma cells proliferation in pre-receptive epithelium of the endometrium and prepare it for implantation • Stathmin was downregulated in receptive endometrium • Expression pattern in a refractory endometrium with an IUD in place is completely reversed, which may inhibit decidualization and interfere with the invasion process

(continued)

Table 49.1 (continued)

Biomarker(s)	Function	Author/study	Research and conclusion
Annexin A2	• Cytoskeleton-related protein • Promotes fibrinolytic activity on surface of vascular endothelial cells. Expressed in amnion epithelial cells, mesenchymal layer, trophoblast, and endothelial cells of blood vessels in the decidua	Dominguez et al. [68]	• Annexin A2 was upregulated in the receptive endometrium • Diminished dramatically in the epithelial cells and absent in stroma cells when an IUD is present, suggesting a lack of functional annexin A2 in the refractory endometrium • Concluded that upregulation of annexin A2 in the receptive endometrium could be important for the changes to prepare the apical pole for the cell-to-cell adhesion needed for embryo implantation
COX enzymes and prostaglandins E2 and F2 alpha	• Prostaglandins increase vascular permeability, are implicated in decidualization of the endometrium, and have a key role in implantation • For prostaglandin synthesis, arachidonic acid is oxidized by cyclooxygenases (COX1 and COX2) to generate PGH2, the precursor for all prostaglandins • In IVF patients, defective endometrial prostaglandin synthesis has been linked with RIF [69]	Achache et al. [70]	• RIF patients expressed reduced levels of cPLA2a and COX-2 compared with controls • Concluded that prostaglandin synthesis appears to be disrupted in patients with repeated IVF failure compared with fertile controls • Reduced prostaglandin synthesis in endometrium may lead to poor endometrial receptivity
		Vilella et al. [69]	• Prior studies showed PGE2 and PGF2α concentrations increased significantly in endometrial fluid during the WOI in natural cycles and IVF patients • Specifically identified PGE2 and PGF2α synthases in the endometrial epithelium being hormonally regulated during the WOI • An in vitro model of embryo adhesion demonstrated that inhibition of PGE2 and PGF2α or PG receptors (EP2 and FP) prevents embryo adhesion, which could be overcome by adding those molecules back or using their agonists • PGE2 and PGF2α concentrations in endometrial fluid 24 h prior to embryo transfer are potential noninvasive biomarkers of receptivity and implantation
IL-6	• Cytokine with a wide range of cellular effects including growth promotion, growth inhibition and cell differentiation to inflammation, and hematopoiesis • Expressed in granulosa cells, corpus luteum and theca cells, endometrium, and preimplantation embryo • Measured in serum and follicular fluid of women undergoing IVF	Altun et al. [71]	• Higher levels of IL-6 were associated with infertility • Increased follicular fluid levels of IL-6 were described in the context of ovarian hyperstimulation syndrome • Found significant positive correlations of IL-6 in follicular fluid with age and estradiol on day of hCG • On adjusted analyses, it is found that IVF patients with IL-6 levels <4.0 pg/ml demonstrated an almost fourfold increase in likelihood for clinical pregnancy • Concluded that lower follicular fluid IL-6 levels in IVF patients are associated with increased likelihood of clinical pregnancy and hypothesized that endometrial receptivity is a likely target for any deleterious influences of elevated IL-6 levels
Leptin	• Adipocyte-derived hormone encoded by the "Ob" gene • Possible marker of adequate nutritional status for reproductive functions • Fluctuates throughout the menstrual cycle	Chakrabarti et al. [72]	• Evaluated leptin in IVF pregnancy outcomes • Found a positive correlation between serum and ovarian follicular fluid leptin • Negative correlation between the serum leptin levels and endometrial thickness • Concluded that elevated leptin may adversely impact pregnancy rate during IVF-ET by modulating uterine receptivity
TGF superfamily and MMP2, MMP9, TIMP1 genes	• TGFβ: multifunctional cytokines, which serve as adhesion molecules and receptors and may increase the receptivity of the endometrium • MMP2: matrix metalloproteinase involved in the breakdown of extracellular matrix and with higher gene expression and activity during the WOI in women with impaired fertility	Skrzypczak et al. [73]	• Examined expression of TGFβ2 and MMP2, MMP9 and TIMP1 in endometrial biopsies of patients with idiopathic infertility, unexplained recurrent SAB, and controls • Biopsy samples done 7–9 days after ovulation: TGFβ2 expression was 2.8× higher in women with idiopathic infertility and 2.1× higher in women with unexplained recurrent SAB compared to controls • No significant difference in MMP2, MMP9, and TIMP1 between study groups and controls • Statistically significant negative correlation between TGFβ2 and MMP9 expression in biopsies from control women • Suggest that dysregulated TGFβ2, MMP2, MMP9, and TIMP1 expression are associated with infertility and early pregnancy loss

Moesin	• Membrane-organizing extension spike protein • Member of the ERM family which includes ezrin and radixin that cross-link between plasma membranes and actin-based cytoskeletons	Martin et al. [74]	• Investigated adhesive features in vitro to simulate embryonic adhesion and studied mRNA expression of ERM proteins in two different cell lines representing receptive uterine endometrium and less receptive endometrium • Concluded that uterine receptivity requires downregulation or absence of moesin, which is a less-polarized actin cytoskeleton
CA-125	• Glycoprotein best known as a tumor marker for epithelial ovarian cancer • Produced by non-ovarian tumors and normal tissues including endometrium • Increased serum levels in patients undergoing ovarian hyperstimulation, although source and production mechanisms are unknown	Brandenberger et al. [75]	• Found that neither CA-125 serum levels nor their increase from day of hCG until the day of ET showed any prognostic significance to the outcome of IVF • Values were not correlated with endometrium thickness or the number of oocytes retrieved or fertilized • Concluded that CA-125 serum levels in conventional IVF cycles were not correlated with IVF outcome

failure after undergoing ERA testing. Although not statistically significant, a nonreceptive endometrium with an altered WOI was present in 25.9% of those with RIF compared to 12% of controls. In the receptive control group, the implantation rate was 55% and pregnancy rate of 81.8%. By comparison, in receptive RIF patients, the implantation rate was 33.9%, and pregnancy rate was 51.7%. In nonreceptive RIF patients who underwent personalized embryo transfer, the implantation rate was 38.5%, and pregnancy rate was 50%. This study suggests that in approximately one fourth of patients with RIF, an endometrial factor exists with a WOI that appears adjustable with the ERA assay [84].

A larger retrospective study of ERA evaluated 3 groups: patients with RIF ($n = 80$), 93 patients with one unsuccessful embryo transfer ($n = 93$), and patients with thin endometrial lining measuring 6 mm or less ($n = 13$). ERA testing revealed a nonreceptive endometrium in 27.5% of the RIF group, significantly higher than the group with one IVF failure (15%, $P = 0.04$). After personalized embryo transfer based on ERA results, the ongoing pregnancy and implantation rates in the RIF group were 42.4% and 33%, respectively. Notably, 75% of those with persistently thin endometrium had a receptive endometrium and overall ongoing pregnancy rate of 66.7% after an ERA-personalized embryo transfer [80]. Though promising, ERA is a relatively new diagnostic tool that is currently undergoing multicenter clinical trials, and additional research outcomes are required to validate its use.

49.8 Controlled Ovarian Hyperstimulation, Progesterone Levels, and the Receptivity Window

While timing of the WOI may vary between women, it can also be altered if a woman is undergoing ART. For patients undergoing COH and IVF, exogenous gonadotropins have been implicated to impair endometrial receptivity due to supraphysiologic estradiol levels and altered endometrial development. Even though COH has not shown a change in endometrial pinopode expression, they appear on average 1–2 days earlier in comparison with natural cycles, which may reflect a shift in the WOI and decreased implantation success in fresh IVF cycles [59].

A number of studies have prospectively evaluated the impact of COH on clinical outcomes. In one randomized control trial comparing fresh ($n = 50$) to frozen blastocyst embryo transfers ($n = 53$), significantly higher implantation rates, clinical pregnancy rates, and ongoing pregnancy rates per transfer were seen in frozen embryo transfers (70.8%, 84%, and 78%, respectively) compared to fresh embryo transfers (38.9%, 54.7%, and 50.9%, $P < 0.001$). These results suggest impaired endometrial receptivity in fresh ET cycles compared to FET cycles with artificial endometrial preparation [85].

In a meta-analysis of 63 studies evaluating 55,199 fresh IVF cycles, including 7,229 frozen-thawed cycles and 1,330 donor/recipient cycles, in cycles with a premature progesterone elevation (PPE), defined using a threshold ≥0.8 ng/ml, there was a decreased probability of pregnancy in women undergoing fresh transfer IVF cycles with PPE of the day of β-hCG administration when compared with those without PPE. The pooled effect sizes based on progesterone level were 0.8–1.1 ng/ml, odds ratio (OR) = 0.79; 1.2–1.4 ng/ml, OR = 0.67; 1.5–1.75 ng/ml, OR = 0.64; 1.9–3.0 ng/ml, OR – 0.68, $P < 0.05$. Interestingly, there was no impact of PPE on pregnancy outcomes from frozen embryo transfer or fresh donor egg recipient cycles [86]. This further support the potential adverse effect of COH with PPE, which is thought to be due to a shift in the window of receptivity, which is in part overcome when performing a frozen embryo transfers (Fig. 49.5).

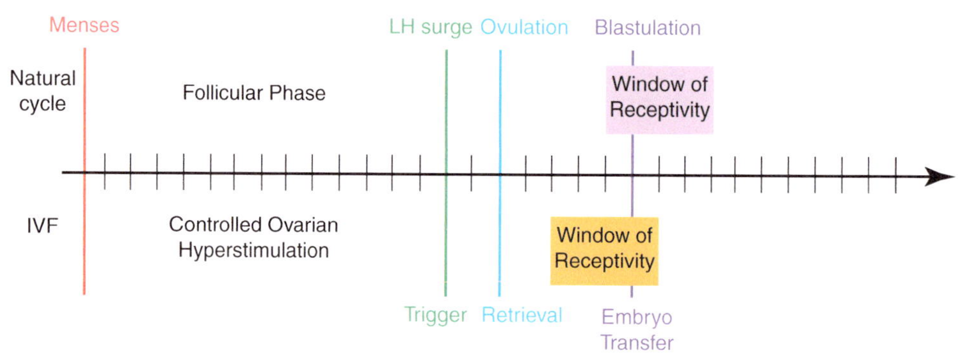

Fig. 49.5 Shift in window of receptivity with controlled ovarian hyperstimulation cycles during in vitro fertilization

49.9 Conclusion

Endometrial receptivity and synchrony between the embryo and the endometrium is essential for an embryo attachment, implantation, and invasion. ART continues to be an inefficient process as many implantation failures occur even in the presence of high-quality genetically normal embryos and appears to be the result of altered endometrial receptivity.

Historically, endometrial biopsy with histologic evaluation has been used to evaluate the WOI. To date, a range of diagnostic tools exist to better assess endometrial receptivity including transvaginal ultrasound, biomarkers, and ERA testing. The adverse effects of COH used in ART cycles have been identified including PPE, which continues to guide decisions about fresh embryo transfer versus embryo freezing due to alterations in the WOI. Further data is needed to further evaluate the endometrial receptivity assay, although preliminary data appears promising. Endometrial receptivity testing elucidates the readiness of the uterine lining to allow for attachment, implantation, and placentation, guiding clinical practice to help optimize and individualize the timing of intercourse, IUI, or embryo transfer and achieve a successful pregnancy.

References

1. Wang H, Dey SK. Roadmap to embryo implantation: clues from mouse models. Nat Rev Genet. 2006;7(3):185–99.
2. Lessey BA. Assessment of endometrial receptivity. Fertil Steril. 2011;96(3):522–9.
3. De Rycke M, Belva F, Goossens V, Moutou C, SenGupta SB, Traeger-Synodinos J, et al. ESHRE PGD consortium data collection XIII: cycles from January to December 2010 with pregnancy follow-up to October 2011. Hum Reprod. 2015;30(8):1763–89.
4. Sharkey AM, Macklon NS. The science of implantation emerges blinking into the light. Reprod Biomed Online. 2013;27(5):453–60.
5. Chen Q, Zhang Y, Lu J, Wang Q, Wang S, Cao Y, et al. Embryo-uterine cross-talk during implantation: the role of Wnt signaling. Mol Hum Reprod. 2009;15(4):215–21.
6. de Ziegler D, Fanchin R, de Moustier B, Bulletti C. The hormonal control of endometrial receptivity: estrogen (E2) and progesterone. J Reprod Immunol. 1998;39(1–2):149–66.
7. Navot D, Scott RT, Droesch K, Veeck LL, Liu HC, Rosenwaks Z. The window of embryo transfer and the efficiency of human conception in vitro. Fertil Steril. 1991;55(1):114–8.
8. Coughlan C, Ledger W, Wang Q, Liu F, Demirol A, Gurgan T, et al. Recurrent implantation failure: definition and management. Reprod Biomed Online. 2014;28(1):14–38.
9. Hawkins SM, Matzuk MM. The menstrual cycle: basic biology. Ann N Y Acad Sci. 2008;1135:10–8.
10. Bulun SEAE. The physiology and pathology of the female reproductive axis. In: Kronenberg HMMS, Polonsky KS, Larsen PR, editors. Williams textbook of endocrinology. 11th ed. Philadelphia, PA: Elsevier; 2009. p. 549–622.
11. Dey SK, Lim H, Das SK, Reese J, Paria BC, Daikoku T, et al. Molecular cues to implantation. Endocr Rev. 2004;25(3):341–73.
12. Lim H, Song H, Paria BC, Reese J, Das SK, Dey SK. Molecules in blastocyst implantation: uterine and embryonic perspectives. Vitam Horm. 2002;64:43–76.
13. Strauss J, Barberi R. Yen and Jaffe's reproductive endocrinology. 6th ed. Philadelphia: Saunders Elsevier; 2009.
14. Garcia E, Bouchard P, De Brux J, Berdah J, Frydman R, Schaison G, et al. Use of immunocytochemistry of progesterone and estrogen receptors for endometrial dating. J Clin Endocrinol Metab. 1988;67(1):80–7.
15. Navot D, Anderson TL, Droesch K, Scott RT, Kreiner D, Rosenwaks Z. Hormonal manipulation of endometrial maturation. J Clin Endocrinol Metab. 1989;68(4):801–7.
16. Remohi J, Gallardo E, Guanes PP, Simon C, Pellicer A. Donor-recipient synchronization and the use of gonadotrophin-releasing hormone agonists to avoid the premature luteinizing hormone surge in oocyte donation. Hum Reprod. 1995;10(Suppl 2):84–90.
17. Michalas S, Loutradis D, Drakakis P, Kallianidis K, Milingos S, Deligeoroglou E, et al. A flexible protocol for the induction of recipient endometrial cycles in an oocyte donation programme. Hum Reprod. 1996;11(5):1063–6.
18. Younis JS, Mordel N, Lewin A, Simon A, Schenker JG, Laufer N. Artificial endometrial preparation for oocyte donation: the effect of estrogen stimulation on clinical outcome. J Assist Reprod Genet. 1992;9(3):222–7.
19. Noyes RW. Uniformity of secretory endometrium; study of multiple sections from 100 uteri removed at operation. Fertil Steril. 1956;7(2):103–9.
20. Psychoyos A, Prapas I. Inhibition of egg development and implantation in rats after post-coital administration of the progesterone antagonist RU 486. J Reprod Fertil. 1987;80(2):487–91.
21. Sarantis L, Roche D, Psychoyos A. Displacement of receptivity for nidation in the rat by the progesterone antagonist RU 486: a scanning electron microscopy study. Hum Reprod. 1988;3(2):251–5.
22. Giudice LC. Microarray expression profiling reveals candidate genes for human uterine receptivity. Am J Pharmacogenomics. 2004;4(5):299–312.
23. Imbar T, Hurwitz A. Synchronization between endometrial and embryonic age is not absolutely crucial for implantation. Fertil Steril. 2004;82(2):472–4.
24. Lessey BA, Yeh I, Castelbaum AJ, Fritz MA, Ilesanmi AO, Korzeniowski P, et al. Endometrial progesterone receptors and markers of uterine receptivity in the window of implantation. Fertil Steril. 1996;65(3):477–83.
25. Tabibzadeh S, Babaknia A. The signals and molecular pathways involved in implantation, a symbiotic interaction between blastocyst and endometrium involving adhesion and tissue invasion. Hum Reprod. 1995;10(6):1579–602.
26. Sharkey AM, Smith SK. The endometrium as a cause of implantation failure. Best Pract Res Clin Obstet Gynaecol. 2003;17(2):289–307.
27. Taylor HS, Arici A, Olive D, Igarashi P. HOXA10 is expressed in response to sex steroids at the time of implantation in the human endometrium. J Clin Invest. 1998;101(7):1379–84.
28. Taylor HS, Igarashi P, Olive DL, Arici A. Sex steroids mediate HOXA11 expression in the human peri-implantation endometrium. J Clin Endocrinol Metab. 1999;84(3):1129–35.
29. Cermik D, Selam B, Taylor HS. Regulation of HOXA-10 expression by testosterone in vitro and in the endometrium of patients with polycystic ovary syndrome. J Clin Endocrinol Metab. 2003;88(1):238–43.
30. Daftary GS, Kayisli U, Seli E, Bukulmez O, Arici A, Taylor HS. Salpingectomy increases peri-implantation endometrial HOXA10 expression in women with hydrosalpinx. Fertil Steril. 2007;87(2):367–72.
31. Rackow BW, Taylor HS. Submucosal uterine leiomyomas have a global effect on molecular determinants of endometrial receptivity. Fertil Steril. 2010;93(6):2027–34.
32. Taylor HS, Bagot C, Kardana A, Olive D, Arici A. HOX gene expression is altered in the endometrium of women with endometriosis. Hum Reprod. 1999;14(5):1328–31.

33. Cavagna M, Mantese JC. Biomarkers of endometrial receptivity - a review. Placenta. 2003;24(Suppl B):S39–47.
34. Paria BC, Reese J, Das SK, Dey SK. Deciphering the cross-talk of implantation: advances and challenges. Science. 2002;296(5576):2185–8.
35. Giudice LC. Potential biochemical markers of uterine receptivity. Hum Reprod. 1999;14(Suppl 2):3–16.
36. Escary JL, Perreau J, Dumenil D, Ezine S, Brulet P. Leukaemia inhibitory factor is necessary for maintenance of haematopoietic stem cells and thymocyte stimulation. Nature. 1993;363(6427):361–4.
37. Yoshida K, Taga T, Saito M, Suematsu S, Kumanogoh A, Tanaka T, et al. Targeted disruption of gp130, a common signal transducer for the interleukin 6 family of cytokines, leads to myocardial and hematological disorders. Proc Natl Acad Sci USA. 1996;93(1):407–11.
38. Illera MJ, Lorenzo PL, Gui YT, Beyler SA, Apparao KB, Lessey BA. A role for alphavbeta3 integrin during implantation in the rabbit model. Biol Reprod. 2003;68(3):766–71.
39. Lessey BA, Damjanovich L, Coutifaris C, Castelbaum A, Albelda SM, Buck CA. Integrin adhesion molecules in the human endometrium. Correlation with the normal and abnormal menstrual cycle. J Clin Invest. 1992;90(1):188–95.
40. Lessey BA, Ilesanmi AO, Lessey MA, Riben M, Harris JE, Chwalisz K. Luminal and glandular endometrial epithelium express integrins differentially throughout the menstrual cycle: implications for implantation, contraception, and infertility. Am J Reprod Immunol. 1996;35(3):195–204.
41. Lessey BA, Castelbaum AJ, Sawin SW, Sun J. Integrins as markers of uterine receptivity in women with primary unexplained infertility. Fertil Steril. 1995;63(3):535–42.
42. Creus M, Ordi J, Fabregues F, Casamitjana R, Ferrer B, Coll E, et al. alphavbeta3 integrin expression and pinopod formation in normal and out-of-phase endometria of fertile and infertile women. Hum Reprod. 2002;17(9):2279–86.
43. Hey NA, Li TC, Devine PL, Graham RA, Saravelos H, Aplin JD. MUC1 in secretory phase endometrium: expression in precisely dated biopsies and flushings from normal and recurrent miscarriage patients. Hum Reprod. 1995;10(10):2655–62.
44. Bergh PA, Navot D. The impact of embryonic development and endometrial maturity on the timing of implantation. Fertil Steril. 1992;58(3):537–42.
45. Mohamed OA, Dufort D, Clarke HJ. Expression and estradiol regulation of Wnt genes in the mouse blastocyst identify a candidate pathway for embryo-maternal signaling at implantation. Biol Reprod. 2004;71(2):417–24.
46. Mohamed OA, Jonnaert M, Labelle-Dumais C, Kuroda K, Clarke HJ, Dufort D. Uterine Wnt/beta-catenin signaling is required for implantation. Proc Natl Acad Sci USA. 2005;102(24):8579–84.
47. Noyes R, Hertig A, Rock J. Dating the endometrial biopsy. Fertil Steril. 1950;1(1):3–25.
48. Coutifaris C, Myers ER, Guzick DS, Diamond MP, Carson SA, Legro RS, et al. Histological dating of timed endometrial biopsy tissue is not related to fertility status. Fertil Steril. 2004;82(5):1264–72.
49. Murray MJ, Meyer WR, Zaino RJ, Lessey BA, Novotny DB, Ireland K, et al. A critical analysis of the accuracy, reproducibility, and clinical utility of histologic endometrial dating in fertile women. Fertil Steril. 2004;81(5):1333–43.
50. Jones HW Jr. Luteal-phase defect: the role of Georgeanna Seegar Jones. Fertil Steril. 2008;90(5):e5–7.
51. Jones GS, Aksel S, Wentz AC. Serum progesterone values in the luteal phase defects. Effect of chorionic gonadotropin. Obstet Gynecol. 1974;44(1):26–34.
52. Smitz J, Devroey P, Faguer B, Bourgain C, Camus M, Van Steirteghem AC. A prospective randomized comparison of intramuscular or intravaginal natural progesterone as a luteal phase and early pregnancy supplement. Hum Reprod. 1992;7(2):168–75.
53. Fatemi HM, Popovic-Todorovic B, Papanikolaou E, Donoso P, Devroey P. An update of luteal phase support in stimulated IVF cycles. Hum Reprod Update. 2007;13(6):581–90.
54. van der Linden M, Buckingham K, Farquhar C, Kremer JA, Metwally M. Luteal phase support for assisted reproduction cycles. Cochrane Database Syst Rev. 2015;(7):Cd009154.
55. Practice Committee of the American Society for Reproductive M. Current clinical irrelevance of luteal phase deficiency: a committee opinion. Fertil Steril. 2015;103(4):e27–32.
56. Nikas G, Drakakis P, Loutradis D, Mara-Skoufari C, Koumantakis E, Michalas S, et al. Uterine pinopodes as markers of the 'nidation window' in cycling women receiving exogenous oestradiol and progesterone. Hum Reprod. 1995;10(5):1208–13.
57. Beier HM, Beier-Hellwig K. Molecular and cellular aspects of endometrial receptivity. Hum Reprod Update. 1998;4(5):448–58.
58. Lessey BA. The role of the endometrium during embryo implantation. Hum Reprod. 2000;15(Suppl 6):39–50.
59. Nikas G, Develioglu OH, Toner JP, Jones HW Jr. Endometrial pinopodes indicate a shift in the window of receptivity in IVF cycles. Hum Reprod. 1999;14(3):787–92.
60. Ordi J, Creus M, Quintó L, Casamitjana R, Cardesa A, Balasch J. Within-subject between-cycle variability of histological dating, alpha v beta 3 integrin expression, and pinopod formation in the human endometrium. J Clin Endocrinol Metab. 2003;88(5):2119–25.
61. Quinn C, Ryan E, Claessens EA, Greenblatt E, Hawrylyshyn P, Cruickshank B, et al. The presence of pinopodes in the human endometrium does not delineate the implantation window. Fertil Steril. 2007;87(5):1015–21.
62. Leach RE, Jessmon P, Coutifaris C, Kruger M, Myers ER, Ali-Fehmi R, et al. High throughput, cell type-specific analysis of key proteins in human endometrial biopsies of women from fertile and infertile couples. Hum Reprod. 2012;27(3):814–28.
63. Kumar S, Zhu LJ, Polihronis M, Cameron ST, Baird DT, Schatz F, et al. Progesterone induces calcitonin gene expression in human endometrium within the putative window of implantation. J Clin Endocrinol Metab. 1998;83(12):4443–50.
64. Aghajanova L, Stavreus-Evers A, Nikas Y, Hovatta O, Landgren BM. Coexpression of pinopodes and leukemia inhibitory factor, as well as its receptor, in human endometrium. Fertil Steril. 2003;79(Suppl 1):808–14.
65. Mikolajczyk M, Skrzypczak J, Wirstlein P. No correlation between pinopode formation and LIF and MMP2 expression in endometrium during implantation window. Folia Histochem Cytobiol. 2011;49(4):615–21.
66. Zanatta A, Rocha AM, Carvalho FM, Pereira RM, Taylor HS, Motta EL, et al. The role of the Hoxa10/HOXA10 gene in the etiology of endometriosis and its related infertility: a review. J Assist Reprod Genet. 2010;27(12):701–10.
67. Bastu E, Mutlu MF, Yasa C, Dural O, Nehir Aytan A, Celik C, et al. Role of Mucin 1 and Glycodelin A in recurrent implantation failure. Fertil Steril. 2015;103(4):1059–64.e2.
68. Dominguez F, Garrido-Gomez T, Lopez JA, Camafeita E, Quinonero A, Pellicer A, et al. Proteomic analysis of the human receptive versus non-receptive endometrium using differential in-gel electrophoresis and MALDI-MS unveils stathmin 1 and annexin A2 as differentially regulated. Hum Reprod. 2009;24(10):2607–17.
69. Vilella F, Ramirez L, Berlanga O, Martinez S, Alama P, Meseguer M, et al. PGE2 and PGF2alpha concentrations in human endometrial fluid as biomarkers for embryonic implantation. J Clin Endocrinol Metab. 2013;98(10):4123–32.
70. Achache H, Tsafrir A, Prus D, Reich R, Revel A. Defective endometrial prostaglandin synthesis identified in patients with repeated implantation failure undergoing in vitro fertilization. Fertil Steril. 2010;94(4):1271–8.

71. Altun T, Jindal S, Greenseid K, Shu J, Pal L. Low follicular fluid IL-6 levels in IVF patients are associated with increased likelihood of clinical pregnancy. J Assist Reprod Genet. 2011;28(3):245–51.
72. Chakrabarti J, Chatterjee R, Goswami S, Chakravarty B, Kabir SN. Overt leptin response to controlled ovarian hyperstimulation negatively correlates with pregnancy outcome in in vitro fertilization--embryo transfer cycle. J Hum Reprod Sci. 2012;5(2):194–9.
73. Skrzypczak J, Wirstlein P, Mikolajczyk M, Ludwikowski G, Zak T. TGF superfamily and MMP2, MMP9, TIMP1 genes expression in the endometrium of women with impaired reproduction. Folia Histochem Cytobiol. 2007;45(Suppl 1):S143–8.
74. Martin JC, Jasper MJ, Valbuena D, Meseguer M, Remohi J, Pellicer A, et al. Increased adhesiveness in cultured endometrial-derived cells is related to the absence of moesin expression. Biol Reprod. 2000;63(5):1370–6.
75. Brandenberger AW, Bersinger NA, Huber PR, Berger E, Glanzmann P, Birkhaeuser MH. CA-125 concentrations in the serum and pregnancy outcome in IVF cycles. J Assist Reprod Genet. 1998;15(6):390–4.
76. Cakmak H, Taylor HS. Implantation failure: molecular mechanisms and clinical treatment. Hum Reprod Update. 2011;17(2):242–53.
77. Tapia A, Gangi LM, Zegers-Hochschild F, Balmaceda J, Pommer R, Trejo L, et al. Differences in the endometrial transcript profile during the receptive period between women who were refractory to implantation and those who achieved pregnancy. Hum Reprod. 2008;23(2):340–51.
78. Ruiz-Alonso M, Blesa D, Diaz-Gimeno P, Gomez E, Fernandez-Sanchez M, Carranza F, et al. The endometrial receptivity array for diagnosis and personalized embryo transfer as a treatment for patients with repeated implantation failure. Fertil Steril. 2013;100(3):818–24.
79. Blesa D, Ruiz-Alonso M, Simon C. Clinical management of endometrial receptivity. Semin Reprod Med. 2014;32(5):410–3.
80. Mahajan N. Endometrial receptivity array: clinical application. J Hum Reprod Sci. 2015;8(3):121–9.
81. Garrido-Gomez T, Ruiz-Alonso M, Blesa D, Diaz-Gimeno P, Vilella F, Simon C. Profiling the gene signature of endometrial receptivity: clinical results. Fertil Steril. 2013;99(4):1078–85.
82. Miravet-Valenciano JA, Rincon-Bertolin A, Vilella F, Simon C. Understanding and improving endometrial receptivity. Curr Opin Obstet Gynecol. 2015;27(3):187–92.
83. Diaz-Gimeno P, Horcajadas JA, Martinez-Conejero JA, Esteban FJ, Alama P, Pellicer A, et al. A genomic diagnostic tool for human endometrial receptivity based on the transcriptomic signature. Fertil Steril. 2011;95(1):50–60.. e1-15
84. Ruiz-Alonso M, Galindo N, Pellicer A, Simon C. What a difference two days make: "personalized" embryo transfer (pET) paradigm: a case report and pilot study. Hum Reprod. 2014;29(6):1244–7.
85. Shapiro BS, Daneshmand ST, Garner FC, Aguirre M, Hudson C, Thomas S. Evidence of impaired endometrial receptivity after ovarian stimulation for in vitro fertilization: a prospective randomized trial comparing fresh and frozen-thawed embryo transfer in normal responders. Fertil Steril. 2011;96(2):344–8.
86. Venetis CA, Kolibianakis EM, Bosdou JK, Tarlatzis BC. Progesterone elevation and probability of pregnancy after IVF: a systematic review and meta-analysis of over 60000 cycles. Hum Reprod Update. 2013;19(5):433–57.

Androgens for Improving Ovarian Response to Stimulation

50

Kayhan Yakin

Poor response to ovarian stimulation is one of the major challenges in reproductive endocrinology and infertility practice. Current efforts fail to hold ovarian aging back or to replenish the ovarian reserve. Nevertheless, throughout the years, a number of empiric therapies have been tested to enhance follicle growth. Among such treatments, the biological plausibility of androgen supplementation, based on the essential role of androgens in ovarian physiology, has drawn a great deal of attention. This chapter presents a critical appraisal of the evidence underpinning the use of androgens and androgen-modulating agents as adjuvants in ovarian stimulation.

50.1 Role of Androgens in Follicle Growth

Androgens appear to be one of the major players involved in the control of early, "gonadotropin-independent" phase of folliculogenesis [1]. While many aspects of the functions and interactions of intraovarian factors remain elusive, there is a growing body of evidence that a critical balance exists between androgens, FSH, AMH, and estradiol for the regulation of optimal follicle growth [2].

The adrenal prohormone dehydroepiandrosterone (DHEA), primarily produced by the adrenal glands, acts as the essential substrate for steroidogenesis in the ovary and other target tissues [3]. DHEA is converted to androstenedione and testosterone determined by the steroidogenic enzymes available in the particular cells, and both can be converted to estrogens by aromatization. Testosterone can also be converted to the much more potent 5α-dihydrotestosterone. Serum levels of both DHEA and testosterone gradually decline with age [4].

Androgens exert their action mainly through the androgen receptors (AR). The AR functions as a ligand-activated nuclear transcription factor, whereas non-genomic effects of androgens have also been reported [3, 5, 6]. AR is expressed at all stages of follicular development, including the oocyte, granulosa, and theca cells [7, 8]. From the primary stage onward, increasing concentrations of AR are detected in granulosa cells, peaking in the antral stage [7–13]. Among AR-induced genes that regulate follicular development in the ovary, only a small number of direct genes including Kit ligand, microRNA-125b, cyclooxygenase-2, amphiregulin, cyclin-dependent kinase inhibitor-1/p21, and liver receptor homolog has been identified [14].

The essential role of androgen receptors was documented in various animal models. Administration of androgens in monkey [15, 16] and ewes [17] was shown to initiate follicular recruitment, stimulate early stages of follicular growth, and increase the number of growing follicles. Moreover, these effects could be blocked by the administration of anti-androgens [10, 18, 19]. Granulosa cell-specific AR knockout mice was characterized with reduced follicle development and ovulation as well as increased follicular atresia and reduced litter size and subfertility [8, 20–22].

Adequate levels of androgens, synergistically with follicle-stimulating hormone (FSH) and through different mechanisms, have been shown to promote follicle growth and development. The proposed mechanisms of action of androgens in folliculogenesis are summarized in Table 50.1. Inadequate androgen levels at the early follicle maturation stages may hamper the process, resulting in increased follicle degeneration and apoptosis. These biological facts have led to the assumption that administration of androgens prior to or concurrent with gonadotropins would improve the ovarian response when follicle growth is impaired, such as in women with low functional ovarian reserve or premature ovarian failure.

K. Yakin (✉)
Department of Obstetrics and Gynecology, Koc University Faculty of Medicine, Istanbul, Turkey
e-mail: kyakin@ku.edu.tr

G. N. Allahbadia et al. (eds.), *Textbook of Assisted Reproduction*, https://doi.org/10.1007/978-981-15-2377-9_50

Table 50.1 Proposed mechanisms of action of androgens

1. Stimulate development of primary, preantral, and antral follicles independent of the gonadotropins [10, 12, 16]
2. Rescue follicles from atresia [23–25]
3. Suppress apoptosis [26]
4. Upregulate FSH receptor expression and prime the follicle for FSH-stimulated growth and maturation [1, 9, 25, 27–29]
5. Show synergistic effect to FSH in follicular recruitment and granulosa cell proliferation [30]
6. Modulate AMH expression and inhibit FSH-induced aromatase expression to maintain a predominantly androgenic intrafollicular milieu [1, 2, 31]
7. Auto-amplify local effects by increasing their own receptor expression and activity [1]
8. Augment the growth-promoting and survival-enhancing effect of IGF-I [32]

Table 50.2 Proposed benefits of DHEA in women with poor ovarian reserve

1. Increased oocyte yield [33–40]
2. Higher fertilization rate [36, 40]
3. Improved embryo morphological grading [36, 37, 40]
4. Increased pregnancy rate [37–42]
5. Lower miscarriage rate when compared to the national IVF statistics [43]
6. Lower aneuploidy rate [44]
7. Improved ovarian reserve markers (AFC, AMH) [39, 45–47]
8. Balanced Th1/Th2 immune response and/or modulation of the types/behavior of T lymphocytes [48]

50.2 DHEA Supplementation

The idea of using DHEA as an adjunct to ovarian stimulation was introduced in 2000 by a case series published by Casson et al., but the interest on the subject climbed sharply after the documentation of a case who had achieved an 18-fold increase in peak estradiol levels and dramatic improvement in ovarian response following self-administration of DHEA [33, 34]. Subsequently, a number of groups have studied the impact of DHEA supplementation on hormonal profile, ovarian reserve, and IVF outcomes. Vast majority of these publications provide low quality of scientific evidence, suggesting potential beneficial effects of DHEA supplementation on reproductive outcomes and ovarian response in women with diminished ovarian reserve. Extrapolation of animal data to clinical practice turned DHEA into a "panacea" being widely marketed as "the first medication to be shown to rejuvenate the ovary to recover its younger functionality, with better quality and quantity of oocytes" [35]. The findings observed following 6–12 weeks of DHEA pretreatment in case series, self-controlled "before and after" trials, historical case-control studies, and non-randomized trials are summarized in Table 50.2. Unfortunately, hardly any of these findings were reproducible in randomized trials.

Despite almost two decades of empirical use in clinical practice, a well-designed, large-scale randomized controlled trial has never been available. A caveat is that perfection cannot be easily achieved in the experimental design of a study on an aggressively marketed oral supplementation, readily found over the counter, because poor responder women would be reluctant to join a randomized trial in which they may be assigned to a placebo group. Nevertheless, until to date, a number of groups managed to perform small-sized randomized trials.

The first, non-blinded RCT ($n = 33$) compared the clinical outcome in 17 poor responder women who completed 26 stimulation cycles following DHEA supplementation with 16 women in the control group who completed 25 cycles. A significant improvement was observed both in embryo quality and live birth rate (23.1% vs. 4.0%; $p < 0.05$) in the DHEA group compared to the controls [49]. However, the study was heavily criticized on methodological and statistical grounds [50, 51]. Therefore, their findings should be treated with caution.

Artini et al. in a small RCT ($n = 24$) reported that 75 mg daily DHEA supplementation for 3 months prior to ovarian stimulation did not confer a significant benefit in terms of the number of oocytes retrieved, fertilization, and clinical pregnancy rates [52]. Another non-blinded RCT [53], comprising the highest number of patients among all published RCTs ($n = 208$), showed that DHEA supplementation failed to increase the number oocytes retrieved and did not improve the pregnancy rate. However, this study was also criticized for carrying high risk of selection, performance, and attrition bias [54, 55].

In a non-blinded RCT [56] ($n = 133$), the use of 75 mg daily DHEA for 12 weeks before ovulation induction was associated with a significant increase in the clinical pregnancy rate per embryo transfer (24.1% vs 21.3%) and per cycle (20.9% vs 15.2%) in younger (<40 years) first-cycle poor responders.

Tartagni et al. analyzed 109 younger women with unexplained infertility in a double-blind, placebo-controlled trial and reported that women who had 8 weeks of DHEA supplementation had similar number of harvested oocytes (8.9 ± 1.8 vs 8.2 ± 2.2) but significantly higher live birth (22% vs 13%) and lower miscarriage rates (0 vs 27.8%) compared to controls [57].

Yeung et al. studied the impact of DHEA supplementation in three different patient populations. In the first double-blind, placebo-controlled trial, 22 women with primary ovarian insufficiency (<40-year-old women with amenorrhea for at least 4 months, sex steroid deficiency, and two recordings of serum FSH in the menopausal range) were analyzed. Higher antral follicle count and ovarian volume but similar AMH and FSH levels were detected in women who had been given 75 mg DHEA for 16 weeks, compared to the control group [58]. In the second RCT including 32 women with anticipated poor response, DHEA supplementation resulted in statistically significant increases in serum DHEAS, free androgen index, and follicular DHEAS levels, but no significant improvement found in ovarian response and clinical outcome parameters [59]. In their third RCT (n = 72), the authors demonstrated that DHEA supplementation for 12 weeks increased serum androgen levels but failed to confer any benefit in terms of ovarian reserve markers or ovarian response in anticipated normal ovarian responders [60].

A double-blind, randomized pilot trial (DITTO: dehydroepiandrosterone intervention to treat ovarian aging) was conducted to test whether DHEA pretreatment would improve clinical outcome in women with anticipated poor ovarian response and to inform the design of a large multicenter DHEA trial [61]. Jayaprakasan et al. presented their findings at the annual meeting of the European Society of Human Reproduction and Embryology in 2015. Sixty women with decreased ovarian reserve as determined with an antral follicle count <10 or serum AMH level < 5 pmol/L, between 23 and 43 years of age, were given 75 mg/day DHEA for up to 16 weeks (median, 12 weeks). Women in the DHEA group had similar number of oocytes collected (median of four oocytes). Clinical pregnancy rate (28.6% vs. 36.0%; relative risk, 0.79) and live birth rate (and 25% vs. 32%; RR, 0.78) were comparable in the study and control groups. Authors concluded that "Successful recruitment for this pilot trial suggests a large definitive trial is feasible, but the lack of effect on IVF outcome—not even a trend—suggests it is a low priority" [62].

On the contrary, the latest non-blinded RCT from Egypt (n = 140) reported significant increases in the number of oocytes retrieved (6.9 ± 3.0 vs 5.8 ± 3.1; p = 0.03), fertilization rate (62.3% ± 27.4 vs 52.2% ± 29.8; p = 0.039), and ongoing pregnancy rate (28.5% vs 12.8%) with 12 weeks of daily 75 mg DHEA pretreatment in Bologna criteria defined poor responder women [63].

One might question whether longer DHEA supplementation might improve IVF outcomes, perhaps by affecting the gonadotropin-responsive follicle pool. The major argument against the use of DHEA for longer durations is that prolonged exposure to high androgen levels in the late follicular phase might cause unfavorable intraovarian environment, reducing the fertilization potential of oocytes harvested from large preovulatory follicles [64, 65]. Some experts would also argue that poor responders, regardless of their age, have similar intrafollicular androgenic concentrations with normal responder women, an observation that would challenge the hypothesis of androgen supplementation [66].

Interpretation of the above data should also take into account the bias introduced by small sample size and major differences in study designs, patient populations, definition of poor response, and ovarian stimulation protocols. A Cochrane review has failed to reveal any benefit when studies at high risk of bias were removed from the meta-analysis [55]. Although findings reported in the literature merit further consideration, the small number of randomized controlled trials does not permit ultimate conclusions regarding the proposed benefits of DHEA supplementation. Until clear benefits are supported by high-quality evidence, DHEA pretreatment to improve ovarian response is regarded as empirical [67].

50.3 Testosterone Pretreatment

Evidence is divided on whether testosterone pretreatment improves ovarian response and clinical outcome in poor responders. The first double-blind, placebo-controlled RCT [68], addressing the use of testosterone gel application (10 mg/day for 15–21 days) in 53 women, showed a nonsignificant increase in the number of cumulus-oophorus complexes (COCs) retrieved as compared with placebo (mean difference, +0.31 COCs; 95% CI, 2.16 to +2.26). Later, in an open-label RCT [68] (n = 110), Kim et al. reported a significant increase in the number of COCs with testosterone pretreatment (12.5 mg/day for 21 days) (mean difference, +1.60 COCs; 95% CI, +0.97 to +2.23) as compared to no pretreatment [69]. The systematic review of these two studies suggested that testosterone pretreatment increased clinical pregnancy and live birth rates by 15% and 11%, respectively [70]. In another RCT, Kim et al. studied the effect of testosterone with respect to duration of pretreatment and showed that statistically significant increase in the number of COCs could be achieved only after 3–4 weeks of application [71].

On the contrary, the latest RCT comprising 48 Bologna criteria defined poor responder women showed that no differences were observed regarding the number of COCs (3.5 versus 3.0), fertilization rates (66.7% vs 66.7%), or live birth rates (7.7% vs 8.3%) with 21 days of pretreatment with transdermal testosterone as compared to no treatment [72].

In summary, published data are conflicting, and it is possible that testosterone pretreatment might be associated with a small increase in the number of oocytes retrieved. Even if the available evidence seems favorable, its efficacy is yet to be proven in large-scale, well-designed randomized trials.

50.4 Adjunctive Use of Aromatase Inhibitors

The rationale behind the use of aromatase inhibitors, as an adjunct to gonadotropins for the stimulation poor responders, is the inhibition of aromatase activity in granulosa cells. This, in turn, not only creates an androgenic ovarian microenvironment but also provides pituitary escape from estrogen feedback, leading to elevated gonadotropins levels. Both anastrozole and letrozole have been used as adjuvant treatments in poor responders as highly potent, reversible aromatase inhibitors.

The implementation of aromatase inhibitors into clinical practice has been hampered due to concerns regarding their teratogenic potential. Biljan et al. called into question the safety of letrozole for infertility treatment, based on their findings showing a higher risk for cardiac and skeletal malformations [73]. This presentation was followed by a statement from the producer, advising against the use of letrozole for indications other than breast cancer therapy. Many experts have argued that it is unlikely for those compounds to exert a teratogenic effect, given their short half-life (45 h), ensuring that complete elimination from the body would occur until the time of conception. However, amidst a growing body of evidence refuting the teratogenic risk of aromatase inhibitors [74, 75], their use in premenopausal women for infertility remains off-label.

The evidence is inconclusive regarding the augmentation of ovarian response by adjunctive use of aromatase inhibitors in poor responders. The first small RCT showed that letrozole + recombinant FSH (rFSH) provides a low-cost regimen alternative for the stimulation of poor responders, achieving comparable pregnancy rates with GnRH agonist + rFSH protocol [76].

Garcia-Velasco et al. 2005 (n = 147) demonstrated that addition of letrozole to GnRH antagonist + gonadotropin stimulation led to significantly higher serum androgen levels, higher number of oocytes retrieved (6.1 vs 4.3; p = 0,033), higher implantation rates (25% vs 9.4%; p = 0.009), but comparable clinical pregnancy rates per cycle (22.4% vs 15.2%) [77]. Likewise, another RCT with a similar design (n = 70) showed no difference in clinical pregnancy rates per embryo transfer (25.8% vs 20%) [78].

Three clinical trials compared GnRH antagonist+FSH + HMG + letrozole stimulation with the microdose flare-up FSH + HMG protocol. In a prospective, nonrandomized controlled trial (n = 534), adjuvant letrozole treatment failed to increase the number of oocytes retrieved (12 ± 6 vs 13 ± 5.3), but it was associated with a lower pregnancy rate (37.9% vs + 51.8%) compared to microdose flare-up regimen [79]. Likewise, another RCT found that adjuvant letrozole treatment resulted in significantly lower number of oocytes (8.5 ± 1.1 vs 9.2 ± 1.2) and pregnancy rate (4.4% vs 12.2%) [80]. The third RCT reported similar number of oocytes in both groups but a lower pregnancy rate (13.3% vs 16.7%) in the letrozole group [81].

In a non-blinded RCT, Lee et al. compared GnRH antagonist protocols with HMG alone and sequential letrozole + HMG administration (n = 53). They showed that letrozole therapy was associated with less gonadotropin use, a shorter period duration, and comparable live birth rates [82].

A recent double-blinded, placebo-controlled RCT (n = 70) in Bologna criteria defined poor responders failed to demonstrate any difference when GnRH antagonist+FSH protocol was coupled with letrozole in terms of the total dose of FSH, duration of induction, number of oocytes retrieved, and clinical pregnancy rate [83].

A critical appraisal of the evidence shows that letrozole shortens the duration of induction, but the assumption that they would augment the follicular response in poor responders has not been confirmed.

50.5 Meta-Analyses and Systematic Reviews

Androgen supplementation in women with diminished ovarian reserve has been the subject of several meta-analyses [55, 70, 84–89]. A comprehensive Cochrane review reported higher ongoing pregnancy rates or live birth rates with the use of DHEA (OR 1.88, 95% CI: 1.30–2.71) and testosterone (OR 2.60, 95% CI: 1.30–5.20) [55]. However, when low-quality studies with high-risk bias were excluded, the suggested benefits of both adjuvants were no longer significant (OR 1.50, 95% CI: 0.88–2.56 for DHEA and OR 2.00, 95% CI: 0.17–23.49 for testosterone) [55].

The evidence provided by the meta-analyses was limited by the heterogeneity between the studies, with regard to difference in study populations; varying definitions of poor ovarian response, type, dose, and duration of androgen supplementation; and ovarian stimulation protocols. Furthermore, imprecision of the calculated treatment effects are reflected by the wide confidence intervals, which result from small sample sizes of the individual primary studies.

50.6 Side Effects of Androgen Therapy

Androgens at the prescribed dosages for 6–16 weeks of supplementation are usually well-tolerated, and the adverse effects are rare. The most frequently reported side effects are related with their virilizing effects, including acne, hair loss, hirsutism, and deepening of voice, some of which may be irreversible [90, 91]. Short-term use of DHEA may be associated with decreased high-density lipoprotein cholesterol levels, insulin resistance, and impaired glucose tolerance [92]. Hepatic dysfunction, hypertension, acute manic symptoms, and seizures in convulsion-prone women have also been reported, albeit rarely [93–96]. DHEA may suppress cytochrome p450 and lead to an increase in serum concentrations of many drugs metabolized by this system [97]. Another concern regarding the prolonged use of androgens is the risk of estrogen- or androgen-dependent malignancies. The risk of breast cancer in premenopausal women was reported to be

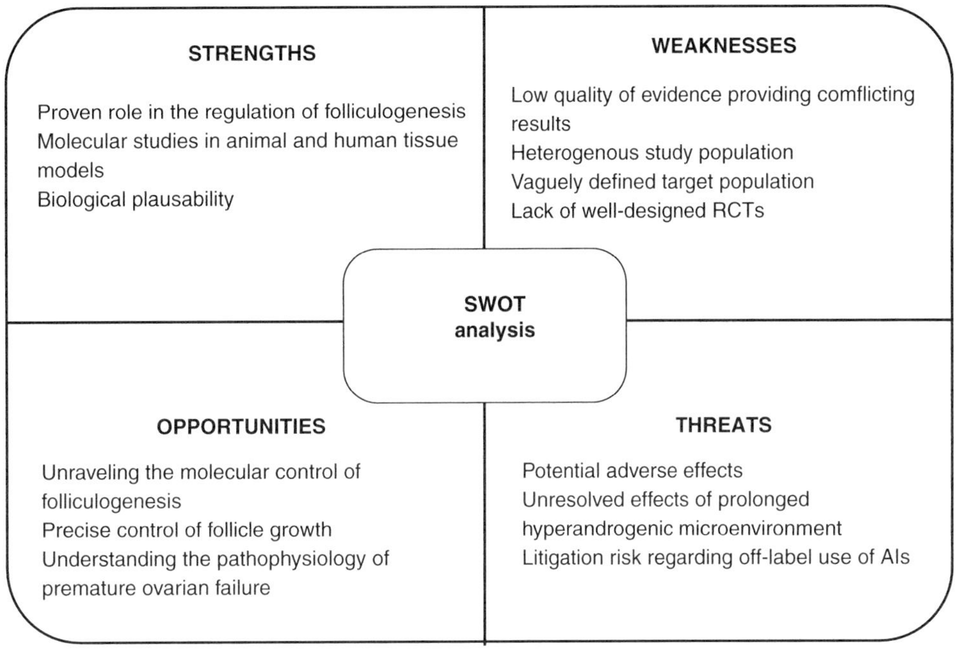

Fig. 50.1 SWOT analysis of the use of androgen and androgen-modulating agents in ovarian stimulation. *RCT*, randomized controlled trial; AI, aromatase inhibitors

positively associated with circulating estrogens and androgens [98].

A Cochrane review on the use of DHEA in the peri- or postmenopausal women failed to show any evidence that DHEA improves quality of life, except slight improvement in sexual function, but there was some evidence that it is associated with androgenic side effects compared with placebo [99].

50.7 Conclusion and Future Directions

Androgen supplementation prior to ovarian stimulation is not supported by the best available evidence (Fig. 50.1). According to the existing animal and human study models, androgens are actively involved in the intraovarian control of folliculogenesis. It is therefore very plausible that increasing the level of androgens in ovarian microenvironment would stimulate development of follicle growth. The hypothesis that they would replenish the follicular pool or augment ovarian response in women with depleted reserves is yet to be proven. Biological plausibility does not justify medical practice in the absence of robust evidence. Clinicians therefore should resist the temptation of offering remedies until they are proven effective in robustly designed clinical studies.

References

1. Lebbe M, Woodruff TK. Involvement of androgens in ovarian health and disease. Mol Hum Reprod. 2013;19:828–37.
2. Dewailly D, Robin G, Peigne M, Decanter C, Pigny P, Catteau-Jonard S. Interactions between androgens, FSH, anti-Mullerian hormone and estradiol during folliculogenesis in the human normal and polycystic ovary. Hum Reprod Update. 2016;22:70–24.
3. Labrie F. DHEA, important source of sex steroids in men and even more in women. Progr Brain Res. 2010;182:97–148.
4. Davison SL, Bell R, Donath S, Montalto JG, Davis SR. Androgen levels in adult females: changes with age, menopause, and oophorectomy. J Clin Endocrinol Metab. 2005;90:3847–53.
5. Gelmann EP. Molecular biology of the androgen receptor. J Clin Oncol. 2002;20:3001–15.
6. Yang JL, Zhang CP, Li L, Huang L, Ji SY, Lu CL, et al. Testosterone induces redistribution of forkhead box-3a and down-regulation of growth and differentiation factor 9 messenger ribonucleic acid expression at early stage of mouse folliculogenesis. Endocrinology. 2010;151.774–82.
7. Rice S, Ojha K, Whitehead S, Mason H. Stage-specific expression of androgen receptor, follicle-stimulating hormone receptor, and anti-Mullerian hormone type II receptor in single, isolated, human preantral follicles: relevance to polycystic ovaries. J Clin Endocrinol Metab. 2007;92:1034–40.
8. Sen A, Hammes SR. Granulosa cell-specific androgen receptors are critical regulators of ovarian development and function. Mol Endocrinol. 2010;24:1393–403.
9. Weil SJ, Vendola K, Zhou J, Adesanya OO, Wang J, Okafor J, et al. Androgen receptor gene expression in the primate ovary: cellular localization, regulation, and functional correlations. J Clin Endocrinol Metab. 1998;83:2479–85.
10. Yang MY, Fortune JE. Testosterone stimulates the primary to secondary follicle transition in bovine follicles in vitro. Biol Reprod. 2006;75:924–32.
11. Cardenas H, Pope WF. Androgen receptor and follicle-stimulating hormone receptor in the pig ovary during the follicular phase of the estrous cycle. Mol Reprod Dev. 2002;62:92–8.
12. Hampton JH, Manikkam M, Lubahn DB, Smith MF, Garverick HA. Androgen receptor mRNA expression in the bovine ovary. Domest Anim Endocrinol. 2004;27:81–8.
13. Juengel JL, Heath DA, Quirke LD, McNatty KP. Oestrogen receptor a and b, androgen receptor and progesterone receptor mRNA

and protein localisation within the developing ovary and in small growing follicles of sheep. Reproduction. 2006;131:81–92.
14. Prizant H, Gleicher N, Sen A. Androgen actions in the ovary: balance is key. J Endocrinol. 2014;222:141–51.
15. Abbott DH, Barnett DK, Bruns CM, Dumestic DA. Androgen excess fetal programming of female reproduction: a developmental aetiology for polycystic ovary syndrome? Hum Reprod Update. 2005;11:357–74.
16. Vendola KA, Zhou J, Adesanya OO, Weil SJ, Bondy CA. Androgens stimulate early stages of follicular growth in the primate ovary. J Clin Invest. 1998;101:2622–9.
17. Smith P, Steckler TL, Veiga-Lopez A, Padmanabhan V. Developmental programming: differential effects of prenatal testosterone and dihydrotestosterone on follicular recruitment, depletion of follicular reserve, and ovarian morphology in sheep. Biol Reprod. 2009;80:726–36.
18. Peluso JJ, Charlesworth J, England-Charlesworth C. Role of estrogen and androgen in maintaining the preovulatory follicle. Cell Tissue Res. 1981;216:615–24.
19. Murray AA, Gosden RG, Allison V, Spears N. Effect of androgens on the development of mouse follicles growing in vitro. J Reprod Fertil. 1998;113:27–33.
20. Hu YC, Wang PH, Yeh S, Wang RS, Xie C, Xu Q, et al. Subfertility and defective folliculogenesis in female mice lacking androgen receptor. Proc Natl Acad Sci USA. 2004;101:11209–14.
21. Walters KA, Middleton LJ, Joseph SR, Hazra R, Jimenez M, Simanainen U, et al. Targeted loss of androgen receptor signaling in murine granulosa cells of preantral and antral follicles causes female subfertility. Biol Reprod. 2012;87:151.
22. Walters KA, Allan CM, Jimenez M, Lim PR, Davey RA, Zajac JD, et al. Female mice haploid insufficient for an inactivated androgen receptor (AR) exhibit age-dependent defects that resemble the AR null phenotype of dysfunctional late follicle development, ovulation, and fertility. Endocrinology. 2007;148:3674–84.
23. Hillier SG, Tetsuka M. Role of androgens in follicle maturation and atresia. Bailliere's Clin Obstet Gynaecol. 1997;11:249–60.
24. Wang H, Andoh K, Hagiwara H, Xiaowei L, Kikuchi N, Abe Y, et al. Effect of adrenal and ovarian androgens on type 4 follicles unresponsive to FSH in immature mice. Endocrinology. 2001;42:4930–6.
25. Sen A, Prizant H, Light A, Biswas A, Hayes E, Lee HJ, et al. Androgens regulate ovarian follicular development by increasing follicle stimulating hormone receptor and microRNA-125b expression. PNAS. 2014;111:3008–13.
26. Otala M, Makinen S, Tuuri T, Sjoberg J, Pentikainen V, Matikainen T, et al. Effects of testosterone, dihydrotestosterone, and 17β-estradiol on human ovarian tissue survival in culture. Fertil Steril. 2004;82(Suppl. 3):1077–85.
27. Weil S, Vendola K, Zhou J, Bondy CA. Androgen and follicle-stimulating hormone interactions in primate ovarian follicle development. J Clin Endocrinol Metab. 1999;84:2951–6.
28. Walters KA, Allan CM, Handelsman DJ. Androgen actions and the ovary. Biol Reprod. 2008;78:380–9.
29. Nielsen ME, Rasmussen IA, Kristensen SG, Christensen ST, Møllgard K, Wreford Andersen E, et al. In human granulosa cells from small antral follicles, androgen receptor mRNA and androgen levels in follicular fluid correlate with FSH receptor mRNA. Mol Hum Reprod. 2011;17:63–70.
30. Feigenberg T, Simon A, Ben-Meir A, Gielchinsky Y, Laufer N. Role of androgens in the treatment of patients with low ovarian response. Reprod BioMed Online. 2009;19:888–98.
31. Narkwichean A, Jayaprakasan K, Maalouf WE, Hernandez-Medrano JH, Pincott-Allen C, Campbell BK. Effects of dehydroepiandrosterone on in vivo ovine follicular development. Hum Reprod. 2014;29:146–54.
32. Vendola K, Zhou J, Wang J, Bondy CA. Androgens promote insulin-like growth factor-I and insulin-like growth factor-I receptor gene expression in the primate ovary. Hum Reprod. 1999;14:2328–32.
33. Casson PR, Lindsay MS, Pisarska MD, Carson SA, Buster JE. Dehydroepiandrosterone supplementation augments ovarian stimulation in poor responders: a case series. Hum Reprod. 2000;15:2129–32.
34. Barad DH, Gleicher N. Increased oocyte production after treatment with dehydroepiandrosterone. Fertil Steril. 2005;84:756.
35. Gleicher N, Weghofer A, Barad DH. Improvement in diminished ovarian reserve after dehydroepiandrosterone supplementation. Reprod Biomed Online. 2010;21:360–5.
36. Barad D, Gleicher N. Effect of dehydroepiandrosterone on oocyte and embryo yields, embryo grade and cell number in IVF. Hum Reprod. 2006;21:2845–9.
37. Sonmezer M, Ozmen B, Cil AP, Ozkavukcu S, Taci T, Olmu H, et al. Dehydroepiandrosterone supplementation improves ovarian response and cycle outcome in poor responders. Reprod Biomed Online. 2009;19(4):508–13.
38. Xu B, Li Z, Yue J, Jin L, Li Y, Ai J, et al. Effect of dehydroepiandrosterone administration in patients with poor ovarian response according to the Bologna criteria. PLoS One. 2014;9(6):e99858.
39. Hyman JH, Margalioth EJ, Rabinowitz R, Tsafrir A, Algur N, Eldar-Geva T. Dehydroepiandrosterone (DHEA) supplementation for poor responders - how does it work? Fertil Steril. 2010;94(4 Supplement):S86.
40. Zangmo R, Singh N, Kumar S, Vanamail P, Tiwari A. Role of dehydroepiandrosterone in improving oocyte and embryo quality in IVF cycles. Reprod Biomed Online. 2014;28:743–7.
41. Barad D, Brill H, Gleicher N. Update on the use of dehydroepiandrosterone supplementation among women with diminished ovarian function. J Assist Reprod Genet. 2007;24:629–34.
42. Fusi FM, Ferrario M, Bosisio C, Arnoldi M, Zanga L. DHEA supplementation positively affects spontaneous pregnancies in women with diminished ovarian function. Gynecol Endocrinol. 2013;29:940–3.
43. Gleicher N, Ryan E, Weghofer A, Blanco-Mejia S, Barad DH. Miscarriage rates after dehydroepiandrosterone (DHEA) supplementation in women with diminished ovarian reserve: a case control study. Reprod Biol Endocrinol. 2009;7:108.
44. Gleicher N, Weghofer A, Barad DH. Dehydroepiandrosterone (DHEA) reduces embryo aneuploidy: direct evidence from preimplantation genetic screening (PGS). Reprod Biol Endocrinol. 2010;8:140.
45. Yilmaz N, Uygur D, Inal H, Gorkem U, Cicek N, Mollamahmutoglu L. Dehydroepiandrosterone supplementation improves predictive markers for diminished ovarian reserve: serum AMH, inhibin B and antral follicle count. Eur J Obstet Gynecol Reprod Biol. 2013;169:257–60.
46. Gleicher N, Weghofer A, Barad DH. The role of androgens in follicle maturation and ovulation induction: friend or foe of infertility treatment? Reprod Biol Endocrinol. 2011;9:116.
47. Vlahos N, Papalouka M, Triantafyllidou O, Vlachos A, Vakas P, Grimbizis G, et al. Dehydroepiandrosterone administration before IVF in poor responders: a prospective cohort study. Reprod Biomed Online. 2015;30:191–6.
48. Zhang J, Qiu X, Gui Y, Xu Y, Li D, Wang L. Dehydroepiandrosterone improves the ovarian reserve of women with diminished ovarian reserve and is a potential regulator of the immune response in the ovaries. Biosci Trends. 2015;9(6):350–9.
49. Wiser A, Gonen O, Ghetler Y, Shavit T, Berkovitz A, Shulman A. Addition of dehydroepiandrosterone (DHEA) for poor-responder patients before and during IVF treatment improves the pregnancy rate: a randomized prospective study. Hum Reprod. 2010;25:2496–500.

50. Yakin K, Urman B. DHEA as a miracle drug in the treatment of poor responders; hype or hope? Hum Reprod. 2011;26:1941–4.
51. Kolibianakis EM, Venetis CA, Tarlatzis BC. DHEA administration in poor responders. Hum Reprod. 2011;26:730–1.
52. Artini PG, Monti M, Matteucci C, Valentino V, Cristello F, Genazzani AR. Vascular endothelial growth factor and basic fibroblast growth factor in polycystic ovary syndrome during controlled ovarian hyperstimulation. Gynecol Endocrinol. 2006;22:465–70.
53. Kara M, Aydin T, Aran T, Turktekin N, Ozdemir B. Does dehydroepiandrosterone supplementation really affect IVF-ICSI outcome in women with poor ovarian reserve? Eur J Obstet Gynecol Reprod Biol. 2014;173:63–5.
54. Haydardedeoglu B. DHEA supplementation and ICSI outcomes: was this really randomized trial? Eur J Obstet Gynecol Reprod Biol. 2016;201:217.
55. Nagels HE, Rishworth JR, Siristatidis CS, Kroon B. Androgens (dehydroepiandrosterone or testosterone) for women undergoing assisted reproduction. Cochrane Database Syst Rev. 2015;26(11):CD009749. https://doi.org/10.1002/14651858.CD009749.pub2.
56. Moawad M, Shaeer M. Long-term androgen priming by use of dehydroepiandrosterone (DHEA) improves IVF outcome in poor-responder patients. A randomized controlled study. Middle East Fertil Soc J. 2012;17:268–74.
57. Tartagni M, Cicinelli MV, Baldini D, Tartagni MV, Alrasheed H, DeSalvia MA, et al. Dehydroepiandrosterone decreases the age-related decline of the in vitro fertilization outcome in women younger than 40 years old. Reprod Biol Endocrinol. 2015;13:13–8.
58. Yeung TW, Li RH, Lee VC, Ho PC, Ng EH. A randomized double-blinded placebo-controlled trial on the effect of dehydroepiandrosterone for 16 weeks on ovarian response markers in women with primary ovarian insufficiency. J Clin Endocrinol Metab. 2013;98:380–8.
59. Yeung TWY, Chai J, Li RHW, Lee VCY, Ho PC, Ng EHY. A randomized, controlled, pilot trial on the effect of dehydroepiandrosterone on ovarian response markers, ovarian response, and in vitro fertilization outcomes in poor responders. Fertil Steril. 2014;102(1):108–15.
60. Yeung T, Chai J, Li R, Lee V, Ho PC, Ng E. A double-blind randomised controlled trial on the effect of dehydroepiandrosterone on ovarian reserve markers, ovarian response and number of oocytes in anticipated normal ovarian responders. BJOG. 2016;123:1097–105.
61. Jayaprakasan K, Narkwichean A, Maalouf WE, Campbell BK. Efficacy of dehydroepiandrosterone to overcome the effect of ovarian ageing (DITTO): a proof of principle randomised controlled trial protocol. BMJ Open. 2014;4:e005767.
62. Jayaprakasan K, Narkwichean A, Maalouf WE, Baumgarten M, Polanski L, Raine-Fenning N, Zujovic L, Thornton J, Campbell BK. Efficacy of dehydroepiandrosterone to overcome the effect of ovarian ageing (DITTO trial): a pilot double blinded placebo controlled randomised controlled trial protocol. 2015; European Society of Human Reproduction and Endocrinology 31th Annual Meeting, Lisbon, Portugal.
63. Kotb MM, Hassan AM, AwadAllah AM. Does dehydroepiandrosterone improve pregnancy rate in women undergoing IVF/ICSI with expected poor ovarian response according to the Bologna criteria? A randomized controlled trial. Eur J Obstet Gynecol Reprod Biol. 2016;200:11–5.
64. Andersen CY, Lossl K. Increased intrafollicular androgen levels affect human granulosa cell secretion of anti-Mullerian hormone and inhibin-B. Fertil Steril. 2008;89:1760–5.
65. Ikeda K, Baba T, Morishita M, Honnma H, Endo T, Kiya T, Saito T. Long-term treatment with dehydroepiandrosterone may lead to follicular atresia through interaction with anti-Mullerian hormone. J Ovarian Res. 2014;7:46.
66. de los Santos MJ, García-Laez V, Beltrán D, Labarta E, Zuzuarregui JL, Alamá P, et al. The follicular hormonal profile in low-responder patients undergoing unstimulated cycles: is it hypoandrogenic? HumReprod. 2013;28:224–9.
67. Garcia-Velasco JA. Poor responders and androgen adjuvant treatment: "still haven't found what I'm looking for…". Reprod Biomed Online. 2014;28:661–2.
68. Massin N, Cedrin-Durnerin I, Coussieu C, Galey-Fontaine J, Wolf JP, Hugues JN. Effects of transdermal testosterone application on the ovarian response to FSH in poor responders undergoing assisted reproduction technique—a prospective, randomized, double-blind study. Hum Reprod. 2006;21:1204–11.
69. Kim CH, Howles CM, Lee HA. The effect of transdermal testosterone gel pretreatment on controlled ovarian stimulation and IVF outcome in low responders. Fertil Steril. 2011;95:679–83.
70. Bosdou JK, Venetis CA, Kolibianakis EM, Toulis KA, Goulis DG, Zepiridis L, et al. The use of androgens or androgen-modulating agents in poor responders undergoing in vitro fertilization: a systematic review and meta-analysis. Hum Reprod Update. 2012;18:127–45.
71. Kim CH, Ahn JW, Moon JW, Kim SH, Chae HD, Kang BM. Ovarian features after 2 weeks, 3 weeks and 4 weeks transdermal testosterone gel treatment and their associated effect on IVF outcomes in poor responders. Dev Reprod. 2014;18:145–52.
72. Bosdou JK, Venetis CA, Dafopoulos K, Zepiridis L, Chatzimeletiou K, Anifandis G, et al. Transdermal testosterone pretreatment in poor responders undergoing ICSI: a randomized clinical trial. Hum Reprod. 2016;31:977–8.
73. Biljan MM, Hemmings R, Brassard N. The outcome of 150 babies following the treatment with letrozole or letrozole and gonadotropins. Fertil Steril. 2005;84:S95.
74. Tatsumi T, Jwa SC, Kuwara A, Irahara M, Kubota T, Saito H. No increased risk of major congenital anomalies or adverse pregnancy or neonatal outcomes following letrozole use in assisted reproductive technology. Hum Reprod. 2017;32:125–32.
75. Tatsumi T, Jwa SC, Kuwara A, Irahara M, Kubota T, Saito H. Pregnancy and neonatal outcomes following letrozole use in frozen-thawed single embryo transfer cycles. Hum Reprod. 2017;32:1244–8.
76. Goswami SK, Das T, Chattopadhyay R, Sawhney V, Kumar J, Chaudhury K, et al. A randomized single-blind controlled trial of letrozole as a low-cost IVF protocol in women with poor ovarian response: a preliminary report. Hum Reprod. 2004;19:2031–5.
77. Garcia-Velasco JA, Moreno L, Pacheco A, Guillen A, Duque L, Requena A, et al. The aromatase inhibitor letrozole increases the concentration of intraovarian androgens and improves in vitro fertilization outcome in low responder patients: a pilot study. Fertil Steril. 2005;84:82–7.
78. Ozmen B, Sonmezer M, Atabekoglu CS, Olmus H. Use of aromatase inhibitors in poor-responder patients receiving GnRH antagonist protocols. Reprod Biomed Online. 2009;19:478–85.
79. Schoolcraft WB, Surrey ES, Minjarez DA, Stevens JM, Gardner K. Management of poor responders: can outcomes be improved with a novel gonadotropin-releasing hormone antagonist/letrozole protocol? Fertil Steril. 2008;89:151–6.
80. Davar R, Oskouian H, Ahmadi S, Firouzabadi RD. GnRH antagonist/letrozole versus microdose GnRH agonist flare protocol in poor responders undergoing in vitro fertilization. Taiwan J Obstet Gynecol. 2010;49:297–301.
81. Mohsen IA, El Din RE. Minimal stimulation protocol using letrozole versus microdose flare up GnRH agonist protocol in women with poor ovarian response undergoing ICSI. Gynecol Endocrinol. 2013;29:105–8.
82. Lee VC, Chan CC, Ng EH, Yeung WSB, Ho PC. Sequential use of letrozole and gonadotrophin in women with poor ovarian

reserve: a randomized controlled trial. Reprod Biomed Online. 2011;23:380–8.
83. Ebrahimi M, Akbari-ASbagh F, Ghalandar-Attar M. Letrozole+ GnRH antagonist stimulation protocol in poor ovarian responders undergoing intracytoplasmic sperm injection cycles: an RCT. Int J Reprod Biomed. 2017;15:101–8.
84. Sunkara SK, Pundir J, Khalaf Y. Effect of androgen supplementation or modulation on ovarian stimulation outcome in poor responders: a meta-analysis. Reprod Biomed Online. 2011;22:545–55.
85. González-Comadran M, Durán M, Solà I, Fábregues F, Carreras R, Checa MA. Effects of transdermal testosterone in poor responders undergoing IVF: systematic review and meta-analysis. Reprod Biomed Online. 2012;25:450–9.
86. Narkwichean A, Maalouf W, Campbell BK, Jayaprakasan K. Efficacy of dehydroepiandrosterone to improve ovarian response in women with diminished ovarian reserve: a meta-analysis. Reprod Biol Endocrinol. 2013;11:44.
87. Li J, Yuan H, Chen Y, Wu H, Wu H, Li L. A meta-analysis of dehydroepiandrosterone supplementation among women with diminished ovarian reserve undergoing in vitro fertilization or intracytoplasmic sperm injection. Int J Gynaecol Obstet. 2015;131:240–5.
88. Zhang M, Niu W, Wang Y, Xu J, Bao X, Wang L, et al. Dehydroepiandrosterone treatment in women with poor ovarian response undergoing IVF or ICSI: a systematic review and meta-analysis. J Assist Reprod Genet. 2016;33:981–91.
89. Qin JC, Fan L, Qin AP. The effect of dehydroepiandrosterone (DHEA) supplementation on women with diminished ovarian reserve (DOR) in IVF cycle: evidence from a meta-analysis. J Gynecol Obstet Biol Reprod. 2016; https://doi.org/10.1016/j.jgyn.2016.01.002.
90. Kroboth PD, Salek FS, Pittenger AL, Fabian TJ, Frye RF. DHEA and DHEA-S: a review. J Clin Pharmacol. 1999;39:327–48.
91. Sadock BJ, Sadock VA. Anabolic—androgenic steroid abuse. Kaplan & Sadock's concise textbook of clinical psychiatry. 3rd ed. Philadelphia: Lippincott Williams & Wilkins; 2008. p. 150–2.
92. Morales AJ, Haubrich RH, Hwang JY, Asakura H, Yen SS. The effect of six months treatment with a 100 mg daily dose of dehydroepiandrosterone (DHEA) on circulating sex steroids, body composition and muscle strength in age-advanced men and women. Clin Endocrinol. 1998;49:421–32.
93. Sahelian R, Borken S. Dehydroepiandrosterone and cardiac arrhythmia. Ann Intern Med. 1998;129:588.
94. Kline MP, Jaggers ED. Mania onset while using dehydroepiandrosterone. Am J Psychiatry. 1999;156:971.
95. Markowitz JS, Carson WH, Jackson CW. Possible dehydroepiandrosterone-induced mania. Biol Psychiatry. 1999;45:241–2.
96. Karp G, Bentov Y, Masalha R, Ifergane G. Onset of late posttraumatic seizure after dehydroepiandrosterone treatment. Fertil Steril. 2009;91:931.
97. Nakamura H, Nakasa H, Ishii I, Ariyoshi N, Igarashi T, Ohmori S, Kitada M. Effects of endogenous steroids on CYP3A4-mediated drug metabolism by human liver microsomes. Drug Metab Dispos. 2002;30:534–40.
98. Hormones E, Breast Cancer Collaborative Group, Key TJ, Appleby PN, Reeves GK, Travis RC, Alberg AJ, et al. Sex hormones and risk of breast cancer in premenopausal women: a collaborative reanalysis of individual participant data from seven prospective studies. Lancet Oncol. 2013;14:1009–19.
99. Scheffers CS, Armstrong S, Cantineau AE, Farquhar C, Jordan V. Dehydroepiandrosterone for women in the peri- or postmenopausal phase. Cochrane Database Sys Rev. 2015; 22:1CD011066.

Part V

Third Party Reproduction

51 Oocyte Donation

Nadine Massiah, Jonathan Briggs, and Meenakshi Choudhary

51.1 Definition

Oocyte donation (OD) is a type of medically assisted reproduction (MAR) through which women voluntarily give their oocytes for the advanced fertility treatment of another woman or for research. 3–23% of MAR cycles for fertility treatment are secondary to oocyte donation [1–6].

51.2 Background

The first oocyte donation (OD) cycle was undertaken in 1982 in Australia [7]. It resulted in pregnancy but ended in miscarriage at 10 weeks gestation. The first live birth following OD cycle was reported in 1984 in the United States [8]. This occurred 6 years after the first IVF baby, Louise Brown, was born in 1978 in the United Kingdom [9]. Currently oocyte donation is an established fertility treatment, but the practice varies worldwide depending on the laws of the country, their ethical perspective and religious beliefs. Internationally, oocyte donation continues to grow in popularity, and in 2014 it was estimated to have resulted in the birth of over 200,000 children [10].

51.2.1 Incidence

Within Europe there is intercountry variation in the incidence of oocyte donor cycles. Between 1997 and 2010, 3% of all ART cycles (n = 178,027) were reported in Europe to be oocyte donation cycles [11]. However, by 2012, this rose to 5.9% of all ART cycles in 26 European countries with most oocyte donor cycles conducted in Spain [6]. The incidence per country varied from 0.0% to 23.9% of ART cycles [6]. The latest figures quote oocyte donor cycles of approximately 1.5% in Australia, 4% in the United Kingdom and Canada, 11.9% in the United States and 17% in Latin America [1–6]. In the United States, oocyte donation accounts for 18% of live births following ART.

51.2.2 Indications

The indications for oocyte donation are summarised in Table 51.1. In a broad context, donor oocyte treatment is an option for women who have non-functioning or absent ovaries and for women with functioning ovaries but having either diminished ovarian reserve, persistent poor quality eggs or poor quality embryos during IVF treatment. It enables these women to carry a pregnancy, experience childbirth and to have a family. Premature ovarian insufficiency (POI) is the main indication for donor oocytes. It is the reduction/loss of ovarian function before the age of 40. Primary ovarian insufficiency occurs in approximately 1% of post-pubertal women [12]. Chromosomal abnormalities such as Turner's syndrome and Fragile X result in gonadal dysgenesis [13]. FSH receptor mutations have also been identified as a cause of ovarian insufficiency [13]. In up to 5% of women with POI, an autoimmune oophoritis (steroidogenic cell autoimmunity) is responsible for their infertility [14]. Secondary iatrogenic causes of ovarian insufficiency include chemotherapy or radiotherapy which irreversibly destroy ovarian tissue, bilateral oophorectomy which may have been undertaken for borderline or malignant ovarian tumours, cancer risk-reduction surgery or other indications such as life-threatening haemorrhagic complications during ovarian cystectomy. Some causes of POI are unknown.

Since the 1980s, in Europe and the United States, the average age at first childbirth has steadily increased [15]. Delayed childbearing has contributed to advanced

N. Massiah · M. Choudhary (✉)
Newcastle Fertility Centre for Life, Newcastle upon Tyne Hospitals NHS Foundation Trust, Biomedicine West Wing, Newcastle upon Tyne, UK
e-mail: meenakshi.choudhary@nuth.nhs.uk

J. Briggs
Royal Victoria Infirmary, Adult Cystic Fibrosis Centre, Newcastle upon Tyne, UK

G. N. Allahbadia et al. (eds.), *Textbook of Assisted Reproduction*, https://doi.org/10.1007/978-981-15-2377-9_51

Table 51.1 Indications for oocyte donation

For treatment purposes
• Women with hypergonadotropic hypogonadism
– Primary ovarian insufficiency, e.g. Turner's syndrome, gonadal dysgenesis
– Secondary ovarian insufficiency, e.g. iatrogenic causes such as post-chemotherapy or radiotherapy, bilateral oophorectomy
• Women with diminished ovarian reserve
– Advanced reproductive age
– Other conditions contributing to low reserve, such as ovarian endometrioma surgery
– Unexplained
• Women with ART factors
– Poor oocyte quality
– Recurrent failed fertilization of oocytes
– Poor embryo quality
– Multiple unsuccessful IVF cycles
• Women with inheritable conditions
– Any significant genetic mutation or carrier state that can result in an affected offspring
• Egg-sharing option
– Women undergoing ART donating some of their eggs as benefit in kind to receive discounted treatment
For research purposes
• Advancing science and technology for clinical translation and improvement such as research into oocyte ageing, genomics and gene editing and mitochondrial replacement techniques
For mitochondrial replacement therapies
• As mitochondrial donation for women affected with cytoplasmic mitochondrial disorders at risk of having high mutation loads in offsprings
• For recurrent implantation failures secondary to poor embryo quality (though still controversial)

reproductive-aged women seeking fertility treatments despite known decline in reproductive outcomes in these women secondary to detrimental effect on egg number, quality and chromosomal segregation errors. Oocyte donation for age-related decline in ovarian reserve is employed to improve live birth outcomes from ART cycles. It was reported that two thirds of the oocyte donor cycles in the United Kingdom were in women aged over 40 [2].

Oocyte donation is also an alternative for those women who wish to prevent transmitting an inheritable severe genetic condition to their offspring as an alternative to pre-implantation genetic diagnosis or prenatal diagnosis. When combined with gestational surrogacy, oocyte donation can enable same-sex male couples to father children biologically related to one parent. Fertility treatment is not the only purpose of donor oocytes. They are utilised for stem-cell and reproductive medicine research. Their use within research enabled the development of mitochondrial replacement therapy aimed at preventing the transmission of mitochondrial disease.

51.2.3 Accessibility

The accessibility of oocyte donation varies around the world. In some countries such as Germany where MAR is legal, oocyte donation is prohibited. In the United States, although oocyte donation is permitted, access to donor oocytes is determined by several factors such as health insurance policy or self-funding capacity. In the United Kingdom, oocyte donation may be funded by the National Health Service with interregional variation in eligibility criteria such as patient age, previous children and number of previous cycles. However the shortage of donors has led to some oocyte recipients waiting for as long as 3 years for donor oocytes. The international disparity in the legality of oocyte donation may contribute to the increased use of cross-border reproductive care.

51.2.4 Categories of Oocyte Donors: Altruistic/Known/Egg Sharing

Oocyte donors for fertility treatment may be altruistic or known donors. An altruistic donor is commonly referred to donors who are not known to the oocyte recipients and give their oocytes benevolently to women whose identity they do not know. Known donors (also referred to as directed donation) give their oocytes to women who they know, such as a friend or family member. In the United States, there are agencies that link potential oocyte donors to recipients. In that setting, a donor and recipient may meet each other and receive identifying information about each other. The donor is then referred to as a known donor rather than an altruistic donor. Altruistic donors are more common than known donors. A questionnaire study reported that 41% of potential oocyte donors thought that they would agree to altruistic donation and 25% to known donation [16].

A controversial reason for oocyte donation is egg sharing, an established practice in some countries where a woman undergoing MAR shares her eggs in exchange for a reduction in the cost of her IVF treatment, commonly regarded as "benefit in kind" [17, 18]. Despite a survey of 234 IVF couples in the United Kingdom reporting that 90% of them were receptive to donating oocytes for fertility treatment of others [16], only 3.8% of women who underwent IVF/ICSI were part of egg-sharing agreements [19]. In 2013, 709 women in the United Kingdom donated oocytes within egg-sharing schemes, with a live birth rate of 38.1% per cycle [19]. Egg sharing for research rather than for treatment of others is an alternative, where eggs are shared for a research project rather than donated to others for creating a baby [20].

51.3 Process of Oocyte Donation

The process of oocyte donation is discussed in this chapter from oocyte donor's perspective. The oocyte recipient will also be required to undergo implications counselling, screening and endometrial preparation regime for oocyte donation cycle. However, it is beyond the remit of this chapter.

51.3.1 Recruitment

The method of recruiting oocyte donors including advertising is influenced by the country's regulation or nonregulation of oocyte donation. Fertility clinics may recruit locally by advertising on their website, local universities and other areas within their community or nationally by advertising in magazines, national newspapers, television and social media. Anonymity and inadequate compensation are often cited as reasons people chose not to donate [21–23]. In the United States commercialisation, anonymity and non-anonymity are allowed, and there is no donor shortage. In Spain, the largest provider of oocyte donor cycles in Europe, commercialisation is not allowed, but anonymity is mandatory. A study of oocyte donors who had received financial compensation reported that altruism was the main reason the women had donated their oocytes. However, the same study reported a significant negative correlation between pre-donation financial motivation and post-donation satisfaction [24]. In countries, where compensation is permitted, the financial reward of oocyte donors has increased, in order to encourage young women to donate their oocytes. Other reasons for the lack of volunteers include fear of complications, time commitment and ethical concerns (Table 51.2).

In the absence of a regulatory body, the American Society for Reproductive Medicine published extensive guidelines for gamete donation in 2012 [25]. Potential donors with or without proven fertility, ideally aged between 21 and 34 years old, may be recruited. The age criteria are comparable in other countries. Donor age under 35 years is associated with reduced risk of chromosomal abnormalities and higher live birth rates. After potential donors are recruited, they are required to undergo rigorous screening and counselling before being approved to go through the actual donation.

Table 51.2 Factors that influence the shortage of oocyte donors

• Time commitment
• Non-anonymity
• Lack of or inadequate compensation
• Potential complications of oocyte donation
• Ethnicity
• Ethical concerns
• Lack of public awareness of need for oocyte donors

51.3.2 Screening Process

The purpose of screening is to identify healthy women who would be suitable oocyte donors. This ensures the safety and welfare of the oocyte donor, oocyte recipient and the donor-conceived child. It also functions to identify women who can undergo the oocyte donation process with minimal risk to their medical well-being. It has been shown than only 17% of potential oocyte donors were considered suitable after medical and genetic screening [26]. Screening can be divided into four categories: (1) medical and family history, (2) physical examination, (3) investigations and (4) psychological assessment. A detailed medical and family history should be taken. Donors should ideally have good general health with no evidence of heritable diseases. Physical examination should include blood pressure and body mass index. The investigations consist of baseline investigations including ovarian reserve tests and screening for genetic and infectious diseases. The genetic screen consists of the karyotype and cystic fibrosis test as a minimum. Some privately run clinics screen for a wide range of genetic diseases. Wallerstein et al. reported that 11% of potential oocyte donors were excluded because of genetic conditions [27]. The infectious diseases screen usually comprises of HIV, hepatitis B and C, syphilis, gonorrhoea, chlamydia and others such as cytomegalovirus, toxoplasmosis and herpes virus. Potential oocyte donors who are from or have visited countries with Zika virus must be screened for Zika virus, to reduce the risk of transmission of this virus [28]. Reasons for exclusion of potential donors can vary among centres. In some centres, potential donors are excluded if they have haemophilia, received an organ transplant, at higher risk for sexually transmitted diseases such as intravenous drug users, had a tattoo within 1 year or have dementia or any degenerative or demyelinating disease [25]. It has been suggested that quarantining of oocytes should be offered to all recipients [25]. The duration of quarantining can be as long as 180 days. Psychological assessment is an approach adopted by some fertility centres to ensure that donors are psychologically capable of undertaking the egg donor process and coping afterwards with their decision.

51.3.3 Egg Donor Cycle

Following a satisfactory history, examination, screening and psychological assessment, donors can be invited to sign oocyte donation consent forms. The consent forms must be signed prior to treatment indicating informed decision process. Blood group and phenotypic characteristics such as height, hair and eye colour are used to match donors to recipients. The number of recipients to one donor cycle can vary based on number of oocytes retrieved and local policy.

A retrospective study of 249 donor oocyte cycles reported a 94% success rate among recipients sharing donor cycles [29]. Following the selection of the oocyte donor, the treatment cycles of the oocyte donor and oocyte recipient are timed together in fresh oocyte donation cycles. The aim is for mature oocytes to be retrieved and fertilized, when the oocyte recipient's endometrium has been optimally prepared for embryo transfer. Controlled ovarian stimulation is initiated for the development of multiple ovarian follicles. Ovarian stimulation following GnRH-antagonist protocols reduce the risk of ovarian hyperstimulation syndrome (OHSS) when compared to GnRH-agonist long downregulation protocols, without affecting live birth rate [30]. Ultrasound monitoring ensures assessment of follicular growth and timing ovulation trigger for oocyte retrieval. Human chorionic gonadotropin (HCG) or GnRH agonist can be used to mimic the endogenous LH surge in natural ovulation [31]. HCG has a longer circulating half-life than GnRH agonists, and the sustained LH receptor activity following HCG increases the risk of OHSS compared to agonist trigger [31]. The donor can withdraw from donating her oocytes until this point though variations do exist. Once the oocytes are obtained and given to the recipient, then the ownership gets transferred to the recipient. In some cases, a recipient may not be lined up for fresh oocyte donation cycles. In these situations, the oocytes donated are cryopreserved (vitrified) for future use by recipients. An oocyte bank works on similar principles where oocytes are batched and frozen to create a stock of donor eggs. Subsequent review of the oocyte donor is recommended to ensure return of menstrual cycles and recovery from the process.

51.3.4 MAR Outcome for OD

Success rates of oocyte donation correlate with the donor age, as opposed to the female recipient's age. It is the most successful treatment option for women aged over 40 years old. The success rate also depends on number of embryos transferred. In Europe, in 2013, pregnancy rates of 49.8%, 46.4% and 38.5% were reported for oocyte donor treatments using fresh embryos, frozen embryo and frozen oocytes, respectively, with a 29.5% live birth rate per embryo transfer [6]. In egg-sharing cycles, live birth rates of 38.1% and 35.0% were observed in donors and recipients, respectively [18]. In countries such as Latin America where restriction doesn't exist on number of embryos transferred, higher live birth rates (42.5%) are reported in conjunction with high multiple pregnancy rates [5]. The Society of Assisted Reproductive Technology (SART) in the United States reported preliminary data of 50% overall live birth rate for fresh donor eggs and 38.4% live birth rate for frozen donor eggs per recipient cycle in 2015. The live birth rate of singleton pregnancies was 36.5% for fresh donor eggs and 29.9% for frozen donor eggs [32]. With the surge of oocyte banks having vitrified donor oocytes, it is recommended that recipients are informed about the slightly lower live birth rate with frozen donor oocytes compared to fresh donor oocytes.

51.3.5 Risks of Oocyte Donation to the Donor

The risks of oocyte donation can be divided into short-term and long-term risks (Table 51.3). The effects of ovarian stimulation include physical risks such as abdominal pain/bloating, mood swings, headaches, nausea, ovarian hyperstimulation syndrome and thrombosis. Allergic reaction to medications can also occur. Moderate to severe ovarian hyperstimulation syndrome occurs in <5% of women undergoing controlled ovarian stimulation. Although uncommon, OHSS can result in serious complications [33]. There is no proven treatment for OHSS; as such it is managed with supportive care, fluid resuscitation and prophylactic anticoagulation [33]. Ultrasound-guided transvaginal oocyte retrieval (TVOR) is considered a safe and effective procedure [34]. Whilst complications are uncommon, they include risks of pelvic pain, bleeding from the vaginal wall, infection, pelvic abscess and injury to local structures such as vessels, bowel or ureters.

There is a paucity of long-term follow-up studies of the oocyte donor population. Whilst the majority of oocyte donors report post-donation satisfaction, some donors have experienced long-term psychological effects [35]. Furthermore, donors may wonder whether their oocytes resulted in the birth of a child or may wonder about the welfare of any children born.

Breast and endometrial cancers are linked to endogenous oestrogen exposure, and hyperstimulation may result in borderline ovarian tumours or malignant transformation [36]. Although plausible, lack of robust evidence precludes one from drawing firm conclusions as regards aftermath of gynaecological cancer risk secondary to oocyte donation per se.

Table 51.3 Risks and complications of oocyte donation

Short term	Effects of the hormones	• Abdominal discomfort/pain • Mood swings • Headaches • Ovarian hyperstimulation syndrome • Thrombosis
	Effects of the oocyte retrieval	• Abdominal/pelvic pain • Vaginal bleeding • Vascular injury • Bowel/bladder injury • Infection
Long term	Effects of the hormones	• Risk of ovarian, endometrial, breast or colon cancers (inconclusive)
	Overall egg donation process	• Psychological problems • Unknown long-term effects

51.3.6 Risks of Oocyte Donation to the Recipient/Child

In an age- and parity-matched study of singleton pregnancies following fresh embryo transfer, donor oocyte pregnancies carried a higher risk of preeclampsia, pregnancy-induced hypertension and caesarean section delivery compared to autologous oocytes [37]. Mascarenhas et al. published a meta-analysis comparing the pregnancy outcomes between oocyte donor pregnancies and autologous oocyte pregnancies following fresh embryo transfers after IVF and found an increased risk of preterm birth and low birth weight in oocyte donor pregnancies compared to autologous pregnancies [38]. It is important to recognise that there is an increased risk of obstetric complications in women with advanced maternal age and Turner syndrome. This could affect findings on the comparison of complications and risks between oocyte donor and autologous pregnancies.

51.4 Facilitators and Barriers to Oocyte Donation

51.4.1 Legal and Regulatory Perspective

The regulation of oocyte donation varies worldwide. In some countries such as Italy and Germany, oocyte donation is illegal. Countries that permit oocyte donation may have legislation on this, and it may be regulated by an official body or authority. Spain was the first country to have a separate law for assisted reproduction, and this was passed in November 1988 [39]. Current Spanish legislation regarding oocyte donation is found under the Assisted Human Reproduction Act, Law 14/2006 and is regulated by the National Commission on Assisted Reproduction [40]. British legislation on oocyte donation is found under the HFEA Act 1990 [41], and oocyte donation is closely regulated by the Human Fertilization Embryology Authority (HFEA). In Greece, the legislation on oocyte donation is found under law 3305/2005 which was implemented in 2005, and the National Authority of Medically Assisted Reproduction regulates IVF treatment including oocyte donation [42]. In the United States, guidelines exist for oocyte donation, but there is no regulatory body. Each state determines whether oocyte donation is permitted. In the United States, there is no state or federal regulation on ART or oocyte donation. The American Society for Reproductive Medicine has produced guidelines on gamete donation [33], and fertility centres can choose whether they wish to follow these guidelines. Similarly, in Japan, there is no legislation on ART or oocyte donation. However, the Japanese Society of Reproductive Medicine has published guidelines which fertility centres may follow [43].

Legal stipulations include the number of families or children that can be formed and single women as recipients. In Spain, oocyte donation from one person is limited to the formation of six families and in the United Kingdom ten families. In Greece, the donations are limited to the formation of ten children. In Spain and in the United Kingdom, it is legal to treat single women, whereas in Greece, it is not permitted.

51.4.2 Anonymity

Donor anonymity is an important factor in the decision of both donors and recipients to participate in oocyte donor treatment. In most countries, donors are anonymous, and their identities will never be known by the donor recipients or donor-conceived children (Table 51.4). This was also the case in the United Kingdom until 2005 when donor anonymity was removed legally. The HFEA recommended that there should be a move toward the removal of donor anonymity based on the findings of a public consultation on the amount of information that should be given to donor offspring [44]. The law now states that at the age of 18, children conceived by oocyte donation have the right to find out the identity of the donor [44]. In Spain, it is possible for medical reasons only, for the donor's identity to be revealed. This can only be obtained through the court. But in the United States, anonymity may or may not be held by prior agreement between the donor, fertility centre and recipient.

51.4.3 Compensation

Variation in financial payment exists between countries (Table 51.4). Some countries such as Israel forbid any financial payment [45] or allow payment for proven expenses. Other countries such as Spain, Greece, France, Belgium and the United Kingdom impose set compensation limits. Oocyte donors are compensated only for their travel expenses and loss of work. The compensation given to the donor varies between 500 and 1000 euros dependent on the decision made by the fertility centre. In the United States, donors may be compensated beyond the coverage of expenses, and it has been reported that donors have been compensated as much as US$8000 [46]. In 2016, the ASRM ethics committee deemed financial compensation to oocyte donors justifiable on the provision that compensation reflects time commitment, inconvenience and discomfort caused by oocyte donation. Further, compensation should not differ based on the number of oocytes retrieved, number of previous donated oocyte cycles, the intended use of the donated oocytes or the donor's characteristics/ethnicity. In a

Table 51.4 Compensation and anonymity of oocyte donors by country

	Compensation	Anonymity
Europe		
France	Expenses only	Anonymous only
Spain	Fixed payment of 900 euros, with some variability	Anonymous only
UK	Fixed cap of £750 set by regulator, per cycle to cover expenses	Anonymous and known donation Donor identity release to offspring at age 18
Netherlands	Fixed amount of 900 euros to cover expenses	Anonymous donation Donor identity release to offspring at age 16
Denmark	Fixed amount to cover expenses	Anonymous and known donation Donor identity release to offspring
Cyprus	Financial compensation, not regulated	Anonymous only
Czech Republic	Payment + expenses	Anonymous only
Greece	Variable financial compensation	Anonymous only
Belgium	Variable but <2000 euros	Known and anonymous donation legal
Portugal	Fixed financial compensation	Anonymous only
Finland	Proven expenses +250 euros fixed payment	Anonymous and known donation Donor identity release to offspring
Sweden	Regional variation	Anonymous and known donation Optional donor identity release to offspring
Ukraine	Payment prohibited	Anonymous and known donation No donor identity release to offspring
Poland	Financial compensation, not regulated	Anonymous only
Austria	Payment prohibited.	Anonymous and known donation Donor identity release to offspring
Switzerland	Financial compensation	Known donation only
Russia	Payment permitted	Anonymous and known donation No donor identity release to offspring
Americas		
Canada	Expenses only	Anonymous and known donation Donor identity release to offspring
USA	Payment recommends up to $5000, >$5000 requires justification	Anonymous and known donation Donor identity release to offspring
Mexico	No information available	Anonymous and known donation
Brazil	Payment prohibited	Anonymous only
Asia		
Australia	Expenses only	Anonymous and known donation Donor identity release to offspring
New Zealand	Expenses only	Anonymous and known donation Donor identity release to offspring
China	Payment prohibited	Only permitted in patients undergoing ART who obtain >20 oocytes. Anonymous only
India	Average $250–500, not regulated	Anonymous donation Donor identity release to offspring
Africa and Middle East		
Israel	Fixed payment to donors of NIS 20 000 (~$5787)	Anonymous only
Iran	Not regulated, commercial OD services exist	Known and anonymous donation permitted
Lebanon	Not regulated	Known and anonymous donation permitted
South Africa	Compensation for time and expenses. Not >5000 R recommended	Known and anonymous donation permitted

survey of 1427 people in the United States, 90% supported payment for oocyte donation, and 90% believed that payment should be less than US$10 000 [47]. Some centres in the United States, including reproductive research centres, ethically object to the provision of large financial compensation and because of this have experienced donor shortage in comparison with other centres [48].

51.4.4 Legal Parenthood

The oocyte donor is not the legal parent of the child and does not have any legal or financial responsibility for the child. The oocyte recipient and her partner are the legal parents of the child. The authors have not identified any country that considers the oocyte donor the legal parent.

51.4.5 Cross-Border Reproductive Care

Cross-border reproductive care (CBRC) or reproductive tourism is on the rise. It is estimated that CBRC accounts for 5% of ART treatment in North America and Europe. Patients choose CBRC for oocyte donation treatment when there is donor shortage in their own country, OD is not permitted in home country, or the cost of oocyte donation is more expensive. In 2013, oocyte donation accounted for 19.4% of CBRC patients across 12 European countries [6]. In the United States, a high proportion of CBRC patients receive treatment with donated oocytes, often due to limited availably of this treatment modality in their home countries. Unfortunately, there is poor data and follow-up on CBRC patients.

51.4.6 Ethical Perspective

Volunteers for oocyte donation are healthy women. An ethical issue is allowing these women to become patients, putting them at risk of harm, although they have no medical problems. Oocyte donation will not improve the health of the oocyte donor but may impair it. Inadequate informed consent is an ethical issue that should not be overlooked. The provision of insufficient information can lead to lack of awareness of the potential risks of oocyte donation. Women need to be fully informed in order to make their decision. Compensation is an ethical issue that has led to worldwide debate [49]. It is known that compensation is a motivating factor for women to donate their oocytes. If potential donors are focused mainly on the financial reward, they may not fully consider the risks and implications of becoming an oocyte donor. They may accept the risks and implications because of their need for money. It has been argued that compensation may also lead to the commodification of the human body, since oocytes are part of the body being exchanged for money [50].

51.4.7 Counselling and Psychosocial Perspective

Counselling is an important element of oocyte donation for both the donors and the recipients. Implications counselling refers to counselling the donors and recipients on the implications of going through the process of egg donation that includes physical and psychosocial consequences. Therapeutic counselling refers to a talking therapy approach where the counsellor listens with empathy and focuses on helping individuals or couples better understand and learn different strategies to cope with their negative thoughts and problematic feelings that they may encounter secondary to oocyte donation process in a confidential manner. The role of the counsellor is not easy. It is essential for the counsellor to be impartial. Ideally the counsellor should not be employed by the fertility centre to minimise bias of the counsellor towards the interests of the fertility centre. This may also be more acceptable to potential oocyte donors and society as a whole.

It is essential that both oocyte donors and recipients receive counselling option. Implications counselling should be mandatory for all going through the process and should be incorporated in the oocyte donation program. However, therapeutic counselling should be an option offered to all if they wish to pursue it. It may be worthwhile for fertility centres to make provisions to offer therapeutic counselling option as a free, confidential service to their oocyte donors and recipients. As counselling is a crucial component of oocyte donation process due to its associated psychosocial and ethical associations, a free counselling service would reduce risk of poor uptake secondary to financial constraints and promote future well-being. In a survey of 217 egg donors and recipients in the United Kingdom, 84% of respondents thought that donors and recipients should be counselled about egg donation [51]. Oocyte donors should be counselled about the physical, psychological and ethical issues surrounding oocyte donation. Psychological issues stem from regret of the decision to donate, failure to conceive themselves in the future, no contact with the donor-conceived child and not knowing whether a child was created. A study reported that 67% of oocyte donors would have liked to know whether the recipient had become pregnant [52]. Another study has shown a negative correlation between pre-donation ambivalence and post-donation satisfaction, suggesting that careful counselling of donors with high levels of pre-donation financial motivation is crucial [53]. The counselling session should also encompass the positive experience that some oocyte donors have reported. A study of 30 altruistic and anonymous oocyte donors found that at 12–18 months post-donation, most oocyte donors were very satisfied and had experienced minimal adverse effects. None of them regretted their decision to donate [52]. A study of 23 oocyte donors found a 91% donor satisfaction rate, and 74% wished to donate their oocytes again. There was also a low report of adverse symptoms [54]. A survey in the United States ($n = 25$) assessed the psychological characteristics and post-donation satisfaction of anonymous oocyte donors. Following oocyte donation, 80% of women stated that they would be willing to donate again [53]. Oocyte recipients should be counselled on the issues of raising a child not genetically related, the decision to disclose to the child that conception was by oocyte donation, presence/absence of anonymity which is dependent on the country that the oocyte donation is conducted and difficulties with having siblings conceived with oocytes from the same donor. The counsellor provides correct information to the recipient but also is someone that the recipient can speak to openly about oocyte donation. A study showed that 80% of oocyte recipients had not told anyone about becoming an oocyte recipient, and 80% did not plan to inform the child [55]. In the United Kingdom, the HFEA has recommended the development of better guidelines on the counselling of donor recipients but also counselling of donor-conceived children. Having a consortium of counsellors specifically trained in the field of providing counselling for oocyte donation and fertility treatments would enable sharing of professional knowledge and expertise. British Infertility Counselling Association is one example of professional society for infertility counsellors in the United Kingdom striving to promote high standards of counselling related to subfertility and assisted conception treatments.

51.5 Other Modalities of Oocyte Donation

51.5.1 Oocyte Donation for Research

The development of medicine and clinical practice is dependent on research. Research centres conduct a variety of studies. These include studies aimed at increasing knowledge in egg function and development and improving the outcomes of reproductive medicine [56]. Research on oocytes is very important since it paves the way for new knowledge to be discovered about fertility problems including ovarian ageing as well as the potential therapeutic targets from this research [57].

51.5.2 Mitochondrial Donation

Mitochondrial donation, also known as mitochondrial replacement therapy (MRT), is a complex development and novel application of in vitro fertilization. The United Kingdom is currently the only country that has granted a licence for a fertility centre to perform MRT for women with mitochondrial disorders [58]. It aims at preventing the transmission of mitochondrial disease from a mother to her offspring as well as future inheritance risk. It uses healthy mitochondria from donor oocytes and can be performed by maternal spindle transfer or pronuclear transfer [59]. Maternal spindle transfer involves transfer of the healthy nucleus of an oocyte with affected mitochondria, into a denucleated donor oocyte with healthy mitochondria. Pronuclear transfer occurs after fertilization of the affected mother's oocyte and donor oocyte. The pronuclei of the embryo containing the mother's mitochondria are transferred to the embryo (fertilized donor oocyte) containing healthy mitochondria. Mitochondrial donation for advanced female age or recurrent implantation failure is highly contentious due to lack of robust evidence to support this and should be deferred till more evidence is available showcasing concept of mitochondrial ageing and its role in ART. Although there have been reports of live births from other countries not regulating this treatment, it is recommended that these new treatments should be offered in a regulated manner where provision for long-term follow-up of MRT-conceived children and their well-being exists.

51.5.3 Double Gamete Donation

Double gamete donation is less common than oocyte donation [60]. It can occur in two ways. The recipient can receive a donated oocyte which is fertilized by a donated sperm, followed by embryo transfer. Alternatively, an embryo can be donated from another couple who underwent IVF treatment. Double gamete donation can be used for the treatment of other couples, research or training of embryologists. Similar to oocyte donors, embryo donors should attend counselling to discuss the implications of embryo donation. The indications for double gamete donation include people with both male and female infertility who require both egg and sperm donations to conceive a child, same-sex couples, single women with low ovarian reserve and older women who are unable to join long waiting lists for donor eggs. Some people may have inheritable diseases that they do not want to pass on to their offspring, for example, a couple where both partners are carriers for autosomal recessive conditions. Alternatives to oocyte donation and double gamete donation are child-free life, adoption or fostering.

51.6 Future Direction of Oocyte Donation

The regulation and process of oocyte donation need to be standardised internationally. Research needs to be done to identify the optimal number of oocytes required for egg sharing. Research is needed to evaluate the effectiveness of counselling on the long-term psychological and social implications of oocyte donation and double gamete donation. Long-term follow-up studies of oocyte donors should be conducted to assess the development of cancer.

51.7 Conclusion

Oocyte donation has a major role in assisted conception (Table 51.5). Ethical concerns have been raised against oocyte donation, but these can be overcome within a well-regulated altruistic service built on a foundation of good clinical practice.

Table 51.5 Clinical pearls: these are the recommendations in relation to oocyte donation

1. All potential oocyte donors should be thoroughly counselled regarding the implications of donating their eggs as well as offered opportunity for therapeutic counselling
2. All oocyte donors should be informed regarding the donor anonymity laws pertinent to the country where the treatment is undertaken.
3. Clinics offering oocyte donation cycles should inform the oocyte donors that they are free to withdraw from the process at any stage until the eggs collected are donated to the recipient.
4. All oocyte donors should be screened for infections and genetic conditions in accordance with the local or national standards
5. Oocyte donor and Zika virus recommendations should be taken into consideration for those living in or visiting a Zika-prone area.
6. Role of infertility specialists is to ascertain a donor-centric approach ensuring their safety and well-being through the oocyte donation process

References

1. Fitzgerald O, Harris K, Paul R, Chambers GM; Assisted reproductive technology in Australia and New Zealand 2015. National Perinatal Epidemiology and Statistics Unit, Sydney. The University of New South Wales, Sydney, Australia. 2017 Oct; 4. npesu.unsw.edu.au. Accessed 4 December 2017.
2. Human Fertilisation and Embryology Authority (HFEA). Oocyte donation statistics. 2014. https://www.hfea.gov.uk/about-us/publications/. Accessed 4 December 2017.
3. Gunby J, Bissonnette F, Librach C, Cowan L. Assisted Reproductive Technologies (ART) in Canada: 2007 results from the Canadian ART register. Fertil Steril. 2011;5(2):542–7.
4. Sunderam S, Chang J, Flowers L, Kulkarni A, Sentelle G, Jeng G, Macaluso M. Assisted Reproductive Technology Surveillance - United States. JSTOR. 2006;58(5):1–25.
5. Zegers-Hochschild F, Schwarze JE, Crosby J, Musri C, Urbina MT, Latin American Network of Assisted Reproduction (REDLARA). Assisted reproduction techniques in Latin America: the Latin American Registry. Reprod Biomed Online. 2017;35(3):287–95.
6. Calhaz-Jorge C, De Geyter C, Kupka MS, de Mouzon J, Erb K, Mocanu E, Motrenko T, Scaravelli WC, Goossens V. Assisted reproductive technology in Europe, 2013: results generated from European registers by ESHRE. Hum Reprod. 2017;32(10):1957–73.
7. Trounson A, Leeton J, Besanko M, Wood C, Conti A. Pregnancy established in an infertile patient after transfer of a donated embryo fertilised in vitro. Br Med J (Clin Res Ed). 1983;286:835.
8. Bustillo M, Buster JE, Cohen SW, Hamilton F, Thorneycroft IH, Simon JA, Rodi IA, Boyers SP, Marshall JR, Louw JA, Seed RW, Seed RG. Delivery of a healthy infant following nonsurgical ovum transfer. JAMA. 1984;251(7):889.
9. Steptoe PC, Edwards RG. Birth after the reimplantation of a human embryo. Lancet. 1978;2(8085):366.
10. Woodriff M, Sauer MV, Klitzman R. Advocating for longitudinal follow-up of the health and welfare of egg donors. Fertil Steril. 2014;102(3):662–6.
11. Ferraretti AP, Nygren K, Nyboe A, Kupka M, Calhaz-Jorge C, Wyns C, Gianaroli L, Goossens V, The European IVF-Monitoring Consortium (EIM), for the European Society of Human Reproduction and Embryology (ESHRE). Trends over 15 years in ART in Europe: an analysis of 6 million cycles. Hum Reprod Open. 2017;34(2):162–5.
12. Tucker EJ, Grover SR, Bachelot A, Touraine P, Sinclair AH. Premature ovarian insufficiency: new perspectives on genetic cause and phenotypic spectrum. Endocr Rev. 2016;37(6):609–35.
13. Kallio S, Aittomäki K, Piltonen T, Veijola R, Liakka A, Vaskivuo TE, Dunkel L, Tapanainen JS. Anti-Mullerian hormone as a predictor of follicular reserve in ovarian insufficiency: special emphasis on FSH-resistant ovaries. Hum Reprod. 2012;27(3):854–60.
14. La Marca A, Marzotti S, Brozzetti A, Stabile G, Artenisio AC, Bini V, Giordano R, De Bellis A, Volpe A, Falorni A, Italian Addison Network. Primary ovarian insufficiency due to steroidogenic cell autoimmunity is associated with a preserved pool of functioning follicles. J Clin Endocrinol Metab. 2009;94(10):3816–23.
15. Mills M, Rindfuss R, McDonald P, te Velde E, ESHRE Reproduction and Society Task Force. Why do people postpone parenthood? Reasons and social policy incentives. Hum Reprod Update. 2011;17(6):848–60.
16. Oskarsson T, Dimitry ES, Mills MS, Hunt J, Winston RM. Attitudes towards gamete donation among couples undergoing in vitro fertilization. Br J Obstet Gynaecol. 1991;98(4):351–6.
17. Bracewell-Milnes T, Saso S, Abdalla H, Thum MY. A systematic review investigating psychosocial aspects of egg sharing in the United Kingdom and their potential effects on egg donation numbers. Hum Fertil. 2017;26:1–11.
18. Glujovsky D, Fiszbajn G, Lipowicz R, Lavolpe M, Sueldo C. Practice of sharing donated oocytes among several recipients. Fertil Steril. 2006;86(6):1786–8.
19. Human Fertilisation and Embryology Authority (HFEA). Fertility treatment 2014 trends and figures. http://ifqtesting.blob.core.windows.net/umbraco-website/1783/fertility-treatment-2014-trends-and-figures.pdf Accessed 04 December 2017.
20. Choudhary M, et al. Egg sharing for research: a successful outcome for patients and researchers. Cell Stem Cell. 2012;10(3):239–40.
21. Brett S, Sacranie RR, Thomas GE, Rajkhowa R. Can we improve recruitment of oocyte donors with loss of donor anonymity? A hospital-based survey. Hum Fertil. 2008;11(2):101–7.
22. Craft I, Flyckt S, Heeley G, Layland S, Thornhill A, Kelada E. Will removal of anonymity influence the recruitment of egg donors? A survey of past donors and recipients. Reprod Biomed Online. 2005;10:325–9.
23. Purewal S, van den Akker OBA. Systematic review of oocyte donation: investigating attitudes, motivations and experiences. Human Reprod Upd. 2009;15(5):499–515.
24. Klock SC, Braverman AM, Rausch DT. Predicting anonymous egg donor satisfaction: a preliminary study. J Women's Health. 1998;7:229–37.
25. American Society for Reproductive Medicine. Recommendations for gamete and embryo donation. A committee opinion. 2013 http://www.asrm.org/globalassets/asrm/asrm-content/news-and-publications/practice-guidelines/for-non-members/recommendations_for_gamete_and_embryo_donation-noprint.pdf. Accessed 04 December 2017.
26. Gorrill MJ, Johnson LK, Patton PE, Burry KA. Oocyte donor screening: the selection process and cost analysis. Fertil Steril. 2001;75(2):400–4.
27. Wallerstein R, Jansen V, Grifo JA, Berkeley AS, Noyes N, Licker J, Licciardi F. Genetic screening of prospective oocyte donors. Fertil Steril. 1998;70:52–5.
28. Food and Drug Administration, Center for Biologics Evaluation and Research. U.S. Department of Health and Human Services. Donor Screening Recommendations to Reduce the Risk of Transmission of Zika Virus by Human Cells, Tissues, and Cellular and Tissue-Based Products. 2016; https://www.fda.gov/downloads/BiologicsBloodVaccines /Guidance ComplianceRegulatoryInformation/Guidances/Tissue/UCM488582.pdf. Accessed 01 January 2018.

29. Moomjy M, Mangieri R, Beltramone F, Cholst I, Veeck L, Rosenwaks Z. Shared oocyte donation: society's benefits. Fertil Steril. 2000;73:1165–9.
30. Shapiro BS, Andersen CY. Major drawbacks and additional benefits of agonist trigger – not ovarian hyperstimulation syndrome related. Fertil Steril. 2015Apr;103(4):874–8.
31. O'Neill KE, Senapati S, Maina I, Gracia C, Dokras A. GnRH agonist with low-dose hCG (dual trigger) is associated with higher risk of severe ovarian hyperstimulation syndrome compared to GnRH agonist alone. J Assist Reprod Genet. 2016;33(9):1175–84.
32. Society of Assisted Reproductive Technology (SART). SART National Summary Report. Preliminary Cumulative Report for donor eggs 2015. https://www.sartcorsonline.com/rptCSR_PublicMultYear.aspx#donor-fresh-egg. Accessed 18 January 2018.
33. Royal College of Obstetricians and Gynaecologists (RCOG). The Management of Ovarian Hyperstimulation Syndrome. Green-top Guideline No. 5. Third edition. 2016 Dec. www.rcog.org.uk/globalassets/documents/guidelines/green-top-guidelines/gtg_5_ohss.pdf. Accessed 04.12.2017.
34. Flood JT, Muasher SJ, Simonetti S, Kreiner D, Acosta AA, Rosenwaks Z. Comparison between laparoscopically and ultrasonographically guided transvaginal follicular aspiration methods in an in vitro fertilization program in the same patients using the same stimulation protocol. J In Vitro Fert Embryo Transf. 1989;3:180–5.
35. Kenney N, McGowan M. Looking back: egg donors' retrospective evaluations of their motivations, expectations, and experiences during their first donation cycle. Fertil Steril. 2010;93(2):455–66.
36. Caligara C, Navarro J, Vargas G, Simón C, Pellicer A, Remohí J. The effect of repeated controlled ovarian stimulation in donors. Hum Reprod. 2001;16(11):2320–3.
37. Tarlatzi TB, Imbert R, Alvaro Mercadal B, Demeestere I, Venetis CA, Englert Y, Delbaere A. Does oocyte donation compared with autologous oocyte IVF pregnancies have a higher risk of preeclampsia? Reprod Biomed Online. 2017;34(1):11–8.
38. Mascarenhas M, Sunkara SK, Antonisamy B, Kamath MS. Higher risk of preterm birth and low birth weight following oocyte donation: a systematic review and meta-analysis. Eur J Obstet Gynecol Reprod Biol. 2017;218:60–7.
39. Gunning J. Oocyte donation: the legislative framework in Western Europe. Hum Reprod. 1998;13(2):98–102.
40. http://www.isciii.es/ISCIII/es/contenidos/fdinvestigacion/SpanishLawonBiomedical ResearchEnglish.pdf. Accessed 04 December 2017.
41. HFEA ACT 2008. http://www.legislation.gov.uk/ukpga /2008/22/pdfs/ukpga _20080022 _en.pdf. Accessed 04 December 2017.
42. Leon G, Papetta A, Spiliopoulou C. Overview of the Greek legislation regarding assisted reproduction and comparison with the EU legal framework. Reprod Biomed Online. 2011;23(7):820–3.
43. Hibino Y, Shimazono Y. Impact of egg donation deliveries from domestic and overseas sources on maternal care: a questionnaire survey of Japanese perinatal physicians. Environ Health Prev Med. 2014;19(4):271–8.
44. Human Fertilisation and Embryology Authority. Disclosure of Donor Information Regulations (2004) Statutory Instrument 2004, No. 1511. London: Stationery Office; 2004.
45. Shalev C, Werner-Felmayer G. Patterns of globalized reproduction: egg cells regulation in Israel and Austria. Isr J Health Policy Res. 2012;1:15.
46. Egg donor compensation. https://www.growinggenerations.com/egg-donor-program/egg-donors/egg-donor-pay/. Accessed 16 January 2008.
47. Lee MS, Farland LV, Missmer SA, Ginsburg ES. Limitations on the compensation of gamete donors: a public opinion survey. Fertil Steril. 2017;107(6):1355–63.
48. Klitzman R, Sauer M. Payment of egg donors in stem cell research in the USA. Reprod Biomed Online. 2009;18(5):603–8.
49. Klein JU, Sauer MV. Ethics in egg donation: past, present, and future. Semin Reprod Med. 2010;28(4):322–8.
50. Almeling R. Gender and the value of bodily goods: commodification in egg and sperm donation. Law Contemp Probl. 2009;72(3):37–58.
51. Ahuja KK, Mostyn BJ, Simons EG. Egg sharing and egg donation: attitudes of British egg donors and recipients. Hum Reprod. 1997;12:2845–52.
52. Soderstrom-Anttila V. Follow-up study of Finnish volunteer oocyte donors concerning their attitudes to oocyte donation. Hum Reprod. 1995;10:3073–6.
53. Klock SC, Braverman AM, Rausch DT. Predicting anonymous egg donor satisfaction: a preliminary study. J Womens Health. 1998;7:229–37.
54. Schover LR, Collins RL, Quigley MM, Blankstein J, Kanoti G. Psychological follow-up of women evaluated as oocyte donors. Hum Reprod. 1991;6:1487–91.
55. Khamsi F, Endman MW, Lacanna IC, Wong J. Some psychological aspects of oocyte donation from known donors on altruistic basis. Fertil Steril. 1997;68:323–7.
56. Lim KS, Chae SJ, Choo CW, Ku YH, Lee HJ, Hur CY, Lim JH, Lee WD. In vitro maturation: clinical applications. Clin Exp Reprod Med. 2013;40(4):143–7.
57. Yamada M, Johannesson B, Sagi I, Burnett L, Kort DH, Prosser R, et al. Human oocytes reprogram adult somatic nuclei of a type 1 diabetic to diploid pluripotent stem cells. Nature. 2014;510:533–6.
58. Human Fertilisation and Embryology Authority (HFEA). HFEA statement on mitochondrial donation.2017. https://www.hfea.gov.uk/about-us/news-and-press-releases/2017-news-and-press-releases/hfea-statement-on-mitochondrial-donation/. Accessed 04 December 2017.
59. Richardson J, Irving L, Hyslop LA, Choudhary M, Murdoch A, Turnbull DM, Herbert M. Concise reviews: assisted reproductive technologies to prevent transmission of mitochondrial DNA disease. Stem Cells. 2015;33(3):639–45.
60. Blázquez A, Vassena R, Rodríguez A, Figueras F, Vernaeve V. Characteristics and clinical outcomes of patients undergoing fertility treatment by double gamete donation. Hum Fertil. 2016;19(3):180–5.

52 Sperm Donation

George Koustas, Peter Larsen, Corey Burke, and Lone Bruhn Madsen

52.1 History of Sperm Donation

The first documented application of a successful artificial insemination is from the 1790s, when the Scotsman Dr. John Hunter performed the first successful homologous insemination in humans using the semen of a husband with hypospadias.

Almost a century later, in 1884, Dr. William Pancoast, of the Jefferson Medical College in Philadelphia, decided to take an alternative approach with one of his patients, a woman who for a long time had been unable to conceive. After numerous examinations, Dr. Pancoast concluded that the fault lay with the low sperm count of her husband. Instead of informing the woman and her husband about the fact that the husband had a low sperm count, Dr. Pancoast summoned the woman to a final "examination." When the woman lay unconscious and chloroformed, the doctor injected into her cervix a syringe full of semen. The semen was freshly donated by one of his medical students. Nine months later the woman gave birth to a healthy boy. Dr. Pancoast never informed the woman what happened to her in the "clinic" that fateful day. It was not until 1909, after the death of Dr. Pancoast, that the truth of the successful donor insemination (DI) became known. At that point one of the students, Dr. Addison Davis Hard, present at the day of insemination, published a letter in the journal *Medical World* containing all the details, and hence, this was the first report of a successful insemination using donor semen.

Starting from this first DI case, several procedures went on to be performed, but they were kept private, and all records were destroyed for privacy reasons. However, it was accepted that sperm donors were used on a regular basis to inseminate women that required semen for fertilization.

In 1953, Dr. Jerome K. Sherman, an American pioneer in sperm freezing, introduced a simple method whereby human sperm could be preserved using glycerol and slow cooling and subsequently freezing in solid carbon dioxide. Moreover, he showed that frozen human sperm, when thawed, could fertilize a human egg and induce normal development. Thus, the first successful human pregnancy with frozen sperm was reported in 1953 [1]. The procedure was debated for several years, and it was considered adultery by many people (and was declared illegal).

However, in 1964, DI was acknowledged in the US state of Georgia, and later it became legal in the entire USA, provided both intended parents gave their written consent. Until 1977, it was estimated that at least 1000 children were born in the USA using frozen sperm [2]. The number of children who have been born today as a result of sperm donation is unknown, but it is probably many hundreds of thousands. Today, many fertility clinics use sperm from central donor sperm banks (see Fig. 52.1), most of which are located in

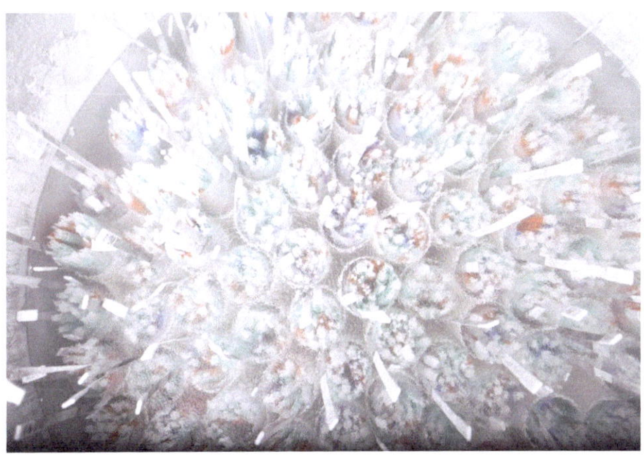

Fig. 52.1 Frozen sperm stored at Cryos International Sperm Bank in liquid nitrogen

G. Koustas
The Agora Clinic, Hove, UK

P. Larsen · L. B. Madsen (✉)
Cryos International, Aarhus, Denmark
e-mail: lbm@cryosinternational.com

C. Burke
Cryos International USA, Orlando, FL, USA

G. N. Allahbadia et al. (eds.), *Textbook of Assisted Reproduction*, https://doi.org/10.1007/978-981-15-2377-9_52

Europe and North America. However, some fertility clinics also use semen donated from their own local donors.

52.2 Regulation of Sperm Donation

The legality and regulation of sperm donation worldwide ranges from no regulation whatsoever to being illegal in some countries. Laws regarding sperm donation generally involve defining donor/recipient rights and obligations, reimbursement, the number of offspring allowed per donor, screening, and donor anonymity.

Donors in most countries are absolved of all parental rights and obligations. However, in many countries donations must be made through sperm banks or fertility clinics to protect donors from these obligations.

The use of the term "sperm donor" implies to many that the donation is an altruistic act. However, most countries allow some amount of payment to donors. In such countries, donor reimbursement is usually defined by law. However, certain countries, such as Italy and France, only allow sperm donation as a voluntary act with no reimbursement, whereas donors in the USA can receive as much as $150 per ejaculate. An alternative approach, as used in the UK, is to allow the donor to be compensated for expenses (e.g., for travel) related to the donation [3].

To minimize the risk of consanguinity, the number of children allowed from a single sperm donor is limited by law in many countries. The number permitted is usually determined by the population of the country in which the sperm is used. Limiting the number of offspring is one of the more difficult challenges faced by sperm banks because there is no universal limit to the number of offspring allowed in the various countries. The USA and Canada have no regulations regarding the number of offspring per donor, and most sperm banks are left to follow guidelines set by the American Society for Reproductive Medicine (ASRM) which recommends a limit of 25 births per population of 850,000 [4]. Other countries, including the UK, Denmark, Germany, Spain, and New Zealand, have a set numbers of offspring that are allowed for each donor, ranging from as few as 6 to as many as 15 [5]. Australia has limits that vary according to the state.

52.3 Sperm Donor Anonymity Versus Non-anonymity

There are two main types of sperm donors: anonymous and non-anonymous. Anonymous sperm donation refers to right of the privacy of anonymity of the donor to the recipient and donor offspring. Recipients select their donor based on non-identifiable information such as physical characteristics, nationality, intelligence, academic achievements, and professional background. Countries such as China, Spain, France, and Greece mostly allow anonymous donation.

Due to an increasing weight to the child's right to know his/her genetic origins under the principle of personal autonomy, there has, over the recent years, been a strong tendency toward non-anonymous open-identity donation. This permits the sperm donor offspring to access the identity of their donor when they reach a certain age, normally 18 years. Following Sweden in 1985, numerous other countries have removed donor anonymity, even though most of the countries did not remove donor anonymity until between 2008 and 2018. A few countries, such as Denmark, allow both anonymous and non-anonymous sperm donation. Table 52.1 lists the status of different countries, regarding donor anonymity, and if the marital status and sexual orientation of a recipient allows her to use donor sperm in a given country.

International studies report that most parents prefer to disclose the nature of conception as early as possible, with homosexual women appearing to be even more positive to disclose, compared to heterosexual couples [6]. Some parents have concerns about informing their children of their biological origin, thinking that it might have a harmful social or psychological effect, or lead to the child rejecting their nonbiological parents. Additionally, some parents may wish not to reveal their male infertility, especially in cultures where sperm donation and assisted conception are not accepted. However, reports indicate that there is no negative impact in the psychological well-being of donor-conceived offspring at the ages of 6, 8, and 12 years, nor on the mental

Table 52.1 Donor anonymity and recipients allowed to use sperm donation in various countries

Donor anonymity	Country	Allowed recipients
Anonymous	France	Heterosexual couples
	China	
	Spain	Single women, homosexual and heterosexual couples
	Greece	
	Belgium	
Non-anonymous	Switzerland	Heterosexual couples
	Germany	Usually heterosexual couples
	The Netherlands	Single women, homosexual and heterosexual couples
	Australia	
	New Zealand	
	UK	
	Sweden	
	Finland	
	Portugal	
Both non-anonymous and anonymous	Denmark	
	USA	

Please note, this information is correct at the time of writing development and parent-child relationships, compared with naturally conceived children [7–12]. Studies also reveal that most sperm donors strongly believe that parents should disclose the use of gamete donation to offspring [13].

A study published in 2014 comparing motivations and attitudes among Danish sperm donors over three decades revealed that the proportion of anonymous donors who would stop their donations if anonymity was abolished was 51% (in 1992), 56% (in 2002), and 67% (in 2012). However, the difference between the various years was not statistically significant [14]. Additionally, it was revealed that 15–22% of the anonymous donors would accept contact from the offspring if anonymity was abolished [14, 15]. In another study investigating an American sample cohort of anonymous donors, 86% of the donors were positive about the prospect of being contacted by their offspring [16]. These differences could potentially be explained by demographic differences and differences in the sample cohort.

Historically, there have been numerous attempts from donor-conceived offspring to access their sperm donor identity. Mahlstedt et al. [17] reported that 25% of sperm donor-conceived offspring wished to request their donors' identities, 36% wished to create a contact, and 26% wished to create a relationship [17]. Specifically, motivations include simple curiosity, investigation of medical risks and consanguineous relationships, and to learn more about the sperm donor [18]. Interestingly, recent data show that compared to egg donors, sperm donors answered more positively for potential involvement with their donor-conceived offspring, perhaps indicating that sperm donors consider the genetic link between parent and child more than egg donors [19]. These interesting findings may indicate the desire of sperm donors to share their "good" genes and wish to procreate [19, 20]. In addition, age is a critical factor, as older sperm donors with children were more positive compared to younger donors (30% vs 9%) [21, 22]. Furthermore, in contrast to heterosexual sperm donors, gay and bisexual donors were more open to being contacted by their offspring, indicating that sexual orientation has an impact [23].

While most studies report positive attitudes toward an offspring's right to information either identifying or non-identifying, little attention has been paid to the donor and donor-offspring potential interaction. Of the scarce current studies published, these tend to highlight an urgent need for donor pre- and post-donation counseling in order to avoid negative long-term consequences in the donors' lives and families [13, 24–26]. Some studies also report that the presence of the donor in the life of the offspring could be a threat to the parents [27].

Moreover, nowadays it is also important to be aware that anonymity cannot be completely guaranteed. Anonymous donors could potentially be traced if their DNA or even the DNA of a relative to the donor is included in a database, which subsequently can be used for genealogy purposes [28].

52.4 Selection and Screening of Sperm Donors

The procedures for selection of sperm donors vary greatly among individual sperm banks. Most banks initially select sperm donors based on a number of parameters, including screening for infectious diseases, genetic screening, and sperm quality. There then follows screening for other traits such as personality, 3–4 generation family history, and age.

52.4.1 Regulations for Screening

In addition to donor/recipient protections, most countries that allow sperm donation also have regulations directed toward health and safety of the sperm. One of the largest regulatory agencies is the Food and Drug Administration (FDA) in the USA.

In 2005, the FDA issued a regulation entitled "21 CFR 1271—Human Cells, Tissues, and Cellular and Tissue-Based Products," a set of federal regulations governing human cells, tissue, and tissue-based products. 21 CFR 1271 contained much broader tissue regulation than previous regulations and included reproductive cells [29]. The focus was to ensure the safety of tissue products against the possible spread of infectious disease. The regulations contain specific requirements for screening donors of all tissues, with many specific requirements for sperm donors. The regulations include the registration of all facilities involved in the collecting, processing, labeling, storage, shipping, and use of donor sperm. Registered facilities are subject to regular inspection by the FDA or the national health authorities in the country where the sperm bank is located.

52.4.2 Screening for Infectious Diseases

Screening of donors under both 21 CFR 1271 and European Union (EU) legislation consists of evaluating donors for risk factors associated with an increased chance of acquiring an infectious disease. This involves a review of relevant medical records and by physical examination of the donor.

Donor interviews then look at family medical history, social behavior, and past medical conditions that may indicate if the donor is at increased risk for a relevant communicable infection. All tissue donors must be screened for HIV I and II, hepatitis B, hepatitis C, syphilis (*Treponema pallidum*), chlamydia (*Chlamydia trachomatis*), and gonorrhea (*Neisseria gonorrhoeae*). Additionally, sperm donors must also be screened for human T-lymphotropic virus (HTLV) types I and II and in many countries also for cytomegalovirus (CMV).

52.4.3 Genetic Screening

Genetic screening of potential sperm donors is a standard component of donor eligibility practiced by most sperm banks, although the level of genetic screening varies. A distinguishing feature of screening compared with diagnostic testing is that screening is usually offered to individuals without any signs or symptoms of a specific health issue and without a priori increased risk.

Screening programs have to meet certain criteria. In many countries, the Wilson and Jungner criteria continue to be the applied standard, although with some adjustments for genetics [30].

The opportunity to minimize the future child's risk of disease is emphasized by most sperm banks, and the screening for inherited diseases will, for many sperm banks, be initiated by a three-generation family history analysis. In the EU, the EU Tissue and Cells Directives must be adhered to [31–33] and further administered in the various member states. This means that potential sperm donor candidates in many countries are assessed using the following criteria:

- Occurrence of severe autosomal dominant or X-linked recessive diseases among first- to third-degree relatives of the potential donor, or in the donor himself
- Occurrence of serious autosomal recessive diseases among first-grade relatives, the potential donor, or the donor himself
- Occurrence of major malformations among first-degree relatives of (including any children of) the potential donor, or in the donor himself
- Prevalence of developmental impairment where the cause is unknown among first- and second-degree relatives to the potential donor
- Occurrence of severe polygenetic or multifactorial disease among first- and second-degree relatives of the potential donor

As a part of a genetic screening program, the majority of commercial sperm banks conduct karyotyping on the sperm donors to ensure that accepted donors have a normal 46,XY karyotype.

Moreover, the sperm donors of most sperm banks are subjected to a carrier screening panel for a certain number of recessively inherited diseases. The number of genes included in the panel varies greatly among sperm banks. Donor candidates who test positive for a pathological mutation are typically rejected.

So far, carrier screening has been conducted for relatively (few) frequent recessive disorders associated with significant morbidity and decreased life expectancy. One example is the screening for cystic fibrosis (CF) which is offered in a variety of countries including the USA, Denmark, and Australia. Another example is beta-thalassemia which has traditionally been offered in countries such as Cyprus, Israel, and Turkey, but also for donors who donate in international sperm banks.

Further screening panels exist for specific disorders which are known to be more frequent in specific communities, such as individuals with an Ashkenazi Jewish background. The disadvantage of ancestry-based screening is that diseases are not limited to specific groups and it is not possible to define who is at risk because of multiethnic backgrounds [34]. There is also increasing evidence that many of the so-called ethnic diseases range past the boundaries of specific ethnic groups [35]. This has, therefore, led to some sperm banks conducting carrier screening using a pan-ethnic approach. This means that all donors who are eligible to donate are screened for all recessive diseases included in the panel at the time of acceptance to become a sperm donor. An expanded carrier screening is carried out, which inevitably leads to the rejection of more donors as more genes are included in the test panels.

Several experimental approaches have led to the same conclusion: every human is a carrier of multiple disease-causing mutations [36–38]. These studies indicate that the real complexity of human reproduction, regardless of the usage of sperm donor, is not just reflected in the standard of care. Since every individual is a carrier of 3–5 recessive diseases, it might be an outdated protocol to reject donors who are carrier positive for a clinically characterized variant without also testing the recipient. This might also lead to a wrong belief among recipients that donors who are included in a donor program are "mutation-free" [39].

One way to achieve the screening goal of protecting future children from a large number of highly heritable diseases is to reflect the genetic reality in the screening approach so that both the donor and recipient are screened for a large number of recessive diseases. This approach is called "matching" and will probably become more utilized in relation to the usage of donated sperm in the future.

52.4.4 Sperm Quality and the Analysis of Sperm

During the selection process of being accepted into a sperm donation program, a semen quality assessment must be performed. Accepted donors must have very good sperm quality.

For potential donors, one or more ejaculates are evaluated for sperm quality, most often after a 2–5 days' abstinence

Table 52.2 The minimum criteria for "normal" semen quality according to the World Health Organization (2010) guidance

Parameter	Lower reference limit
Semen volume (ml)	1.5 (1.4–1.7)
Total sperm number (million per ejaculate)	39 (33–46)
Sperm concentration (million per ml)	15 (12–16)
Total motility (progressive + non-progressive, %)	40 (38–42)
Progressive motility (progressive, %)	32 (31–34)
Vitality (live spermatozoa, %)	58 (55–63)
Sperm morphology (normal forms, %)	4 (3.0–4.0)

Note the reference limits are for the lower level of "normality"

interval. The sample should be examined after liquefaction not more than 1 h after ejaculation to minimize the time the sperm are exposed to seminal plasma. The liquefaction process usually takes less than 15 min but can take up to an hour [40].

There are no uniformly accepted standards for selecting donors based on sperm quality, but the minimum criteria for normal semen quality according to the World Health Organization (WHO) can be applied [40] (Table 52.2).

All ejaculates donated to a sperm bank undergo processing (e.g., gradient centrifugation, washing and addition of cryoprotectants, cryopreservation, test thawing) which will inevitably lead to a loss of motile sperm. This means that the sperm quality of donor samples must be very good, if the end product is to meet the requirements by the recipient and be suitable for artificial insemination.

At fertility clinics, a semen analysis is typically performed on patients for diagnostic purposes, to collect information so that an appropriate fertility treatment can be chosen. This means that the sperm analysis is very comprehensive and includes several macroscopic and microscopic examination steps.

- The macroscopic examination usually consists of assessing volume, pH, appearance, liquefaction, and viscosity.
- The microscopic examination consists of assessing sperm, concentration, motility, morphology, vitality, aggregation, and agglutination. Additionally, testing for antibody coating of sperm and interaction assays between sperm and cervical mucus may be performed. Some clinics also perform DNA integrity tests such as sperm chromatin structure assay (SCSA) [41].

At sperm banks, the semen analysis is less comprehensive, as the donors are healthy young men with no history of infertility. Here, the semen analysis is not used as a diagnostic tool, but rather as a way to determine the quality of the sample. Volume, motility, and concentration are the main parameters assessed in all sperm banks. Morphology is also often a part of the semen analysis, at least in the initial evaluation process.

In 2011, Ping et al. demonstrated the acceptance criteria for Chinese sperm banks related to semen parameters. This group stated that fresh donor semen is required to have a liquefaction time <60 min, sperm concentration ≥60 million per ml, motility (rapid and slow progressive sperm) ≥60%, normal morphology >30%, post-thaw sperm motility ≥40%, number of motile sperm per vial ≥12 million, and frozen-thaw survival rate ≥60%. The study also demonstrated that inadequate semen parameters were the most common rejection rate (55%) [42].

In 2014, Thijssen et al. [43] reported a substantial difference in acceptance criteria between sperm banks in Belgium:

> The lower limit for native sperm concentration ranges from 15 up to 60 million spermatozoa per ml. Additionally, the threshold for good forward progressive motility has to be at least 30% in one centre and up to 70% in another centre. Minimum criteria for sperm morphology range from 4% to 25% morphologically normal spermatozoa.

The sperm bank Cryos International (Aarhus, Denmark), only accepts donors with a total number of progressive motile cells of at least 100 million per ml.

North American and European sperm banks typically offer a few different qualities. The quality of the available specimens is often defined as "MOT," meaning the concentration of motile sperm cells per ml. For example, a "MOT30" sample contains 30 million motile sperm cells per ml. Most sperm banks offer volumes of 0.5 ml in vials or straws.

The MOT quality is defined post-thaw, where an aliquot of the processed semen sample is thawed after freezing and then reanalyzed. During processing, including freezing and thawing, a loss of motility is unavoidable, meaning that a post-thaw motility assessment is important. This post-thaw motility assessment determines the quality of the commercially available specimen. The result of the analysis of the aliquot will therefore define the quality of the entire sample; hence, thorough mixing is essential.

Commonly different qualities are offered including unprocessed semen with the addition of cryoprotectant media for use in intracervical insemination (ICI) treatment, or density gradient centrifugated and washed sperm for use in intrauterine insemination (IUI) treatment. Some sperm banks offer lower MOT qualities for IVF or ICSI treatment. Large-scale sperm banks have developed factory-like settings to be able to analyze and process as many samples as possible throughout the day. A Makler Counting Chamber (Sefi-Medical Instruments, Haifa, Israel) is often used when manually assessing motility and concentration in a sperm bank. It is accepted that a Makler Counting Chamber may cause an overestimation of concentration and motility, but the use is very fast and simple, which is the main reason why it is used at many sperm banks and fertility clinics [44].

Some sperm banks are now using computer-assisted sperm analysis (CASA) [45], particularly if there are many

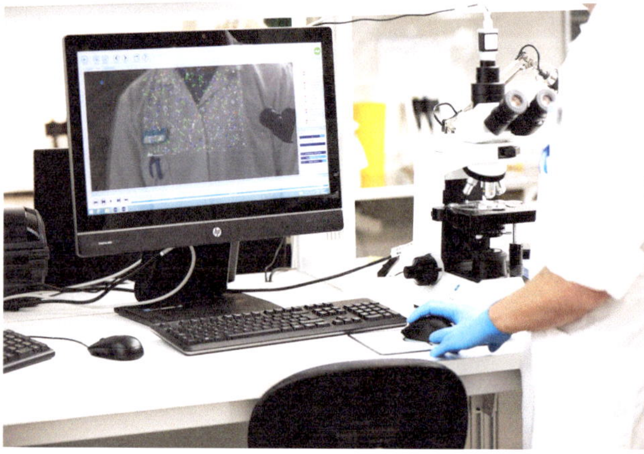

Fig. 52.2 Computer-assisted sperm analysis (CASA). Sperm quality may be analyzed using a CASA to minimize subjectivity among andrologists and enable standardization of the semen sample assessment

laboratory technologists and several collection sites. CASA can help to minimize subjectivity and intra- and interpersonal variation and enables standardization and documentation which is a part of ensuring the most optimal sperm samples for the use in ART procedures (Fig. 52.2).

52.5 Summary

The use of sperm donation is not new, and donor semen is today widely used to assist heterosexual couples to conceive in cases of severe male factor subfertility, as well as single women and lesbian couples where no male partner is present. Historically, sperm donation and conception have remained secretive. However, in recent years, there has been an increasing international trend supporting openness. In some countries, a recipient can choose between anonymous and non-anonymous donors, where the use of the latter ensures that the future child receives the possibility to know the identity of the sperm donor. In other countries, only the use of either anonymous or non-anonymous sperm donors is allowed.

The sperm donation process is usually regulated by law, which means that sperm donors are screened in order to decrease the risk for transferring infectious and genetic diseases. Testing for genetic diseases is an area with an increasing awareness, especially due to the growing knowledge and technical possibilities within genetic compatibility. Another key aspect of sperm donation is ensuring a high sperm quality, which means that ensuring highly motile sperm samples upon freeze-thawing is a key element in the processing of the sperm. Taken together, the various procedures within the sperm donation process will enable that the most optimal sperm samples are available for insemination or other assisted reproduction procedures.

References

1. Ombelet W, Van Robays J. Artificial insemination history: hurdles and milestones. Facts Views Vis Obgyn. 2015;7(2):137–43.
2. Jackson MC, Richardson DW. The use of fresh and frozen semen in human artificial insemination. J Biosoc Sci. 1977;9(2):251–62.
3. authority HFE. Donor compensation, reimbursement and benefits in kind 2017. Available from: http://www.hfea.gov.uk/6177.html
4. Practice Committee of the American Society for Reproductive Medicine; Practice Committee of the Society for Assisted Reproductive Technology. 2006 guidelines for gamete and embryo donation. Fertil Steril. 2006;86(5 Suppl 1):S38–50.
5. Limitations on the use of gametes (or embryos created using gametes) from an individual donor. HEFA Practice Guidance Note: Human Fertilisation and Embryology Authority; 2006.
6. Sawyer N, Blyth E, Kramer W, Frith L. A survey of 1700 women who formed their families using donor spermatozoa. Reprod Biomed Online. 2013;27(4):436–47.
7. Amuzu B, Laxova R, Shapiro SS. Pregnancy outcome, health of children, and family adjustment after donor insemination. Obstet Gynecol. 1990;75(6):899–905.
8. Golombok S. New families, old values: considerations regarding the welfare of the child. Hum Reprod. 1998;13(9):2342–7.
9. Jadva V, Freeman T, Kramer W, Golombok S. The experiences of adolescents and adults conceived by sperm donation: comparisons by age of disclosure and family type. Hum Reprod. 2009;24(8):1909–19.
10. Pennings G. Disclosure of donor conception, age of disclosure and the well-being of donor offspring. Hum Reprod. 2017;32(5):969–73.
11. Blake L, Jadva V, Golombok S. Parent psychological adjustment, donor conception and disclosure: a follow-up over 10 years. Hum Rep. 2014;29(11):2487–96.
12. Ilioi E, Blake L, Jadva V, Roman G, Golombok S. The role of age of disclosure of biological origins in the psychological wellbeing of adolescents conceived by reproductive donation: a longitudinal study from age 1 to age 14. J Child Psychol Psychiatry. 2017;58(3):315–24.
13. Hammarberg K, Johnson L, Bourne K, Fisher J, Kirkman M. Proposed legislative change mandating retrospective release of identifying information: consultation with donors and government response. Hum Reprod. 2014;29(2):286–92.
14. Bay B, Larsen PB, Kesmodel US, Ingerslev HJ. Danish sperm donors across three decades: motivations and attitudes. Fertil Steril. 2014;101(1):252–7.e1.
15. Ernst E, Ingerslev HJ, Schou O, Stoltenberg M. Attitudes among sperm donors in 1992 and 2002: a Danish questionnaire survey. Acta Obstet Gynecol Scand. 2007;86(3):327–33.
16. Jadva V, Freeman T, Kramer W, Golombok S. Sperm and oocyte donors' experiences of anonymous donation and subsequent contact with their donor offspring. Hum Reprod. 2011;26(3):638–45.
17. Mahlstedt PP, LaBounty K, Kennedy WT. The views of adult offspring of sperm donation: essential feedback for the development of ethical guidelines within the practice of assisted reproductive technology in the United States. Fertil Steril. 2010;93(7):2236–46.
18. Ravelingien A, Provoost V, Pennings G. Open-identity sperm donation: how does offering donor-identifying information relate to donor-conceived offspring's wishes and needs? J Bioeth Inq. 2015;12(3):503–9.
19. Svanberg AS, Lampic C, Gejervall AL, Gudmundsson J, Karlstrom PO, Solensten NG, et al. Gamete donors' motivation in a Swedish national sample: is there any ambivalence? A descriptive study. Acta Obstet Gynecol Scand. 2012;91(8):944–51.
20. Riggs DW, Russell L. Characteristics of men willing to act as sperm donors in the context of identity-release legislation. Hum Reprod. 2011;26(1):266–72.

21. Godman KM, Sanders K, Rosenberg M, Burton P. Potential sperm donors', recipients' and their partners' opinions towards the release of identifying information in Western Australia. Hum Reprod. 2006;21(11):3022–6.
22. Daniels KR, Kramer W, Perez-y-Perez MV. Semen donors who are open to contact with their offspring: issues and implications for them and their families. Reprod Biomed Online. 2012;25(7):670–7.
23. Freeman T, Jadva V, Tranfield E, Golombok S. Online sperm donation: a survey of the demographic characteristics, motivations, preferences and experiences of sperm donors on a connection website. Hum Reprod. 2016;31(9):2082–9.
24. Kirkman M, Bourne K, Fisher J, Johnson L, Hammarberg K. Gamete donors' expectations and experiences of contact with their donor offspring. Hum Reprod. 2014;29(4):731–8.
25. Isaksson S, Skoog-Svanberg A, Sydsjo G, Linell L, Lampic C. It takes two to tango: information-sharing with offspring among heterosexual parents following identity-release sperm donation. Hum Reprod. 2016;31(1):125–32.
26. Isaksson S, Sydsjo G, Skoog Svanberg A, Lampic C. Preferences and needs regarding future contact with donation offspring among identity-release gamete donors: results from the Swedish study on gamete donation. Fertil Steril. 2014;102(4):1160–6.
27. Hertz R, Nelson MK, Kramer W. Sperm donors describe the experience of contact with their donor-conceived offspring. Facts Views Vis ObGyn. 2015;7(2):91–100.
28. Harper JC, Kennett D, Reisel D. The end of donor anonymity: how genetic testing is likely to drive anonymous gamete donation out of business. Hum Reprod. 2016;31(6):1135–40.
29. CFR Title 21 Part 1271 -Human Cells, Tissue, and Cellular and Tissue Based Products (2005).
30. Andermann A, Blancquaert I, Beauchamp S, Dery V. Revisiting Wilson and Jungner in the genomic age: a review of screening criteria over the past 40 years. Bull World Health Org. 2008;86(4):317–9.
31. European Directive 2004/23/DC, (2004).
32. European Directive 2006/17/EC, (2006).
33. European Directive 2006–86-EC, (2006).
34. Edwards JG, Feldman G, Goldberg J, Gregg AR, Norton ME, Rose NC, et al. Expanded carrier screening in reproductive medicine-points to consider: a joint statement of the American College of Medical Genetics and Genomics, American College of Obstetricians and Gynecologists, National Society of Genetic Counselors, Perinatal Quality Foundation, and Society for Maternal-Fetal Medicine. Obstet Gynecol. 2015;125(3):653–62.
35. Lazarin GA, Haque IS, Nazareth S, Iori K, Patterson AS, Jacobson JL, et al. An empirical estimate of carrier frequencies for 400+ causal Mendelian variants: results from an ethnically diverse clinical sample of 23,453 individuals. Genet Med. 2013;15(3):178–86.
36. Bell CJ, Dinwiddie DL, Miller NA, Hateley SL, Ganusova EE, Mudge J, et al. Carrier testing for severe childhood recessive diseases by next-generation sequencing. Sci Transl Med. 2011;3(65):65ra4.
37. Xue Y, Chen Y, Ayub Q, Huang N, Ball EV, Mort M, et al. Deleterious- and disease-allele prevalence in healthy individuals: insights from current predictions, mutation databases, and population-scale resequencing. Am J Hum Genet. 2012;91(6):1022–32.
38. Henn BM, Botigue LR, Bustamante CD, Clark AG, Gravel S. Estimating the mutation load in human genomes. Nat Rev Genet. 2015;16(6):333–43.
39. Callum P, Iger J, Ray M, Sims CA, Falk RE. Outcome and experience of implementing spinal muscular atrophy carrier screening on sperm donors. Fertil Steril. 2010;94(5):1912–4.
40. World Health Organization DoRHaR. WHO laboratory manual for the examination and processing of human semen. 5th ed. Geneva: WHO Press; 2010. p. 287.
41. Bungum M, Bungum L, Giwercman A. Sperm chromatin structure assay (SCSA): a tool in diagnosis and treatment of infertility. Asian J Androl. 2011;13(1):69–75.
42. Ping P, Zhu WB, Zhang XZ, Li YS, Wang QX, Cao XR, et al. Sperm donation and its application in China: a 7-year multicenter retrospective study. Asian J Androl. 2011;13(4):644–8.
43. Thijssen A, Dhont N, Vandormael E, Cox A, Klerkx E, Creemers E, Ombelet W. Artificial insemination with donor sperm (AID): heterogeneity in sperm banking facilities in a single country (Belgium). Facts Views Vis Obgyn. 2014;6(2):57–67.
44. Peng N, Zou X, Li L. Comparison of different counting chambers using a computer-assisted semen analyzer. Syst Biol Reprod Med. 2015;61(5):307–13.
45. Dearing CG, Kilburn S, Lindsay KS. Validation of the sperm class analyser CASA system for sperm counting in a busy diagnostic semen analysis laboratory. Hum Fertil (Camb). 2014;17(1):37–44.

53 Embryo Donation

Jody Lyneé Madeira

Since embryo cryopreservation emerged as a viable technology in the early 1980s, it has simultaneously improved medically assisted reproduction (MAR) treatment by improving cumulative pregnancy rates and facilitating elective single embryo transfer [1]. But with these advances have come new, potentially difficult decisions. While couples now routinely preserve surplus embryos, they also need to choose a disposition for those remaining after their families are complete or in the event that they or their spouses die or divorce. Given that fresh embryos are used in over 80% of IVF cycles, patients frequently have surplus embryos [2].

While choosing embryo dispositions can be difficult for couples, it also presents challenges for social policy and legal regulation. Certain disposition options, like discarding embryos or donating them to stem cell research, have generated extensive debate and controversy. Moreover, there is the question of what to do about the large number of "abandoned" embryos, which according to recent estimates is over 1 million in the USA alone [3]. For clinics and storage facilities, cryopreserving large numbers of embryos is "expensive and time-consuming" and has been described as an "ethical and practical problem" [4]. Although some countries have enacted legislative limits on how long embryos can be stored, the USA has no such regulatory scheme; instead, facilities discourage long-term storage by raising fees [5]. Thus, patients might feel pressure to choose a disposition option when they no longer want to pay cryostorage fees, which they often name as a decisional influence [5].

For most patients, the major disposition options include using embryos for personal reproductive use, donating them for scientific research or embryologist training, donating them to another couple for reproductive use, discarding or destroying them, or keeping them cryopreserved [2]. Other less common options include compassionate transfer into a woman's uterus when she is unlikely to become pregnant (preferred by a "significant minority" of patients according to Lyerly et al. [2]) and a disposal ceremony. Lyerly et al. reported that these last alternatives are offered at fewer than 5% of American fertility clinics [2].

The process of choosing a disposition option is made more complex by the fact that patients' attitudes toward their embryos change over the course of their treatment experiences. Patients may initially regard cryopreserved embryos as conceptive resources, a means to the end of a healthy baby [6]. Embryos might seem like an "insurance policy," to preserve fertility or as a safeguard lest anything happen to existing children [7]. Later, they may view them very differently, especially if their cryopreserved embryos are effectively the siblings of their existing children [5, 8]. Patients might even feel more attached to their embryos after they receive a picture of their embryos before transfer [6, 9]. At any point, they may feel quasi-parental feelings of responsibility or "an obligation to protect the welfare and the interests of the potential offspring" [6, 9].

Though patients likely affirm and implement their chosen dispositions years or even decades after undergoing their first IVF cycle, these decisions about what should happen to surplus embryos in the event of death, divorce, nonpayment, and loss of contact should be made prior to their first IVF cycle to adequately protect their legal interests as well as those of the clinic. Surprisingly, however, Lyerly et al. reported that patients are "often" not asked about their preferences prior to freezing, but only upon donation or disposal [2]. Furthermore, giving patients only one meaningful opportunity to select a disposition decision does not accord with best practices [2].

This essay will review how patients choose disposition decisions, why these decisions are difficult, and what happens when they break down. It first explores factors affecting which dispositions patients elect and the reasons why certain options are more popular or controversial. This essay then describes why the disposition decision can be difficult and

J. L. Madeira (✉)
Center for Law, Society and Culture, Indiana University Bloomington, Bloomington, IN, USA
e-mail: jmadeira@indiana.edu

G. N. Allahbadia et al. (eds.), *Textbook of Assisted Reproduction*, https://doi.org/10.1007/978-981-15-2377-9_53

interrogates the growing problem of abandoned embryos. Finally, it discusses potential solutions that might improve the ease and quality of patients' disposition decisions.

53.1 How Patients Choose Dispositions

Patients evaluate embryo disposition options according to their availability and acceptability and prioritize finding a meaningful and respectful disposition [2]. Several factors influence disposition decisions, including demographics, family and personal issues, perceptions of embryos' moral status (as human or nonhuman), perceived responsibility toward their embryos, perceived responsibility toward society, the adequacy of disposition information, the acceptability of options, and trust in medical professionals [10]. For instance, Lyerly et al. found that patients who had no children or few children or who attribute high moral status to embryos were more likely to use or store them for future reproduction, but patients whose embryos had been cryopreserved for over 5 years, who believed embryos had low moral status, and who were highly concerned about the welfare of their embryo, future fetus, or child were more likely to discard them or store them indefinitely [2].

In choosing an embryo disposition, patients often first determine their ideal family size; those who want additional children usually keep their embryos for their own reproductive use. Family size is in turn dependent on patients' age, finances, and health, although cryopreserved embryos make age less determinative, since they might function as a "security blanket" [10]. Patients might not be willing to allocate financial resources toward frozen embryo transfers, or they could be cautious about how future cycles would affect their health. If patients are uncertain about their family size or are certain they will not use their embryos, they face more difficult disposition choices.

Disposition choices often depend on how much trust patients repose in medical professionals. Trust might be more influential for some disposition decisions, like donation to research, than others, like disposal. Patients may be reluctant to donate embryos to research if they lack confidence in medicine; they might fear that professionals would misuse the embryos or allow them to develop into children [11]. Conversely, those who do donate their embryos to research describe positive treatment experiences and trusting treatment relationships [5]. Diminished trust may be linked to inadequate information. Patients who thought they lacked information about certain options often could be dissuaded from donating embryos to research by "generalized fears about science" like "embryo misplacement, disposal, or use in the creation of chimeras, for eugenic purposes, or having embryos 'grown into babies'" [5]. Although Samorinha et al. found that patients likely receive more information about donation to research than other options, they still might lack details about particular research objectives [12].

Patients' disposition decisions might also be influenced by whether they accord embryos' moral or human status; this status might merit special protective efforts like ensuring embryos are gestated or, alternatively, prevented from developing further [13, 14]. Couples might liken the disposition decision to other reproductive choices like adoption, pregnancy termination, and tissue donation; couples electing donation to research over disposal might feel their choice is more like donating tissue than terminating a pregnancy, but those who discard their embryos could feel they were protecting potential children from being adopted or given away [14]. Religious beliefs might either intensify or alleviate decisional conflict, dictating particular dispositions (like gestating each embryo) or ruling out others [11]. Feelings that embryos have a symbolic meaning, like being representative of a couple's relationship, can also influence disposition choices [6].

Research suggests that patients' viewpoints on embryos' moral status is usually less important than the patients' feelings of responsibility toward the embryos [10, 15]. Patients who are genetically related to their embryos might feel a procreative responsibility that manifests as concern for the welfare of the embryo or potential child, eliciting fears that potential children could be raised by strangers and subject to unknown dangers [10]. This genetic relationship is so important that comparatively few couples are willing to consider donating their surplus embryos to others for reproductive use; according to one Australian study, only 22% of couples were even willing to consider it, and only 4% considered themselves likely to donate their embryos [16]. Patients might be more willing to donate embryos created with donor oocytes [17].

Donating embryos to research is a popular option for patients who want their embryos to be of use to others but who do not want others to raise the children they might become. These individuals may feel responsible toward and protective of their embryos, yet also feel an altruistic obligation to give back to society through their embryo disposition. They might feel their embryos have a "high instrumental value," and regard destruction as wasteful [11, 14]. Donation to research, then, allows patients to both protect embryos and use them for social good, illustrating how embryos can be "simultaneously … epistemic or medical objects for research and clinical practices, and ontological objects for reproduction, with an instrumental value that should not be wasted" [12]. Patients who elect this disposition are likely optimistic that it involves minimal risk and can improve MAR techniques, public health, and/or clinical treatment of disease [12]. According to Samorinha et al., patients were more likely to donate their embryos to research if they were older than 40 years, had higher levels of education, and were

Caucasian; they were less likely to donate to research if they believed their embryos were life or a potential child, had high moral status, or symbolized the couples' relationship [12]. But Deniz et al. found that some patients felt they lacked sufficient information on this option and were unaware of "how research initiatives were chosen and the amount of the information on the study they would receive"—potential barriers to choosing donation to research [18].

The least popular disposition option is donation to another couple or individual for reproductive use; Lyerly et al. found that only 7% of patients stated that they were very likely to choose this option, while 59% indicated they were very unlikely to choose it [2]. Some countries ban donation to another couple outright because of its many "emotional, ethical, legal and psychosocial aspects" [19]. It is permitted in countries such as Australia, Belgium, Brazil, Canada, Finland, France, the Netherlands, Portugal, Russia, Spain, the UK, and some states in the USA [19]. Even in countries that do permit it, regulations differ substantially, and "few clinicians ... have clear guidelines for the procedure" [19]. In the USA, the ASRM has promulgated professional guidelines for embryo donation that require counseling for both donors and recipients and prohibit compensation for embryo donors, and embryo donors usually do not know of their donated embryos' outcomes [20].

Finally, embryo destruction is often regarded as unattractive, often because of an altruistic desire to "give back to society and to help others" [2]. But it might seem an appropriate disposition option for low-quality embryos, or might be the best option for parents who do not want their embryos used for research or donated to another couple for reproductive use. Again, a lack of knowledge about the procedures for ethical disposal might discourage patients from choosing this option [18].

53.2 Difficulty Selecting a Disposition and the Problem of Abandoned Embryos

Numerous researchers have found that patients often have difficulty choosing a disposition decision [10, 11, 21] although few couples disagree [1], particularly because life circumstances and perceptions of embryos change across the treatment journey. Nonetheless, selecting a disposition might feel less like an ideal outcome and more like the "least uncomfortable alternative" [6, 14].

Since most patients initially choose a disposition before undergoing MAR, they might not know whether they will have any embryos to freeze and are certainly not anticipating that they will die or divorce. Patients might feel unprepared to choose a disposition if they lack information about cryopreservation before IVF or feel overwhelmed by what information they have received [10]. Or they might be focused on their procreative chances at that time and unlikely to consider disposition options other than their own reproductive use. Once patients have begun treatment, they might view their embryos differently, particularly after they have more information about embryo numbers and quality, after children are born, or after certain embryo "batches" proved successful or unsuccessful [10]. Nachtigall et al. found that patients were very interested in embryo quality and how long cryopreserved embryos could be viable; those having few or poor-quality embryos "questioned whether it would be worth the emotional and/or financial investment to attempt additional frozen embryo transfers" [5].

Delayed disposition decisions can be agonizing for patients and difficult for those institutions responsible for storing or disposing of potentially abandoned embryos [2]. Patients experiencing decisional conflict might postpone their choices for 5 years or more, or keep their embryos perpetually frozen [22]. Because attitudes toward embryos change over time, patients' relief over having surplus embryos may eventually become weariness, reluctance to commit to a disposition decision, and even regret [9, 22]. Those who are initially confident about their disposition decisions might experience great indecision later on, when it is time to implement them.

Fortunately, empirical research has identified a number of factors that can predict when patients will experience decisional conflict over embryo disposition. Patients who are unsure whether their families are complete are likely to have high decisional conflict, as are those who are sure that they are done; these groups know that they must confront the disposition decision sooner rather than later. In contrast, patients who know they want more children tend to have low decisional conflict [22]. Moreover, patients who assign either full or no moral status to their embryos are also likely to have low decisional conflict; most patients fall in between these positions, however, and find their decisions more challenging, particularly if they assign high but not full moral status to their embryos [22].

Couples' disposition decisions are even harder when their desired option is unavailable. Women might desire choices like a disposal ceremony or compassionate transfer that are offered by very few clinics [10]. Patients wishing to donate their embryos to another couple for reproductive use can face additional difficulties. Bankowski et al. reported that most clinics that offered embryo donation had actually had not completed donation cycles [1], and Nachtigall et al. observed that some patients who were initially interested in embryo donation ultimately selected another disposition because their clinics lacked the infrastructure to facilitate donation [5]. And those whose embryos were frozen before the US Food and Drug Administration (FDA) promulgated its most recent policy requiring infectious disease testing for gamete providers might be unable to donate at all [2]. When acceptable disposition options are unavailable, patients might choose instead to keep their embryos frozen [10].

The worst disposition option is when patients intentionally or unintentionally abandon their embryos. Abandoned embryos are defined as those kept in storage for long time periods without clear written disposition instructions from their progenitors, who either cannot be contacted to provide a disposition or intentionally fail to do so [4]. Patients move, change their marital status, fail to make decisions by a certain deadline, or neglect to make decisions at all [23]. Clinics and storage facilities may be reluctant to carry out clear disposition instructions when progenitors have not affirmed their choices [4].

According to Sweet et al., an increased risk of embryo abandonment correlated with several patient characteristics, including low education level, having more children at home, storing embryos for a long period, owing a large debt to their fertility practice, having partial or complete insurance coverage for IVF, a primary diagnosis of tubal or peritoneal infertility or endometriosis, and having a large number of frozen embryos [24]. Sweet et al. reported that, for each year patients paid cryopreservation storage fees, the risk of abandonment increased by 7.8% [24]. Abandonment may also occur when surplus embryos lose their original perceived value after patients decide they will not use them [25].

Abandoned embryos raise several ethical questions, from what acceptable disposition options might be to who can make these decisions [25]. The ASRM Ethics Committee recommends that a center may discard embryos after 5 years of no contact with the patients and after significant contact attempts [26].

53.3 Strategies for Improving Disposition Decisions

Despite the difficulty of the disposition decision, practitioners can help patients make more expeditious and informed decisions. Reproductive medicine professionals influence the timing and outcome of patients' disposition choices and affect their attitudes toward stored embryos' viability [5]. Correspondingly, patients rank clinic information provision and support very important in making these choices; they expect medical professionals to be primary sources of information regarding cryopreservation and disposition and even believe that clinics have an obligation to assist in this decision [5].

But these informational needs and expectations may not be met. While patients trust physicians and feel that they have the greatest access to relevant information, some report that communication with their clinics "decreased drastically" once they had conceived, and others note that they received much more information about IVF than about embryo disposition [5]. Many patients want detailed information, but find the written material they are given to be "impersonal" or of low "impact" or "importance" [26]. Information about disposition options is especially critical when certain possibilities, like donation to research or another couple, are inherently more opaque or complex, and patients need more details about what these options involve.

Both patients and researchers have identified solutions to ease disposition decisions and ultimately reduce large numbers of cryopreserved embryos. Patients have recommended the opportunity to participate in a follow-up educational seminar or support group, or the chance to consult trained counselors who can provide assistance in choosing among disposition options or offer emotional support [5]. Researchers like Nachtigall et al. recommend providing patients with "comprehensible and detailed" information about disposition options before cryopreservation and regularly thereafter, expansive information about stored embryos' number and viability as well as storage fees and terms (including fee increases), and access to a knowledgeable medical expert or counselor [5]. Lyerly et al. suggest that "improv[ed] information and support" will likely "alleviate distress and facilitate informed and reasoned decisions and closure" [22]. Finally, Samorinha et al. recommend decision-making guidelines incorporating "psychosocial care … that should be sensitive to … age, religion, trait anxiety, and conceptualization of cryopreserved embryos" [12].

Informed consent provides a logical opportunity to deliver relevant information about embryo disposition and becomes especially crucial when patients are likely to experience high decisional conflict and when they are ready to implement a disposition decision. It is undeniably crucial to require patients to choose a disposition prior to undergoing MAR, since an estimated one-third of patients will not return to affirm their initial disposition choices [18]. At that time, however, patients' attention is largely on other matters, and they might spend an average of less than 1 h contemplating the decision [18]. For this reason, patients should be given other, later opportunities to revisit the disposition decision. Lyerly et al. propose "revisit[ing] discussions about disposition preferences at regular intervals, to engage with patients later on … when they themselves can engage with the complexity of embryo disposition decisions and consider them in the contexts of their lives" [22]. This could be as simple as enclosing updated information on disposition options in patients' billing correspondence [22]. Models of shared decision-making provide support for patient counseling about disposition options, help patients to reflect upon and develop informed disposition preferences through healthy clinical relationships, allow patients to express their viewpoints, and give them relevant information that can reduce decisional conflict [27].

Implementing such evidence-based solutions transforms a one-stage informed consent process into a patient-centered process consisting of two or three stages, based not only on rational and autonomous decision-making but also on trust and treatment relationships [28]. Emphasis is placed not on the initial consent opportunity but on subsequent posttreatment contacts, when patients are less stressed and have lower anxiety [12]. Revisiting patients' disposition preferences at regular intervals posttreatment might better accord with how patients cognitively approach these decisions. In the beginning, many might not even have "settled moral views or reflective preferences about their embryos"; instead, they formulate them through their treatment experiences [10].

If the informed consent process were altered to better reflect patients' own disposition decision-making trajectories, informed consent's initial goal would be "not to secure a patient's commitment to a particular course of action regarding 'spare' embryos, but to communicate that embryo cryopreservation may have untoward consequences" [10]. Periodically revisiting the subject of embryo disposition may also prevent patients from being surprised when storage terms are up, or other changes occur [25]. Of course, this increases clinics' administrative burdens [25]. Apte et al. found that staff members in one clinic that contacted patients with stored embryos had to send many patients multiple letters; more than one letter was required for 26.7% of patients who had stored embryos for 1 year and for 50% of patients who were in the final year of storage [23]. Nonetheless, this contact policy allowed the clinic to more effectively discard nonresponding patients' embryos, reducing the burden of abandoned embryos [23].

For these reasons, best practices dictate that, in addition to requiring patients to complete an advanced disposition directive, clinics should maintain contact with patients at regular intervals and request that they confirm their initial disposition choice. This strategy both provides a "safety net for patients as imperfect decision makers" and allows clinics to dispose of embryos when patients cannot be reached [25]. One randomized controlled trial which offered the experimental group a meeting with a mental health professional to discuss disposition options and provide additional support found that this group had "increased awareness knowledge of embryo donation to research and possibly an increased tendency towards donation" as compared with a control group that received standard care [29].

Finally, developing new educational options is another promising option for improving disposition decisions. Clinics can facilitate peer discussions among patients so that couples in the early stages of treatment can benefit from veteran patients' advice and experiences about decision-making and emotional challenges [27]. Technology also offers new options for educating patients. New multimedia e-learning applications could be developed that educate patients, better preparing them to choose dispositions for their surplus embryos [30].

References

1. Bankowski BJ, Lyerly AD, Faden RR, Wallach EE. The social implications of embryo cryopreservation. Fertil Steril. 2005;84(4):823–32.
2. Lyerly AD, Steinhauser K, Voils C, Namey E, Alexander C, Bankowski B. Fertility patients' views about frozen embryo disposition: results of a multi-institutional U.S. survey. Fertil Steril. 2010;93(2):499–509.
3. Cohen IG, Adashi EY. Embryo disposition disputes: controversies and Case Law. Hastings Cent Rep. 2016;46(4):13–9.
4. Cattapan A, Baylis F. Frozen in perpetuity: 'abandoned embryos' in Canada. Reprod Biomed Soc Online. 2016;1:104–12.
5. Nachtigall RD, MacDougall K, Lee M, Harrington J, Becker G. What do patients want? Expectations and perceptions of IVF clinic information and support regarding frozen embryo disposition. Fertil Steril. 2010 November;94(6):2069–72.
6. Provoost V, Pennings G, De Sutter P, Gerris J, Van de Velde A, De Lissynder E, Dhont M. Infertility patients' beliefs about embryos and their disposition preferences. Hum Reprod. 2009;24(4):896–905.
7. Goswami M, Murdoch A, Haimes E. To freeze or not to freeze embryos: clarity, confusion, and conflict. Hum Fertil. 2015 June;18(2):113–20.
8. Madeira JL. Taking baby steps: how patients and fertility clinics collaborate in conception. Berkeley: University of California Press; 2017.
9. Nactigall RD, Becker G, Friese C, Butler A, MacDougall K. Parents' conceptualization of their frozen embryos complicates the disposition decision. Fertil Steril. 2005 August;84(2):2094–6.
10. Lyerly AD, Steinhauser K, Namey E, Tulsky JA, Cook-Deegan R, Sugarman J. Factors that affect infertility patients' decisions about disposition of frozen embryos. Fertil Steril. 2006 June;85(6):1623–30.
11. Fuscaldo G, Russell S, Gillam L. How to facilitate decisions about surplus embryos: Patients' views. Hum Reprod. 2007 December;22(12):3129–38.
12. Samorinha C, Severo M, Alves E, Machado H, Figueredo B, Silva S. Factors associated with willingness to donate embryos for research among couples undergoing IVF. Reprod Biomed Online. 2015 February;32(2):247–56.
13. de Lacey S. Parent identity and 'virtual children': why patients discard rather than donate unused embryos. Hum Reprod. 2005 June;20(6):1661–9.
14. de Lacey S. Decisions for the fate of frozen embryos: fresh insights into patients' thinking and their rationales for donating or discarding embryos. Hum Reprod. 2007 April;22(6):1751–8.
15. Laruelle C, Englert Y. Psychological study of in vitro fertilization-embryo transfer participants' attitudes towards the destiny of their supernumerary embryos. Fertil Steril. 1995 May;63(5):1047–50.
16. McMahon CA, Saunders DM. Attitudes of couples with stored frozen embryos toward conditional embryo donation. Fertil Steril. 2009;91(1):140–7.
17. Juliá CR, Sobrino JM, Vives MT, Peruchet AS, Aizpitarte AC, Guerrero OR. Embryo donation: is it a good option for surplus frozen embryos? Fertil Steril. 2013 September;100(3 Suppl):1147.
18. Deniz SG, Hughes EG, Neal MS, Faghih M, Amin S, Karnis MF. Are health care providers adequately educating couples for embryo disposition decisions? Fertil Steril. 2016 March;105(3):684–9.
19. Wanggren K, Alden J, Bergh T, Skoog SA. Attitudes towards embryo donation among infertile couples with frozen embryos. Hum Reprod. 2013;28(9):2432–9.
20. Ethics Committee of the American Society for Reproductive Medicine. Recommendations for gamete and embryo donation: a committee opinion. Fertil Steril. 2013 January;99(1):47–62.
21. Hammarberg K, Tinney L. Deciding the fate of supernumerary frozen embryos: a survey of couples' decisions and the factors influencing their choice. Fertil Steril. 2006;86:86–91.

22. Lyerly AD, Nakagawa S, Kuppermann M. Decisional conflict and the disposition of frozen embryos: implications for informed consent. Hum Reprod. 2011 March;26(3):646–54.
23. Apte M, Gibson SH, Blanchette-Porter M, Stern JE. Disposition of frozen embryos: one program's experience with contacting patients about embryos in storage. JFIV Reprod Med Genet. 2015;3:157.
24. Sweet CR, Papkov G, Wiedman-Klayum KC, Norton EL, Miles KF. The number of children living at home and the duration of embryo cryopreservation are significant risk factors for cryopreserved embryo abandonment. Fertil Steril. 2016;106(3):e71.
25. Provoost V, Pennings G, De Sutter P, Dhont M. The frozen embryo and its nonresponding parents. Fertil Steril. 2011 May;95(6):1980–4.
26. Ethics Commitee of the American Society for Reproductive Medicine. Disposition of abandoned embryos: a committee opinion. Fertil Steril. 2013;99(7):1848–9.
27. Quinn GP. Peer counseling to improve shared decision making in surplus embryo decisions. Fertil Steril. 2016 March;105(3):601.
28. Samorinha C, Silva S. A patient-centred approach to embryo donation for research. Israel J Health Policy Res. 2016;5:44.
29. Zimon A, Shepard DS, Prottas J, Rooney KL, Sakkas D, Oskowitz SP. Development and implementation of a clinic-based procedural intervention to enhance embryo donation: a randomized controlled trial. Fertil Steril. 2013 September;100(3):S96.
30. Martens M. An online educational program on the disposition options of cryopreserved embryos. Fertil Steril. 2016 October;106(3):e116–7.

Gestational Surrogacy

54

Virginia Mensah, Reeva Makhijani, and Carol Wheeler

The ability to use a surrogate to have a child has been possible for centuries and was described in the bible when Sarah, who was barren, gave her servant Hagar to Abraham to bear a child [1]. The advent of medically assisted reproduction (MAR) has made it possible to utilize a gestational surrogate, also referred to as a gestational carrier (GC), which differs from the traditional surrogacy described in the bible. In traditional surrogacy, the surrogate provides her own oocyte and conceives with insemination (or coitus) with the intended father's sperm. Because of the risk of regret and complicated legal issues, many ART programs no longer offer traditional surrogacy arrangements. Alternatively, a gestational surrogate or carrier does not have a genetic connection to the child but carries the child for another individual or couple. In both situations, the "intended parents" (intended mother(s) and/or father(s)) will ultimately be both the social and legal parents of the child or children.

When using a gestational carrier, the gamete providers (source of egg and sperm) may or may not be the intended parents. This complicated legal and ethical relationship for the child born of this process may thus involve as many as five individual parent relationships: the GC provides the uterus to carry the child; the intended parents are the legal and rearing family; the gametes and/or embryos may come from a source other than the GC or the intended parents.

Gestational surrogacy requires in vitro fertilization (IVF) for conception, and, in general, a number of gestational surrogacy cycles are increasing over time. The US Center for Disease Control tracks fresh gestational carrier cycles, and, in 2013, 86% of IVF programs offered gestational carrier programs with <1% of 190,777 cycles utilizing gestational carriers [2]. Outside of the United States, gestational surrogacy is often severely limited or outlawed by many countries, particularly when there is payment to the carrier for her services. This has led to an increase in cross-border reproduction resulting in intended parents and/or carriers coming to the United States (or other countries with more liberal laws) for treatment and delivery [3].

This chapter will review the indications for gestational carrier use and describe the process for the use of a GC, including carrier selection, evaluation, and management. It will also discuss the evaluation of gamete providers, who may or may not be the same as the intended parents. Lastly, the success rates, costs, and ethical issues surrounding the process of gestational surrogacy will also be reviewed.

54.1 Indications for the Intended Parent

When it comes to gestational surrogacy, there is a variable range of practices and criteria for whom this method of reproduction is indicated. From more obvious indications such as women lacking a uterus or having mullerian disorders to more subtle reasons such as recurrent implantation failure, no current standard of care dictates what women may utilize a gestational carrier to achieve pregnancy. However, here we review generally accepted evidence-based indications for the use of GCs with emphasis on three groups: women who "cannot carry," women who "fail to carry," and the unique situations of same sex female and male partnerships or single males [4].

54.1.1 Women Who "Cannot Carry": Altered or Absent Mullerian Anatomy

54.1.1.1 Turner Syndrome (45 X0)

Women born with Turner Syndrome generally lack functional gonads capable of gametogenesis and therefore have very limited autologous reproductive potential. Additionally, although these women have uteri and thus can experience menstrual cycles with hormone replacement, they often have

V. Mensah
Reproductive Science Center of New Jersey, Eatontown, NJ, USA

R. Makhijani · C. Wheeler (✉)
Women & Infants' Fertility Center, Providence, RI, USA
e-mail: cawheeler@wihri.org

G. N. Allahbadia et al. (eds.), *Textbook of Assisted Reproduction*, https://doi.org/10.1007/978-981-15-2377-9_54

significant cardiac comorbidities which preclude pregnancy (i.e., aortic root abnormalities) [5]. Consequently, these women are often recommended to avoid pregnancy and instead use gestational surrogacy to conceive.

54.1.1.2 MRKH/Mullerian Agenesis

Mullerian agenesis is a failure of proper development of the female reproductive tract resulting in absent or abnormal formation of the vagina, cervix, and/or uterus. These women generally lack a uterus and, as a result, lack the ability to carry a pregnancy. Given the failure of development only affects the uterus, women with mullerian agenesis are capable of reproducing using their own gametes via in vitro fertilization and GC cycles [6].

54.1.1.3 Women Status Post Hysterectomy

Hysterectomy is the second most commonly performed gynecologic procedure in the United States. Though the majority is completed after a woman has completed childbearing, for some women, hysterectomy is performed at an early age for indications such as fibroids, endometriosis, and severe chronic pelvic pain [7]. Therefore in these women, if childbearing is desired, gestational surrogacy may be the preferred option to achieve parenthood.

54.1.1.4 Women with Significant Medical or Pregnancy-Related Comorbidities or Complications

There are a number of cardiovascular conditions which confer significant risk of morbidity and mortality in pregnancy [8]. Consequently, if pregnancy is desired, the use of a GC is often strongly recommended. Similarly, women with medical conditions that require use of powerful and potentially teratogenic medications may consider use of a GC. For these women, gestational surrogacy offers the opportunity to continue their medical treatment uninterrupted while pursuing pregnancy without harm to the developing fetus. Finally, pregnancy-related complications may provide some women with an indication to pursue gestational surrogacy. For example, a woman with a history of several prior poor obstetric outcomes (including preterm deliveries or stillbirths) due to severely shortened cervix who previously failed vaginal or abdominal cerclage may benefit from use of a gestational carrier.

54.1.2 Women Who "Fail to Carry": Recurrent Miscarriage and Issues of Uterine Receptivity

54.1.2.1 Recurrent Implantation Failure (RIF)

Although there is no universally accepted definition of RIF in the IVF literature, it is a condition marked by repeated failures of an embryo to implant within the endometrium. The etiology of such implantation failures is largely unknown but is usually attributed to aberrations within the gametes, the embryo, or the endometrium [9]. If RIF is apparent after several cycles of IVF, the use of a gestational carrier offers a solution for concerns regarding endometrial receptivity.

54.1.2.2 Recurrent Pregnancy Loss (RPL)

Per ASRM guidelines, an evaluation for RPL can be undertaken as soon as two or more pregnancy losses have occurred. In approximately 50% of cases, the etiology is identifiable and potentially correctable. Therefore, a gestational carrier may not be necessary. Examples include cases of endocrinopathies (abnormal TSH or glucose studies), uterine malformations (uterine septum), parental genetic translocations, and aberrations in coagulation (antiphospholipid antibody syndrome) [10]. In the case of unexplained RPL, however, the use of a GC may address a potential unidentified issue with endometrial receptivity.

54.1.2.3 Women with Severe Asherman Syndrome

Asherman syndrome is the significant loss of normal endometrium and replacement of it with abnormal scar tissue within the uterus. Risk factors include infection and aggressive curettage, which denudes the endometrial lining. Scar tissue formation may render the endometrial cavity incapable of embryo apposition and implantation. Thus, women with severe Asherman syndrome can have difficulty achieving pregnancy.

54.1.3 Unique Considerations

54.1.3.1 Same Sex Female Couples (Reciprocal IVF)

Though both partners may have the necessary reproductive structures to carry a pregnancy, any of the abovementioned situations can apply to same sex female couples and therefore may warrant this unique situation of gestational surrogacy. On the other hand, in the case of elective "reciprocal IVF," no specific medical indication exists wherein the gamete donor is unable to carry the gestation. However, the decision to proceed with such a cycle may derive from a desire for both partners to contribute in some way to the pregnancy.

54.1.3.2 Same Sex Male Couples or Single Males

Same sex male couples or single males who desire to conceive fundamentally lack the total complement of reproductive structures to do so. As such, gestational surrogacy combined with oocyte donation affords an excellent option for reproduction. Additionally, same sex male couples have the option of using either one or both partner's sperm as the male gamete source, which allows both partners to potentially contribute to a given pregnancy.

54.2 Evaluation and Treatment

54.2.1 Carrier Requirements/Screening/Evaluation

As discussed in the introduction, the majority of the gestational surrogacy arrangements made in the United States use a GC rather than a traditional surrogate. GCs are typically a directed carrier, which means her identity is known to the intended parents prior to becoming a GC. She may be provided by an agency, and the intended parents do not know her identity prior to her being their carrier. Directed GCs may be family members or friends of the intended parents who have volunteered to carry the pregnancy. The most cited reasons for why couples use directed carriers include trying to preserve a familial link and reducing both costs and waiting times [11]. For example, a sister acting as a GC is unlikely to request payment, which can yield huge financial savings for the intended parents.

The usual baseline requirements for a GC are that she is between the ages of 21 and 45, has ideally had a prior uncomplicated pregnancy, and delivered a live-born term infant [12, 13]. Of course, one must also consider that use of a GC of advanced maternal age poses a number of potential risks to the pregnancy, such as higher rates of preeclampsia and diabetes. As gestational surrogacy also confers a number of unique physical and emotional stresses on the carrier, it is also preferable if the GC has a stable and supportive home life. Per ASRM practice guidelines, the carrier also should not have had more than five vaginal deliveries or three cesarean sections, as there is an increased risk of postpartum hemorrhage and abnormal placentation, respectively (Table 54.1).

In selecting a GC, counseling should include information about the preliminary required work up, which involves a battery of infectious disease tests. It should also discuss the medical treatments and procedures that will be performed. Additionally, counseling should include the more unique demands of gestational surrogacy to decide whether the potential carrier is truly suitable and willing to take on the challenges. These issues include the ability to relinquish or separate from the offspring after birth, the risks of multiple pregnancy including preterm birth and the need for prolonged hospitalization, possible need to abstain from sexual intercourse, and also decisions about pregnancy termination, multifetal reduction, and invasive prenatal testing.

Table 54.1 Gestational carrier relative exclusion criteria

Five prior vaginal deliveries
Three cesarean sections
Presence of significant psychopathology/abnormal psychological testing
Current use of psychoactive medications/substance abuse
Impaired cognitive functioning or mental impairment
History of sexual or physical abuse without professional treatment
Excessive stress and/or chaotic lifestyle
High-risk sexual practices
Significant medical problems that preclude pregnancy
Evidence of financial or emotional coercion
Current marital or relationship instability
Inability to maintain respectful relationship with intended parents
Evidence of emotional inability to separate from child at birth
Child-to-parent collaboration is generally prohibited

Unsurprisingly, it is strongly recommended that a mental health professional who is experienced in dealing with third-party reproduction be involved in the selection and evaluation of GCs. The mental health assessment should include both a clinical interview and psychological testing. If any factors warrant further investigation, the clinician should refer the potential carrier for further psychiatric evaluation. The clinician should counsel the patient on the aforementioned considerations and also discuss the impact being a GC may have on the relationships the carrier has with her family and other people in her life. It should also be clear what relationship the GC will have with the intended parents, the plan for disclosure or nondisclosure of the GC to the offspring, and the plan for future contact, if any.

In addition to a mental health evaluation, screening and evaluation of the GC should include a complete medical history with a detailed personal and sexual history to identify individuals at high risk for HIV, STIs, and other infections that may be transmissible to the fetus. The potential carrier should be evaluated by a qualified medical provider and be cleared for pregnancy. A thorough physical exam should follow to identify physical evidence of current or past sexually transmitted or other infectious diseases, evidence of illicit drug use, and inspection of recently obtained tattooed or piercings where sterile technique may have not been used. Laboratory testing should be done to rule out any current infectious diseases in the patient or partner as well as pertinent preconception testing (Table 54.2).

Lastly, given the conflict of interests between parties involved in these incredibly complex arrangements, the GC should have independent legal counsel who will draw up the gestational surrogacy contract. This contract should address informed consent, payment, psychological support, access to medical treatment, and also contingency plans for all foreseeable hazards or scenarios.

Table 54.2 Recommended laboratory testing for the gestational carrier

HIV-1 and HIV-2 antibody as well as NAT
HIV group O antibody
Hepatitis C antibody and NAT
Hepatitis B surface antigen
Hepatitis B core antibody (IgG and IgM)
Serologic test of syphilis
CMV IgG and IgM
Gonorrhea and chlamydia cultures
Blood type and Rh factor
Pap smear
Mammogram if indicated by age-based screening guidelines
Varicella titer
Rubella titer
Urine drug screen—if indicated
Male partner of the GC—gonorrhea, chlamydia, HLTV-1, HLTV-2, CMV IgG and IgM

Table 54.3 Conditions that confer FDA ineligible status for gamete donors

Evidence of sexually transmitted infection (i.e., genital ulcerative lesions, HSV, chancroid, urethral discharge)
Risk for or evidence of syphilis, N. gonorrhea, or C. trachomatis[a]
Positive serum testing for HIV (1, 2, or group 0), Hepatitis B or C, HTLV-1 or HTLV-2
Evidence of anal intercourse in the male partner (history or physical evidence, including perianal condylomata)
Evidence of non-medical percutaneous drug use
Evidence of recent tattooing, ear piercing, or body piercing within the last 12 months where sterile technique was not used
Disseminated lymphadenopathy
Unexplained oral thrush
Evidence of Kaposi sarcoma
Unexplained jaundice, hepatomegaly, or icterus
Recent history or evidence of (large scab) smallpox immunization
Eczema vaccinatum, generalized vesicular rash, severely necrotic lesion (vaccinia necrosum), or corneal scarring (vaccinial keratitis)

[a]Ineligible for use in GC for 12 months but should be treated, retested, and, if successful treatment is documented after 12 months with no active evidence of infection, may be reconsidered for use

54.2.2 Intended Parents (IPs) Screening/Gamete Donor Screening

An important consideration for GC cycles involves the distinction of the intended parent and gamete source, who may not necessarily be the same. In fact, according to recent CDC/NASS data, a majority of GC cycles use donor oocytes [14]. Thus, the oocyte source can either be the intended female parent or an oocyte donor, and likewise the sperm source can be either the intended male parent(s) or donor sperm. In the case of the latter, the intended parents (if both male) may elect to use sperm specimens from both partners to inseminate donor eggs. Not surprisingly, these permutations of traditional-assisted reproduction cycles can sometimes complicate the social, legal, and ethical ramifications of GC cycles.

Regardless of whether autologous IP gametes or donor gametes are selected, the gamete source requires appropriate evaluation prior to initiation of an assisted reproduction cycle. These individuals must undergo a thorough evaluation with a complete history and physical examination within 6 months of creation of embryos to ensure appropriate fitness for assisted reproductive procedures. Additionally, genetic screening of the gamete source should be performed to minimize genetic risks to offspring. This evaluation should include appropriate genetic testing based on personal/family history and ethnic background. In addition, ACOG recommends universal screening for cystic fibrosis and spinal muscular atrophy.

Furthermore, it is recommended that the IPs have psychosocial education and counseling prior to undertaking a GC cycle. The assessment at a minimum should include a clinical interview by a qualified mental health professional and may or may not also involve psychological testing [12, 13]. Important areas to address include the impact of the pregnancy on family and community dynamics, the nature of the relationship between IPs and GC, as well as plans for disclosure or future contact [12, 13].

54.2.3 Food and Drug Administration (FDA) Eligibility for Gamete Donors

In the United States, it is important to understand the terminology FDA eligible versus FDA ineligible, which are likewise used in the donor literature. The former implies all mandated screening has taken place, and the intended parent or gamete donor has no positive findings based either on screening questionnaire or serum testing (Table 54.3). On the contrary, FDA ineligible indicates a positive finding during screening or testing; it is important to note, however, that this status does NOT preclude use of the gametes. Rather, in the case of FDA ineligible IPs or donors, embryos created can be transferred into a GC so long as (1) the tissue is labeled to indicate any associated increased risks and (2) physicians transferring the embryos are aware of the results [12, 13]. ASRM also recommends that all parties involved in a GC cycle undergo appropriate informed consent.

54.2.4 Lab Testing

In addition to minimizing risk to the embryo or fetus, the goal of lab testing is to minimize transmission of disease to the GC. However, no method completely mitigates the risk. The FDA requires testing within 30 days of oocyte retrieval and within 7 days of sperm collection with negative results documented before gametes are deemed eligible for transfer (Table 54.4). In addition to the tests mandated by the FDA, ASRM recommends both IPs undergo testing for blood type and Rh factor.

All positive tests should be confirmed and subsequently managed by or referred to the appropriate provider for coun-

Table 54.4 FDA recommended lab testing for gamete donors

HIV-1 and HIV-2 antibody as well as NAT HIV group O antibody Hepatitis C antibody and NAT Hepatitis B surface antigen Hepatitis B core antibody (IgG and IgM) Serologic test of syphilis Neisseria gonorrhea and chlamydia trachomatis NAT on urine or swab
Additional testing for male gamete donor: CMV IgG and IgM HTLV-1 and HTLV-2
Additional testing recommended by ASRM: Blood type and Rh factor

seling and management. Furthermore, the FDA requires records pertaining to each IP be maintained for at least 10 years. The GC should be offered the option of cryopreserving and quarantining embryos derived from IPs for 180 days, with release of embryos following IP re-testing and confirmed negative results. In the event of seroconversion of an IP, the GC should be counseled appropriately.

54.2.5 Cycle Synchronization and Management

In the management of a GC cycle, the first question pertains to whether the cycle will be completed in a fresh or frozen cycle and whether autologous IP or donor oocytes are to be used. A recent retrospective review of CDC/NASS data that revealed most GC cycles to date completed in the United States is in a frozen cycle, with more than half using donor oocytes [14]. In general, frozen cycle coordination is simpler than fresh cycle, as no cycle synchronization is usually required.

For a frozen cycle, once embryos have been created and cryopreserved, a GC can undergo either embryo transfer following a natural unstimulated cycle or synthetic cycle with estrogen and progesterone supplementation. In either case, the endometrial lining of the GC is typically evaluated between CD11-14 for adequate thickness and structure (i.e., trilaminar). After the GC endometrial lining appears appropriate for transfer, embryo thaw and transfer are coordinated with lab staff accordingly.

On the other hand, a fresh GC cycle requires synchronization of the IP/oocyte donor stimulation with the GC stimulation and thus falls along similar lines as a fresh oocyte donor-recipient cycle. This requires a coordination of cycles based on type of stimulation protocol planned for the IP/oocyte donor. Initial coordination can be accomplished through use of oral contraceptive pills and/or GnRH agonist to ensure both GC and IP/donor are in synchronous cycles. The prevailing principles governing this timing are to optimize likelihood of implantation by harnessing the optimal window of endometrial receptivity and achieving embryo and endometrial synchrony.

The GC typically initiates a synthetic estrogen several days prior to the IP/donor initiating exogenous gonadotropins. This ensures the GC endometrium is sufficiently exposed to estrogen before progesterone supplementation commences. If the IP/donor does not meet criteria for oocyte trigger by 12–14 days of stimulation, the GC can be maintained on her synthetic estrogen dose. The optimal duration of estrogen exposure before progesterone supplementation has not been established, and successful pregnancies have been reported in stimulated cycles with estrogen exposure lasting between days and weeks [15]. The endometrial thickness of the GC should be monitored during this time to ensure adequate thickness and appearance. The adequacy of endometrial thickness varies by IVF program, and some evidence supports that a lining less than 7 mm is associated with lower live birth rates [16]. Studies also suggest a trilaminar pattern is optimal and has been associated with higher implantation rates than a homogenous hyperechogenic pattern [17]. Progesterone supplementation for the GC usually begins on the day of the oocyte retrieval in the IP/donor. This timing of progesterone start is intended to enhance the synchronization between embryo development and receptivity of the secretory endometrium. Estrogen and progesterone supplementation is then continued for upward of 8–12 weeks per individual clinic protocol.

54.2.6 Financial Considerations

It is difficult to estimate the cost of using a GC as it depends largely on the clinic/program the intended parents choose as well as the type of GC. Several fertility clinic websites quote that, on average, intended parents who plan to use a GC should budget $75,000 to $140,000. The basic components that make up the cost include compensation to the carrier, agency fee, cost of health insurance for the carrier, legal fees, cost of psychological services, and cost for possible travel. The total cost may be higher or lower depending on whether the intended parents use their own or donor gametes, the number of IVF cycles and embryo transfers required to achieve pregnancy, as well as any pregnancy-related complications.

54.3 Outcomes

54.3.1 Success Rates

The pregnancy success rate in gestational surrogacy treatment is dependent on a number of factors but is overall very high compared to other ART treatments. The most significant contribution comes from the age of the oocyte source. If the intended mother is the oocyte source, the ultimate success rate will depend on her age. The SART (Society of Assisted Reproductive Technology) reported preliminary primary outcomes for intended retrievals in 2014 with a live birth rate of 50.5% for women < age 35 years but only 9.5% for women >age 42 years [18]. The use of healthy donor oocytes leads to higher success rates. These statistics do not take into account the sperm quality, which also may impact pregnancy rates. It also does not take into account the characteristics of the GC; assuming she was selected based on the criteria noted earlier, this would presumably have little impact on overall success rates.

Beyond pregnancy and delivery rates, there must be consideration of the impact on the intended parents and, ultimately, the children. A recent systematic review on the ultimate impact on the children born from surrogacy arrangements reveals that the incidence of low birth weight and birth defects is no different than that after fresh IVF or donor oocyte use [19].

In addition, this same review showed no psychological differences in the children at the age of 10 years.

Parents of children conceived with a GC have marital relationships similar to those conceived naturally by the time the children are 3 years old [20]. There are no psychological differences in the mothers of children born through surrogacy compared to natural conception [19]. Gay men who have become parents through surrogacy show lower levels of stress and depression associated with parenting than heterosexual families [21]. In terms of outcomes for the carrier, most studies have shown no detrimental psychological concerns, but there can be relinquishing issues which can persist, emphasizing the need for careful carrier selection and psychological evaluation [19].

54.3.2 Ethical and Legal Issues

There are a number of ethical concerns that come up during the process of gestational surrogacy. Since compensation for carriers is controversial, with some countries not allowing paid carriers, the payment for the GC is quite variable. The financial compensation may entice women who are of lower socioeconomic status to be carriers leading to differences in the status of carriers and typically higher socioeconomic status intended parents. This compensation may be viewed as coercive with the carrier having to participate in procedures which she may not otherwise feel comfortable with such as amniocentesis and pregnancy termination in the presence of an abnormal fetus. Others may view this as "baby selling" and recommend limits on compensation to only the carrier's direct expenses.

In the case of a known carrier, it is important to explore the motivations of the carrier for participating to ensure there is no underlying financial or emotional coercion. This is challenging as relatives may feel an obligation to help their family members and accept more risk than they otherwise would. That is why some feel that a certain level of emotional distance may be required to truly gain informed consent [22].

Pregnancy entails medical risk to the carrier, particularly if she has multiple embryos transferred and conceives a multiple gestation. The pregnancy may impact the carrier's ability to care for her own family and specifically her own children should complications arise. Spouses or partners should be included in any decision-making for the carrier. Although in general no significant impact on the emotional health of the carrier has been identified, the research is quite limited [23]. Pregnancy hormonal changes and unexpected issues can lead to emotionally charged and legally complicated situations.

Legality of gestational surrogacy varies by both country and state. Any legal counsel involved in gestational surrogacy contracts should be familiar with the laws surrounding gestational surrogacy in the state or country in both where the arrangement is being made and where the carrier may deliver. Some states entirely ban surrogacy contracts, whereas others allow them with certain regulations [24]. With international or "cross-border" surrogacy arrangements, the legal advice is the responsibility of the local practitioner including possible conflicts in the intended parents' home country [25]. Disagreements between a carrier and the intended parents are not unusual and may require extensive legal counsel to achieve resolution. Ideally, these should be anticipated in advance and be spelled out in the legal agreements.

Gestational surrogacy is a complicated process, replete with ethical and legal issues. In general, the medical management is fairly straightforward and allows individuals and couples the opportunity to have a family when they otherwise would not be able. Programs that provide these services need to focus on the best interests of all of the parties involved to insure healthy family relationships in the future.

References

1. Jacob B, Jacob E, Jacob W. The first book of the bible, genesis. New York: KTAV Publishing House; 2007.
2. Centers for Disease Control and Prevention. Assisted Reproductive Technology (ART) Data: National Data [Internet]. Atlanta (GA). Centers for Disease Control and Prevention; 2016. [cited 2016 Oct 3]. Available from: https://nccd.cdc.gov/drh_art/rdPage.aspx?rdReport=DRH_ART.ClinicInfo&ClinicId=9999&ShowNational=1
3. Ethics Committee of the American Society for Reproductive Medicine. Cross-border reproductive care: an Ethics Committee

opinion. Fertil Steril. 2016; https://doi.org/10.1016/j.fertnstert.2016.08.038.
4. Dar S, Lazer T, Swanson S, Silverman J, Wasser C, Moskovtsev SI, et al. Assisted reproduction involving gestational surrogacy: an analysis of the medical, psychosocial and legal issues: experience from a large surrogacy program. Hum Reprod. 2015;30(2):345–52.
5. Oktay K, Giuliano B, Berkowitz K, Bronson R, Kashani B, McGovern P, Pal L, Quinn G, Rubin K. Fertility preservation in women with Turner Syndrome: a comprehensive review and practical guidelines. J Pediatr Adolesc Gynecol. 2016;29:409–16.
6. Friedler S, Grin L, Liberti G, Saar-Ryss B, Rabinson Y, Meltzer S. The reproductive potential of patients with Mayer-Rokitansky-Kuster-Hauser syndrome using gestational surrogacy: a systematic review. Reprod Biomed Online. 2016;32:54–61.
7. Whiteman MK, Hillis SD, Jamieson DJ, Morrow B, Podgornik MN, Brett KM, Marchbanks PA. Inpatient hysterectomy surveillance in the United States, 2000-2004. Am J Obstet Gynecol. 2008;198(1):34.e1–7.
8. Brikner ME. Cardiovascular management in pregnancy: congenital heart disease. Circulation. 2014;130:273–82.
9. Coughlan C, Ledger W, Wang Q, Liu F, Demirol A, Gurgan T, Cutting R, Ong K, Sallam H, Li TC. Recurrent implantation failure: definition and management. Reprod Biomed Online. 2014;28(1):14–38.
10. Practice Committee of American Society for Reproductive Medicine. Evaluation and treatment of recurrent pregnancy loss: a committee opinion. Fertil Steril. 2012;98(5):1103–11.
11. Ethics Committee of the American Society for Reproductive Medicine. Using family members as gamete donors or surrogates. Fertil Steril. 2012 Oct 31;98(4):797–803.
12. Ethics Committee of the American Society for Reproductive Medicine. Consideration of the gestational carrier: a committee opinion. Fertil Steril. 2013 June;99(7):1838–41.
13. Practice Committee of American Society for Reproductive Medicine and Practice Committee of Society for Assisted Reproductive Technology. Recommendations for practices utilizing gestational carriers: a committee opinion. Fertil Steril. 2015;103(1):e1–8.
14. Perkins KM, Boulet SL, Jamieson DJ, Kissin DM. Trends and outcomes of gestational surrogacy in the United States. Fertil Steril. 2016 Apr 14; https://doi.org/10.1016/j.fertnstert.2016.03.050.
15. Teh WT, McBain J, Rogers P. What is the contribution of embryo-endometrial asynchrony to implantation failure? J Assist Reprod Genet. 2016;33(11):1419–30.
16. Kasius A, Smit JG, Torrance HL, Eijkemans MJ, Mol BW, Opmeer BC, Broekmans FJ. Endometrial thickness and pregnancy rates after IVF: a systematic review and meta-analysis. Hum Reprod Update. 2014;20:530–41.
17. Franchin R, Righini C, Ayoubi J-M, Olivennes F, de Ziegler D, Frydman R. New look at endometrial echogenicity: objective computer assisted measurements predict endometrial receptivity in in vitro fertilization-embryo transfer. Fertil Steril. 2000;74:274–81.
18. Society for Assisted Reproductive Technology. SART: National Summary Report [Internet]; 2016. [Cited 2016 Oct 3]. Available from: https://www.sartcorsonline.com/Csr/Public?ClinicPKID=0#patient-first-attempt
19. Söderström-Anttila V, Wennerholm UB, Loft A, Pinborg A, Aittomäki K, Romundstad LB, et al. Surrogacy: outcomes for surrogate mothers, children and the resulting families - a systematic review. Hum Reprod Update. 2016;22(2):260–76.
20. Blake L, Casey P, Jadva V, Golombok S. Marital stability and quality in families created by assisted reproduction techniques: a follow-up study. Reprod Biomed Online. 2012;25(7):678–83.
21. Golombok S, Mellish L, Jennings S, Casey P, Tasker F, Lamb ME. Adoptive gay father families: parent-child relationships and Children's psychological adjustment. Child Dev. 2014;85(2):456–68.
22. American College of Obstetricians and Gynecologists' Committee on Ethics. ACOG Committee Opinion No. 660: family building through gestational surrogacy. Obstet Gynecol. 2016 March;127:e97–e103.
23. Braverman AM, Corson SL. A comparison of oocyte donors' and gestational carriers/surrogates' attitudes towards third party reproduction. J Assist Reprod Genet. 2002;19(10):462–9.
24. Center for American Progress. Guide to State Surrogacy Laws [Internet]. 2016; [cited 3 Oct 2016]. Available from: https://www.americanprogress.org/issues/women/news/2007/12/17/3758/guide-to-state-surrogacy-laws/
25. Shenfield F, Pennings G, De Mouzon J, Ferraretti AP, Goossens V. ESHRE's good practice guide for cross-border reproductive care for centers and practitioners. Hum Reprod. 2011 Jul 1;26(7):1625–7.

Uterus Transplantation: An Experimental Approach

55

Mats Brännström and Jana E. C. Pittman

Absolute uterine factor infertility (AUFI) was considered untreatable until recently, when uterus transplantation (UTx) proved its potential as an effective treatment [1]. In 2014, live births were reported after transplantation, using an altruistic living donor [1] and a recipient's mother [2] as the uterus donors.

Women with AUFI have either absence of a uterus (congenital/surgical) or abnormalities (anatomic/functional) that prevent embryo implantation or further pregnancy. The uterine absence can occur from birth as part of the Mayer-Rokitansky-Kuster-Hauser (MRKH) syndrome, affecting around 1:4000 girls [3]. This is the predominant group where UTx attempts have been performed but represent less than 3% of women with AUFI. The MRKH girls have an absence of the vagina above the hymen and absence of a uterus. The uterus may be replaced by rudimentary tissue above the vaginal dimple and bilaterally on the pelvic sidewalls by two small buds of myometrial tissue. A large proportion of women with MRKH have additional malformations in the urinary/renal system, with unilateral renal agenesis being the most prevalent co-malformation. The first recipient to give birth after UTx had a single kidney, and this may have been a major underlying cause of preeclampsia [4] that she developed [1].

The most prevalent cause of AUFI is uterine absence after a hysterectomy, which is the most frequent major gynecological surgical procedure that women may undergo. Hysterectomy during fertile age could be secondary to benign disease (leiomyoma or endometriosis), malignancy (cervical or endometrial cancer), or postpartum complications (massive obstetric bleeding because of uterine atony, uterine rupture, or invasive placentation).

Anatomical uterine abnormalities that preclude pregnancy are present in every case of hypoplastic uterus as well as in women with the unification defects such as unicornuate or bicornuate uterus. While there is no difference in conception rates in bicornuate/unicornuate uteri, in comparison with normal uteri, increased rates of first-trimester miscarriage occur [5]. Increased rates of preterm labor and fetal malpresentation later in pregnancy are also more common in these uterine malformations [5].

Other causes of uterine factor infertility relate to the presence of adenomyosis or radiation injury of the uterus, with secondary repeated miscarriage/implantation failure. Uterus transplantation may provide a treatment for these women, as well as for women with no obvious uterine disease on radiology imaging but with repeated miscarriage/implantation failure despite high-quality oocytes/embryos.

Intrauterine adhesions, most commonly following curettage or endometritis, are usually treatable by hysteroscopic resection. However, despite repeated hysteroscopy, almost 70% of those with severe intrauterine adhesions stage 3 and 4 remain infertile [6]. Uterus transplantation will then be the only infertility treatment for these women.

The overall prevalence of AUFI is estimated to be around 20,000 women of fertile age in a population of 100 million [7].

Previously, the two options for women with AUFI to acquire motherhood were adoption or use of a gestational carrier. Adoption is not acceptable in all societies and if accepted often excludes lesbian couples or single mothers. Gestational surrogacy may be practiced either as an altruistic or commercial arrangement. In most countries, this procedure is not allowed due to legal, religious, and/or ethical reasons. Uterus transplantation would be the only solution for AUFI that provides full motherhood concerning genetics, gestation, and legal aspects. Moreover, the typical risks of pregnancy (thromboembolism, hypertension, preeclampsia, diabetes, etc.) and those associated with delivery, such as pelvic floor dysfunction, are taken by the mother and not by

M. Brännström (✉)
Department of Obstetrics and Gynecology, Sahlgrenska Academy, University of Gothenburg, Gothenburg, Sweden

Stockholm IVF, Stockholm, Sweden
e-mail: brannstrom@obgyn.gu.se

J. E. C. Pittman
Western Sydney University School of Medicine, Campbelltown, NSW, Australia

G. N. Allahbadia et al. (eds.), *Textbook of Assisted Reproduction*, https://doi.org/10.1007/978-981-15-2377-9_55

a third person as in gestational surrogacy. However, it should be acknowledged that in live donor UTx, the woman donating her womb to the woman with AUFI is also at risk.

Thirty-six UTx attempts have been performed from 2013 and until November 2017, with around half of them published as scientific reports (Table 55.1). Previous to 2013, two failed attempts were performed in settings with no surgical preparation or research prior to the procedure. The first human UTx case in the world was performed (2000) in Saudi Arabia using a live donor [8]. Shortly after transplantation a necrotic uterus was removed. The second UTx attempt in the world occurred in Turkey (2011), which involved a deceased donor UTx procedure [9]. Around 2 years after UTx, two early miscarriages occurred [10], but at 6 years after a successful UTx, delivery of a healthy child has not yet been reported.

Modern, animal-based research on UTx was initiated around the millennium shift. Initial research included rodents, which was followed by domestic species and subsequently by nonhuman primate models. The models were used to investigate surgery, tolerability to ischemia, detection of rejection, immunosuppression, and fertility [12, 13]. This research-based approach follows the established Moore criteria [14] and IDEAL recommendations [15] for introduction of surgical innovations.

In this review article, the UTx animal research with fertility outcome as end point and all published human cases from 2013 and onward are covered in detail.

55.1 Animal UTx Research on Fertility

Aspects of fertility post-UTx have been studied in several animal species, and the experiments have included models with autologous, syngeneic, and allogeneic models. The syngeneic and autologous UTx models only test the results of UTx surgery, altering supply and outflow of blood to the uterus and changing fixations or position of the uterus. Additional allogeneic UTx models test the effects of immunosuppression and possible rejection episodes before and during pregnancy.

55.1.1 Fertility in Macaque UTx Model

A nonhuman primate model, such as the macaque, is the final preclinical stage with most relevance to the human setting. The first, and so far only, offspring reported in a nonhuman primate species was after autologous UTx in the macaque [16]. In that report, two cynomolgus macaques underwent autotransplantation with unilateral preservation of the oviduct and the ovary. In one case, pregnancy and delivery were achieved, and in that animal the anastomoses were between the uterine arteries and the external iliac arteries bilaterally, and venous outflow was only on the side of the preserved ovary-oviduct, by one deep uterine vein and the ovarian vein. Anastomoses were end-to-side of the small graft vessels, with a diameter of 1–2.5 mm, to the external iliac vessels with use of 12–0 sutures. In the animal with subsequent pregnancy, the complicated surgery took a total of 13.5 h, with almost 5 h of warm ischemia, to accomplish the four vascular connections. Spontaneous menstruation restarted after 3 months, and natural mating occurred. At gestational week 5, a viable intrauterine pregnancy was confirmed. The pregnancy was uneventful until day 143, when genital bleeding occurred. A caesarean section was preformed, due to signs of partial placental abruption, and a live offspring was delivered but with fetal respiratory distress. No attempts were made to secure further survival of the fetus. No studies exist on fertility after allogeneic UTx in a nonhuman primate species.

55.1.2 Fertility in Sheep UTx Model

The UTx model in the sheep has been tested by numerous UTx teams worldwide and is a good model to conduct preclinical training. Both the autologous and the allogeneic UTx models have been tested concerning fertility after UTx.

The autologous UTx model was with uterine-tubal-ovarian transplantation and end-to-side vascular anastomoses of the uterine artery, utero-ovarian vein, and the ovarian artery, including an aortic patch, to the external iliacs [17]. Around 3 months after auto-UTx, five ewes were placed with rams for mating which occurred in 4/5 ewes. Three of these conceived and delivered normal size offspring via cesarean section around 2 weeks before term (145 days). The offspring were not followed up after birth.

The allogeneic sheep UTx model involved hysterectomy with short vascular pedicles of the uterine artery and vein, divided above the ureteric level [18]. The same surgery was done in parallel in the recipient, and the uteri could be shifted between the outbred sheep. Transplantation was by bilateral end-to-end anastomosis of the uterine arteries and veins, as well as attachment of the vaginal rim of the graft to the open vaginal vault of the recipient. Twelve transplanted ewes received maintenance immunosuppression of cyclosporine with addition of prednisone during the first post-UTx week. Around 3 months after UTx, embryo transfer (ET) was performed in five ewes receiving donor, single fresh cleavage-stage ET in three cases, and frozen blastocyst ET in two cases. Three of these resulted in pregnancy; one was an ectopic gestation, one carried to 105 days, and the third delivered a premature but fully developed lamb with normal for gestational

Table 55.1 Uterus transplant experience as of September 2017 divided into publish cases and those communicated by personal communications

City, country	Publication/personal communication	Year	Donor type	Surgery donor	Birth/pregnancy
Jeddah, Saudi Arabia	Pub [8]	2000	LD (x1)	Laparotomy	
Antalya, Turkey	Pub [9, 10]	2011	DD (x1)	Laparotomy	
Gothenburg, Sweden	Pub [1, 2, 11]/personal comm	2013	LD (x9)	RAL	8 births
Xian, China	Pub	2017	LD (x2)	Laparotomy	
Prague, Czech Republic	Personal comm	2016	DD (x4), LD (x4)	Laparotomy	
Cleveland, USA	Pub	2016	DD (x1)	Laparotomy	
Sao Paulo, Brazil	Pub	2016	DD (x2)	Laparotomy	1 pregnant
Dallas, USA	Pub	2016–2017	LD (x6), DD (x1)	Laparotomy	
Tubingen, Germany	Personal comm	2016–2017	LD (x2)	Laparotomy	
Belgrade, Serbia	Personal comm	2017	LD (x1) monozygotic twins	Laparotomy	1 pregnant
Guangzhou, China	Personal comm	2017	LD (x1)	Laparotomy	
Pune, India	Personal comm	2017	LD (x2)	Laparotomy	

LD Live Donor, *DD* Deceased Donor

age markers [18]. This demonstrated success of UTx in an allotransplanted large animal model for the first time.

55.1.3 Fertility in Rabbit UTx Model

Only one study has examined fertility after UTx in the rabbit model. Nine allogeneic UTx procedures were done in New Zealand white rabbits with proven fertility of both donors and recipients [19]. The uterus with the entire vascular tree including uterine vessels, internal iliacs, as well as the lower abdominal parts of the caval vein and aorta was surgical isolated. The two anastomoses were aorto-aortic and cavo-caval end-to-side. Immunosuppression was with tacrolimus. After a post-transplantation recovery period of 2 months, vitrified donor morulae-stage embryos were transferred into one rabbit after ovulation-induction with hCG. A total of 17 embryos were thawed and placed inside the two uterine horns during a laparotomy procedure. Nine days after ET, ultrasound detected a fetal sac with a pregnancy and heartbeat, which continued to grow for 7 more days [19]. However, spontaneous abortion with fetal resorption then occurred. The cause of the pregnancy arrest could not clearly be identified, but did not seem to be related to diminished blood flow, since at autopsy, the size of the anastomosis opening of the internal iliac artery of the graft was normal.

55.1.4 Fertility in Rat UTx Model

The rat UTx model was extensively used in the early preclinical trials. Fertility was tested both after syngeneic and allogeneic UTx. In syngeneic UTx, inbred Lewis rats were used as both donors and recipients [20]. The model was with orthotopic UTx, after hemi-hysterectomy of the left uterine horn, and with anastomoses end-to-end between the right common iliacs of the graft and the recipient. A vaginal-vaginal end-to-end anastomosis was achieved with the upper part of the right uterine anastomosed to the tip of the uterine graft to allow for normal fertilization by spontaneous mating. Controls were with left-sided hemi-hysterectomy. The pregnancy rate was similar in UTx animals as in controls, and there was no difference in pups per pregnancy. Growth trajectory, up to 60 days after birth, was similar in offspring from animals of the UTx group and the sham-operated control group.

The first ever report of fertility after allogeneic UTx explored this in the rat model [21]. The uterus donors were of the Dark Agouti strain, and the recipients were Lewis rats, with discordance of two major histocompatibility sites (RT1, RT2). Tacrolimus immunosuppression was given via mini-osmotic pumps to prevent rejection. As predetermined in the ethics approval, the experiments were terminated by cesarean sections at 2/3 through pregnancy. The pregnancy rates (number of pregnant females/total number of females within group) were similar and around 60% in the UTx group and in the tacrolimus-control group that had been sham-operated and also received tacrolimus. Moreover, median ranges of fetus per animal were similar in these two groups but lower than in the non-tacrolimus control group, with animals that had been sham-operated but had not received tacrolimus treatment. This demonstration of pregnancy after allogeneic UTx for the first time in any species was a fundamental proof of the concept of UTx, as a possible future treatment of AUFI in humans.

In a follow-up study, the allogeneic combination of Lewis rats, as uterus donors, and Piebald-Virol-Glaxo rats, as recipients, was used and with tacrolimus as maintenance immunosuppression [22]. The pregnancy rate was somewhat lower in the UTx group, as compared to the two sham-operated control groups, with one of them also receiving tacrolimus. Birth weights of UTx offspring were the same as controls, and up to 16 weeks, the growth trajectory of the pups was also unaltered in comparison with controls. This data indicated for the first time that allogeneic UTx may be regarded as safe in terms of perinatal outcome, at least in a rodent species.

55.1.5 Fertility in Mouse UTx Model

The first ever UTx with successful implantation was in the mouse, with a syngeneic donor uterus transplanted into a heterotopic position and the cervix of the uterine graft positioned intra-abdominally [23]. The transplantation model was with vascular anastomoses of the caval vein and the aorta of the graft coupled end-to-side to the mid-abdominal parts of the aorta and vena cava of the recipient, using microsurgery to anastomose the vessels with 11–0 sutures. Due to this being a syngeneic transplantation between inbred female of C57BL76xCBA/ca F-1 hybrids, no immunosuppression was required as immunological rejection would not occur. In the initial report of pregnancies after ET, accomplished by a transmyometrial approach through a small midline abdominal incision, only occasional early pregnancies were seen [23]. The low implantation rate was most likely due to the fact that the uterine cavity accumulated fluid, secondary to the intra-abdominally positioned cervix developing mucous clogging inside the canal.

In subsequent mouse UTx models, the procedure was modified to avoid intrauterine fluid accumulation by exteriorizing the uterine cervix as a cervical cutaneous stoma, allowing for drainage of uterine/cervical mucus [24]. The mouse was used as its own control with the native uterus kept in the transplanted animals, to compare implantation rate and pregnancy rate. Three to six blastocysts were transferred (transmyometrial through a mini-midline incision) into each of the grafted and native uteri. Pregnancy rate per uterus was similar in the transplanted uteri as compared to the native control uteri within the same animals and when compared to the uteri of non-transplanted animals with sham operations. The offspring were of normal birth weight, and the growth trajectory up to adulthood followed the normal curves. Both male and female offspring from transplanted uteri showed normal fertility.

An additional study in the syngeneic mouse model focused on the effect of ischemic time, between organ harvesting and transplantation. Live offspring was demonstrated after cold ischemic conditions for 24 h but not after 48 h [25], indicating that the uterus is greatly tolerable to ischemic conditions. There are no studies testing fertility after allogeneic UTx in the mouse.

55.2 Clinical Trials

The human UTx attempts performed within the context of proper clinical trials and with published data are reported below. That will not include the first two cases, from 2000 [8] to 2011 [9, 10], that are not registered as clinical trials or resulted in any live birth.

55.2.1 The Swedish Clinical Trial and Results

Nine LD UTx procedures were performed in Sweden in 2013, within an observational clinical trial [26]. Eight recipients had MRKH, and one had undergone hysterectomy for cervical cancer. Comprehensive medical and psychological investigations were completed on donors, recipients, and partners of recipients [27]. All donors had achieved normal pregnancies, and none had a history of repeated miscarriages or pre-/post-term delivery. The uterus recovery, with dissection of the uterus with bilaterally vascular pedicles including segments of the internal iliacs, had durations of 10.5–13 h [26]. The perioperative outcomes of the donors were favorable, and no patient needed blood transfusion. One donor acquired a ureteric-vaginal fistula, presenting 2 weeks after hysterectomy, possibly due to thermic injury from diathermy. Repair of the fistula was conducted 3 months post uterus donation with reimplantation of the ureter. That patient and all other donors were in good psychological and medical health, at the 1-year follow-up after surgery [28].

The recipient surgery was initiated prior to final graft retrieval and back-table preparation. Surgical preparation, including dissection of the external iliacs and vaginal vault with separation from the bladder and rectum, was done prior to the removal of the uterus from the recipient. This vaginal vault preparation was somewhat more cumbersome in patients with MRKH as opposed to the patient that had undergone hysterectomy, possibly because of the shorter vagina in the MRKH patients and variations in the anatomy of the uterine rudiment above the vaginal vault. After graft procurement in the donor and back-table preparation, the chilled and flushed uterus was positioned inside the recipient's pelvis. Anastomosis was by bilateral end-to-side anastomoses to the external iliacs of the uterine pedicles that included uterine vessels and the anterior iliac arteries as well as patches/segments of the internal iliac veins. Surgical duration was 4–5 h, and the patients stayed in the hospital for up to 9 days. The immunosuppression regimen was induction with two perioperative doses of thymoglobulin plus methylprednisolone. From the day of surgery, tacrolimus and mycophenolate mofetil (MMF) were also given daily, and oral glucocorticoids were given for 4 days [26]. After 8 months, MMF was discontinued if no or only one rejection episode had occurred during this period, but in patients with several rejection episodes, MMF was replaced with azathioprine. The 6-month outcome [26] was that seven out of nine uteri were still in place. Two uterine grafts were removed within the first 4 months. The causes were bilateral thrombotic occlusion of the uterine vessels in one case and persistent intrauterine infection, developing into an intrauterine abscess, in the other case [26].

During the first post-UTx year, uterine artery blood flow was within normal ranges in all seven patients [29]. Interestingly, protocol cervical biopsies revealed that five out of seven women had subclinical, mild rejection episodes during the first year, but all episodes of rejection were reversed with brief courses of corticosteroids or increments of tacrolimus [11, 29]. The psychological outcomes of recipients and partners were overall optimism, with only minor anxiety concerning graft survival during the first 3 months post-UTx [30].

According to the study protocol, around 12 months after UTx, single ETs were performed. The first live birth after UTx took place in Sweden, on September 4, 2014 [1], after becoming pregnant on their first ET with a cleavage stage embryo. By definition, this was the first successful UTx procedure, since the final goal of every UTx is a healthy baby. However, the patient was the fifth woman to undergo UTx in the Swedish trial [26] and the seventh UTx case worldwide [8, 9, 26]. In this successful UTx case [1], a rejection episode at gestational week 18 was diagnosed, which was effectively reversed by an intermittent increase in corticosteroids. The pregnancy was uneventful from then on, and she worked full time up until 31 full weeks and 5 days when she acquired a strong headache and was admitted to the hospital with preeclampsia. During the following morning, a cesarean section was performed, and a healthy baby boy with normal weight for gestational age (1775 g; −11%) was delivered.

The second UTx baby [2] was delivered in November 2014 by an elective caesarean section, planned for 35 + 0, but it was brought forward 3 days due to cholestasis. This pregnancy was also successful on the first ET, which in this case was a blastocyst. The baby was of normal (+4%) birth weight. The uniqueness of this case is that the donor was the mother of the woman that delivered the child. Therefore, the same uterus had been used to bridge three generations.

These first [1] and second [2] UTx children, as well as the six children [11] that were delivered in 2014–2017, are all healthy. The take-home baby rate among the seven UTx women that have undergone ET attempts is now 6/7, and the clinical pregnancy rate is 7/7, with one recipient having had miscarriages as late as gestational week 15. This substantial efficiency of UTx, at this initial experimental stage, clearly indicates that UTx will have a future clinical role as an established treatment for AUFI.

In Sweden, a second UTx trial with the live donor concept has been initiated. So far, two cases have been completed using robotic-assisted laparoscopy for donor surgery, with surgically favorable outcomes in the donor and graft survival for several months in the recipient. In 2018, the plan is to complete an additional six to eight cases and start ET attempts in the first two cases.

55.2.2 The Chinese Clinical Trial and Results

The twelfth UTx attempt in the word occurred in China in late 2015 [31]. The case utilized robotic-assisted laparoscopy for the uterus retrieval in the 42-year-old premenopausal mother who donated the uterus to her 22-year-old daughter with MRKH. The surgery followed the general principles used in the Swedish trial [26] but with one major difference. The secured uterine outflow was not through the uterine veins but through the utero-ovarian veins. The reason for this is unclear, but it is stated in the paper [31] that the uterine veins were difficult to identify. The use of the utero-ovarian veins necessitated oophorectomy in the 42-year-old donor, who may have been around a decade away from menopause. Naturally, this raises concerns of long-term medical consequences for the donor in relation to osteoporosis and cardiovascular disease. However, the surgical duration in the donor was substantially reduced due to avoidance of the complicated dissection of the uterine veins that are firmly attached to the ureters, with several communicating branches between the deep and superficial uterine veins. The retrieval of the graft was through the vagina. The donor surgery was by laparotomy, with bilateral end-to-side anastomosis to the external iliac vessels [31]. It is unclear whether there would be sufficient lengths of the utero-ovarian veins in a future pregnancy. After this kind UTx procedure, the outflow and attachment of the veins would be through the external iliac vessels of the pelvis, instead of the upper abdominal parts of the caval vein and the left renal veins. During pregnancy, the uterine inlets of the utero ovarian veins move toward the upper abdomen with the increase in uterine size. This may lead to stretching of these veins and compromised blood flow.

The duration of the recipient surgery was two times that of the Swedish trial, indicating that the anastomosis of the utero-ovarian veins, with minimal thickness of the vascular walls, is far more difficult than when using a patch/segment of the internal iliac vein [26]. This prolonged warm ischemic time did not seem to influence the function of the uterus since the patient had spontaneous and regular menstruations from around 1.5 months after UTx. In the report [31] that presents the results at 1 year after UTx, it was stated that ten spontaneous menses had occurred and that ET attempts would start during the second post-transplantation year. The patient only experienced one rejection episode (after 2.5 weeks), which was diagnosed by clinical symptoms (low backache, fatigue, and fever) and confirmed by increased

CD4/CD8 ratio. The rejection resolved by iv corticosteroid treatment for 3 days. Reports of results of ET, pregnancy, and live birth are expected to come in 2018. The results will be of interest in the future development of robotic-assisted uterine retrieval with exclusive usage of the ovarian veins as outflow blood vessels.

55.2.3 The US Clinical Trials and Results

Two UTx trials have been initiated in the USA. The first study involved using a deceased donor UTx procedure and is presently underway at Cleveland Clinic. The first case that took place in February 2016 unfortunately ended in graft removal around 2 weeks later and has been presented both in the media and mentioned in a scientific report [32]. There was a long cold ischemic time of more than 8 h, since the graft had to be transported interstate. A fungal vaginal infection was present in the donor, and this was not diagnosed at retrieval. This fungus contamination later affected also the vascular tree of the graft, and the graft was removed due to an infectious aneurysm of the internal iliac artery of the graft.

The second UTx trial in the USA was a live donor trial that was initiated in Dallas in September 2016 [33]. The results of the first five attempts have been reported. A similar laparotomy technique as in the Swedish trial [26] was used, with surgical durations of around 8 h for retrieval. The first three cases failed, due to vascular complications that were related to both inflow and outflow problems [33]. In these three initial cases, the grafts were removed during the initial 2 weeks. In the subsequent two cases, graft survival for 3 and 6 months has been reported.

55.2.4 The Brazilian Clinical Trial and Results

The third deceased UTx case in the world was completed in Sao Paulo, Brazil, in September 2016 [34]. It involved one UTx procedure from a deceased donor to a young woman with MRKH. The procurement process was purposely prolonged to avoid vascular leakage on the back-table and at reperfusion after unclamping in the recipient. The postoperative recovery has been fine with regular menstruations. As of September 2017, a 20-week long pregnancy was reported. This is a promising result and may become the first live birth following a deceased donor UTx.

55.3 Conclusion

Uterus transplantation is the first available treatment for AUFI. As a consequence of meticulous research preparations in a variety of animal models, the initial human clinical trials in 2013 have been successful with several births that occurred during 2014–2017 period. A number of new trials are underway in all continents. Uterus transplantation should stay at this experimental stage for several years, as this will allow time to optimize the procedure further and ensure that it is safe concerning long-term medical and psychological effects for donors, recipients, and children.

References

1. Brännström M, Johannesson L, Bokström H, Kvarnström N, Mölne J, Dahm-Kähler P, et al. Live birth after uterus transplantation. Lancet. 2015;385:607–16.
2. Brännström M, Bokström M, Dahm-Kähler P, Diaz-Garcia C, Ekberg J, Enskog A, et al. One uterus bridging three generations; first live birth after mother-to-daughter uterus transplantation. Fertil Steril. 2016;107:261–6.
3. Oppelt P, Renner SP, Kellermann A, Brucker S, Hauser GA, Ludwig KS, et al. Clinical aspects of Mayer-Rokitansky-Kuester-Hauser syndrome: recommendations for clinical diagnosis and staging. Hum Reprod. 2006;21:792–7.
4. Brännström M, Diaz-Garcia C, Johannesson L, Dahm-Kähler P, Bokström H. Live birth after uterus transplantation – authors' reply. Lancet. 2015;385:2352–3.
5. Chan YY, Jayaprakasan K, Tan A, Thornton JG, Coomarasamy A, Raine-Fenning NJ. Reproductive outcomes in women with congenital uterine anomalies: a systematic review. Ultrasound Obstet Gynecol. 2011;38:371–81.
6. Fernandez H, Al-Najjar F, Chauveaud-Lambling A, Frydman R, Gervaise A. Fertility after treatment of Asherman's syndrome stage 3 and 4. J Minim Invasive Gynecol. 2006;13:398–402.
7. Sieunarine K, Zakaria FB, Boyle DC, Corless DJ, Noakes DE, Lindsay I, et al. Possibilities for fertility restoration: a new surgical technique. Int Surg. 2005;90:249–56.
8. Fageeh W, Raffa H, Jabbah H, Marzouki A. Transplantation of the human uterus. Int J Gynaecol Obstet. 2002;76:245–51.
9. Özkan Ö, Akar ME, Özkan Ö, Erdogan O, Hadimioglu N, Yilmaz M, et al. Preliminary results of the first human uterus transplantation from a multiorgan donor. Fertil Steril. 2013;99:470–6.
10. Erman Akar M, Özkan Ö, Aydinuraz B, Dirican K, Cincik M, Mendilcioglu I, et al. Clinical pregnancy after uterus transplantation. Fertil Steril. 2013;100:1358–63.
11. Mölne J, Broecker V, Ekberg J, Nilsson O, Dahm-Kähler P, Brännström M. Monitoring of human uterus transplantation with cervical biopsies: a provisional scoring system for rejection. Am J Transplant. 2017;17:1628–36.
12. Brännström M, Diaz-Garcia C, Hanafy A, Olausson M, Tzakis A. Uterus transplantation: animal research and human possibilities. Fertil Steril. 2012;97:1269–76.
13. Brännström M. The Swedish uterus transplantation project; the story behind the project. Acta Obstet Gynecol Scand. 2015;94:675–9.
14. Moore FD. Ethical problems special to surgery. Arch Surg. 2000;135:14–6.
15. McCulloch P, Altman DG, Campbell WB, Flum DR, Glasziou P, Marshall JC, et al. No surgical innovation without evaluation: the IDEAL recommendations. Lancet. 2009;374:1105–12.
16. Mihara M, Kisu I, Hara H, Iida T, Araki J, Shim T, et al. Uterine autotransplantation in cynomolgus macaques: the first case of pregnancy and delivery. Hum Reprod. 2012;27:2332–40.
17. Wranning CA, Marcickiewicz J, Enskog A, Dahm-Kähler P, Hanafy A, Brännström M. Fertility after autologous ovine uterine-tubal-ovarian transplantation by vascular anastomosis to the external iliac vessels. Hum Reprod. 2010;25:1973–9.

18. Ramirez ER, Ramirez Nessetti DK, Nessetti MB, Khatamee M, Wolfson MR, Shaffer TH, et al. Pregnancy and outcome of uterine allotransplantation and assisted reproduction in sheep. J Minim Invasive Gynecol. 2011;18:238–45.
19. Saso S, Petts G, David AL, Thum MY, Chatterjee J, Vicente JS, et al. Achieving an early pregnancy following allogeneic uterine transplantation in a rabbit model. Eur J Obstet Gynecol Reprod Biol. 2015;85:164–9.
20. Wranning CA, Akhi SN, Diaz-Garcia C, Brännström M. Pregnancy after syngeneic uterus transplantation and spontaneous mating in the rat. Hum Reprod. 2011;26:553–8.
21. Diaz-Garcia C, Akhi SN, Wallin A, Pellicer A, Brännström M. First report on fertility after allogeneic uterus transplantation. Acta Obstet Gynecol Scand. 2010;89:1491–4.
22. Diaz-Garcia C, Johannesson L, Shao R, Bilig H, Brännström M. Pregnancy after allogeneic uterus transplantation in the rat: perinatal outcome and growth trajectory. Fertil Steril. 2014;102:1545–52.
23. Racho El-Akouri R, Kurlberg G, Dindelegan G, Mölne J, Wallin A, Brännström M. Heterotopic uterine transplantation by vascular anastomosis in the mouse. J Endocrinol. 2002;174:157–66.
24. Racho El-Akouri R, Kurlberg G, Brännström M. Successful uterine transplantation in the mouse: pregnancy and postnatal development of offspring. Hum Reprod. 2003;18:2018–23.
25. Racho El-Akouri R, Wranning CA, Mölne J, Kurlberg G, Brännström M. Pregnancy in transplanted mouse uterus after long-term cold ischaemic preservation. Hum Reprod. 2003;18:2024–30.
26. Brännström M, Johannesson L, Dahm-Kähler P, Enskog A, Mölne J, Kvarnström N, et al. The first clinical uterus transplantation trial: a six months report. Fertil Steril. 2014;101:1228–36.
27. Järvholm S, Johannesson L, Brännström M. Psychological aspects in pre-transplantation assessments of patients prior to entering the first uterus transplantation trial. Acta Obstet Gynecol Scand. 2015;94:1035–8.
28. Kvarnström N, Järvholm S, Johannesson L, Dahm-Kähler P, Olausson M, Brännström M. Live donors of the initial observational study of uterus transplantation-psychological and medical follow-up until 1 year after surgery in the 9 cases. Transplantation. 2017;101:664–70.
29. Johannesson L, Kvarnström N, Mölne J, Dahm-Kähler P, Enskog A, Diaz-Garcia C, et al. Uterus transplantation trial: 1-year outcome. Fertil Steril. 2015;103:199–204.
30. Järvholm S, Johannesson L, Clarke A, Brännström M. Uterus transplantation trial: psychological evaluation of recipients and partners during the post-transplantation year. Fertil Steril. 2015;104:1010–5.
31. Wei L, Xue T, Tao KS, Zhang G, Zhao GY, Yu SQ, et al. Modified human uterus transplantation using ovarian veins for venous drainage: the first report of surgically successful robotic-assisted uterus procurement and follow-up for 12 months. Fertil Steril. 2017;108:346–56.
32. Flyckt RL, Farrell RM, Perni UC, Tzakis AG, Falcone T. Deceased donor uterine transplantation; innovation and adaption. Obstet Gynecol. 2016;128:837–42.
33. Testa G, Koon EC, Johannesson L, McKenna GJ, Anthony T, Klintmalm GB, et al. Living donor uterus transplantation: a single center's observations and lessons learned from early setbacks to technical success. Am J Transplant. 2017;17:2901–10.
34. Soares JM, Ejzenberg D, Andraus W, D'Albuquerque LA, Baracat EC. First Latin uterine transplantation: we can do it! Clinics (Sao Paulo). 2016;71:627–8.

Part VI

Fertility Preservation

Semen Cryopreservation: A Practical Guide

56

Charlene A. Alouf, Gerard F. Celia, and Grace Centola

56.1 Introduction

Although first noted as a rudimentary observation in 1776, the initial report of successful sperm cryopreservation by Sherman and colleagues was in the 1950s [1, 2], with the first birth resulting from artificial insemination with cryopreserved sperm reported in 1953 [3, 4]. As methods for sperm freezing evolved leading to improved recoveries, pregnancy, and live birth rates, the use became commonly widespread as a successful method to preserve fertility in patients with spermatogenic failure, severe oligozoospermia, anatomical deviations, or for those at risk of iatrogenic sterilization from medical procedures or treatment. Frequently patients also exercise the right to bank sperm as an insurance policy prior to vasectomy, or even following a successful reversal, as the vas deferens can fibrose after the vasovasostomy, leading to a reduction in sperm concentration [5]. Sperm cryopreservation and long-term storage have also been recommended prior to military travel, testicular surgery, or hormonal replacement therapy [6–8]. More recently, sperm banking has been recommended as insurance against the effects of aging on male reproduction, which includes increased risks of autism and schizophrenia with increased paternal age [9–12]. Sperm banking may also provide the potential for fertility chemotherapy or surgical treatments [13, 14]. Freezing and storage of testicular tissue has been suggested in those with azoospermia, severe oligozospermia, and Kleinfelter's condition, for example.

C. A. Alouf (✉)
Invitae, San Francisco, CA, USA

Chelsea Fertility, New York, NY, USA

Reproductive Science Center of NJ, Eatontown, NJ, USA

South Jersey Fertility Center, Marlton, NJ, USA
e-mail: charlene.alouf@gmail.com

G. F. Celia
The Jones Institute for Reproductive Medicine, Norfolk, VA, USA

Dominion Fertility, Arlington, VA, USA

G. Centola
Reproductive Laboratory and Tissue Bank Consultant, Port St. Lucie, FL, USA

Dadi, Inc., New York, NY, USA

Regarding ART, it is common to bank sperm for short-term storage as a backup for infertility treatment if the partner is absent on the day of retrieval, or there is a history of ejaculatory or collection issues [15–18]. Testicular tissue and epididymal aspirates may be frozen and stored for future use in ART cycles, to avoid repeated biopsies or the difficulties of synchronizing surgical removal of sperm with the timing of oocyte retrieval [1, 8, 9, 17–22].

The donor sperm industry accounts for most of the annual sperm freezing within the US. Trends in donor sperm use have increased in SART reported cycles alone, as shown by Gerkowicz and colleagues [23]. This abstract examined SART surveillance data reported between 1996 and 2014, with 4.4% of fresh and embryo banking cycles using frozen-thawed donor sperm (74,892 cycles). An increasing trend was observed through 2011 and remained constant through 2014. Based on these trends, much of the safety and efficacy of the sperm cryopreservation process have been established through the numerous reports with the use of donor sperm. There have been several milestones reported for the length of sperm storage prior to use leading to pregnancy with live births following both artificial insemination and IVF from sperm stored for more than 20 years [24, 25]. The greatest length of storage of sperm leading to a live birth was reported to date in 2012 with a semen specimen that was donated almost 41 years prior, suggesting the success of the process even in its earlier years [26].

As expected, the safety with the use of cryopreserved sperm has been demonstrated by larger scale donor sperm cycle analyses. Gerkowicz and colleagues found similar perinatal outcomes between donor (frozen) and non-donor, predominantly fresh sperm after adjusting for patient and cycle variables [23]. In a similar analysis of SART data, between 2012 and 2013 specifically, in which 2186 donor sperm cycles were analyzed, there were no significant differences in mis-

G. N. Allahbadia et al. (eds.), *Textbook of Assisted Reproduction*, https://doi.org/10.1007/978-981-15-2377-9_56

carriage rate, gestational age at delivery, or birth weight from the use of donor sperm [27]. A study in Denmark examined the outcomes of 1881 singletons born from donor IUI (IUI-D) compared with 4281 singletons born from IUI with husbands' sperm (IUI-H) [28]. Although the main goal of the report was to compare outcome data to spontaneous conception and that of IUI when results were adjusted for confounding variables, natural conception rates were very similar to the IUI group. There was no difference in perinatal mortality between the singletons born from either IUI-H or IUI-D. Similarly, several publications have reported the safe use of frozen surgically retrieved sperm [19, 29–31].

For specimens with parameters within normal limits at the time of the pre-freeze semen analysis, it is generally acceptable to expect approximately a 50% recovery of total motile sperm. Loss in these samples has very little impact on ICSI or conventional IVF insemination. The effect of sperm cryopreservation and thawing can be seen in all parameters of the post-thaw analysis including untoward alterations in mitochondrial function and DNA [32, 33]. Sperm recovery post-thaw depends on the quality of the sperm initially frozen [34, 35]. Recoveries from specimens frozen with low starting concentrations (<100,000 total sperm) or from specimens that were obtained through surgical removal can demonstrate complete cellular loss that can present an unexpected challenge on the day of ICSI, especially if there is not an option for donor sperm backup. Although infrequent and with a small sample size, Kathrins et al. reported a complete loss of sperm in ~7% of ejaculated samples and in 5.8% from surgically removed samples [35]. Although fresh sperm samples from TESE and from patients with severe male factor are preferred for oocyte injections, it is still in the best interest of the couple to freeze ahead of time to avoid cancellation of the retrieval or oocyte freezing in the event of azoospermia on the day of oocyte retrieval.

56.2 The Cryopreservation Process

The methods of sperm cryopreservation have evolved over the decades to promote improved recovery of motile sperm post thaw. Successful sperm cryopreservation, not only requires a basic understanding of the principles of cryobiology but also a facility with skilled laboratory staff and adequate facilities [16, 36]. Cryopreservatives are used to mitigate intracellular ice formation and osmotic shock during freeze-thaw process [1, 16]. A standard cryopreservative for sperm freezing is glycerol, either alone, or with extenders such as an appropriate buffer or a protein such as egg yolk [1, 6, 16]. Currently, most cryobanks use a combination of glycerol with egg yolk, commercially available as TEST-yolk-glycerol (TYB) freezing medium. Following slow addition of the cryopreservative with the semen specimen in order to avoid osmotic effects on the sperm cells, the specimen is aliquoted into labeled cryovials or plastic straws at a volume of 0.5 ml [6, 16, 17, 36]. Cryovials have been preferred since the vials provide a larger surface area to volume ratio for uniform sample cooling, are easily handled in the lab, and are easily labeled [36].

The freezing process involves slow or rapid cooling using a programmable freezer or a manual cooling and freezing method. Generally, the thaw rate should match the freeze rate [1, 16, 36]. The specimens can be frozen using either a programmable freezer or manual freezing. For the manual process, the vials are cooled at refrigerated temperature for approximately 30–45 min, followed by exposure to liquid nitrogen temperature by suspending the vials in liquid nitrogen vapor, followed by plunging the vials directly into a liquid nitrogen storage tank [6, 17]. Alternately, a metal cane holding the vials can be placed directly into a LN dry shipper that is charged with LN vapor for 30 min followed by plunging directly into liquid nitrogen [6]. A test vial is generally thawed by 24–48 h to determine cryosurvival.

Semen can be cryopreserved as raw, neat semen, or the motile sperm can removed from the seminal fluid utilizing gradient or simple wash-centrifugation procedures followed by freezing in liquid nitrogen [6]. Following either of these processes, the sperm are placed into a nutrient fluid, and the cryopreservative added to complete the freezing process [6]. The thawed raw semen will be further processed for intrauterine insemination or IVF/ICSI when thawed. If the specimen is processed prior to freeze, it is ready for an intrauterine insemination immediately upon thaw.

Post-thaw test results for each banked semen specimen are provided to the ART facility in advance of use of the specimen. The sperm bank client must consent for the transfer of specimens to an ART facility for the use in ART. The ART laboratory can then determine what method of processing should be used to yield adequate numbers of normal motile or viable sperm for use in standard treatments, such as intrauterine insemination, standard IVF oocyte insemination or ICSI. In each case, specific laboratory processing of the thawed semen is used to optimize recovery of the viable sperm. The laboratory will determine the number of vials to be thawed based on the recipient treatment regimen and estimated number of recoverable oocytes in the upcoming cycle. The laboratory must be attentive to the procedure used since the thawed sperm are more labile to osmotic stresses and centrifugation than fresh sperm. Generally, following thaw of the vial(s), the semen is slowly diluted with nutrient medium (to avoid osmotic shock), and then centrifuged at low speed for a maximum of 10 min. The pellet can then be resuspended and used directly for intrauterine insemination. Alternately, the washed sperm can be subjected to a swim-up or migration procedure to further extract the motile sperm for oocyte insemination or ICSI.

56.3 Surgically Obtained Sperm

Prior to the advent of ICSI (intracytoplasmic sperm injection), surgically retrieval of sperm for ART procedures was an extreme measure requiring only the highest quality specimens for a reasonable chance of success [37]. However, surgical retrieval has become a relatively common procedure, with many clinics reporting fertilization rates approaching that of freshly ejaculated specimens [38–41]. This trend has given hope that patients presenting with azoospermia may father their own biological offspring without resorting to donor samples. It has also, however, raised a number of logistical concerns for reproductive clinics and laboratories in terms of when, and for multiple cycles, how often, a sample must be obtained.

56.4 Causes of Azoopsermia

Azoospermic patients who may benefit from surgery fall into two categories: obstructive and non-obstructive. Obstructive azoospermia occurs when a physical blockage, either congenital or acquired, prevents the ejaculation of otherwise normal sperm. Congenital azoospermia can be caused by conditions such as cystic fibrosis, congenital absence of the vas deferens, or other anatomical defects. Obstructive azoospermia may also be acquired later in life through vasectomy (or failure of a vasectomy reversal), infection such as *Chlamydia trachomatis* or prostatitis, or acute injury to the reproductive tract [42]. Collectively, men with obstructive azoospermia may still show normal or reduced spermatogenesis, which allows for sperm to be obtained relatively easily by surgical means [42, 43].

In contrast, non-obstructive azoospermia is caused by a disruption of spermatogenesis. The etiologies of non-obstructive azoospermia encompass physical deformations such as varicocele; genetic disorders, such as Klinefelter's syndrome; and developmental abnormalities one of which is Sertoli cell-only syndrome (SCO), which is characterized by the lack of sperm producing cells in the testicle and thus no sperm. Due to the wide variation in potential causes, surgical approaches to obtaining sperm are often more invasive and have a lower incidence of success, in part due to the heterogeneous spermatogenesis. Despite this, surgical approaches still offer hope in even the most severe of cases [42]. It should also be noted that in some instances both obstructive and non-obstructive factors result in azoospermia, although these cases typically are treated in the same manner as pure non-obstructive azoospermia.

56.5 Surgical Approaches to Obtaining Sperm from Azoospermic Patients

There are five common methods of surgically obtaining sperm from a patient: percutaneous epididymal sperm aspiration (PESA), micro-surgical epididymal sperm aspiration (MESA), testicular sperm aspiration (TESA), testicular sperm extraction (TESE), and micro-dissection testicular sperm extraction (Micro-TESE). There are many excellent references detailing the performance and benefits of each procedure, so for this review we will limit the scope to a brief description of each and its most common application. PESA and MESA are simple puncture techniques used to aspirate sperm directly from the epididymis [42]. The specimen obtained tends to be predominantly tissue free with minimal erythrocytes. This method is used mainly in obstructive azoospermia cases, wherein the patient has adequate spermatogenesis.

Similarly, TESA is a simple puncture procedure of the testicle whereby suction is used to remove a small sample of the seminiferous tubules. As a result, TESA samples typically contain tissue that, unlike PESA and MESA, may require further processing to isolate usable sperm. This procedure is most often used in obstructive cases or as a diagnostic procedure. TESE and Micro-TESE are far more invasive procedures and are more appropriate for non-obstructive cases or as a backup to failed aspiration-based attempts [42–44]. Both of these procedures involve a surgical biopsy of the either or both testicles, resulting in a significant amount of tissue that must be processed to isolate spermatozoa. Furthermore, as the cells are obtained directly from the seminiferous tubules, they display a range of maturity and often have not undergone spermiation. Motility is typically very low and characterized by twitching or slow circling rather than forward progression. Despite this, when viable sperm are identified for ICSI, they demonstrate appreciable fertilization and pregnancy rates [40, 41, 45].

56.6 Specimen Processing

The goal of processing a specimen once it enters the reproductive laboratory is to achieve reasonable refinement, concentration, and an adequate number of aliquots, for embryologists to apply the sample to an ART procedure. Quantification of these endpoints is difficult, as laboratories vary widely in both what is expected, as well as what is tolerated. Laboratories with extensive experience using surgically obtained specimens usually prefer less refined samples and can easily recover sperm from specimens with very few sperm as compared to technical staff with less experience. For this reason, it is critical that each group defines its own standards and conducts quality control measures such that these standards may be defended. Once parameters have been established, there are numerous approaches to processing samples, each with specific advantages and drawbacks. Additionally, the time between sample retrieval and cryopreservation may vary widely by both laboratory and specimen quality. Numerous reports have shown extended culture, ranging from hours to days prior to processing, may result in a higher yield of motile sperm [45–47]. Whether this impacts final outcomes has yet to be determined.

The most basic method of processing is simple centrifugation, resulting in a concentrated pellet that is resuspended to achieve appropriate sperm-rich aliquots. This method is useful for aspirate samples that contain relatively little debris, erythrocytes, and tissue. Prior to centrifugation, the total motile count in the initial sample should be calculated so that the volume of media and/or cryoprotectant used to resuspend the pellet may be adjusted to achieve the desired final density. Although there is little consensus, studies indicate the best results are achieved with spin times less than 10 min, at no more than 800 g [48, 49]. Anecdotal reports suggest 300–400 g is optimal.

Samples with a large number of sperm and relatively high motility may also benefit from gradient centrifugation as described for ejaculated samples to remove non-motile sperm and debris [50]. Similar to basic centrifugation, this process is most effective when the sample is relatively clean, although it is further recommended that the specimen be divided onto multiple gradient columns with no more than 1 ml of the original specimen on each column. Column preparation and use should be per individual manufacturer's protocol. After centrifugation, pellets should be combined, resuspended in 0.5 ml of media, and counted to determine concentration and motility. This is then aliquoted for cryopreservation with consideration toward expected concentration at thaw.

Biopsy samples derived from TESA, TESE, and Micro-TESE are typically tissue rich. This requires the spermatozoa to be separated from the tissue prior to use and/or cryopreservation. A number of methods have been described for isolating sperm in these cases, although the most common are mincing, mechanical maceration, extrusion, and enzymatic digestion [51].

Mincing is the simplest and most common means of processing biopsy samples. The sample is first placed in a medium size petri dish (100 mm is common) in a suspension of sperm washing medium. Utilizing a scalpel or sterile razor blade the tissue is diced under a stereomicroscope into a fine suspension that can then be inspected for the presence of viable free spermatozoa using an inverted microscope. This method is simple and effective for processing sperm-rich tissue, although it may require enzymatic digestion to obtain usable sperm from poorer quality tissue samples [51–53].

Maceration is a more aggressive means of mechanically separating sperm from tissue. This method utilizes a mortar and pestle style tissue grinder in place of a blade to generate a much finer suspension of the biopsy sample. It is much faster than mincing and more effective at freeing sperm into solution; however it also poses a greater risk of damaging mature sperm. Following maceration, the sample is placed in a petri dish and a high power inverted microscope should be used to determine the presence and concentration of viable sperm.

Extrusion is a highly effective mechanical means of separating mature sperm from a biopsy sample [51]. In order to apply this technique the seminiferous tubules should be relatively intact; therefore excessive processing by the surgeon should be discouraged. Samples are placed in a dish and the tubules are initially teased away from connective tissue using small needles—insulin syringes work well. Following separation, one end of each tubule is held against the bottom of the dish, while the luminal contents are gently extruded using gentle pressure along the length of the tubule with a blunt tool. Glass Pasteur pipettes bent at a 30°–90° angle, as well as sterile microscope slides are commonly utilized for this procedure. After each tubule has been carefully processed, the dish should be searched for the presence of viable sperm. Mincing or maceration of the remaining tissue may then be performed in order to optimize recovery.

Regardless of the method used to mechanically isolate sperm from a biopsy sample, the goal is to produce a sample with as little contamination as possible. In order to optimize the separation of viable sperm from tissue, the media and final suspension in the dish should be aspirated, with care given to avoiding tissue fragments, and placed in a conical centrifuge tube. The tissue remaining should be cryopreserved in a separately labeled vial in the event additional processing is needed in the future. The suspension is then pelleted by centrifugation and may either be processed for cryopreservation as described for fresh ejaculates or exposed to 2 to 4 ml of erythrocyte lysing buffer (155 mM NH_4Cl, 10 mM $KHCO_3$, and 2 mM EDTA; pH 7.2) for 10 min at room temperature for further refinement [54]. Erythrocyte lysing buffer has been shown to greatly improve the ease with which the sample maybe used for an ICSI procedure upon thawing. Following treatment, the suspension is once again pelleted and then processed for cryopreservation as previously described.

Enzymatic digestion utilizing collagenase types IA and type IV has been shown to effectively recover sperm from samples with little or no sperm after mechanical processing [52, 53]. This method relies on incubation with the enzyme of choice for several hours in a gas controlled, humidified incubator, followed by centrifugation and resuspension of the resulting pellet, which may be then processed for cryopreservation as previously described. A potential disadvantage to this method may be the alteration of sperm membrane proteins, although the use of ICSI renders this concern largely moot [53].

56.7 Aliquoting

Decisions about the type of cryovessel to be used and the number of aliquots possible from a sample are highly dependent on individual lab practices. Factors to be considered are the anticipated number of viable sperm in the thawed sample, number of oocytes anticipated for ICSI, and the ease of recovering viable sperm. The number of viable sperm upon thaw can be estimated as approximately 50% of initial and should be verified by a test-thaw prior to use. While it is difficult to predict the number of sperm needed for a given procedure, common practice dictates that fewer sperm are needed for natural cycle IVF, minimal-stimulation IVF, and diminished ovarian reserve patients, while younger, male-factor only patients are likely to yield large numbers of mature ova requiring fertilization. The most critical factor is ease of recovery. This will vary depending on the degree of pre-freeze processing, percent motile, and of course the total number of viable sperm in the biopsy. For extremely low yield cases, individual sperm may be isolated prior to cryopreservation and novel vitrification techniques employed to ensure acceptable recovery [55]. More abundant samples should be divided into usable volumes, utilizing 0.25 cc straws, 0.5 cc vials, 0.5 cc vials, and 1.0 cc vials as carriers.

56.8 Post-Thaw

Thawing procedures should match freezing protocols as previously described. Generally, vials or straws are removed from the holding tank and placed at room temperature on the lab bench for 10–15 min. The vial can then be mixed by gentle flicking, and the vial or straw should be placed into a 37 °C incubator for an additional 10–15 min. It is important to remove viable sperm from the cryopreservative within 30 min of thaw, as extended exposure to glycerol can be detrimental to sperm vitality.

Post-thaw processing depends on the quality and nature of the sample. Sperm-rich samples with high motility may be pelleted to remove excess cryoprotectant, while more coarse samples with low motility should be diluted with pre-warmed washing media to avoid further loss of viable sperm. Incubation in a humidified, warmed incubator for 2–4 h is often beneficial in recovering motility prior to use. In the complete absence of motility, various approaches may be used to identify viable sperm, including hypo-osmotic swelling, pliability testing, or chemical treatment [51].

56.9 Informed Consent, Disposition, and Advanced Directives

State laws may vary regarding informed consent and reproductive tissue banking, including disposition. Therefore the process should be compliant with the standards and public policy of both local and national accrediting agencies and state and federal regulations including particulars regarding directed donation. The hospital or practice legal team should review and approve consent verbiage prior to use. Consent language should be reviewed annually and amended as necessary as a means to proactively reflect current legal precedent.

The content of any consent for medical or laboratory services can be rather complex and challenging even for the most informed patient. The FDA and the Joint Commission have published general requirements for informed consent in clinical research and healthcare treatments to ensure effective communication and dissemination of information [56, 57]. Additionally, in 2003 Shuster et al. published recommendations and guidance for inclusions in consents and disposition agreements [58]. Obtaining consent should not merely involve providing a signature but the opportunity to introduce a process of communication of the intentions of the laboratory and practice, of the cryopreservation procedure itself and the responsibilities of both parties, the clinic/laboratory and the male patient [56–58]. Consents should be written at the eighth grade level, with easy readability, as healthcare literacy can be low. The consent should be informative to the patient/client depositor and outline the options or plan with the signature witnessed by a laboratory or practice member or by that of a notary if signed externally. Consent should be available for review by all regulatory agencies for every specimen stored in the reproductive tissue bank [56–58].

Unlike embryos that can be the "property" of two partners, autologous sperm is the sole property of the male patient/client depositor. The contents of the consent for cryopreservation should minimally include:

- The name and address of hospital or practice.
- The date of consent.
- The printed name and signature of the client depositor/patient.
- The printed name and signature of witness.
- The name of procedure (i.e., short-term or long-term sperm cryopreservation)
- An explanation and term of short- or long-term storage and associated costs.
- The duration of the disposition agreement (quarterly, annually etc.).
- The potential risks (equipment failure, poor recovery).
- A general release of facility/practice liability.
- There is no guarantee for survival or pregnancy resulting from the use of the frozen-thawed specimen in ART and no method to predict recovery without thawing a test/QC vial as all specimens may vary within an individual at various time intervals.
- That the patient/client depositor accepts the responsibility of maintaining current contact information with the clinic/sperm bank for purposes of billing and consent renewal. An acceptable alternate contact should be provided in case the laboratory cannot contact the client depositor.

- The client must specify disposition in the event of abandonment, including attempted contact at last known address or alternative contact address via certified mail. Terms of abandonment and disposition in the event including provisions for transfer out of the facility and its associated costs should be defined within the consent.
- That the specimen(s) will be used in ART processes for intimate partner, donor oocytes or for directed donation. The specimen(s) are not for use for insemination of anonymous recipients.
- For directed donation, consents should include clear directives or stated inclusions/exclusions of use such as the number of cycles or the number of children born and in the case of a married couple in the event of divorce.
- The disposition in the event of death, incapacitation, divorce which can include:
  - Destruction.
  - Donation to research. Research should be qualified as use for QA, QC or clinical assay development. Reproductive tissues or embryos resulting from such research will not be transferred into animals or humans.
  - Directed donation with the same parameters for use as samples initially stored for directed donation.
  - Continued maintenance for use in partner ART procedures.
  - Released to another authorized, accredited facility for storage or use.
- Posthumous use must be clearly stated with intent of support [59].
- A provisional statement indicating that consent can be altered or withdrawn at any time with written notification in the presence of clinic/laboratory personnel or an outside notary.

The consent can include an information sheet for clarity and to introduce technical terminology and procedures including information related to the cryopreservation process, recoveries, and storage in liquid nitrogen or its vapors. Additionally, either the information sheet or the informed consent should outline the required minimal infectious disease work up required prior to cryopreservation. Minimally, for the protection of all specimens stored within the cryogenic tank, the patient/client depositor should be tested for:

- HIV-1 and HIV-2
- RPR with reflex
- Hepatitis B surface antigen
- Hepatitis B core antibody
- Hepatitis C
- CMV (IgG and IgM)

The communicable disease testing should be recommended even when the specimen is planned for use with an intimate partner. If a gestational carrier might need to be employed, or if the embryos might be donated in the future, additional testing would be required for FDA compliance. Furthermore, same-sex male couples may elect to use the specimens in a surrogate who is not a sexually intimate partner, and thus communicable disease testing is required by FDA regulations.

56.10 General Reproductive Tissue Bank Laboratory Practice

Cryogenic tanks should be maintained according to the laboratory quality control schedule. Liquid nitrogen levels should measure within manufacturers range or within acceptable range as established by the laboratory. It is good laboratory practice to have each tank alarmed with an established back up plan in the event of tank failure. Cryogenic tanks should not be used for clinical specimens outside of the time period of recommended use. Unless it is a "quarantine" tank, specimens should be fully immersed in the liquid phase at all times. Quarantine tanks are maintained as vapor tanks with the vials on canes located only in the upper portion of the tank to prevent liquid transfer between vials. These tanks can demonstrate a wide degree of temperature fluctuation within the vapor phase as the liquid phase evaporates. To avoid thermal fluctuations, which may impact sample integrity, there should be a more stringent minimal acceptable range for the liquid phase in vapor storage tanks.

The tank inventory should be maintained in both digital and hard copy forms and updated as samples are added and removed. Additionally a physical inventory should be performed and documented annually. Any inventory inconsistencies or missing samples should be reported to the Laboratory Director immediately.

56.11 Eye to the Future

History has revealed that the normal parameter specimen is quite resilient. Even under suboptimal conditions of freezing and storage there is minimal impact on the functionality of the sample, perhaps a result of the total number of motile sperm compensating for any loss. Challenges, however, still remain under conditions of severe impairment or near complete azoospermia, wherein individual cells risk being unrecoverable. As conventional methods are not refined enough for reliable use of these specimens in ART procedures, there are clear opportunities for advancement in this field.

More recently the methods of freeze-drying and single human sperm freezing have been introduced [60, 61]. These methods hold promise for lower concentration specimens including the minimal post rehydration or thawing processing, which may limit loss.

References

1. Shehata F, Chian RC. Cryopreservation of sperm: an overview. In: Chian RC, Quinn P, editors. Fertility cryopreservation. New York: Cambridge University Press; 2010. p. 39–45.
2. Sherman JK. Synopsis of the use of frozen human semen since 1964: state of the art of human semen banking. Fertil Steril. 1973;24:397–412.
3. Bunge RG, Sherman JK. Fertilizing capacity of frozen human spermatozoa. Nature. 1953;172:767–8.
4. Fader, S. Sperm banking a reproductive resource. California Cryobank 1993. Available from https://cryobank.com/learning-center/sperm-banking-101/sperm-banking-history/
5. Silber S. Microscopic vasectomy reversal. Fert Steril. 1997;28:1191–202.
6. Centola GM. Sperm banking, donation, and transport in the age of assisted reproduction: Federal and state regulation. In: Carrell DT, Peterson CM, editors. Reproductive endocrinology and infertility: integrating modern clinical and laboratory practice. New York: Springer; 2010. p. 509–16.
7. Ranganathan P, Mahran AM, Hallak J, et al. Sperm cryopreservation for men with nonmalignant, systemic disease: a descriptive study. J Androl. 2001;23:71–5.
8. Pacey AA. Referring patients for sperm banking. In: Pacey AA, Tomlinson MJ, editors. Sperm banking: theory and practice. Cambridge: Cambridge University Press; 2009. p. 30–40.
9. Kong FML, Masson G, Besenbacher S, Sulem P, Magnusson G, Gudjonsson SA, Sigurdsson A, et al. Rate of de novo mutations and the importance of father's age to disease risk. Nature. 2012;488:471–5.
10. D'Onofrio BM, Rickert ME, Frans E, Kuja-Halkola R, Almqvist C, Sjolander A, Larsson H, Lichtenstein P. Paternal age at childbearing and offspring psychiatric and academic morbidity. JAMA Psychiat. 2014;71(4):432–8.
11. Centola GM, Blanchard A, Demick J, Li S, Eisenberg M. Decline in sperm count and motility in young adult men from 2003-2013: observations from a U.S. sperm bank. Andrology. 2016:4(3), 270–6.
12. Sharma R, Agarwal A, Rohra VK, Assidi M, Abu-Elmagd M, Turki RF. Effects of increased paternal age on sperm quality, reproductive outcome and associated genetic risks to offspring. Reprod Biol Endocrinol. 2015;13:35.
13. Wyns C, Curaba M, Vanabelle B, Van Langendonckt A, Donnez J. Options for fertility preservation in prepubertal boys. Hum Reprod Update. 2010;16(3):312–28.
14. Van Saen D, Gies I, De Schepper J, Tournaye H, Goossens E. Can pubertal boys with Klinefelter syndrome benefit from spermatogonial stem cell banking? Hum Reprod. 2012;27(2):323–30.
15. Witt MA. Sperm banking. In: Lipshultz LI, Howards SS, editors. Infertility in the male. 3rd ed. St. Louis: Mosby Year Book; 1997. p. 501.
16. Wald M, Prins GS. Sperm banking: indications and techniques. In: Infertility in the male. 4th ed. Cambridge: Cambridge University Press; 2009. p. 596–602.
17. DiSanto M, Tarozzi N, Nadalini M, Borini A. Human sperm cryopreservation: Update on techniques, effect on DNA integrity and implications for ART. Adv Urol. 2012; https://doi.org/10.1155/2012/854837.
18. Jensen JR, Morbeck DE, Coddington CC III. Fertility preservation. Mayo Clin Proc. 2011;86(1):45–9.
19. Shin DH, Turek PJ. Sperm retrieval techniques. Nat Rev Urology. 2013;10:723–30.
20. Anger JT, Gilbert BR, Goldstein M. Cryopreservation of sperm: indications, methods and results. J Urol. 2003;170:1079–84.
21. Frydman R, Grynberg M. Male fertility preservation: innovations and questions. Fertil Steril. 2015;105:247–8.
22. Practice Committee of American Society for Reproductive Medicine; Practice Committee of Society for Assisted Reproductive Technology. Fertility preservation in patients undergoing gonadotoxic therapy or gonadectomy: a committee opinion. Fertil Steril. 2013;100:1214–23.
23. Gerkowicz SA, Crawford S, Hipp H, Boulet S, Kissin DM, Kawwass JF. Assisted reproductive technology with donor sperm: national trends and perinatal outcomes. Fertil Steril. 2017;108(3):e72.
24. Feldschuh J, Brassel J, Durso N, Levine A. Successful sperm storage for 28 years. Fertil Steril. 2005;84:1017.
25. Ome G, Atkinson AD, Pease EH, Logue JP, Brison DR, Lieberman BA. Live birth with sperm cryopreserved for 21 years prior to cancer treatment: case report. Hum Reprod. 2004;19:1488–9.
26. Szell AZ, Bierbaum RC, Hazelrigg WB, Chetkowski RJ. Live births from frozen human semen stored for 40 years. J Assist Reprod Genet. 2013;30:743–4.
27. Fritz R, Jindal S, Yu B, Vega M, Buyuk E. Does donor sperm affect birth weight, preterm birth, and miscarriage rates in fresh autologous in vitro fertilization cycles? Analysis of 46.061 cycles reported to SART. Fertil Steril. 2017;107:3.
28. Malchau SS, Loft A, Henningsen A-K, Andersen AN, Pinborg A. Perinatal outcomes in 6338 singletons born after intrauterine insemination in Denmark, 2007 to 2012: the influence of ovarian stimulation. Fertil Steril. 2014;102:1110–6.
29. Devroey P, Silber S, Nagy Z, Liu J, Tournaye H, Joris H, et al. Ongoing pregnancies and births after intracytoplasmic sperm injection with frozen-thawed epididymal spermatozoa. Hum Reprod. 1995;10:903–6.
30. Fischer R, Baukloh V, Naether OGJ, Schulze W, Salzbrunn A, Benson DM. Pregnancy after intracytoplasmic sperm injection of spermatozoa extracted from frozen-thawed testicular biopsy. Hum Reprod. 1996;11:2197–9.
31. Gil-Slamon M, Romeo J, Mingues Y. Pregnancies after intracytoplasmic sperm injection with cryopreserved testicular sperm. Hum Reprod. 1996;11:1309–13.
32. O'Connell M, McClure N, Lewis SEM. The effects of cryopreservation on sperm morphology, motility and mitochondrial function. Hum Reprod. 2002;17:704–9.
33. Gandini L, Lombardo F, Lenzi A, Spano M, Dondero F. Cryopreservation and sperm DNA integrity. Cell Tissue Bank. 2006;7:91–8.
34. Degl'Innocenti S, Filimberti E, Magini A, Krausz C, Lombardi G, Fino MG, et al. Semen cryopreservation for man banking for oligospermia, cancers and other pathologies: prediction of post thaw outcome using basal semen quality. Fertil Steril. 2013;100:1555–63. e1-3.
35. Kathrins M, Abhyankar N, Shoshany O, Liebermann J, Uhler M, Prins G, et al. Post-thaw recovery of rare or very low concentrations of cryopreserved human sperm. Fertil Steril. 2017;107:1300–4.
36. Tomlinson MJ. Sperm processing and storage. In: Pacey AA, Tomlinson MJ, editors. Sperm banking: theory and practice. Cambridge: Cambridge University Press. p. 86–104.
37. Temple-Smith PD, Southwick GJ, Yates CA, Trounson AO, Kretser DM. Human pregnancy by in vitro fertilization (IVF) using sperm aspirated from the epididymis. J In Vitro Fert Embryo Transf. 1985;2:119–22.
38. Abhyankar N, Kathrins M, Niederberger C. Use of testicular versus ejaculated sperm for intracytoplasmic sperm injection among men with cryptozoospermia: a meta-analysis. Fertil Steril. 2016;105:1469–75.
39. Zini A, Bach PV, Al-Malki AH, Schlegel PN. Use of testicular sperm for ICSI in oligozoospermic couples: how far should we go? Hum Reprod. 2017;32:7–13.

40. Yalcin I, Berker B, Sukur YE, Kahraman K, Ates C. Comparison of intracytoplasmic sperm injection with testicular spermatozoa success in infertile men with obstructive and non-obstructive azoospermia; a retrospective analysis. Hum Fertil. 2016;20:186–91.
41. Nagy Z, Liu J, Cecile J, Silber S, Devroey P, Steirteghem AV. Using ejaculated, fresh, and frozen-thawed epididymal and testicular spermatozoa gives rise to comparable results after intracytoplasmic sperm injection. Fertil Steril. 1995;63:808–15.
42. Schlegel PN. Causes of azoospermia and their management. Reprod Fertil Dev. 2004;16:561–72.
43. Coward RM, Mills JN. A step-by-step guide to office-based sperm retrieval for obstructive azoospermia. Transl Androl Urol. 2017;6:730–44.
44. Donoso P, Tournaye H, Devroey P. Which is the best sperm retrieval technique for non-obstructive azoospermia? A systematic review. Hum Reprod Update. 2007;13:539–49.
45. Wu B, Wong D, Lu S, Dickstein S, Silva M, Gelety TJ. Optimal use of fresh and frozen-thawed testicular sperm for intracytoplasmic sperm injection in azoospermic patients. J Assist Reprod Genet. 2005;22:389–94.
46. Hosseini A, Khalili MA. Improvement of motility after culture of testicular spermatozoa: the effects of incubation timing and temperature. Transl Androl Urol. 2017;6:271–6.
47. Schiewe MC, Rothman C, Spitz A, Werthman PE, Zeitlin SI, Anderson RE. Validation-verification of a highly effective, practical human testicular tissue in vitro culture-cryopreservation procedure aimed to optimize pre-freeze and post-thaw motility. J Assist Reprod Genet. 2016;33:519–28.
48. Fredricsson B, Kinnari S. Vitality and morphology of human spermatozoa studies on the resistance to storage and centrifugation and on the removal of dead spermatozoa. Andrologia. 1979;11:135–41.
49. Shekarriz M, Dewire D, Thomas JAJ, Agarwal A. A method of human semen centrifugation to minimize the iatrogenic sperm injuries caused by reactive oxygen species. Eur Urol. 1995;28:31–5.
50. Henkel RR, Schill WB. Sperm preparation for ART. Reprod Biol Endocrinol. 2003;1:108.
51. Popal W, Nagy Z. Laboratory processing and intracytoplasmic sperm injection using epididymal and testicular spermatozoa: what can be done to improve outcomes? Clinics. 2013;68:125–30.
52. Salzbrunn A, Benson D, Holstein A, Schulze W. A new concept for the extraction of testicular spermatozoa as a tool for assisted fertilization (ICSI). Hum Reprod. 1996;11:752–5.
53. Crabbe E, Verheyen G, Tournaye H, Steirteghem AV. The use of enzymatic procedures to recover testicular germ cells. Hum Reprod. 1997;12:1682–7.
54. Nagy ZP, Verheyen G, Tournaye H, Devroey P, Steirteghem AV. An improved treatment procedure for testicular biopsy specimens offers more efficient sperm recovery: case series. Fertil Steril. 1997;68:376–9.
55. Desai NN, Blackmon H, Goldfarb J. Single sperm cryopreservation on cryoloops: an alternative to hamster zona for freezing individual spermatozoa. Reprod Biomed Online. 2004;9:47–53.
56. Informed consent: more than getting a signature. https://www.jointcommission.org/assets/1/23/Quick_Safety_Issue_Twenty-One_February_2016.pdf
57. Gearhart, J. The FDA's consent from language – understandable or not? 2014. https://www.quorumreview.com/fdas-consent-form-language-understandable-not/
58. Shuster TG, Hickner-Cruz K, Ohl DA, Goldman E, Smith G. Legal considerations for cryopreservation of sperm and embryos. Fertil Steril. 2003;80:61–6.
59. Ethics Committee of the American Society of Reproduction. Posthumous collection and use of reproductive tissue: a committee opinion. Fertil Steril. 2013;99:1842–5.
60. Patrizio P, Natan Y, Barak Y, Levi Setti P. A simple new method for the freeze-drying and storage of human sperm. Fertil Steril. 2016; https://doi.org/10.1016/j.fertnstert.2016.07.871.
61. Tanaka A, Nagayoshi M, Tanaka I, Yamaguchi T, Ichiyama T, Ohno M, et al. Single human sperm freezing technique for cryptozoospermia or non-obstructive azoospermia patients. Fertil Steril. 2017;107:1148–52.

Cryopreservation of Human Embryos: Basic Principles and Current Considerations

57

Helen Hunter, Natalie Getreu, Maureen Wood, and Barry Fuller

Over the past 40 years, the ability to manipulate reproductive cells in vitro to correct problems of infertility has become both remarkable and now routine practice. One key facilitation to this whole process has been the successful application of cryopreservation to 'stop biological time'. This has been particularly so in embryo cryopreservation, where good quality preimplantation embryos, supernumerary to fresh transfer, can be selected and stored for up to several years. This improves patient management in particular conditions and increases the overall cumulative success rate of infertility treatment [1, 2].

Knowledge about fundamental cryobiology developed in parallel with in vitro embryological studies, because embryos provided good models whereby the biophysical events encountered in cryopreservation could be tested in systems which had clearly defined criteria for survival and continued development after thawing [3–5]. This chapter will outline the recent knowledge of the scientific basis for embryo cryopreservation and discuss current trends in application of the technologies in infertility treatment.

H. Hunter
Department of Reproductive Medicine, Old St Mary's Hospital, Manchester, UK

N. Getreu
Institute of Reproductive Health, Division of UCL, London, UK

M. Wood
Department of Obstetrics and Gynaecology, University of Aberdeen, Aberdeen, UK

B. Fuller (✉)
Division of Surgery & Interventional Science, UCL Medical School, Royal Free Hospital, London, UK
e-mail: b.fuller@ucl.ac.uk

57.1 Contributions of Fundamental Cryobiology to Embryo Cryopreservation

57.1.1 Some Historical Aspects of Applied Cryobiology

The development of robust cryopreservation protocols in infertility services has depended on an understanding of cryobiology, which is itself a young science. It was in the 1960s when 'cryobiology' became an accepted term, and in 1963 the International Society for Cryobiology was founded. It is now accepted that cryopreservation means the maintenance of cells, alive but in a suspended state, at the necessary cryogenic temperatures of around −170 °C to −196 °C (the latter being the temperature of liquid nitrogen).

It has taken decades to understand the importance of this low temperature requirement (e.g. why other temperatures such as −80 °C are not sufficient). Also, we now know that successful cryopreservation can be achieved by application of a number of different biophysical protocols (see below). For example, two commonly used techniques for embryo cryopreservation are fast-rate vitrification and controlled slow-rate cooling (CRSC), which both deliver similar modifications on cell and molecular architectures. For the purposes of this chapter, the term 'cryopreservation' is used to cover all of these variants.

Scientists have been fascinated with the effects of low temperatures on biology for centuries. They easily identified that the phase change of water to form ice during cooling was both a dramatic and inescapable challenge for death or survival in biological systems. In the 1890s, the freezing process in plant tissues was observed by Molisch using a microscope system modified with a stage to allow freezing [6]. He noticed that as ice formation began, the plant cells trapped pure water. This caused the liquid volume to shrink, concentrating the solutes that had previously existed in the original aqueous environment. The resulting exposure of cells to

G. N. Allahbadia et al. (eds.), *Textbook of Assisted Reproduction*, https://doi.org/10.1007/978-981-15-2377-9_57

hypertonic surroundings is one of the central problems with ice formation.

Some plant cells have evolved an ability to endure freezing temperature by synthesising of high levels of certain sugars and solutes, as first recognised by Maximov [7]. We now understand that this mechanism counteracts the damage that can be induced by the formation of ice (known as 'freeze dehydration') and that the solutes that protect against cellular damage are called 'osmolytes'. As such, osmolytes might also be protective if they could be applied to other systems to yield 'cryoprotection'—thus allowing the survival of cells when exposed to ice.

When it comes to reproductive cryobiology, these collected strands of knowledge undoubtedly influenced Polge and colleagues in 1949 in their search for solutes which would allow survival of fowl spermatozoa during deep freezing [8]. They witnessed successful cryoprotection by addition of glycerol as the nontoxic osmolyte, and this kick-started the modern era of applied cryopreservation.

57.1.2 The Challenges of the Water-Ice Phase Transition for Embryos

To understand how protocols have been developed to allow embryos to survive deep cryogenic temperatures, it is worth making a few comments about the phase where water transitions into ice. We know that biological reactions require water in its liquid state [9] and that if this essential liquid is removed during ice formation, then this poses extreme survival challenges, irrespective of the lowering of temperature per se.

Several reviews have discussed this in detail in relation to cryopreservation [10, 11]. In brief, water exists in the liquid state as a collection of randomly orientated molecules, connected to one another via hydrogen bonds to form a matrix, accepting that this timescale for association is extremely fleeting. For most biological processes, this enables solvent molecules to interact with vital solutes and ions and provides stability to the structure of macromolecules. As the temperature decreases, the rotations of the molecules of water are slowed. The resulting water-water self-association leads to longer-lived intermolecular connections which, at the appropriate low temperature (the freezing point), result in the formation of ice nuclei with hexagonally arranged water molecules. These multiply repetitively throughout the aqueous milieu to yield hexagonal ice, which is the commonly observed form of ice.

As the network begins to stabilise, energy is released. This is known as the 'latent heat of ice formation' and can be measured directly using a thermocouple. This reliable marker for the point of ice nucleation has been a critical factor in the improvement of protocols for cryopreserving embryos.

The open lattice nature of the network causes a slight difference in the densities of liquid water compared to ice. This is why ice is mostly seen to accumulate at the top of the sample during CRSC. The ice lattice excludes solutes, which transfer from the original solution into the residual liquid volume. This is because freezing is not an instantaneous event: as the temperature decreases, there is a steady growth in the amount of ice forming within the aqueous portion of the solution. This results in an ever-increasing concentration of solutes trapped in the residual solution, providing an accumulating osmotic stress on the cells as cooling progresses. If this were a linear continuum occurring all the way down to the essential deep cryogenic temperatures, it is unlikely that embryos could survive cryopreservation and long-term storage.

Fortunately, chemistry and physics intervene in a helpful way. At a certain deep cryogenic temperature (see below), solidification takes place for all of the matrix. The system is then 'locked' into a configuration which is incapable of further change and remains stable over many years. As might be imagined, for cells to experience such extremities of dehydration can be traumatic: cell membranes can destabilise and the cytosol can be damaged due to pH changes, damage to proteins and impairment to organelles essential for life. All of this can be fatal to the embryo [10, 11].

These events occur as a consequence of osmosis, causing water to move from the cells to the surrounding residual liquid fraction, which has a high osmotic potential. During CRSC, cell membranes have a partial role in stopping the initial growth of ice crystals, with nucleation taking place in the surrounding freezing solution instead.

There is, however, another potential source of injury other than osmotic damage, which can occur. This can take place if the cytoplasm has managed to keep enough molecules of residual water, which might then be capable of nucleating intracellular ice. This might occur if the biophysical aspects of cooling have not maintained osmotic equilibrium throughout the system. This is most commonly seen if cooling has progressed too quickly during CRSC. As a result, unstable 'pockets' of intracellular liquid water remain to inescapably nucleate intracellular ice crystals, and this almost invariably produces lethal embryo injury.

Many of these events during embryo cryopreservation have been described and mechanistically explained with the aid of cryomicroscopes, which allow direct visual assessment of the process of freezing [5, 12].

57.1.3 Cryoprotection: How Can Embryos Survive Cryogenic Storage?

The preceding comments have made it clear that any cells, including the blastomeres in embryos, cannot survive cryogenic storage unless the essential cell water compartments can be managed to mitigate or prevent ice transition on an osmo-kinetic basis. In both cases, there is an associated extreme dehydration of cell macromolecules. This is true regardless of the cryopreservation method (CRSC or vitrification).

57.1.4 Cryoprotectants

For certain nontoxic osmolytes, if they can be safely incorporated prior to the actual cooling process, then they may be useful to the processes of cryopreservation. This is the realm of cryoprotectants (CPA), solutes which can modify the water structure during cryopreservation and thawing (the removal of water from the embryos quickly after thawing is equally important!).

Following on from Polge's ground-breaking report about how glycerol can be used as a CPA [8], studies showed that solutes such as sugars or other polyols could also have useful CPA properties, provided there is strong tendency for hydrogen bond formation with water. This is because, as the temperature cools, these solutes can affect the way in which ice crystal forms. From a kinetic perspective, protection is thereby offered in the early stages of cooling, prior to the 'lockdown' phase, when everything becomes solid (as discussed above). Once cells are solidified, no further damage can take place if the temperature continues to decrease.

The need to balance the inescapable osmotic stress during cooling also explains why CPAs are required in such relatively high concentrations. These concentrations are much higher than if they were acting in ways typical of pharmacological agents, for example.

Embryos in standard culture media experience isotonic conditions (effectively close to 0.15 M sodium chloride). Once ice formation proceeds, salt concentrations will rise to about 3.51 M in the residual liquid portion by freezing to about −5 °C. However, in the presence of 1 M CPA, e.g. glycerol, the molarity increase in salts is mitigated. The CPA is so effective that even when the temperature reduces to less than −30 °C, the molarity is manageable [11]. This property became known in cryobiology as the colligative effect of CPA [13].

In the search for other successful CPAs, the compound dimethyl sulphoxide [DMSO] was proposed by Lovelock and Bishop in the 1960s [13] as a water-modifying solute with low toxicity. Nowadays, DMSO is a commonly used CPA, with a range of applications. It wasn't until a decade later that the term 'cryoprotectant' was formally adopted, based on the studies from Karow et al. [14]. Since that time, there have been very few other solutes put forward that have the required water-modifying property to be effective primary CPAs. Interestingly, embryo cryopreservation is one area where there has been a shift away from accepting DMSO as the universal CPA, in favour of a different polyol, propylene glycol (1,2-propanediol; PrOH), which has become predominant in CRSC.

In order to protect cellular macromolecules, primary CPAs have to reach the intracellular sites. Some CPAs (e.g. DMSO and glycerol) are able to protect the cytosol, since they can traverse membranes. Alternative water-modifying agents (e.g. sugars or polymers) cannot cross membranes and are less effective, although they can still provide some CPA effects. As a result, CPAs were classified according to their ability to permeate cells [15–18].

Numerous studies have indicated that in almost every case, embryos require intracellular CPA protection during cryopreservation. The growth of extracellular ice crystals can be modulated by non-permeating CPAs, which can help to reduce effects on osmosis. However, primary cryoprotection cannot be provided by non-permeating CPAs [16, 17]. For example, in embryo cryopreservation by CRSC, PrOH is often supplemented with sucrose and trehalose, to enhance orderly redistribution of liquid water from within intracellular spaces and lessen the later likelihood that ice might form intracellularly [19]. For vitrification, again sugars and polymers such as ficoll may be included in the solute mix [20], to modify water by their nonideal physicochemical properties (restricting water molecule mobility on a kinetic basis such that ice nuclei cannot grow during rapid deep cryogenic cooling).

Given the relatively high concentrations of CPA required for effective cryoprotection, and the fact that they directly impact on cell water relationships (at any temperature), it is unsurprising that embryos may encounter CPA toxicity when exposed to these solutes unless protocol conditions are optimised. Since CPA toxicity affects a wide range of cell and molecular targets [16, 21], CPA exposure prior to cryopreservation and the temperatures used have to be defined as the minimum conditions to achieve effective cryoprotection.

Another confounding challenge is the CPA-related osmotic stress which results from loading of the solutes into the cell, largely by simple transmembrane diffusion processes [16, 22]. This requires a finite time, yet transmembrane water diffusion takes place at a much faster pace. Thus, when embryos are introduced to CPA loading solutions, where the concentration may be ≥0.5 M, the blastomeres initially shrink as a result of water leaving the cells. The CPA and associated water molecules then enter intracellular space, to re-equilibrate and restore the cell volume [5, 23].

Using lower temperatures for CPA loading can mitigate CPA chemical toxicity but can also lead to a more prolonged exposure time. For example, a longer exposure time of up to twice the duration may be needed to achieve good intracellular permeation, if the CPA exposure temperature is reduced (e.g. to ≤10 °C) [24]. There are equally important chemico- and osmo-toxicity considerations for the steps to dilute out

CPA at the end of cryopreservation. This is why stepwise, time-controlled protocols have been routinely applied in embryo cryopreservation to minimise all the associated risks.

Predictive modelling can be used, incorporating variables such as the cell membrane permeability coefficients of water or CPA [25]. However, practical testing is needed to verify the optimal CPA protocols to achieve high rates of success post-thawing.

By now, the relevance of CPAs as water-modifying agents to reduce cellular stress should be clear, accepting that this may simultaneously impair cellular function. Almost all normal biological processes are influenced if a cytosol experiences an unusually high level of a particular solute. This is of paramount importance if toxicity results, which can injure the cell prior to ice formation.

Problems can also occur for osmosis. For example, if a relatively high concentration of a permeating CPA is needed, it will take a slower period of time to traverse a cell membrane compared to the movement of water.

Temperature is also critical, as higher temperatures (e.g. 37 °C) will lead to faster CPA permeation of mammalian oocytes than ambient temperature [26], but there is an increased risk of toxicity from the accelerated CPA influx. Lower temperatures (such as <10 °C) can mitigate chemical toxicity but require longer periods of exposure [24].

57.1.5 Relevance of Cooling Protocols for Embryo Cryopreservation

For efficacious embryo cryopreservation, the rate of cooling must control interconnected biophysical events. Controlled changes to temperature are critical for both CRSC and vitrification, accepting that they differ. The two approaches are often seen as mutually exclusive, but this is not the case when viewed from the biophysical changes which need to be achieved within the cells to survive the process.

57.1.6 Embryo Cryopreservation by CRSC Methods

Early success in embryo cryopreservation was achieved using CRSC [3, 27], where the 'slow' rate was about -0.3 °C min^{-1}. Based on this success, a 'two-factor hypothesis' was proposed by Mazur and his team [27] to illustrate two different scenarios whereby injury could occur at different cooling rates. Mazur's hypothesis proposes that to survive cryopreservation, cells must be optimally dehydrated to such a level that there is no chance of any free liquid water within the cytosol which can transition into ice.

At temperatures less than or equal to -40 °C, the thermodynamic imperative for water molecules is to nucleate ice [28]. On the other hand, cells cannot normally withstand such extreme dehydration, which affects not only metabolic interactions but also the many molecular structures (such as cell membrane bilayers and organelles and down to the level of macromolecules such as proteins or DNA). Irreversible disruption may result [29, 30] unless ultra-low temperatures can be reached: in essence, it is a 'catch 22' situation.

The presence of CPAs can go some way to mitigate the problems of ice nucleation but cannot completely remove the requirement for control of cooling rate. Applications of CRSC were facilitated by the manufacture of reliable cryo-coolers using the vapour of liquid nitrogen (LN2) as the coolant [31, 32]. During CRSC, ice formation itself is the essential dehydrative driving force but in the extracellular space. Thus, ice formation can be either friend or foe, depending on the location.

Mazur's hypothesis suggests that cells require optimal dehydration to remove the risk of ice forming intracellularly, as this can cause lethal cell injury in most instances [33] (Table 57.1). At an optimal slow cooling rate of -0.3 °C min^{-1}, the added CPA protects the ultrastructure of the embryo, to allow dehydration during ultra-low cooling until such time that cryogenic temperatures are reached. At this point, another important phase change (see below) takes place – the 'glassy transition' range (T_g). Beyond T_g, no further molecular changes are possible, and all components of the blastomeres are 'locked stable' for prolonged periods of time which even now are not fully quantified but are in the realms of decades if not centuries.

If intracellular dehydration is crucial to survival, then reliable ice nucleation in the external medium is a critical step. This is achieved by the various mechanisms of 'seeding ice' in the embryo straws [22, 35]. For optimised extreme embryo dehydration, intracellular water needs to continually be removed as the external ice burden progressively increases [36] (pragmatically down to temperatures in the region of

Table 57.1 Mazur's two-factor injury hypothesis [22, 34]

Mazur's injury factor 1 was associated with very slow cooling (much slower than the optimal rate). With this, embryos would be exposed to the extreme ice-related dehydration for intolerably long times. Even in the presence of CPAs, before reaching the safety of T_g, lethal injury would ensue
Mazur's injury factor 2 was associated with fast cooling rates (much faster than the optimal rate), providing conditions where intracellular free water did not have sufficient time to leave the embryos in response to the growing extracellular osmotic potential provided by the external ice milieu and so could nucleate intracellular ice which is invariably lethal

These descriptions oversimplify the complex biophysical processes occurring during cryopreservation, many of which remain to be fully elucidated. However, Mazur's two-factor hypothesis does tend to fit the observed outcomes for CRSC of embryos over the past three decades [22, 34]. The hypothesis also explains the rationale for some of the steps in embryo CRSC which are now standard

−40 °C). Below this, essential dehydration is almost complete – so CRSC can be modified to cool at somewhat faster rates taking the embryos down to T_g – again a protocol step commonly used in the clinical setting.

Several studies now show that temperatures less than −100 °C are essential to maintain cryopreserved embryos in the long term [37, 38]. However, a T_g from −120 °C to −130 °C is needed to impart true long-term cryogenic stability, where there is complete solidification of embryos within the cryopreserved matrix of ice, solutes and CPAs. The temperature of LN2 (at −196 °C) or LN2 vapour (at about −170° C) for embryo storage is safely below T_g and should provide a 'safety net' for any minor fluctuations in storage temperature (e.g. when filling storage vessels).

The protection provided by the T_g range is quickly lost if large temperature fluctuations are permitted, which is why protocol checks and records for embryo storage temperatures are of high importance.

57.1.7 Vitrification as a Strategy for Embryo Cryopreservation

For vitrification, ultra-low temperatures through T_g and extreme dehydration are equally important for embryo survival. It has been known for more than 60 years that ice nucleation can be fully prevented at ultra-low temperatures by using different approaches [39, 40]. For common aqueous solutions, this suppression was achievable only by cooling at extremely high rates (several 1000° C min^{-1}). By doing this, water molecules retained the state characteristic of liquid water, even after passing through T_g, to effectively yield a glass without any crystalline structure.

Cryobiologists struggled to develop this into a practical way for storage of cell systems, until the seminal work undertaken by Rall and Fahy [41] on mouse embryos. They postulated that very high CPA concentrations would allow the glassy state to be reached at lower cooling rates (now in the ranges of −100° Cs min^{-1}) and also provide the essential extreme dehydration required for embryo survival during cryogenic storage. However, the required high toxicity levels of CPA concentrations >60% w/v were a concern. Therefore, attention was placed on identifying the least toxic CPA and use of combinations of CPAs, where each individual CPA was under the threshold level of toxicity [42].

This method was applied cautiously to human embryo cryopreservation, using high CPA concentrations in vitrification solutions (VS) without toxicity [43–46]. The high cooling rates required were too fast for use of traditional embryo vials or straws, so alternative devices were introduced, e.g. pulled straws and cryo-loops, holding only small liquid samples (<10 μl containing the embryo). This allowed embryos to reliably attain the 'glassy state' [47, 48], whereby the embryo samples effectively 'outran' the propensity of water molecules to form ice nuclei before reaching T_g. An example of commercially available vitrification device is shown in Fig. 57.1.

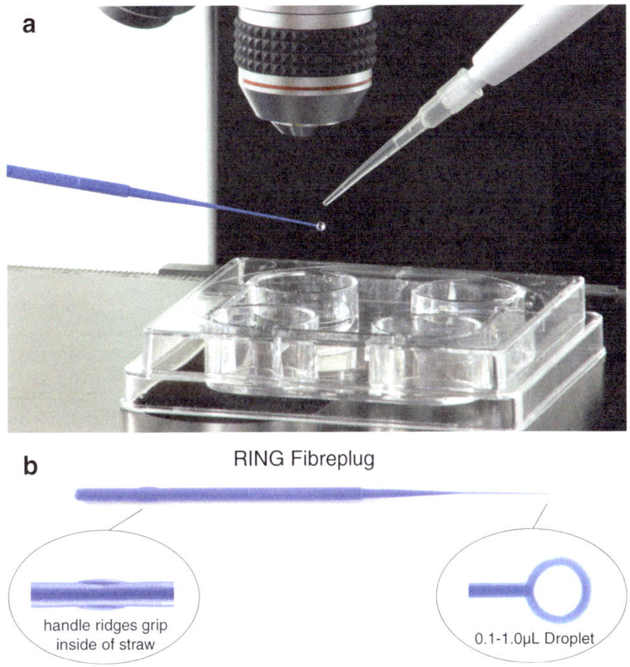

Fig. 57.1 (**a**) Adding embryo to Fibreplus. (**b**) RING Fibreplug (courtesy of CryoLogic Ply Ltd., Blackburn, Victoria, Australia)

Over the past 5 years, vitrification has become increasingly popular for clinical embryo cryopreservation, and many IVF clinics now use this [20, 49, 50]. Furthermore, clinics have gradually improved the vitrification protocols such that post-warm embryo survival surpasses CRSC outcomes [51–53]. However, some of these comparisons are retrospective, and it is difficult to produce prospective trials in this area.

Vitrification obviates the need for use of cryo-cooling machines, and the cooling step can be performed rapidly, avoiding the time required for slow cooling. However, the vitrification process requires an increase in the number of essential skilled manipulations to be undertaken, particularly if several embryos need to be cryopreserved on a particular day. Nevertheless, many centres have invested the efforts required to make vitrification a success [50].

57.1.8 Importance of Warming Protocols

Warming protocols are just as important as cooling protocols, as suboptimal warming puts a cryopreserved embryo at risk. When a cryopreserved embryo is warmed above the T_g range (around −120 °C), an accumulation of high solutes can cause damage. At above −110 °C water molecules start to mobilise, even in vitrified embryos [54]. As embryos warm, any existing ice crystals may grow and reorganise themselves, in a process known as Ostwald ripening [55]. Numerous tiny intracellular ice nucleation centres that may have formed during cooling can dissolve and redeposit onto larger ice crystals. This is more likely in frozen aqueous solutions if warming rates are slow [55] but can also take place after vitrification. During cooling, provided T_g has been safely passed, these are not a source of immediate injury. However, during warming, if mobile water becomes available, ice crystal may grow from these nucleation centres. This concept is known as 'freezing during thawing' [56].

The biophysics related to the speed of warming has yet to be fully understood [57]. In theory, slow warming allows time for osmotic re-equilibration [3], as the ice matrix first melts and liquid water becomes available for the shrunken cells. Carefully controlled CPA dilution steps aim to prevent reverse osmosis and harmful blastomere swelling [5, 58]. Inclusion of osmotic buffers, such as sucrose, during the dilution phase has been found to be helpful in mitigating injury [59]. However, slow warming has been shown to cause injury to blastocysts [60].

For vitrified embryos, fast warming rates are essential [61, 62]. Osmotic injury is possible during the CPA dilution phase, as high CPA concentrations will initially exist intracellularly.

57.1.9 Essential Aspects of Robust Cryogenic Storage for Cryopreserved Embryos

Cryo-attrition is highly likely if embryos are stored at temperatures above T_g. It is therefore pragmatic to impose a 'storage shelf life' on cryopreserved cells, taking into account their 'product stability'. For example, in the USA, the Food and Drugs Administration (FDA) has imposed a shelf life of 10 years for red blood cells stored at −80 °C [63, 64].

On a physicochemical basis, reports of possible detrimental effects linked to storage duration [65] are unlikely, provided storage has been maintained below T_g.

Cryopreserved embryos can be subjected to fluctuations in storage temperature, e.g. if there has been a delayed time for filling with LN2 or if neighbouring samples are removed from storage. For example, 'deep-frozen' samples store in racks can be subjected to a temperature change from −135 °C to −60 °C within a few minutes, when lifted out of storage [66]. Unsurprisingly, repeated temperature changes through the range for T_g can impact on viability [66].

There has been a trend from LN2 to LN2 vapour phase storage for some cell types, following concern that infectious agents could be transmitted through liquid LN2 [67]. Safety concerns have particular relevance to 'open' devices used for embryo vitrification, where samples may be exposed directly to LN2, and thus use of closed embryo containers has been proposed [68].

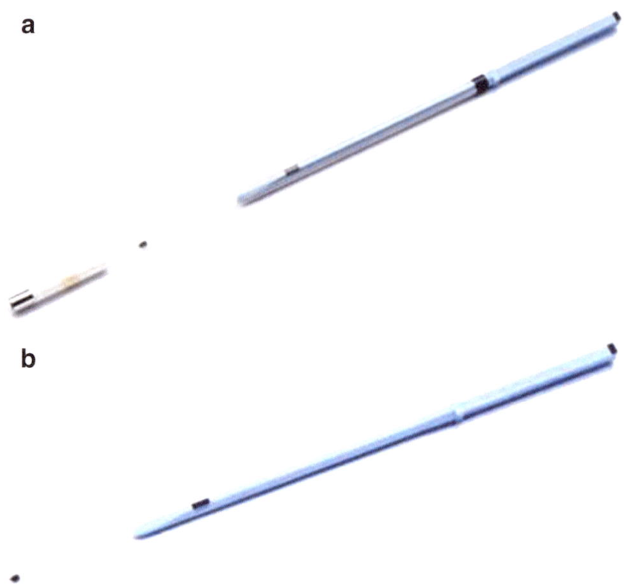

Fig. 57.2 (**a**, **b**) Cryotop vitrification (courtesy of Kitazato Corporation, Tokyo, Japan)

Whilst LN2 vapour phase storage provides −150° to −170 °C storage, the vessels may be prone to rapid changes in temperature, e.g. when the vessel is opened. Aluminium racking within the storage tank can provide some thermal stability as a 'cold sink' [69].

However, in the majority of IVF clinics, the preferred storage option remains immersed in the liquid phase of LN2, because of concerns over temperature fluctuations in the vapour phase. Embryos are typically stored as small volume samples in sheathed vitrification devices (Fig. 57.2) and not in direct contact with cold aluminium racks, so the safety net of a large thermal mass provided by the aluminium is not available.

The potential for loss of embryo viability following temperature fluctuations during storage or transport, particularly for vitrified embryos, has to be balanced by the risks of cross-infection resulting directly from the LN2 [70]. In all situations, for optimal storage of cryopreserved embryos, there should be protocols to manage and monitor the cryostore.

57.2 Embryo Cryopreservation in Clinical Practice

This section aims to provide an overview of current practice in a large NHS IVF Unit in the UK, with some reflection on the rationales of these practices and regulation.

57.2.1 Why Is Embryo Cryopreservation Important?

In a clinic with robust protocols and skilled embryologists, results suggest that supernumerary potentially viable embryos can be stored safely, without significant loss of implantation potential after thawing or warming [49]. Being able to store embryos successfully for future use increases the acceptability to patients of the option to transfer a single embryo, which can help to reduce the multiple pregnancy rates [71].

Elective embryo cryopreservation (i.e. when a fresh transfer is not planned) has an important role in patient management and fertility preservation. Embryo cryopreservation allows patients with an ovarian hyperstimulation (OHSS) risk to be managed [72] and has also allowed the development of services for pre-implantation genetic testing (PGT). Blastocysts can be tested and then vitrified; screened embryos can be warmed for transfer in a subsequent cycle, allowing sufficient time for advanced testing and patient counselling.

Fertility preservation for medical reasons is another emerging field. The British Fertility Society has published policy and practice guidelines for fertility preservation for medical reasons in girls and women [73]. Furthermore, for women who have cryopreserved embryos prior to chemo-/radiotherapy, the live birth rates following FET are similar to those for age-matched controls [74].

57.2.2 How, What and When to Cryopreserve in Clinical Practice?

There is no absolute consensus or regulation governing the choice of laboratory protocols or policies on embryo cryopreservation. Whilst various professional bodies have published consensuses [75, 76], a broad spectrum of methods used for CRSC and vitrification continues. A meta-analysis by Rienzi and her team [77] showed that vitrification appeared to provide better clinical results when compared to CRSC but with the caveat that the quality of evidence was mostly low when comparing clinical outcomes.

Guidelines on embryo grading and selection for transfer and cryopreservation have been produced [76, 78]. Clinics with very strict freezing criteria tend to report better embryo survival and FET success rates but may also conduct fewer FET cycles per oocyte collection, and hence, their cumulative pregnancy rates per fresh cycle may be lower when compared to clinics with a more lenient approach to cryopreservation [2].

In recent years, a debate has arisen about whether prospective elective cryopreservation of all embryos produced within a fertility cycle should take place, on the basis that clinical outcomes may be improved [79–81]. However, caution has been expressed about such an approach until further evidence is accumulated [82] (Table 57.2) [75–77, 83, 84].

Table 57.2 Embryo cryopreservation: the experience of St. Mary's IVF clinic, Manchester, UK, where both CRSC (for pronucleate and early cleavage-stage embryos) and vitrification (for oocytes and blastocysts) take place

Pronucleate stage (PN) freezing
Elective 'freeze-all' cycles are performed at PN stage, using CRSC. This policy gives flexibility when thawing embryos (allowing patients to take advantage of possible future developments in culture techniques); maximises the chance of ET (as all zygotes are cryopreserved); and avoids any concern of unknown long-term stability of vitrified embryos. Whilst the potential embryo quality is unknown at the time of cryopreservation, the clinical pregnancy rate per FET cycle is similar to that of our vitrified blastocyst transfers (Hunter, unpublished data). Slow freezing continues to be preferred due to extensive expertise and good experiences with this method. Additionally (and importantly), often large numbers of embryos require freezing within a narrow time window (i.e. before the PN fade) which makes vitrification logistically difficult in a busy laboratory
Early cleavage (EC) stage
Since the advent of extended culture, cryopreservation rarely takes place at the EC stage. When it does, slow freezing is performed rather than vitrification, although the evidence for superiority of either cryostorage technique is relatively poor [77]. Either approach can be used for cryopreservation at this stage of embryo development, depending on local logistics
Blastocyst stage
Blastocyst cryopreservation is exclusively performed by vitrification, without blastocoel collapse, and with survival rates of around 92% and implantation rates of 30% (compared to a fresh implantation rate of 37%) (H Hunter unpublished data). Some laboratories report good results with CRSC, but they are in the minority (75,76, M Wood personal communication). Current clinical data may not justify collapsing the blastocoel [83], but data are still limited, and this should be reviewed by each centre in the light of their own practice and results
Storage duration
In the UK, embryos can only remain in storage both up to a legal time limit (specified at the time of consent and whilst both gamete providers continue to consent. At the time of writing, the standard statutory period of up to 10 years from the date of storage for ART cycles has been extended to 12 years due to the COVID-19 pandemic [84]

57.2.3 Warming and Thawing Embryos in the Clinical Context

Cleavage-stage embryos are deemed to have survived warming/thawing if half of the blastomeres appear intact [76]. For blastocysts, at least 75–90% of cells should be intact in the warmed embryo [76].

A consensus report from the UK's Association of Clinical Embryologists [75] emphasised that thawing/warming protocols must be matched to the cryopreservation protocol, and transferring embryos between centres may compromise viability. This is not only due to the risks in moving the cryopreserved material, but it was also considered that the best survival rate is most likely if the same clinic that cryopreserved the embryos then thawed/warmed the embryos. At the very least, the same solutions, carrier systems and protocols should be used for thawing/warming. Patients should be made aware of the risk of compromise to the outcome by moving embryos between centres [70].

57.3 Conclusion

The technology and understanding of embryo cryopreservation have developed rapidly in 30 years since the first reports of pregnancy and live births following FET [85, 86]. From what was initially considered to be a research technology, embryo cryopreservation has become a mainstream component of infertility treatments on a global scale. In the past decade, new approaches, notably vitrification, are making significant impact on the practice of embryo cryopreservation. However, routine application should not deflect from the need for high-level staff training and continued professional development in this area, as is acknowledged to be essential good practice in any clinical endeavour.

A fundamental understanding of all the principles involved in embryo cryopreservation is essential, as each step can potentially impact on whether the embryo survives. These concerns have recently been expressed in an editorial comment [70] where specific risks associated with embryo cryopreservation were identified in situations where non-optimised procedures can have negative impact.

References

1. Brown JR, Modell E, Obasaju M, King YK. Natural cycle in-vitro fertilization with embryo cryopreservation prior to chemotherapy for carcinoma of the breast. Hum Reprod. 1996 Jan;11(1):197–9.
2. Wong KM, Mastenbroek S, Repping S. Cryopreservation of human embryos and its contribution to in vitro fertilization success rates. Fertil Steril. 2014 Jul;102(1):19–26.
3. Whittingham DG, Leibo SP, Mazur P. Survival of mouse embryos frozen to -196 degrees and -269 degrees C. Science. 1972;178(4059):411–4.
4. Leibo SP. Cryobiology: preservation of mammalian embryos. Basic Life Sci. 1986;37:251–72.
5. Leibo SP. Cryopreservation of oocytes and embryos: optimization by theoretical versus empirical analysis. Theriogenology. 2008 Jan 1;69(1):37–47.
6. Molisch H. Scientific Literature: Untersuchungen uber das Erfrieren der Pflanzen. Science. 1897;6(157):1002–3.
7. Maximov NA. Chemical protective agents of plants against freezing injury concerning the nature of the protective effect. Berichte Dtsch Bot Geselschafft. 1912;30:504–16.
8. Polge C, Smith AU, Parkes AS. Revival of spermatozoa after vitrification and dehydration at low temperatures. Nature. 1949 Oct 15;164(4172):666.
9. Chaplin M. Do we underestimate the importance of water in cell biology? Nat Rev Mol Cell Biol. 2006;7(11):861–6.
10. Mazur P. Principles of cryobiology. In: Barry J, Fuller NL, Benson EE, editors. Life in the frozen state. Boca Raton, FL: CRC Press; 2004. p. 3–65.
11. Muldrew K, Elliott J, McGann L, Fuller B, Benson E, State LN. The water to ice transition: implications for living cells. In: Fuller BJ, Lane N, Benson EE, editors. Life in the frozen state. Boca Raton, FL: CRC Press; 2004. p. 67–108.
12. Toner M, Cravalho EG, Stachecki J, Fitzgerald T, Tompkins RG, Yarmush ML, et al. Nonequilibrium freezing of one-cell mouse embryos. Membrane integrity and developmental potential. Biophys J. 1993 Jun;64(6):1908–21.
13. Lovelock JE, Bishop MW. Prevention of freezing damage to living cells by dimethyl sulphoxide. Nature. 1959;183(4672):1394–5.
14. Karow AM. Cryoprotectants—a new class of drugs. J Pharm Pharmacol. 1969;21(4):209–23.
15. Fuller B, Paynter S. Fundamentals of cryobiology in reproductive medicine. Reprod Biomed Online. 2004 Dec;9(6):680–91.
16. Elliott GD, Wang S, Fuller BJ. Cryoprotectants: a review of the actions and applications of cryoprotective solutes that modulate cell recovery from ultra-low temperatures. Cryobiology. 2017 Jun;76:74–91.
17. Fuller BJ. Cryoprotectants: the essential antifreezes to protect life in the frozen state. Cryo Lett. 25(6):375–88.
18. Fuller B, Gonzalez-Molina J, Erro E, De Mendonca J, Chalmers S, Awan M, et al. Applications and optimization of cryopreservation technologies to cellular therapeutics. Cell Gene Ther Insights. 2017;3(5):359–78.
19. Lassalle B, Testart J, Renard JP. Human embryo features that influence the success of cryopreservation with the use of 1,2 propanediol. Fertil Steril. 1985;44(5):645–51.
20. Mukaida T, Oka C. Vitrification of oocytes, embryos and blastocysts. Best Pract Res Clin Obstet Gynaecol. 2012 Dec;26(6):789–803.
21. Best BP. Cryoprotectant toxicity: facts, issues, and questions. Rejuvenation Res. 18(5):422–36.
22. Fuller BJ, Paynter SJ. Cryopreservation of mammalian embryos. Methods Mol Biol. 2007;368:325–39.
23. Jackowski S, Leibo SP, Mazur P. Glycerol permeabilities of fertilized and unfertilized mouse ova. J Exp Zool. 1980;212(3):329–41.
24. Paynter SJ, O'Neil L, Fuller BJ, Shaw RW. Membrane permeability of human oocytes in the presence of the cryoprotectant propane-1,2-diol. Fertil Steril. 2001;75(3):532–8.
25. Paynter SJ, McGrath JJ, Fuller BJ, Shaw RW. A method for differentiating nonunique estimates of membrane transport properties: mature mouse oocytes exposed to glycerol. Cryobiology. 1999;39(3):205–14.
26. Paynter SJ, Cooper A, Gregory L, Fuller BJ, Shaw RW. Permeability characteristics of human oocytes in the presence of the cryoprotectant dimethylsulphoxide. Hum Reprod. 1999;14(9):2338–42.
27. Leibo SP, Mazur P. The role of cooling rates in low-temperature preservation. Cryobiology. 1971 Oct;8(5):447–52.
28. Morris GJ, Acton E. Controlled ice nucleation in cryopreservation—a review. Cryobiology. 2013;66(2):85–92.
29. Rudolph AS, Crowe JH. Membrane stabilization during freezing: the role of two natural cryoprotectants, trehalose and proline. Cryobiology. 1985 Aug;22(4):367–77.
30. Zhang M, Oldenhof H, Sieme H, Wolkers WF. Freezing-induced uptake of trehalose into mammalian cells facilitates cryopreservation. Biochim Biophys Acta Biomembr. 2016 Jun;1858(6):1400–9.
31. Hayes AR, Pegg DE, Kingston RE. A multirate small-volume cooling machine. Cryobiology. 1974;11(4):371–7.
32. Sperling S. A simple apparatus for controlled rate corneal freezing II. Acta Ophthalmol. 1981;59(1):134–41.
33. Leibo SP, McGrath JJ, Cravalho EG. Microscopic observation of intracellular ice formation in unfertilized mouse ova as a function of cooling rate. Cryobiology. 1978 Jun 1;15(3):257–71.
34. Liu W-X, Luo M-J, Huang P, Yue L-M, Wang L, Zhao C-Y, et al. Comparative study between slow freezing and vitrification of

mouse embryos using different cryoprotectants. Reprod Domest Anim. 2009;44(5):788–91.
35. Fahning ML, Garcia MA. Status of cryopreservation of embryos from domestic animals. Cryobiology. 1992 Feb;29(1):1–18.
36. Mazur P. Equilibrium, quasi-equilibrium, and nonequilibrium freezing of mammalian embryos. Cell Biophys. 1990 Aug;17(1):53–92.
37. Liu Q, Lian Y, Huang J, Ren X, Li M, Lin S, et al. The safety of long-term cryopreservation on slow-frozen early cleavage human embryos. J Assist Reprod Genet. 2014 Apr 28;31(4):471–5.
38. Yao Y-C, Qi M-Y, Lu M-H, Wang S-M, Li W, Han H-B. Long-term cryopreservation had no adverse effect on viability of embryos and their offspring in sheep. Anim Reprod Sci. 2012 Dec;136(1–2):42–6.
39. Luyet BJ, Gehenio PM. Thermoelectric recording of ice formation and of vitrification during ultra-rapid cooling of protoplasm. Fed Proc. 1947;6(1 Pt 2):157.
40. Wowk B. Thermodynamic aspects of vitrification. Cryobiology. 2010 Feb;60(1):11–22.
41. Rall WF, Fahy GM. Ice-free cryopreservation of mouse embryos at -196 degrees C by vitrification. Nature. 1985;313(6003):573–5.
42. Fahy GM, Wowk B. Principles of cryopreservation by vitrification. Methods Mol Biol. 2015;1257:21–82.
43. Son W-Y, Yoon S-H, Park S-J, Yoon H-J, Lee W-D, Lim J-H. Ongoing twin pregnancy after vitrification of blastocysts produced by in-vitro matured oocytes retrieved from a woman with polycystic ovary syndrome: case report. Hum Reprod. 2002 Nov;17(11):2963–6.
44. El-Danasouri I, Selman H. Successful pregnancies and deliveries after a simple vitrification protocol for day 3 human embryos. Fertil Steril. 2001 Aug;76(2):400–2.
45. Vanderzwalmen P, Bertin G, Debauche C, Standaert V, van Roosendaal E, Vandervorst M, et al. Births after vitrification at morula and blastocyst stages: effect of artificial reduction of the blastocoelic cavity before vitrification. Hum Reprod. 2002 Mar;17(3):744–51.
46. Kasai M, Mukaida T. Cryopreservation of animal and human embryos by vitrification. Reprod Biomed Online. 2004 Aug;9(2):164–70.
47. Lane M, Schoolcraft WB, Gardner DK. Vitrification of mouse and human blastocysts using a novel cryoloop container-less technique. Fertil Steril. 1999 Dec;72(6):1073–8.
48. Kuwayama M. Highly efficient vitrification for cryopreservation of human oocytes and embryos: the Cryotop method. Theriogenology. 2007 Jan 1;67(1):73–80.
49. Edgar DH, Archer J, McBain J, Bourne H. Embryonic factors affecting outcome from single cryopreserved embryo transfer. Reprod Biomed Online. 2007 Jun;14(6):718–23.
50. Vajta G. Vitrification in human and domestic animal embryology: work in progress. Reprod Fertil Dev. 2013;25(5):719–27.
51. Balaban B, Urman B, Ata B, Isiklar A, Larman MG, Hamilton R, et al. A randomized controlled study of human day 3 embryo cryopreservation by slow freezing or vitrification: vitrification is associated with higher survival, metabolism and blastocyst formation. Hum Reprod. 2008 Jun 20;23(9):1976–82.
52. Kolibianakis EM, Venetis CA, Tarlatzis BC. Cryopreservation of human embryos by vitrification or slow freezing: which one is better? Curr Opin Obstet Gynecol. 2009 Jun;21(3):270–4.
53. Konc J, Kanyó K, Kriston R, Somoskői B, Cseh S. Cryopreservation of embryos and oocytes in human assisted reproduction. Biomed Res Int. 2014;2014:1–9.
54. Kirichek O, Soper A, Dzyuba B, Callear S, Fuller B. Strong isotope effects on melting dynamics and ice crystallisation processes in cryo vitrification solutions. PLoS One. 2015 Mar 27;10(3):e0120611.
55. Karlsson JO, Toner M. Long-term storage of tissues by cryopreservation: critical issues. Biomaterials. 1996;17(3):243–56.
56. Rall WF, Polge C. Effect of warming rate on mouse embryos frozen and thawed in glycerol. J Reprod Fertil. 1984 Jan;70(1):285–92.
57. Leibo SP, Pool TB. The principal variables of cryopreservation: solutions, temperatures, and rate changes. Fertil Steril. 2011 Aug;96(2):269–76.
58. Byrd W. Cryopreservation, thawing, and transfer of human embryos. Semin Reprod Med. 2002 Feb;20(1):37–43.
59. Wood MJ, Mollison J, Harrild K, Ferguson E, McKay T, Srikantharajah A, et al. A pragmatic RCT of conventional versus increased concentration sucrose in freezing and thawing solutions for human embryos. Hum Reprod. 2011 Aug 1;26(8):1987–96.
60. Hochi S, Akiyama M, Minagawa G, Kimura K, Hanada A. Effects of cooling and warming rates during vitrification on fertilization of in vitro-matured bovine oocytes. Cryobiology. 2001 Feb;42(1):69–73.
61. Seki S, Jin B, Mazur P. Extreme rapid warming yields high functional survivals of vitrified 8-cell mouse embryos even when suspended in a half-strength vitrification solution and cooled at moderate rates to -196°C. Cryobiology. 2014 Feb;68(1):71–8.
62. Desai N, Blackmon H, Szeptycki J, Goldfarb J. Cryoloop vitrification of human day 3 cleavage-stage embryos: post-vitrification development, pregnancy outcomes and live births. Reprod Biomed Online. 2007 Feb;14(2):208–13.
63. Meryman HT. Red cell freezing by the American National Red Cross. Am J Med Technol. 1975;41(7):265–82.
64. Scott KL, Lecak J, Acker JP. Biopreservation of red blood cells: past, present, and future. Transfus Med Rev. 2005;19(2):127–42.
65. Desrosiers P, Légaré C, Leclerc P, Sullivan R. Membranous and structural damage that occur during cryopreservation of human sperm may be time-related events. Fertil Steril. 2006;85(6):1744–52.
66. Germann A, Oh Y-J, Schmidt T, Schön U, Zimmermann H, von Briesen H. Temperature fluctuations during deep temperature cryopreservation reduce PBMC recovery, viability and T-cell function. Cryobiology. 2013;67(2):193–200.
67. Grout BWW, Morris GJ. Contaminated liquid nitrogen vapour as a risk factor in pathogen transfer. Theriogenology. 2009;71(7):1079–82.
68. Vajta G, Rienzi L, Ubaldi FM. Open versus closed systems for vitrification of human oocytes and embryos. Reprod Biomed Online. 2015 Apr;30(4):325–33.
69. Hunt CJ, Pegg DE. Improved temperature stability in gas-phase nitrogen refrigerators: use of a copper heat shunt. Cryobiology. 1996;33(5):544–51.
70. Alikani M. Cryostorage of human gametes and embryos: a reckoning. Reprod Biomed Online. 2018 Jul 1;37(1):1–3.
71. Maheshwari A, Griffiths S, Bhattacharya S. Global variations in the uptake of single embryo transfer. Hum Reprod Update. 17(1):107–20.
72. Devroey P, Polyzos NP, Blockeel C. An OHSS-free clinic by segmentation of IVF treatment. Hum Reprod. 2011;26(10):2593–7.
73. Yasmin E, Balachandren N, Davies MC, Jones GL, Lane S, Mathur R, et al. Fertility preservation for medical reasons in girls and women: British fertility society policy and practice guideline. Hum Fertil. 2018 Jan 2;21(1):3–26.
74. Cardozo ER, Thomson AP, Karmon AE, Dickinson KA, Wright DL, Sabatini ME. Ovarian stimulation and in-vitro fertilization outcomes of cancer patients undergoing fertility preservation compared to age matched controls: a 17-year experience. J Assist Reprod Genet. 2011;32(4):587–96.
75. Brison D, Cutting R, Clarke H, Wood M. ACE consensus meeting report: oocyte and embryo cryopreservation Sheffield 17.05.11. Hum Fertil. 2012 Jun 23;15(2):69–74.
76. Alpha. The alpha consensus meeting on cryopreservation key performance indicators and benchmarks: proceedings of an expert meeting. Reprod Biomed Online. 2012 Aug;25(2):146–67.
77. Rienzi L, Gracia C, Maggiulli R, LaBarbera AR, Kaser DJ, Ubaldi FM, et al. Oocyte, embryo and blastocyst cryopreservation in ART:

systematic review and meta-analysis comparing slow-freezing versus vitrification to produce evidence for the development of global guidance. Hum Reprod Update. 23(2):139–55.

78. Harbottle S, Hughes C, Cutting R, Roberts S, Brison D, Association of Clinical Embryologists & The (ACE) British Fertility Society (BFS). Elective single embryo transfer: an update to UK best practice guidelines. Hum Fertil (Camb). 18(3):165–83.
79. Roque M. Freeze-all policy: is it time for that? J Assist Reprod Genet. 2015 Feb 27;32(2):171–6.
80. Magdi Y, El-Damen A, Fathi AM, Abdelaziz AM, Abd-Elfatah Youssef M, Abd-Allah AA-E, et al. Revisiting the management of recurrent implantation failure through freeze-all policy. Fertil Steril. 2017 Jul;108(1):72–7.
81. Chang J-C, Chen M-J, Guu H-F, Chen Y-F, Yi Y-C, Kung H-F, et al. Does the "freeze-all" policy allow for a better outcome in assisted reproductive techniques than the use of fresh embryo transfers? - A retrospective study on cumulative live birth rates. Taiwan J Obstet Gynecol. 2017 Dec;56(6):775–80.
82. Rinaudo PF, Hsu J. To freeze or not to freeze: heating the debate but cooling the practice? J Assist Reprod Genet. 2017 Feb 14;34(2):187–9.
83. Van Landuyt L, Stoop D, Verheyen G, Verpoest W, Camus M, Van de Velde H, et al. Outcome of closed blastocyst vitrification in relation to blastocyst quality: evaluation of 759 warming cycles in a single-embryo transfer policy. Hum Reprod. 2011;26(3):527–34.
84. HFEA. Code of practice, 8th edn. London; 2009.
85. Trounson A, Mohr L. Human pregnancy following cryopreservation, thawing and transfer of an eight-cell embryo. Nature. 1983;305(5936):707–9.
86. Zeilmaker GH, Alberda AT, van Gent I, Rijkmans CM, Drogendijk AC. Two pregnancies following transfer of intact frozen-thawed embryos. Fertil Steril. 1984 Aug;42(2):293–6.

Fertility Preservation in Prepubertal Children

58

Leslie Coker Appiah

Over the last 25 years, the incidence of cancer has risen slowly to 1.7 million new cases in 2017. Of those cases, 10,270 occurred in the pediatric population and 70,000 in adolescents and young adults (AYA) ages 15 to 39 [1]. Fortunately, due to early detection and advancements in treatment, cancer mortality has decreased significantly with a 5-year survival of 80–85% in the pediatric population. Unfortunately, survival rates for AYA have not seen as dramatic an improvement, with 5-year survival rates remaining at 70% [2]. Reasons for lower AYA survival rates include differences in tumor biology, fewer clinical trials, lack of comprehensive insurance coverage, and barriers to access such as underemployment and educational pursuits. Nonetheless, by 2020, there are estimated to be 500,000 childhood cancer survivors of reproductive age who will experience late effects of survivorship. The scope of care in survivors has thus broadened to include quality of life in survivorship. Parenthood in survivorship is now well-established as an important quality-of-life indicator with survivors describing this as one of the most important aspects of their survivorship [3]. In a study of health outcomes in 1713 survivors of childhood cancer between the ages of 18–60, the prevalence of primary ovarian insufficiency was 12% in females receiving fertility-harming therapies. The prevalence in males was higher with 66% of at-risk males experiencing germ cell dysfunction and 12% experiencing Leydig cell function [4]. Given these findings, preserving fertility prior to gonadotoxic therapy is a critically important aspect of cancer care.

National and international efforts have increased exponentially to bring disciplines together to care for the fertility and reproductive health needs of individuals receiving treatments that affect fertility [5, 6]. Disciplines include gynecology, urology, oncology, endocrinology, reproductive endocrinology and infertility, ethics, and basic science research teams within the respective fields. Evidence-based practice guidelines and consensus statements for fertility preservation in individuals receiving gonadotoxic agents are now well-established. Guidelines from the American Society of Clinical Oncology (ASCO) and the American Society of Reproductive Medicine (ASRM) describe the risks to fertility from cancer treatments, the current state of fertility preservation counseling, and circumstances under which standard and investigational fertility preservation should be offered [7, 8]. These guidelines have been endorsed by the American College of Obstetrics and Gynecology (ACOG), the American Academy of Pediatrics (AAP), and the Association of Pediatric Hematology Oncology Nurses (APHON) [9–11]. Despite pervasiveness of these guidelines, there has only been a slight gain from less than 50% to now 60% in individuals who recall discussing fertility risks prior to cancer [12–15], and the range of individuals counseled who undergo fertility preservation therapies remains 2% to 50% [16, 17]. The challenge is not in concurring with the guidelines, but in overcoming the barriers to fertility preservation. This challenge proves even more salient in the prepubertal individual where options are limited.

Several factors should be taken into account when counseling individuals and families regarding risk to fertility and include age, type of treatment, treatment dose, disease location, and underlying conditions that compromise baseline fertility. Females are born with a finite number of follicles at approximately two to four million. Over time, through predominantly atresia and secondarily ovulation, the follicle count is depleted with approximately 400,000 or 10% of follicles remaining at puberty [18]. When the follicle count reaches 1000 at age 50, menopause ensues. Fecundity naturally decreases approximately 10 years before the menopause in healthy women [19]. Chemotherapeutic agents affect the growing follicles through disruption of cell

L. C. Appiah (✉)
Department of Obstetrics and Gynecology, Nationwide Children's Hospital, Pediatric and Adolescent Gynecology, The Ohio State University College of Medicine, Columbus, OH, USA

The Fertility Preservation and Reproductive Health Program, OSU Comprehensive Cancer Center, James Cancer Hospital and Solove Research Institute, Columbus, OH, USA
e-mail: appiah.30@osu.edu

G. N. Allahbadia et al. (eds.), *Textbook of Assisted Reproduction*, https://doi.org/10.1007/978-981-15-2377-9_58

division, resulting in apoptosis and amenorrhea. However, upon discontinuation of therapy, folliculogenesis resumes and in most cases, menses return. Alkylating agents and radiation are non-cell cycle specific and therefore not only affect the growing follicles but also damage the resting pool or ovarian reserve. The younger the individual, the larger the pretreatment resting pool and the higher the posttreatment reserve. The decrease in ovarian reserve paradoxically results in an accelerated loss of follicles. Consequently, although individuals may resume menses, ovarian insufficiency (previously termed premature ovarian failure) can occur significantly earlier than the expected age of natural fertility decline. Ovarian insufficiency is referred to as acute ovarian failure (AOF) when complete absence of menses occurs within 2 years of treatment. The definition is often extended to 5 years to include those individuals who resume and then cease menses within 5 years posttreatment [20].

Males have an almost infinite ability to produce sperm. However, risk of infertility increases after paternal age 45 due to increased risk of spontaneous abortion, late fetal deaths, birth defects, and developmental/behavioral abnormalities in offspring [21]. Males receiving alkylating agents are at greatest risk of infertility with azoospermia occurring in >90% of individuals receiving therapies for Hodgkin lymphoma that include nitrogen mustard, procarbazine, and cyclophosphamide. Permanent azoospermia is seen in 30% of males receiving CHOP. Normospermia can be expected in greater than 95% of males receiving combination chemotherapies that reduce the cumulative doses of alkylating agents. Chemotherapy regimens in bone marrow transplants result in azoospermia in greater than 95% of individuals. Individuals with testicular cancer receiving cisplatin and carboplatin-based therapy can expect normospermia in 50% at 2 years and 80% at 5 years [22] (Table 58.1).

Intracranial, total body, and pelvic irradiation have significant deleterious effects on fertility. In females, age confers protection, with prepubertal ovaries tolerating higher doses of pelvic radiation (≤ 15 Gy) than postpubertal (≤ 10 Gy) or adult (≤ 6 Gy) ovaries before experiencing AOF [23]. Studies have established however that as low as 2 Gy of radiation to the ovaries results in a 50% decrease in ovarian function. Pelvic and total body irradiation to the uterus ≥30 Gy result in irreversible damage from cortical fibrosis, whereas injury from smaller radiation doses may be corrected with high-dose estrogen therapy [24]. Uterine injury results in miscarriage, preterm delivery, and low-birth-weight infants. In males, prepubertal status is not protective of gonadal injury. Male germ cells are highly sensitive to the effects of radiation with infertility reported at >1.2 Gy of radiation. Leydig cells are more resistant to the effects of radiation with androgen deficiency occurring at upwards of 20 Gy [25]. Intracranial radiation results in infertility in males and females through direct injury to the hypothalamus and pituitary gland with subsequent hypogonadotropic hypogonadism. Although the ovary and testis may function normally, lack of stimulation by gonadotropins requires assisted reproductive technologies with gonadotropins for conception.

Table 58.1 Effects of chemotherapy on spermatogenesis

Diagnosis and treatment	Fertility posttreatment
Hodgkin disease	
MVPP	Azoospermia in >90%
MOPP	Azoospermia in >90%
ChlVPP/EVA hybrid	Azoospermia in >90%
COPP	Azoospermia in >90%
ABVD	Temporary azoospermia with normal sperm count in all at 18 months
Non-Hodgkin lymphoma	
CHOP	Permanent azoospermia in 30%
VAPEC-B	Normospermia in >95%
VACOP-B	Normospermia in >95%
MACOP-B	Normospermia in >95%
VEEP	Normospermia in >95%
Bone marrow transplant for a variety of malignancies	
Cyclophosphamide alone	FSH raised in 40%
Busulfan and cyclophosphamide	FSH raised in 80%
CBV	FSH raised in >95%
High-dose melphalan	FSH raised in >95%
BEAM	FSH raised in >95%
Testicular cancer	
Cisplatin/carboplatin	Normospermia in 50% at 2 years-based therapy and 80% at 5 years

MVPP mustine, vinblastine, procarbazine, and prednisolone, *MOPP* mustine, vincristine, procarbazine, and prednisolone, *ChlVPP/EVA* chlorambucil, vinblastine, prednisolone, procarbazine, doxorubicin, vincristine, and etoposide, *COPP* cyclophosphamide, vincristine, procarbazine, and prednisolone, *ABVD* doxorubicin hydrochloride, bleomycin, vinblastine, and dacarbazine, *CHOP* cyclophosphamide, doxorubicin, vincristine, and prednisolone, *VAPEC-B* vincristine, doxorubicin, prednisolone, etoposide, cyclophosphamide, and bleomycin, *VACOP-B* vinblastine, doxorubicin, prednisolone, vincristine, cyclophosphamide, and bleomycin, *MACOP-B* mustine in place of vinblastine, *VEEP* vincristine, etoposide, epirubicin, and prednisolone, *CBV* cyclophosphamide, carmustine, and etoposide, *BEAM* carmustine, etoposide, Ara-C, and melphalan, and *FSH* follicle-stimulating hormone

From Howell SJ, Shalet SM. Spermatogenesis after cancer treatment: damage and recovery. J Natl Cancer Inst Monogr 2005;34:12–17, with permission

To adequately counsel individuals on fertility preservation options, accurate risk stratification is required. Estimating risk, however, is exceedingly challenging due to a lack of robust long-term follow-up data of survivors. Only recently has this information become more available, although not comprehensive of all treatment regimens. The current risk stratification models categorize low risk <20%, intermediate risk 30–70%, and high risk >80% likelihood of complete ovarian failure after gonadotoxic treatment [26]

Table 58.2 Fertility risk stratification

Subfertility/infertility risk		
High risk >80%	Medium risk 30–70%	Low risk <20%
Conditioning for BMT Hodgkin's: w/ alkylators Soft-tissue sarcoma: metastatic Ewing's sarcoma: metastatic Localized pelvic or testicular radiation	AML Hepatoblastoma Osteosarcoma Ewing's sarcoma: nonmetastatic Soft-tissue sarcoma: stage II/III Neuroblastoma Non-Hodgkin lymphoma Hodgkin's: alternating alkylator tx Craniospinal radiation >24Gy	ALL Wilms' tumor Soft-tissue sarcoma: stage I Retinoblastoma Germ-cell tumors (Fertility sparing)

(Table 58.2). Agents that fall in the low-risk category include methotrexate, vincristine, radioactive iodine, anthracyclines, and multi-agent therapies with an overall decreased cumulative dose of alkylating agents. As alkylating agents are most toxic to the gonads, risk stratification models have been developed based on these agents. The cyclophosphamide equivalent dose (CED) and alkylating agent dose (AAD) scoring systems are both now well-established means of quantifying individuals at high risk of reduced fecundity after treatment. The AAD describes the cumulative dose effects of alkylating agents on fertility and was developed for two case-control studies conducted by the Late Effects Study Group [27, 28]. Gonadal toxicity was determined by comparing drug dose distribution of the study population in first, second, and third, tertiles, with the highest doses distributed in the third tertile. The CED was subsequently developed as the AAD is specific only to the study population and cannot be used for comparisons across populations [29]. In males, a CED $\geq$ 4000 - < 8000 mg/m^2 is associated with a hazard ratio (HR) of pregnancy among partners of 0.72 (CI 0.55–0.95, p 0.019). A CED $\geq$ 8000–<12,000 correlates with a HR 0.49 (CI 0.36–0.68, $p < 0.001$). In correlation, a summed AAD in the third tertile denotes an almost 50% (HR 0.48, CI 0.36–0.65) reduced likelihood of siring a pregnancy. In females, a CED $\geq$ 4000–< 8000 mg/m^2 denotes a relative risk (RR) of nonsurgical premature menopause of 2.74 (CI 1.13–6.61, p 0.025). A CED $\geq$ 8000 confers a 4.19 (CI 2.18–8.08, $p < 0.001$) RR of nonsurgical premature menopause. An AAD in the third tertile corresponds to a RR 4.99 (2.53–9.84, $p < 0.001$) of nonsurgical premature menopause. In clinical practice, individuals should be counseled to consider standard fertility preservation options of sperm, oocyte, and embryo cryopreservation when receiving chemotherapeutic agents with a CED of $\geq$4000 mg/m^2 or an AAD in the third tertile. Individuals receiving chemotherapeutic agents with a CED of $\geq$8000 mg/m^2 should also consider investigational therapies such as ovarian tissue freezing with concomitant in vitro maturation of aspirated oocytes and testicular tissue freezing when standard therapies are not available due to time or cost constraints.

Limitations of the AAD and CED are that the models are restricted to the effects of well-established alkylating agents on fertility and do not encompass the wide range of newer agents of unknown gonadal toxicity. These newer agents include nonclassical alkylators such as temozolomide, taxanes including paclitaxel and docetaxel, tyrosine kinase inhibitors such as imatinib, topoisomerase inhibitors such as irinotecan, immunotherapies including the monoclonal antibodies bevacizumab and trastuzumab and the newest of these agents to be approved in children, and immune checkpoint inhibitors such as pembrolizumab. Agents that historically have resulted in low (< 20%) and moderate (30–70%) risk to fertility also need to be better characterized to allow personalized risk stratification. Ultimately, models based on age, baseline fertility status, genetic differences in ovarian and testicular biology, and chemotherapeutic and radiation agents received would provide the best estimate of risk across treatments and ages.

58.1 Female Fertility Preservation Options

It is imperative that counseling about fertility options occur *prior* to initiating cancer therapies. Once chemotherapy has been initiated, no standard options are available, and investigational options are limited. Standard options for fertility preservation in adult females include mature oocyte cryopreservation, embryo cryopreservation, and ovarian shielding and transposition. Sperm cryopreservation via ejaculation, testicular aspiration and extraction, and testicular shielding are standard therapies in males. Investigational options for adults include immature oocyte cryopreservation, in vitro maturation, and ovarian and testicular tissue cryopreservation. Investigational options for prepubertal females include immature oocyte cryopreservation, in vitro maturation, and in vivo activation, the newest technology. In prepubertal males testicular cryopreservation is the only option and is investigational [30].

58.1.1 Standard Options

Mature egg freezing is now a standard option for infertility with success rates of 35–60% depending on age and underlying concomitant causes of infertility [31]. The benefit of mature oocyte cryopreservation is that no partner is required, making it a viable option for children and young adults. Historically, oocyte stimulation for retrieval required 14 days, and individuals were required to be within the early follicular phase, days 2–4 of menses. Advancements in technology have now allowed for random start cycles that may occur in either the follicular or luteal phase, with an average of 10–11 days for stimulation [32–34].

Stimulation in the prepubertal individual is not feasible due to negative inhibition of the hypothalamic-pituitary axis, which is not released until puberty by mechanisms that are not fully understood. However several centers around the country have begun to successfully stimulate early postpubertal individuals at risk of acute ovarian failure [35–37]. Stimulation in adolescents requires finesse and sensitivity as these individuals are typically unable to tolerate transvaginal ultrasound and may require higher doses of gonadotropins. Transabdominal ultrasound is typically performed for follicle surveillance with sedation and transvaginal ultrasound for retrieval. Higher gonadotropin doses may increase the risk of ovarian hyperstimulation syndrome (OHSS), potentially placing individuals at risk of fluid extravasation, hypercoagulation, and PE with a consequent delay in cancer treatment [38]. Studies have also suggested that oocyte yield may be lower in postpubertal individuals. Given the 28% probability of live birth with two oocytes thawed after vitrification in young women less than age 25 and 31% with six oocytes, a greater number of eggs are required to improve fertility rates [39]. Subjecting adolescents to ovarian stimulation (OS) must therefore be justified by retrieval of an adequate number of oocytes for successful pregnancy.

Embryo cryopreservation is reserved for individuals age 18 and older due to legal considerations in embryo creation. The upper age limit for most IVF programs is 42 due to significantly decreased success rates thereafter with success rates averaging 40% for women less than age 35 [40]. The requisite 10–12 days is required for stimulation and retrieval. The limitations of embryo cryopreservation are that a partner or sperm donor is required and ovarian function is not preserved. Embryo ownership concerns exist, and legal counseling and documentation are necessary prior to assisted reproduction.

Ovarian transposition (OT) is becoming increasingly more utilized with the development of formal fertility preservation programs. Success rates of preservation of ovarian function are high at 65–95%, depending on the mode of radiation used. Specifically, meta-analyses suggest that OT in pelvic brachytherapy and external beam radiotherapy have ovarian preservation rates of 94% and 65%, respectively [41]. Concerns with OT include loss of blood flow and difficulty conceiving due to the transposed location of the ovary. It is thus recommended to maintain the relationship between the ovary and the fallopian tube to minimize risk of infertility and the need for IVF. It is not necessary for the ovary to be transposed back into the pelvis, and pregnancies may be achieved through spontaneous conception and more commonly IVF. Ovarian shielding involves blocking the ovaries during pelvic radiation. Success rates with the technique are underreported, and scatter effect remains a concern. This may be due in part to the fact that concomitant chemotherapy is administered making it challenging to separate the effect of the two treatments on fertility.

58.1.2 Investigational Options

Investigational options include ovarian tissue cryopreservation, immature oocyte freezing, ovarian suppression with gonadotropin-releasing hormone agonists (GnRHa), and in vivo activation. Ovarian tissue cryopreservation (OTC) is currently the most successful investigational therapy for fertility preservation across age groups with a clinical pregnancy rate of 57.5% and live birth rate of 37% after tissue transplantation [42, 43]. There remains some debate regarding which individuals should pursue OTC due to the risk, albeit low, of surgical harvesting. The Edinburgh criteria for OTC in the setting of malignant disorders have been utilized in Europe since 1996 [44, 45]. Using the criteria, OTC is recommended when individuals have a $\geq$ 50% risk of gonadal failure after cancer treatment, absence of previous high gonadotoxic chemotherapy, and absence of surgical contraindication and negative infectious serology. Ovarian tissue cryopreservation is also offered to individuals with nonmalignant disorders, differences in gender and sex diversity, and those with a genetic predisposition to accelerated follicular loss. In the USA, infectious serology is not a contraindication to OTC, with storage protocols designed to isolate infectious samples. Currently there are 130 live births from OTC worldwide [46, 47]. Ages at retrieval range from adolescent to mid-30s with two reports of live births in individuals who underwent OTC prior to menarche. One individual was prepubertal and the other peri-pubertal [48, 49]. Pregnancies have occurred through both spontaneous conception and assisted reproductive technologies. Given the proven success of this technology, several investigators have suggested that OTC no longer be considered experimental. Transplanted tissue has been shown to be viable for up to 10 years [43].

Immature oocyte retrieval via in vitro maturation and cryopreservation is an investigational therapy that is attractive in that no stimulation is required and no partner is needed. Similar to egg and embryo freezing, it is a surgical procedure involving sedation, and there is no preservation of ovarian function. Follicles may be aspirated in both the follicular and luteal phases of the menstrual cycle. The major limitation of immature oocyte cryopreservation is that very few follicles may be aspirated due to the lack of stimulation. IVM has proven to be successful in individuals with polycystic ovaries with live birth rates approximating 20–35% [50–52]. With the advent of OTC, retrieval of immature oocytes with subsequent in vitro maturation and freezing at the time of ovarian tissue harvesting is now widely practiced. There remains concern that IVM from follicles retrieved from the prepubertal ovary are suboptimal for fertilization due to the presence of abnormal nongrowing follicles with slow in vitro growth and maturation. Reassuringly, these follicles show the ability to grow and acquire maturation complexes with ovarian tissue transplantation [52].

GnRHa therapy for ovarian protection has been the most controversial investigational option. Reasons include the use of different agonists in studies and a preponderance of retrospective and prospective studies with short follow-up periods and inaccurate markers of fecundity such as return of menstrual function and FSH and estradiol levels. Recent studies acknowledge that although menses, FSH, and estradiol may reflect current ovarian function, these markers do not predict future function or likelihood of fertility and live birth. Endpoints in current literature more accurately reflect ovarian function and include pregnancy and longer follow-up periods up to 3 years [53, 54]. In a meta-analysis of 29 randomized controlled trials, 10 met inclusion criteria with final analysis showing preservation of ovarian function after GnRHa therapy OR 1.83 (1.34, 2.49) [55]. The majority of studies have been performed in the breast cancer population; therefore the use of GnRHa therapy for ovarian protection in other cancer populations should occur only after clear and transparent discussion with the individual about the benefits. GnRHa therapy is often used for menstrual suppression during cancer treatment and has a low side-effect profile of hot flushes, irritability, and decreased bone mineral density, all of which can be ameliorated by add-back therapy with norethindrone acetate or estradiol [56, 57]. Consequently, individuals may be counseled that as they are receiving GnRHa therapy for menstrual suppression, there may be a secondary benefit of ovarian protection. Furthermore, the updated ASCO guidelines reflect the current knowledge stating "when proven fertility preservation methods such as oocyte, embryo, or ovarian tissue cryopreservation are not feasible, and in the setting of young women with breast cancer, GnRHa may be offered to individuals in the hope of reducing the likelihood of chemotherapy-induced ovarian insufficiency" [58].

In vitro activation is the newest emerging investigational option for individuals with POI due to any cause [59]. To date, the studies have been performed in women diagnosed with idiopathic POI and have not been extended to cancer survivors. After harvesting ovarian tissue, the tissue undergoes fragmentation of ovarian strips into cubes. The ovarian cubes are then stimulated with phosphatidylinositol 3 K (PI3k). The PI3k-stimulated cubes are then autotransplanted followed by ovarian stimulation with gonadotropins, retrieval, and IVF. The proposed mechanism of action is stimulation of primordial follicle growth by PI3k stimulation and growth of secondary follicles by ovarian cubing. To date, embryo transfer has led to four live births.

58.2 Male Fertility Preservation Options

58.2.1 Standard Options

Sperm banking is the only standard fertility preservation option in males. Sperm production is viable in male individuals as young as age 11 (Tanner stage II-III). For males who are unable to produce a specimen, sperm may be produced through ejaculation or with the assistance of vibratory stimulation and electro-ejaculation or testicular sperm aspiration, extraction, or biopsy [60, 61]. Electro-ejaculation is performed under anesthesia by placing a probe in the rectum and transmitting an electrical current that simulates the prostate gland and seminal vesicles to produce an ejaculate [62, 63]. Side effects include burning of the rectum and pain. Success rates for testicular sperm aspiration (TESA), extraction (TESE), and microdissection testicular sperm extraction (micro-TESE) are 15–50%, 20–60%, and 40–67%, respectively.

58.2.2 Investigational Options

Investigational options prior to treatment exist through cryopreservation of testicular tissue or testicular cell suspensions and include autologous SSC transplantation, testicular tissue grafting (autotransplantation), and in vitro spermatogenesis. Sperm extracted through aspiration from the testis or harvested testicular tissue can be processed by enzymatic digestion and cryopreserved. In prepubertal boys, there are no mature sperm to harvest; however, spermatogonial stem cells are present and may be used for investigational therapies. Prepubertal testicular tissue cryopreservation may be offered to males from birth through age 13 (under Tanner stage III) under an IRB-approved protocol. Testicular cryopreservation in prepubertal boys is an unproven technology, but research indicates the potential to produce viable sperm in the future [64]. Testicular biopsy for harvesting involves excision of up to 25% of testicular parenchyma. Testicular biopsy should not be considered with acute leukemia not in remission due to the theoretical risk of introducing leukemic cells into the testes at the time of the biopsy. It is important to note that the duration of sperm integrity after an initial course of chemotherapy is currently unknown [65–67]. Therefore, the standard of care is to collect sperm or tissue prior to starting therapy to optimize sample quantity and minimize the risk of sperm damage, which may lead to pregnancy loss and/or birth defects. Experimental options during treatment include testicular shielding during radiation therapy and temporary gonadal relocation. Locations for relocation of testes include the anterior abdominal wall before radiation therapy of the pelvis or perineum [68]. Hormonal suppression with gonadotropin agonists for fertility preservation in men has not been shown to be beneficial for recovery of spermatogenesis and is not recommended.

58.3 Decision-Making and Ethics

The physician-patient dyad becomes a triad when caring for children as the child's contribution to shared decision-making is valued. It is necessary to have an understanding of decision-making and ethical considerations in this population, particularly as relates to enrollment in investigational studies [69]. Shared decision-making requires the use of terminology that the child and family can understand as well as an appreciation that there may be a difference in values. Time is necessary to allow full understanding of treatment options and short- and long-term implications. Involvement of ethicists prior to implementation of investigational protocols in children allows thoughtful consideration of potential challenges to study approval and recruitment that may be addressed preemptively. The lower age of competence for assent is 9–10 years with most authorities acknowledging that children under age 9 are unable to participate in informed assent. Children ages 10–12 may provide verbal assent, whereas children ages 12–17 typically are required to provide written assent for investigational studies. Recent authors challenge the notion of informed assent in adolescents, suggesting that children 12 and older may instead provide written consent [70]. Involvement of child-life services during the assent process can ameliorate anxiety and improve the experienced of child-parent-physician.

58.4 Survivorship

The National Cancer Institute (NCI) defines a cancer survivor as an individual from the time of cancer diagnosis through the balance of his or her life and encompasses cancer-free survival, chronic or intermittent disease, and palliative care [71]. Survivorship care should thus be incorporated into the individual's care continuum at diagnosis. Fertility and reproductive aspects of survivorship include posttreatment fertility assessment, hormone insufficiency, sequelae from pelvic radiation, and timing of conception.

58.4.1 Assessment of Ovarian Reserve

Assessment of ovarian reserve after cancer treatment in female survivors of childhood remains an area of debate. Antral follicle count (AFC) is the most reliable and direct measure of ovarian reserve and is obtained by averaging the follicles measuring 2–10 mm in both ovaries via transvaginal ultrasound. Consequently, AFC is challenging to obtain in adolescents who cannot tolerate transvaginal ultrasound. An AFC < 5 is considered diminished ovarian reserve [72]. Anti-Mullerian hormone (AMH) serum testing is an indirect measure of ovarian reserve and thus is more widely used than AFC. AMH has a bimodal expression with levels falling after birth, rising at age 4, and falling again at age 8. Levels then rise a second time to plateau at age 25 when levels begin to slowly fall to the menopause [73]. An AMH less than 0.5 ng/ml is consistent with impending onset of premature menopause and predicts low ovarian response to ovarian stimulation. Values between 0.5 and 1.0 ng/ml suggest a limited egg supply and diminished reserve as well as a shortened reproductive window. Normal testing ranges between >1.0 and < 3.5, and elevated AMH >3.5 ng/ml is typically consistent with polycystic ovaries and risk of OHSS [74] (Table 58.3). Despite well-established cutoffs for diminished ovarian reserve, the predictive accuracy of AMH for live birth after IVF remains poor [75].

Elchuri et al. are the first to attempt to characterize the utility of AMH *after cancer treatment* in the pediatric population [76]. They stratify AMH levels into 5th, 50th, and 95th percentiles based on age to provide a nomogram to define diminished ovarian reserve. In this stratification model, diminished ovarian reserve is defined as AMH less than the 5th percentile. Conversely, assessment of *pretreatment* AMH levels as predictors of posttreatment ovarian function has been widely studied. A recent study has shown that individuals with pretreatment AMH levels greater than 2 ng/ml recovered their AMH levels at a rate of 11.9% per month after chemotherapy. Individuals with AMH <2 ng/ml recovered at a rate of 2.6% per month [77]. Importantly, AMH has been shown to decrease before the onset of irregular cycles and before the rise of FSH levels [78].

Studies show that childhood cancer survivors with spontaneous menses more than 5 years after diagnosis have a 13-fold higher risk of premature menopause. Further studies show that these survivors had a significantly decreased pregnancy rate with 38% (30% for males and 46% of females) reporting having a pregnancy compared to 62% of control. Approximately 13% of survivors required more than

Table 58.3 Anti-Mullerian hormone (AMH) and ovarian reserve

[1]AMH ng/ml	Clinical situation	Implications
Very low (0.5)	Impending onset of premature menopause	Predicts low ovarian response to stimulation
Low (<1.0)	Limited egg supply	Shortened reproductive window
Mid-range (1–3.5)	Normal testing	Consider preservation of high-risk chemotherapy
Elevated (>3.5)	PCO or PCO-like ovaries	Risk of OHSS

12 months of attempts to achieve pregnancy compared to 8.3% of sibling controls [20, 79].

There are currently no guidelines to recommend fertility preservation based on pretreatment FSH, AMH or AFC, or posttreatment monitoring in the absence of clinical signs of ovarian insufficiency. The Children's Oncology Group recommends posttreatment referral of all postpubertal individuals treated with a potentially gonadotoxic regimen without any signs or symptoms of POI who desire assessment for future fertility and those with POI who require HRT for pubertal induction [80]. Recommendations include baseline FSH, LH, and estradiol at age 13 as well as baseline FSH, LH, and estradiol with abnormal menses and in the setting of signs of estrogen deficiency [81]. AMH testing is not yet considered standard of care in individuals < age 25 years; however, several authors describe an algorithm to utilize posttreatment AMH. Dillon et al. illustrate that individuals with pretreatment AMH levels greater than 2 ng/ml recovered their AMH levels at a rate of 11.9% per month after chemotherapy. Individuals with AMH <2 ng/ml recovered at a rate of 2.6% per month [77]. Guzy and Demeestere suggest baseline AMH testing to assess ovarian reserve prior to cancer treatment with serial AMH yearly to follow rate of decline. Referral should be made to REI for fertility pretreatment when levels fall below norms for age or if individual desires preservation [82]. Given findings that AMH has been shown to decrease before the onset of irregular cycles and before the rise of FSH levels, yearly monitoring of AMH and FSH is a reasonable approach with referral to REI if AMH less than reference range for age or FSH >10 [78].

58.4.2 Assessment of Testicular Reserve

Assessment of testicular function includes evaluation of both spermatogenesis from germ cells lining the seminiferous tubules and testosterone production from the Leydig cells. As previously described, germ cell function is impaired at lower chemotherapeutic doses compared to Leydig cell function. Evaluation of spermatogenesis is not typically performed in childhood; however, semen analysis may be performed at any age postpuberty. Studies consistently show time to recovery after pelvic radiation and chemotherapy to be 12–72 months [25, 83]. Consequently, in practice, semen analysis is typically reserved until an individual is interested in conception and is at least 12–24 months posttreatment. The COG long-term follow-up (LTFU) guidelines recommend yearly evaluation of pubertal onset and tempo and sexual function by erections, nocturnal emissions, and libido [80, 84]. Physical examination should include Tanner staging and testicular volume by Prader orchiometer. It is recommended to assess baseline testosterone at age 14 and as clinically indicated in patients with delayed or arrested

Table 58.4 Symptoms of low testosterone

Sexual	Constitutional	Cognitive
Diminished sexual drive	Anemia	Depression
Delayed orgasm	Decreased muscle	Decreased motivation
Decreased nocturnal erection	Decreased bone density	Decreased sense of overall Well-being
Erectile dysfunction	Hot flashes	Insomnia
		Irritability
		Lethargy
		Short-term memory loss

puberty and/or clinical signs and symptoms of testosterone deficiency. Recently, evidence has supported the usefulness of AMH, inhibin B, and testicular volume for the early diagnosis of puberty disorders and primary testicular damage [85]. Symptoms of low testosterone include sexual, constitutional, and cognitive disturbances (Table 58.4). Long-term consequences of low testosterone include an estimated doubling in mortality risk comparted with men with normal testosterone levels [86]. Hormone replacement therapy is typically provided by a pediatric or adult endocrinologist or reproductive urologist. The recommendation is that individuals be treated with replacement when total testosterone is below 230–300 ng/dl and/or free testosterone is approximately 5–9 ng/dl [87]. Close monitoring is required to assess response to testosterone replacement for pubertal induction or as replacement in adolescents and young adults.

58.4.3 Reproductive Health Concerns

Reproductive health concerns for survivors of pediatric cancers include gonadal insufficiency, infertility, diminished bone density and early onset dementia, genitourinary symptoms, sexual dysfunction, and graft-versus-host disease (GVHD) in females [88]. Radiation therapy to the female pelvis increases risk of miscarriage, preterm labor, and low birth weight. Vaginal fibrosis, stenosis, and fistula formation occur at ≥90–100 [89]. In individuals without hormone-sensitive tumors, vasomotor and genitourinary symptoms may be managed with hormonal and nonhormonal therapies. HRT is indicated for pubertal induction in children or as replacement doses in adolescents and young adults experiencing ovarian insufficiency or AOF [90]. Transdermal HRT is the preferred method of add-back therapy and provides continuous physiologic doses of HRT which avert the first-pass effect through the liver [91, 92]. Administration of progestin for uterine protection and completion of breast development are often challenging. Options include oral progestin therapy daily for 12 days each month, continuous therapy with one pill daily, or use of the levonorgestrel intrauterine system. There are no well-controlled studies comparing the options for uterine protection. However, levonorgestrel IUD is used for the treatment of endometrial hyperplasia and uterine protection against the recurrence of endometrial cancer [93]. As most survivors of pediatric cancers do not often develop hormone-sensitive tumors, nonhormonal and investigational therapies to manage genitourinary syndrome such as DHEA, ospemifene, a selective estrogen receptor modulator, and CO_2 laser are typically not indicated in the pediatric population.

Genital GVHD after stem cell transplantation (SCT) in females is of significant concern. Genital GVHD usually occurs in combination with systemic disease with an incidence of 25–49%. Distribution is typically 68% vulvar and 28% vulvovaginal with onset typically 7–10 months after SCT. Late disease can occur 1–2 years later, and recurrence rate is unknown. The presentation of GVHD includes redness of the vulva, erosions, sores and fissures as well as tenderness of vulvar glands, and ultimately scarring, if left untreated [94, 95]. This is in comparison with genital atrophy which presents as pale pink vaginal tissue, easy bleeding on contact, and thin labia which may fuse. The recommendation is early evaluation of all allogeneic HSCT individuals for GVHD for early diagnosis and prevention of vaginal stenosis and narrowing. Vaginal stenosis may be managed by dilator therapy or surgical repair. Management should include primarily topical immunosuppressive agents such as corticosteroids, tacrolimus, or cyclosporine. Topical estrogen may be used as supportive care for concomitant hypoestrogenism but should not be considered the first-line therapy [96, 97].

Sexual dysfunction should be assessed in adolescent survivors after cancer treatment similarly to adults. There are well-established screening tools for males but no gold-standard screening tools for females; thus a combination of tools may be indicated [98]. Individuals should be referred to a therapist specializing in this area upon positive screening. Studies show that adolescent cancer survivors are as interested in sexual activity as their peers and engage in risky sexual behavior at rates equivalent to sibling controls [99]. It is important to recognize that due to the nature of FP counseling, individuals often equate "increased risk of infertility" with "infertility" and do not consider contraception. Assessment of sexual activity and contraceptive needs during treatment and in survivorship is therefore critical.

58.5 Conclusion

Advancements in cancer treatment have significantly improved the future outlook for individuals diagnosed with cancer and other life-threatening conditions now treated with chemotherapeutic agents. Survivors require and expect a quality-of-life commensurate with these breakthroughs. As attention is given to improve cardiac, renal, pulmonary, and neurologic function in survivorship, so must there also be continued focus on fertility and parenthood after treatment. The approach to the prepubertal child with cancer must be comprehensive and include fertility risk assessment with implementation of fertility preservation options as available, assessment of gonadal function pre- and posttreatment with HRT as indicated, and attention to the reproductive concerns in survivorship that are often underappreciated. Interventions to remove barriers include parental awareness, provider knowledge, increased number of referral sites, legislative efforts to cover fertility preservation therapies, and reduced overall cost. In doing this, we provide an opportunity for life after cancer that is reflective of the great achievements in cancer treatment.

References

1. Siegel RL, Miller KD, Jemal A. Cancer statistics, 2018. CA Cancer J Clin. 2018;68(1):7–30.
2. Lewis DR, et al. Adolescent and young adult cancer survival. J Natl Cancer Inst Monogr. 2014;2014(49):228–35.
3. Taylor JF, Ott MA. Fertility preservation after a cancer diagnosis: a systematic review of adolescents', parents', and providers' perspectives, experiences, and preferences. J Pediatr Adolesc Gynecol. 2016;29(6):585–98.
4. Hudson MM, et al. Clinical ascertainment of health outcomes among adults treated for childhood cancer. JAMA. 2013;309(22):2371–81.
5. Lambertini M, et al. Cancer and fertility preservation: international recommendations from an expert meeting. BMC Med. 2016;14:1.
6. Woodruff TK. Oncofertility: a grand collaboration between reproductive medicine and oncology. Reproduction. 2015;150(3):S1–S10.
7. Lee SJ, et al. American Society of Clinical Oncology recommendations on fertility preservation in cancer patients. J Clin Oncol. 2006;24(18):2917–31.
8. Loren AW, et al. Fertility preservation for patients with cancer: American Society of Clinical Oncology clinical practice guideline update. J Clin Oncol. 2013;31(19):2500–10.
9. No Authors Listed. Committee opinion no. 607: Gynecologic concerns in children and adolescents with cancer. Obstet Gynecol. 2014;124(2 Pt 1):403–8.
10. Fallat ME, et al. Preservation of fertility in pediatric and adolescent patients with cancer. Pediatrics. 2008;121(5):e1461–9.
11. Barbara Carr R, et al. APHON position paper on fertility preservation for pediatric and adolescent young adult (AYA) cancer patients.
12. Quinn GP, Vadaparampil ST, Fertility Preservation Research Group. Research, fertility preservation and adolescent/young adult cancer patients: physician communication challenges. J Adolesc Health. 2009;44(4):394–400.
13. Quinn GP, et al. Physician referral for fertility preservation in oncology patients: a national study of practice behaviors. J Clin Oncol. 2009;27(35):5952–7.
14. Niemasik EE, et al. Patient perceptions of reproductive health counseling at the time of cancer diagnosis: a qualitative study of female California cancer survivors. J Cancer Surviv. 2012;6(3):324–32.
15. Chin HB, et al. Which female cancer patients fail to receive fertility counseling before treatment in the state of Georgia? Fertil Steril. 2016;106(7):1763–1771 e1.

16. Lawrenz B, et al. Fertility preservation in >1,000 patients: patient's characteristics, spectrum, efficacy and risks of applied preservation techniques. Arch Gynecol Obstet. 2011;283(3):651–6.
17. Gwede CK, et al. The role of radiation oncologists and discussion of fertility preservation in young cancer patients. Pract Radiat Oncol. 2012;2(4):242–7.
18. Douglas NL. Roger, reproductive endocrinology: neuroendocrinology, gonadotropins, sex steroids, prostaglandins, ovulation, menstruation, hormone assay. In: Lobo RA, editor. Comprehensive Gynecology. Philadelphia, PA: Elsevier; 2017. p. 77–107.
19. Wallace WH, Kelsey TW. Human ovarian reserve from conception to the menopause. PLoS One. 2010;5(1):e8772.
20. Chemaitilly W, et al. Acute ovarian failure in the childhood cancer survivor study. J Clin Endocrinol Metab. 2006;91(5):1723–8.
21. Bray I, Gunnell D, Davey Smith G. Advanced paternal age: how old is too old? J Epidemiol Community Health. 2006;60(10):851–3.
22. Howell SJ, Shalet SM. Testicular function following chemotherapy. Hum Reprod Update. 2001;7(4):363–9.
23. Wallace WH, et al. Predicting age of ovarian failure after radiation to a field that includes the ovaries. Int J Radiat Oncol Biol Phys. 2005;62(3):738–44.
24. Critchley HO, Wallace WH. Impact of cancer treatment on uterine function. J Natl Cancer Inst Monogr. 2005;34:64–8.
25. Meistrich ML. Effects of chemotherapy and radiotherapy on spermatogenesis in humans. Fertil Steril. 2013;100(5):1180–6.
26. Levine J, Canada A, Stern CJ. Fertility preservation in adolescents and young adults with cancer. J Clin Oncol. 2010;28(32):4831–41.
27. Tucker MA, et al. Bone sarcomas linked to radiotherapy and chemotherapy in children. N Engl J Med. 1987;317(10):588–93.
28. Tucker MA, et al. Leukemia after therapy with alkylating agents for childhood cancer. J Natl Cancer Inst. 1987;78(3):459–64.
29. Green DM, et al. The cyclophosphamide equivalent dose as an approach for quantifying alkylating agent exposure: a report from the Childhood Cancer Survivor Study. Pediatr Blood Cancer. 2014;61(1):53–67.
30. Javed A, et al. Options for fertility preservation in children. Pediatr Endocrinol Rev. 2018;15(3):223–33.
31. Practice Committees of American Society for Reproductive Medicine, Society for Assisted Reproductive Technology. Mature oocyte cryopreservation: a guideline. Fertil Steril. 2013;99(1):37–43
32. Cakmak H, et al. Effective method for emergency fertility preservation: random-start controlled ovarian stimulation. Fertil Steril. 2013;100(6):1673–80.
33. Cakmak H, Rosen MP. Random-start ovarian stimulation in patients with cancer. Curr Opin Obstet Gynecol. 2015;27(3):215–21.
34. Kim JH, et al. Efficacy of random-start controlled ovarian stimulation in cancer patients. J Korean Med Sci. 2015;30(3):290–5.
35. Srikanthan A, et al. Fertility preservation in post-pubescent female cancer patients: A practical guideline for clinicians. Mol Clin Oncol. 2018;8(1):153–8.
36. Oktay K, Bedoschi G. Oocyte cryopreservation for fertility preservation in postpubertal female children at risk for premature ovarian failure due to accelerated follicle loss in Turner syndrome or cancer treatments. J Pediatr Adolesc Gynecol. 2014;27(6):342–6.
37. Reichman DE, et al. Fertility preservation using controlled ovarian hyperstimulation and oocyte cryopreservation in a premenarcheal female with myelodysplastic syndrome. Fertil Steril. 2012;98(5):1225–8.
38. Boothroyd C, et al. Consensus statement on prevention and detection of ovarian hyperstimulation syndrome. Aust N Z J Obstet Gynaecol. 2015;55(6):523–34.
39. Cil AP, Bang H, Oktay K. Age-specific probability of live birth with oocyte cryopreservation: an individual patient data meta-analysis. Fertil Steril. 2013;100(2):492–9.. e3
40. Wong KM, Mastenbroek S, Repping S. Cryopreservation of human embryos and its contribution to in vitro fertilization success rates. Fertil Steril. 2014;102(1):19–26.
41. Gubbala K, et al. Outcomes of ovarian transposition in gynaecological cancers; a systematic review and meta-analysis. J Ovarian Res. 2014;7:69.
42. Jensen AK, et al. 86 successful births and 9 ongoing pregnancies worldwide in women transplanted with frozen-thawed ovarian tissue: focus on birth and perinatal outcome in 40 of these children. J Assist Reprod Genet. 2017;34(3):325–36.
43. Jensen AK, et al. Cryopreservation of ovarian tissue for fertility preservation in a large cohort of young girls: focus on pubertal development. Hum Reprod. 2017;32(1):154–64.
44. Wallace WH, Anderson RA, Irvine DS. Fertility preservation for young patients with cancer: who is at risk and what can be offered? Lancet Oncol. 2005;6(4):209–18.
45. Wallace WH, et al. Fertility preservation for girls and young women with cancer: population-based validation of criteria for ovarian tissue cryopreservation. Lancet Oncol. 2014;15(10):1129–36.
46. Pacheco F, Oktay K. Current success and efficiency of autologous ovarian transplantation: a meta-analysis. Reprod Sci. 2017;24(8):1111–20.
47. Donnez J, Dolmans MM. Fertility preservation in women. N Engl J Med. 2017;377(17):1657–65.
48. Demeestere I, et al. Live birth after autograft of ovarian tissue cryopreserved during childhood. Hum Reprod. 2015;30(9):2107–9.
49. Walsh F, Woman has baby using ovary frozen in childhood. BBC News. 2016.
50. Shirasawa H, Terada Y. In vitro maturation of human immature oocytes for fertility preservation and research material. Reprod Med Biol. 2017;16(3):258–67.
51. Chian RC, Uzelac PS, Nargund G. In vitro maturation of human immature oocytes for fertility preservation. Fertil Steril. 2013;99(5):1173–81.
52. Prasath EB, et al. First pregnancy and live birth resulting from cryopreserved embryos obtained from in vitro matured oocytes after oophorectomy in an ovarian cancer patient. Hum Reprod. 2014;29(2):276–8.
53. Moore HC, et al. Goserelin for ovarian protection during breast-cancer adjuvant chemotherapy. N Engl J Med. 2015;372(10):923–32.
54. Hickman LC, et al. Preservation of gonadal function in women undergoing chemotherapy: a systematic review and meta-analysis of the potential role for gonadotropin-releasing hormone agonists. J Assist Reprod Genet. 2018;35(4):571–81.
55. Lambertini M, et al. Gonadotropin-releasing hormone agonists during chemotherapy for preservation of ovarian function and fertility in premenopausal patients with early breast cancer: a systematic review and meta-analysis of individual patient-level data. J Clin Oncol. 2018;36(19):1981–90.
56. DiVasta AD, et al. Practice-based quality improvement collaborative to increase chlamydia screening in young women. Pediatrics. 2016;137(5):e20151082.
57. Chu MC, et al. Formation of ethinyl estradiol in women during treatment with norethindrone acetate. J Clin Endocrinol Metab. 2007;92(6):2205–7.
58. Oktay K, et al. Fertility preservation in patients with cancer: ASCO clinical practice guideline update. J Clin Oncol. 2018;36(19):1994–2001.
59. Kawamura K, Kawamura N, Hsueh AJ. Activation of dormant follicles: a new treatment for premature ovarian failure? Curr Opin Obstet Gynecol. 2016;28(3):217–22.
60. Katz DJ, et al. Fertility preservation strategies for male patients with cancer. Nat Rev Urol. 2013;10(8):463–72.
61. Jurewicz M, et al. Fertility preservation in pubertal and pre-pubertal boys with cancer. Pediatr Endocrinol Rev. 2018;15(3):234–43.

62. Adank MC, et al. Electroejaculation as a method of fertility preservation in boys diagnosed with cancer: a single-center experience and review of the literature. Fertil Steril. 2014;102(1):199–205 e1.
63. Hovav Y, et al. Electroejaculation before chemotherapy in adolescents and young men with cancer. Fertil Steril. 2001;75(4):811–3.
64. Orwig KE, Schlatt S. Cryopreservation and transplantation of spermatogonia and testicular tissue for preservation of male fertility. J Natl Cancer Inst Monogr. 2005;34:51–6.
65. Balduzzi A, et al. Fertility preservation issues in pediatric hematopoietic stem cell transplantation: practical approaches from the consensus of the Pediatric Diseases Working Party of the EBMT and the International BFM Study Group. Bone Marrow Transplant. 2017;52(10):1406–15.
66. Choy JT, Brannigan RE. The determination of reproductive safety in men during and after cancer treatment. Fertil Steril. 2013;100(5):1187–91.
67. Meistrich ML. Potential genetic risks of using semen collected during chemotherapy. Hum Reprod. 1993;8(1):8–10.
68. Acosta JM, et al. Temporary relocation of testes to the anterior abdominal wall before radiation therapy of the pelvis or perineum. J Pediatr Surg. 2002;37(8):1232–3.
69. Tates K, Meeuwesen L. Doctor-parent-child communication. A (re) view of the literature. Soc Sci Med. 2001;52(6):839–51.
70. Hein IM, et al. Assessing children's competence to consent in research by a standardized tool: a validity study. BMC Pediatr. 2012;12:156.
71. National Cancer Policy Board. From cancer patient to cancer survivor: lost in transition. Washington, DC: National Academies Press; 2005.
72. Scheffer GJ, et al. The number of antral follicles in normal women with proven fertility is the best reflection of reproductive age. Hum Reprod. 2003;18(4):700–6.
73. Hagen CP, et al. Serum levels of anti-Mullerian hormone as a marker of ovarian function in 926 healthy females from birth to adulthood and in 172 Turner syndrome patients. J Clin Endocrinol Metab. 2010;95(11):5003–10.
74. Toner JP, Seifer DB. Why we may abandon basal follicle-stimulating hormone testing: a sea change in determining ovarian reserve using antimullerian hormone. Fertil Steril. 2013;99(7):1825–30.
75. Iliodromiti S, et al. The predictive accuracy of anti-Mullerian hormone for live birth after assisted conception: a systematic review and meta-analysis of the literature. Hum Reprod Update. 2014;20(4):560–70.
76. Elchuri SV, et al. Low anti-Mullerian hormone in pediatric cancer survivors in the early years after gonadotoxic therapy. J Pediatr Adolesc Gynecol. 2016;29(4):393–9.
77. Dillon KE, et al. Pretreatment antimullerian hormone levels determine rate of posttherapy ovarian reserve recovery: acute changes in ovarian reserve during and after chemotherapy. Fertil Steril. 2013;99(2):477–83.
78. Grynnerup AG, Lindhard A, Sorensen S. The role of anti-Mullerian hormone in female fertility and infertility: an overview. Acta Obstet Gynecol Scand. 2012;91(11):1252–60.
79. Chow EJ, et al. Pregnancy after chemotherapy in male and female survivors of childhood cancer treated between 1970 and 1999: a report from the Childhood Cancer Survivor Study cohort. Lancet Oncol. 2016;17(5):567–76.
80. Curesearch Children's Oncology Group. Long-term follow-up guidelines for survivors of childhood, adolescent and young adult cancers. Monrovia, CA: Children's Oncology Group; 2013.
81. van Dorp W, et al. Recommendations for premature Ovarian insufficiency surveillance for female survivors of childhood, adolescent, and young adult cancer: a report from the international late effects of childhood cancer guideline harmonization group in collaboration with the PanCareSurFup Consortium. J Clin Oncol. 2016;34(28):3440–50.
82. Guzy L, Demeestere I. Assessment of ovarian reserve and fertility preservation strategies in children treated for cancer. Minerva Ginecol. 2017;69(1):57–67.
83. Howell SJ, Shalet SM. Spermatogenesis after cancer treatment: damage and recovery. J Natl Cancer Inst Monogr. 2005;34:12–7.
84. Kremer LCM, et al. A worldwide collaboration to harmonize guidelines for the long-term follow-up of childhood and young adult cancer survivors: a report from the international late effects of childhood cancer guideline harmonization group. Pediatr Blood Cancer. 2013;60(4):543–9.
85. Condorelli RA, et al. Evaluation of testicular function in prepubertal children. Endocrine. 2018;62(2):274–80.
86. Tivesten A, et al. Low serum testosterone and estradiol predict mortality in elderly men. J Clin Endocrinol Metab. 2009;94(7):2482–8.
87. Bhasin S, et al. Testosterone therapy in men with androgen deficiency syndromes: an Endocrine Society clinical practice guideline. J Clin Endocrinol Metab. 2010;95(6):2536–59.
88. Faubion SS, Loprinzi CL, Ruddy KJ. Management of hormone deprivation symptoms after cancer. Mayo Clin Proc. 2016;91(8):1133–46.
89. Jackson SE, et al. Sexuality after a cancer diagnosis: a population-based study. Cancer. 2016;122(24):3883–91.
90. Nelson LM, Covington SN, Rebar RW. An update: spontaneous premature ovarian failure is not an early menopause. Fertil Steril. 2005;83(5):1327–32.
91. Bondy CA, Turner Syndrome G. Study, care of girls and women with Turner syndrome: a guideline of the Turner Syndrome Study Group. J Clin Endocrinol Metab. 2007;92(1):10–25.
92. Delemarre EM, Felius B, de Waal HA D-v. Inducing puberty. Eur J Endocrinol. 2008;159(Suppl 1):S9–15.
93. Jareid M, et al. Levonorgestrel-releasing intrauterine system use is associated with a decreased risk of ovarian and endometrial cancer, without increased risk of breast cancer. Results from the NOWAC Study. Gynecol Oncol. 2018;149(1):127–32.
94. Stratton P, et al. Vulvovaginal chronic graft-versus-host disease with allogeneic hematopoietic stem cell transplantation. Obstet Gynecol. 2007;110(5):1041–9.
95. Majhail NS, et al. Recommended screening and preventive practices for long-term survivors after hematopoietic cell transplantation. Biol Blood Marrow Transplant. 2012;18(3):348–71.
96. Spiryda LB, et al. Graft-versus-host disease of the vulva and/or vagina: diagnosis and treatment. Biol Blood Marrow Transplant. 2003;9(12):760–5.
97. Hamilton BK, et al. Clinical management of genital chronic GvHD. Bone Marrow Transplant. 2017;52(6):803–10.
98. Jones LR. The use of validated questionnaires to assess female sexual dysfunction. World J Urol. 2002;20(2):89–92.
99. Klosky JL, et al. Risky sexual behavior in adolescent survivors of childhood cancer: a report from the Childhood Cancer Survivor Study. Health Psychol. 2014;33(8):868–77.

59 Fertility Preservation for Prepubertal Boys at Risk of Infertility

Rod T. Mitchell and Federica Lopes

For prepubertal boys at risk of infertility, there are currently no established options for fertility preservation. The possibility for future fertility in these individuals is dependent on survival of the spermatogonial stem cell population during prepuberty testis. These stem cells will ultimately give rise to mature gametes following the onset of spermatogenesis at puberty. In this chapter we will describe the important changes that occur in the testis during prepuberty and the clinical situations in which fertility may be compromised during this period, with a particular focus on the effects of cancer treatment during childhood. We will discuss the present options for cryopreserving testicular tissue from prepubertal boys at risk of infertility and the experimental approaches that are under investigation as future clinical strategies for fertility restoration.

59.1 The Seminiferous Epithelium of the Testis in Prepubertal and Adolescent Males

The timing of the onset of puberty is variable across mammalian species, with a pronounced interval between birth and initiation of puberty in primates. In humans, puberty usually starts between the ages of 9–13 years and lasts for about 2–4 years before the accomplishment of full sexual competency. During this long prepubertal period, testicular volume remains fairly constant (0.57 mls from birth to 1.5 mls at 10 years of age) [1], leading to the widely held hypothesis that this period represents a quiescent stage. Nevertheless, several studies have shown that testicular tissue in children is far from being dormant [2, 3], although the precise details of the cellular and molecular modifications that occur during this period require further investigation.

The first important period of postnatal testicular development occurs in the first 6 months of life during the so called minipuberty, when a sixfold increase in Sertoli cell number and a threefold increase in germ cell number are observed [4]. This results in a doubling of testis volume, although such an increment does not appear to be detectable by clinical evaluation [5]. More recently, it has been reported that the majority of this initial testicular growth occurs within the first 4 weeks of life [3], as a possible consequence of hormonal adaptation to extrauterine life. At birth, the majority of the germ cells are spermatogonia, having differentiated from gonocytes during foetal life. During the infantile period, the remainder of the gonocytes differentiate to spermatogonia which represent the only germ cell population present for the majority of the prepubertal period [6].

Morphological studies show that seminiferous tubules in the childhood testis are represented by solid cords (60–65 μm in diameter), with a lumen forming only around the age of 8–9 years [7]. These tubules are populated predominantly by immature Sertoli cells (>90%; more than 20 cells per cross-section) and spermatogonia in early stages of development [8].

Sertoli cells, in addition to being the most abundant, are also the most actively proliferating cells during childhood: such exponential increment in Sertoli cell number is responsible for the increase in length of the seminiferous tubules, coupled with an increase in number and volume of peritubular myoid cells. This proliferation of Sertoli cells is faster during the first few months of life and slower during childhood [9]. As the seminiferous cords are elongating, the number of Sertoli cells per cross-section reduces; however, the total number per testis increments.

Sertoli cells are epithelial cells, which need to be anchored to the basal lamina, therefore, as a consequence of their proliferation, seminiferous tubules elongate. During childhood, due to their abundant number coupled with the scarcity of germ cells, Sertoli cells appear to form a pseudostratified

R. T. Mitchell (✉)
MRC Centre for Reproductive Health, University of Edinburgh, The Queen's Medical Research Institute, Edinburgh, UK
e-mail: rod.mitchell@ed.ac.uk

F. Lopes
Centre for Discovery Brain Sciences, University of Edinburgh, Hugh Robson Building, Edinburgh, UK

G. N. Allahbadia et al. (eds.), *Textbook of Assisted Reproduction*, https://doi.org/10.1007/978-981-15-2377-9_59

epithelium. Since a mature Sertoli cell will have the ability of nurturing only a certain number of germ cells in adulthood [10–20] during spermatogenesis, this prepubertal phase of somatic cell proliferation is of major importance for future fertility [21].

Germ cells also proliferate during childhood, however, at a much lower rate compared with Sertoli cells, therefore, even if germ cell number per testis increases, quantitative studies showed that the number of germ cells expressed per Sertoli cell or per tubule cross-section reduces [1, 22]. An important subset of germ cells is represented by the spermatogonial stem cell (SCC) pool. SSCs possess the ability to self-renew or differentiate to undergo spermatogenesis. SSCs are located on the basal membrane of the seminiferous tubules surrounded by Sertoli cells in the SSC niche, the characteristics of which remain poorly understood in humans [23]. It is likely that intrinsic and extrinsic factors will be involved in the maintenance of this unique cell population within its microenvironment. SSCs represent the key spermatogonial population that must be preserved during prepuberty in order for future fertility to be possible.

At the onset of puberty, Sertoli cells enter mitotic arrest and start to undergo further maturation, forming the blood-testis barrier and developing cytoplasmic processes [8], while, concurrently, germ cells start to proliferate. Spermatogonial proliferation is responsible for the increase in seminiferous tubule diameter, which in turn produces a significant and clinically appreciable increase in testis volume. As a consequence, Sertoli cells are spread out in a columnar layer (about ten cells per cross-section) along the seminiferous tubules, which are now mainly populated by germ cells at different stages of development.

Although the appearance of early spermatocytes is associated with the start of puberty, occasional primary spermatocytes can be found in the prepubertal testis, and in rare cases, spermatids may also be identified from as early as 4 years of age, although spermatozoa are not produced during this stage [7]. The presence of these cell types is believed to represent initial trials of completing spermatogenesis, ending with cell death. Similarly, during the first few years from the onset of puberty, initial waves of spermatocytes inevitably degenerate, and only when cell death is reduced, coupled with increased proliferation rate, germ cells will progressively become capable of completing spermatogenesis [3]. Similarly, the first appearance of spermatozoa does not mean the accomplishment of full sexual maturity: the full process will only be achieved 2–4 years after it begins [8].

During prepubertal life, scarce immature Leydig cells can be found in the interstitial space [2]. However, during early puberty, prior to the development of secondary sex characteristics or any clinically appreciable increase in testis volume, Leydig cell precursors will become able to respond to luteinising hormone (LH) and synthetise testosterone. This increase in testicular testosterone coincides with the kick-start of spermatogonial proliferation and reduction in apoptosis, incremental increase in seminiferous tubules diameter, Sertoli cell maturation and ultimately puberty.

From ~9 years of age onward, LH and follicle-stimulating hormone (FSH) start to rise concomitantly with the increase in testicular volume. After the age of 13, hormones levels increase dramatically, with testes reaching a size close to the final adult volume of $\geq$12mls. During prepuberty and puberty, high levels of FSH and testosterone induce Sertoli cell proliferation and maturation (cytoplasmic organelle changes, tight junction formation and reduction in anti-Mullerian hormone secretion), while Leydig cell proliferation and maturation are under the control of LH. During puberty and early post-puberty, spermatogenesis progresses efficiently, although spermatozoa abnormalities are not infrequent.

59.2 Young Males at Risk of Infertility

Infertility affects up to 15% of males of reproductive age, and approximately 50% of these cases are considered idiopathic [24]. For those cases for which a cause can be identified, this may be the result of events that occur during foetal, prepubertal or adult life. The aetiologies for male factor infertility are numerous and include genetic, non-genetic and environmental causes [25].

Whilst the majority of males with infertility are identified as adults, there are many conditions associated with infertility that may be identified at birth or during childhood. Genetic causes such as Klinefelter syndrome and many disorders of sex development (DSD) are associated with impairment of germ cell development [25]. A testicular dysgenesis syndrome (TDS) has also been described which is believed to arise as a result of genetic and/or environmental impacts during foetal life [26]. In addition to effects on fertility, TDS includes a number of associated abnormalities including cryptorchidism, hypospadias and testicular cancer. For such individuals with impairment of germ cell development prior to adulthood who fail to establish normal spermatogenesis, there are no established options to preserve or restore fertility, and any attempt to develop such strategies would need to overcome the underlying impairment of germ cell development.

In addition to those individuals in which infertility results from a disorder of testis development, there is an important group of individuals in whom infertility is a consequence of receiving gonadotoxic therapies during childhood. This primarily includes childhood cancer patients in whom the use of regimens involving chemotherapy and/or radiotherapy are standard. In the majority of these individuals, testicular function is considered normal prior to treatment, and the risk of subsequent infertility relates primarily to the treatment that the patient

Table 59.1 Gonadotoxicity of chemotherapeutic agents

	Class	Agent
High/moderate risk	Alkylating agents	Cyclophosphamide
		Busulphan
		Melphalan
		Ifosfamide
		Procarbazine
	Platinum	Cisplatinum
		Carboplatin
Low risk	Antimetabolites	Methotrexate
		Cytarabine
		Mercaptopurine
	Antitumour antibiotics	Bleomycin
		Dactinomycin
		Doxorubicin
	Vinca alkaloids	Vincristine
		Vinblastine
	Others	Etoposide
		Asparaginase

receives, although in some cases there may be some contribution by the underlying disease [27]. The risk of infertility will depend largely on the type of treatment that they will receive.

59.2.1 Chemotherapy

Whilst all chemotherapeutic drugs can affect fertility, the effect can vary depending on the individual agents used (Table 59.1). In addition, the dose, frequency and duration are also important factors [28]. The chemotherapeutics considered to be associated with the highest degree of gonadotoxicity include procarbazine and alkylating agents such as cyclophosphamide, in addition to platinum agents, e.g. cisplatin [28, 29]. For cyclophosphamide treatment during childhood, whilst it is clear that there is a dose response for the risk of subsequent infertility, an upper threshold cumulative dose that will result in azoospermia, or a lower cumulative dose below which azoospermia will not occur, has not been established [30].

59.2.2 Radiotherapy

Irradiation involving the gonadal region can also result in damage to the seminiferous epithelium and is dependent on dose, field and fractionation schedule (reviewed in Mitchell [18]). Whilst low-dose single fraction radiotherapy (2–4 Gy [Gy is the acronym for grey, the SI unit of ionising radiation. 1 Gy is the absorption of one joule of radiation energy per kilogram]) in men may be associated with recovery of spermatogenesis, doses in excess of 6 Gy have been shown to result in azoospermia lasting at least 2 years, and doses as high as 20–24 Gy lead to the total eradication of germ cells and permanent azoospermia. For men treated with fractionated total body irradiation (TBI), gonadal recovery has been reported to occur in less than 20% of patients [31].

Most childhood cancer treatments involve the use of multiple chemotherapeutics and/or radiotherapy, and therefore the risk of infertility is dependent on the overall regimen rather than an individual agent. Standard treatment for acute lymphoblastic leukaemia, the most common paediatric malignancy, can be considered relatively low risk (<20% infertility), whilst treatment for Hodgkin's lymphoma with alkylating agents is considered high-risk (>80% infertility) treatment [28]. Whilst in some cases patients may initially receive low-risk treatment, they may subsequently be reclassified into high risk in the case of relapse requiring treatment with highly gonadotoxic agents [32]. This would include stem cell transplantation, which is frequently used for relapsed cancers in childhood, in addition to several other non-oncological chronic conditions. Conditioning for stem cell transplantation is associated with a high risk of germ cell failure (>85% azoospermia) which relates to the specific regimen (e.g. busulphan or cyclophosphamide versus TBI) used [32].

For individuals in whom testicular development and function is considered normal but who are at high risk of subsequent infertility, e.g. prior to highly gonadotoxic therapy, there is the option of performing a testicular biopsy and cryopreserving tissue for potential future clinical use. However, it must be emphasised that this should be regarded as experimental due to the lack of an established clinical option to restore fertility using cryopreserved testicular tissue.

59.3 Fertility Preservation

59.3.1 Preservation of Fertility by Protection of the Prepubertal Testis

One approach to preserving fertility involves leaving the gonads in situ and modifying treatment regimens to involve less gonadotoxic agents. Such an approach has been demonstrated in adult men with Hodgkin's lymphoma in whom the use of a regimen containing procarbazine was compared to another regimen containing dacarbazine. Azoospermia was demonstrated in 86% of men receiving the former, whereas all of the men receiving the latter had recovery of spermatogenesis [33].

Where gonadotoxic therapies are required, an option may be co-administering treatments to protect the testis. Hormonal therapies to suppress the hypothalamic-pituitary-gonadal axis have been proposed. These have been supported by a number of experimental studies in rodents demonstrating that hormonal treatments (e.g. GnRH antagonists, sex steroids) can protect the testis from chemotherapy-induced damage and even restore fertility when administered several weeks after the chemotherapy is given [34]. However, this has not been successfully translated into primate models, and the limited evidence in humans does not support this approach for clinical application [29].

Recent studies involving administration of granulocyte colony-stimulating factor (G-CSF) have demonstrated a degree of protection of fertility in animal models, including rhesus monkeys. However, this approach has also not yet been translated into humans [35].

59.3.2 Preserving Fertility Through Testicular Tissue Cryopreservation

Adolescent boys at risk of infertility can opt for the well-established technique of sperm cryostorage in order to fulfil their future desire for parenthood. However, for those unable to provide a semen sample and for prepubertal patients where this is not yet possible, there are only experimental strategies in place to preserve their fertility. Nevertheless, animal studies have demonstrated that spermatogenesis can be restored when cryopreserved testicular cells are transplanted into seminiferous tubules of sterilised recipient animals [35]. Moreover, the compelling evidence of success in restoring fertility in women and girls affected by iatrogenic sterility using re-implantation of cryopreserved ovarian cortex [36] provides support for the development of techniques to cryopreserve testicular biopsies and cells, for potential future restoration of fertility in young male patients.

59.3.3 Testicular Tissue Cryopreservation in Prepubertal Males

Testicular tissue cryopreservation remains experimental, and as such should be conducted as part of an ethically approved research study. Currently, a limited number of centres have in place strategies to cryopreserve testicular tissue of young male patients, when compared with those offering fertility preservation options to adult men, women and girls [37]. For instance, until 2013 in Switzerland, 19 out of 19 oncological centres performing ovarian cortex cryopreservation in prepubertal girls had never performed testicular cryopreservation [37].

Nevertheless, an increasing number of centres worldwide are cryopreserving sperm specimens from adolescents and men at risk of infertility, and others are implementing their research plans including cryopreservation of testicular biopsies. Cryopreservation of sperm is common practice in many centres worldwide, and the number of young men opting for sperm freezing is steadily rising.

A French survey, performed over four decades, showed an increase in the percentage of patients under 18 referred to sperm banks, as well as a progressive reduction in age, with the youngest patient in which it was possible to collect sperm sample aged 12 years old [38]. Before 2012, half of the European and Israeli hospitals (7 out of 14) that responded to a questionnaire from the European Society for Human Reproduction and Embryology (ESHRE) reported that they offer testicular cryopreservation to young patients at risk of infertility, with the rest planning to establish it in the future [39]. A degree of variability in the fertility preservation options offered to young patients has been highlighted in several countries [38, 40, 41].

A particular effort is now devoted by various parties to harmonise and coordinate clinical practice and increase knowledge exchange between centres and countries with regard to fertility preservation in cancer patients. The Oncofertility Consortium, established in the USA (Northwestern University in Chicago), includes centres from 19 different countries across the world and provides a networking platform for an interdisciplinary approach to fertility issues in oncological patients [42].

59.3.4 Methods for Testicular Tissue Cryopreservation

The efficacy of storing mature testicular cells (spermatozoa) using extremely low temperatures (at liquid nitrogen [LN2] temperature of −196 °C) is well established. In pubertal boys, a sperm sample is usually obtained by masturbation. Sperm can also be obtained by electroejaculation, penile vibratory stimulation or, more invasively, by surgical sperm retrieval from the epididymis or testicles which can be performed at the same time as another planned procedure [43, 44]. In all those conditions where a semen sample can be obtained or mature cells are found during the analysis of a testicular biopsy of a young patient, established protocols for sperm freezing are used, primarily using glycerol as cryoprotectant at concentrations of 6–15% (Fig. 59.1).

However, for biopsies obtained from younger boys, where tissue collected contains only immature spermatogonia, alternative protocols have been developed for cryopreservation. Importantly, these new approaches aim to preserve the viability of the SSCs, the cells potentially capable of restoring spermatogenesis by repopulating seminiferous tubules.

Two main methods for cryopreservation have been investigated, slow-freezing and vitrification. Taking advantage of knowledge gained from ovarian cortex cryopreservation for fertility preservation in women, initial freezing methods for prepubertal testicular tissue involved controlled slow-freezing, and this remains the most widely used method [45]. Freezing is performed in computerised freezers, with temperatures reduced at a designated rate. The time-temperature regimen is often represented by several steps of cooling by ~1–2 °C/min until it reaches a certain temperature (often −8-9 °C), holding

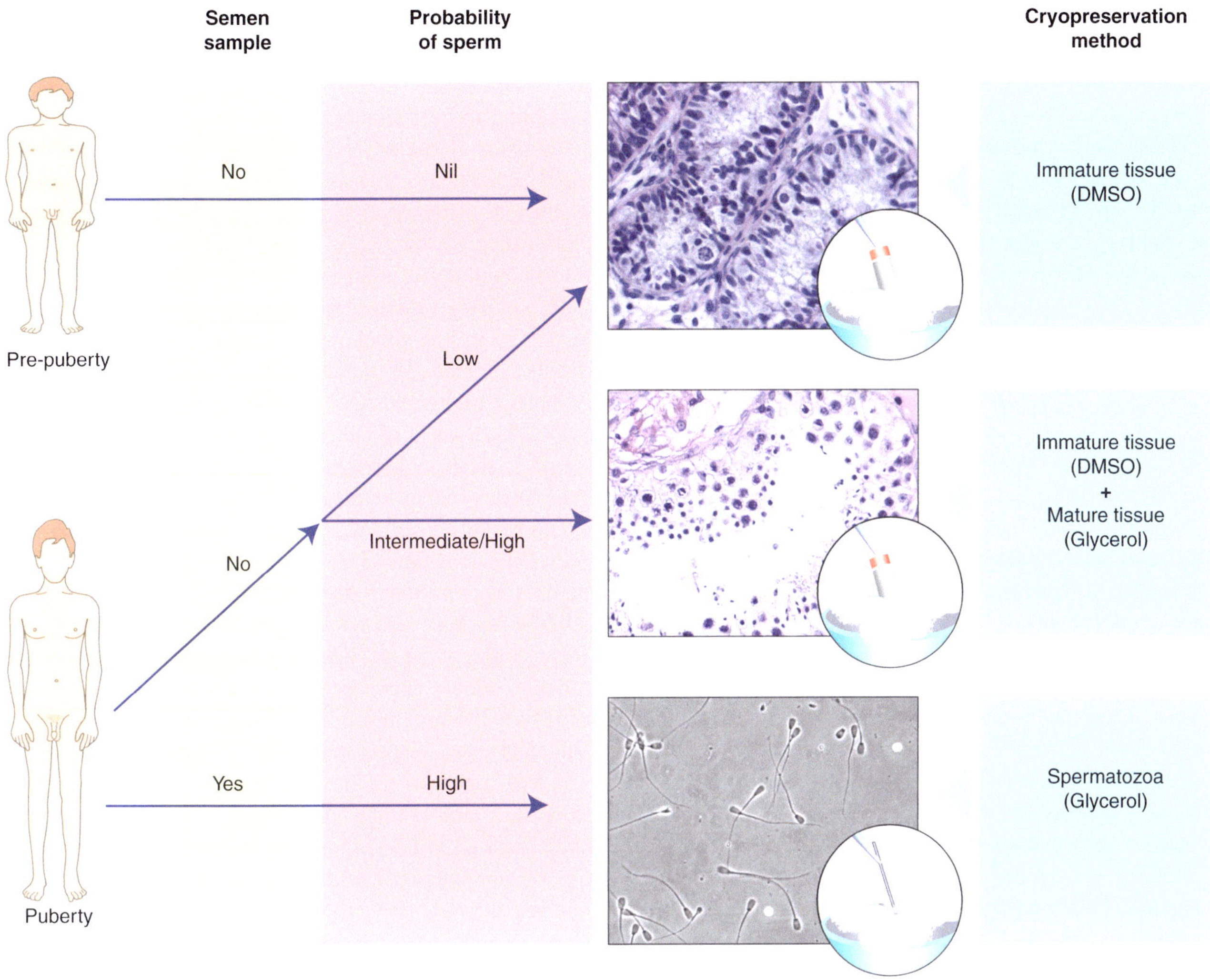

Fig. 59.1 Semen sample protocols for sperm freezing

at the designated temperature for 5 min and cooling again until tissues are moved into LN2 (reviewed in Onofre et al. [46]).

Alternative slow-freezing methods have been used in an uncontrolled fashion. Tissue fragments are placed into cryovials, which are in turn allocated into a small container, filled with isopropyl alcohol. Afterwards, the cryovials are placed in −80 °C freezer. It is predicted that this system decreases the temperature of the tissues at 1 °C/min speed, which enables an estimation of the time needed for the tissues to reach −80 °C. Eventually, cryovials with tissues are transferred to LN2 for long-term storage [47]. This method is less time-consuming, avoids the economic burden of buying expensive equipment, and yields similar results to controlled slow-freezing, which makes it useful when the collection point is distant from tissue bank or in developing countries.

Vitrification is an ultrarapid method which provides an alternative option to slow-freezing. The fast cooling speed avoids intracellular ice crystal formation preventing membrane insults. Vitrification can be used either as an open or closed solid-surface system.

Since the water-ice passage is the most difficult step that cells and tissues undergo during cryopreservation, cryoprotectant agents (CPAs) are often used in order to lower the temperature at which intracellular ice crystals form and to stabilise cellular membranes during dehydration/rehydration to preserve cellular integrity and cell-to-cell interaction.

In general, slow-freezing methods require lower concentrations of CPAs in comparison with vitrification, therefore reducing their potential cytotoxic effects. The main cryoprotectant agent utilised for testicular tissues containing immature cells is the permeating agent dimethyl sulphoxide (DMSO; Fig. 59.1). Concentrations of 0.7–3 M of DMSO have been satisfactorily used so far to freeze adult testis and proved to be efficient also in preserving prepubertal human testicular tissue [46]. However, ethylene glycol has also been used with success by some [45]. Furthermore, the addition of

0.1 M sucrose, a non-permeating CPA, seemed to improve spermatogonial proliferation after thawing [48].

By contrast, vitrification requires higher concentrations of CPAs, and, in some instances, a cocktail of agents can be used in order to reduce the cytotoxicity of each individual agent. Whilst the presence of spermatogonia has been demonstrated in prepubertal tissue following cryopreservation, the viability and functional capacity of these cells for spermatogenesis and fertilization have not been established.

59.3.5 Patient Selection and Consent for Testicular Tissue Cryopreservation

The majority of individuals for whom testicular tissue cryopreservation is considered are those receiving gonadotoxic therapies for malignant or non-malignant disease [39]. Testicular tissue cryopreservation remains experimental, and therefore this practice should be conducted as part of an ethically approved study [27].

Criteria for selection of patients should be clearly defined and depends on a variety of factors (Table 59.2). Factors specific to the patient include general health and psychological well-being. Health status may be affected by the underlying disease or by its treatment. Specifically, chemotherapy often increases the risk of infection and bleeding, both of which would be risk factors for complications following a surgical testicular biopsy. Extrinsic factors may also influence patient selection. This includes the risk of gonadotoxicity for the proposed treatment.

Whilst most centres consider a testicular biopsy only for those considered 'high-risk' for gonadotoxicity, this is not universally the case. Availability of expertise is also an important aspect as currently testicular tissue cryopreservation is only offered in a limited number of centres [39]. A key-limiting factor is the time available to conduct the biopsy, as cancer treatment often commences within days of a diagnosis which means that there is a narrow time to counsel, consent and conduct a biopsy in these patients.

Table 59.2 Factors that determine suitability for testicular cryopreservation in prepubertal males including 'Edinburgh criteria' for patient selection

Extrinsic factors
Expertise and facilities (e.g. clinical tissue storage facility)
Ethical/regulatory approval for testicular cryopreservation
Time available before treatment begins
Patient selection criteria
Age 0–16 years
A high risk of infertility (>80%)
Unable to produce a semen sample by masturbation
No clinically significant pre-existing testicular disease (e.g. cryptorchidism)
Fit for surgery (general health, low risk of infection and bleeding)
Informed consent (parent and, when possible, patient)
Negative HIV, syphilis and hepatitis serology

Selection criteria have been established following ethical review and approval and should be regarded as a starting point for future discussion, research and refinement. According to the Edinburgh selection criteria (Table 59.2) for gonadal tissue cryopreservation, patients are selected based on several factors which include a 'high-risk' (>80%) of infertility as a result of their treatment. Individuals with significant pre-existing testicular damage are also considered not suitable for this procedure [27].

Importantly, testicular tissue cryopreservation should not be offered to individuals who are able to produce a semen sample as semen cryopreservation followed by insemination, IVF or ICSI are well-established methods for fertility preservation. Assessment of pubertal status is therefore important. For post-pubertal patients with adult testicular volumes (≥12 mls), production of a semen sample by masturbation should be considered, whilst for prepubertal individuals with a testicular volume (≤3 mls), testicular cryopreservation is the only option. For those individuals in mid-puberty, it is unlikely that they will be able to produce a semen sample. However, due to the fact that there may be sperm in the testis, testicular biopsy may be performed and the tissue stored using two different methods designed to preserve spermatogonia and sperm respectively [39] (Fig. 59.1).

A key aspect of the process involves ensuring adequate counselling and consent. All individuals undergoing treatments that may affect fertility should receive fertility counselling by an individual with the experience to discuss the relative risks and present the options for fertility preservation, where applicable. It is recognised that the provision of adequate fertility counselling can vary across centres and that even for established methods of fertility preservation, such as semen cryopreservation, the provision for patients can be very low [49]. For patients in whom testicular cryopreservation is being considered, this should include discussion of the risks and benefits of the procedure in addition to informing on the experimental nature of this form of fertility preservation with no current options to restore fertility using the tissue.

Fully informed consent must be obtained from the patient according to the legal requirements surrounding competence to give consent and in cases where the patient is not deemed competent to consent, this should be sought from the individual's legal guardian(s) with patient assent, with the underlying principle of safeguarding the best interests of the child [39].

59.4 Restoring Fertility

59.4.1 Restoring Fertility from Cryopreserved Testicular Tissue

To date there have been no reports of clinical applications that can be used to restore fertility in males using cryopreserved prepubertal testis tissue. However, over recent years there have been successful cases of restoration of fertility in females using cryopreserved ovarian cortex which has resulted in >60 live births worldwide [36]. This includes a case in which ovarian tissue was removed and cryopreserved from a prepubertal girl and transplanted back to the patient in adulthood resulting in a spontaneous pregnancy and live birth.

Although this approach cannot be directly translated into the male, primarily because of important differences in the stage of maturation of the germ cells in prepubertal ovary and testis, it does support the general concept that fertility preservation may be possible for prepubertal males. Indeed, a number of experimental approaches in animal models have demonstrated proof of principle for several approaches that may be applicable for fertility preservation in prepubertal males.

59.4.2 Testicular Tissue Transplantation

Testicular transplantation has been shown in animal studies to be successful in permitting the differentiation of germ cells from spermatogonia to elongated spermatids capable of fertilizing oocytes and generating progeny [50]. This was first demonstrated using testis tissue from neonatal mice grafted subcutaneously under the dorsal skin of immunocompromised mice [10]. Since then, there have been successful transplantations using xenografts of tissue from several other species including primates, with generation of spermatozoa capable of generating blastocysts using ICSI [10].

Despite this, there are some species for which xenografting has not been successful, the most notable being humans. Experimental attempts to xenograft testis tissue from foetal, neonatal, and prepubertal human testis result in differentiation from spermatogonia to early meiotic germ cells (pachytene spermatocytes), but no further development towards haploid gametes [11].

The importance of the host species for the success of testis tissue grafting has been demonstrated in marmoset monkeys. Immature marmoset testis, xenografted into an immunocompromised mouse host, did not result in spermatogenesis; however, when grafted autologously into a marmoset testis, full spermatogenesis was achieved [12]. This suggests that autologous transplantation of human tissue may be successful despite the lack of success with xenografting. Indeed, autologous grafting is more likely to be an acceptable method for future clinical application given potential concerns with xenografting, such as virus transmission, DNA damage, and epigenetic modification [29].

Should such an approach prove to be successful, there are some important factors that should be taken into consideration before it could be used in clinical practice. Firstly, although the tissue may produce sperm, it is unlikely that this would allow for restoration of natural fertility due to the fact that the transplanted tissue would not connect to the seminiferous tubules of the remaining testis. Therefore, sperm would need to be extracted from the tissue that had been matured by transplantation and used for ART. Secondly, and more importantly, the use of such a technique must avoid the possibility of reintroduction of malignancy. This is more likely to be a potential risk for individuals with haematological malignancy. Research is ongoing to develop strategies to ensure that malignant infiltration can be excluded or eradicated from testis tissue biopsies [32].

59.4.3 Spermatogonial Stem Cell (SSC) Isolation and Transplantation

Whilst testicular tissue transplantation is unlikely to result in restoration of spermatogenesis in the remaining testis, transplantation of SSCs from cryopreserved tissue may offer such an option. This has been successful in experiments involving several animal models.

SSCs isolated from neonatal mouse testes and injected directly into the seminiferous tubules of a germ cell ablated mouse have been successful in generating functional gametes that can produce progeny [13]. SSC transplantation has also been successfully performed in rhesus monkeys for generating sperm that are capable of fertilization using ICSI [35].

However, to date, no successful use of this method has been described for humans. Only one study has reported using this approach in patients [14]. This study involved men ($n = 11$) with Hodgkin's lymphoma for whom testicular tissue was taken prior to treatment and cryopreserved. A cell suspension was then transplanted back into the rete testis for five of these men, but no restoration of spermatogenesis has been reported. Although disappointing, this could relate to several factors that may be overcome. Firstly, the cryopreservation method may have been suboptimal for retaining the viability of the SSCs. Secondly, the cells that were injected were in a crude cell suspension, and it is not clear how many SSCs were in the samples. Thirdly, the efficiency of seminiferous tubule colonisation was not determined. Given that SSCs are thought to represent ~1:3000 of total spermatogonia, this method may require in vitro propagation of SSCs prior to transplantation, in addition to refinement of the injection technique [29].

59.4.4 In Vitro Spermatogenesis

In vitro generation of sperm from immature male germ cells has been explored by scientists since the early 1900s (Martinovitch, 1937; Steinberger and Steinberger 1970, reviewed in Song and Wilkinson 2012 [15, 16]); however, it is only in recent years that this has been shown to work in a murine model [11]. This study demonstrated full spermatogenesis in vitro using testicular tissue from neonatal (postnatal day 6) mice. Testicular fragments were cultured on agarose pillars at the liquid-gas interphase in humidified atmosphere with 5%CO_2 at 34 °C. Haploid elongated spermatids were generated which were capable of fertilizing oocytes via microinjection and producing viable offspring [11]. Although successful, the efficiency and consistency of Sato's culture system are relatively low, indicating that refinement of the technique would be required in order for it to be utilised to study mammalian spermatogenesis or for translation into human applications for fertility preservation [17]. Therefore, several studies have been devoted to improving the culture systems [17, 18]. Several factors have been identified that enhance the efficiency of in vitro spermatogenesis. These include melatonin, FSH, LH and retinol [17, 19].

Although organ culture represents a promising approach, several groups have been trying to mature sperm using immortalised germ cells in co-culture with somatic Sertoli cells [20]. These studies produced some evidence suggesting germ cell maturation to the spermatid stage; however, there was no demonstration of their competence [51]. Whilst progress has been made in developing these techniques, they have not yet been translated into human for clinical applications. Only one group has reported live births after intracytoplasmic injection of elongated spermatids differentiated in vitro from meiotic germ cells [52]; however, these results have not been reproduced by other groups [16], and, as a result, they must be interpreted with caution.

59.5 Conclusion

Unlike the situation for post-pubertal and adult men at risk of infertility, who can benefit from the well-established options of sperm cryostorage and assisted reproductive technologies, methods aiming to protect fertility of prepubertal boys are in an early experimental stage. Cryopreservation of testicular tissue/cells is increasingly offered to selected children, albeit that currently no evidence has been provided for their future usefulness in restoring fertility. Current research is aimed at ensuring that testis tissue cryopreservation methods are optimal to ensure the viability and safety of the tissue for future clinical use. Strategies for reimplantation of tissue or in vitro spermatogenesis are also being developed as part of ongoing experimental research. The attainment of full spermatogenesis and offspring using such approaches in several animal species, coupled with the success in restoring female fertility after transplantation of cryopreserved ovarian cortex from adult and prepubertal females, offer the promise for future clinical options for fertility preservation in prepubertal boys at risk of infertility.

References

1. Nistal M, Abaurrea MA, Paniagua R. Morphological and histometric study on the human Sertoli cell from birth to the onset of puberty. J Anat. 1982;134:351–63.
2. Chemes HE. Infancy is not a quiescent period of testicular development. Int J Androl. 2001;24:2–7.
3. Berensztein EB, Sciara MI, Rivarola MA, Belgorosky A. Apoptosis and proliferation of human testicular somatic and germ cells during prepuberty: high rate of testicular growth in newborns mediated by decreased apoptosis. J Clin Endocrinol Metab. 2002;87:5113–8.
4. Muller JAND, Skakkebaek NE. Quantification of germ cells and seminiferous tubules by stereological examination of testicles from 50 boys who suffered from sudden death. Int J Androl. 1983;6:143–56.
5. Burr IM, Sizonenko PC, Kaplan SL, Grumbach MM. Hormonal changes in puberty. I. Correlation of serum luteinizing hormone and follicle stimulating hormone with stages of puberty, testicular size, and bone age in normal boys. Pediatr Res. 1970;4:25–35.
6. Mitchell RT, Cowan G, Morris KD, Anderson RA, Fraser HM, Mckenzie KJ, Wallace WH, Kelnar CJ, Saunders PT, Sharpe RM. Germ cell differentiation in the marmoset (*Callithrix jacchus*) during fetal and neonatal life closely parallels that in the human. Hum Reprod. 2008;23:2755–65.
7. Paniagua R, Nistal M. Morphological and histometric study of human spermatogonia from birth to the onset of puberty. J Anat. 1984;139(Pt 3):535–52.
8. Rey RA, Campo SM, Bedecarras P, Nagle CA, Chemes HE. Is infancy a quiescent period of testicular development? Histological, morphometric, and functional study of the seminiferous tubules of the cebus monkey from birth to the end of puberty. J Clin Endocrinol Metab. 1993;76:1325–31.
9. Cortes D, Muller J, Skakkebaek NE. Proliferation of Sertoli cells during development of the human testis assessed by stereological methods. Int J Androl. 1987;10:589–96.
10. Honaramooz A, Snedaker A, Boiani M, Scholer H, Dobrinski I, Schlatt S. Sperm from neonatal mammalian testes grafted in mice. Nature. 2002;418:778–81.
11. Sato Y, Nozawa S, Yoshiike M, Arai M, Sasaki C, Iwamoto T. Xenografting of testicular tissue from an infant human donor results in accelerated testicular maturation. Hum Reprod. 2010;25:1113–22.
12. Luetjens CM, Stukenborg JB, Nieschlag E, Simoni M, Wistuba J. Complete spermatogenesis in orthotopic but not in ectopic transplants of autologously grafted marmoset testicular tissue. Endocrinology. 2008;149:1736–47.
13. Brinster RL, Zimmermann JW. Spermatogenesis following male germ-cell transplantation. Proc Natl Acad Sci U S A. 1994;91:11298–302.
14. Radford J, Shalet S, Lieberman B. Fertility after treatment for cancer. Questions remain over ways of preserving ovarian and testicular tissue. BMJ. 1999;319:935–6.
15. Steinberger A, Steinberger E. Tissue culture of male mammalian gonads. In Vitro. 1970;5:17–27.
16. Song HW, Wilkinson MF. In vitro spermatogenesis: a long journey to get tails. Spermatogenesis. 2012;2:238–44.
17. Chapin RE, Winton T, Nowland W, Danis N, Kumpf S, Johnson K, Coburn A, Stukenborg JB. Lost in translation: the search for an

in vitro screen for spermatogenic toxicity. Birth Defects Res B Dev Reprod Toxicol. 2016;107:225–42.
18. Komeya M, et al. Long-term ex vivo maintenance of testis tissues producing fertile sperm in a microfluidic device. Sci Rep. 2016;6:21472.
19. Arkoun B, Dumont L, Milazzo JP, Way A, Bironneau A, Wils J, Mace B, Rives N. Retinol improves in vitro differentiation of prepubertal mouse spermatogonial stem cells into sperm during the first wave of spermatogenesis. PLoS One. 2015;10:e0116660.
20. Hofmann MC, Hess RA, Goldberg E, Millan JL. Immortalized germ cells undergo meiosis in vitro. Proc Natl Acad Sci U S A. 1994;91:5533–7.
21. Orth JM, Gunsalus GL, Lamperti AA. Evidence from Sertoli cell-depleted rats indicates that spermatid number in adults depends on numbers of Sertoli cells produced during perinatal development. Endocrinology. 1988;122:787–94.
22. Clermont Y, Perey B. Quantitative study of the cell population of the seminiferous tubules in immature rats. Am J Anat. 1957;100:241–67.
23. Ogawa T, Ohmura M, Ohbo K. The niche for spermatogonial stem cells in the mammalian testis. Int J Hematol. 2005;82:381–8.
24. Esteves SC. Novel concepts in male factor infertility: clinical and laboratory perspectives. J Assist Reprod Genet. 2016;33:1319–35.
25. Tournaye H, Krausz C, Oates RD. Novel concepts in the aetiology of male reproductive impairment. Lancet Diabetes Endocrinol. 2016;5(7):544–53.
26. Skakkebaek NE, Rajpert-de Meyts E, Main KM. Testicular dysgenesis syndrome: an increasingly common developmental disorder with environmental aspects. Hum Reprod. 2001;16:972–8.
27. Anderson RA, Mitchell RT, Kelsey TW, Spears N, Telfer EE, Wallace WH. Cancer treatment and gonadal function: experimental and established strategies for fertility preservation in children and young adults. Lancet Diabetes Endocrinol. 2015;3:556–67.
28. Wallace WH, Anderson RA, Irvine DS. Fertility preservation for young patients with cancer: who is at risk and what can be offered? Lancet Oncol. 2005;6:209–18.
29. Mitchell RT, Saunders PT, Sharpe RM, Kelnar CJ, Wallace WH. Male fertility and strategies for fertility preservation following childhood cancer treatment. Endocr Dev. 2009;15:101–34.
30. Green DM, et al. Cumulative alkylating agent exposure and semen parameters in adult survivors of childhood cancer: a report from the St Jude Lifetime Cohort Study. Lancet Oncol. 2014;15:1215–23.
31. Socie G, Salooja N, Cohen A, Rovelli A, Carreras E, Locasciulli A, Korthof E, Weis J, Levy V, Tichelli A. Nonmalignant late effects after allogeneic stem cell transplantation. Blood. 2003;101:3373–85.
32. Jahnukainen K, Mitchell RT, Stukenborg JB. Testicular function and fertility preservation after treatment for haematological cancer. Curr Opin Endocrinol Diabetes Obes. 2015;22:217–23.
33. Viviani S, Santoro A, Ragni G, Bonfante V, Bestetti O, Bonadonna G. Gonadal toxicity after combination chemotherapy for Hodgkin's disease. Comparative results of MOPP vs ABVD. Eur J Canc Clin Oncol. 1985;21:601–5.
34. Shetty G, Meistrich ML. Hormonal approaches to preservation and restoration of male fertility after cancer treatment. J Natl Cancer Inst Monogr. 2005;2005:36–9.
35. Hermann BP, et al. Spermatogonial stem cell transplantation into rhesus testes regenerates spermatogenesis producing functional sperm. Cell Stem Cell. 2012;11:715–26.
36. Donnez J, Dolmans MM. Ovarian cortex transplantation: 60 reported live births brings the success and worldwide expansion of the technique towards routine clinical practice. J Assist Reprod Genet. 2015;32:1167–70.
37. Diesch T, Von der Weid NX, Szinnai G, Schaedelin S, De Geyter C, Rovo A. Fertility preservation in pediatric and adolescent cancer patients in Switzerland: a qualitative cross-sectional survey. Cancer Epidemiol. 2016;44:141–6.
38. Daudin M, et al. Sperm cryopreservation in adolescents and young adults with cancer: results of the French national sperm banking network (CECOS). Fertil Steril. 2015;103:478–486.e471.
39. Picton HM, et al. A European perspective on testicular tissue cryopreservation for fertility preservation in prepubertal and adolescent boys. Hum Reprod. 2015;30:2463–75.
40. Glaser AW, Phelan L, Crawshaw M, Jagdev S, Hale J. Fertility preservation in adolescent males with cancer in the United Kingdom: a survey of practice. Arch Dis Child. 2004;89:736–73.
41. Neal MS, Nagel K, Duckworth J, Bissessar H, Fischer MA, Portwine C, Tozer R, Barr RD. Effectiveness of sperm banking in adolescents and young adults with cancer: a regional experience. Cancer. 2007;110:1125–9.
42. Ataman LM, et al. Creating a global community of practice for oncofertility. J Glob Oncol. 2016;2:83–96.
43. Katz DJ, Kolon TF, Feldman DR, Mulhall JP. Fertility preservation strategies for male patients with cancer. Nat Rev Urol. 2013;10:463–72.
44. Moss JL, Choi AW, Fitzgerald Keeter MK, Brannigan RE. Male adolescent fertility preservation. Fertil Steril. 2016;105:267–73.
45. Kvist K, Thorup J, Byskov AG, Hoyer PE, Mollgard K, Yding AC. Cryopreservation of intact testicular tissue from boys with cryptorchidism. Hum Reprod. 2006;21:484–91.
46. Onofre J, Baert Y, Faes K, Goossens E. Cryopreservation of testicular tissue or testicular cell suspensions: a pivotal step in fertility preservation. Hum Reprod Update. 2016;22:744–61.
47. Baert Y, Van Saen D, Haentjens P, In't Veld P, Tournaye H, Goossens E. What is the best cryopreservation protocol for human testicular tissue banking? Hum Reprod. 2013;28:1816–26.
48. Wyns C, Van Langendonckt A, Wese FX, Donnez J, Curaba M. Long term spermatogonial survival in cryopreserved and xenografted immature human testicular tissue. Hum Reprod. 2008;23:2402–14.
49. Schover LR, Brey K, Lichtin A, Lipshultz LI, Jeha S. Oncologists' attitudes and practices regarding banking sperm before cancer treatment. J Clin Oncol Off J Am Soc Clin Oncol. 2002;20:1890–7.
50. Arregui L, Dobrinski I. Xenografting of testicular tissue pieces: 12 years of an in vivo spermatogenesis system. Reproduction. 2014;148:R71–84.
51. Feng LX, Chen Y, Dettin L, Pera RA, Herr JC, Goldberg E, Dym M. Generation and in vitro differentiation of a spermatogonial cell line. Science. 2002;297:392–5.
52. Tesarik J, Bahceci M, Ozcan C, Greco E, Mendoza C. Restoration of fertility by in-vitro spermatogenesis. Lancet. 1999;353:555–6.

Recent Advances in Fertility Preservation

60

Shrenik Shah and Wendy Vitek

Fertility is a concern for the majority of young men and women diagnosed with cancer, as many will face infertility as a consequence of surgery, chemotherapy, radiation therapy, and delayed childbearing. Fertility concerns can impact quality of life as well as treatment decisions, adherence to therapy, and possibly survival [1]. Therefore, fertility preservation counseling is an important aspect of comprehensive cancer care for young men and women. Recent advances in fertility preservation techniques, such as oocyte, embryo, and ovarian tissue cryopreservation, have expanded the options available to prepubescent girls and young women, though long-term outcome data is limited. While semen cryopreservation is an established option for men, advances in testicular tissue cryopreservation may lead to an option for prepubescent boys. Future advances will expand our understanding of the risk of infertility with newer cancer therapies and the long-term safety and efficacy of current fertility options. In addition, the possibility of in vitro maturation of gametes and the development of artificial gametes may create options for individuals with cancer who are unable to bank gametes prior to treatment [2].

60.1 Advances in Fertility Preservation Counseling

Individualized risk assessment is an advance in fertility preservation counseling. The risk of infertility is dependent on factors related to the cancer, treatment, and the individual [3]. For example, cancers arising from the reproductive organs may necessitate surgery that would limit fertility though fertility sparing surgical techniques may be offered to select patients depending on their prognosis and desire for future fertility [4]. Treatment factors, such as the chemotherapeutic agent, dose, and combination of therapies, are factored into the risk assessment. Alkylating agents and pelvic radiation pose the greatest risk for gonadotoxicity. Finally, individual characteristics such as age, gender, and genetic factors further modify the risk of gonadotoxicity. As ovarian reserve declines with age, lower doses of alkylating agents and radiation can precipitate premature ovarian insufficiency. In addition to age, gender further modifies the risk. For example, prepubescent boys are more susceptible to gonadotoxicity from chemotherapy and radiation than are girls at the same age [5]. Genetic factors, such as BRCA mutations, may also contribute to the risk of infertility given the association of BRCA mutations with reduced ovarian reserve [6]. Online risk assessment tools that factor in cancer diagnosis, treatment, age, and gender can be used to quantify an individualized risk of infertility [7]. Future advances in fertility preservation counseling will be understanding the fertility risk posed by immunotherapies used to treat cancer patients.

60.2 Advances in Fertility Preservation for Women

Fertility preservation options through oocyte, embryo, and ovarian tissue cryopreservation can be offered to women who are at risk for infertility or women facing an uncertain risk of infertility (Fig. 60.1). Oocyte and embryo banking require controlled ovarian hyperstimulation and oocyte retrieval, while ovarian tissue cryopreservation requires a laparoscopic partial or complete oophorectomy. Timing, safety, and success rates factor into the decision to pursue these options.

Advances in ovarian hyperstimulation protocols allow for oocyte and embryo banking to occur quickly after the fertility preservation consultation. Conventional ovarian hyperstimulation protocols start in the early follicular phase of the menstrual cycle. Depending on the phase of the menstrual

S. Shah
Department of Obstetrics and Gynecology, University of Rochester School of Medicine & Dentistry, Rochester, NY, USA

W. Vitek (✉)
UR Medicine – Strong Fertility Center, Rochester, NY, USA
e-mail: wendy_vitek@urmc.rochester.edu

G. N. Allahbadia et al. (eds.), *Textbook of Assisted Reproduction*, https://doi.org/10.1007/978-981-15-2377-9_60

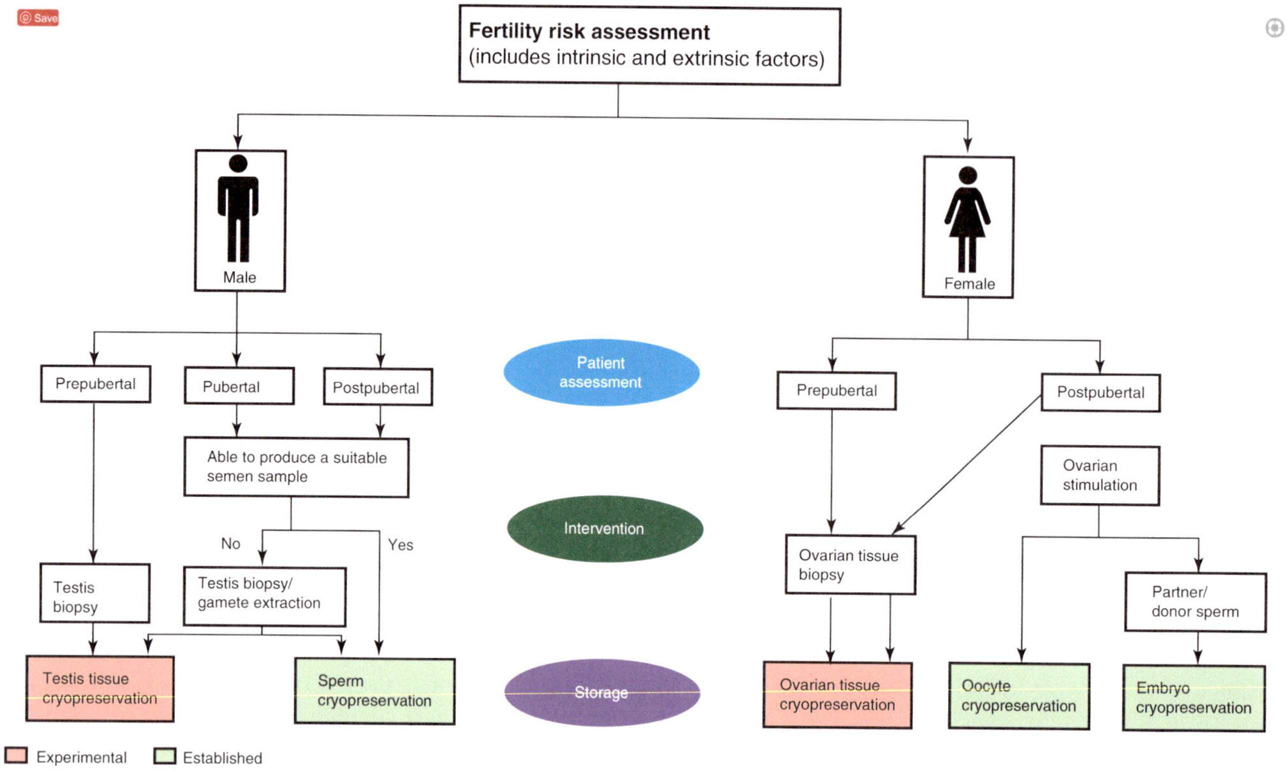

Fig. 60.1 Established and experimental fertility preservation options for males and females with cancer based on pubertal status. (From Anderson RA, Mitchell RT, Kelsey TW, Spears N, Telfer EE, Wallace WH. Cancer treatment and gonadal function: experimental and established strategies for fertility preservation in children and young adults. Lancet Diabetes Endocrinol. 2015 Jul;3 (7):556–67, with permission)

cycle that the patient presents in, completion of an oocyte or embryo banking cycle could take 2–6 weeks, which introduce an unacceptable delay in starting cancer therapy. Random-start ovarian hyperstimulation protocols can be initiated in the late follicular phase and luteal phase of the menstrual cycle and appear to have comparable outcomes to the conventional protocols that start in the early follicular phase [8]. Random-start ovarian hyperstimulation protocols reduce the time to complete oocyte or embryo banking to 2 weeks and avoid delaying the initiation of neoadjuvant or adjuvant chemotherapy [9]. Ovarian tissue cryopreservation is an alternative option for women who cannot delay the start of cancer therapy by 2 weeks. Laparoscopic partial or complete oophorectomy for ovarian tissue cryopreservation can be performed at the time of port placement to minimize cost and anesthetic risks [2]. Ovarian tissue cryopreservation is the only option for prepubescent girls who cannot undergo oocyte banking.

Safety of oocyte, embryo, and ovarian tissue banking is a top concern of patients and providers. Supra-physiologic estradiol and progesterone levels encountered during and after controlled ovarian hyperstimulation for oocyte or embryo banking can be a concern for women with hormone-sensitive cancers. Several adjustments can be made to conventional and random-start ovarian hyperstimulation protocols to minimize estradiol and progesterone levels. Letrozole, an aromatase inhibitor, can be taken during controlled ovarian hyperstimulation and immediately after oocyte retrieval to lower estradiol levels. This approach results in a similar number of oocytes and embryos banked when compared to controlled ovarian hyperstimulation without letrozole and significantly lower peak serum estradiol levels among women treated with letrozole [10]. The safety of letrozole ovarian hyperstimulation protocols has been examined in a study comparing 79 breast cancer patients, 81% of whom had an estrogen receptor-positive cancer, with 136 control patients who did not undergo ovarian stimulation. The median follow-up time of the study was 2 years, ranging from 23 months in the letrozole group to 33 months in the control group. During this time period, there were 3 (4%) recurrences in the letrozole group and 11 (8%) in the control group. There was no significant difference in relapse-free survival between the groups. This study was not randomized so selection bias is possible, but the experimental and control groups were similar with respect to age and prognostic markers for cancer recurrence. Long-term follow-up data is not yet available although recurrence risk is generally thought to be highest during the first 2 years after treatment [11]. Another adjustment to minimize peak estradiol and progesterone levels is to utilize a GnRH agonist to induce final oocyte maturation in preparation for oocyte retrieval instead of a standard HCG trigger [12]. A GnRH agonist triggers an LH surge, but does not support sustained release of LH in the luteal phase. The lack of LH support induces lysis of the multiple corpora lutea that are a consequence of controlled ovarian hyperstimulation. Luteolysis leads to a rapid decline in estradiol and progesterone levels post retrieval, which minimizes supra-physiologic hormone exposure in women with hormone-sensitive cancers without compromising the number or quality of oocyte or embryo banked. This approach also nearly eliminates the risk of ovarian hyperstimulation syndrome, which is a rare but serious complication of oocyte and embryo banking. Ovarian tissue cryopreservation is considered experimental given concerns regarding safety and efficacy. Laparoscopic partial or complete oophorectomy allows for isolation of the ovarian cortical tissue, which is comprised of primordial follicles. The cortical strips are dissected into small fragments and cryopreserved. Autotransplantation of the thawed ovarian cortical tissue to the residual ovary or the pelvic side wall has resulted in spontaneous and in vitro fertilization pregnancies among women with various malignancies [3]. Although there have been no reported cases of recurrent cancer after ovarian tissue autotransplantation, there is concern that transplanted ovarian tissue could be contaminated with cancer cells, particularly in cancers such as breast cancer which can metastasize to the ovary [13]. In vitro maturation of primordial follicles would avoid the need for, and risks of, ovarian tissue cryopreservation. This approach has been successful in animal models but has not yet produced a live birth in humans [14]. Mature oocyte and immature oocytes have been retrieved from ovarian tissue at the time of partial or complete oophorectomy in unstimulated patients [15]. Mature oocytes have been fertilized and embryo cryopreservation has been performed. Immature oocytes can be in vitro matured using culture media treated with gonadotropins, and mature oocytes have been cryopreserved from this technique. These strategies have resulted in live births among women with ovarian cancers which are a contraindication to controlled ovarian hyperstimulation and autotransplantation of thawed cryopreserved ovarian tissue. While these cases demonstrate evidence that this approach can result in live birth, this option is not widely offered, given that the efficiency of oocyte recovery is not known.

Success rates, defined as a live birth, after oocyte, embryo, and ovarian tissue cryopreservation preformed prior to chemotherapy of women with cancer are based on limited data. Women with cancer are typically counseled on their chance of a live birth based on their age at the time of oocyte or embryo banking and the chance of live birth is extrapolated from women of a similar age who underwent IVF for infertility-related diagnoses [16]. Success rates for ovarian tissue cryopreservation and subsequent autotransplantation have been reported as 57.5% live birth rate in a meta-analysis comprised 309 cases, of which 78% had been diagnosed with a malignancy with a mean age of 29.3 years at the time of ovarian tissue cryopreservation and mean age of 33.0 years at the time of autotransplantation [17]. There have been case reports of successful pregnancy with prepubescent ovarian tissue cryopreservation and subsequent autotransplantation [18]. Future advances in fertility preservation options will be in vitro maturation of primordial follicles, the development of artificial gametes from primordial germ cells, or pluripotent stem cells and long-term safety and outcome data for oocyte, embryo, and ovarian tissue cryopreservation in women with cancer [2].

60.3 Advances in Ovarian Protection During Cancer Therapy

Maintaining endocrine function of the ovaries, as well as fertility, is important for quality of life and overall wellbeing in reproductive age women with cancer. GnRH agonist co-treatment during chemotherapy has been proposed for ovarian protection. Chemotherapies such as cyclophosphamide induce apoptosis of growing follicles, resulting in less negative feedback by estradiol and inhibin B and an increase in follicle-stimulating hormone (FSH)-driven follicular recruitment and accelerated folliculogenesis. GnRH agonists have been hypothesized to preserve ovarian reserve through several mechanisms. Depot GnRH agonist induces downregulation of FSH production 7–10 days post administration, which leads to suppression of the hypothalamic-pituitary-ovarian axis. The lower circulating levels of FSH diminish the accelerated loss of ovarian reserve mediated by FSH-driven follicular recruitment. Another possible protective mechanism is that GnRH agonists decrease ovarian perfusion, reducing delivery of the chemotherapeutic agent to the ovaries. Side effects of GnRH agonists related to the induced hypoestrogenic state include hot flashes, vaginal dryness, and bone loss. Norethindrone acetate is a progestin with estrogenic properties and has been shown to preserve bone mass and significantly reduce vasomotor symptoms without increasing the rate of vaginal bleeding, but may not be appropriate in women with hormone-sensitive cancers. Given the challenge of conducting research that is powered to compare and track long-term outcomes such as fertility, there are limited randomized data on fertility-related outcomes such as fecundity, miscarriage rate, and maternal and neonatal outcomes after co-treatment with a GnRH agonist during chemotherapy. As a result, most GnRH agonist co-treatment studies are designed to show a difference in the rate of resumption of menses or premature ovarian insufficiency at 1–2 years after chemotherapy. More recent studies have examined the endpoint of diminished ovarian reserve as measured by changes in ovarian reserve markers such as anti-Müllerian hormone (AMH) and antral follicle count (AFC). To date, 12 randomized controlled trials have been published on co-treatment with a GnRH agonist or chemotherapy alone in women with breast cancer. A recent meta-analysis found a significant reduction in the odds of developing premature ovarian insufficiency in women with breast cancer who were co-treated with a GnRH agonist during chemotherapy compared to women who received chemotherapy alone with an odds ratio that favors GnRH agonist co-treatment of 0.34 and a 95% confidence interval of 0.025–0.46 and a P value of 0.026 [19]. Despite a possible 34% reduction in premature ovarian insufficiency in women with breast cancer who are co-treated with an GnRH agonist during chemotherapy, neither the American Society for Reproductive Medicine (ASRM) nor the American Society of Clinical Oncology (ASCO) recommends GnRH agonist co-treatment as a primary means of fertility preservation, possibly due to the limited efficacy and limitations in the data [20, 21]. Both societies recommended that GnRH agonist co-treatment be offered as a means of fertility preservation in addition to, but not instead of, oocyte, embryo, or ovarian tissue cryopreservation. Future advances in ovarian protection will include understanding if GnRH agonist can preserve ovarian function in women treated for cancers other than breast cancer and the development of fertility-protective agents that prevent follicle loss without interacting with cancer therapies [2].

60.4 Advances in Fertility Preservation for Men

Sperm cryopreservation is a fertility preservation option for postpubescent men at risk for infertility or when the risk is uncertain (Fig. 60.1). Sperm banking may also be indicated if a couple is interested in conceiving in the short term as most experts recommend waiting at least 9–12 months after chemotherapy or radiation treatment before attempting pregnancy [22]. Ideally, sperm banking is performed prior or shortly after the initiation of cancer therapy. Men capable of masturbation and ejaculation can provide fresh semen for cryopreservation. In the event that a man is unable to collect, assisted ejaculation methods such as penile vibratory stimulation or electroejaculation may be attempted. An alternative option is epididymal aspiration or testicular sperm extraction (TESE) to retrieve sperm for cryopreservation. TESE can be performed at the time of orchiectomy in men with testicular cancer (who are azoospermic based on ejaculated samples) with high rates of recovery of sperm for cryopreservation reported [23]. Success rates with cryopreserved sperm vary depending on a number of factors including motile count post-thaw and use of the specimen for insemination or in vitro fertilization/intracytoplasmic sperm injection (IVF/ICSI). Couples undergoing IVF/ICSI for the indication of male cancer appear to have a higher live birth rate than couples undergoing IVF/ICSI for other indications [24].

Testicular tissue cryopreservation is an experimental option for prepubescent boys who are unable to sperm bank [2]. Testicular tissue can be harvested by testis biopsy, and the tissue and spermatogonial stem cells can be cryopreserved. In the future, it is hoped that the testicular tissue may be autotransplanted in order to restore fertility or possibly undergo in vitro maturation in order to produce sperm in quantities sufficient for IVF/ICSI. Neither approach has been attempted for human reproduction at this time. Future advances in male fertility preservation will include developing a viable option for prepubescent boys through safe autotransplantation, in vitro maturation, or artificial gametes from spermatogonial stem cells or pluripotent stem cells.

60.5 Conclusion

Women with cancer have safe and effective options for fertility preservation through random-start and modified controlled ovarian hyperstimulation protocols for oocyte and embryo cryopreservation, ovarian tissue cryopreservation with autotransplantation, and GnRH agonist co-treatment during chemotherapy. Ovarian tissue cryopreservation with autotransplantation at a later date is in an option for prepubescent girls with cancer. Men with cancer can undergo sperm cryopreservation through masturbation, assisted ejaculation methods, or surgical sperm extraction for future insemination or IVF/ICSI. Prepubescent boys with cancer can be offered testicular tissue cryopreservation as an experimental fertility preservation option. Knowledge of cancer therapy-related infertility risks and long-term safety and outcome data will advance fertility preservation counseling, while the development of in vitro maturation, artificial gametes, and fertility-protective agents will advance fertility preservation options.

References

1. Llarena NC, Estevez SL, Tucker SL, Jeruss JS. Impact of fertility concerns on tamoxifen initiation and persistence. J Natl Cancer Inst. 2015;107(10):djv202.
2. Martinez F. International Society for Fertility Preservation–ESHRE–ASRM Expert Working Group. Update on fertility preservation from the Barcelona International Society for Fertility Preservation-ESHRE-ASRM 2015 expert meeting: indications, results and future perspectives. Fertil Steril. 2017;108(3):407–15.
3. Donnez J, Dolmans MM. Fertility preservation in women. Nat Rev Endocrinol. 2013 Dec;9(12):735–49.
4. Denschlag D, Reed NS, Rodolakis A. Fertility-sparing approaches in gynecologic cancers: a review of ESGO task force activities. Curr Oncol Rep. 2012 Dec;14(6):535–8.

5. Ogilvy-Stuart AL, Shalet SM. Effect of radiation on the human reproductive system. Environ Health Perspect. 1993;1010(2):109–16.
6. Lin W, Titus S, Moy F, Ginsburg ES, Oktay K. Ovarian aging in women with BRCA germline mutations. J Clin Endocrinol Metab. 2017 Oct 1;102(10):3839–47.
7. https://www.teamlivestrong.org/we-can-help/fertility-services/risks/ Accessed 5 Jan 2018.
8. Cakmak H, Katz A, Cedars MI, Rosen MP. Effective method for emergency fertility preservation: random-start controlled ovarian stimulation. Fertil Steril. 2013;100(6):1673–80.
9. Baynosa J, Westphal LM, Madrigrano A, Wapnir I. Timing of breast cancer treatments with oocyte retrieval and embryo cryopreservation. J Am Coll Surg. 2009;209:603–7.
10. Oktay K, Hourvitz A, Sahin G, Oktem O, Safro B, Cil A, Bang H. Letrozole reduces estrogen and gonadotropin exposure in women with breast cancer undergoing ovarian stimulation before chemotherapy. J Clin Endocrinol Metab. 2006;91(10):3885–90.
11. Azim A, Costantini-Ferrando M, Oktay K. Safety of fertility preservation by ovarian stimulation with letrozole and gonadotropins in patients with breast cancer: a prospective controlled study. J Clin Oncol. 2008;26(16):2630–5.
12. Anderson RA, Kinniburgh D, Baird D. Preliminary experience of the use of a gonadotrophin-releasing hormone antagonist in ovulation induction/in-vitro fertilization prior to cancer treatment. Hum Reprod. 1999;14(10):2665–8.
13. Bastings L, Beerendonk CC, Westphal JR, et al. Autotransplantation of cryopreserved ovarian tissue in cancer survivors and the risk of reintroducing malignancy: a systematic review. Hum Reprod Update. 2013;19:483–506.
14. Smitz J, Dolmans MM, Donnez J, et al. Current achievements and future research directions in ovarian tissue culture, in vitro follicle development and transplantation: implications for fertility preservation. Hum Reprod Update. 2010;16:395–414.
15. Prasath EB, Chan ML, Wong WH, Lim CJ, Tharmalingam MD, Hendricks M, et al. First pregnancy and live birth resulting from cryopreserved embryos obtained from in vitro matured oocytes after oophorectomy in an ovarian cancer patient. Hum Reprod. 2014;29:276–8.
16. Oktay K, Turan V, Bedoschi G, Pacheco FS, Moy F. Fertility preservation success subsequent to concurrent aromatase inhibitor treatment and ovarian stimulation in women with breast Cancer. J Clin Oncol. 2015 Aug 1;33(22):2424–9.
17. Pacheco F, Oktay K. Current success and efficiency of autologous ovarian transplantation: a meta-analysis. Reprod Sci. 2017 Aug;24(8):1111–20.
18. Demeestere I, Simon P, Dedeken L, Moffa F, Tsépélidis S, Brachet C, Delbaere A, Devreker F, Ferster A. Live birth after autograft of ovarian tissue cryopreserved during childhood. Hum Reprod. 2015 Sep;30(9):2107–9.
19. Lambertini M, Ceppi M, Poggio F, Peccatori FA, Azim HA Jr, Ugolini D, Pronzato P, Loibl S, Moore HC, Partridge AH, Bruzzi P, Del Mastro L. Ovarian suppression using luteinizing hormone-releasing hormone agonists during chemotherapy to preserve ovarian function and fertility of breast cancer patients: a meta-analysis of randomized studies. Ann Oncol. 2015;26(12):2408–19.
20. Ethics Committee of ASRM. Fertility preservation and reproduction in patients facing gonadotoxic therapies: a committee opinion. Fertil Steril. 2013;100(5):1224–31.
21. Loren AW, Mangu PB, Beck LN, Brennan L, Magdalinski AJ, Partridge AH, Quinn G, Wallace WH, Oktay K, American Society of Clinical Oncology. Fertility preservation for patients with cancer: American Society of Clinical Oncology clinical practice guideline. J Clin Oncol. 2013;31(19):2500–10.
22. Holoch P, Wald M. Current options for preservation of fertility in the male. Fertil Steril. 2011 Aug;96(2):286–90.
23. Furuhashi K, Ishikawa T, Hashimoto H, Yamada S, Ogata S, Mizusawa Y, Matsumoto Y, Okamoto E, Kokeguchi S, Shiotani M. Onco-testicular sperm extraction: testicular sperm extraction in azoospermic and very severely oligozoospermic cancer patients. Andrologia. 2013 Apr;45(2):107–10.
24. García A, Herrero MB, Holzer H, Tulandi T, Chan P. Assisted reproductive outcomes of male cancer survivors. J Cancer Surviv. 2015 Jun;9(2):208–14.

Prevention of Gonadotoxicity

61

Zeev Blumenfeld

61.1 Scope of the Problem

The incidence of malignant diseases has increased in children, adolescents, and young adults by 0.6% every year in the last four decades [1–5]. Indeed, malignancy is a cardinal public health issue worldwide and is one of the two leading causes of mortality in the USA [1]. On the other hand, mortality has continuously deteriorated, from 6.5/100,000 persons, in 1970, to 2.4/100,000 in 2012, a decrease of 63% (65% in children and 60% in adolescents) [1–5]. This reduction is attributed to an improvement in the 5-year survival for all cancers from 58% for children during the years 1975 to 1977 to 83% for those diagnosed during 2005–2011 [1–9]. These changes have brought about an almost three times increment in the rate of cancer survivors, in the last five decades [10]. The percentage of the US population that has survived a diagnosis of malignancy has increased from 1.5% in 1971, to 3.5% in 2001, and to 3.9% in 2007 [10]. Extrapolation of this trend to the present would come to over 4% cancer survivors, about 1:25 in the general population! Indeed, several estimations based on cancer statistics have speculated that between 1 in 49 to 1 in 250 women younger than 40, in the USA, have or would suffer cancer [11, 12]. Others speculated that 1 in 250 to 1000 people at 20–30 years are cancer survivors, whereas some publications have reported an incidence of 7% malignancy in reproductive-age women with an increasing 5-year survival in the last decade [13–15]. About 790,000 to 1,665,540 new cancers are diagnosed every year in females in the USA, and in the last years, almost 1 in 7 diagnosed patients are reproductive-age women [1–3, 16]. Whereas more than a million of cancer survivors are patients of reproductive age in the USA and many millions worldwide, it is a global ubiquitous interest to attempt fertility preservation to these patients [16–26].

Whereas 5% or more of the patients diagnosed with malignancy are in the reproductive age [1–3], the late sequelae of chemo- and radiotherapy, affecting so many survivors, have become a major medical problem. Long-term survivors may suffer several remote sequelae, such as premature ovarian insufficiency (POI), previously called premature ovarian failure (POF),, subfertility, adverse pregnancy outcomes, and health morbidity in offspring [13–15]. The POF/POI and associated infertility are unfortunate sequelae of gonadotoxic chemotherapy for the patients who, having survived the malignancy, look forward to a normal reproductive life. Indeed, the last three decades have witnessed an exponential increase in the publications on preservation of fertility in spite of the gonadotoxic chemo- and radiotherapy in young adults and prepubertal children. Therefore, the increasing incidence in malignancy in the young age and the significant improvement in the long-term survival have been associated with worldwide interest in fertility preservation in young patients facing gonadotoxic radio- and/or chemotherapy among gynecologists, hematologists, oncologists, reproductive endocrinologists, pediatricians, rheumatologists, endocrinologists, general practitioners, family physicians, and almost all subspecialty physicians. The interest in preservation of fertility has ubiquitously increased, presently representing standard of care for children and reproductive age patients exposed to gonadotoxic radio- and/or chemotherapy. Combating the remote effects of gonadotoxic treatment is a universal priority in medicine aiming at improving and preserving the survivors' life quality including their future fertility and gonadal function. The new coined "oncofertility" specialty and fertility preservation have affected reproductive endocrinology and many other medical specialties, such as oncology, assisted reproduction, and subfertility treatment [20–30].

Z. Blumenfeld (✉)
Rappaport Faculty of Medicine, Reproductive Endocrinology, Obsterics/Gynecology, Technion – Israel Institute of Technology, Haifa, Israel
e-mail: z_blumenfeld@rambam.health.gov.il

G. N. Allahbadia et al. (eds.), *Textbook of Assisted Reproduction*, https://doi.org/10.1007/978-981-15-2377-9_61

The main current methods for preservation of fertility in the postpubertal female exposed to gonadotoxic treatments are [20–30]:

- Controlled ovarian stimulation and egg retrieval for in vitro *fertilization* (IVF) for married patients and those with a male spouse/partner and embryo cryopreservation, or cryopreservation of unfertilized metaphase-II ova, for single women, without a male partner
- Biopsy and cryopreservation of ovarian tissue
- Ovariopexy-surgical displacement of one ovary (or both), from the irradiation field
- Temporary, endocrine suppression during the gonadotoxic chemotherapy, by a long-acting gonadotropin-releasing hormone agonist (GnRHa)

61.2 Suppression of Ovarian Function Before Gonadotoxic Chemotherapy

61.2.1 The Logic Behind Suppression Using GnRH Analogues

As previously stated, the chances of gonadal function preservation following gonadotoxic chemotherapy are much better for prepubertal girls than for prepubertal boys [29–31]. Since ovarian function was preserved in most long-term female survivors treated prepubertally for lymphoma [31], compared to only half of the similarly treated adult women [20], it is clinically rational and therefore tempting to induce a reversible and temporary hypogonadotropic, prepubertal milieu in adult females before and during the gonadotoxic insult [25–31]. In line with this rationale, many centers have used GnRHa cotreatment for amelioration and minimizing the effects of gonadotoxic chemotherapy [25–31], by simulating a prepubertal hormonal milieu, with the philosophy that POI prevention in survivors is preferred to treating it after its occurrence, following the rule of "an ounce of prevention is worth a pound of cure."

61.2.2 Previous and Current Experience Using GnRH Agonists for Preservation of Fertility

The administration of a noninvasive adjuvant cotreatment that may decrease chemotherapy-induced gonadotoxicity is tempting [20, 25–30]. Glode et al. [32] have examined this hypothesis, almost 40 years ago, in a murine model suggesting that GnRHa protected male mice from the cyclophosphamide-induced gonadotoxicity. However, later studies found that the GnRHa cotreatment was ineffective in the male, as opposed to females [20, 25–31]. It has been hypothesized [20, 25–32] that metabolically inactive primordial follicles fare better than dividing, actively growing follicles [30]. Prepubertal girls fare much better than prepubertal boys in their chances of preserving gonadal function following gonadotoxic chemotherapy [20, 25–33]. Since ovarian function was preserved in over 90% of long-term female survivors who were prepubertally treated for lymphoma, but only in a minority of similarly treated adult women [31], preclinical and clinical studies have induced a temporary and reversible prepubertal hypogonadotropic milieu in reproductive-age women and female adolescents before and during gonadotoxic chemotherapy [20, 25–31].

The only published study assessing the ovarian histology before and after GnRHa cotreatment in parallel to gonadotoxic chemotherapy, which obviously cannot be conducted clinically in women, has been performed in female primates, over 30 years ago [34]. This randomized prospective study demonstrated that GnRHa can protect the ovary against cyclophosphamide-induced gonadotoxicity [34]. Cotreatment with GnRHa from before and along cyclophosphamide has significantly decreased the daily rate of follicular decline, from 0.12 ± 0.012% to 0.057 ± 0.019% ($P < 0.05$), and the number of primordial follicles lost during the gonadotoxic chemotherapeutic, from 64.6 ± 2.8% to 28.9 ± 9.1% ($P < 0.05$), versus the control group of cyclophosphamide without GnRHa cotreatment [34].

In the clinical setting, many groups of clinicians have used GnRHa cotreatment along chemotherapy for fertility preservation and minimizing the gonadotoxic effects of chemotherapy [6–10], with the philosophy that preventing POF in survivors is more advantageous to treating it, following the rationale: "an ounce of prevention is better than a pound of cure" [20, 25–30, 35–60]. Therefore, this noninvasive and inexpensive cotreatment has gained worldwide popularity and investigation, and many groups of physicians have been using it in the last decade [20, 25–30, 35–60]. Up to date 24 studies (16 retrospective and 8 RCT) have reported on over 3000 patients treated with GnRHa prior to and in parallel to chemotherapy, demonstrating a significant decrease in POI rate in survivor's vs. eight publications including 350 patients, where the GnRHa cotreatment did not bring about a significant decrease in POI rate [20, 25–30, 35–70]. The GnRHa adjuvant co-treated patients along the gonadotoxic chemotherapy resumed regular menses and normal ovarian function in almost 90% of cases as compared to about 50% in the chemotherapy only group [20, 25–30, 35–64]. However, resuming cyclic ovarian function (COF), normal gonadotropins, and other sex hormonal levels, such as estradiol, progesterone, and AMH, and even antral follicle count (AFC), are only surrogate markers of fertility. It is, therefore, most correct to compare the spontaneous PR in the survivors, in the GnRHa-treated patients compared to the controls, untreated with GnRHa adjuvant [20, 25–30, 35–64]. Indeed, spontaneous conceptions in the GnRHa adjuvant co-treated survivors ranged from 23% to 88%, compared to 11–35% ($P < 0.05$) in the control groups who received chemotherapy without the GnRHa cotreatment [20, 25–30, 35–64].

Fourteen meta-analyses of RCT's and 4 recent international expert consensus meetings [44, 45], along numerous smaller studies, have critically summarized the efficiency of GnRHa cotreatment, concluding that this cotreatment along chemotherapy can significantly decrease the POI risk and increases conceptions in survivors [20, 25–30, 35–64]. Three convincing, recent, large, prospective RCT's were published in the last years [50, 51, 72]. The POEMS-SWOG S0230 study enrolled HR-negative breast cancer patients [50], whereas most patients in the PROMISE-GIM6 [51] study were HR positive. All these three RCTs have demonstrated a statistically significant decrease in POI rate in the GnRHa arms (OR: 0.28–0.30; $P = 0.04$). Moreover, the conception rate was significantly increased by the GnRHa cotreatment (OR: 2.45; $P = 0.03$) [50, 51]. Furthermore, long-term evaluation of the survivors, with a median follow-up of 7.3 years (range, 5–8.2 years) [51], has shown a 5-year cumulative COF resumption of 72.6% (95% CI, 65.7%–80.3%) in the GnRHa group compared to 64% (95% CI, 56.2%–72.8%) among the controls (age-adjusted HR, 1.48 (95% CI, 1.12–1.95); $P = 00.006$), with no difference in the 5-year disease-free survival (DFS) [51].

The POEMS-SWOG S0230 study was a NIH-sponsored, prospective RCT, where 257 premenopausal breast cancer patients were treated with either chemotherapy alone or chemotherapy with GnRHa [50]. The GnRHa-treated arm has shown an improved COF rate across multiple endpoints and higher pregnancy rate compared to the control group [50]. Unexpectedly, the GnRHa cotreatment arm had better overall survival (OS) and disease-free survival (DFS) rates compared to the only chemotherapy arm [50]. Two years after chemotherapy, the POI rate was 22% in the chemotherapy alone arm compared to only 8% in the GnRHa co-treated patients (OR = 0.30, 95% CI (0.09, 0.97); $P < 0.04$) [50]. Successful pregnancy was achieved by 12 of the 18 survivors who were interested in conceiving in the chemotherapy alone group compared with 22 patients who successfully conceived of the 25 survivors who attempted conception in the GnRHa arm (adjusted OR 2.45; $P < 0.03$) [50]. Moreover, the GnRHa co-treated survivors gave birth to 18 healthy neonates compared to only 12 in the chemotherapy only group [50]. Furthermore, the authors found that the 4-year mortality rate in the GnRHa group was significantly lower than in the chemotherapy without GnRHa group ($P = 0.05$), a finding defined as surprising and unexpected [50].

Very relevant to this controversial issue is a publication [53] from one of the past opponents to the GnRHa use for fertility preservation, which concluded that the GnRHa adjuvant cotreatment has significantly increased the pregnancy rate in survivors of Hodgkin lymphoma (HL) (*OR = 12.8; P (0=.001*. Moreover, these previous opponents to the GnRHa cotreatment [53] have "adjusted the analysis to a high degree and nevertheless…found surprisingly *strong (OR (12<indirect evidence supporting the prophylactic use of GnRHa* in women receiving therapy for early unfavorable HL." Thus, these investigators [53], have therefore, concluded "…the multivariate analysis in the present study reveals that the use of GnRH analogues during therapy is a *strong, independent, and a highly significant predictor of pregnancies*." This study supports the use of GnRHa adjuvant cotreatment in HL female patients for preservation of ovarian function and fertility [53].

We have demonstrated that the GnRHa cotreatment, in parallel to chemotherapy, has significantly increased the rate of spontaneous pregnancies in survivors ($P < 0.006$), in addition to preserving COF (OR = 6.87) in a large group of young women followed up for over 20 years [37]. Ninety one patients (62.7%) conceived 179 times in the GnRHa group vs. only 32 patients experiencing 56 pregnancies (41.6%) in the controls ($P < 0.003$), generating 132 and 42 newborns ($P < 0.01$), respectively [37]. Spontaneous pregnancies occurred in 58% of the survivors in the GnRHa group, compared to only 35% in the control arm ($P = 0.006$) [37]. These favorable results are in keeping with the results of the three large recent RCT's publications [50, 51, 72], which similarly found significant reduction in POI in the GnRHa-treated patients vs. controls (OR: 0.28–0.3; $P < 0.001$–0.04).

Whereas the definitive gold standard of fertility preservation is conceptions, it is important to put forward the high pregnancy rates after GnRHa adjuvant cotreatment demonstrated in three different publications from three continents:

- In Wong et al. study [55], in the UK, 71% survivors conceived after GnRHa and chemotherapy.
- In the POEMS-SWOG study, [50], in the USA, 88% survivors conceived after GnRHa+ chemotherapy.
- In our study, [37], in Israel 62% of the survivors spontaneously conceived.

Moreover, GnRHa adjuvant cotreatment was also effective in decreasing POI and protecting COF rate, not only in patients treated with conventional chemotherapy but also in survivors after bone marrow transplantation, who were treated with aggressive conditioning gonadotoxic chemotherapy [59, 60].

Three recent international consensus meetings support the use of GnRHa for fertility preservation including the 2015 St. Gallen International Expert Consensus panel [44] and the National Comprehensive Cancer Network guidelines (www.nccn.org), [45, 71]. The 14th St. Gallen international conference and expert consensus [44] supports the use of GnRHa in breast cancer patients concluding that

GnRHa therapy during chemotherapy "proved effective to protect against POF and preserve fertility" in young patients with ER-negative breast cancer undergoing chemotherapy [44]. This consensus states that the GnRHa cotreatment also increased the rate of subsequent successful conceptions without compromising the disease outcomes [44]. The second expert consensus meeting, the National Comprehensive Cancer Network guidelines (www.nccn.org), summarized ten concluding recommendations [45]. The recommendations were graded according to the evidence levels and grades of recommendation (according to the ESMO Clinical Practice Guidelines) for fertility preservation in cancer patients [45]. The only conclusion (out of the ten) that received the highest grading, IA, according to the ESMO classification was the conclusion regarding GnRHa [45]. This conclusion states: "Ovarian suppression with the use of LHRHa during chemotherapy should be considered a reliable strategy to preserve ovarian function and fertility, at least in breast cancer patients, given the availability of new data suggesting both the safety and the efficacy of the procedure have become available (IA)" [45]. The third international consensus meeting, the second international consensus guidelines for breast cancer in young women [71], also concluded that the use of GnRHa in young patients with both hormone receptor (HR) positive and negative breast cancer is beneficial and bears a protective role against POI. The conclusions of the three international expert meetings [44, 45, 71] are incompatible with most meta-analyses of RCTs and recent summaries and, including the Cochrane collaboration analysis [47], supporting the use of GnRHa cotreatment and concluding that it was associated with a decreased risk of POI and significantly increased conception rate. Also, of important clinical impact, the use of GnRHa along chemotherapy can significantly abolish the thrombocytopenia-associated menometrorrhagia in the thrombocytopenic patients [20, 25–30, 35–64].

The largest and recent meta-analysis [42] concluded:

- Overall, 12 RCTs including 1231 breast cancer patients were eligible for evaluation.
- The GnRHa cotreatment along chemotherapy was associated with a significant reduced risk of POI (OR 0.36, 95% CI 0.23–0.57; $P < 0.001$) but with significant heterogeneity ($P = 0.026$ for heterogeneity).
- In eight studies evaluating amenorrhea 1 year after chemotherapy, the GnRHa use diminished the POI risk (OR 0.55, 95% CI 0.41–0.73, $P < 0.001$) with no heterogeneity ($P = 0.936$ for heterogeneity).
- In five studies assessing PR, more patients treated with GnRHa successfully conceived (33 versus 19 survivors; OR 1.83, 95% CI 1.02–3.28, $P = 0.041$; $P = 0.629$ for heterogeneity).
- In three studies no difference was observed in disease-free survival (DFS), (HR 1.00, 95% CI 0.49–2.04, $P = 0.939$; $P = 0.044$ for heterogeneity).

More recently, Leonard et al. [72] summarized the outcome of the prospective Anglo Celtic group OPTION trial, a prospective, RCT on 227 patients randomized to GnRHa in parallel to chemotherapy vs. chemotherapy alone in stage I–III B breast cancer patients. GnRHa reduced amenorrhea between 1 and 2 years to 22% compared to 38% in the control group ($P = 0.015$) and POI to 18.5% versus 34.8% in the controls ($P = 0.048$). FSH levels were lower in GnRHa arm at both 1 and 2 years ($P = 0.027$, $P = 0.001$, respectively). This RCT concluded that GnRHa could reduce the POI risk in early breast cancer, with particular efficiency in patients below the age of 40 years.

61.2.3 The Possible Mechanisms of GnRHa Fertility Preservation

Five possible mechanisms were suggested to possibly elucidate the effect of GnRHa in ameliorating the detrimental effect of gonadotoxic chemotherapy [28–30].

61.2.3.1 Simulating a Prepubertal, Hypogonadotropic Milieu

The hypogonadotropic state, induced by the GnRHa administration, creates a prepubertal hormonal milieu. The gonadotoxic chemotherapy destroys many follicles resulting in diminished concentration of sex hormones and inhibins [26–30]. The decreased serum levels of steroid sex hormones and inhibin negatively feedback on the hypothalamus and pituitary to increase the secretion of gonadotropins, mainly follicle-stimulating hormone (FSH). The high FSH concentrations may increase the recruitment and maturation rate of resting preantral follicle enhancing the unidirectional process of folliculogenesis. Thus, since these growing follicles and their dividing granulosa cells have an active metabolism during folliculogenesis, they may be highly subjected to the gonadotoxic effects of chemotherapy, resulting in an enhanced rate of follicular demise [26–30]. Similarly, Meirow's group [73, 74] coined the "burnout" hypothesis, to describe the accelerated follicular demise due to enhanced folliculogenesis in the gonad subjected to gonadotoxic chemotherapy. They hypothesized that alkylating agents may enhance protein phosphorylation, through the phosphatidylinositol 3-kinase (PI3K) signaling route, which upregulates the activation of primordial follicles (PMF), resulting in the "burnout effect" and follicle demise [73, 74].

Morgan et al. [75] explained the mechanisms of chemotherapy-associated gonadotoxicity, suggesting that POI results from PMF demise through both a direct effect and also due to an accelerated rate of folliculogenesis to replace the damaged growing follicles [75]. The gonadotoxic effect is not only direct damage to oocytes but also indirectly through a gonadotoxic effect on the granulosa cells [75]. The rate of PMF recruitment to exit the non-active, resting pool is affected by the absence or presence of the larger, gonadotropin-dependent, growing follicles [75]. Thus, GnRHa administration may possibly interrupt the destructive vicious cycle by desensitizing of GnRH receptors in the hypophysis, interfering with the negative feedback-generated increase in FSH secretion in spite of low inhibins and estrogen plasma concentrations [26–30, 75].

Others [76, 77] have put forward a possible detrimental effect of high gonadotropin levels on the resting pool of PMF. Mice, transgenic for β-LH, where LH levels are significantly increased, possess at birth a comparable number of follicles as the wild-type controls [77]. However, several weeks later, chronic exposure to the significantly higher LH concentrations bring about a significant loss in the primordial and primary follicle pool, supporting the notion that high gonadotropins may be detrimental to the follicle pool compatible with the suggested pathophysiologic vicious cycle [26–30].

Although, canonically, the nondividing follicular pool, mainly primordial follicles, is believed to be gonadotropin independent, several publications have suggested that primary and PMF may express messenger RNA (mRNA) for FSH and LH receptors [78, 79]. These publications are in keeping with the concept that even primordial and primary, immature follicles may not be gonadotropin independent [80–82].

Patel et al. [83] have reported that FSH can modulate ovarian germinative stem cells (OGSCs), such as pluripotent, very small embryonic-like stem cells (VSELs), and their "progenitors," located in the adult mammalian gonadal surface epithelium. Four FSH receptors (FSHR) isoforms have been reported, but only FSH-R_1 and FSH-R_3 isoforms are biologically active. Patel et al. [83] examined the effect of FSH on FSH-R_1 and FSH-R_3 isoforms and on Oct-4A and Sox-2, stem cell-specific markers for VSELs, and OGSCs (Oct-4) in ovine ovaries. They have found an increase in FSH-R_3 mRNA transcripts, but FSH-R_1 did not increase after FSH incubation [83]. FSH-R_1, a member of the GPR superfamily of receptors, is a 75 kDa protein, expressed on granulosa cells of growing follicles, and its activation by ligand stimulation brings about steroidogenesis through cAMP signal transduction [81, 83]. FSH-R_3, expressed by OSE and granulosa cells, is a 39 kDa protein and a growth factor receptor which can promote DNA synthesis leading to proliferation via MAPK pathway, specifically the extracellular-regulated kinase (ERK) [81, 83]. These two isoforms, FSH-R_1 and FSH-R_3 transcripts, are different in exons 9–11, whereas FSH-R_1 lacks exon 11 and possesses exons 9 and 10 and FSH-R_3 possesses exon 11 but lacks exons 9 and 10 [81, 83].

According to the above, assuming that FSH-R_3 (lacking exon 10) is the key player modulating FSH effect on the ovarian germinative stem cells to induce neo-oogenesis during postnatal life, it is possible to explain why the previous experiments in search of mutations in exon 10 of the FSH receptor failed to yield any results and concluded, therefore, that PF do not possess FSH receptors [81–83]. The studies that failed to detect FSH receptors on PF's used rtPCR primers selected from exon 10 of the FSH-R_1 receptor, whereas the study that did find active FSH receptors on the ovarian germinative cells demonstrated FSH-R_3 that lacks exon 10 on PF and GSC [81–83]. Thus, it was concluded that FSH modulates ovarian stem cells through the FSH-R_3 to undergo self-renewal, clonal expansion, and differentiation into oocytes and follicles [81–83]. For those who still remain unconvinced and persistently hold the canonical dogma that PMF are gonadotropin independent, an alternative theoretic explanatory mechanism may be suggested [26–30]. Even if they may be gonadotropin independent, the primordial and primary follicles are unequivocally dependent on growth factors (GFs) such as bone morphogenetic proteins (BMP's)–4, −7, and − 9 activins and many others [80]. These and possibly other GFs which are secreted by the more advanced and gonadotropin-dependent follicles may induce the exit of PMF from the nondividing, dormant, inactive pool [80]. Thus, FSH stimulates the secretion of these GFs by the more advanced stages of ovarian follicles [80]. The GnRHa cotreatment causes initially a flare-up and within 7–10 days induces pituitary downregulation through receptors desensitization leading to decreased FSH secretion. The decreased FS levels prevent the secretion of GFs by the FSH-dependent follicles and therefore prevent PMF activation by GF's resulting in more PMF remaining in the uncommitted, "dormant" stage and minimizing their ultimate destruction by alkylating agents [26–30, 80]. Thus, even for those who believe that the activation of PMF the early stages of folliculogenesis, and their exit from the dormant state may be gonadotropin independent, FSH may affect early folliculogenesis through GF's secreted by the more advanced, GN-dependent follicles [84, 85]. Indeed, the canonical dogma that PM, primary follicles, and early folliculogenesis are totally gonadotropin independent may need reevaluation and reconsideration [30].

61.2.3.2 Possible Direct Effect on GnRH Receptors

The human ovary also contains GnRH receptors, similar to rodents' gonads although at a lower concentration [30, 86–88]. Activation of the receptor by the GnRH ligand may possibly decrease apoptosis [86]. Imai et al. [89] have shown that GnRHa may decrease the in vitro gonadotoxic effect of doxorubicin, regardless of gonadotropins concentrations. They have demonstrated a direct in vitro protective effect from chemotherapy-induced GC damage by GnRHa [89]. Most recently, the group of Del Mastro and Lambertini have shown a direct, anti-apoptotic effect of GnRHa on cumulus cells [106, 107].

61.2.3.3 Decreased Perfusion of the Ovary

Estrogens increase the utero-ovarian perfusion [89]. An additional put forward mechanism to possibly explain the GnRHa cotreatment beneficial effect in minimizing the chemotherapy-associated gonadotoxicity is the decrease in utero-ovarian perfusion resulting from the hypoestrogenic milieu generated by pituitary-gonadal desensitization down-regulation [30, 89, 90]. High estrogen levels were shown to increase the ovarian perfusion in a rat model of ovarian stimulation, and GnRHa administration has significantly alleviated this increase in a dose-dependent manner [89]. This decrease in the utero-ovarian perfusion generated by the hypoestrogenic milieu due to GnRHa-induced hypophysiary desensitization may possibly decrease the cumulative exposure of the ovaries to the chemotherapeutic agents, secondarily resulting in a decreased gonadotoxic effect. Such a possibility immediately raises the question whether this decreased exposure of the internal genital organs may be associated with an increased risk of metastases to the internal genitalia, in patients treated with GnRHa in addition to chemotherapy. Up to date, the overall survival and DFS of the GnRHa co-treated women were not different from those of controls [30, 40–48], and in one RCT, the DFS was even significantly improved [50].

61.2.3.4 Sphingosine-1-Phosphate (S-1-P)

It has been put forward that sphingosine-1-phosphate (S-1-P) and its agonistic analogues, such as Fingolimod (FTY720), may be possibly associated with chemotherapy-induced oocyte apoptosis [30, 91–93]. The S-1-P molecule has many different activities and is a pleiotropic lipid mediator involved in cell growth and cancer progression in addition to cell viability, angiogenesis and vascular maturation, invasion, survival, inflammation, allergy, and asthma [30, 91–93]. The balance between sphingosine kinases that synthesize the molecule and S-1-P lyases and phosphatases, which degrade it [30, 91–93], determines its intracellular concentration. It has been suggested that GnRHa may possibly upregulate the ovarian S-1-P and thus decrease the chemotherapy-induced follicular demise [30]. Disruption of the Bax gene, Bcl-2, in rodents, or targeted expression of the Bax antagonist, to the female mouse germ line can prevent the gonadotoxic effect of doxorubicin and protect the oocytes from destruction, either in vivo or in vitro [30, 91–93]. Oocytes deficient of acid sphingomyelinase, which degrades S-1-P and generates ceramide, are resistant to the apoptosis induced in vitro by doxorubicin [30, 91–93]. Administration of S-1-P into the murine periovarian bursa prevented the irradiation-induced ovarian follicles destruction [30, 91–93]. Zelinsky et al. [94] have shown that administration of FTY720 or S-1-P to female macaque monkeys by direct intraovarian cannulation for a week before ovarian irradiation maintained the ovarian follicles and resumed menstrual cycles [94]. FTY720 had a more potent effect than S-1-P on fertility preservation [94]. Even more convincing, not only ovarian follicles were preserved but also fertility and spontaneous conception. The offsprings conceived and delivered by the radio-protected females developed normally and showed no evidence of genomic instability [94]. Adult human ovarian cortical slices pretreated with S-1-P before being xenografted into nude mice lost significantly less PMF than the untreated controls [94]. Moreover, S-1-P protected the female germ cells from irradiation without a discernible propagation of genomic damage [95]. Obviously, the long-term ovarian cannulation for S-1-P or FTY720 infusion during the long chemo- or radiotherapy period is impractical, in women with malignant diseases. Future endeavors should challenge the methodology of gonadal administration of S-1-P, without systemic absorption, in order to minimize follicular loss and not jeopardize the ability of chemo- and radiotherapy to fight systemically the neoplastic cells. Nevertheless, the hypothesis that the GnRHa adjuvant cotreatment beneficial effect may be possibly associated with an intraovarian increase in S-1-P or similar anti-apoptotic molecule(s) is tempting [30]. This hypothesis of GnRHa possibly upregulating intraovarian S-1-P effect is speculative and awaits validation.

61.2.3.5 Protection of the Germinative Stem Cells

Over a decade ago, Tilly's group [96, 97] revolutionized the canonical concept by publishing data whereby rodent gonads may possess mitotically active germ cells that undergo continuous mitosis and replication. They [96, 97] suggested that these germinative stem cells (GSC) can rejuvenate the ovarian PMF reserve. Their publications challenged the canonical dogma of reproductive endocrinology, whereby mammalian females are delivered with a fixed and nonincreasing of follicular reserve and lose the capacity for germ-cell renewal during intrauterine life [96–99]. The dogma that de novo oogenesis does not exist after birth in mammals was established and upheld for over 60 years. The suggested revolutionary concept ignited an ongoing dispute whether the mammalian ovary is capable, or not, of generating ovarian follicles de novo postnatally [96–102]. More recent publications suggested that oocyte-producing GSC may indeed exist and can be isolated from ovaries of adult rodents and even humans [100–102]. Following these revolutionary publications, one may speculate that GnRHa administration may possibly protect the undifferentiated GSCs, which ultimately generate de novo PMF [29, 30]. In keeping with such a possibility, we have measured increased, menopausal FSH and undetectable AMH levels, in about a third of our patients treated with GnRHa from before and in parallel to chemotherapy, for up to 1 year [20, 25–30]. However, about a year after the gonadotoxic chemotherapy and GnRHa cotreatment, the FSH levels decreased to normal, AMH increased in 90% of those patients, and more than 60% of those who were interested, spontaneously conceived [20, 25–30, 35–41]. We speculate that most, if not all the growing follicles, were destroyed by the gonadotoxic chemotherapy, and the GSC, preceding the primordial follicles, were possibly protected by the GnRHa cotreatment [20, 25–30, 35–41]. Whereas folliculogenesis, from the stage of GSC to mature Graafian follicle, may last somewhere between 6 and 12 months, it is understandable why it lasted almost a year to rejuvenate the ovaries in these patients. The protected GSC started folliculogenesis, maturation, secretion of AMH, and estrogens, and the latter fed back to decrease FSH levels to normal [20, 25–30, 35–41]. Again, this hypothesis needs further data, and it remains to be validated whether this mechanism can be attributed to the GnRHa administration.

61.2.4 The Debate Pros and Cons

Up to date, 38 publications (12 RCTs, 25 non-RCTs, and 14 meta-analyses) have reported on over 3000 patients treated with GnRHa along chemotherapy, demonstrating a significant decrease in POI rate in survivors of malignant diseases or those receiving cyclophosphamide pulses for autoimmune diseases such as systemic lupus erythematosus (SLE) nephritis [20, 25–30, 35–41, 108]. However, there are also ten publications not supporting the GnRHa as an effective modality of fertility preservation [20, 25–30, 35–41, 108]. For several years the pendulum switched from a negative to a positive conclusion regarding the ability of GnRHa to minimize gonadotoxicity and preserve fertility. It seems that in the last few years, the pendulum tends toward a positive conclusion, ending the debate and suggesting the GnRHa adjuvant cotreatment may indeed preserve ovarian function and fertility (higher PR) without an adverse effect on OS or DFS [20, 25–30, 35–41, 108].

61.3 Alternative Noninvasive Methods for Fertility Preservation and New Endeavors

Only GnRHa has been clinically shown to preserve fertility and reduce chemotherapy-induced gonadotoxicity in human. However, many other agents have been suggested as possible beneficial agents to prevent gonadotoxicity in preclinical, animal, or in vitro studies [103–105, 109]:

- GnRH antagonists
- Oral contraceptive (OC) pills
- Sphingosine-1-phosphate/FTY720 (S1P analogue, Fingolimod)
- AS101 – ammonium trichloro(dioxoethylene-O,O′) tellurate
- AMH
- G-CSF
- Imatinib
- Dexrazoxane (ICRF-187)
- Luteinizing hormone (LH)
- In vitro generation of oocytes from induced pluripotent stem cells (ipSCs)

61.4 Conclusions

It is recommended to offer all the young women facing gonadotoxic chemotherapy all the options for fertility preservation: GnRHa cotreatment along chemotherapy and cryopreservation of oocytes, embryos, or ovarian tissue [20, 25–30], even in high-risk patients with leukemia. This optimistic policy hopes that in a few years, the "artificial ovary"–IV technology of growing PMS to Graafian follicles containing M-II fertilizable oocytes, may turn clinically possible, bypassing the need of ovarian autotransplantation, in those patients suffering POI following the gonadotoxic insult. Although this technology is not ripe and unavailable yet in human, the preliminary success in rodents, and the three-dimensional follicle culture in alginate gel, may hopefully become clinically available in a few years. Therefore, all the avenues for fertility preservation should be put forward and offered to young women facing gonadotoxic chemotherapy [108, 109].

References

1. Siegel RL, Miller KD, Jemal A. Cancer statistics, 2016. CA Cancer J Clin. 2016;66:7–30.
2. Miller KD, Siegel RL, Lin CC, Mariotto AB, Kramer JL, Rowland JH, Stein KD, Alteri R, Jemal A. Cancer treatment and survivorship statistics. CA Cancer J Clin. 2016;66:271–89.
3. Surveillance, Epidemiology, and End Results (SEER) Program. 2015 SEER* Stat Database: Mortality-All COD, Aggregated With State, Total US (1969–2012) <Katrina/Rita Population Adjustment>. Bethesda, MD: National Cancer Institute, Division of Cancer Control and Population Sciences, Surveillance Research Program, Cancer Statistics Branch; underlying mortality data provided by National Center for Health Statistics; 2015.
4. Wingo PA, Cardinez CJ, Landis SH, Greenlee RT, Ries LA, Anderson RN, Thun MJ. Long-term trends in cancer mortal-

ity in the United States, 1930-1998. Cancer. 2003;97(suppl 12):3133–275.

5. Murphy SL, Kochanek KD, Xu J, Heron M. Deaths: final data for 2012. Natl Vital Stat Rep. 2015;63(9):1–117.
6. Hudson MM, Meyer WH, Pui CH. Progress born from a legacy of collaboration. J Clin Oncol. 2015;33:2935–7.
7. Quaresma M, Coleman MP, Rachet B. 40-year trends in an index of survival for all cancers combined and survival adjusted for age and sex for each cancer in England and Wales, 1971-2011: a population-based study. Lancet. 2015;385:1206–18.
8. Trudgen K, Ayensu-Coker L. Fertility preservation and reproductive health in the pediatric, adolescent, and young adult female cancer patient. Curr Opin Obstet Gynecol. 2014;26:372–80.
9. Noyes N, Knopman JM, Melzer K, Fino ME, Friedman B, Westphal LM. Oocyte cryopreservation as a fertility preservation measure for cancer patients. Reprod BioMed Online. 2011;23:323–33.
10. Alterkruse SF, Kosary CL, Krapcho M, editors. SEER cancer statistics review, 1975–2007. Bethesda, MD: National Cancer Institute; 2010.
11. Jemal A, Siegel R, Xu J, Ward E. Cancer statistics, 2010. CA Cancer J Clin. 2010;60:277–300.
12. Blatt J. Pregnancy outcome in long-term survivors of childhood cancer. Med Pediatr Oncol. 1999;33:29–33.
13. Horner MJ, Ries LAG, Krapcho M, Neyman N, Aminou R, Howlader N, Altekruse SF, Feuer EJ, Huang L, Mariotto A, et al., editors. SEER Cancer statistics review, 1975–2006. Bethesda, MD: National Cancer Institute; 2011.. http://seer.can-cer.gov/faststats/selections
14. Alvarez RM, Ramanathan P. Fertility preservation in female oncology patients: the influence of the type of cancer on ovarian stimulation response. Hum Reprod. 2016 Jul 1. Pii: dew158. [Epub ahead of print].
15. Howlader N, Noone AM, Krapcho M, Garshell J, Miller D, Altekruse SF, Kosary CL, Yu M, Ruhl J, Tatalovich Z, editors. SEER Cancer statistics review, 1975–2012. Bethesda, MD: National Cancer Institute; 2015.. http://seer.cancer.gov/csr/1975_2012/
16. Trudgen K, Ayensu-Coker L. Fertility preservation and reproductive health in the pediatric, adolescent, and young adult female cancer patient. Curr Opin Obstet Gynecol. 2014;26:80.
17. Oeffinger K, Mertens AC, Sklar C, Kawashima T, Hudson MM, Meadows AT, Friedman DL, Marina N, Hobbie W, Kadan-Lottick NS, Schwartz CL, Leisenring W, Robison LL, Childhood Cancer Survivor Study. Chronic health conditions in adult survivors of childhood cancer. N Engl J Med. 2006;355:1572–82.
18. Thomson AB, Critchley HOD, Kelnar CJH, Wallace WHB. Late reproductive sequelae following treatment of childhood cancer and options for fertility preservation. Best Pract Res Clin Endocrinol Metab. 2002;16:311–34.
19. Meirow D, Schiff E. Appraisal of chemotherapy effects on reproductive outcome according to animal studies and clinical data. J Natl Cancer Inst Monogr. 2005;34:21–5.. Review
20. Blumenfeld Z, Katz G, Evron A. 'An ounce of prevention is worth a pound of cure': the case for and against GnRH-agonist for fertility preservation. Ann Oncol. 2014;25:1719–28.
21. De Vos M, Smitz J, Woodruff TK. Fertility preservation in women with cancer. Lancet. 2014;384:1302–10.
22. Waimey KE, Duncan FE, Su HI, Smith K, Wallach H, Jona K, Coutifaris C, Gracia CR, Shea LD, Brannigan RE, Chang RJ, Zelinski MB, Stouffer RL, Taylor RL, Woodruff TK. Future directions in oncofertility and fertility preservation: a report from the 2011 oncofertility consortium conference. J Adolesc Young Adult Oncol. 2013;2:25–30.
23. Wallace WHB, Anderson RA, Irvine DS. Fertility preservation for young patients with cancer: who is at risk and what can be offered? Lancet Oncol. 2005;6:209–18.
24. Linkeviciute A, Boniolo G, Chiavari L, Peccatori FA. Fertility preservation in cancer patients: the global framework. Cancer Treat Rev. 2014;40:1019–27.
25. Blumenfeld Z. Chemotherapy and fertility. Best Pract Res Clin Obstet Gynaecol. 2012;26:379–90.. Review
26. Blumenfeld Z, Evron A. Endocrine prevention of chemotherapy-induced ovarian failure. Curr Opin Obstet Gynecol. 2016;28:223–9.
27. Blumenfeld Z, Dann E, Avivi I, Epelbaum R, Rowe JM. Fertility after treatment for Hodgkin's disease. Ann Oncol. 2002;13(Suppl 1):138–47.
28. Blumenfeld Z, Avivi I, Ritter M, Rowe JM. Preservation of fertility and ovarian function and minimizing chemotherapy-induced gonadotoxicity in young women. J Soc Gynecol Investig. 1999;6:229–39.
29. Blumenfeld Z. How to preserve fertility in young women exposed to chemotherapy? The role of GnRH agonist cotreatment in addition to cryopreservation of embrya, oocytes, or ovaries. Oncologist. 2007;12:1044–54.
30. Blumenfeld Z, von Wolff M. GnRH-analogues and oral contraceptives for fertility preservation in women during chemotherapy. Hum Reprod Update. 2008;14:543–52.
31. Ortin TT, Shostak CA, Donaldson SS. Gonadal status and reproductive function following treatment for Hodgkin's disease in childhood: the Stanford experience. Int J Radiol Oncol Biol Phys. 1990;19:873–80.
32. Glode LM, Robinson J, Gould SF. Protection from cyclophosphamide induced testicular damage with an analogue of gonadotropin-releasing hormone. Lancet. 1981;1:1132–4.
33. Johnson DH, Linde R, Hainsworth JD, Vale W, Rivier J, Stein R, Flexner J, Van Welch R, Greco FA. Effect of a luteinizing hormone releasing hormone agonist given during combination chemotherapy on posttherapy fertility in male patients with lymphoma: preliminary observations. Blood. 1985;65:832–6.
34. Ataya K, Rao LV, Laurence E, Kimmel R. Luteinizing hormone-releasing agonist inhibits cyclophosphamide induced ovarian follicular depletion in rhesus monkeys. Biol Reprod. 1995;52:365–72.
35. Blumenfeld Z, Avivi I, Eckman R, et al. Gonadotropin releasing hormone agonist decreases chemotherapy induced gonadotoxicity and premature ovarian failure in young female patients with Hodgkin lymphoma. Fertil Steril. 2008;89:166–73.
36. Blumenfeld Z. GnRH-agonists in fertility preservation. Curr Opin Endocrinol Diabet Obes. 2008;15:523–8.
37. Blumenfeld Z, Zur H, Dann EJ. Gonadotropin-releasing hormone agonist cotreatment during chemotherapy may increase pregnancy rate in survivors. Oncologist. 2015;20:1283–9.
38. Blumenfeld Z, Evron A. Preserving fertility when choosing chemotherapy regimens – the role of gonadotropin-releasing hormone agonists. Expert Opin Pharmacother. 2015;16:1009–20.
39. Blumenfeld Z. Pregnancy rate and preservation of cyclic ovarian function with gonadotropin-releasing hormone agonist Cotreatment during chemotherapy. JAMA Oncol. 2016;2:545–6.
40. Blumenfeld Z. Preservation of ovarian function and fertility despite gonadotoxic chemotherapy. Expert Rev Endocrinol Metab. 2012;7:567–76.
41. Blumenfeld Z. Critical care for young women before chemotherapy: preserving fertility using gnrh agonists. Crit Care Obst & Gyne. 2016;2:23–8.
42. Lambertini M, Ceppi M, Poggio F, Peccatori FA, Azim HA Jr, Ugolini D, Pronzato P, Loibl S, Moore HC, Partridge AH, Bruzzi P, Del Mastro L. Ovarian suppression using luteinizing hormone-releasing hormone agonists during chemotherapy to preserve ovarian function and fertility of breast cancer patients: a meta-analysis of randomized studies. Ann Oncol. 2015;26:2408–19.

43. Lambertini M, Ginsburg ES, Partridge AH. Update on fertility preservation in young women undergoing breast cancer and ovarian cancer therapy. Curr Opin Obstet Gynecol. 2015;27:98–107.
44. Coates AS, Winer EP, Goldhirsch A. Tailoring therapies improving the management of early breast cancer: St Gallen international expert consensus on the primary therapy of early breast cancer. Ann Oncol. 2015;26:1533–46.
45. Lambertini M, Del Mastro L, Pescio MC. Cancer and fertility preservation: international recommendations from an expert meeting. BMC Med. 2016;14:1.
46. Del Mastro L, Ceppi M, Poggio F. Gonadotropin-releasing hormone analogues for the prevention of chemotherapy induced premature ovarian failure in cancer women: systematic review and meta-analysis of randomized trials. Cancer Treat Rev. 2014;40:675–83.
47. Chen H, Xiao L, Li J, Cui L, Huang W. Adjuvant gonadotropin-releasing hormone analogues for the prevention of chemotherapy-induced premature ovarian failure in premenopausal women. Cochrane Database Syst Rev. 2019;3:CD008018.
48. Del Mastro L, Giraudi S, Levaggi A, Pronzato P. Medical approaches to preservation of fertility in female cancer patients. Expert Opin Pharmacother. 2011;12:387–96.
49. Woodruff TK. Preserving fertility during cancer treatment. Nat Med. 2009;15:1124–5.
50. Moore HCF, Unger JM, Phillips KA, Boyle F, Hitre E, Porter D, Francis PA, Goldstein LJ, Gomez HL, Vallejos CS, POEMS/S0230 Investigators. Goserelin for ovarian protection during breast-cancer adjuvant chemotherapy. N Engl J Med. 2015;372:923–32.
51. Lambertini M, Boni L, Michelotti A, Gamucci T, Scotto T, Gori S, Giordano M, Garrone O, Levaggi A, Poggio F, GIM Study Group. Ovarian suppression with Triptorelin during adjuvant breast Cancer chemotherapy and long-term ovarian function, pregnancies, and disease-free survival: a randomized clinical trial. JAMA. 2015;314:2632–40.
52. Munhoz RR, Pereira AA, Sasse AD. Gonadotropin- releasing hormone agonists for ovarian function preservation in premenopausal women undergoing chemotherapy for early- stage breast cancer: a systematic review and meta-analysis. JAMA Oncol. 2016;2:65–73.
53. Behringer K, Thielen I, Mueller H. Fertility and gonadal function in female survivors after treatment of early unfavorable Hodgkin lymphoma (HL) within the German Hodgkin Study Group HD14 trial. Ann Oncol. 2012;23:1818–25.
54. Demeestere I, Brice P, Peccatori FA, Kentos A. Gonadotropin-releasing hormone agonist for the prevention of chemotherapy-induced ovarian failure in patients with lymphoma: 1-year follow-up of a prospective randomized trial. J Clin Oncol. 2013;31:903–9.
55. Wong M, O'Neill S, Walsh G, Smith IE. Goserelin with chemotherapy to preserve ovarian function in pre-menopausal women with early breast cancer: menstruation and pregnancy outcomes. Ann Oncol. 2013;24:133–8.
56. Recchia F, Saggio G, Amiconi G, Di Blasio A, Cesta A, Candeloro G, Rea S. Gonadotropin-releasing hormone analogues added to adjuvant chemotherapy protect ovarian function and improve clinical outcomes in young women with early breast carcinoma. Cancer. 2006;106:514–23.
57. Recchia F, Candeloro G, Rosselli M, Bratta M, Pasta V, D'Orazi V, Fumagalli LA, Rea S. Adjuvant ovarian suppression, high-dose chemotherapy and immunotherapy for premenopausal patients with high-risk breast cancer. Anticancer Res. 2015;35:6847–53.
58. Recchia F, Necozione S, Bratta M, Rosselli M, Guerriero G, Rea S. LH-RH analogues in the treatment of young women with early breast cancer: long-term follow-up of a phase II study. Int J Oncol. 2015;46:1354–60.
59. Blumenfeld Z, Patel B, Leiba R, Zuckerman T. Gonadotropin-releasing hormone agonist may minimize premature ovarian failure in young women undergoing autologous stem cell transplantation. Fertil Steril. 2012;98:1266–70.
60. Blumenfeld Z, Zuckerman T. Repeated spontaneous pregnancies and successful deliveries after repeated autologous stem cell transplantation and GnRH-agonist. Oncologist. 2010;15:59–60.
61. Hickman LC, Valentine LN, Falcone T. Preservation of gonadal function in women undergoing chemotherapy: a review of the potential role for gonadotropin-releasing hormone agonists. Am J Obstet Gynecol. 2016;215:415–22.
62. Nitzschke M, Raddatz J, Bohlmann MK, et al. GnRH analogs do not protect ovaries from chemotherapy-induced ultrastructural injury in Hodgkin's lymphoma patients. Arch Gynecol Obstet. 2010;282:83–8.
63. Del Mastro L, Ceppi M, Poggio F, Bighin C, Peccatori F, Demeestere I, Levaggi A, Giraudi S, Lambertini M, D'Alonzo A, et al. Gonadotropin-releasing hormone analogues for the prevention of chemotherapy-induced premature ovarian failure in cancer women: systematic review and meta-analysis of randomized trials. Cancer Treat Rev. 2014;40:675–83.
64. Del Mastro L, Lambertini M. Temporary ovarian suppression with gonadotropin-releasing hormone agonist during chemotherapy for fertility preservation: toward the end of the debate? Oncologist. 2015;20:1233–5.
65. Gerber B, von Minckwitz G, Stehle H, Reimer T, Felberbaum R, Maass N, Fischer D, Sommer HL, Conrad B, Ortmann O, Fehm T, Rezai M, Mehta K, Loibl S, German Breast Group Investigators. Effect of luteinizing hormone-releasing hormone agonist on ovarian function after modern adjuvant breast cancer chemotherapy: the GBG 37 ZORO study. J Clin Oncol. 2011;29:2334–41.
66. Elgindy EA, El-Haieg DO, Khorshid OM, Ismail EI, Abdelgawad M, Sallam HN, Abou-Setta AM. Gonadatrophin suppression to prevent chemotherapy-induced ovarian damage: a randomized controlled trial. Obstet Gynecol. 2013;121:78–86.
67. Elgindy E, Sibai H, Abdelghani A, Mostafa M. Protecting ovaries during chemotherapy through gonad suppression: a systematic review and meta-analysis. Obstet Gynecol. 2015;126:187–95.
68. Yang B, Shi W, Yang J, Liu H, Zhao H, Li X, Jiao S. Concurrent treatment with gonadotropin-releasing hormone agonists for chemotherapy-induced ovarian damage in premenopausal women with breast cancer: a meta-analysis of randomized controlled trials. Breast. 2013;22:150–7.
69. Demeestere I, Brice P, Peccatori FA, Kentos A, Dupuis J, Zachee P, Casasnovas O, Van Den Neste E, Dechene J, De Maertelaer V, Bron D, Englert Y. No evidence for the benefit of gonadotropin-releasing hormone agonist in preserving ovarian function and fertility in lymphoma survivors treated with chemotherapy: final long-term report of a prospective randomized trial. J Clin Oncol. 2016;34:2568–74.
70. Munster PN, Moore AP, Ismail-Khan R, Cox CE, Lacevic M, Gross-King M, Xu P, Carter WB, Minton SE. Randomized trial using gonadotropin-releasing hormone agonist triptorelin for the preservation of ovarian function during (neo)adjuvant chemotherapy for breast cancer. J Clin Oncol. 2012;30:533–8.
71. Paluch-Shimon S, Pagani O, Partridge AH, Bar-Meir E, Fallowfield L, Fenlon D, Friedman E, Gelmon K, Gentilini O, Geraghty J, Harbeck N, Higgins S, Loibl S, Moser E, Peccatori F, Raanani H, Kaufman B, Cardoso F. Second international consensus guidelines for breast cancer in young women (BCY2). Breast. 2016;26:87–99.
72. Leonard R, Adamson D, Bertelli G, Mansi J, Yellowlees A, Dunlop J, Thomas GA, Coleman RE, Anderson RA, Anglo Celtic Collaborative Oncology Group and National Cancer Research Institute Trialists. GnRH agonist for protection against ovarian toxicity during chemotherapy for early breast cancer: the Anglo Celtic Group OPTION trial. Ann Oncol. 2017;28:1811–6.
73. Kalich-Philosoph L, Roness H, Carmely A, Fishel M, Ligumsky H, Paglin S, Wolf I, Kanety H, Sredni B, Meirow

D. Cyclophosphamide triggers follicle activation causing ovarian reserve 'burn out'; AS101 prevents follicle loss and preserves fertility. Sci Transl Med. 2013;15:185.
74. Gavish Z, Peer G, Roness H, Cohen Y, Meirow D. Follicle activation and 'burn-out' contribute to post-transplantation follicle loss in ovarian tissue grafts: the effect of graft thickness. Hum Reprod. 2014;29:989–96.
75. Morgan S, Anderson RA, Gourley C, Wallace WH, Spears N. How do chemotherapeutic agents damage the ovary? Hum Reprod Update. 2012;18:525–35.
76. Lobo RA. Potential options for preservation of fertility in women. N Engl J Med. 2005;353:64–73.. Review
77. Flaws JA, Abbud R, Mann RJ, Nilson JH, Hirshfield AN. Chronically elevated luteinizing hormone depletes primordial follicles in the mouse ovary. Biol Reprod. 1997;57:1233–7.
78. Patsoula E, Loutradis D, Drakakis P, Michalas L, Bletsa R, Michalas S. Messenger RNA expression for the follicle-stimulating hormone receptor and luteinizing hormone receptor in human oocytes and preimplantation-stage embryos. Fertil Steril. 2003;79:1187–93.
79. Zheng W, Magid MS, Kramer EE, Chen YT. Follicle-stimulating hormone receptor is expressed in human ovarian surface epithelium and fallopian tube. Am J Pathol. 1996;148:47–53.
80. Knight PG, Glister C. TGF-beta superfamily members and ovarian follicle development. Reproduction. 2006;132:191–206.
81. Babu PS, Danilovich N, Sairam MR. Hormone-induced receptor gene splicing: enhanced expression of the growth factor type I follicle-stimulating hormone receptor motif in the developing mouse ovary as a new paradigm in growth regulation. Endocrinology. 2001;142:381–9.
82. Adriaens I, Cortvrindt R, Smitz J. Differential FSH exposure in preantral follicle culture has marked effects on folliculogenesis and oocyte developmental competence. Hum Reprod. 2004;19:398–408.
83. Patel H, Bhartiya D, Parte S, Gunjal P, Yedurkar S, Bhatt M. Follicle stimulating hormone modulates ovarian stem cells through alternately spliced receptor variant FSH-R3. J Ovarian Res. 2013;6:52.
84. Edson MA, Nagaraja AK, Matzuk MM. The mammalian ovary from genesis to revelation. Endocr Rev. 2009;30:624–712.
85. Webb R, Garnsworthy PC, Gong JG, Armstrong DG. Control of follicular growth: local interactions and nutritional influences. J Anim Sci. 2004;82(Suppl E):E63–74.
86. Grundker C, Emons G. Role of gonadotropin-releasing hormone (GnRH) in ovarian cancer. Reprod Biol Endocrinol. 2003;1:65–71.
87. Harrison GS, Wierman ME, Nett TM, Glode LM. Gonadotropin-releasing hormone and its receptor in normal and malignant cells. Endocr Relat Cancer. 2004;11:725–48.
88. Leung PC, Cheng CK, Zhu XM. Multi-factorial role of GnRH-I and GnRH-II in the human ovary. Mol Cell Endocrinol. 2003;202:145–53.
89. Imai A, Sugiyama M, Furui T, Tamaya T, Ohno T. Direct protection by a gonadotropin-releasing hormone analog from doxorubicin-induced granulosa cell damage. Gynecol Obstet Investig. 2007;63:102–6.
90. Kitajima Y, Endo T, Nagasawa K, Manase K, Honnma H, Baba T, Hayashi T, Chiba H, Sawada N, Saito T. Hyperstimulation and a gonadotropin releasing hormone agonist modulate ovarian vascular permeability by altering expression of the tight junction protein claudin-5. Endocrinology. 2006;147:694–9.
91. Paris F, Perez GI, Fuks Z, Haimovitz-Friedman A, Nguyen H, Bose M, Ilagan A, Hunt PA, Morgan WF, Tilly JL, Kolesnick R. Sphingosine-1 phosphate preserves fertility in irradiated female mice without propagating genomic damage in offspring. Nat Med. 2002;8:901–2.
92. Perez GI, Knudson CM, Leykin L, Korsmeyer SJ, Tilly JL. Apoptosis associated signaling pathways are required for chemotherapy-mediated female germ cell destruction. Nat Med. 1997;3:1228–32.
93. Morita Y, Perez GI, Paris F, Miranda SR, Ehleiter D, Haimovitz-Friedman A, Fuks Z, Xie Z, Reed JC, Schuchman EH, Kolesnick RN, Tilly JL. Oocyte apoptosis is suppressed by disruption of the acid sphingomyelinase gene or by sphingosine-1-phosphate therapy. Nat Med. 2000;6:1109–14.
94. Zelinski MB, Murphy MK, Lawson MS, Jurisicova A, Pau KY, Toscano NP, Jacob DS, Fanton JK, Casper RF, Dertinger SD, Tilly JL. In vivo delivery of FTY720 prevents radiation-induced ovarian failure and infertility in adult female nonhuman primates. Fertil Steril. 2011;95:1440-5.e1–7.
95. Paris F, Perez GI, Kolesnick RN, Tilly JL. Suppression of oocyte apoptosis by sphingosine-1 phosphate therapy in vivo preserves fertility following radiotherapy. Proc 83rd Ann meeting endocrine Soc Denver CO, 2001.
96. Johnson J, Canning J, Kaneko T, Pru JK, Tilly JL. Germline stem cells and follicular renewal in the postnatal mammalian ovary. Nature. 2004;428:145–50.
97. Johnson J, Bagley J, Skaznik-Wikiel M, Lee HJ, Adams GB, Niikura Y, Tschudy KS, Tilly JC, Cortes ML, Forkert R, Spitzer T, Iacomini J, Scadden DT, Tilly JL. Oocyte generation in adult mammalian ovaries by putative germ cells in bone marrow and peripheral blood. Cell. 2005;122:303–15.
98. Gargett CE. Review article: stem cells in human reproduction. Reprod Sci. 2007;14:405–24.
99. Telfer EE, Gosden RG, Byskov AG, Spears N, Albertini D, Andersen CY, Anderson R, Braw-Tal R, Clarke H, Gougeon A, McLaughlin E, McLaren A, McNatty K, Schatten G, Silber S, Tsafriri A. On regenerating the ovary and generating controversy. Cell. 2005;122:821–2.
100. Woods DC, Telfer EE, Tilly JL. Oocyte family trees: old branches or new stems? PLoS Genet. 2012;8:e1002848.
101. Tilly JL, Telfer EE. Purification of germline stem cells from adult mammalian ovaries: a step closer towards control of the female biological clock? Mol Hum Reprod. 2009;15:393–8.
102. Byskov AG, Faddy MJ, Lemmen JG, Andersen CY. Eggs forever? Differentiation. 2005;73:438–46.
103. Roness H, Kashi O, Meirow D. Prevention of chemotherapy-induced ovarian damage. Fertil Steril. 2016;105:20–9.
104. Rossi V, Lispi M, Longobardi S, Mattei M, Rella FD, Salustri A, De Felici M, Klinger FG. LH prevents cisplatin-induced apoptosis in oocytes and preserves female fertility in mouse. Cell Death Differ. 2017;24:72–82.
105. Xiao S, Zhang J, Romero MM, Smith KN, Shea LD, Woodruff TK. In vitro follicle growth supports human oocyte meiotic maturation. Sci Rep. 2015;5:17323.
106. Poggio F, Lambertini M, Bighin C, Conte B, Blondeaux E, D'Alonzo A, Dellepiane C, Buzzatti G, Molinelli C, Boccardo F, Del Mastro L. Potential mechanisms of ovarian protection with gonadotropin-releasing hormone agonist in breast cancer patients: a review. Clin Med Insights Reprod Health. 2019;13 https://doi.org/10.1177/1179558119864584.
107. Scaruffi P, Stigliani S, Cardinali B, Massarotti C, Lambertini M, Sozzi F, Dellepiane C, Merlo DF, Anserini P, Mastro LD. Gonadotropin releasing hormone agonists have an anti-apoptotic effect on cumulus cells. Int J Mol Sci. 2019;20(23):E6045. https://doi.org/10.3390/ijms20236045.
108. Blumenfeld Z. Fertility preservation using GnRH agonists: rationale, possible mechanisms, and explanation of controversy. Clin Med Insights Reprod Health. 2019;13:1179558119870163. https://doi.org/10.1177/1179558119870163.. eCollection 2019. Review
109. Blumenfeld Z. Fertility preservation in women with malignancy: future endeavors. Clin Med Insights Reprod Health. 2019;13:117. https://doi.org/10.1177/1179558119872490.

Ovarian Tissue Cryopreservation

62

Pankaj Talwar and Pooja Awasthi

The improvements in the early diagnosis and significant advancements in the surgical procedures, radiotherapy, and chemotherapy have drastically improved the survival rate of not only cancer patients but also of numerous other diseases (autoimmune disease, ovarian diseases, bone marrow transplantation, adjunctive oophorectomy). Advancement also has immensely enhanced the rate of cure in case of both children and young adults. According to a study published in united states (January 2016), the number of cancer survives are on increasing side, and the rate of increase is estimated by 31% (15.5 million in 2016 to 20.3 million in 2026). Common cancer sites of our generation include breast cancer (female, 3.6 million), approximately 3.3 million prostate cancer, 1.3 million gynaecological, 1.5 million colorectal, and melanoma 1.2 million [1–3]. Von Wolff M et al. (2015) documented more than 1000 patients in Europe, who had undergone OTC [4]. As per ESHRE working group on oocytes in 2017, 12 of 17 EU countries had performed OTC, during 2010–2015, and 7 countries were reported for carrying out OTT. On 5529 patients, OTC was performed, and 237 were undergone for OTT. Among all the countries, Germany scored the highest number of OTC/ OTT patients (1895/85), France scored second place with 1373 OTC patients, and Belgium with 727 OTC patients [5] was at third place.

The increased survival rate post-cancer treatment especially in young women impacts the ovarian reserve leading to POF and POI [6]. However, to deal with iatrogenic infertility, various fertility preservation techniques like oophoropexy, ART, oocyte freezing, follicle culture, and in vitro maturation are available to the reproductive biologists. Cryopreservation of the ovarian cortex is a technique which facilitates the preservation of gonadal function in cancer patients of reproductive ages. Associated risks of cancer therapy including radiotherapy and chemotherapy have detrimental effects on the reproductive health. The first live birth was reported by Donnez [7] after ovarian tissue cryopreservation and transplantation. According to the resent data, the rate of live birth rate has been achieved around 30% by transplantation of frozen-thawed ovarian tissue, and nearly 100 live birth have been reported worldwide [8].

62.1 Ovarian Reserve

Ovarian reserve which at foetal mid-gestational period is around 6–8 million, reduces to 1–2 million at birth, and further falls to 300,000 by the onset of puberty and further drops to 25,000 by the age of 37–38 years and are left with only 1000 or less by the stage of menopause. Figure 62.1 represents the number of follicles at different stages of life.

62.2 Historical Background

Hovatta et al. did the initial work in ovarian tissue cryopreservation on humans. He validated that human ovary is cryo-resistant to frozen-thaw protocol because the primordial follicles present in the cortex are immature, dormant, less differentiated, and without zona. Lack of zona and cortical granule makes these immature oocytes tolerant to cryoprotectant [9–11]. Figure 62.2 shows a timeline that contains the name of the scientists with their scientific studies.

62.3 Indication for Ovarian Tissue Cryopreservation

Ovarian tissue cryopreservation is an option for patients who require immediate gonadotoxic treatment for aggressive malignancies when there is insufficient time to allow the woman to undergo ovulation induction, oocyte retrieval, and cryopreservation of oocytes or embryos. The only option

P. Talwar
ART Centre, Army Hospital (Research and Referral), Delhi, India

P. Awasthi (✉)
Origin IVF & Fertility Centre, Ghaziabad, Uttar Pradesh, India

G. N. Allahbadia et al. (eds.), *Textbook of Assisted Reproduction*, https://doi.org/10.1007/978-981-15-2377-9_62

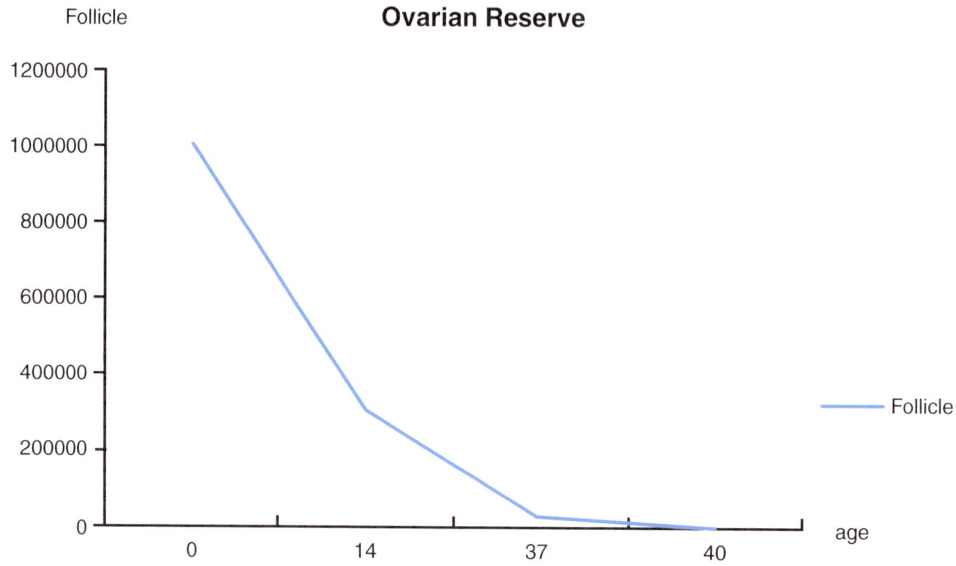

Fig. 62.1 The number of follicles at different stages of life

available for fertility preservation in prepubertal girls [12–17] or in women who have hormone-sensitive malignancies [18] is ovarian tissue cryopreservation. The decrease in both antral follicle count (AFC) and ovarian volume with chemotherapy have been documented by Andersen et al. Rapid fall in AMH and inhibin B were also reported by them during chemotherapy although E_2 levels remain same [19]. Figure 62.3 summarizes the indications for ovarian tissue cryopreservation.

62.4 Recommended Guidelines for Ovarian Tissue Banking [20, 21]

1. Patient's age (<37)
2. Status of the ovarian reserve and function (AMH level, AFC, premenopausal by FSH)
3. A detailed discussion between oncologist and patient about cancer treatment plan and prognosis
4. Informed consent from the adult patients should be taken
5. Ovarian transposition: Ovarian transposition (oophoropexy) can be offered when pelvic radiation is performed as the cancer treatment
6. Oocyte cryopreservation should be performed when embryo cryopreservation is not possible
7. The experimental nature and potential risks of cancer cell transmission should be explained to the patient
8. Through patient counselling
9. The desire to have children in future (before 50)
10. High risk of POF
11. Prepubertal girls, who do not have any other option
12. When embryo and oocyte freezing is not indicated. (Sensitive to hormonal stimulation and ATR is not allowed)

62.5 Ovarian Damage Due to Cancer Treatment

At any age, ovarian follicles are vulnerable to agents that lead to DNA damage, including ionizing radiation and chemotherapy. Such anticancer treatments affect the ovarian follicle reserve in a dose-dependent manner and can eventually cause amenorrhea and premature ovarian failure [22].

62.5.1 Radiotherapy and Ovarian Damage

Cancer patients, who are scheduled to undergo abdominal, pelvic, and total body irradiation, are at risk for infertility, reduced gonadal age, and premature ovarian failure due to the loss of primordial follicles. Elderly women are at higher risk of ovarian failure as the degree of ovarian damage is determined by the total irradiation dose, location, fractionation schedule, and age at the time of treatment. Radiosensitivity of the human ovary that leads to the loss of 50% of primordial follicles (LD50) is estimated to be 2 Gy [23] (Table 62.1).

62.5.2 Chemotherapy and Ovarian Damage

Most of the drugs used in chemotherapy work in a more or less similar fashion, that is, creating DNA cross-links, which in turn cause DNA breaks, eventually triggering apoptosis. Only the taxanes are microtubule-stabilizing agents and different from DNA-damaging drugs [25–27].

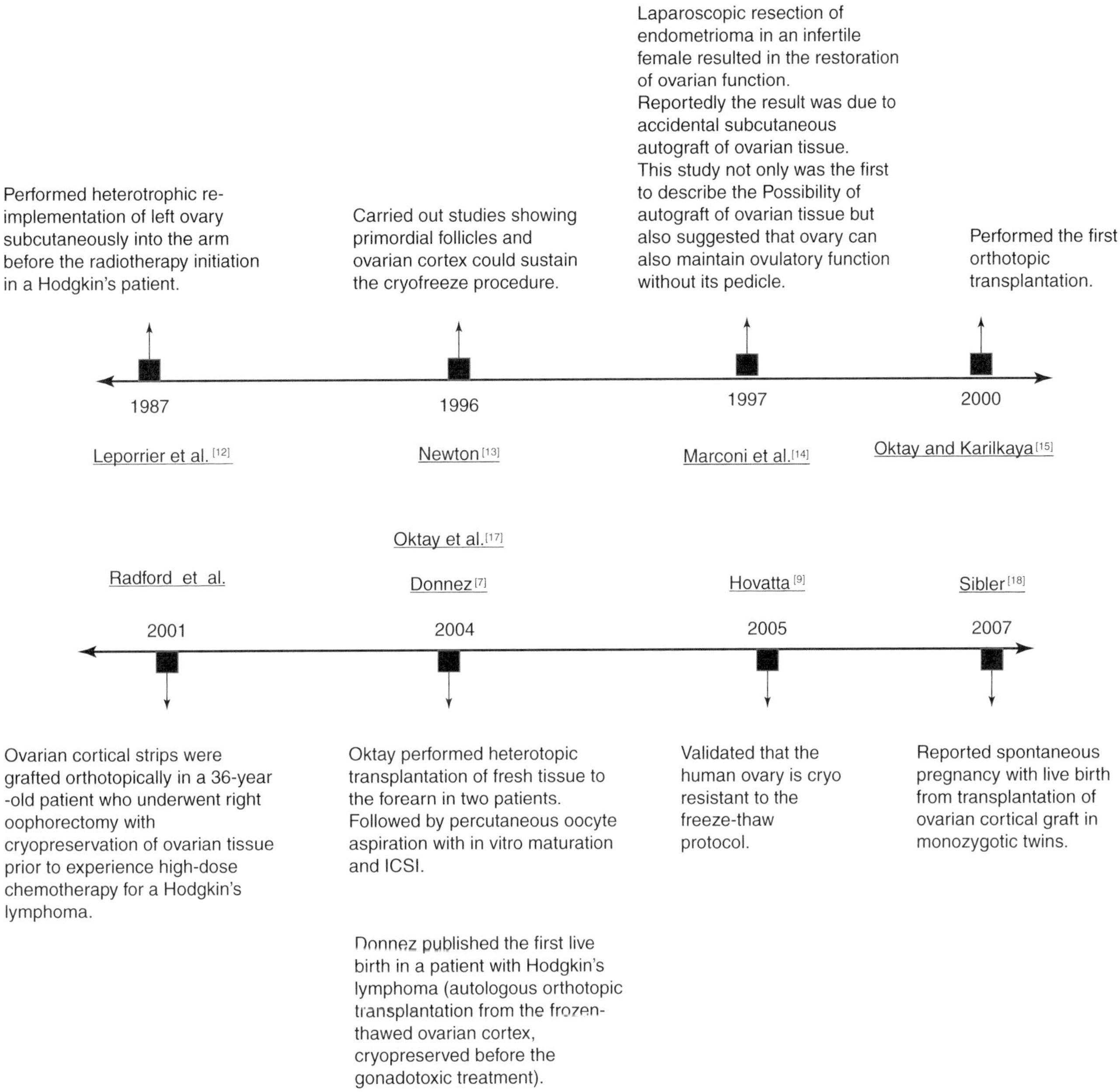

Fig. 62.2 Timeline of ovarian tissue freezing scientists with their scientific studies

Table 62.2 summarizes the drugs, their mode of action, and how they affect the oocyte quality. Figure 62.4 summarizes the level of toxicity of different chemotherapy drugs.

62.6 Various Fertility Methods in Females with Cancer

Various fertility methods are in practice for patients with cancer, depending upon the type and severity of malignancy. Table 62.3 summarizes the various fertility preservation methods in females with cancer.

62.7 Techniques of Ovarian Tissue Cryopreservation

Follicular viability and integrity of tissue compartments and cell-to-cell contacts must be indemnified by the cryopreservation techniques [9, 30]. Thus, studies investigating the most favourable cooling rates and dehydration times have been conducted. It is now well established that for obtaining satisfactory results, adequate penetration of cryoprotectant through the stroma and granulosa cells to the oocytes is required [9]. Choosing optimal freezing must minimize ice crystal formation.

Fig. 62.3 Indications for ovarian tissue cryopreservation

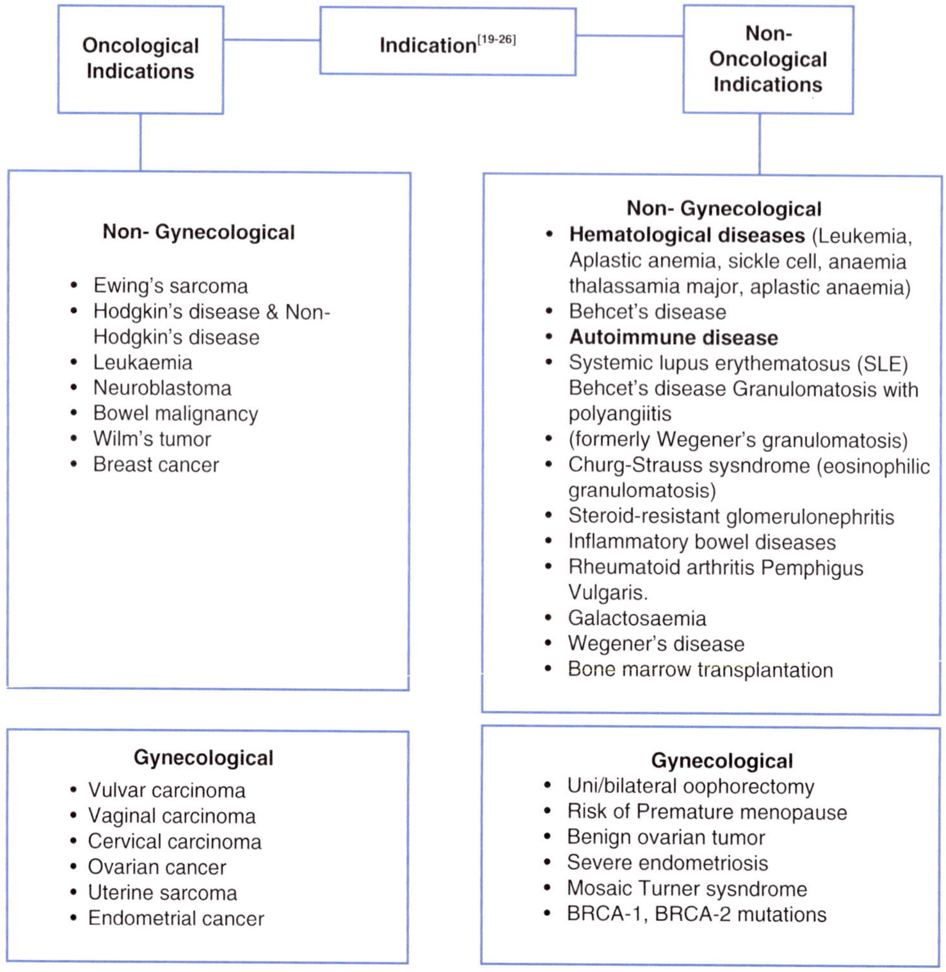

Table 62.1 Age-related effective sterilizing dose (ESD) [23, 24]

Age	Effective sterilizing dose
At birth	20.3 Gy
At 10 years	18.4 Gy
At 20 years	16.5 Gy
At 30 years	14.3 Gy

Table 62.2 Summarizes the level of toxicity of different chemotherapy drugs

Name of drug	Mode of action	How it affects oocyte quality
Cyclophosphamide	Damages the DNA (cross-linking of DNA, acts on the adjacent N-7 position of guanine)	Causes DNA strand breaks, leading to abnormal base pairing. Inhibits the cell division and consequently leads to apoptosis. Cyclophosphamide exposure in paediatric systemic lupus erythematous is associated with reduced serum AMH [28]
Busulphane	Damages the DNA	Increases the number of mature atrophied follicles and causes cell shrinkage, chromosomal and cytoplasm fragmentation fallowed by apoptosis [29]
Anthracycline	Damages the DNA	Blocks DNA replication and leads to double-stranded (ds) DNA breaks; it also induces apoptosis in the stroma and the granulosa cells of growing follicles subsequently
Taxanes	Acts on beta-tubulin, anti-mitotic agent	Disruption of microtubule functions, thereby inhibiting the process of cell division
Cytarabine	Chromosomal damage	Damages the DNA and consequently leads to apoptosis
Platinum complexes	Damages the DNA (crosslinking of DNA, acts on the adjacent N-7 position of guanine)	Causes DNA strand breaks, leading to abnormal base pairing. Inhibits the cell division and consequently leads to apoptosis

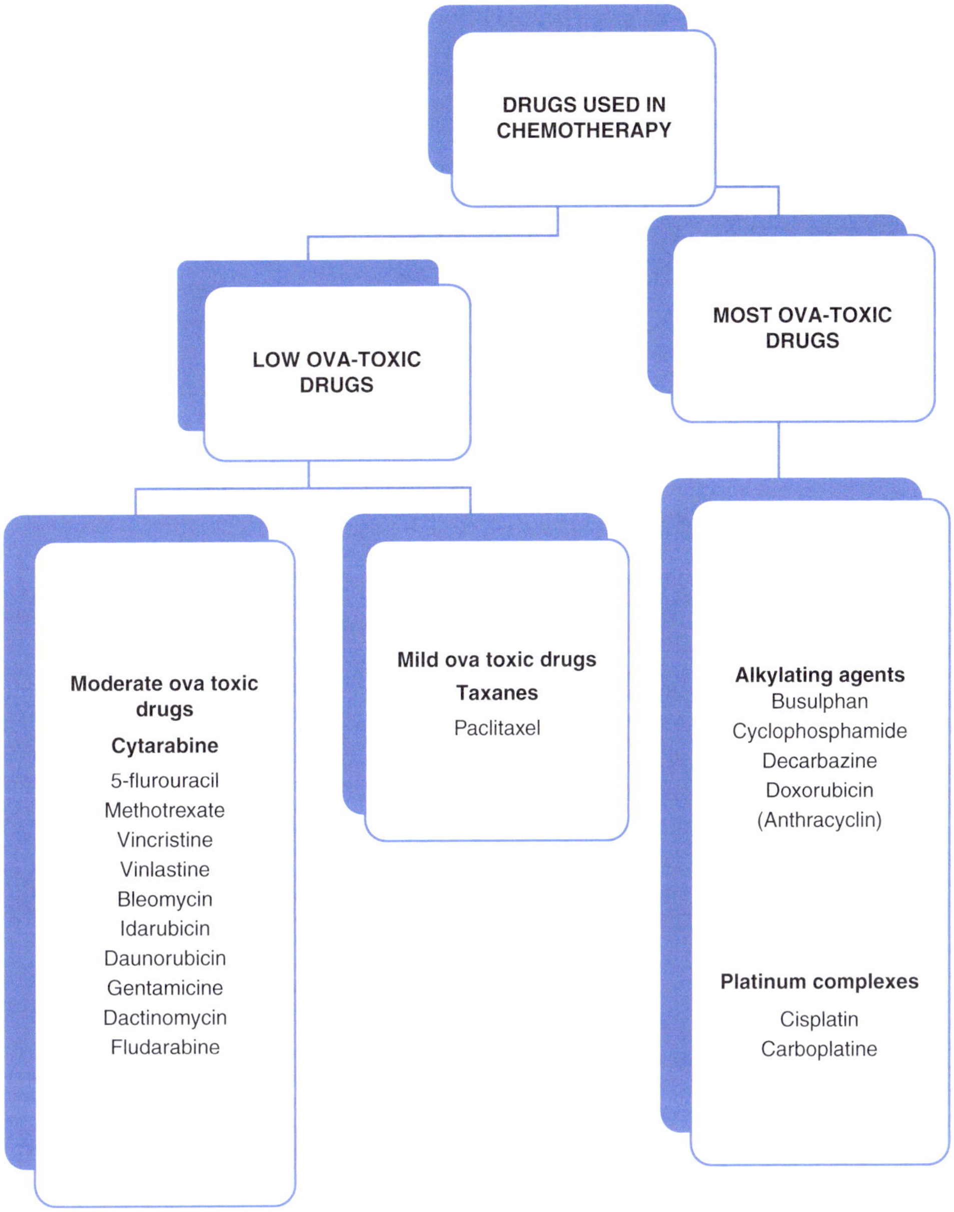

Fig. 62.4 Summary of the levels of toxicity of different chemotherapy drugs

Table 62.3 Fertility preservation techniques in females with cancer

Fertility preservation techniques	Requirement of ovarian stimulation	Does the procedure delay the definitive cancer therapy	Requirement of the male partner	Success rates	Special considerations
Use of long activity of GnRH agonist	Does not require	Does not delay	Not required	Not documented	Controversial
Oocyte cryopreservation	Required	Yes, it delays	Not required	Pregnancy rate per cycle of 50.2% or per embryo transfer 55.4%	Nil
Embryo freezing	Required	Yes, it delays (advent)	Yes	Cumulative pregnancy rate of 66% among women with cancer	Nil
In vitro maturation	Does not require	Does not delay	Not required	Not documented	Nil
Ovarian cortex cryopreservation	Does not require	Does not delay	Not required	Pregnancy rate of 25% among women with cancer	No indication when high risk of ovarian metastases

Adapted from Muñoz M, Santaballa A, Seguí M A, et al. SEOM Clinical Guideline of fertility preservation and reproduction in cancer patients. Clin Transl Oncol. 2016; 18(12): 1229–1236, with permission

62.7.1 Collection of Ovarian Tissue [31]

1.	Early follicular phase is the best time for the tissue collection to avoid large ovarian follicles/cyst or corpus luteum. Being hyper vascular and space occupying, these causes anatomic distortion.
2.	The tissues should be transported to the laboratory on ice, in a 4-(2-hydroxyethyl)-1- piperazineethane-sulfonic acid (HEPES)-buffered medium.
3.	Ovarian tissue is collected by laparoscopy under general anaesthesia since it has better and early recovery.
4.	Electrocoagulation of the ovary should be avoided as it can lead to thermal damage to primordial follicles in the ovarian cortex.

62.7.2 Cryoprotectant Preparation

Dimethylsulphoxide (DMSO), propanediol, and ethylene glycol-based solutions are all equally effective for human ovarian tissue freezing.

We do not add protein supplement due to its antigenicity.

62.7.3 Preparation of Required Cryoprotectants [31]

- **Step 1.** To DMSO 1.06 ml, sucrose 0. 1 M solution 1 ml and patients serum 1 ml add 6.94 ml of bicarbonate media to a final volume of 10 ml.
- **Step 2.** This is then filter-sterilized through a 0.22 um filter and cocktail is refrigerated.
- **Step 3.** Pour 4 ml of cryoprotective solution in 60 mm dish, and place it on the ice at least 30 min so that the solution is ice-cooled before the specimen is put in it for equilibration.
- **Step 4.** Put 1 ml of the solution in cryovial and ice cool it.

62.7.4 Thickness of Cortical Slices

Thin slices of 1 mm, thick with the surface area from 2 × 2 mm to 5 × 5 mm, the tissue is preferred to facilitate equilibration of the cryoprotectant [32–35].

62.7.5 Histological Analysis

Randomly chosen one representative sample of the ovarian cortex, for every patient, should be sent for histopathological examination. The specimens should be fixed in formaldehyde and embedded in paraffin.

Five µm sections are cut perpendicularly to the ovarian surface and stained with haematoxylin-eosin. All follicles are systematically counted. Serial sections are useful for follicle classification.

62.8 Freezing Protocols

Freezing of ovarian tissue can be carried out either by slow freezing or by vitrification (Fig. 62.5).

62.8.1 Slow Freezing vs Vitrification

Documented studies of slow-programmed freezing show comparatively poor survival of the ovarian stroma. The study has been validated by transmission-electron microscopy [35], a technique that precisely evaluates cryoinjury of membranes, mitochondria, and other organelles.

Vitrification is a reliable cryopreservation method in which the tissue is first exposed to high concentrations of permeating cryoprotectants for a short interval and then plunged directly into liquid nitrogen. This induces a glass-like state in the cells and evades the formation of destructive ice crystals [36]. OTC through vitrification has been demonstrated to improve the viability of all tissue compartments. However, survival rate of follicles remains similar to that after slow freezing, the integrity of ovarian stroma, and blood vessels were largely improved. All the factors are summarized in Table 62.4.

62.8.2 Slow Freezing

Slow freezing involves the addition of cryoprotectants and programmed cooling (vapour phase to -196 °C) (Figs. 62.6, 62.7, 62.8, 62.9, 62.10, and 62.11).

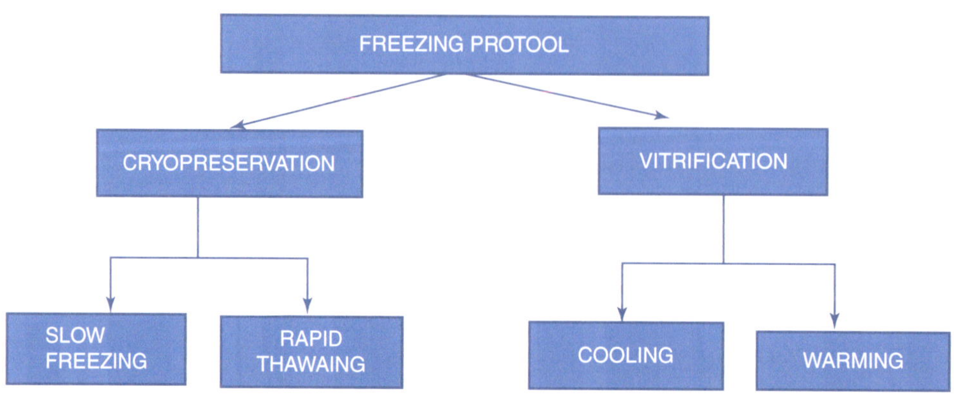

Fig. 62.5 Freezing protocols

Table 62.4 Vitrification vs slow freezing

Factors	Vitrification	Slow freezing
Equipment	Inexpensive	Expensive
CPA concentration	High	Low
Ice crystallization	No	Yes
Cooling rate	High	Low
Chemical damage	More	Less
Mechanical damage	Less or none	More
Time consumed	Less	More
Survival	Better	Poor

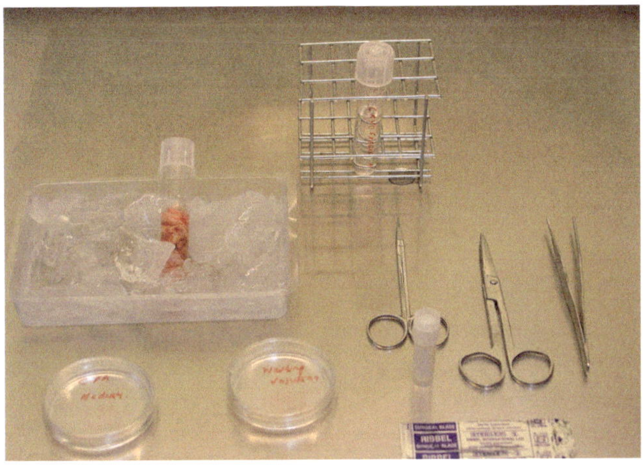

Fig. 62.6 Preparation for the slow freezing (all the instruments required, ovaries and freezing cocktail). Ovary has been kept on ice and freezing media consisting of DMSO, and sucrose has been kept at room temperature

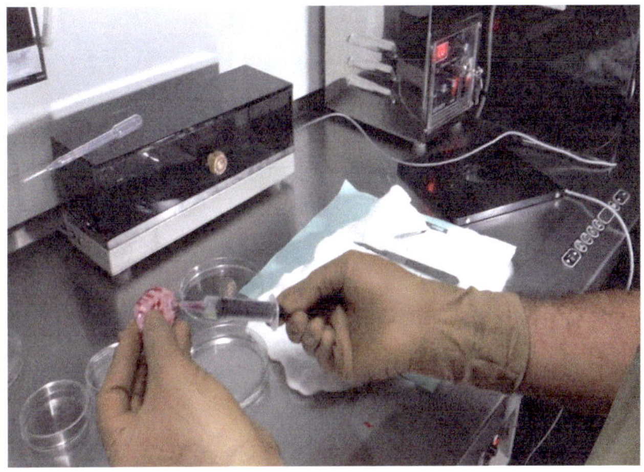

Fig. 62.7 The antral follicles on the ovaries are aspirated, and if any immature oocytes are recovered, they are cultured for in vitro maturation. This is a common step in both the techniques

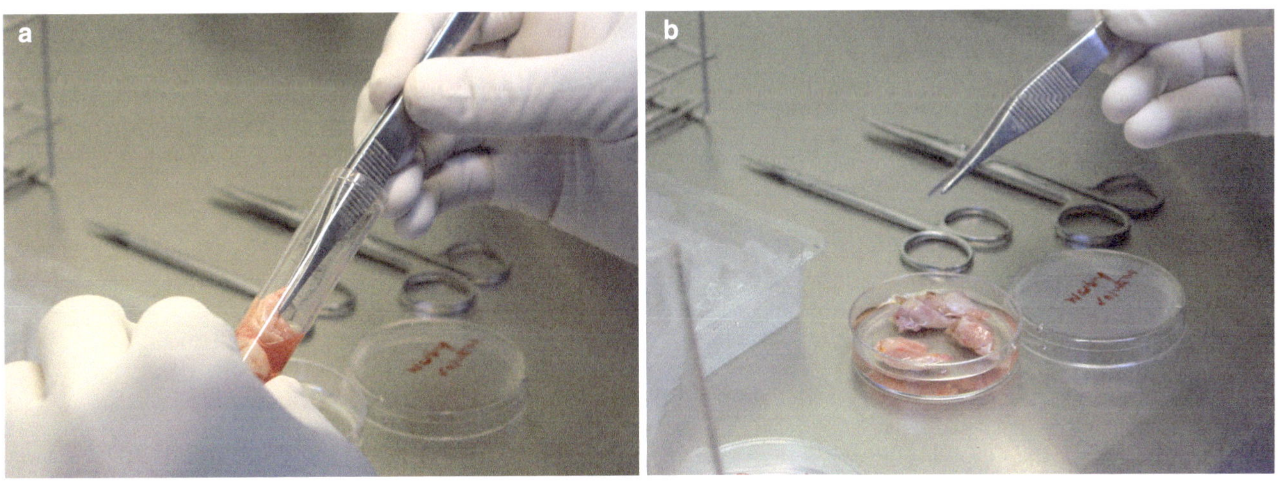

Fig. 62.8 (**a** and **b**) Ovary specimen has been shifted to the 60 mm Falcon IVF plate containing HEPES buffered media at 4*C. Ovary has been bisected in two halves for easy handling

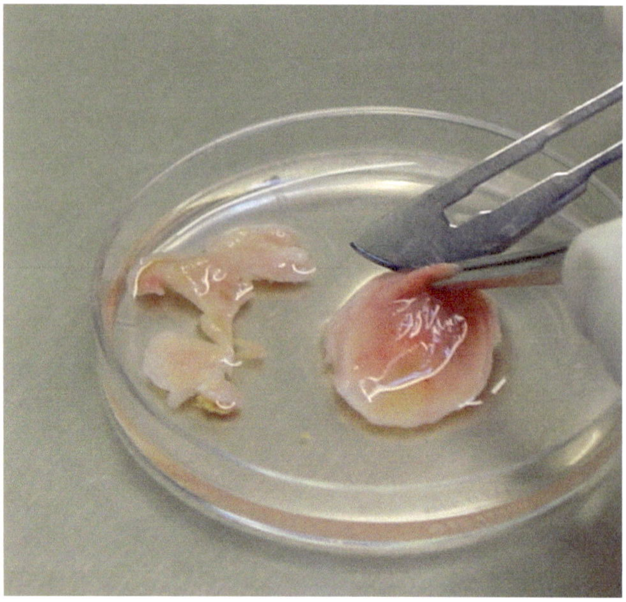

Fig. 62.9 Ovarian tissue is held carefully using a coarse dissecting forceps, and medulla is gradually shaved off from the cortex. Ensure that the medulla is completely removed leaving behind white tunica albuginea

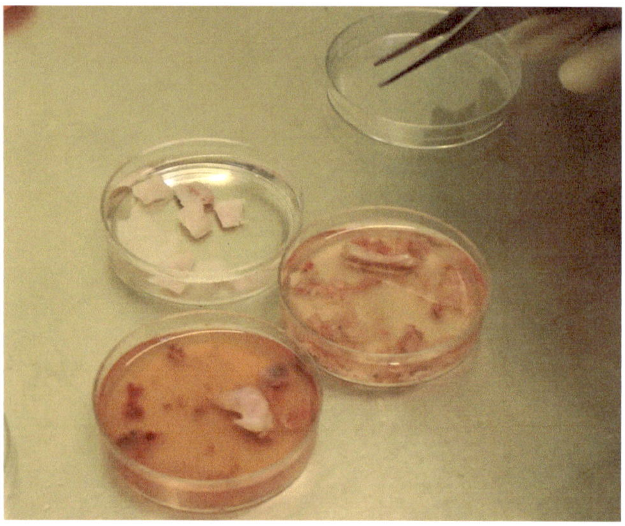

Fig. 62.10 The carved ovarian cortex bits are moved through different plates having washing media to clean all the debris and blood

62.8.3 Slow Freezing (Equilibration Procedure) [37, 38]

Tissue slices of 1 mm thickness should be placed in the ice-cold cryoprotectant solution.

Place the slices in 60 mm falcon dish filled with cold cryoprotectant solution.

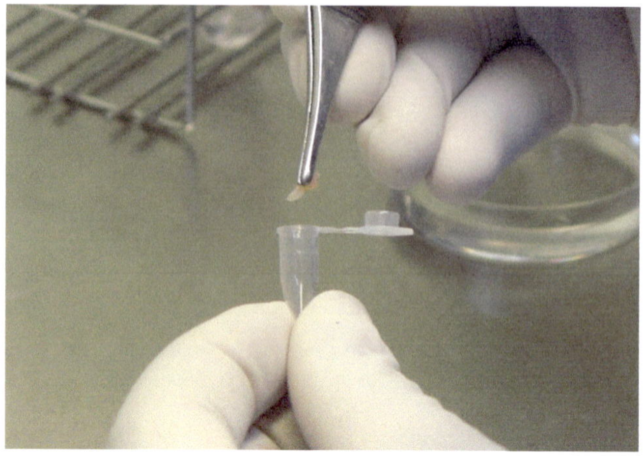

Fig. 62.11 After washing them thoroughly, these are loaded in a cryovials containing the freezing media and kept at 4*C for 30–40 min for soakage. Use a shaker if available. Always send a small specimen of cortex and medulla each, for PCR and histopathological studies

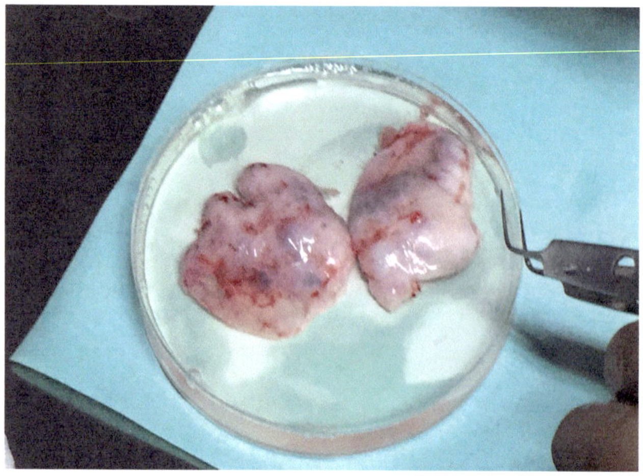

Fig. 62.12 The ovary is bisected in two halves for easy handling

62.8.4 Rapid Thawing

1. The cryovials are removed from the liquid nitrogen. Thaw the vials at room temperature for 30 s.
2. The cryovials are removed from the liquid nitrogen. Thaw the vials at room temperature for 30 s.
3. Wash tissue in progressively lower concentrations of sucrose.
4. Perform the last wash in 10% autologous serum.
5. Cortex is ready for transplantation.

62.8.5 Vitrification

Vitrification enables the instant freezing of the cells by using the cryoprotectants and turns them into amorphous solid or glass-like structure without ice crystal formation (Figs. 62.12, 62.13, 62.14, and 62.15).

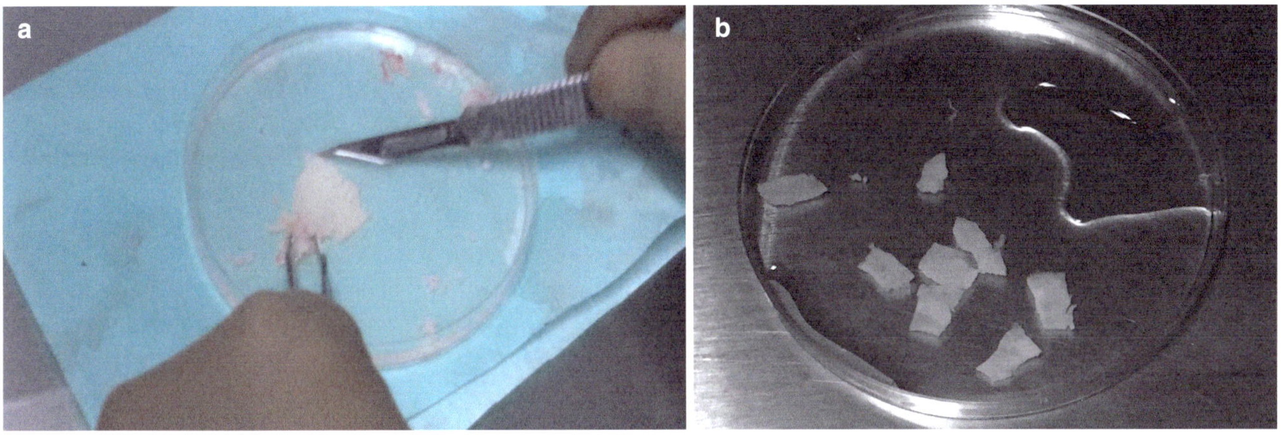

Fig. 62.13 (**a** and **b**) Using fine instruments, remove the complete medulla and at the end properly carved cortex should be thin and transparent. Preparation for vitrification is more challenging

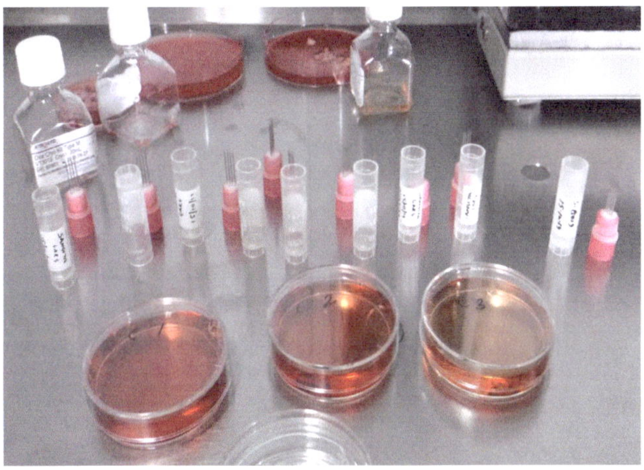

Fig. 62.14 Move the cortical bits through the Kitazato ovarian cortex Vitrification media. Equilibrate the cortex in the media for 5 min each at room temperature

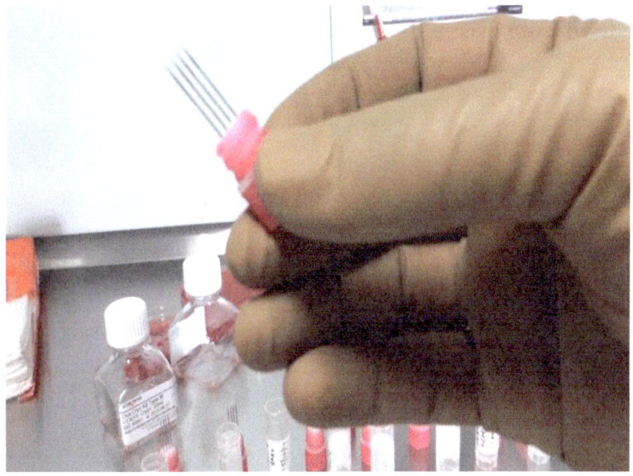

Fig. 62.15 Prepare the Cryo M devices for loading the cortex bits. Do proper labelling of the vials as these are to be cryopreserved for long duration of time

62.9 Cooling

1. Ultra-thin slices of the tissue are required for the cryopreservation, as well as rapid revascularization after grafting.
2. Bring ES and VS to room temperature (25 ~ 27 °C). Pour the full contents of ES vial (15 ml) into a 60 mm dish.
3. Place the extracted tissue on the dish and wait for 25 min.
4. Pour the full contents of VS vial (15 ml) into a 60 mm dish. Transfer the tissue in ES to the surface of VS using tweezers.
5. Wait for 15 min.
6. After the equilibration to VS, place the tissue on the Cryo M device. Plunge the Cryo M device into fresh liquid nitrogen quickly.
7. Check whether the tissue is translucent. Insert the Cryo M device into the cap and twist it. Make sure if it is completely sealed.
8. The cortical bits equilibrate in the media for 5 min each and then loaded on the Cryo M device and then immersed in liquid nitrogen and store.

This procedure is adapted from Kitazato ovarian cortex vitrification manual [39].

62.9.1 Warming (Vitrification)

1. Take out the tissue from liquid nitrogen;quickly immerse it into Thawing Solution warmed to 37 °C) within 1 s.

2. Leave the tissue in Thawing Solutions for 1 min after immersing.
3. Pour the Dilution solution (DS) (15 ml) into a 60 mm dish. Pour the Thawing Solution (TS) with the tissue into a 90 mm dish.
4. Transfer the tissue in TS to DS using tweezers. Wait for 3 min.
5. Pour the washing solution (WS_1) (15 ml) and WS_2 (15 ml) into 60 mm dishes. Do this preparation while waiting for dilution is done.
6. Transfer the tissue from DS to WS_1. Wait for 5 min.
7. Transfer the tissue in WS_1 to WS_2. Wait for 5 min.
8. After 5 min in WS_2, immediately transplant or culture the tissues.

This procedure is adapted from Kitazato ovarian cortex vitrification manual. Refer to Related Picture for Vitrification in Appendix 1 of Kitazato website [39].

62.10 Transplantation

The objective of ovarian tissue cryopreservation is to re-implant a couple of thawed cortical strips into the patient (i.e., auto-transplantation) once the patient is disease-free and desires pregnancy (Fig. 62.16). [40] Re-implantation of cryopreserved ovarian tissue in the pelvic cavity is routinely done by laparoscopy. Fortuitous, if at least one ovary is present [10].

Each site has distinct advantages and disadvantages. However both heterotopic and orthotopic sites were studied for the transplantation of cryopreserved ovarian tissue despite the remaining menopausal ovary having been cited as the most popular site (in orthotopic studies) [10, 34].

Primarily two techniques are performed in case of orthotopic re-implantation of cortical stripes: (1) either slices of frozen-thawed ovarian tissue are fixed on the decorticated medulla(in the presence of remaining ovary) [41] (2) or pushed by a small incision under the cortical capsule. In the absence of ovary, the cortical slices could be placed in a peritoneal window [7, 42–44]. The advantages of ovarian tissue re-implantation at orthotopic sites are (a) natural conception and (b) the favourable condition for follicular development (O2, pressure, and the presence of peritoneal fluid).

Ovarian function and spontaneous pregnancy in a female, earlier treated for bone marrow transplantation, were reported in 2006 by Demeestere I et al., after the transplantation of ovarian tissue at combined heterotopic and orthotopic sites [34].

A female, menopausal for 2.5 years, resulted in spontaneous pregnancy followed by birth of a healthy baby post-ovarian tissue transplantation 3 months of autologous heterotopic transplantation of ovarian tissue to a supra pubic site [45]. Demonstrated studies showed that the OTC is a feasible and safe option for paediatric patients too.

In adults, 4–5 ovarian cortical biopsies (1*0.5 *1.5 mm thick) are usually taken. However, left oophorectomy should be performed because of the small size of the ovaries.

A paper published very recently by Gellert SE et al. documented 360 ovarian tissue transplantations (OTT) in 318 women. 95% women resumed the normal ovarian endocrine function. 50% of the newborn were from natural conception and healthy (except one with chromosomal anomaly derived from family disposition). In nine women, recurrence of malignancy was seen post-OTT, but not because of transplantation [46].

62.11 Outcomes of Ovarian Tissue Grafting

Donnez in 2015 presented a study on the rate of live births of OTC re-implantation of 111 women. According to the survey, 29% LBH (n = 32) women conceived. Two women delivered 3 babies each and listed 33 (+4) live birth and

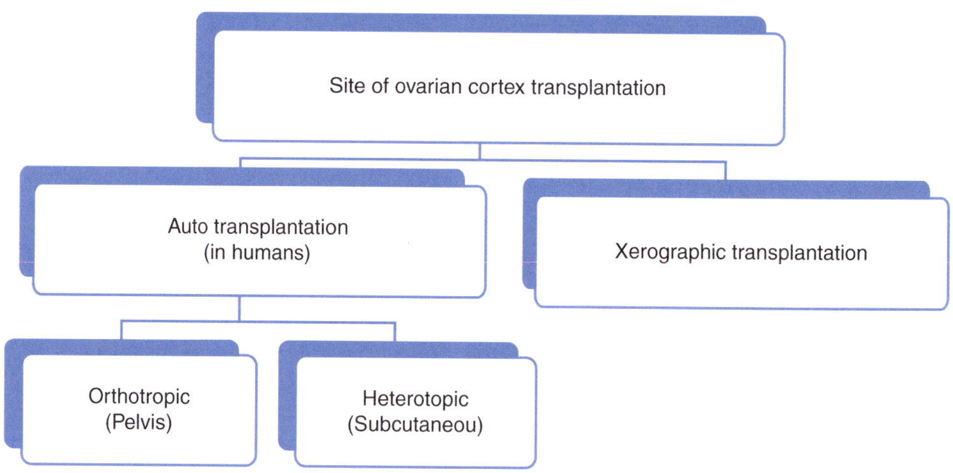

Fig. 62.16 The objective of ovarian tissue cryopreservation is to re-implant a couple of thawed cortical strips into the patient

Table 62.5 Outcomes of ovarian tissue grafting

Scientist name	Year	Study
Restoration of ovarian activity		
Oktay and Karlikaya [47]	2000	Documented orthotopic transplantation of ovarian tissue resulted in follicular development in response to menopausal gonadotropin stimulation
Oktay et al. [45]	2004	Reported heterotopic transplantation of the ovarian cortex to the forearm, after stimulation with gonadotropins, yields three oocytes
Dunlop CE et al. [48]	2016	Reported the successful natural conception and birth of a healthy male infant after orthotropic re-implantation of ovarian cortex, which was cryopreserved 10 years before, the treatment of a high dose chemotherapy. Patient was a 32-year-old woman and underwent for haematopoietic stem cell transplantation for Wilm's tumour. She ovulated 15 and 29 weeks post-laparoscopic orthotopic transplantation with AMH detectable
Live birth		
Roux C et al. [49]	2010	Reported the live birth in a sickle cell anaemia patient after autografting of ovarian tissue. The reported study opens up the new perspective in case of non-malignant diseases
Muller A [50]	2012	Reported first live birth from re-transplantation of frozen-thawed ovarian tissue in Germany
Revelli et al. [51]	2013	Reported the spontaneous conception and live birth in Italy, post-orthotopic grafting of the frozen-thawed autologous ovarian issue
Stern C.J and Gook D [52]	2013	Reported first pregnancy through heterotopic grafting of frozen-thawed cortical strips in a female post-bilateral oophorectomy.
Prasath et al. [53]	2014	Reported first pregnancy and live birth from cryopreserved embryos through IVM after oophorectomy in an ovarian cancer patient
Suzuki N et al. [54]	2015	Reported two live births in Japan after vitrification of cortical stripes followed by in vitro activation. The vitrified-warmed cortical strips transplanted beneath the serosa of fallopian tube in a patient with the history of POI for more than 1 year
Jensen et al. [55]	2017	Reported approximately 86 live birth and nine ongoing pregnancies worldwide in women transplanted with frozen-thawed ovarian tissue
Animal studies		
Godsen et al. [55]	1994	Reported the live birth of lambs post autographic frozen-thawed ovarian tissue in sheep
Salle B et al [56]	2002	Documented (two twin and two singleton) pregnancies after transplantation (autografting) of frozen-thawed hemi-ovary into the hilum of previously removed ovary before grafting. (Only three out of six lambs survived)
L Lillu et al. [57]	2008	Reported the possibility of fertility restoration after orthotopic grafting of frozen-thawed ovarian tissue in mice

ongoing pregnancies, proving the efficacy of technique and restoration of gonadal functions to reproduce naturally in future [40]. Table 62.5 summarizes the outcomes of tissue grafting in both humans and animals.

62.12 Future of Ovarian Cortex Preservation

The successful live births after transplant from both orthotopic and heterotopic sites along with newer techniques of culturing the primordial follicles, in vitro maturation, and the chances of in vitro activation (IVA) suggest more fertility alternatives for the number of girls and women. Several pregnancies and few live births have also documented through vitrification of ovarian tissue as it is an efficient and more economical technique with minimal tissue damage. Additionally, various methods of transplantation have demonstrated important advancements in fertility preservation like transplantation through the artificial ovary with an extracellular tissue matrix (ECTM) scaffolding, besides the consequences of sphingosine-1-phosphate (SIP) and a vascular endothelial growth factor (VEGF) and fibrin modified with heparin-binding peptide (HBP), heparin [58].

Primordial follicles are noticeably less vulnerable to the injury caused by cryoprotectants compared to oocytes due to (a) size, (b) slow metabolic rates, and c) lack of the zona.

Recent practices for cryopreservation of ovarian tissues are:

1. Ovarian cortical strips cryopreservation
2. Whole ovary cryopreservation
3. IVM
4. Follicle culture

62.12.1 Whole Ovary Cryopreservation

Recently, whole ovary cryopreservation using multi-gradient freezing device has been reported [59–63].

Although the outcomes are inspiring, confirmed refurbishment of fertility by whole ovary transplantation in human is yet to be reported. However, the risk of reintroduction of malignancy is also associated with this technique.

62.12.2 In Vitro Maturation (IVM)

In vitro maturation is the method which allows the maturation of ovarian follicles "in-vitro." The combination of OTC and IVM, along with vitrification of oocytes, can be a promising technique to preserve the fertility in females with cancer. Abir R, Grynberg M, et al., and Prasath reported successful live births through IVM [53, 64–66].

62.12.3 Follicular Culture

Apart from ovarian tissue cryopreservation, follicle culture can also be considered as the promising method in preserving fertility [67].

- Especially for young patients without partners
- Patients with the risk of ovarian hyper stimulation for embryo/oocyte cryopreservation
- Patients, with an associated risk of reintroduction of cancerous cells, preclude transplantation

62.13 Conclusion

In case of malignancy, ovarian tissue freezing can be the most appropriate fertility preservation method as cryopreserving the cortex containing primordial follicles offers a more beneficial option than oocyte and embryo freezing. Thus, delay in cancer treatment can be avoided. Although for young women, cryopreservation of oocyte and embryo are the promising FP methods, they have their limitations. Cryopreservation of ovarian tissue (OTC) is a COS (controlled ovarian stimulation) independent method and has a larger application providing an extended fertility window, and patients can immediately undergo for cancer treatment. Currently, for paediatric patients and patients with hormone-dependent diseases, it is the only fertility preservation option [68].

References

1. Miller KD, Siegel RL, Lin CC, Marito AB, et al. Cancer treatment and survival statistics. CA Cancer J Clin. 2016;66:271–89.
2. Siegel RL, Miller KD, Jemal A. Cancer statistics. CA Cancer J Clin. 2017 Jan;67(1):7–30.
3. American Cancer Society. Cancer treatment & survivorship facts & figures 2016–2017. Atlanta: American Cancer Society; 2016.
4. Von Wolff M, Dittrich R, Liebenthron J, Nawroth F, Schüring AN, Bruckner T, et al. Fertility-preservation counselling and treatment for medical reasons: data from a multinational network of over 5000 women. Reprod BioMed Online. 2015;31:605–12.
5. Shenfield F, Mouzon JD, Scaravelli G, Kupka M, Ferratti AP, The ESHRE Working Group on Oocyte Cryopreservation in Europe, et al. Oocyte and ovarian tissue cryopreservation in European countries: statutory background, practice, storage and use. Hum Reprod Open. 2017;1:1–9.
6. Meirow D, Nugent D. The effects of radiotherapy and chemotherapy on female reproduction. Hum Reprod Update. 2001;7:535–43.
7. Donnez J, Dolmans MM, Demylle D, et al. Live birth after orthotopic transplantation of cryopreserved ovarian tissue. Lancet. 2004;364:1405–10.
8. Suzuki N. Ovarian tissue cryopreservation and transplantation using thawed ovarian cortex for fertility preservation. Onco Fertil J. 2018;1(1):3–8.
9. Hovatta O. Methods of cryopreservation of human ovarian tissue. Reprod BioMed Online. 2005;10(6):10729–34.
10. Kim SS, Battaglia DE, Soules MR. The future of human ovarian cryopreservation and transplantation: fertility and beyond. Fertil Steril. 2001;75(6):1049–56.
11. Kim SS. Fertility preservation in female cancer patients: current developments and future directions. Fertil Steril. 2006;85(1):1–11.
12. Donnez J, Bassil S. Indications for cryopreservation of ovarian tissue. Hum Reprod Update. 1998;4:248–59.
13. Meirow D, Ben Yehuda D, Prus D, Poliak A, Schenker JG, et al. Ovarian tissue banking in patients with Hodgkin's disease: is it safe? Fertil Steril. 1998;69:996–8.
14. Oktay K, Newton H, Aubard Y, Salha O, Gosden RG. Cryopreservation of immature human oocytes and ovarian tissue: an emerging technology? Fertil Steril. 1998;69:1–7.
15. Donnez J, Dolmans MM, Martinez-Madrid B, Demylle D, van Langendonckt A. The role of cryopreservation for women prior to treatment of malignancy. Curr Opin Obstet Gynecol. 2005;17:333–8.
16. Ott J, Nouri K, Stogbauer L, Fischer EM, Lipovac M, Promberger R, et al. Ovarian tissue cryopreservation for nonmalignant indications. Arch Gynecol Obstet. 2010;281:735–9.
17. Talwar P. Fertility preservation in female cancer patients. ISRN Obstet Gynecol. 2009;1(3):5–11.
18. Albani E, Bracone G, Biccari SD, Vitobello D, Fattizzi N, Levi-Setti PE. Human ovarian tissue cryopreservation as fertility reserve. In: Mohan R, editor. Topics in cancer survivorship. Rijeka: InTech; 2012. p. 215.
19. Andersen RA, Themmen APN, Al-Qahtani A, Groome NP, Cameron DA. The effects of chemotherapy and long-term gonadotrophin suppression on the ovarian reserve in premenopausal women with breast cancer. Hum Reprod. 2006;21(10):2583–92.
20. Kim SS. Recommendations for fertility preservation in patients with lymphoma, leukaemia, and breast cancer. J Assist Reprod Genet. 2012;29:465–8.
21. Muñoz M, Santaballa A, Seguí MA, et al. SEOM clinical guideline of fertility preservation and reproduction in cancer patients. Clin Transl Oncol. 2016;18(12):1229–36.
22. Meirow D. Reproduction post-chemotherapy in young cancer patients. Mol Cell Endocrinol. 2000;169:123–31.
23. Wallace WH, Thomson AB, Saran F, Kelsey TW. Predicting age of ovarian failure after radiation to a field that includes the ovaries. Int J Radiat Oncol Biol Phys. 2005;62:738–44.
24. Meirow D, Biederman H, Anderson RA, Wallace W. Toxicity of chemotherapy and radiation on female reproduction. Clin Obstet Gynecol. 2010;53:727–39.
25. Stumm S, Meyer A, Lindner M, Bastert G, Wallwiener D, Guckel B. Paclitaxel treatment of breast cancer cell lines modulates Fas/

Fas ligand expression and induces apoptosis which can be inhibited through the CD40 receptor. Oncology. 2004;66:101–11.
26. Lopes F, Smith R, Anderson RA, Spears N. Docetaxel induces moderate ovarian toxicity in mice, primarily affecting granulosa cells of early growing follicles. Mol Hum Reprod. 2014;20:948–59.
27. Roti REC, Leisman SK, Abbott DH, Salih SM. Acute doxorubicin insult in the mouse ovary is cell- and follicle-type dependent. PLoS One. 2012;7(8):e42293.
28. Isgro J, Nurudeen SK, Imundo LF, Sauer MV, Douglas NC. Cyclophosphamide exposure in pediatric systemic lupus erythematosus is associated with reduced serum anti-Müllerian hormone levels. J Rheumatol. 2013;40(6):1029–31.
29. Pazhuhi H, Pousty I, Tajik P, Bokaie S. Protective effect of melatonin on mature ovarian follicle structure in an adult mice treated with Busulphan. IJBPAS. 2015;4(9):5833–47.
30. Fuller B, Paynter S. Fundamentals of cryobiology in reproductive medicine. Reprod BioMed Online. 2004;9:680–91.
31. Talwar P, Awasthi P. Chapter 18: Principal and practice of assisted reproductive technology. Kamini A. Rao, Howard Carp, Robert Fischer, (eds). Laboratory aspects of IVF & Andrology. 2nd ed. New Delhi: Jaypee, 2018. 196–206.
32. Huang JY, Tulandi T, Holzer H, Lau NM, MacDonald S, Tan SL, et al. Cryopreservation of ovarian tissue and in vitro matured oocytes in a female with mosaic turner syndrome the case report. Hum Reprod. 2008;23:336–9.
33. Gook DA, Edgar DH, Stern C. Effect of cooling rate and dehydration regimen on the histological appearance of human ovarian cortex following cryopreservation in 1,2-propanediol. Hum Reprod. 1999;14:2061–8.
34. Demeestere I, Simon P, Buxant F, Robin V, Fernandez SA, Centner J, et al. Ovarian function and spontaneous pregnancy after combined heterotopic and orthotopic cryopreserved ovarian tissue transplantation in a patient previously treated with bone marrow transplantation the case report. Hum Repord. 2006;21:2010–4.
35. Schmidt KL, Ernst E, Byskov AG, et al. Survival of primordial follicles following prolonged transportation of ovarian tissue prior to cryopreservation. Hum Reprod. 2003;18:2654–9.
36. Newton H, Aubard Y, Rutherford A, et al. Low-temperature storage and grafting of human ovarian tissue. Hum Reprod. 1996;11:1487–91.
37 Hovatta O, et al. Cryopreservation of human ovarian tissue using di-methyl-sulphoxide and propanediol-sucrose as cryoprotectants. Hum Reprod. 1996;11(6):1268–72.
38. Gandolfi F, Paffoni A, Papasso Brambilla E, Bonetti S, Brevini TA, Ragni G. Efficiency of equilibrium cooling and vitrification procedures for the cryo- preservation of ovarian tissue: comparative analysis between human and animal models. Fertil Steril. 2006;85:1150–6.
39. https://www.kitazato-dibimed.com/cryotop-vitrification/ovarian-tissue-vitrification/
40. Donnez J, Dolmans MM, Diaz C, Pellicer A. Ovarian cortex transplantation: time to move on from experimental studies to open the clinical application. Fertil Steril. 2015;104(5):1097–8.
41. Donnez J, Dolmans MM. Fertility preservation in women. Nat Rev Endocrinol. 2013;9:735–49.
42. Andersen CY, Rosendahl M, Byskov AG, Loft A, Ottosen C, Dueholm M, et al. Two successful pregnancies following autotransplantation of frozen/thawed ovarian tissue. Hum Reprod. 2008;23(10):2266–72.
43. Meirow D, Levron J, Eldar-Geva T, Hardan I, Fridman E, Zalel Y, et al. Pregnancy after transplantation of cryopreserved ovarian tissue in a patient with ovarian failure after chemotherapy. N Engl J Med. 2005;353(3):318–21.
44. Donnez J, Jadoul P, Pirard C, Hutchings G, Demylle D, Squifflet J, et al. Live birth after transplantation of frozen-thawed ovarian tissue after bilateral oophorectomy for benign disease. Fertil Steril. 2012;98(3):720–5.
45. Oktay K, Buyuk E, Veeck L, et al. Embryo development after heterotopic transplantation of cryopreserved ovarian tissue. Lancet. 2004;363:837–40.
46. Gellert SE, Pors SE, Kristensen SG, Andersen CY, et al. Transplantation of frozen-thawed ovarian tissue: an update on worldwide activity published in peer-reviewed papers and on the Danish cohort. J Assist Reprod Genet. 2018 Apr;35(4):561–70.
47. Oktay K, Karilkaya G. Ovarian function after transplantation of frozen, banked autologous ovarian tissue. N Engl J Med. 2000;342:1919.
48. Dunlop CE, et al. Re-implantation of cryopreserved ovarian cortex resulting in restoration of ovarian function, natural conception and successful pregnancy after hematopoietic stem cell transplantation for Wilms tumor. J Assist Reprod Genet. 2016;33(12):1615–20.
49. Roux C, Amiot C, Agnani G, Aubard Y, Rohrlich PS, Piver P. Live birth after ovarian tissue autograft in a patient with sickle cell disease treated by allogeneic bone marrow transplantation. Fertil Steril. 2010;93(7):2413.
50. Muller A, Keller K, Wacker J, Dittrich R, Keck G, Montag M, et.al. Re-transplantation of cryopreserved ovarian tissue: the first live birth in Germany. Dtsch Arztebl Int 2012; 109(1–2):8–13.
51. Revelli A, Marchino G, Dolfin E, Molinari E, Delle Piane L, Salvagno F, et al. Live birth after orthotopic grafting of autologous cryopreserved ovarian tissue and spontaneous conception in Italy. Fertil Steril. 2013;99(1):227–30.
52. Stern CJ, Gook D, Hale LG, Agresta F, Oldham J, Jobling GRT. First reported clinical pregnancy following heterotopic grafting of cryopreserved ovarian tissue in a woman after a bilateral oophorectomy. Hum Reprod. 2013;28(11):2996–9.
53. Prasath EB, Chan ML, Wong WH, Lim CJ, Tharmalingam MD, Hendricks M, et al. First pregnancy and live birth from cryopreserved embryos obtained from in vitro matured oocytes after oophorectomy the ovarian cancer patient. Hum Reprod. 2014;29:276–8.
54. Suzuki N, Yoshioka N, Takae S, Sugishita Y, Tamura M, Hashimoto S, et al. Successful fertility preservation following ovarian tissue vitrification in patients with primary ovarian insufficiency. Hum Reprod. 2015;30(3):608–15.
55. Jensen AK, Macklon KT, Fedder J, Humaidan P, Andersen CY. 86 successful births and 9 ongoing pregnancies worldwide in women transplanted with frozen-thawed ovarian tissue: focus on birth and perinatal outcome in 40 of these children. J Assist Reprod Genet. 2017;34(3):325–36.
56. Salle B, Demirci B, Franck M, Rudigoz RC, Guerin JF, Lornage J. Normal pregnancies and live births after autograft of frozen-thawed hemi-ovaries into ewes. Fertil Steril. 2002;77:403–8.
57. Liu L, Wood GA, Morikawa L, Ayearst R, Fleming C, McKerliel C. Restoration of fertility by orthotopic transplantation of frozen adult mouse ovaries. Hum Reprod. 2008;23(1):122–8.
58. Ladanyi C, et al. Recent advances in the field of ovarian tissue cryopreservation and opportunities for research. J Assist Reprod Genet. 2017;34(6):709–22.
59. Qi S, Ma A, Xu D, Daloze P, Chen H. Cryopreservation of the vascularized ovary: an evaluation of histology and function in rats. Microsurgery. 2008;28:380–6.
60. Oktay K. Ovarian tissue cryopreservation and transplantation: preliminary findings and implications for cancer patients. Hum Reprod Update. 2001;7:526–34.
61. Martinez MB, Dolmans MM, Van Langendonckt A, Defrere S, Donnez J. Freeze-thawing intact human ovary with its vascular pedicle with a passive cooling device. Fertil Steril. 2004;82:1390–4.
62. Gosden RG. Ovary and uterus transplantation. Reproduction. 2008;136(6):671–80.
63. Jadoul P, Donnez J, Dolmans MM, Squifflet J, Lengele B, Martinez-Madrid B. Laparoscopic ovariectomy for whole human ovary cryopreservation: technical aspects. Fertil Steril. 2007;87:971–5.
64. Abir R, Ben-Aharon I, Garor R, Yaniv I, Ash S, Stemmer SM, et al. Cryopreservation of in-vitro matured oocytes in addition to

ovarian tissue freezing for fertility preservation in pediatric female cancer patients before and after cancer therapy. Hum Reprod. 2016;31(4):750–62.

65. Grynberg M, Peltoketo H, Christin-Maître S, Poulain M, Bouchard P, Fanchin R. First birth achieved after in-vitro maturation of oocytes from a woman endowed with multiple antral follicles unresponsive to follicle-stimulating hormone. J Clin Endocrinol Metab. 2013;98(11):4493–8.
66. Chian RC, Uzelac PS, Nargund G. In-vitro maturation of human immature oocytes for fertility preservation. Fertil Steril. 2013;99(5):1173–81.
67. Telfer EE, Zelinski MB. Ovarian follicle culture: advances and challenges for human and non-human primates. Fertil Steril. 2013;99(6):1523–33.
68. Talwar P. Fertility preservation, ovarian tissue cryo preservation (OTC) revisited. Fertil Sci Res Issue. 2016;3(1):2–5.

Effects of Ethnicity on Ovarian Stimulation and Fertility Preservation

63

Heather Skanes-DeVold, Ashley Wiltshire, and Sana M. Salih

Chapter Objectives

At the end of this chapter, the reader should be familiar with:

1. Current knowledge on the effects of ethnicity on ovarian stimulation
2. Healthcare disparities in the utilization and outcomes of assisted reproduction
3. Effect of race and ethnicity on fertility preservation in cancer patients

63.1 Introduction

Approximately 12.1% of women aged 15–44 years old suffer from infertility or decreased fecundity according to the National Health Statistics Report 2013 [1]. Only about half of the women diagnosed with infertility, 6.9% of women ages 15–44, reported ever using any assisted reproductive services. Many have criticized assisted reproductive technology (ART) as a medical option for only a privileged minority of women. The biggest barrier to ART is cost [2]. In addition to financial obstacles, there may be geographical barriers. A recent cross-sectional study found that geographic access is limited or absent for more than 25 million women of reproductive age in the USA [3].

Racial and ethnic variation in the timing of puberty and symptoms of perimenopause has been documented [4]. Similar to other fields of medicine, there are ethnic disparities with regard to access and utilization of ART. The National Health Statistics Report showed that non-Hispanic black women were more likely to experience infertility than non-Hispanic Caucasian women [1]. However, despite having higher infertility rates, African Americans were less likely to seek fertility treatments than their Caucasian counterparts and were less likely to utilize Advanced Reproductive Technologies (ART), Fig. 63.1 [5]. The inequity in the utilization of assisted reproduction services is often attributed to differences in socioeconomic status among ethnicities. A retrospective cohort study by the Department of Defense of 1457 women undergoing their first cycle of ART found that in equal access to care setting, African-American women were four times more likely to utilize assisted reproductive services [6].

Despite the cost and healthcare disparities, the overall number ART treatment cycles have increased over the past decade by 26% [7]. As access to healthcare increases and infertility awareness rises, new populations of women are seeking treatment in an effort to fulfill their desire for motherhood. This evolving patient population has led to new questions about treatment protocols and ovarian response. One of the most controversial questions is whether or not ethnicity is a major contributor to ovarian response to fertility treatments.

63.2 Ovarian Response Assessment

63.2.1 Ovarian Response

Controlled ovarian stimulation to ensure proper ovarian response for a reasonable likelihood of pregnancy while avoiding the dangers of ovarian hyperstimulation syndrome is a critical part of infertility therapy. While there have been several proposed criteria for inadequate ovarian response, there is no widely accepted standard. The need for the development of a standardized definition has come to the forefront of current literature; this definition will help practitioners identify and anticipate "poor responders" in a consistent fashion and will allow for research studies to be compared and results applied appropriately.

H. Skanes-DeVold · A. Wiltshire
Department of Obstetrics and Gynecology, Morehouse School of Medicine, Atlanta, GA, USA

S. M. Salih (✉)
RMA of Central Pennsylvania at PinnacleHealth, Mechanicsburg, PA, USA

G. N. Allahbadia et al. (eds.), *Textbook of Assisted Reproduction*, https://doi.org/10.1007/978-981-15-2377-9_63

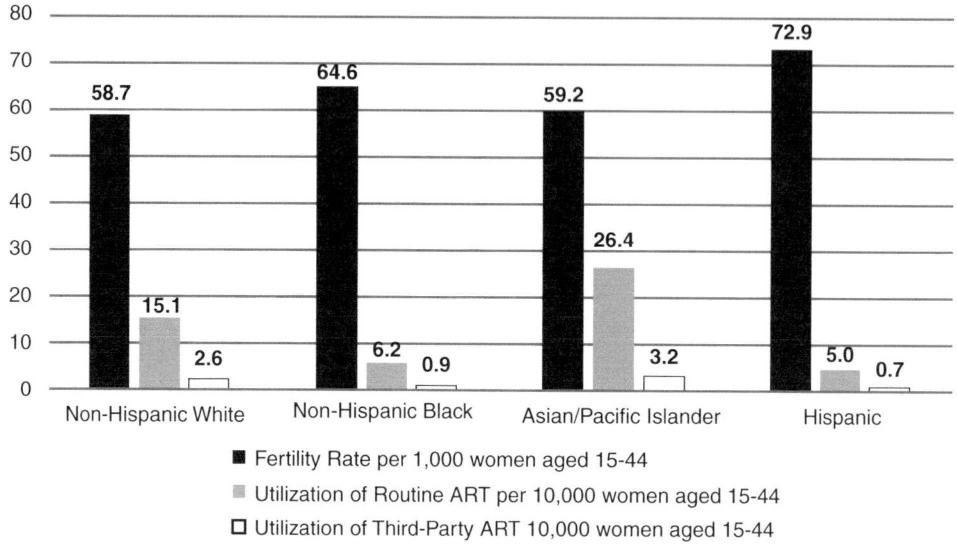

Fig. 63.1 Fertility rates per 1000 women aged 15–44 in 2013 were relatively high among Hispanic and Black women compared to White and Asian women; while utilization of one or three cycles of ART was highest in Asian and White women compared to Hispanic and Black women. (From Shapiro AJ, Darmon SK, Barad DH, Albertini DF, Gleicher N, Kushnir VA. Effect of race and ethnicity on utilization and outcomes of assisted reproductive technology in the USA. Reprod Biol Endocrinol 2017; 15:44, with permission)

Ovarian response has been measured using anti-Mullerian hormone (AMH), antral follicle count (AFC), basal follicle stimulating hormone (FSH), and estradiol, inhibin B, ovarian volume, and multivariate prediction models. Of these current methods, AFC and AMH have the highest specificity and sensitivity but still have a 10–20% false-positive rate [8]. The major limitations to AFC are timing (due to intra-cycle variability), inter-center variation, cost, and inadequate estimations due to increasing body habitus, inclusion of atretic follicles, and the skill level of the ultrasonographer. The major limitation to AMH is the lack of standardization across assays [9]. A large, retrospective analysis of two randomized, controlled, multicenter trials found AMH to be superior to AFC, noting that AMH had a higher correlation with oocyte yield than AFC, regardless of whether women achieved a pregnancy [10].

In general, poor response can be defined as failure to respond to standard ovarian stimulation protocols and to recruit an adequate number of follicles [11]. Some studies have defined poor ovarian response as <3–5 follicles after stimulation, peak estradiol <300–500 pg/ml, day 3 FSH > 7–15 mIU/mL, or previous cancelled cycle(s) [8]. In 2010, The ESHRE Consensus meeting developed the Bologna criteria (Table 63.1). These criteria require at least one previous stimulation cycle in addition to two of the following: advanced maternal age, a previous poor ovarian response, or an abnormal ovarian reserve test [8]. Despite the establishment of these consensus criteria, there is still debate over their reliability. The main criticisms are a lack of homogeneity of the population, suggested cut-offs for age, AFC, and AMH values, focus on oocyte quantity rather than quality, evidence to support included risk factors, possibility of overdiagnosis, and lack of large scale validation of the criteria [12].

Table 63.1 Bologna criteria for ovarian reserve

Bologna criteria for poor ovarian response	
Must have a one stimulated cycle in order to have a diagnosis of poor ovarian response[a] in addition to at least two of the following:	
1. Advanced maternal age (>40 years old) or any other risk factor for poor ovarian response	Risk factors include genetic conditions (e.g., Turners, FMR1 premutation), pelvic infection, endometriosis, history of chemotherapy, etc.
2. A previous poor ovarian response (< or = 3 oocytes with conventional stimulation protocol	
3. An abnormal ovarian reserve test	AFC <5–7 follicles OR AMH < 0.5–1.1 ng/ml

From Ferraretti AP, La Marca A, Fauser BC, Tarlatzis B, Nargund G, Gianaroli L, Definition EwgoPOR. ESHRE consensus on the definition of "poor response" to ovarian stimulation for in vitro fertilization: the Bologna criteria. Hum Reprod 2011; 26:1616–1624, with permission

[a]Patient >40 with abnormal ovarian reserve test may be considered poor ovarian responders and this may substituted for a stimulation cycle

63.2.2 Ethnicity and Ovarian Response Measurements

Recent studies have shown conflicting results with regard to ethnicity and ovarian response. Multiple studies have shown that there are significant ethnic differences about ovarian reserve, aging, and response (Table 63.2). One prospective cohort study of 229 Spanish and 236 Indian women, under age 42, undergoing their first or second round of IVF, found that the ovaries of Indian women aged 6 years faster than those of Spanish women. In addition, this study found that younger age, higher BMI, lower AMH, higher FSH, and

Table 63.2 Live birth rates in black women compared to Caucasian women

	Ratio	95% CI	*P* value	References
RR	0.63	0.44–0.90		[6]
OR	0.55	0.35–0.85 $P = 0.007$		[13]
OR	0.62	0.55–0.71	$p < 0.001$	[14]
ARR	1.31	1.26–1.37	$p < 0.001$	[15]
AOR	0.62	0.56–0.68	$p < 0.0001$	[16]
AOR	0.73	0.57–0.92	$p = 0.008$	[17]
AOR	0.60	0.51–0.72	$p < 0.05$	[18]
RR	0.74	0.63–0.91		[19]
OR	0.30	0.10–0.89	$p = 0.035$	[20]

RR relative risk, *OR* odd ratio, *ARR* adjusted relative risk, *AOR* adjusted odds ratio

longer duration of infertility were all associated with Indian ethnicity, which may reflect differences in early diagnostic capacity of diminished ovarian reserve [21]. Another prospective longitudinal study of 809 women found that even after controlling for age, BMI, HIV status, and smoking, black women had an average decrease of AMH value that was significantly more steep, − 25.2% (95% CI −43.0 to −1.9, $p = 0.037$) than that of Caucasian women [22]. However, a large retrospective cohort study of 2308 infertile women using 32 ancestry informative markers to classify women as European, African, Central/South Asian, or East Asian concluded that there was no difference in ovarian reserve or response markers including FSH, AMH, AFC, and oocyte yield (P values 0.16, 0.12, 0.22, and 0.26, respectively) [23]. This study suggests that reliance on self-reported ethnicity may explain, or at least contribute to, conflicting studies regarding ethnic and ovarian performance. However, it is important to note that patients in the study accurately self-reported ethnicity 88.9% of the time [23].

63.3 Art Outcomes in Minorities

For those patients who are able to produce an adequate ovarian response and proceed with IVF, it is important to note that there continue to be differences in outcomes between ethnic groups. The Society of Assisted Reproductive Technology (SART) holds a national database for ART outcomes in the USA. Ninety-five percent of IVF cycles are reported through the SART registry. SART has published multiple studies looking into racial trends over the years via retrospective cohort studies. Shapiro et al. analyzed data on 1,132,844 women undergoing IVF between 2004 and 2013. They reported a recent decline in fertility rates in all ethnic groups that was most pronounced in Hispanic and Non-Hispanic Black women and an increase in the utilization of autologous ART in all ethnic groups, but the increase was least pronounced among Hispanic and Non-Hispanic Black women (Fig. 63.2) [5]. A recent report of racial trends of IVF outcomes is a comparison between 1999–2000 and 2004–2006 [15]. This study examined 158,693 IVF cycles using non-donor embryos. SART also found that the rate of live births per cycle increased across all ethnic groups. This is to be expected as ART continues to evolve with more advanced techniques such as recombinant gonadotropins, intracytoplasmic sperm injection, and preimplantation genetic screening. Consistent with what has been described earlier in this chapter, SART data found increase in the diagnosis of diminished ovarian reserve among all women, but the increase was higher in African-American women (from 7.5% to 14.4%; $P \leq 0.001$). In addition, there was an overall greater increase in live births for Caucasian women, further implicating the widening disparities within in ART live birth outcome between black and Caucasian women (22.2% vs. 32.3%; $P \leq 0.001$) [15]. On the other hand, the outcome of frozen blastocyst transfer appears to be similar between African-American and white women despite a higher peak level of estradiol during the IVF stimulation [20].

Studies have shown that this outcome variation is not strictly black versus Caucasian. McQueen found similar results in a retrospective analysis of women undergoing their first autologous IVF cycle in Illinois [24]. The study was performed between January of 2010 and December of 2012. Of the 4045 total female subjects, there were 3003 Caucasian, 213 black, 541 Asian, and 288 Hispanic women. McQueen's study showed that both African-American and Asian women had significantly lower odds of clinical pregnancy rate, Black 0.63 (95% CI 0.44–0.88) and Asian 0.73 (95% CI 0.60–0.90); lower odds for live birth rate, Black 0.50 (95% CI 0.33–0.72) and Asian 0.64 (95% CI 0.51–0.80); as well as higher odds of spontaneous miscarriage compared to white women. Decreased live birth rates with higher rates of miscarriage have also been found among women of Middle Eastern/North African (MENA) descent in the USA when compared to Caucasian women. In a retrospective cohort study of 190 MENA and 200 Caucasian women undergoing their first autologous IVF cycle between May 2006 and May 2014, MENA women experienced significantly fewer live births, OR 0.55 (95% CI 0.35–0.85, $P = 0.007$) and experienced miscarriage at a significantly higher rate, OR 2.55, (95% CI 1.04–6.27; $P = 0.036$) than Caucasian women, after controlling for age and BMI [13]. Disparities in IVF outcomes have also revealed an increase infant morbidity. Moderate and severe growth restriction and preterm birth were increased among singletons for infants in all three minority groups when compared to Caucasian [16].

There have been numerous studies outside of the USA that are consistent with these findings. Dhillon, et al.'s retrospective cohort study, conducted in the UK, compared IVF outcomes of 13,473 first cycles to meta-analyzed data from 16 countries [14]. Black women were found to have significantly lower clinical pregnancy rates, OR 0.41 (95% CI 0.25

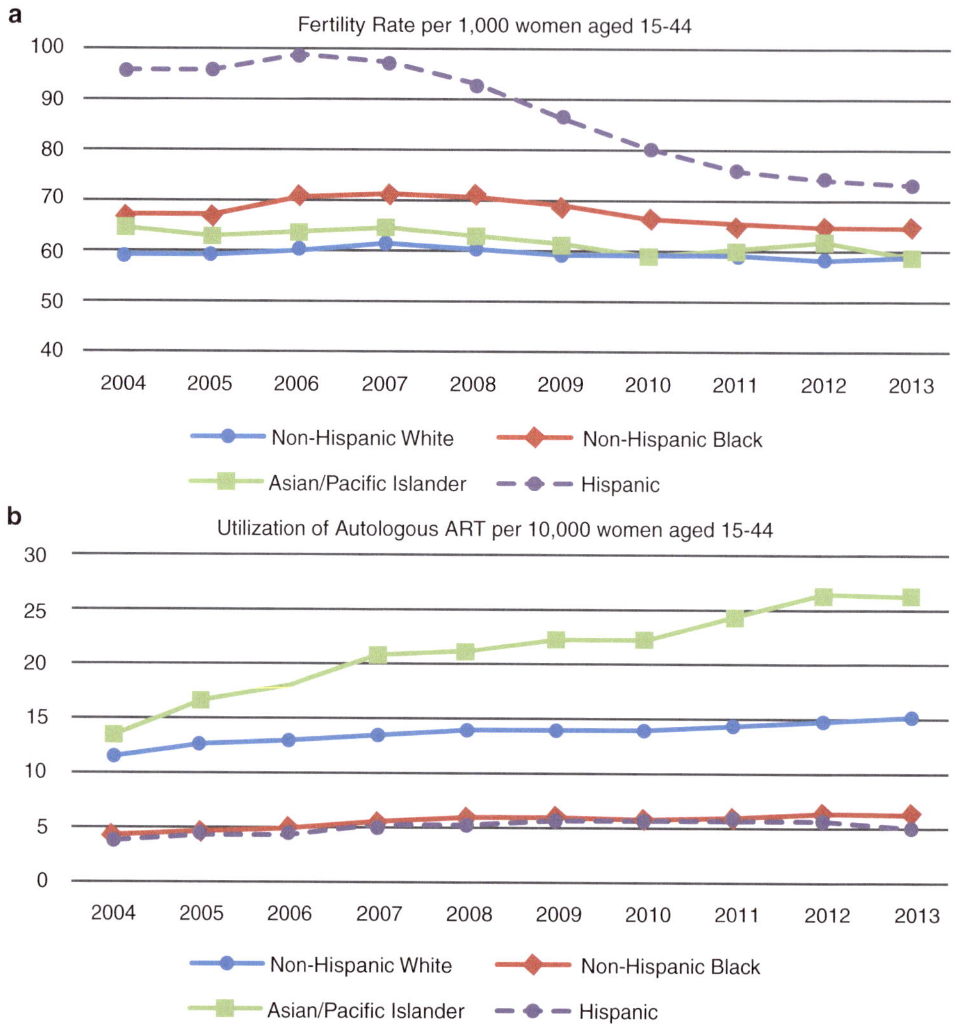

Fig. 63.2 (**a**) Fertility rates declined in all groups after 2007; this decrease was most pronounced among Hispanic women. (**b**) Utilization of one or three ART cycles increased among all groups; this increase was most pronounced among Asian women. (From Shapiro AJ, Darmon SK, Barad DH, Albertini DF, Gleicher N, Kushnir VA. Effect of race and ethnicity on utilization and outcomes of assisted reproductive technology in the USA. Reprod Biol Endocrinol 2017; 15:44, with permission)

to 0.67; $P < 0.001$), and lower live birth rates, OR 0.42 (95% CI 0.25 to 0.70; $P = 0.001$), when compared with Caucasian women, which is consistent with prior studies. Additionally, their research showed that South Asian women also had significantly reduced odds of live birth, OR 0.80 (95% CI 0.65 to 0.99; $P = 0.04$), when compared with Caucasian women. Controlled factors within this study included age, BMI, infertility etiology, infertility duration, previous live birth, previous spontaneous abortion, and number of embryos transferred [14]. In an observational study using the UK's National ART database, 38,709 women undergoing their first fresh IVF/ICSI cycle from 2000–2010 were compared [25]. Jayaprakason et al. found significantly lower odds of live birth for the ethnic minority group (Caucasian Irish, Indian, Bangladeshi, Pakistani, Black African, and Asian women) in comparison to Caucasian British women, OR 0.59 (95% CI 0.42–0.82; $P \leq 0.01$). Interestingly, there was a trend, but no significant difference in live birth outcome in the South East Asian, African-Caribbean, and Middle Eastern populations in comparison to Caucasian British women, OR 0.86 (95% CI 0.71–1.05; $P = 0.15$), 0.53 (95% CI 0.28–1.02; $P = 0.06$), and 0.49 (95% CI 0.18–1.34; $P = 0.16$), respectively [25].

Table 63.3 Causes for decreased ART success in ethnic minorities

Causes	References
Uterine factor	[5, 6, 15, 16, 18, 20, 26]
Tubal factor	[5, 13, 15, 16, 18–20, 27]
Obesity	[26, 28, 29]
Spontaneous abortion	[5, 13, 15, 28, 30]

With the multitude of studies concluding that race/ethnicity may be a significant factor for ovarian reserve and ART outcome, the next question is "why" (Table 63.3). Some believe the origin of these racial/ethnic differences could be due to environmental/developmental factors. A retrospective study comparing immigrants from Bangladesh currently living in the UK examined 179 healthy women between ages 35 and 59 years old [31]. They examined markers of ovarian reserve between those who migrated as an adult versus as a child. Main outcome measures included serum AMH, inhibin B, FSH, and E2, anthropometrics derived from biomarkers. They also used reproductive, demographic, and health variables from structured questionnaires. Results revealed that those who spent a substantial amount of time in Bangladesh before immigrating (i.e., immigrating as an adult) had lower ovarian reserve markers than those who came to the UK early, as children [31]. This study strongly suggests that environmental factors may have a strong influence on ovarian response and thereby on ART outcome as well. Premature progesterone elevation may contribute to racial disparity in IVF outcomes. Elevated progesterone level is associated with decreased live birth rate in IVF cycles. A study found that premature progesterone >2 ng/ml occurred in only 2.3% of cycles in white women compared with 6.3% in Hispanic, 5.9% in Asian, and 4.4% in African-American women, thus adding to the inferior outcome of IVF in ethnic minorities.

Another possible cause for the differing ART outcomes between races may be the racial differences in infertility etiology. A systematic review found that infertility diagnosis, spontaneous abortion, and obesity could explain some of the lower clinical pregnancy rates and live birth rates after IVF in ethnic minorities when compared with white women [32]. Studies showed that black women have higher prevalence of tubal factor and uterine factor infertility including fibroids compared to Caucasian women [5, 6, 15]. Based on the previously cited SART cohort study of racial trends, from 2004 to 2006, African-American women who had no prior ART experience were 2.5 times more likely to have tubal factor than Caucasian women (45% vs. 17.9%;$P < 0.001$) [15]. There was a significant decrease of tubal factor infertility in all women who underwent their first ART between 1999–2000 and 2004–2006, but the decrease was less discernible in African-American women. Tubal factor infertility decreased from 63% to 45% ($P < 0.001$) among African-American women and from 28.2% to 17.9% ($P < 0.001$) among Caucasian women. Although both groups had a significant decrease in tubal factor, the difference in the rate of tubal factor between the groups significantly widened ($P = 0.015$). Between 1999–2000 and 2004–2006, African women also continued to be three times more likely than Caucasian women to have uterine factor diagnosed as a cause of their infertility, (12.4% vs. 3.9%, $P < 0.001$), respectively [15]. Fibroids were three times more prevalent in black women leading to reduced ART success in an equal-access-to-care environment [6]. With the vast array of factors that can impact one's fertility, it is quite likely that the cause of differing ovarian response and ART outcomes is multifactorial as a culmination of race, environmental and developmental factors, medical and gynecologic history, and anatomical factors.

63.3.1 Fertility Preservation in Minorities

Despite the 2006 ASCO report recommending that all female cancer patients receive oncofertility counseling before initiating therapy, there is still an enormous gender gap in counseling rates. While 60% of both men and women are advised that cancer treatment may adversely affect their fertility, a recent report by Armuand et al. reveals that only 14% of women receive counseling for oncofertility treatment options, compared to 68% of men [33]. Preserving fertility in men is accomplished through the relatively simple and noninvasive process of sperm banking. The procedures for women are much more expensive and invasive, and they can significantly delay cancer treatment by up to 2 to 3 weeks due to the hormonal treatments required; all these factors contribute to the small percentage of women who are offered fertility preservation. Among women who are offered treatment, there are further disparities based on education level, economic status, and race [28, 34–36]. The expensive and invasive methodologies are complicated, can delay cancer treatment, require adequate information and referral to a reproductive endocrinologist, and are often not covered by insurance [37, 38]. While oncologists appear to mention the risk of infertility to all patients, Blacks, Hispanics, and Asian women are less likely to seek a follow-up consultation with an endocrinologist compared to white patients. Counseling and preservation services were less likely in women who didn't attend college, had lower household income, and weren't white [38]. One study showed Latino women were 80% less likely than white women to have taken steps to preserve fertility before cancer treatment, while none of the African-American women who answered the survey had received fertility preservation services before cancer treatment [28]. Education level and economic status also contribute significantly to the disparities in who gets treated.

63.4 Controversy and Conclusions

Given that African-American women are a small fraction of the population seeking infertility treatment and also have the worse treatment outcomes, it is reasonable to believe that the current database of literature may not be generalizable to this sub-group of patients. African Americans are also more likely to have medical conditions such as fibroids and history of tubal factor, which may exclude them from research studies [39]. The lack of inclusion in the current research may lead to sub-adequate treatment protocols, which thus resulted in decreased live birth rates seen after treatment. In addition, difficulty in identifying ethnicity by both patient and provider may cause misrepresentation in the current studies that seek to evaluate ethnicity.

Under the assumption that the reproductive liberty is a negative human right, the United Nations has recommended that countries "ensure that family planning, medical, and related social services aim not only at the prevention of unwanted pregnancies but also at the elimination of involuntary sterility and subfecundity in order that all couples may be permitted to achieve their desired number of children, and that child adoption may be facilitated" [40]. Understanding potential differences among ethnicities with regard to reproductive health is one way to implement this goal of eliminating barriers to fertility. Determining whether ethnic differences in ovarian response truly exist may assist in further development of treatment protocols, improve the live birth rates of minority populations, and aid in developing new ways to predict poor responders.

References

1. Chandra A, Copen CE, Stephen EH. Infertility and impaired fecundity in the United States, 1982–2010: data from the national survey of family growth. Natl Health Stat Rep. 2013;11:1–18.
2. Katz P, Showstack J, Smith JF, Nachtigall RD, Millstein SG, Wing H, et al. Costs of infertility treatment: results from an 18-month prospective cohort study. Fertil Steril. 2011;95:915–21.
3. Harris JA, Menke MN, Haefner JK, Moniz MH, Perumalswami CR. Geographic access to assisted reproductive technology health care in the United States: a population-based cross-sectional study. Fertil Steril. 2017;107:1023–7.
4. Butts SF, Seifer DB. Racial and ethnic differences in reproductive potential across the life cycle. Fertil Steril. 2010;93:681–90.
5. Shapiro AJ, Darmon SK, Barad DH, Albertini DF, Gleicher N, Kushnir VA. Effect of race and ethnicity on utilization and outcomes of assisted reproductive technology in the USA. Reprod Biol Endocrinol. 2017;15:44.
6. Feinberg EC, Larsen FW, Catherino WH, Zhang J, Armstrong AY. Comparison of assisted reproductive technology utilization and outcomes between Caucasian and African American patients in an equal-access-to-care setting. Fertil Steril. 2006;85:888–94.
7. Centers for Disease Control and Prevention A, Society for Assisted Reproductive Technology. Assisted reproductive technology national summary report. Atlanta (GA): US Dept of Health and Human Services; 2016. Available at http://www.cdc.gov/art/pdf/2014-report/art-2014-national-summary-report.pdf - page=9
8. Ferraretti AP, La Marca A, Fauser BC, Tarlatzis B, Nargund G, Gianaroli L, et al. ESHRE consensus on the definition of 'poor response' to ovarian stimulation for in vitro fertilization: the Bologna criteria. Hum Reprod. 2011;26:1616–24.
9. Fleming R, Seifer DB, Frattarelli JL, Ruman J. Assessing ovarian response: antral follicle count versus anti-Mullerian hormone. Reprod BioMed. 2015;31:486–96.
10. Nelson SM, Klein BM, Arce JC. Comparison of antimullerian hormone levels and antral follicle count as predictor of ovarian response to controlled ovarian stimulation in good-prognosis patients at individual fertility clinics in two multicenter trials. Fertil Steril. 2015;103:923–30.. e921
11. Badawy A, Wageah A, El Gharib M, Osman EE. Prediction and diagnosis of poor ovarian response: the dilemma. J Reprod Infertil. 2011;12:241–8.
12. Younis JS, Ben-Ami M, Ben-Shlomo I. The Bologna criteria for poor ovarian response: a contemporary critical appraisal. J Ovarian Res. 2015;8:76.
13. Salem WH, Abdullah A, Abuzeid O, Bendikson K, Sharara FI, Abuzeid M. Decreased live births among women of middle eastern/north African ethnicity compared to Caucasian women. J Assist Reprod Genet. 2017;34:581–6.
14. Dhillon RK, Smith PP, Malhas R, Harb HM, Gallos ID, Dowell K, et al. Investigating the effect of ethnicity on IVF outcome. Reprod BioMed. 2015;31:356–63.
15. Seifer DB, Zackula R, Grainger DA, Society for Assisted Reproductive Technology Writing Group R. Trends of racial disparities in assisted reproductive technology outcomes in black women compared with white women: society for assisted reproductive technology 1999 and 2000 vs. 2004–2006. Fertil Steril. 2010;93:626–35.
16. Fujimoto VY, Luke B, Brown MB, Jain T, Armstrong A, Grainger DA, et al. Racial and ethnic disparities in assisted reproductive technology outcomes in the United States. Fertil Steril. 2010;93:382–90.
17. Luke B, Brown MB, Grainger DA, Cedars M, Klein N, Stern JE. Practice patterns and outcomes with the use of single embryo transfer in the United States. Fertil Steril. 2010;93:490–8.
18. Maalouf W, Maalouf W, Campbell B, Jayaprakasan K. Effect of ethnicity on live birth rates after in vitro fertilisation/intracytoplasmic sperm injection treatment: analysis of UK national database. BJOG. 2017;124:904–10.
19. McCarthy-Keith DM, Schisterman EF, Robinson RD, O'Leary K, Lucidi RS, Armstrong AY. Will decreasing ART costs improve utilization and outcomes among minority women? Fertil Steril. 2010;94(7):2587–9.
20. Csokmay JM, Hill MJ, Maguire M, Payson MD, Fujimoto VY, Armstrong AY. Are there ethnic differences in pregnancy rates in African-American versus white women undergoing frozen blastocyst transfers? Fertil Steril. 2011;95:89–93.
21. Iglesias C, Banker M, Mahajan N, Herrero L, Meseguer M, Garcia-Velasco JA. Ethnicity as a determinant of ovarian reserve: differences in ovarian aging between Spanish and Indian women. Fertil Steril. 2014;102:244–9.
22. Seifer DB, Golub ET, Lambert-Messerlian G, Benning L, Anastos K, Watts DH, et al. Variations in serum mullerian inhibiting substance between white, black, and Hispanic women. Fertil Steril. 2009;92:1674–8.
23. Olcha M, Franasiak JM, Shastri S, Molinaro TA, Congdon H, Treff NR, et al. Genotypically determined ancestry across an infertile population: ovarian reserve and response parameters are not influenced by continental origin. Fertil Steril. 2016;106:475–80.
24. McQueen DB, Schufreider A, Lee SM, Feinberg EC, Uhler ML. Racial disparities in in vitro fertilization outcomes. Fertil Steril. 2015;104:398–402.. e391
25. Jayaprakasan K, Pandian D, Hopkisson J, Campbell BK, Maalouf WE. Effect of ethnicity on live birth rates after in vitro fertilisation or intracytoplasmic sperm injection treatment. BJOG. 2014;121:300–7.
26. Pandey S, Maheshwari A, Bhattacharya S. The impact of female obesity on the outcome of fertility treatment. J Hum Reprod Sci. 2010;3(2):62–7.
27. Sharara FI, McClamrock HD. Differences in in vitro fertilization (IVF) outcome between white and black women in an inner-city, university-based IVF program. Fertil Steril. 2000;73(6):1170–3.
28. Letourneau JM, Smith JF, Ebbel EE, Craig A, Katz PP, Cedars MI, et al. Racial, socioeconomic, and demographic disparities in access to fertility preservation in young women diagnosed with cancer. Cancer. 2012;118:4579–88.
29. Jungheim ES, Travieso JL, Hopeman MM. Weighing the impact of obesity on female reproductive function and fertility. Nutr Rev. 2013;71(1):10.

30. Seifer DB, Frazier LM, Grainger DA. Disparity in assisted reproductive technologies outcomes in black women compared with white women. Fertil Steril. 2008;90:1701–10.
31. Begum K, Muttukrishna S, Sievert LL, Sharmeen T, Murphy L, Chowdhury O, et al. Ethnicity or environment: effects of migration on ovarian reserve among Bangladeshi women in the United Kingdom. Fertil Steril. 2016;105:744–54.. e741
32. Humphries LA, Chang O, Humm K, Sakkas D, Hacker MR. Influence of race and ethnicity on in vitro fertilization outcomes: systematic review. Am J Obstet Gynecol. 2016;214:212.e1.
33. Armuand GM, Rodriguez-Wallberg KA, Wettergren L, Ahlgren J, Enblad G, Hoglund M, et al. Sex differences in fertility-related information received by young adult cancer survivors. J Clin Oncol. 2012;30:2147–53.
34. Blinder VS, Griggs JJ. Health disparities and the cancer survivor. Semin Oncol. 2013;40:796–803.
35. Goodman LR, Balthazar U, Kim J, Mersereau JE. Trends of socioeconomic disparities in referral patterns for fertility preservation consultation. Hum Reprod. 2012;27:2076–81.
36. Kim J, Deal AM, Balthazar U, Kondapalli LA, Gracia C, Mersereau JE. Fertility preservation consultation for women with cancer: are we helping patients make high-quality decisions? Reprod BioMed. 2013;27:96–103.
37. Campo-Engelstein L. Consistency in insurance coverage for iatrogenic conditions resulting from cancer treatment including fertility preservation. J Clin Oncol. 2010;28:1284–6.
38. Flink DM, Sheeder J, Kondapalli LA. A review of the oncology Patient's challenges for utilizing fertility preservation services. J Adolesc Young Adult Oncol. 2017;6:31–44.
39. Johnstone E, Sandler JR, Addauan-Andersen C, Sohn SH, Fujimoto VY. Asian women are less likely to express interest in infertility research. Fertil Steril. 2010;94:1249–53.
40. United Nations Department of Economic and Social Affairs. Population division economic. Reproductive rights. http://www.un.org/en/development/desa/population/theme/rights/ (cited 2017 June 30).

64 Managing a Sperm Cryobank

Karla Turner and Paul Wilson

64.1 Introduction

Sperm banking is offered to men in need of fertility preservation, primarily prior to undertaking medical or surgical procedures that could render them infertile. However, requests for sperm banking are also becoming increasingly common for other reasons, including areas of medicine involving the use of cytotoxic medicines, immunological conditions such as rheumatoid arthritis, those involved in high risk occupations (e.g. members of the armed forces) as well as those about to electively undertake sterilizing procedures or gender reassignment. Cryobanking also takes place for men who agree to donate their sperm.

This chapter aims to give a brief overview of the main areas to be considered by any storage facility wishing to offer a sperm cryobanking service.

64.2 The Person Who Wants to Store Sperm

Sperm cryobanking is a relationship between the clinic and the person who wishes to store sperm. Identifying that the storing individual is the most important party within this relationship is the first step to providing a successful cryobanking service. Although the individual's wishes must be permissible within the legislative framework set out by the country of storage and be feasible within the constraints of the storing clinic, the clinic's primary purpose is to provide an efficient, lawful service meeting the needs of the storing individual, often at a time of great personal difficulty.

As a service user, the responsibilities of the storing individual are essentially limited to:

- Complying with any pre-storage blood-borne virology screening that is required
- Attending at agreed appointment times (either on- or off-site)
- Producing at least one sample for storage
- Completing the necessary consent forms
- Providing contact details and agreeing to remain contactable for the duration of storage
- Honouring any other specific terms and conditions held within any contract which may exist between the individual and the storing clinic, such as the agreement to pay ongoing storage fees (if this is required)

It is the responsibility of the clinic, its staff and associated professionals involved in the care pathway to ensure procedures are in place to facilitate the above, ensuring the provision of a quality service to achieve the patient-specific wishes as far as is possible and a 'good patient experience'.

Understanding the reason for sperm storage helps the cryobank to provide a bespoke service regarding the provision of relevant information and the accurate completion of any appropriate consent forms required by regulation. It may also aid decision-making about future sample utilization and help in maintaining contact with the individual.

All processes and procedures leading to the provision of a storage service for referred individuals should be dealt with sensitively and empathetically. Individuals referred to the clinic may have recently received potentially life-changing news, e.g. a terminal diagnosis if they have been referred from an oncology clinic. Attending adolescents may feel embarrassed at the thought of discussing very personal issues such as masturbation with complete strangers, perhaps with their parents present in the consultation.

Consideration should also be given as to how gender reassignment individuals might wish to be addressed when attending appointments. Staff members may have to deal with transwomen who are anxious or angry about having to complete consent forms which focus on their 'maleness', as this can be emotionally difficult. In the UK, the Human

K. Turner (✉) · P. Wilson
Bristol Centre for Reproductive Medicine, Southmead Hospital, Bristol, UK
e-mail: karla@bcrm.org.uk

G. N. Allahbadia et al. (eds.), *Textbook of Assisted Reproduction*, https://doi.org/10.1007/978-981-15-2377-9_64

Fertilization and Embryology Authority (HFEA) has addressed this issue by including a gender 'neutral' designation on consent forms.

The initial consultation should include information giving prior to the taking of appropriate consent. This should entail efforts by the staff to understand the specific circumstances of that particular individual. Assumptions should not be made based on the individual's marital status or perceived sexual orientation. All options should be explored in order to ensure the consent recorded is an accurate reflection of the individual's wishes. Such discussions should prompt staff to consider not only the practicalities of sample production but also how the sperm may be used for future treatment services, should this be requested.

Depending upon the circumstances, additional consent forms may be required, e.g. those required to permit future surrogacy arrangements and/or any additional associated screening tests. Additional consents may be also be needed for people who are about to undertake gender reassignment treatments or for homosexual men.

There may be a need for swift access to the cryobank, e.g. in the event of an urgent need to proceed to storage. In such instances, care must be taken to ensure the quality of the service, and the information provided is not compromised, as this may increase the risk of future difficulties for both the cryobank and the individual or their partner. Where complex situations arise, or are envisaged, the cryobank should not hesitate to seek specific clarification from its regulating body and/or independent legal advice as appropriate, as this may mitigate future risk for the cryobank in the event of legal challenge.

The information provided to the individual prior to filling out a consent form ensures that the consent obtained is 'informed consent'. Informed consent is based on the premise of patient autonomy, namely, that the individual has the right to make decisions about their own health. To achieve this, the information provided must allow the individual to make informed decisions and understand the purpose, benefits and risks and any other implications of the proposed treatment. This may be difficult to achieve, since the implications of the treatment to be undertaken may not be known at the time of cryobanking.

Individuals who are uncertain about which decisions to take should be advised to provide consent which does not restrict their future choices, e.g. posthumous use. As each person is unique, blanket policies or approaches within the cryobank may lead to future difficulties and should be avoided.

If the individual is a minor, this person should be assessed to check if they are able to give valid consent. This can be performed via a Gillick competence check [1]. If the child is not Gillick competent, parental permission may be required.

Gillick Competence

Gillick competence is a term used in medical law in England and Wales to determine whether a child under the age of 16 years has the intelligence and maturity needed to make decisions regarding their own medical treatment without the need for parental permission.

As has been demonstrated by publicized legal cases in the UK [2–6], a failure to provide adequate information/counselling to the individual at the time of consent taking may have the same consequences as failing to complete the consent form at all. In such instances, this may mean that the consent given is legally invalid. It is therefore recommended that a written record is kept of all information provided to the individual (with document version numbers, if appropriate) to evidence that appropriate information was given before consent was taken and samples stored.

Regardless of the reason for storage, it is the cryobank's duty to ensure that the samples are stored safely and lawfully, and any consent taken accurately reflects the wishes of the individual concerned. It is entirely reasonable for the storing individual to expect that such a service will be provided.

64.3 The Cryobank Facility

Managing a cryobank may, on the surface, appear relatively straightforward. The individual is referred to the cryobank, an appointment is organized, consent forms are completed, and a sample is produced, processed and stored for possible use at a later date.

In practice, the delivery of a comprehensive service is rarely so simple. Problems may exist because:

- Urgent requests for storage may be needed, but the virology status has not yet been determined.
- Individuals may be unable to produce samples on request due to anxiety or illness.
- An off-site consultation is requested, as the individual is unable to attend the facility.
- Translation services may be needed to understand the complex issues before being able to give informed consent.
- Maintaining contact with the individual may become difficult if the patient's address/contact details change and the cryobank isn't informed.
- The cryobank may receive requests to export samples to a different cryobank, either nationally and internationally.
- As the cryobank is likely to store samples for extended time periods (potentially decades), regulations or protocols may change, such that they could significantly differ from the information and consent at the time of storage.

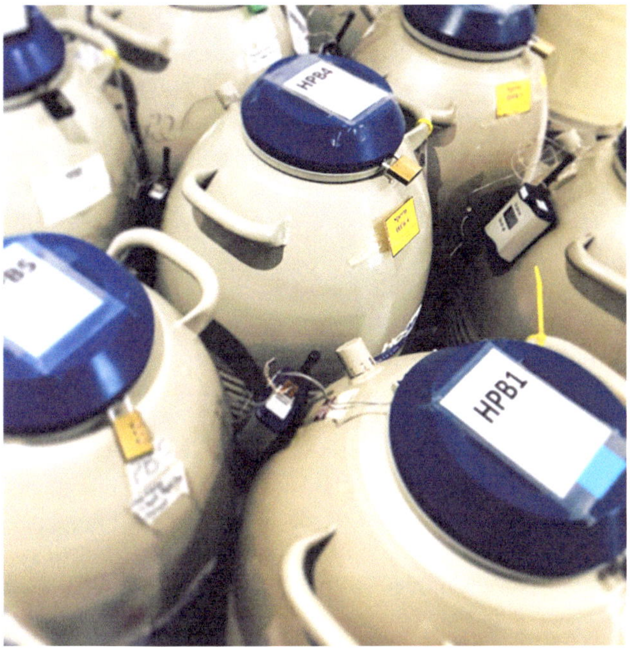

Fig. 64.1 Liquid nitrogen dewars in a cryobank. All dewars are individually padlocked and fitted with low level liquid nitrogen alarms to ensure samples are always maintained in a safe environment. Image courtesy of the Bristol Centre for Reproductive Medicine, Bristol, UK

These scenarios illustrate that cryobank management requires careful planning and a real understanding of the task and potential issues and outcomes. The service must therefore be adequately resourced and staffed by well-trained, competent and empathetic individuals who are adaptable enough to provide a professional and easily accessible service for all users. It is imperative the all staff have a sound knowledge of the legal framework set out by any regulator to ensure that samples are stored lawfully (Fig. 64.1).

64.3.1 Staff

Responsibility for the processing and storage of the sample should fall to an appropriately trained scientist or technician. A decision must be taken as to who should assist in the completion of the necessary consent forms and provide the required counselling. These roles require an in-depth knowledge and understanding of any regulatory framework and the complexities of any consent forms to be completed. Counselling should be available to the patient not only at the time of sperm banking but also during the storage period, and the counsellor should have experience in both therapeutic and implications counselling.

Proper training, with regular update training, should be provided to the staff members involved. They must also be aware that patient decisions in relation to the cryobanking and future use may also affect the patient's partner, family and any children that may subsequently be conceived. Staff dealing with adolescents should allow them the opportunity to discuss the process away from the parent/guardian if they feel this is appropriate.

64.3.2 Cryobank Facilities

The cryobank will be required to comply with the prevailing regulatory environment, as well as ensuring professional guidelines are followed for processing and storage. Best practice guidelines by professional societies and regulators can help to ensure a quality service is provided, e.g. those published by the Association of Biomedical Andrologists [7] and the Association of Clinical Embryologists [8] in the UK; the American Society for Reproductive Medicine [9] and the American Society of Clinical Oncology [10] in the USA; the European Society of Human Reproduction and Embryology [11] in Europe; and the National Institute for Health and Care Excellence [12] and the HFEA [13].

In the UK, to obtain a storage licence, the cryobank is required to adhere to the guidelines set out in the HFEA Code of Practice [13] and is inspected on a regular basis to ensure compliance. The timing of HFEA inspections can be pre-agreed or unannounced. Adherence to published guidelines should ensure that samples are processed safely and stored in a manner where risks are minimized, although individual clinics should review and risk assess their own procedures on a regular basis.

For sample security, cryobank access should be restricted to authorized personnel only. Continuous monitoring with alarms should be in place for all samples, and these should be linked to an on-call facility/autodialler to provide 24-hour cover (Fig. 64.2).

64.3.3 Storage Consent and Contracts

Following referral, information relating to the patients should be taken prior to storage and should be as comprehensive as possible. The information collected is essential for maintaining future patient contact and should include:

- The patients full name (and any former names by which the patient has been known)
- Formal evidence of identity, ideally including a photographic image of the patient, e.g. passport or driving licence where possible
- Information relating to the patient's partner and/or other next of kin information
- Information relating to the patient's referring clinician and details of their general practitioner
- Telephone contact information

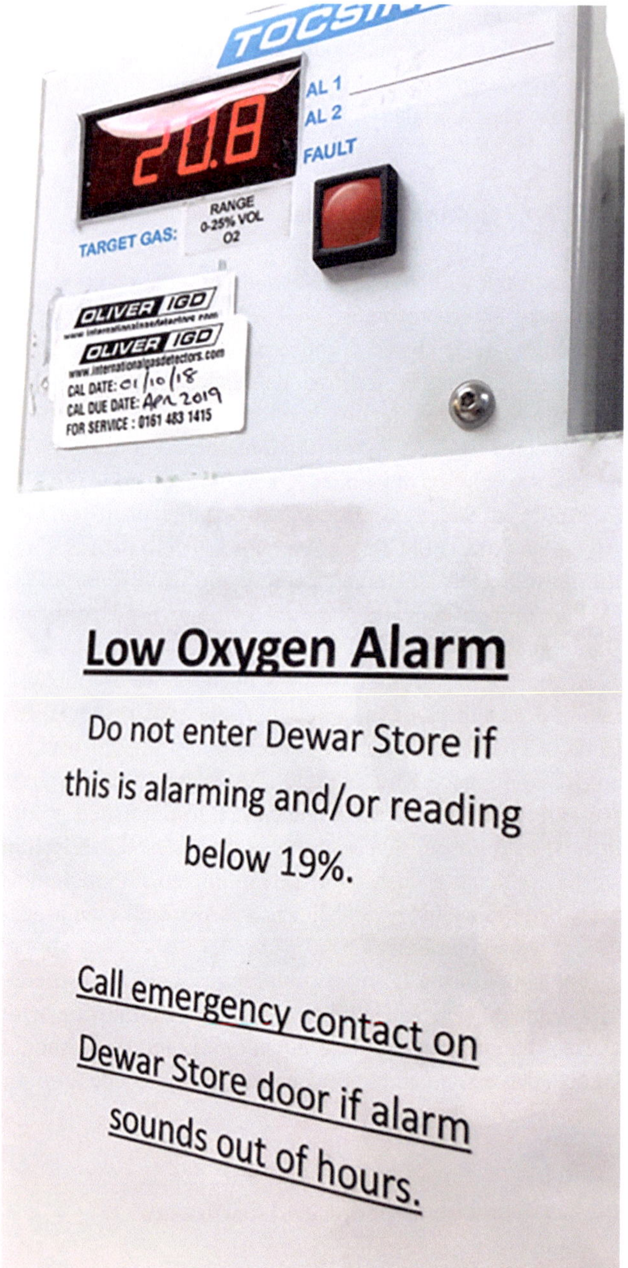

Fig. 64.2 Low oxygen alarms are essential in the cryobank to ensure staff safety. All alarms should be regularly maintained to ensure good working order, and there should be clear signage to alert staff regarding action to take if the alarm is triggered. Image courtesy of the Bristol Centre for Reproductive Medicine, Bristol, UK

- Email addresses, with a corresponding agreement relating to the possible risks of communication by this method

Statutory consent forms should be completed as required, prior to sample production. Local contracts should also be in place to reinforce any local terms and conditions associated with the storage of samples at that cryobank, including terms relating to storage charges. A local contract ensures the responsibilities of each party are clear from the beginning of the storage period. This not only helps to protect the clinic in the event of unforeseen circumstances but also helps to ensure that patients have been properly informed of their own responsibilities relating to storage periods. It is up to individual clinics to decide what the contract should entail, but it is suggested that any contract should include the following:

- The responsibilities and limitations of the clinic about the care of the samples, e.g. it may be useful to have a statement about the possibility of unforeseen circumstances which may lead to sample loss or unforeseen changes to any legislation.
- The responsibilities of the patient about remaining contactable, complying with the terms and conditions pertaining to storage and the possible consequences of not doing so, including the potential removal from the cryobank. This may or may not include the implications of non-payment of any storage charges due.

It is important to state that it is the cryobank's responsibility to ensure that the terms of the contract are lawful and compliant with any national legislation and legally binding or enforceable should the need arise. Independent legal advice should be sought regarding the drafting of any local clinic contract (Fig. 64.3).

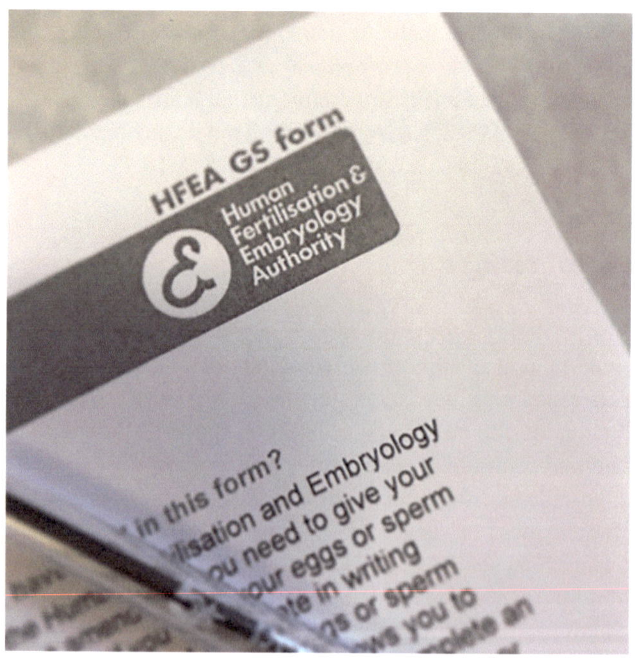

Fig. 64.3 Statutory consent forms should be completed prior to sample production. In the UK, the Human Fertilization and Embryology Authority (HFEA) provides a "Gamete Storage (GS) form" for this purpose. Image courtesy of the Bristol Centre for Reproductive Medicine, Bristol, UK

64.3.4 Sample Production, Processing and Storage

The provision of an appropriate sample production room is considered essential. Expecting a patient to use a facility not intended for sample production is unacceptable and does not represent a quality service. The production room should be in a quiet area, away from excessive noise and public areas, and should be equipped with a sink for washing, comfortable chair or bed and a lockable door. Decontamination of the room in-between patients is required and must be considered when selecting furnishings. Room size and access is also important, as some service users may be bedbound or wheelchair users.

Provision of pornography to facilitate sample production is permissible but remains a controversial topic, both from a financial and moral perspective [14]. Some consider that spending healthcare funds on pornography is wasteful. Conversely however, if a patient is unable to produce a sample without some form of stimulation, the appointment could be abandoned which is also a waste of resources, not to mention deeply distressing for the patient (Fig. 64.4).

The practicalities of providing adult material are somewhat complex. Providing material to satisfy all patient groups is difficult without causing offence. The format must satisfy infection control requirements, which precludes magazines. DVDs may be expensive and require the provision of a monitor, as well as soundproofing or headphones (which must be cleanable) to provide discretion. The provision of Internet access to allow patients to select their own material may present difficulties for the Internet provider if the patient is found to have accessed inappropriate or illegal Internet content. Thought also needs to be given to patients who may be minors and any laws surrounding child protection or the supply of adult material to minors. Each cryobank must therefore decide how to manage the provision of adult material by carefully considering the advantages and disadvantages of each option or scenario and national laws (Fig. 64.5).

Following production, samples should be processed and packaged in a manner which maximizes their future treatment potential. The number of viable sperm present in the ejaculate will inform the strategy to be used. This also needs to take into account whether the patient is able to produce further samples for storage, particularly if this is prior to the initiation of potentially fertility-reducing therapy.

Decisions regarding the sample container, cryoprotectant and cryopreservation method must also be made. Options include ampoules and straws (sealed or open), and the carrier must be labelled appropriately in accordance with local regulations, which usually include the use of several separate identifiers and in a manner which will remain functional for many years (Fig. 64.6).

Individual samples, where considered irreplaceable, should be divided and stored in separate tanks alongside samples which have been screened to an equivalent level.

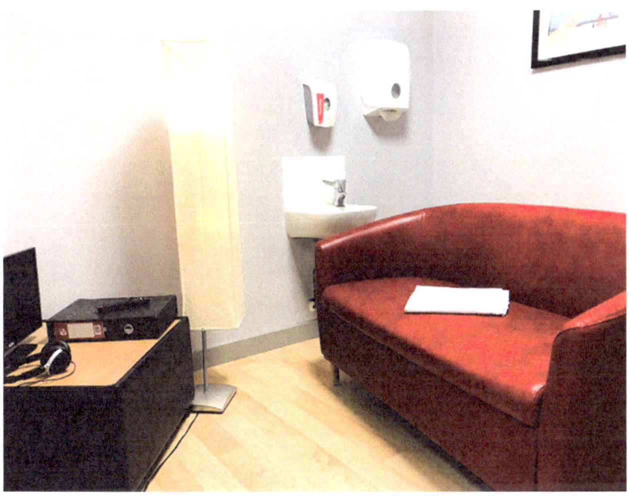

Fig. 64.4 The men's sample production room. This room should contain suitable furnishings, which are easily cleaned, a sink for washing, and a lockable door. Image courtesy of the Bristol Centre for Reproductive Medicine, Bristol, UK

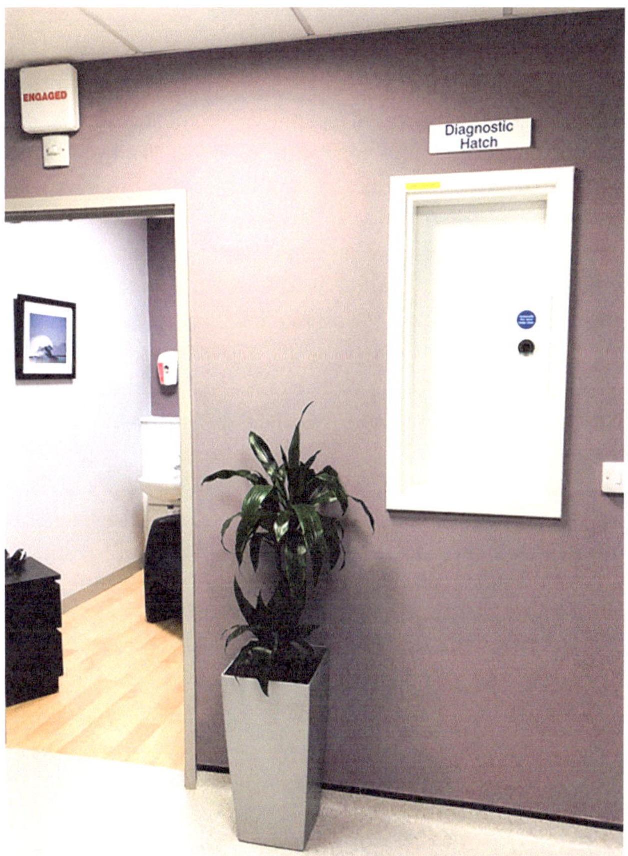

Fig. 64.5 Hatch for handing over semen samples. The hatch should be close to the production room to ensure the sample is passed to the andrologist immediately after production. Image courtesy of the Bristol Centre for Reproductive Medicine, Bristol, UK

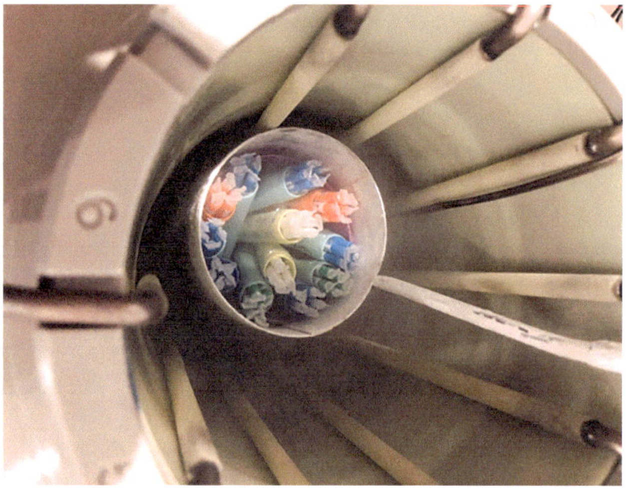

Fig. 64.6 Storing semen samples. Semen is cryopreserved in heat-sealed high security straws. Each straw is uniquely labelled and the same color straw is used for an individual patient. This helps ease of recognition when removing straws or performing audits of stored material. Image courtesy of the Bristol Centre for Reproductive Medicine, Bristol, UK

This offers protection against the risks associated with tank failure.

The choice of whether to store in vapour or liquid phase nitrogen lies with the cryobank. Liquid phase storage is simple and utilizes well-tested technology requiring little, if any, ongoing maintenance. Monitoring of levels of liquid nitrogen (LN2) is key and may allow advanced warning of tank performance deterioration. However, LN2 may be considered to have a higher risk of cross-contamination compared to vapour phase [15]. There is also an increased risk to the samples if physical audits are required, since access to LN2 tanks is usually via a narrow neck.

Vapour phase storage reduces the risk of cross-contamination, but the equipment is of higher complexity and ongoing running costs may be higher due to maintenance costs and increased LN2 use when compared to liquid phase storage. An advantage of some vapour phase storage systems is that samples may also be audited without removal from the tank, reducing handling risks.

Whichever system is chosen, a suitable reserve of LN2 should also be held locally, to protect the clinic against any supply issues which may arise.

64.3.5 Record Keeping and Management

Choosing an appropriate inventory system is imperative to allow easy access and minimize disruption and risk to other samples during audit or sample removal. The use of colour-coding helps to provide a quick visual aid, thus limiting the amount of time samples are exposed to suboptimal temperature conditions. Technology, including the use of radio frequency identification (RFID) tags on sample containers, may further enhance sample identification and audit procedures.

Creation of a computerized database from the outset is essential to ensure the smooth cryobank running. Recommended fields include:

- Patient identifiers
- Number of receptacles in storage
- Storage date
- Consent period expiry date
- Funded storage period expiry date (if applicable)
- Free text fields to allow information relevant to the ongoing management of the samples to be recorded (e.g. 'patient only contactable by email', 'patient lost to contact', 'patient now wishes to be known as…', 'patient seeking further funding'

Using this format should allow the easy generation of lists in date order to facilitate patient contact in order of priority and alert staff when a sample is approaching the consented or funding expiry date.

To assist with patient contact, it may also be useful to include fields documenting the last time communication was made or attempted. Although this information should be recorded in the patient records, it is useful to be able to view such information at a glance.

Databases should be backed up and secure, to ensure patient confidentiality is maintained. Regular housekeeping should also be carried out to ensure any data entry errors are identified and rectified. Such errors can lead to complications during audit and list generation. Historical computerised records should be reviewed regularly to ensure they are held in an easily accessible format.

64.3.6 Maintaining Contact with the Individual and Audit of Samples

Cryobanks should regularly audit stored material and associated records to confirm the purpose and duration of storage, reconcile paper and electronic records with the stored material and identify any action needed. An effective 'bring forward' system is also recommended in order to ensure regular contact takes place between the facility and the individual for whom samples are in storage.

A 'Bring Forward' System for Cryobank Management

A 'bring forward' system ensures that all samples are held within their consent period. Such a system is usually digital and allows the generation of chronological lists ensuring the cryobank is aware of impending expiry dates.

The aim of this contact is to ensure the patient's wishes remain accurately recorded and that should the end of the legal consent period be approaching, the individual has the time to make informed decisions about cryopreserved samples. For some patients, being reminded that they have sperm in storage may be a painful reminder of a time in their lives they would rather not revisit. However, failing to contact a patient for prolonged periods of time undoubtedly increases the chance that contact will not be possible.

Cryobanks in the UK are required to take 'reasonable' steps to maintain contact with patients. However, this is poorly defined and sperm banks may lose contact with patients for many reasons, including changes of address, a conscious decision by the patient to not respond or possibly because the patient has died.

Establishing a regular pattern of contact may depend on how long the patient has consented to store his samples. If the consent is for just 1 year, it may be prudent to make contact at 6 months to set out the options available. If the consent is for 10 years, annual or biennial contact may be deemed more appropriate.

Given that samples can remain in storage for many years, this part of the process generally affords an ever-increasing workload and should be staffed appropriately. Even a relatively small storage facility with one storage case a week could find themselves with up to 52 letters to write at the end of year one, but up to 520 letters by the end of a storage period of 10 years.

The management of the samples of patients lost to contact is problematical for the storing clinic and may prove to be a drain on resources and so must be carefully considered. The clinic should ensure that any decision to remove samples from storage has been carefully risk assessed and, where necessary, independent legal advice sought to clarify any potential liability on a case-by-case basis.

64.3.7 Methods of Contact

Clinics should not rely on just one method to maintain contact with individuals but should be mindful of confidentiality issues and any regulatory restrictions which may apply. Additionally, the cryobank should allow the individual sufficient time to consider options and respond.

Telephone contact is often quicker than a letter. However, the patient may not be in an appropriate location to answer the call, either due to confidentiality issues or the emotional response the call may create. Details of any attempts at telephone contact should be recorded in the patient records to ensure continuity of care and inform decision-making. This is particularly important if contact is considered to be 'lost'.

Contacting a patient by letter removes the concerns about the ability to speak without being overheard and also provides a written record from the clinic. A copy of the letter should also be included in the patient records for continuity. A drawback with written contact is its cost and reliability, as the intended recipient may not receive the letter, even where registered or signed postal services are employed.

Contact by email has also become more common in recent years. Email is fast, reliable and usually free. However, concerns arise surrounding confidentiality. Before embarking on this method of communication, both the patient and storing clinic must be aware of the potential threat to confidentiality and take the necessary steps to minimize the risks involved. Clinics should also ensure they are aware of the relevant legislation surrounding forms of contact, e.g. in Europe the EU General Data Protection Regulation was implemented in 2018 [16].

Staff should be mindful of the risk of revealing sensitive information to the wrong person, by whichever method of contact is used. Confidentiality breaches may be more likely with emails due to auto-completion functions within such services. Although a paper envelope sent through the regular post may seem less secure, there are, in some countries, laws surrounding the opening of mail by anyone other than the addressee [17]. Unfortunately, the nature of emails makes it difficult to prevent messages from being read by anyone other than the intended recipient.

Clinics must also decide where limits should be drawn regarding attempts at contact. The increasing use of social media poses an interesting dilemma in this situation. Whilst social media may offer further avenues to explore ways to achieve contact, it should be remembered that the loss of contact may have been a conscious deliberate decision by the individual.

64.3.8 Information to Provide When Making Contact

Making regular patient contact ensures that the samples continue to be stored legally and reflect the patient's latest circumstances or wishes. The following information may be included in any correspondence:

- A record of what the patient has cryobanked, including the number of storage receptacles (e.g. straw or vials)
- The original date of cryobanking
- The expiration date of the current consent period
- The expiration date of storage payment (if applicable)
- Any partner named for posthumous use
- Information detailing the options available with regard to:
  - Extending the current consent period
  - Obtaining further funding for storage or how to self-fund

- Amending or removing a named partner
- Updating contact information
- Removing the samples from storage (e.g. to allow to perish)
- Making any other changes to the current consent

It is important to ensure the information is given clearly and concisely to aid understanding and compliance. It may be practical to provide a short questionnaire with a return envelope allowing patients to indicate their wishes quickly and easily.

64.3.9 Dealing with Non-compliance

Despite all attempts to have the correct systems in place, unfortunately cryobank-patient communication may, on occasion, break down. For the cryobank, storage of samples outside of the consented period may constitute a criminal offence and lead to prosecution or revocation of the facilities licence. However, disposal of a potentially irreplaceable, precious sample should never be carried out nonchalantly. Rather, each disposal should be risk assessed on a case-by-case basis. The cryobank must be confident that, should contact be lost and a decision taken to remove samples from storage, it could confidently state that it had been reasonable in its endeavours to make contact and in allowing the individual sufficient time to respond. Evidence of all attempts at communication, and the risk assessment, should be kept in the patient's notes.

64.3.10 Removal from Storage and Disposal Protocols

Robust, locally approved procedures for the ethical disposal of samples identified for removal from the cryobank should be in place, including the double witnessing of all paperwork and permissions associated with the case to ensure the removal from storage is appropriate.

64.4 Legal and Ethical Considerations

International regulations pertaining to cryobanking vary considerably, ranging from an absence of any national laws to detailed legislation. Legal and ethical issues relating to cryobanking include adequate documentation of consent and ownership issues. Furthermore, given that sperm can essentially be cryobanked indefinitely, this theoretically allows genetic offspring to be conceived long after the sperm provider's death, and issues surrounding the posthumous use of stored samples need to be considered. The latter may be considered to be the area which gives rise to the most complex issues.

It is beyond the scope of this chapter to examine in detail the legal, ethical and moral issues which arise because of sperm banking. Therefore, it is recommended that readers seek more specific guidance concerning the legal framework applicable to their specific circumstances.

64.4.1 Consent

In many countries, consent must be provided in writing. This should give clear detail of the sperm provider's wishes in the event of death or mental incapacitation. Individuals consenting to cryobanking should be offered counselling about the nature of the consent given, as it may have serious consequences for both their own and their partner's reproductive future. Regarding consent relating to posthumous use, this cannot be changed after the sperm provider's death. Should the patient find it difficult, or be unwilling, to provide consent relating to anything beyond the initial storage of the samples, it must be clearly explained to the patient that this may restrict the ability for the sperm to be used for future treatment should circumstances change.

64.4.2 Posthumous Collection and Posthumous Use of Stored Sperm

It is now accepted that viable sperm, capable of resulting in pregnancy and live birth, may be retrieved and stored for later use following a man's death, provided the sperm are retrieved within a limited period after death. However, legislation regarding posthumous collection varies greatly between countries: in some places it remains illegal, whilst other countries have no specific legislation. Currently, requests for posthumous sperm collection remain rare, and it is far more common for sperm banked prior to the gamete provider's death to lead to requests for posthumous use. Complex issues arise from the ability to use sperm collected posthumously and include considerations of ownership, legal parentage and inheritance.

64.4.3 Notable Legal Cases

Problems with sperm banking have resulted in legal cases, related to the collection and storage of sperm, or the use (including posthumous) of stored sperm [18–22]. These generally centre on the following issues:

- The failure to obtain or accurately record consent prior to surgical retrieval or storage
- Lack of competence of the practitioner and clinic when taking and recording consent

- Failure of the storage facility
- Ambiguous ownership of samples following the death of the provider

It is clear from the judgements in these cases, that it is of paramount importance to document the consent of the gamete provider in detail. Furthermore, evidence must be available to demonstrate that the person who sperm was cryobanked was given the correct information to allow informed consent. Covering both of these issues reduces the likelihood of any legal challenge regarding their samples in the event of death or mental incapacity.

64.5 Conclusion

The successful delivery of any cryobanking service, and the subsequent management of samples held in storage, requires a harmonious relationship between the patient, the cryobank and the legal framework in place under which the facility operates.

At best, the consequences of a poorly run system could, for the cryobank, result in financial penalty and/or reputational damage. At worst, it could result in licence revocation and potentially lead to its suspension or closure. For the patient, a poor sperm banking service could lead to an inadvertent reduction in sample viability, an inability to use the samples in the manner intended or possibly the loss of irreplaceable samples. Such incidents could lead to lifelong psychological damage, for which there is no comparable compensation.

Such risks can be significantly reduced by ensuring consideration is given to all aspects of a sperm storage service. Attention to detail can help to ensure the provision of a high-quality service and the best possible patient experience.

References

1. Gillick v West Norfolk and Wisbech Area Health Authority. 1985. 2 All ER 402.
2. Warren v Care Fertility (Northampton) Ltd & Anor. 2014. EWHC 602 (Fam) (sperm storage linked to payment).
3. Case V (Human Fertilisation and Embryology Act 2008). 2016. EWHC 2356 (Fam) (legal parenting).
4. HFEA 2008 (Cases A, B, C, D, E, F, G and H Declaration of Parentage). 2015. EWHC 2602 (Fam) (legal parenting).
5. Human Fertilisation and Embryology Authority (HFEA). Chairs Letter (CH15 (01): April update to the Code of Practice and consent forms [Online]. 2015. Available at https://portal.hfea.gov.uk/knowledge-base/chairs-letters/916. Accessed 3 May 2019.
6. Human Fertilisation and Embryology Authority (HFEA). Consent workshop summary report: November 2014. [Online]. 2014. Available at https://ifqlive.blob.core.windows.net/umbraco-portal/1131/consent_workshop_report.pdf. Accessed 3 May 2019.
7. Tomlinson MJ, Harbottle SJ, Woodward BJ, Lindsay KS, Association of Biomedical Andrologists, et al. Hum Fertil. 2012;15(4):156–73.
8. Hughes C, Association of Clinical Embryologists. Association of clinical embryologists – guidelines on good practice in clinical embryology laboratories 2012. Hum Fertil. 2012 Dec;15(4):174–89.
9. Ethics Committee of American Society for Reproductive Medicine. Fertility preservation and reproduction in patients facing gonadotoxic therapies: a committee opinion. Fertil Steril. 2013;100:1224–31.
10. Loren AW, Mangu PB, Beck LN, Brennan L, Magdalinski AJ, Partridge AH, Quinn G, Wallace WH, Oktay K, American Society of Clinical Oncology. Fertility preservation for patients with cancer: American Society of Clinical Oncology clinical practice guideline update. J Clin Oncol. 2013 Jul 1;31(19):2500–10.
11. De los Santos MJ, et al. Revised guidelines for good practice in IVF laboratories (2015). ESHRE Guideline Group on Good Practice in IVF Labs. Hum Reprod. 2016;31(4):685–6.
12. National Institute for Health and Clinical Excellence (NICE). Fertility problems: assessment and treatment Clinical Guidelines [CG156, 1.16]. 2013. [Online].Available at https://www.nice.org.uk/guidance/cg156/chapter/Recommendations#people-with-cancer-who-wish-to-preserve-fertility. Accessed 3 May 2019
13. Human Fertilisation and Embryology Authority (HFEA) 9th Code of Practice, 2019. [Online]. Available at https://www.hfea.gov.uk/media/2793/2019-01-03-code-of-practice-9th-edition-v2.pdf. Accessed 3 May 2019
14. Manning, J. Who said pornography was acceptable in the workplace? 2020Health.org. 2010. Available at http://www.2020health.org/2020health/Publications/Publications-2010/porn.html. Accessed 3 May 2019.
15. Tedder RS, et al. Hepatitis B transmission from contaminated cryopreservation tank. Lancet. 1995 Jul 15;346(8968):137–40.
16. European Parliament and Council of the European Union. The General Data Protection Regulation 2016/679.
17. Postal Services Act, 2000. (C.26), UK.
18. Human Fertilisation and Embryology Authority Ex p. Blood, R v. 1997. CA.
19. Mrs U v Centre for Reproductive Medicine. 2002. EWCA Civ 565.
20. Yearworth v. North Bristol NHS Trust. 2009. EWCA Civ 37.
21. Edwards J. Re the estate of the late Mark Edwards. 2011. NSWSC 478.
22. Bazley v Wesley Monash IVF Pty Ltd. QSC 118; 2 Qd R 207 (10/2731) White J. 2010. Accessed 21 Apr 2010.

65 Managing an Embryo Cryobank

Eleanor Taylor

With increasing acceptance of elective single embryo transfer (eSET), it is now commonplace for supernumerary in vitro embryos to be created during a single-assisted conception treatment cycle with superovulation and IVF treatment [1]. It has therefore become important for fertility clinics to invest in a successful embryo cryopreservation programme. Indeed, the ability to successfully cryopreserve embryos allows clinics to tailor each treatment cycles to meet the unique needs of patients. For example, a fresh embryo transfer may not be the most appropriate course of action for every patient, and cryopreservation offers the opportunity to have a single embryo replaced at a more conducive time [2].

A well-organised, optimal-functioning cryobank is therefore essential. Consideration should be paid to the design and the layout of the cryobank. Good design can minimise the health and safety risks associated with using liquid nitrogen (LN2) and can also support the safe handling of cryopreserved embryos within the facility.

The importance of providing high-quality staff training cannot be understated. Poor-quality staff training will lead to poor quality clinical activity, which will ultimately be to the detriment of the patient. Risk assessments should be performed for all cryobank activities, and appropriate SOPs should be developed for staff members to follow. Inadequate staff training will not only have a negative impact on service provision but will also increase the risk of a work-place incident occurring. Clinical incidents involving cryopreserved samples generally have devastating consequences, and every effort should be made to minimise the risk of such an incident occurring [3].

Ultimately, it is the duty of the clinic to ensure that every sample within the cryobank is stored safely with full traceability. When an adverse clinical event does occur, the contributing factors should be identified, and measures put in place to reduce the risk of a similar incident occurring in the future. Clinics should continuously strive to improve their services by performing procedural audits to assess whether appropriate standards are being met and whether improvements can be made. This chapter explores all aspects of the embryo cryobank, from the initial design through to the daily management.

65.1 Cryobank Design

The cryobank should be designed to support the safe and efficient handling of the clinic's cryopreserved material and consideration should be given to the regulatory legislation that the clinic must adhere to. The cryobank should be of a sufficient size to accommodate:

- Storage tanks (LN2-based vessels or vapour phase vessels in which to store cryopreserved gametes and embryos)
- Bulk LN2 vessels (used as a source of LN2 for cryopreservation activities and for maintaining LN2 levels within the storage tanks)
- Controlled-rate freezers (if required)
- Personal protective equipment (PPE)
- Equipment used for the handling of LN2 and/or the handling of cryopreserved samples
- Work space for handling cryopreserved samples and processing laboratory paperwork

65.1.1 Number of Storage Tanks

The following factors will influence the required storage capacity of the cryobank:

- The number of treatment cycles performed
- The clinic's embryo cryopreservation policy

E. Taylor (✉)
The Hewitt Fertility Centre, Liverpool Women's NHS Foundation Trust, Liverpool, UK
e-mail: Eleanor.Taylor@lwh.nhs.uk

G. N. Allahbadia et al. (eds.), *Textbook of Assisted Reproduction*, https://doi.org/10.1007/978-981-15-2377-9_65

- The storage capacity of each tank
- Whether the clinic treats patients with a known viral infection as these will require separate 'viral-positive' storage tanks

It is recommended that clinics should also have a 'reserve' storage tank for use in emergency situations. This tank should be kept filled with LN2 in a 'ready-to-use' state in case there is a suspected storage tank failure.

65.1.2 Bulk LN2 Vessels

Some clinics may have the opportunity to store their bulk LN2 vessels externally to the cryobank and install pipework to connect the LN2 supply to a dispensing device in the clinical area. The length of the connecting pipes is often a limiting factor as to whether this is a viable option for the clinic. As pipe length increases, so does the time and volume of LN2 required to prime the temperature of the pipework prior to LN2 dispensation in the cryobank, which may not be cost-effective (Fig. 65.1).

Some clinics may opt to install a generator to produce LN2 on-site to reduce their reliance on LN2 deliveries. LN2 generators can also be used to generate N2 gas for use in low oxygen incubators. However, the initial cost of installing the generator can be prohibitively expensive.

For deliveries of LN2, bulk vessels should be easily accessed by the LN2 supply company. If the vessels need to be moved in order to be filled, a manual handling risk assessment and appropriate training should be performed (Fig. 65.2). Where vessel movement requires use of an elevator, it is important that safety measures are put in place to ensure that the elevator is never accessed by anybody else, including the general public, when LN2 tanks are being transported.

It is recommended that a working third party agreement is established between the clinic and the LN2 supply company to specify the frequency of the deliveries. Specific plans should be made regarding delivery schedules over public holidays to ensure that the clinic never runs out of LN2. The clinic should also have a contingency plan in place for unexpected events such as a missed delivery due to unforeseen circumstances, e.g. adverse weather. Laboratory staff should have a checking system in place to confirm that each expected delivery has arrived.

65.1.3 Flooring

The cryobank floor should be made from a LN2-resistant material. Flooring which has not been specifically designed to withstand the low temperatures (e.g. lino or PVC covering) may crack over time, creating trip hazards or compromising the structural integrity of the floor.

65.1.4 Oxygen Monitoring

LN2 is converted into nitrogen gas at temperatures above −196 °C. Since nitrogen displaces oxygen from the atmosphere, the use of LN2 within the restricted space of a cryobank could potentially create an oxygen-deficient environment. Due to the asphyxiation risk, appropriate safety measures should be incorporated.

All areas within the cryobank should be well-ventilated and fitted with low oxygen sensors (Fig. 65.3), at a height of around 1 m from the floor. The sensors activate an audio-

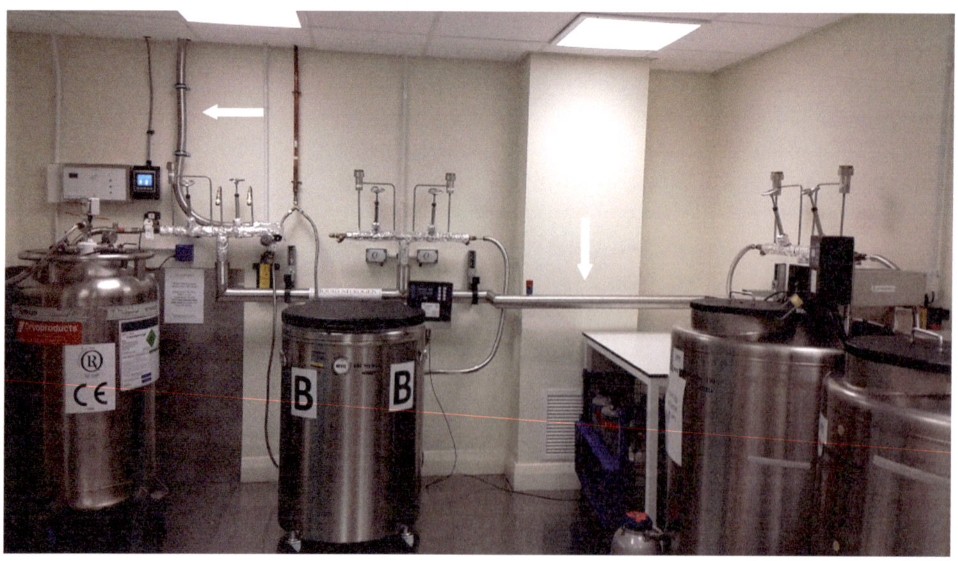

Fig. 65.1 Cryobank pipework. The arrows indicate the pipework required to connect an external LN2 source to multiple vapour phase storage tanks within the cryobank. (Image courtesy of the Knutsford Hewitt Fertility Centre, Liverpool Women's NHS Foundation Trust, Liverpool, UK)

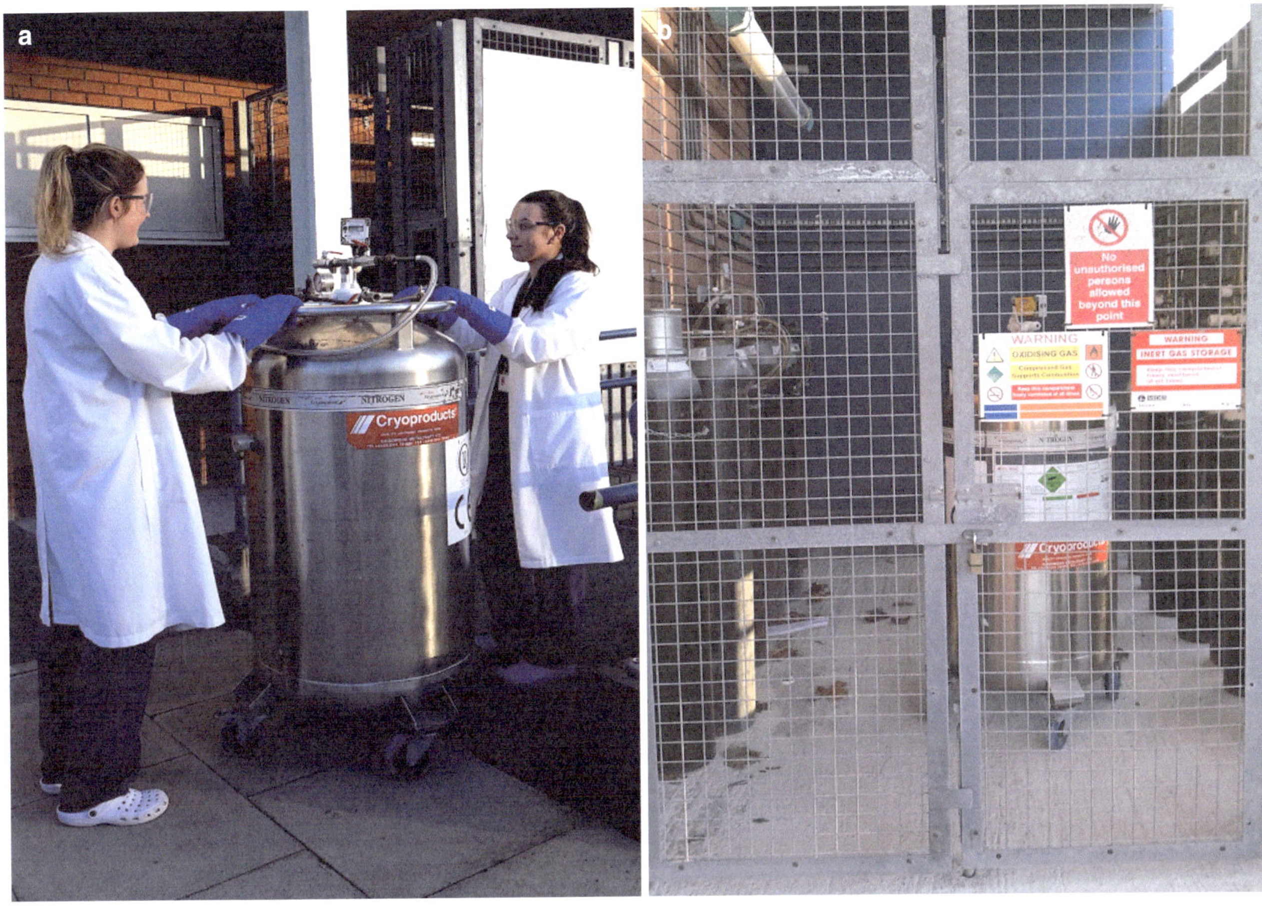

Fig. 65.2 (**a**) Clinic staff moving a bulk LN2 tank between the cryobank and a secure outdoor storage area (**b**) which can be accessed by the LN2 supply company. (Courtesy of the Knutsford Hewitt Fertility Centre, Liverpool Women's NHS Foundation Trust, Liverpool, UK)

visual alarm system at two different oxygen concentrations: an initial alarm activates at an oxygen level of 19.5% and a further alarm activates at an oxygen concentration of 18% (this varies according to the device).

The alarm system should be linked to an extraction system to help restore the oxygen concentration within the cryobank. Any staff must exit the cryobank if an oxygen alarm activates and not re-enter the room until the alarm ceases. Portable oxygen sensors can be used, but caution is advised as staff may fail to realise that they are entering an oxygen-deficient environment and collapse before their personal alarm is activated.

65.1.5 Servicing of Equipment

All equipment within the cryobank needs to be serviced regularly to reduce the risk of unexpected equipment failure. Servicing should only be performed by qualified individuals, and all service reports should be retained by the clinic.

65.1.6 Cryobank Security

Sample security is of the upmost importance and access to the cryopreserved samples should be strictly limited to laboratory personnel. This can be achieved by employing a fob/key card or locked entry system to prevent unauthorised individuals from entering the cryobank. Each storage tank within the cryobank should also be secured with a separate padlock to prevent inappropriate access to the stored material (Fig. 65.4).

65.1.7 Storage Tank Management

LN2-based storage tanks are typically favoured for the storage of cryopreserved oocytes and embryos (Fig. 65.5a). The use of LN2 creates an internal core temperature of −196 °C which is uniformly maintained throughout the tank.

Nevertheless, some clinics may opt to store their cryopreserved samples within a vapour phase vessel (Fig. 65.5b) at a temperature between −180 °C and −190 °C. However, the

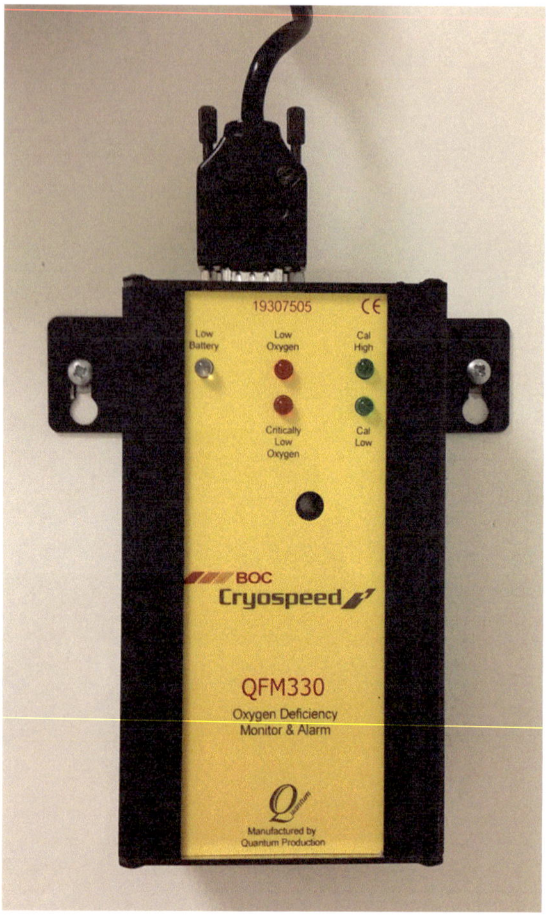

Fig. 65.3 An example of an oxygen monitoring device that can be used within the cryobank to detect low atmospheric oxygen. (Courtesy of the Knutsford Hewitt Fertility Centre, Liverpool Women's NHS Foundation Trust, Liverpool, UK)

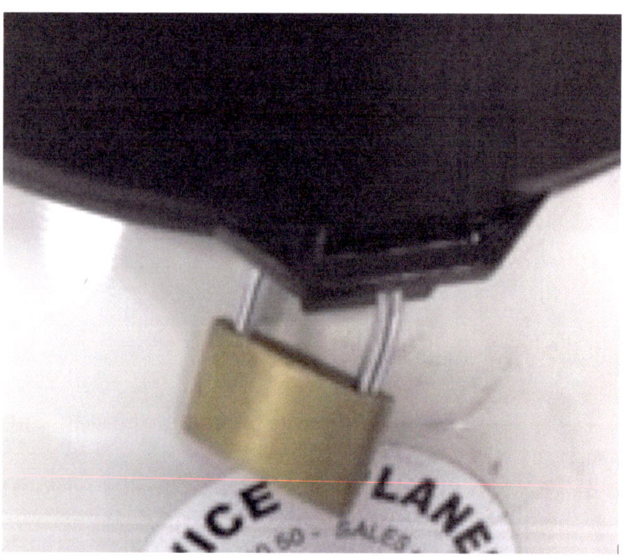

Fig. 65.4 Liquid nitrogen tanks should be securely locked to prevent inappropriate access to the stored material (Image courtesy of the Assisted Conception Service, Glasgow Royal Infirmary, Glasgow, UK)

potential for vertical temperature gradients to form within the vessel should be considered. Vapour phase vessels also require a power source to run their auto-fill function. As such, a back-up generator should be available to support the functioning in the event of a power outage. Vitrified embryos are particularly susceptible to temperature fluctuations, and sample viability may be compromised if the storage vessel temperature fluctuates above −150 °C.

Monitoring the temperature of the storage tanks is critical, as warming (e.g. via an accident, physical damage or poor practice) could have devastating consequences, with perhaps loss of irreplaceable samples for hundreds of patients.

It is recommended that all storage tanks are fitted with devices that continuously record the internal tank temperatures, either directly with a temperature probe or indirectly with a device that monitors the tank weight. Monitoring devices are activated if the temperature of the storage tank deviates outside of the acceptable working range. This triggers an alarm system to alert staff so that any deviation in vessel temperature can be quickly resolved. A robust out-of-hours on-call system should be in place so that staff can cover emergency call-out procedures, e.g. if all samples need to be moved from a faulty tank to the reserve tank as quickly as possible.

If alarms are triggered, it is important to establish the root cause. Some alarms may be 'false' and may result from the improper functioning of the probe. By contrast, a 'true' alarm may result from an insufficient LN2 reserve within the tank and could be quickly remedied by adding more LN2 to the vessel. However, if the tank temperature cannot be stabilised by manually increasing the LN2 level, cryopreserved samples should be transferred to another tank as soon as possible, as the vacuum of the storage vessel could be compromised.

It is important that safety measures are observed when dealing with a tank with a suspected vacuum failure. The cryobank should not be entered if the low oxygen alarm is active and one working in the cryobank is not acceptable out of hours.

Clinics are recommended to follow rigid schedules for maintaining LN2 levels to reduce the risk of the cryopreserved samples becoming damaged through the unexpected warming. Rather than allowing LN2 levels to fall dangerously low prior to filling, there should be a comfortable margin built into the tank filling schedule to accommodate unexpected delays, such as a missed LN2 delivery.

Care should be taken when moving the tanks within the cryobank. Impact-based damage to the storage vessel could compromise the vacuum surrounding the core, which in turn could result in vessel warming. The presence of 'cold spots' or ice on the outer shell of a storage tank is indicative of a failing vacuum. The simplest and safest way to move tanks is

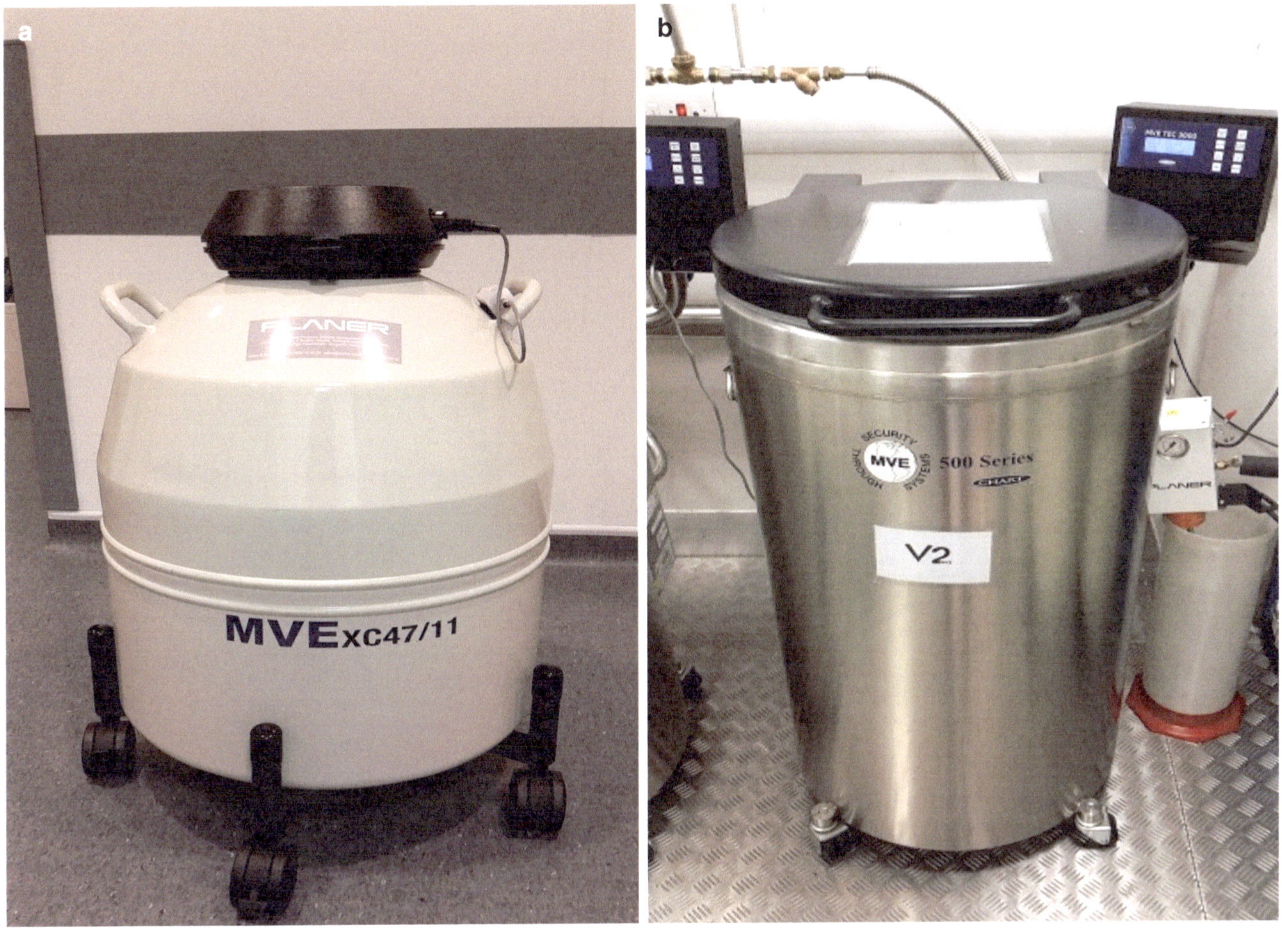

Fig. 65.5 (**a**) Example of a liquid-nitrogen based storage tank. (**b**) Example of vapour phase storage tank. (Courtesy of the Assisted Conception Service, Glasgow Royal Infirmary, Glasgow, UK)

by mounting them on movable bases with lockable wheels. However, all movement should be carefully undertaken.

65.1.8 Staff Training

Since working with LN2 poses a serious safety risk, training should be provided for all staff that could be at risk of direct or indirect exposure to LN2. Staff should understand about the hazardous properties of cryogenic liquids, the measures to take to protect themselves from LN2-associated injuries, and the action to take in the event of an injury or in an emergency.

Direct contact with LN2, or non-insulated equipment that has been exposed to LN2, can result in cryogenic burns. Personal protective equipment (PPE) should therefore be available for use within the cryobank and staff should be trained in how to use this equipment appropriately (Fig. 65.6). A face visors or goggles should be used for eye protection from LN2 splashes. Non-absorbent, insulated gloves should be used to protect the hands and protective aprons to protect the torso. LN2 will rapidly penetrate porous material due to its low viscosity, and as such, non-specialised clothing will not provide sufficient protection against cryogenic burns. Footwear should not contain holes, and trousers should not be tucked into boots to protect the feet from LN2 exposure. All personnel should understand the first aid procedures that should be followed if a cryogenic burn is sustained.

65.2 Managing the Storage of Cryopreserved Embryos

65.2.1 Obtaining Patient Consent

Prior to any cryopreservation, it is important to confirm if the patient has consented for cryopreservation to take place. Some patients may not want embryo cryopreservation if they do not wish to embark on any further treatment or object on ethical grounds. Patients that do consent to embryo cryopreservation may have specific requests. For example, some patients may only consent to cryopreservation of pronuclear-stage embryos,

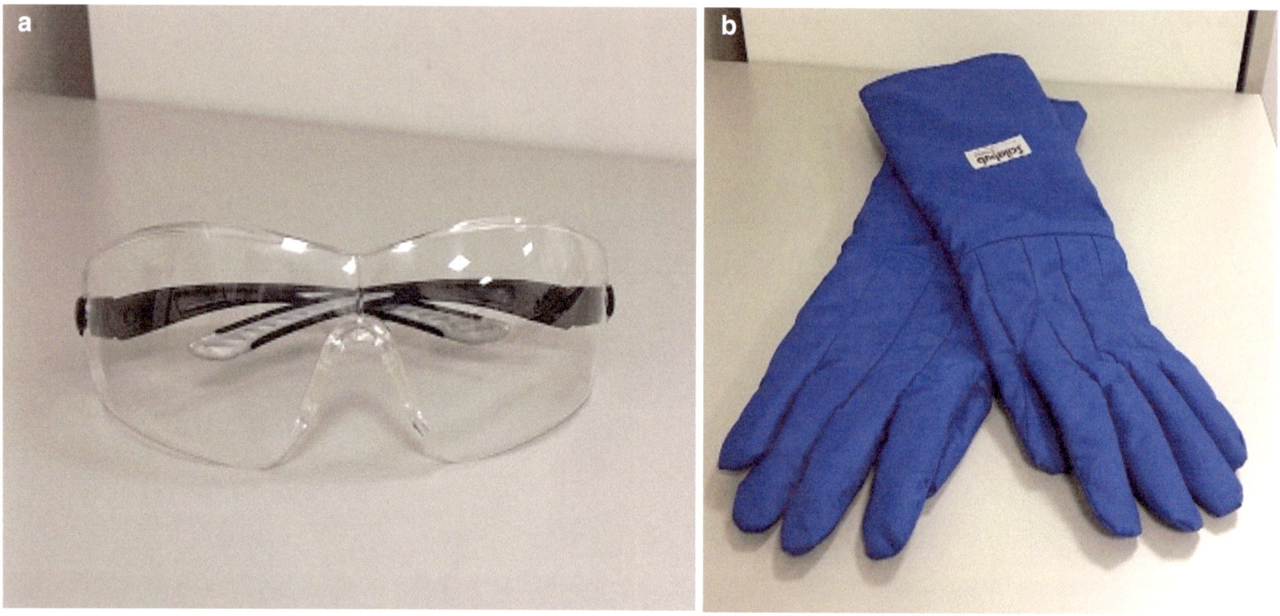

Fig. 65.6 Examples of Personal Protective Equipment (PPE) for use with LN2 and cryopreserved material. (**a**) Protective Glasses. (**b**) Insulated gloves. (Courtesy of the Assisted Conception Service, Glasgow Royal Infirmary, Glasgow, UK)

and/or some patients may wish to place a limit on the length of time that their embryos are kept in storage.

All patients should be informed of the risks associated with embryo cryopreservation, the responsibilities of both the clinic and the patient during embryo storage and any regulatory limitations. It should be made clear if there are fees associated with embryo storage and what action will be taken by the clinic if this fee is not paid or if the clinic is unable to contact the patient.

Obtaining patient consent in a written format is considered best practice. Verbal information may be misinterpreted or inaccurately recorded. Retaining a copy of the patient's written treatment consent may also help to resolve any complaints or legal disputes that occur following treatment.

All patients should have the opportunity to update their storage consent should their wishes change. It is important that measures are put in places to ensure that any consent changes are rapidly communicated to the laboratory staff so that appropriate action can be implemented immediately.

65.2.2 Selecting an Embryo Storage Device

There are many different types of embryo storage device that are commercially available for clinical use. A number of factors relating to cryobank management should be considered when first choosing a storage device:

- The dimensions of the storage device and the number of embryos that can be stored per storage tank.
- The number of storage tanks that the cryobank can accommodate.
- Whether the storage device is available in different colours to facilitate the patient identification.
- The ease with which patient identification information present on the storage device can be visualised.
- The ease with which the storage device can be removed from the storage tank.
- The robustness of the storage device.

65.2.3 Labelling the Embryo Storage Device

Embryo traceability is of paramount importance within the cryobank. Use of a comprehensive system for labelling storage devices will facilitate embryo traceability and minimise the risk of mistakes occurring when cryopreserved samples are removed from storage.

Best practice dictates that storage devices should be labelled with three patient identifiers, one of which should be a unique identifier. This is usually achieved by including the patient's name, date of birth and unique clinic number on the device label. The process of locating the correct embryo within the cryobank can be performed with accuracy if the device label also includes the date of the cryopreservation procedure, a unique storage device number and the number and developmental stage of the embryo(s) stored.

The numbering of storage devices is essential for embryos that are undergoing pre-implantation genetic testing (PGT). Embryos that are diagnosed as genetically suitable for transfer need to be located with absolute accuracy.

Device labelling can be performed manually using marker pens with indelible ink or with an automated label maker. Where handwritten labels are to be used, it is important that the transcribed information is legible and that an appropriate ink source is utilised so that the labels can withstand a prolonged period of exposure to LN2 or LN2 vapour. For automated labels, it is important to use an appropriate font size to ensure that the label information can be read quickly and easily. All labels need to be firmly fixed to the storage device to prevent the patient identifying information from being lost during storage.

The labelling of the storage device is a key step in establishing embryo traceability, and all labels should be checked by two members of staff before use to identify any inaccuracies. Where an automated labelling device has been used, it is recommended that an additional 'reference' label is printed and attached to the patient record.

65.2.4 Adding Embryos to the Cryobank

Storage tanks can be segregated into specific locations within the cryobank according to the tank type and contents. Typical storage arrangements involve the use of numbered canisters or racks which are subdivided into goblets, canes and/or visotubes (Fig. 65.7). All storage locations within the tank should be identifiable without any ambiguity.

Two staff members should be present when placing samples into storage. One staff member should physically move the cryopreserved embryo(s) from the holding location into the tank, with the second member of staff acting as a witness for the procedure. The second staff member can then verify that the embryo has been moved into the desired location and confirm that the correct storage location has been recorded on the patient record. This is important since errors that occur when recording the final storage location can create difficulties in the future. For example, entire storage tanks may need to be searched to locate an embryo, which can be time-consuming and place the samples stored within the tank at unnecessary risk.

Oocytes or embryos that have been stored for fertility preservation reasons should be split evenly between two storage tanks; this mitigates the risk that such patients could lose all cryopreserved material in the event of a catastrophic storage tank failure. Whilst the method of 'splitting samples' can be used for all cryopreserved embryos, clinics may prefer to store all of the embryos for 'low-risk' patients in a single location.

All patients should undergo viral screening prior to assisted conception treatment. Clinics that offer treatment to patients that test positive for HIV, hepatitis B (HBV) and/or hepatitis C (HCV) should ensure that any cryopreserved embryos derived from 'viral positive' gametes are stored separately from embryos created for patients with 'viral negative' screening results. Cross-contamination is

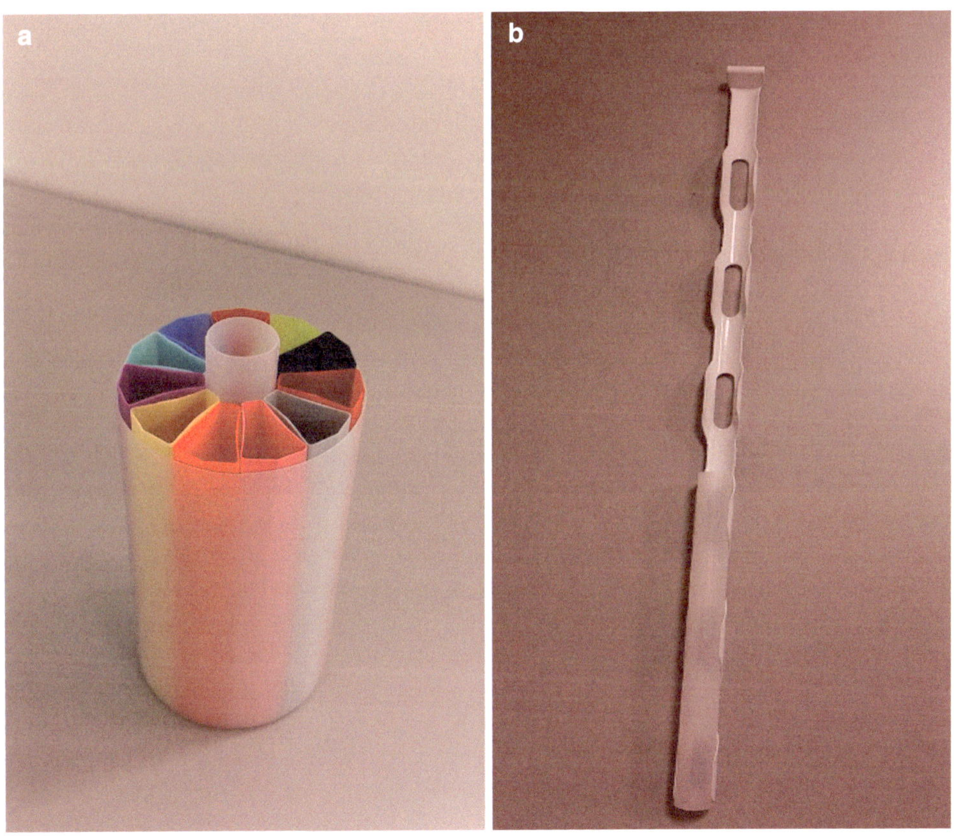

Fig. 65.7 Examples of storage device holders for use within a storage tank. (**a**) A storage goblet containing 12 storage locations (11 triangular surrounding 1 circular) of differing colour. (**b**) A single visotube attached to a cane. (Courtesy of the Assisted Conception Service, Glasgow Royal Infirmary, Glasgow, UK)

theoretically possible, even though no incidents of disease transmission between cryopreserved embryos have been reported to date, and the probability is extremely low. At least three separate storage tanks should therefore be available for viral positive samples: one for HIV-positive samples, one for HBV-positive samples and one for HCV-positive samples. Smaller storage tanks may also be required to house samples from patients that test positive for more than one virus.

65.2.5 Removal of Embryos from Storage

Whilst many patients opt to use their cryopreserved embryos, some patients may request that their embryos are removed from storage and allowed to perish, donated to another individual/couple requiring fertility treatment or donated to licenced research.

At the time of removal, two members of the laboratory team should perform an identity check. The identifying details on the patient record should be crossed-checked against the storage inventory and the patient identifying information on the storage device. The embryo(s) should only be removed after these checks have taken place.

The storage inventory system should be updated after embryo removal. It is recommended that one team member is responsible for this task. Periodic storage audits will also help to identify any problems linked to embryo removal. Due to the devastating consequences that misidentification errors can produce, it is recommended that such audits take place at least annually.

Whilst many patients maintain good communication with the clinic, some patients need to be prompted to specify what their intentions are for their stored embryos, and unfortunately some patients will lose contact with the clinic altogether. The latter situation may occur more frequently if the cost of storing the embryos is covered by a third party, such as a national healthcare system or an insurance company. The risk of losing contact with a patient also increases with the length of the time that the embryos have been kept in storage [4]. Annually sending out letters to patients reduces the ris of loss of patient contact; this letter should inform the patient of their treatment options and remind the patient to update the clinic should they change their address. It is recommended that copies of all letters are filed in the patient's clinical notes as a record of the clinic's attempt to contact them.

National regulatory bodies may stipulate the maximum length of time that a clinic can keep an embryo in storage, e.g. the HFEA has a limit of 10 years in the UK, unless the patient is storing embryos for fertility preservation purposes. Patients can also request a reduced length of storage.

65.2.5.1 A Bring-Forward System for Embryos in Storage

Each clinic should have a process in place to identify embryos that are due to reach the end of their storage period: this is known as a 'bring-forward' system.

This can be achieved via an electronic database which sorts the cryobank contents by storage expiry date. Patients should be informed of the upcoming storage expiry date and provided with options for the fate of their stored embryos, e.g. use in personal treatment, removal or donation. Due to the varying length in time it takes to prepare a patient for treatment, it can be beneficial to contact the patient 12 months prior to the expiry date to ensure that any requested treatment can be performed before the embryos need to be remove from storage in line with regulatory legislation.

Failure of the clinic to identify embryos that are due to 'expire' may result in embryos being kept in storage after their legal expiry date. This could result in patients being unable to use their stored embryos in treatment and potentially the suspension/revocation of the clinic's treatment licence! It is therefore important that a robust system for monitoring embryo storage expiry dates is developed and maintained.

65.2.5.2 Managing the Cryobank in the Future

As ART success rates improve, clinics should invest in developing an efficient cryobank management system from the outset. The size of the team responsible for managing the contents of the cryobank should be large enough to ensure that:

- All embryos due to reach their storage expiry are identified approximately 12 months in advance
- Patients are contacted about the upcoming storage expiry date of their embryos in a timely manner
- Patients have sufficient time to decide how they wish their stored embryos to be used and to have the opportunity to undergo treatment if desired
- Appropriate measures are taken to contact 'lost' patients
- Embryos are removed from storage promptly at the point of storage expiry

Clinics also need to have specific protocols in place to define how cryopreserved embryos should be managed if (a) a couple separate, (b) a couple differ in their wishes for the fate of their frozen embryo(s) and (c) the clinic is notified that a patient has died.

Typically, an embryo should only be used in treatment if both members of a couple agree to the treatment; however, this situation can become more complicated if donor gametes were used to create the embryo. Distressing situations can also occur if embryos were created for fertility preservation reasons and the couple subsequently separate. In the UK, the HFEA recommends a 1-year 'cooling off' period for couples who disagree on the fate of their cryopreserved embryos in the hope that over time a resolution will be achieved. If a decision has not been agreed by the end of the 'cooling off' period, the embryos should be removed from storage and allowed to perish. The cryopreserved embryos of a deceased patient should only remain in storage if the patient had explicitly consented to their posthumous use.

Where embryos are to be removed from storage and allowed to perish, a formal procedure should be in place to ensure this act is performed in a respectful manner. Some patients may request that their embryos receive some form of funeral, and clinics should work with these patients to formulate a procedure that meets both the legal requirements and patient wishes. Clinic staff should keep in mind that couples can equate removal of embryos from a cryobank as a form of child abandonment [5].

65.3 Storage Audit

The cryopreserved embryos stored within the cryobank should be audited periodically to confirm that the electronic and/or paper storage records accurately reflect the physical contents of the storage tanks. This allows the clinic to determine whether their SOPs for adding to and removal from the cryobank are appropriate and being followed. Any discrepancies that are identified should be corrected wherever possible and investigated to determine the root cause.

Different national regulations often specify how often an audit should be performed. For example, the HFEA states that all licenced fertility clinics in the UK should perform a storage audit at least once every 2 years. However, the performance of a full storage audit can be extremely time-consuming. Some large-scale clinics may decide to audit a proportion of their cryopreserved samples in the first instance and only expand to performing a full audit if there are discrepancies that indicate that it would be of benefit to do so.

Two staff members should perform the physical audit, with the first leading the audit and the second acting as a witness. Training is important for handling cryopreserved samples during the physical audit. Cryopreserved embryos are extremely sensitive to fluctuations in temperature. Staff members must therefore endeavour to protect the cryopreserved material from undergoing uncontrolled thawing/warming during the physical audit, which might compromise future embryo viability. Extra care should be taken when handling vitrified embryos, since the small volume of media that embryos are vitrified in renders them more susceptible to temperature fluctuations than slow-frozen embryos.

65.3.1 Performing a Physical Audit

An example of a successful audit procedure is described below:

1. Collect the clinical case notes for all patients that have cryopreserved embryos stored within the same location of a storage tank, i.e. the same canister.
2. Cross-check the freeze paperwork stored in the patient's clinical case notes against the electronic storage database and/or the inventory paperwork for the storage tank. Check the following details for any discrepancies:
   (a) Patient name
   (b) Patient date of birth
   (c) Clinic registration number
   (d) The number of embryos cryopreserved
   (e) The stage at which the embryos were cryopreserved
   (f) The date of cryopreservation
   (g) The location of the embryo(s) within the storage tank
3. The patient's consent forms should be checked to confirm that appropriate written consent for embryo storage has been obtained. The length of time that the patients have consented to embryo storage should also be cross-checked against the electronic database and/or paper inventory to confirm that the recorded storage expiry date is correct and has not been exceeded.
4. Where possible, the physical contents of each sub-location should be examined during the same audit session to prevent excessive movement of the stored contents. The embryos stored for each patient should be cross-checked against the inventory paperwork for the:
   (a) Number of devices in storage
   (b) Number of embryos in storage
   (c) Colour and style of the storage device(s)
   (d) Identifying information on the label of the storage device
5. Any discrepancies should be discussed with the laboratory team leader and amended where possible. Any changes made to the paperwork should be clearly marked as an outcome of the storage audit and initialled by the person who has made the amendment.

Discrepancies identified during a storage audit can be wide ranging. Possible discrepancies include:

- Absence of storage consent or invalid storage consent.
- Embryos that have exceeded their storage expiry date.
- Errors on the storage device label.
- Transcription errors on the freeze documentation/inventory paperwork/electronic database such as incorrect storage device colour.

- Fewer storage devices present in the storage location than expected; this may result from poor record keeping, such as the absence of embryo thaw details on the paperwork. However, this discrepancy may also result from the breakage of a storage device or the loss of a storage device within the tank.

The nature of the identified discrepancies will indicate whether a change in SOP is required or whether the laboratory staff would benefit from a period of retraining.

65.4 Transporting Embryos Between Clinics

Cryopreserved embryos and oocytes can be transferred between fertility clinics using a specialist transport vessel known as a dry shipper (Fig. 65.8). The central cavity of the dry shipper, which houses the cryopreserved samples during transit, is surrounded by an absorbent material that can be 'charged' with LN2. If the dry shipper has been primed appropriately, the samples to be transferred will be maintained in their cryopreserved state by the resultant LN2 vapour.

The time period over which a dry shipper can maintain a stable temperature (static hold time) varies depending on the style and size of the vessel. It can be beneficial to use a data logger to record the temperature during transportation; however, clinics should be mindful that data logger use can reduce the static hold time. The dry shipper should be housed in a sturdy protective case to prevent damage to the vessel during transportation and should remain in an upright position throughout transit. All dry shippers used for international transfers must meet the requirements set by the International Air Transport Association (IATA).

The arrangement of the transfer process requires the two participating clinics to liaise closely with one another. Good communication needs to also be established with the patients, the courier service and regulatory or government agencies. Some countries and regions have specific regulations in place to govern the movement of samples between clinics, and it is essential that all regulatory requirements are met and approved to ensure that the transfer is performed in a lawful manner.

A generic import/export protocol is described below:

1. Patients register their intent to transfer their cryopreserved embryos to/from the clinic.
2. Patients are informed of the risks, costs and the process involved in embryo import/export. The patients complete transport consent forms acknowledging and accepting the risks associated with transferring embryos in a dry shipper.

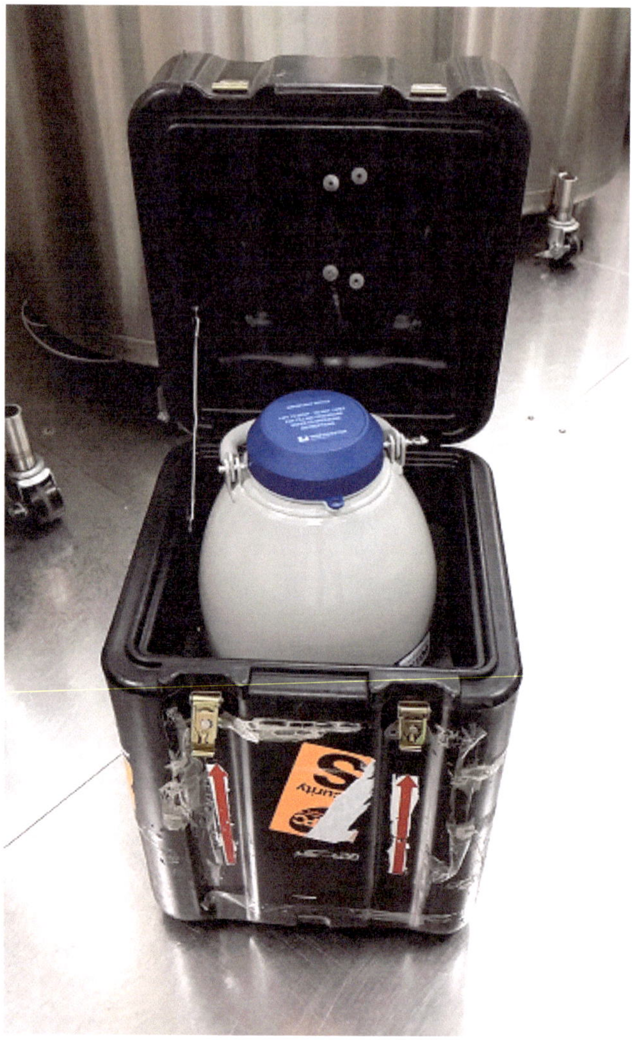

Fig. 65.8 A dry shipper. This specialist transport vessel is used to transport cryopreserved material between fertility clinics within the same country or internationally. (Courtesy of the Assisted Conception Service, Glasgow Royal Infirmary, Glasgow, UK)

3. Documents relating to the creation and cryopreservation of the patient's embryos, including the consent to embryo storage, are sent to the receiving clinic.
4. Where required, licencing and accreditation documents are shared between the sending and the receiving clinics, and approval for the transfer is sought from the regulatory/licencing body.
5. A date for embryo shipment is agreed upon by the two clinics and the courier company.
6. Priming of the dry shipper commences 1–2 days prior to the transfer date.
7. On the day of the transfer, the embryos are removed from their storage tank and transferred to the dry shipper; this process should be performed by two staff members to ensure that the correct samples are exported.

Documentation describing to the contents of the dry shipper should be included in the shipment.

8. The courier company collects the dry shipper, and the receiving clinic should be notified that the shipment is in progress.
9. Upon the receipt of the dry shipper, two members of staff at the receiving clinic should transfer the embryos into their new storage tank and verify that the identifying information present on the storage devices is consistent with the laboratory paperwork.
10. The receiving clinic should inform both the patients and the sending clinic that the embryos have been safely received and the cryobank inventory of both ART clinics should be updated to reflect the occurrence of the import/export event.

65.5 Conclusion

This chapter has explored all aspects of the clinical embryo cryobank. The design has been described, including how to decide on the type and number of vessels, the equipment needed and how safety and security should be managed. The processes of adding and removing embryos from the cryobank have been covered, including tips on how to manage a cryobank containing many embryos via a 'bring-forward' system. Embryo cryopreservation is commonplace in ART, and this trend will likely continue for the foreseeable future. Thus, the cryobank has a pivotal role in delivering successful outcomes for our patients.

References

1. Kemper JM, Wang R, Vuong LN, Mol BW. Single embryo transfer with frozen transfer of all remaining embryos without further embryonic testing should be the standard of care in IVF. BJOG. 2019 Jan;126(2):142–4. https://doi.org/10.1111/1471-0528.15486.
2. Zacà C, Bazzocchi A, Pennetta F, Bonu MA, Coticchio G, Borini A. Cumulative live birth rate in freeze-all cycles is comparable to that of a conventional embryo transfer policy at the cleavage stage but superior at the blastocyst stage. Fertil Steril. 2018 Sep;110(4):703–9. https://doi.org/10.1016/j.fertnstert.2018.05.012.
3. Tomlinson M, Morroll D. Risks associated with cryopreservation: a survey of assisted conception units in the UK and Ireland. Hum Fertil (Camb). 2008 Mar;11(1):33–42. https://doi.org/10.1080/14647270701553280.
4. Apte M, Gibson SH, Blanchette-Porter M, et al. Disposition of frozen embryos: one program's experience with contacting patients about embryos in storage. JFIV Reprod Med Genet. 2015;3:3.
5. Melamed RM, Bonetti TC, Braga DP, Madaschi C, Iaconelli A, Borges E. Deciding the fate of supernumerary frozen embryos: parents' choices. Hum Fertil (Camb). 2009;12(4):185–90.

Part VII

Counselling

Psychological Aspects of Infertility

66

Julianne E. Zweifel and Angela K. Lawson

It is common wisdom that "pregnancy begins psychologically long before it occurs physiologically" [1]. In short, the quest for pregnancy is a complex intertwining of physiology and psychology. This means that high-quality care of fertility patients necessitates awareness of the psychosocial aspects of infertility. In contrast to other fields of medical care where patients seek alleviation of maladies, patients presenting for fertility care are seeking the opportunity to be a parent. More specifically, they are seeking a loving relationship with a child, the experiences and fulfillment inherent in parenting, carrying out the natural instinct of reproduction, the continuance of family relationships and lineage, and the opportunity to enrich parental relationships [2]. Couples seeking fertility treatment may also be motivated to alleviate potential negative experiences including the stigma of childlessness, marital insecurity, and exclusion from child-related social activities and relationships [2]. Thus, there are multiple psychosocial factors at stake for those seeking fertility care.

Infertility is generally an unexpected crisis that threatens the dream of parenthood and one's anticipated life agenda. An individual's sense of self-determination and physiological competence may be threatened, and for many, this will be the first experience at not being able to attain a life goal through hard work. As a result, patients are highly motivated to identify and rectify factors (real or otherwise) that may be contributing to their infertility.

The experience of infertility treatment also carries with it many burdens including the discomfort of discussing sexual and reproductive health issues, complex treatment regimens, uncertain outcomes, financial strain, frequent clinic visits, physical discomfort, and potential moral/ethical dilemmas [3]. Given the totality of the infertility experience, it is not surprising that clinically significant depression and anxiety is an associated struggle for many infertility patients. The prevalence of depression, anxiety, and general distress among infertility patients has led some to argue that, rather than a consequence of infertility, distress is a cause of infertility.

The goal of this chapter is to prepare clinicians to support the psychological needs of their patients through sensitive care that recognizes the emotional/psychological concerns of the patient. The chapter will first provide a foundation for patient education on the relationship of stress and infertility and will then present a practical model for providing routine proactive psychological support within a fertility clinic.

66.1 Psychological Stress and Infertility

For generations, scientists have worked to discover and effectively treat the causes of infertility. There are many identified medical causes of infertility; however, a large number of patients have no identified medical cause for their infertility. For patients without a medical answer for their infertility (and even for those with a medical diagnosis), many may turn to alternative explanations and nonmedical treatments for their infertility. This is likely related to historical and inaccurate beliefs about the relative ease of achieving pregnancy and resulting belief that if pregnancy is not easily attained, the intended parents have done something wrong and can make behavioral changes to correct the problem. Historic examples exist of beliefs that a woman's behavior, in particular her level of stress, affects whether or not she gets pregnant and whether or not she carries a pregnancy to term. Anecdotes about women relaxing and getting pregnant abound, whereas anecdotes about women relaxing and not getting pregnant are notably

J. E. Zweifel (✉)
Department of Obstetrics and Gynecology, University of Wisconsin School of Medicine & Public Health, Madison, WI, USA
e-mail: julianne.zweifel@uwmf.wisc.edu

A. K. Lawson
Departments of Clinical Obstetrics and Gynecology and Psychiatry, Northwestern University Feinberg School of Medicine, Chicago, IL, USA

G. N. Allahbadia et al. (eds.), *Textbook of Assisted Reproduction*, https://doi.org/10.1007/978-981-15-2377-9_66

absent. As a result, women commonly lament being told by well-meaning family and friends to "relax" in order to improve pregnancy chances. Such comments reinforce the woman's belief that it is her fault that she is not conceiving and often result in women's increased focus on reducing their level of stress.

66.1.1 What Is Stress and How Could It Affect Fertility?

Stress is the result of automatic physiological responses to an internal or external noxious stimulus. Individual reactions to stress vary but can lead to either positive (eustress) or negative (distress) outcomes [4]. These reactions have been described as the "the fight or flight response" and in times of acute or chronic stress results in the activation of the sympathetic nervous system via the sympathetic adrenal medullary axis (SAM) as well as the hypothalamic pituitary adrenal axis (HPA) in times of chronic stress. The activation of the HPA and SAM axes results in the release of neurotransmitters (e.g., epinephrine and norepinephrine) and stress hormones (e.g., cortisol and α-amylase). This cascade effect serves to help defend the body against harm and return it to a state of homeostasis [5, 6].

Stress-related stimulation of the HPA axis may be viewed as particularly relevant to the biological plausibility of a relationship between stress and infertility. This is because activation of the HPA axis is hypothesized to inhibit the hypothalamic-pituitary-gonadal (HPG) axis which is responsible for the production of hormones vital to reproduction (e.g., luteinizing hormone; LH and follicle-stimulating hormone; FSH) [7]. However, the activation of the sympathetic nervous system has been found to result in reduced activity, but not complete obstruction, in the parasympathetic nervous system which is responsible for reproduction among other biological processes [8].

66.1.2 Support for Stress as a Cause of Infertility

Some research suggests that psychological stressors play a role in reproductive processes such as delayed pubertal onset and functional hypothalamic amenorrhea [7]. However, this research is limited by use of animal models, inconclusive research with humans, as well as limited control for the role of environmental factors such as food insecurity and excessive exercise on these processes. More recent research on the relationship between psychological stressors and infertility focuses on elevated stress hormones (e.g., α-amylase and cortisol) and infertility.

66.1.3 Stress Hormones

Studies of salivary-α amylase (s-αA) and cortisol in women attempting to conceive have found that, among fertile and infertile women, higher stress hormone levels were generally not associated with overall probability of becoming pregnant despite an association with lower daily conception chances in first month of attempting pregnancy or increases in overall time to pregnancy. One study of IVF patients did find a relationship between cortisol levels on day of oocyte retrieval and day of pregnancy test (prior to delivery of test results) and chance of pregnancy success [9]. The findings of this study are unclear particularly in light of research findings which show a positive relationship between cortisol and perimenopausal changes (e.g., increasing FSH and decreased estradiol) but no relationship between cortisol and distress levels [10, 11]. It is therefore unclear if this relationship between cortisol and pregnancy results was related to patient's differential exposure to exogenous FSH during IVF, baseline FSH levels, low peak E_2 reflecting a poor stimulation response, and/or temporal proximity to perimenopause.

Overall, the outcomes of these studies are limited by the fact that no attempt was made to assess for the cause(s) of increased hormone levels and no formal fertility evaluation took place [5, 12, 13]. Thus, research on the relationship between stress and s-αA or cortisol are difficult to interpret as these hormone levels may be influenced by many variables other than stress (e.g., diet, substance use, medication, coping strategies, exercise, circadian rhythm, variability in sample collection and storage techniques, etc.) [14–16].

It should also be noted that some have postulated, without sufficient empirical support, that stress is the cause of at least some medically unexplained miscarriages. The proposed biological mechanism is similar to that of stress and infertility in that it is hypothesized that increases in stress hormones can cause immunological changes and/or inflammation in the uterus which may lead to miscarriage [17]. Limitations to the length of this chapter prevent a full exploration of relevant research. However, the research on stress and miscarriage are inconsistent at best and more rigorous research with appropriate control variables is needed. [18]

66.2 Survey-Based Assessment of Psychological Stress and Infertility

A great deal of research has also focused on participant's perceptions of stress and any associated negative fertility-related outcomes. Although some researchers have identified a relationship between psychological stress or negative life events and fertility treatment outcomes [19, 20], others have not. [21, 22] Unfortunately, many survey-based studies of stress and infertility are limited by lack of relevant control variables, use of empirically valid measures of distress, small sample sizes, and inappropriate statistical analyses. Further, limited research exists which explores men's perceptions of stress and fertility outcomes, but this research has also resulted in inconsistent findings [23]. Finally, survey research on the relationship between perceived stress and fertility, while providing insight into participant's experiences of distress, is inherently limited and ultimately unable to provide data regarding causation.

66.2.1 Distress Reduction and Fertility

Given the ethical and other difficulties in designing a rigorously designed randomized controlled trial to assess stress exposure and fertility outcomes, another research approach has been to assess changes in pregnancy following relaxation inducing or otherwise stress reducing activities.

66.2.1.1 Complementary and Alternative Medicine

Acupuncture is hypothesized to serve as both a treatment for infertility and as a stress-reduction activity [24]. As with much of the research on stress and infertility, the research on acupuncture and fertility is inconsistent. However, acupuncture has generally not been found to be harmful to patients and indeed may result in emotional benefits; therefore use of acupuncture during fertility treatment is not prohibited [25].

Mindfulness meditation and other mind/body interventions including yoga have also been examined as ways to improve patient's emotional well-being and pregnancy chances [26–28] Nonetheless, research is inconclusive and often marked by design flaws but finds that such interventions may improve emotional well-being and thus may continue to be utilized by patients who are attempting to conceive.

66.2.1.2 Psychotherapy

A large body of research has examined the relationship between psychological counseling and distress reduction among infertility patients. Many studies have found that counseling is associated with improvements in emotional well-being [29]. Results of research on psychological counseling and improved pregnancy rates are less consistent. [30–32] As with most research on stress reduction interventions, psychotherapy does not appear to harm patients and is often well-received by patients and thus continued appropriate referrals for psychological support appears warranted.

66.2.1.3 Adoption

Although on the surface adoption would not appear to be a stress reduction strategy, anecdotally, many patients report hearing stories of friends or family members who adopted and subsequently conceived. Anecdotal stories which contradict any relationship between adoption and conception are less frequently shared. Overall, research on adoption and spontaneous conception finds that although some women can conceive after adoption, most do not [33, 34].

66.2.1.4 Stopping or Starting Fertility Treatment

It has been hypothesized that the cessation of fertility treatment and/or the intention to begin such treatment is associated with a reduction in stress that may increase rates of spontaneous conception. Although some women can spontaneously conceive after the end or before the start of fertility treatment, it appears that the likely cause of such conceptions are related to those women's younger age, shorter duration of infertility, and less severe fertility diagnoses. Further, women who pursue fertility treatment often do not have a 0% chance of spontaneous conception, and some women may have been misdiagnosed as infertile; thus spontaneous conception among fertility patients would not be unexpected [35]. Regardless of the reason for spontaneous conception, there is no strong link between stress and spontaneous conception among patients starting or stopping fertility treatment.

66.2.2 Support for Infertility as a Cause of Distress

It is accepted that the experience of infertility and infertility treatment serve as psychological stressors for women and men that may lead to mild to severe levels of emotional distress. Infertile patients have frequently been found to report symptoms of depression and anxiety, marital discord, and other personal and social symptoms of distress. Research also supports that these symptoms of distress may worsen throughout the course of failed fertility treatments, may result in premature treatment termination, and may rise to the severity of distress seen among cancer patients [36–38].

In summary, given the inconsistent and at best weak relationship between stress and infertility, as well as the distress caused by infertility and infertility treatment, it seems best to offer high-quality care with appropriate emotional support to patients while avoiding telling patients to "relax."

66.3 A Model for Routine Psychological Care in Fertility Treatment

High-quality care refers to a treatment approach that is effective, safe, patient-centered, timely, efficient. and accessible [39]. Adoption of the term "high-quality ART" into the vernacular of reproductive endocrinology and infertility care reflects the evolution of fertility care beyond live birth rates to include consideration of overall patient well-being while in treatment. Studies of patient-centered care indicate that clinics' and providers' ability to educate, communicate, and convey respect to patients translates into lowered concerns about treatment and lowered overall anxiety [40]. Patients value psychosocial support being offered through fertility clinics before, during, and after ART and providing this element of care may address the fact that the burden of psychosocial factors is a primary reason for discontinuing fertility treatments [40]. Further, consideration of well-being in treatment also factors into patients' selection of treatment programs and providers [41]. While it is important for each member of a clinic team to be sensitive to the psychosocial experience of patients and to provide effective patient education, communication, and respect, the mental health provider (MHP) on the team has a unique opportunity to impact these aspects of patient care.

66.3.1 Wisconsin/Northwestern University Model of Care

The fertility programs at the University of Wisconsin School of Medicine and Public Health and Northwestern University Feinberg School of Medicine share a unique model of infertility care that routinely incorporates psychological services. While patients are offered supportive psychotherapy as a venue to process mood, relationship issues, and treatment decisions, all patients pursing IVF, third-party reproduction, and fertility preservation are required to participate in a pretreatment psychological consultation with an MHP who is embedded in the clinic. Resistance to the consult is mitigated by presenting the consult as a routine component of care, and studies suggest that pre-IVF counseling is acceptable to most participants [3].

66.4 Pretreatment Psychological Consultation

The broad goals of the psychological consultation associated with fertility care include (a) screening to identify patients who have mental health or psychosocial concerns that may necessitate additional pretreatment considerations; (b) preparing patients for treatment including discussion of psychological and ethical factors in care; (c) introducing coping and communication strategies; (d) providing a venue for supportive discussion regarding patients' infertility experience; and (e) discussion of situation/treatment-specific concerns [1, 3]. Structured examples of psychological consults in fertility care are available for review [42] but are beyond the scope of this chapter; however, primary points will be discussed below. Though the psychological consult is conducted by the team MHP, familiarity with the content and purpose of the consult allows all team members to better support the psychosocial experience of patients.

66.4.1 Psychosocial Screen

Although patients presenting for fertility care often experience stress, depressed mood, and anxiety, their underlying psychological health is typically sound. Most will report good relationship stability and few if any conflicts related to their fertility treatment plans. However, at times the psychological consult reveals problems that necessitate their physician postponing or denying treatment. Postponement of care for psychological reasons is appropriate when the concern can be remedied or effectively managed by additional services such as psychological/psychiatric interventions. Physicians may also choose to deny fertility care for psychological reasons, based on MHP recommendations regarding identified psychosocial contraindications to treatment (Table 66.1) [3].

66.5 Preparation for Treatment and Discussion of Psychological/ Ethical Factors in Care

Effective patient preparation in fertility care has been shown to decrease infertility specific anxiety and stress [40]. Patient preparation is a team effort, and although medical providers routinely discuss treatment regimens, clinic policies, potential complications, and success rates, patients often require multiple discussions to absorb all of the information provided to them [3]. Within the psychological consult, the MHP has an opportunity to not only re-present information but also to identify when patients are failing to comprehend information or holding on to unrealistic treatment expectations. Furthermore, the topics of unsuccessful treatment, number of embryos to transfer, patient preference for twins or sex selection, high-order pregnancy, multi-fetal pregnancy reduction,

Table 66.1 Psychosocial contraindications to infertility treatment

- Treatment or pregnancy may significantly worsen an active psychiatric illness
- Active substance dependence with concomitant chaotic lifestyle
- One partner is coercing the other to proceed with treatment
- One or both partners are unable or unwilling to provide consent for the treatment
- Decisions about privacy and disclosure in third-party reproduction cannot be resolved
- Use of a family member gamete donor would cause significant familial discord
- Custody arrangements for the potential child of a known gamete donor have not been agreed to by all parties
- Serious marital discord

age limits in care/older parenting, posthumous reproduction, futility of care, and disposition of excess embryos involve psychological, relationship, social, ethical, religious, and moral complexities that benefit from discussion in a therapeutic setting. Many of these topics are distressing and patients are often taken aback by the profound nature of the risks and decisions associated with treatment. Forecasting these issues prior to initiating care is an element of an effective informed consent process and also may enable patients to cope more effectively when faced with these challenges.

66.5.1 Introduce Coping and Communication Strategies

The psychological consult is also an opportunity to introduce effective coping and communication strategies. Studies have demonstrated that cognitive behavioral therapy, relaxation training, and psychoeducational interventions are typically effective in reducing psychological distress with fertility patients [43, 44]. While it is not possible to provide in-depth coping skills training within the consult, some simple strategies such as breathing techniques and restructuring catastrophic thoughts can be implemented during the consult. Furthermore, helping patients to recognize that stress levels increase during an IVF cycle, with peaks during oocyte retrieval, embryo transfer, and the waiting period before pregnancy testing, allows for advance planning and use of coping strategies [40]. In addition, introduction of effective communication of feelings during times of high stress may reduce marital discord and improve emotional well-being.

66.5.2 Providing a Venue for Support

Finally, the psychological consult provides an initial therapeutic encounter where patients have an opportunity to discuss feelings associated with their fertility experience. For many this will be their first experience with an MHP. Meeting the MHP and demystifying the therapeutic experience may facilitate patients seeking supportive psychotherapy. Further, research shows that embedding an MHP into medical practices increases the probability of patients obtaining psychological support [45]. This is particularly important following unsuccessful treatment or reproductive loss when the depression experience can intensify [40].

66.5.3 Third-Party, Single, LGBT Patients

Psychological consults with single patients, LGBT patients, and patients in third-party reproduction necessitates addressing additional, situation specific, issues. A full detailing of these issues is beyond the scope of this chapter but a brief summary can be helpful. Those interested in a broader understanding of the psychological issues specific to these populations as well as treatment recommendations are encouraged to review relevant published texts as well as relevant ASRM ethics and practice documents [46–50].

66.5.3.1 Third-Party

Generally, individuals approach family building with the expectation of using their own gametes to conceive. Although patients may recognize the logic associated with using donated oocytes/sperm, many will struggle with feelings of loss, sadness, anger, worry, fear, and shame. Patients often harbor fears that their relationship with a non-genetic child will be less than it would have been with a genetic child. Similarly, many express concern that the child's parenting/family experience may somehow be lesser due to a lack of a genetic link [51]. The psychological consult provides an opportunity to normalize these concerns and to share research which has suggested that children conceived through third-party reproduction have positive relationships with their parents and are as well-adjusted as their naturally conceived peers [52]. Importantly, the consult is also an opportunity to discuss patients' views and concerns related to disclosure/secrecy, identity-release donors, closed-identity donors, and the prospect of future contact with the donor or donor siblings.

66.5.3.2 Single Parents

Increasingly single women, and to a lesser extent, single men, are pursuing parenting. Generally research has focused on single mother families. These studies suggest no differences in parent-child relationships or child adjustment for single-mother families compared to two-parent families [53]; however, regardless of the type of family structure, child-adjustment is impacted by the family's economic and social resources. Typically single mothers presenting for care are well-educated, economically stable professionals in their late 1930s or early 1940s. The majority indicate that they are saddened that they do not have a partner; however, due to age-related time pressure and the lack of a suitable partner, they elect to go forward on their own [53].

In addition to issues discussed above, the psychological consult with prospective single parents will review decision-making regarding single parenthood and anticipated social support. Occasionally prospective single parents choose not to tell family/friends about their reproductive plans or report poor family/friend support. This may indicate practical or psychosocial difficulties and merits further discussion. Finally, as with all third-party reproductive plans, the psychological consult is a venue for discussing choice of, and comfort with use of, a gamete donors, disclosure to the child, and the child's potential interest in the donor and donor siblings.

66.5.3.3 LGBT Patients

In many respects, fertility care with lesbian, gay, bisexual, and transgender (LGBT) women and men is very similar to that of heterosexual non-transgender patients. Further, LGBT patients are equally at risk of infertility, failed treatment cycles, and reproductive loss as non-LGBT patients. However LGBT patients face additional challenges including legal uncertainties, social biases, and hetero-normative terminology/policy within the clinic. Further, they may face additional decisions regarding whose egg/sperm to use and who will carry the pregnancy. All psychological consults should convey respect for patients, reassure that the consult is not an assessment of fitness for parenting, and convey sensitivity to the psychosocial experience of the patient; however, given the biases and discrimination commonly experienced by LGBT patients, this approach is essential. It is also important that all members of the clinic team be aware that parental sexual orientation and gender identity have not been found to negatively impact the development and psychological adjustment of children [46].

In addition to the more general topics addressed above, in the psychological consult with LGBT patients, the mental health provider encourages discussion of the implications of patients' choices, helps them feel supported in their care, and highlights the importance of legal counsel for parentage.

66.6 Conclusions

Overall research findings on the relationship between stress and infertility are inconsistent, marked by design flaws, and ultimately may only result in a minor delay in time to pregnancy but not in overall pregnancy chances. Although anecdotal data is widely shared, it appears that only anecdotes which support the relationship between stress and fertility are shared, thus creating a confirmation bias which likely supports what patients and others may want to believe: that we as human beings have a great deal of control over our fertility. It is likely the fear that we do not have control over our fertility and that fertility is inherently unfair, and not as easy as we would hope, results in the symptoms of anxiety and depression found among fertility patients. Further, for generations, women in particular have suffered in silence following infertility and miscarriage out of fear that they would be blamed by others for causing these outcomes by being too stressed. Given the psychological sequelae of infertility and fertility treatments, high-quality fertility care should include embedded mental health professionals trained in reproductive health to improve patient mood and coping, to improve the informed consent process, and to reduce premature treatment termination.

References

1. Van den Broeck U, Emery M, Wischmann T, et al. Counselling in infertility: individual, couple and group interventions. Patient Educ Couns. 2010;81:422–8.
2. Cassidy T, Sintrovani P. Motives for parenthood, psychosocial factors and health in women undergoing IVF. J Reprod Infant Psychol. 2008;26:4–17.
3. Klock SC. Psychosocial evaluation of the infertile patient. In: Covington SN, Burns LH, editors. Infertility counseling a comprehensive handbook for clinicians. New York: Cambridge University Press; 2006. p. 83–96.
4. Hargrove MB, Quick JC, Nelson DL, et al. The theory of preventative stress management: a 33-year review and evaluation. Stress Health. 2011;27:182–93.
5. Lynch CD, Sundaram R, Maisog JM, et al. Preconception stress increases the risk of infertility: results from a couple-based prospective cohort study--the LIFE study. Hum Reprod. 2014;29:1067–75.
6. Lawson AK. Psychological stress and fertility. In: Stevenson EL, Hershberger PE, editors. Fertility and assisted reproductive technology (ART): theory, research, policy, and practice for health care practitioners. New York, NY: Springer; 2016. p. 65–86.
7. Whirledge S, Cidlowski JA. A role for glucocorticoids in stress-impaired reproduction: beyond the hypothalamus and pituitary. Endocrinology. 2013;154:4450–68.
8. McCorry LK. Physiology of the autonomic nervous system. Am J Pharm Educ. 2007;71:78.
9. An Y, Sun Z, Li L, et al. Relationship between psychological stress and reproductive outcome in women undergoing in vitro fertilization treatment: psychological and neurohormonal assessment. J Assist Reprod Genet. 2013;30:35–41.
10. Butler L, Santoro N. The reproductive endocrinology of the menopausal transition. Steroids. 2011;76:627–35.
11. Woods NF, Mitchell ES, Smith-Dijulio K. Cortisol levels during the menopausal transition and early postmenopause: observations from the Seattle midlife Women's health study. Menopause. 2009;16:708–18.
12. Tiplady S, Jones G, Campbell M, et al. Home ovulation tests and stress in women trying to conceive: a randomized controlled trial. Hum Reprod. 2013;28:138–51.
13. Nouri K, Litschauer B, Huber JC, et al. Saliva cortisol levels and subjective stress are not associated with number of oocytes after controlled ovarian hyperstimulation in patients undergoing in vitro fertilization. Fertil Steril. 2011;96:69–72.
14. Stegmann BJ. Other nonstress influences can alter salivary alpha-amylase activity. Fertil Steril. 2011;95:2190–1.
15. Rohleder N, Nater UM. Determinants of salivary alpha-amylase in humans and methodological considerations. Psychoneuroendocrinology. 2009;34:469–85.
16. Garde AH, Persson R, Hansen AM, et al. Effects of lifestyle factors on concentrations of salivary cortisol in healthy individuals. Scand J Clin Lab Invest. 2009;69:242–50.
17. Beydoun H, Saftlas AF. Physical and mental health outcomes of prenatal maternal stress in human and animal studies: a review of recent evidence. Paediatr Perinat Epidemiol. 2008;22:438–66.
18. Nelson DB, Grisso JA, Joffe MM, et al. Does stress influence early pregnancy loss? Ann Epidemiol. 2003;13:223–9.
19. Quant HS, Zapantis A, Nihsen M, et al. Reproductive implications of psychological distress for couples undergoing IVF. J Assist Reprod Genet. 2013;30:1451–8.
20. Williams KE, Marsh WK, Rasgon NL. Mood disorders and fertility in women: a critical review of the literature and implications for future research. Hum Reprod Update. 2007;13:607–16.

21. Boivin J, Griffiths E, Venetis CA. Emotional distress in infertile women and failure of assisted reproductive technologies: a meta-analysis of propsective psychosical studies. Br Med J. 2011;23:1–9.
22. Matthiesen SM, Frederiksen Y, Ingerslev HJ, et al. Stress, distress and outcome of assisted reproductive technology (ART): a meta-analysis. Hum Reprod. 2011;26:2763–76.
23. Hall E, Burt VK. Male fertility: psychiatric considerations. Fertil Steril. 2012;97:434–9.
24. Anderson B, Rosenthal L. Acupuncture and in vitro fertilization: critique of the evidence and application to clinical practice. Complement Ther Clin Pract. 2013;19:1–5.
25. Meldrum DR, Fisher AR, Butts SF, et al. Acupuncture--help, harm, or placebo? Fertil Steril. 2013;99:1821–4.
26. Galhardo A, Cunha M, Pinto-Gouveia J. Mindfulness-based program for infertility: efficacy study. Fertil Steril. 2013;100:1059–67.
27. Domar AD, Rooney KL, Wiegand B, et al. Impact of a group mind/body intervention on pregnancy rates in IVF patients. Fertil Steril. 2011;95:2269–73.
28. Valoriani V, Lotti F, Vanni C, et al. Hatha-yoga as a psychological adjuvant for women undergoing IVF: a pilot study. Eur J Obstet Gynecol Reprod Biol. 2014;176:158–62.
29. Wischmann T. Implications of psychosocial support in infertility--a critical appraisal. J Psychosom Obstet Gynaecol. 2008;29:83–90.
30. Hammerli K, Znoj H, Barth J. The efficacy of psychological interventions for infertile patients: a meta-analysis examining mental health and pregnancy rate. Hum Reprod Update. 2009;15:279–95.
31. Frederiksen Y, Farver-Vestergaard I, Skovgard NG, et al. Efficacy of psychosocial interventions for psychological and pregnancy outcomes in infertile women and men: a systematic review and meta-analysis. BMJ Open. 2015;5:e006592.
32. de Liz TM, Strauss B. Differential efficacy of group and individual/couple psychotherapy with infertile patients. Hum Reprod. 2005;20:1324–32.
33. Wischmann TH. Psychogenic infertility--myths and facts. J Assist Reprod Genet. 2003;20:485–94.
34. de La Rochebrochard E, Quelen C, Peikrishvili R, et al. Long-term outcome of parenthood project during in vitro fertilization and after discontinuation of unsuccessful in vitro fertilization. Fertil Steril. 2009;92:149–56.
35. Troude P, Bailly E, Guibert J, et al. Spontaneous pregnancies among couples previously treated by in vitro fertilization. Fertil Steril. 2012;98:63–8.
36. Lawson AK, Klock SC, Pavone ME, et al. Prospective study of depression and anxiety in female fertility preservation and infertility patients. Fertil Steril. 2014;102:1377–84.
37. Gameiro S, Boivin J, Peronace L, et al. Why do patients discontinue fertility treatment? A systematic review of reasons and predictors of discontinuation in fertility treatment. Hum Reprod Update. 2012;18:652–69.
38. Verhaak CM, Smeenk JMJ, Evers AWM, et al. Women's emotional adjustment to IVF: a systematic review of 25 years of research. Hum Reprod. 2007;13:27–36.
39. Benoga R, Kawar R, Key P, et al. Quality of care: a process for making strategic choices in health systems. Geneva: WHO Press; 2006.
40. Gameiro S, Boivin J, Dancet E, et al. ESHRE guideline: routine psychosocial care in infertility and medically assisted reproduction-a guide for fertility staff. Hum Reprod. 2015;30:2476–85.
41. van Empel IW, Dancet EA, Koolman XH, et al. Physicians underestimate the importance of patient-centredness to patients: a discrete choice experiment in fertility care. Hum Reprod. 2011;26:584–93.
42. Covington SN, Burns LH. Infertility counseling: a comprehensive handbook for clinicians. 2nd ed. New York: Cambridge University Press; 2006.
43. Cousineau TM, Green TC, Corsini E, et al. Online psychoeducational support for infertile women: a randomized controlled trial. Hum Reprod. 2008;23:554–66.
44. Faramarzi M, Pasha H, Esmailzadeh S, et al. The effect of the cognitive behavioral therapy and pharmacotherapy on infertility stress: a randomized controlled trial. Int J Fertil Steril. 2013;7:199–206.
45. van Eeghen C, Littenberg B, Holman MD, et al. Integrating behavioral health in primary care using lean workflow analysis: a case study. J Am Board Fam Med. 2016;29:385–93.
46. Ethics Committee of the American Society for Reproductive Medicine. Access to fertility treatment by gays, lesbians, and unmarried persons: a committee opinion. Fertil Steril. 2013;100:1524–7.
47. Ethics Committee of the American Society for Reproductive Medicine. Access to fertility services by transgender persons: a committee opinion. Fertil Steril. 2015;104:1111–5.
48. Ethics Committee of the American Society for Reproductive Medicine. Interests, obligations, and rights in gamete donation: a committee opinion. Fertil Steril. 2014;102:675–81.
49. Ethics Committee of the American Society for Reproductive Medicine. Oocyte or embryo donation to women of advanced reproductive age: a committee opinion. Fertil Steril. 2016;106:e3–7.
50. The Practice Committee of the American Society for Reproductive Medicine and the Practice Committee of the Society for Assisted Reproductive Technology. Recommendations for gamete and embryo donation: a committee opinion. Fertil Steril. 2013;99:47–62.
51. Iloi E, Blake L, Jadva V, et al. The role of age of disclosure of biological origins in the psychological well being of adolescents conceived by reproductive donation: a longitudinal study from age 1 to age 14. J Child Psychol Psychiatry. 2017;58:315–24.
52. Iloi E, Golombok S. Psychological adjustment in adolescents conceived by assisted reproduction techniques: a systematic review. Hum Reprod Update. 2015;21:84–96.
53. Golombok S, Zadeh S, Imrie S, et al. Single mothers by choice: mother-child relationships and children's psychological adjustment. J Fam Psychol. 2016;30:409–18.

Counselling Prior to Medically Assisted Reproduction

67

Jody Lyneé Madeira

Patient counselling is an integral process that continues for the duration of an assisted reproductive technology (ART) or medically assisted reproduction (MAR) treatment cycle. It might be thought of as the "informed" component within informed consent to medical treatment, a legal and ethical imperative that requires that providers educate patients and obtain their consent prior to medical treatment. Informed consent is connected to the four moral principles of medical ethics: autonomy (respect for persons), beneficence (do good), nonmaleficence (doing no harm), and justice (being fair) [1].

This chapter will provide an overview of patient counselling in MAR. It will first discuss how patient counselling and its broader corollary, informed consent, are ethical and legal mandates within medical treatment. It will then explain the unique dimensions of patient counselling with MAR. Finally, it will explore possibilities for improving patient counselling in MAR in the future.

67.1 Patient Counselling and Informed Consent as an Ethical Imperative and Legal Doctrine

In general, patient counselling prior to MAR is designed to convey material information that competent patients might use to evaluate treatment options and make medical decisions. This includes information about a procedure's purpose and elements as well as its risks, benefits, side effects, odds of success, alternatives, and costs and a provider's treatment recommendation [1, 2]. The American Society for Reproductive Medicine (ASRM) has outlined specific recommendations for what information should be conveyed to ART patients and best practices for doing so [3]. These include advising that all consents be in writing, signed by all parties, and witnessed, recommending that couples be fully informed about all alternative procedures and nonmedical options for managing infertility [3]. Patients should also have an opportunity to ask questions as well as time to evaluate the information and come to a decision. Predictably, it can be difficult to determine exactly how much information patients need, since informational needs can vary from individual to individual. While too much information may overwhelm some patients, too little may leave them unprepared to make informed treatment decisions and expose providers to legal liability.

Informed consent is a comparatively recent historical addition to medical treatment relationships. Rooted in the need to safeguard human dignity, it grew in importance following the human experimentation atrocities of the Nazi regime [4, 5] and others like the Tuskegee Syphilis Study [6]. These events culminated in two influential resources: the Nuremberg Code of 1947 [4] and the 1978 Belmont Report [7]. The Nuremberg Code set up basic international standards for medical research that have since been incorporated into ethical guidelines within the social sciences. The Belmont Report explicated ethical principles for human subjects research, including informed consent, risk-benefit assessment, and subject selection.

Patient counselling and informed consent typically occur in a predictable sequence of acts. First, a patient is provided with information (usually in the form of documents) that describe the treatment procedure, risks, and benefits, either with or without an explanatory conversation with the provider. The patient then reviews and signs a document to affirm that she gives consent to treatment — a procedure typically known as "legal" informed consent. This paperwork is frequently lengthy and saturated with medical and legal jargon, and various experts have questioned whether patients read or understand their consent forms prior to signing [8]. Ideally, patients are given a chance to ask questions or request changes to the existing treatment procedure. Patients might review informed con-

J. L. Madeira (✉)
Center for Law, Society and Culture, Indiana University Bloomington, Bloomington, IN, USA
e-mail: jmadeira@indiana.edu

G. N. Allahbadia et al. (eds.), *Textbook of Assisted Reproduction*, https://doi.org/10.1007/978-981-15-2377-9_67

sent documents in a number of environments, from their homes to providers' offices, and at a variety of times, from weeks before to the day of treatment. Of course, in some circumstances, like emergencies, it is not possible to give patients adequate time to read forms and formulate and ask questions [8].

Though informed consent is an ethical imperative, it is also a legal mandate, and it is these concerns that have been increasingly prioritized in recent decades by medical administrators and, by implication, practitioners in recent decades.

67.1.1 Legal Perspectives on Informed Consent

Though it is undisputable rooted in ethics, over the course of the twentieth century, informed consent became increasingly defined by courts of law, where patients who alleged their physicians had violated informed consent principles could seek redress.

In the United States, state courts have identified various legal informed consent standards. The most popular of these are the "reasonable patient" and the "reasonable physician" standards, which require a provider to disclose all information that either a "reasonable patient" [9] or a "reasonable physician" [10] would deem important to a treatment decision. Currently, the majority of states adhere to the "reasonable physician" standard [11]. There are a few exceptions to the informed consent obligation, including emergency circumstances that preclude a patient from consenting and the therapeutic privilege, which allows a provider to withhold information out of concern that full disclosure would psychologically harm the patient or cause the patient to forego an essential treatment [12]. Once a patient consents, a physician can perform only those procedures within the "scope of consent," barring an emergency that occurs during the consented-to procedure.

These legal standards have profoundly influenced patient counselling and informed consent routines in American medical practice. Failure to disclose material information exposes a provider to a civil claim of negligence sounding in tort law; a plaintiff patient must prove that her physician failed to disclose information as required by the relevant legal standard, as proven by expert testimony, and that this failure caused the plaintiff a legal injury. A plaintiff patient might need to prove that, if properly informed, she would not have consented to that procedure or that the harm that she suffered was not disclosed even though most doctors would have disclosed that risk. A patient could also sue a provider for battery for carrying out a procedure to which she did not consent; in one famous early informed consent case, a plaintiff successfully sued her doctor for operating on her left ear after she had consented to an operation on her right ear [13].

In 2008, the American Bar Association's Family Law Section, Committee on Reproductive and Genetic Technology, created a "Model Act Governing Assisted Reproductive Technology" out of concern that new reproductive technologies have "created a host of novel legal issues" that previously could not be satisfactorily resolved due to "confusion and contradictions in the application of a body of existing statutory and common law" [14]. The Model Act establishes "legal standards for the use, storage, and other disposition of gametes and embryos by addressing societal concerns about ART," like a lack of health insurance coverage for infertility, and "legal standards for informed consent, reporting, and quality assurance" [14]. This Model Act is intended to provide a "flexible framework" by which to resolve current and future controversies [14]. It requires that informed consent be given orally and in writing; its other requirements will be discussed subsequently.

67.1.2 Counteracting Informed Consent's Increasing Legalization

While informed consent is both an ethical and legal imperative, some experts have noted that legal concerns have gradually taken priority over the past several decades. Beauchamp and Childress have criticized informed consent's increasing legalization — what they term "informed consent-as-disclosure" — for being "unduly influenced by medical convention and malpractice law" and for incorporating "dubious assumptions about medical authority, physician responsibility, and legal theories of liability" that focus informed consent away from human understanding [1]. Instead, they claim, informed consent should center around and support patients' autonomous choice [1]. When it does not, informed consent is in tension with providers' interests, with adverse consequences for both patients and providers. In a moral sense, informed consent concerns are supposed to facilitate patients' autonomous choices, not professionals' liability for nondisclosure.

To counteract this overemphasis on informed consent's legal dimensions, Beauchamp and Childress have proposed a more comprehensive definition of informed consent, under which it is comprised of *threshold* elements like patients' ability to understand and competency to make a voluntary decision, *information* elements such as disclosing material information and treatment recommendation, and *consent* elements like deciding upon a treatment plan and giving authorization [1]. When executed correctly, informed consent can satisfy both providers' and patients' informational and security needs, as well as encourage innovation and deliver patient-centered medical care [8].

Thus, patient counselling cannot be reduced to a signed document, and patient understanding, not legal liability, should be its primary goal. In this light, informed consent is a dialogic process that ideally begins, while a patient is actually considering various treatment options and continues until treatment is complete. At the heart of this process is an open, trusting, and communicative treatment relationship between patient and provider. The patient counselling process may involve documents, but it should begin and end with conversation. This approach to patient counselling and informed consent is supported by a growing body of research on effective treatment relationships and interactions, especially those focusing on patient-centered care and shared decision-making [15, 16].

Perhaps because of its importance to both ensuring patient understanding and in limiting providers' professional liability, experts are concerned that traditional routines of patient counselling and informed consent might diminish providers' liability without increasing patient comprehension or promote informed decision making. Patients might have trouble understanding medical documents and consent forms that include legal and medical jargon, [17] particularly if their literacy level is low or English is not their native language (consent forms are often supposed to be written at an eighth-grade level) [18]. Medical consent forms are lengthy, being on average 12 pages long [18]; consent forms for ART procedures often fill whole binders. Moreover, there are more incentives for physicians to include as much information as possible than there are incentives to make the forms shorter and less comprehensive but perhaps more comprehensible. But more information is not always better for patients, who might feel this information is overwhelming or irrelevant to her circumstances [19]. Furthermore, patients may disregard documents if they feel that consent processes and aids, like consent forms, are designed to protect providers rather than educate patients or if they regard them as bureaucratic rituals and not meaningful opportunities for learning and asking questions [20]. Informed consent today may be analogized to a race that begins with a signature and ends in an operating room, more an experience of "getting it done and quickly" or "an activity performed out of necessity" [21] than an ongoing relational and communicative process between patient and provider.

As a corollary to its role in bioethics and patient-centered care, patient counselling and informed consent are perhaps best defined as both processes and as relationships [21]. How patients regard consent forms need not define how they regard the patient counselling project as a whole. The relationship component of patient counselling is particularly important when patients find information to be emotionally threatening due to its content or ambiguity [8]. Perhaps the first stage in helping advance these qualities of patient counselling is to acknowledge that "'getting through' and 'being moved along' are the lived experiences of consent," particularly when "the discretion of debating, changing, supplementing, or discarding the form is not available to them" [21]. Prioritizing patient counselling as a relationship over patient counselling as a legal mandate is the first step toward emphasizing an interactive, trusting medical relationship over one that is suspicious, adversarial, and litigious [8].

67.2 Unique Aspects of Patient Counselling and Informed Consent in Art

There has been surprisingly little empirical scholarship on generalized informed consent within ART, despite the many technological advances that have been implemented since the turn of the century [8]. Instead, researchers have addressed consent issues in third party reproduction, particularly for egg donors. Within legal scholarship, experts routinely speculate that patients' strong desire for a child may jeopardize informed consent but cite no studies in support of that claim [22–24]. For instance, Reame has cautioned that, because "competition for patients is intense and the pressure to keep published pregnancy rates high, critics have warned that the process of obtaining informed consent to assisted reproduction is seriously deficient, particularly with respect to the risks associated with multiple births" [25]. Zeiselman also observed that, according to the infertility advocacy group RESOLVE, "given the physical, financial, and emotional stress infertile individuals are experiencing, they may be deceived easily by misleading advertising, so heightened sensitivity and caution on the part of the in vitro fertilization (IVF) practitioner is required" [26].

Empirical research has only recently begun to address these questions. Patient counselling needs may well be different in ART; ART patients are generally more well-educated and wealthy compared to other patient populations and might have different orientations to the importance of consent information as well as diverse informational needs and informed consent preferences. Recent research, for instance, suggests that the vast majority of IVF patients do read and understand information in consent forms but still repose more trust and confidence in provider informed consent consultations [20]. Because ART is a non-emergent field, patients have more time to read and fully consider consent information. And it suggests that informed consent and patient counselling processes are more robust than in other medical fields, providing more information and deeper discussion, despite the overall lower health risks of ART procedures [20].

Moreover, research confirms that ART patients are highly motivated and eager to begin treatment and prioritize being informed. In a 2009 study, Frazier et al. found that 71.8% of women patients and 67.7% of male partners wanted to know about rare side effects [27]. Moreover, 69.1% of women and

42.7% of men desired information about possible but unproven side effects. These informational desires were correlated with older age in women, a preference for twins/triplets, transferring more than two embryos, and receiving care in a larger city (Chicago, IL) rather than a smaller city (Witchita, KS). Patients also preferred to make their treatment decisions jointly with the IVF team in shared decision-making.

Within ART, the landscapes of patient counselling and informed consent are constantly unfolding as treatment outcomes yield ever more health information and diagnoses, enabling patients to access more involved reproductive technologies. ART patients routinely consent to several reproductive procedures as part of one treatment cycle, including in vitro fertilization (IVF) surgical procedures, embryo transfer, embryo cryopreservation, and embryo disposition, as well as more specialized techniques like preimplantation genetic diagnosis (PGD) and intracytoplasmic sperm injection (ICSI) and assisted hatching (AH). Even more counselling and documentation are needed in third-party reproduction scenarios involving donor gametes and surrogacy. Many providers also believe that informed consent in ART is different because of different risks and ethical questions [20]. Furthermore, reproductive medicine professionals enjoy a wide range of discretion in consenting patients and might disagree on whether certain practices are acceptable, like transferring certain numbers of embryos or whether to use gamete donors with certain characteristics or a family history of serious mental illness. This discretion can lead to inconsistency in patient counselling efforts. Finally, consent to an ART procedure like IVF is an agreement to embark on an uncertain journey, where patients proceed on the basis of educated guesses since it is unclear how medications will affect patients' ovaries, how embryos will fertilize, and how many embryos will be transferred.

In ART, then, patient counselling is especially critical because the treatment decisions involved in procedures like IVF often extend far beyond medical concerns and can implicate moral, ethical, and religious values and lifestyle concerns. Decisions made at the time of treatment affect not just patients and their partners but future offspring and potentially third-party reproductive collaborators like gamete donors and surrogates. Moreover, although informed consent decisions must be made prior to treatment to protect all participants' legal interests, this timing means that patients might perceive these decisions as premature. When they make these choices, patients are not directly confronting troubling circumstances and might not seriously believe they could or will occur. In IVF, for example, couples must make decisions about cryopreserved embryos that do not yet exist; they might initially regard these embryos as conceptive resources but later view them as potential siblings of children already born.

Thus, the most difficult and complicated parts of patient counselling in ART — and its weaknesses — are most likely to be those subjects that extend beyond surgical and invasive procedures. Patients are likely more able to comprehend what egg retrieval involves than what happens to the risks of a multiple pregnancy. ART patients might disregard those risks that seem more contingent and potential outcomes that, while serious, seem unlikely to occur.

To respond to the unique concerns in ART, ASRM and the ABA have created professional models of informed consent and patient counselling guidelines: the ASRM Model Consent Forms and the American Bar Association's Model Act Governing Assisted Reproductive Technology [14]. In 2006, the ASRM outlined in detail what aspects of ART procedures had to be included in consent forms, and in 2008, the ASRM promulgated a Model Informed Consent Form for IVF, ICSI, AH, and embryo cryopreservation.

Under the 2008 American Bar Association Model Act, patients should be told that they can withdraw consent at any time prior to gamete or embryo transfer, as well as an ART procedure's various risks, consequences, and benefits including the inherent risks of embryo loss, hormones and other drugs, egg retrieval, multiple pregnancies, and selective reduction. Section 201 of the Act recommends that patients be advised to seek legal counsel concerning these matters and informed about confidentiality protections, access to medical records, possession and control of stored embryos, embryo disposition, and provider policies on numbers of embryos transferred and other ASRM or Society for Assisted Reproductive Technology (SART) guidelines [14]. Informed consent must be documented in a "record" that uses plain language, is dated and signed by providers and participants, clarifies parental rights in collaborative reproduction circumstances, states that disclosures have been made and will remain in effect for a stated time period, and informs patients that they can receive a copy. Under Section 203 of the Model Act, certain disclosures must be made, including the health risks of ovarian stimulation and retrieval and information about drugs used, possible embryo dispositions, the right to transport embryos to other providers, and an embryo transfer disclosure including embryo quality [14]. Other sections of the Model Act have to do with donor limitations (Section 204) and Posthumous Reproduction (Section 205) [14]. Finally, the Model Act requires that "all participants known to the ART provider must undergo a mental health consultation" as outlined in ASRM and SART standards, which cannot be used to arbitrarily deny any patients the right to procreate [14]. During this consultation, Section 301 of the Model Act requires that providers offer additional counselling, but patients' acceptance of this offer is voluntary [14]. Under Section 302, however, patients using donor gametes or embryos or gestational surrogacy must have a mental health evaluation, as does the surrogate, prior to transfer [14].

Although these models are helpful, they must be continually updated as new reproductive technologies are developed and implemented, spurring modifications in patient counselling. If important details of newer technologies are left out, patients are inadequately informed, and providers are exposed to legal liability. For example, in recent litigation concerning PGD, patients have argued that they were not informed of facilities' inexperience in performing PGD, its associated errors, or the option of obtaining PGD [11, 28–30]. However, such cases rarely result in litigation; Amagwula et al. report that, of 15,125 PGD cycles in over 10 years, "only 24 cases of misdiagnosis and adverse outcomes were reported to the ESHRE [European Society of Human Reproduction and Embryology] PGD Consortium" [11]. Though practices may have little choice whether to offer technologies such as PGD, liability may be minimized by "properly informing patients of the inherent inaccuracies of PGD as part of a thorough informed consent process are crucial in helping deter liability" [11].

Innovations in accessing reproductive technologies, like certain financing arrangements, may also warrant additional counselling. In 2016, the ASRM Ethics Committee published guidelines concerning "risk-sharing" or "refund" programs, which "offer patients a payment structure under which they pay a higher initial fee but provide reduced fees for subsequent cycles and may receive a refund if they do not become pregnant or deliver a baby" [31]. Often, these programs have certain criteria for including patients, and patients' participation in these programs can be terminated. These programs present possible conflicts of interests between patients who want to become pregnant while retaining funds for other alternative family-building options like adoption and providers' financial interests [31]. The ASRM Ethics Committee thus advised that patients must be "fully informed of the financial costs, advantages, or disadvantages of the programs" as well as alternatives, "clearly informed" about their chances of success, and advised that the program does not guarantee pregnancy or delivery [31]. One study alleged that practitioners often did not disclose inclusion or termination criteria and participation risks and benefits [32].

67.3 The Future of Patient Counselling and Informed Consent in Art

Currently, patients undergoing ART procedures like IVF receive and are asked to review lengthy informed consent forms — sometimes, whole binders of information — prior to consenting to medical treatment. Short of reviewing these documents with patients in detail, providers have no way of ascertaining whether or not patients read or understand their contents, or maintaining quality in patient counselling, ensuring that consent disclosures are consistent from patient to patient. Though research suggests that most IVF patients report reading and understanding these documents, [20] technology is providing better and more comprehensive alternatives to traditional paper consent forms [8].

As a supplement to face-to-face patient counselling, some reproductive medicine practices have begun to use a multimedia e-learning application, EngagedMD, the first within reproductive medicine. EngagedMD consists of approximately 13 videos on topics from genetic prescreening to reproductive science and ART procedures to pregnancy risks and the health of an IVF-conceived baby, each of which is under 10 min and is followed by a brief quiz. Incorrect quiz answers generate a "pop-up" response with brief explanations as to why another answer was correct. Videos respond to a variety of patient learning styles, permit patients to view processes like egg retrieval procedures and embryology techniques they would not otherwise see, allow patients to review consent information at a time and place of their choosing, and enable them to review information multiple times. Providers can use the program to monitor each patient's progression through the video series and use their quiz scores to identify areas to focus on during informed consent conversations. According to EngagedMD's creators, this product is more efficient than traditional consent forms, more effective at educating patients, and improves treatment relationships and patient satisfaction. Because EngagedMD has only been recently implemented in clinic environments, it will take time before empirical research methods like randomized controlled trials can ascertain how EngagedMD impacts patient counselling and informed consent [33].

Regardless of how technological developments enhance patient counselling, face-to-face consent conversations will likely remain most the most useful patient counselling medium, simultaneously enhancing patient knowledge, personalizing treatment, and building relational trust. On the one hand, one danger of multimedia consent technologies is that providers will use them as replacements for, not supplements to, interpersonal conversations, weakening treatment relationships and positioning patients like mere products on an assembly line [33]. On the other, however, alternative methods of ensuring informed consent compliance, such as reviewing consent documents with patients line by line, might be equally ineffective. Any patient questions left unresolved remain unasked or are answered later by nurses or other staff members tasked with responding to patients' phone calls. Given the brevity of physician appointments, the time that patients and physicians have together is precious. While there is no substitution for genuine engagement between physicians and their patients, innovative media platform products may help to increase and provide evidence of compliance and utilize appointment time more effectively. Such technologies can answer patients' basic questions, generate new ones, and allow them to prioritize which needs and concerns to resolve when they are face-to-face with their physicians. If used inappropriately, however, these technologies can distance patients from their providers — a critical error given reproductive medicine's range of complex impacts and outcomes, the manifest importance of patient compliance, and the invaluable benefits of a trusting treatment relationship.

In conclusion, patient counselling and informed consent have both legal and ethical dimensions, which can be in tension with one another when an emphasis on completing consent forms supplants a focus on effective treatment conversations. Patient counselling is best understood as both a process and a relationship that lasts for the duration of the patient's treatment experience. Patient counselling is especially critical within ART, where treatment decision-making entails many unique choices that go beyond medical decisions, such as determining prior to treatment what should happen to surplus embryos, should patients die or become divorced. Although consent forms have traditionally been the most frequently counselling aid, patients might find them too bureaucratic or overwhelming due to length or jargon; other alternatives to consent forms, such as multimedia e-learning applications, may help to improve patient education and counselling.

References

1. Beauchamp TL, Childress JF. Principles of biomedical ethics. 5th ed. New York: Oxford University Press; 2001.
2. Kass NE, Sugarman J, Medley AM, Fogarty LA, Taylor HA, Ckea D. An intervention to improve cancer patients' understanding of early-phase clinical trials. IRB. 2009 May–June;31(3):1–10.
3. Practice Commitee of the American Society for Reproductive Medicine. Elements to be considered in obtaining informed consent to ART. Fertil Steril. 2006 November;86(5 (Supp. 1)):S272–3.
4. Annas GJ, Grodin MA. The Nazi doctors and the Nuremberg code: human rights in human experimentation. New York: Oxford University Press; 1995.
5. Lifton RJ. The Nazi doctors: medical killing and the psychology of genocide. New York: Basic Books; 2017.
6. Jones JH. Bad blood: the Tuskegee syphilis experiment. New York: Free Press; 1993.
7. United States, National Commission for the Protection of Human Subjects of Biomedical and Behavioral Research. The Belmont report: ethical principles and guidelines for the protection of human subjects of research. Ann Arbor: University of Michigan Press; 1978.
8. Madeira JL, Andraka-Christou B. Paper trails, trailing behind. J Law Biosci. 2016 January;3(1):2–38.
9. Arato v. Avedon: 858 P.2d 598; Cal. 1993.
10. Nathanson v. Kline: 350 P.2d 1093; Kan. 1960.
11. Amagwula T, Chang PL, Hossain A, Tyner J, Rivers AL, Phelps JY. Preimplantation genetic diagnosis: a systematic review of litigation in the face of new technology. Fertil Steril. 2012 November;98(5):1277–82.
12. Nishi v. Hartwell: 473 P.2d 116; Hawaii 1970.
13. Mohr v. Williams: 104 N.W. 12; Minn. 1905.
14. American bar association model act governing assisted reproductive technology. Chicago: American Bar Association, Section on Family Law's Committee on Reproductive and Genetic Technology; 2008.
15. Stewart M, Brown JB, Weston W, McWhinney IR, McWilliam CL, Freeman T. Patient-centered medicine. 3rd ed. London: Radcliffe Publishing; 2013.
16. Gerteis M, Edgman-Levitan S, Daley J, Delbanco TL, editors. Through the patient's eyes: understanding and promoting patient-centered care. San Francisco: Jossey-Bass; 2002.
17. Willis G. Cognitive interviewing as a tool to improve the informed consent process. J Empir Res Hum Res Ethics. 2006 March;1(1):9–24.
18. Getz KA. In search of informed consent improvement. Appl Clin Trials. 2007 November;16(11):42–5.
19. Schenker Y, Meisel A. Informed consent in clinical care: practical considerations in the effort to achieve ethical goals. J Am Med Assoc. 2011 March;305(11):1130–1.
20. Madeira JL. Taking baby steps: how patients and fertility clinics collaborate in conception. Berkeley: University of California Press; 2017.
21. Jacob MA. Form-made persons: consent forms as consent's blind spot. POLAR. 2007;30(2):249–68.
22. Madeira JL. Woman scorned?: resurrecting infertile women's decision-making autonomy. Maryland Law Rev. 2012;71(2):339–410.
23. Strong C. Too many twins, triplets, quadruplets, and so on: A call for new priorities. J Law Med Ethics. 2003;31(2):272–82.
24. Waldman E. Disputing over embryos: of contracts and consents. Arizona State Law J. 2000;32:897–940.
25. Reame N. Informed consent issues in assisted reproduction. J Obstet Gynecol Neonatal Nurs. 1998 December;28:331–8.
26. Zeiselman K. Infertility, advertising, and choice: a consumer advocate's perspective. Womens Health Issues. 1997;7:180–5.
27. Frazier LM, Grainger DA, Jain T, Ahlers-Schmidt CR, Klemp JR, Miller VA. Desire by IVF patients for information about rare or uncertain risks and for shared decision-making. Fertil Steril. 2009 October;92(3):149.
28. Bergero V. USC Keck School of Medicine; CA 2nd App. District Div. 8, April 9, 2009.
29. Paretta V. Medical Offices of Human Reproduction: 760 N.Y.S.2d 639; NY Sup. Ct. 2003.
30. Coggeshell V. Reproductive Endocrine Associates of Charlotte: 656 S.E.2d 476; SC 2007.
31. Ethics Committee of the American Society for Reproductive Medicine. Financial 'risk-sharing' or refund programs in assisted reproduction: an ethics committee opinion. Fertil Steril. 2016 October;106(5):e8–e11.
32. Hawkins J. Financing infertility. Harv J Legis. 2010;47:115–65.
33. Madeira JL, Coyne K, Jaeger AS, Parry JP, Lindheim SR. Inform and consent: more than just sign here. Fertil Steril. 2017 July;108:40.

Part VIII

Genetic Testing

Noninvasive Prenatal Testing (NIPT): Current Status

68

K. Aparna Sharma and Neerja Bhatla

68.1 History

The concept of circulating fetal cells in the mother was first discussed by a German pathologist, Georg Schmorl, who identified fetal trophoblasts in lungs of eclamptic women on autopsy in 1893 [1]. After this suggestion there was a hiatus of nearly 100 years before any development could be made in the field. Gradually, with the development of cell sorting techniques, separation of single cells was possible, and the further development of PCR and FISH techniques allowed the analysis of single cells. In the 1990s, there was a lot of interest in various methods for noninvasive prenatal diagnosis (NIPT) [2]. It was then that the paper on cell-free fetal DNA by Lo et al. generated great enthusiasm among the proponents of NIPT [3]. In this landmark study, circulating male fetal DNA was detecting in 80% of women carrying male fetuses using a sensitive Y-PCR assay. This paved the way for a revolution leading to its present day status having an undisputed stand among the tests for prenatal diagnosis.

68.2 Technical Aspects and Types of NIPT

68.2.1 Cell-Free DNA (cfDNA)

Cell-free DNA is normally found in all individuals. This originates from dead cells and is found in a concentration of 10–100 ng/mL. The length of these fragments could be between 100–300 base pairs (bp) with a concentration of 10^{11} fragments per mL. The turnover time is rather rapid with a half-life of only 15 min.

K. A. Sharma (✉) · N. Bhatla
Department of Obstetrics and Gynaecology, All India Institute of Medical Sciences, New Delhi, India

68.2.2 Cell-Free Fetal (cff) DNA

In a pregnant woman, 5–40% of free DNA fragments have a fetal origin from the placenta resulting from the apoptosis of the syncytiotrophoblasts, which leads to the release of DNA fragments [4]. Being placental in origin, cfDNA increases in conditions of abnormal placentation like abruption and is not detectable within hours after delivery [5]. It can be reliably detected after 7 weeks of gestation [6]. Using specific enzymes (CG nuclease), it is possible to degrade only the maternal DNA at the sites where its methylation differs from the fetus' and hence differentiate maternal from fetal DNA [7].

68.2.3 The Noninvasive Prenatal Test (NIPT)

NIPT is the detection of fetal DNA circulating in the mother's blood to diagnose various fetal conditions. High-throughput DNA sequencing technology (massive parallel genomic sequencing (MPS) or NGS) is used to sequence millions of DNA molecules in parallel [8]. There are three commonly used methods for performing the tests.

68.2.3.1 Whole Genome Sequencing

In this test, the entire fetal DNA is sequenced in short reads and referenced in comparison to a standard human genomic database such that every sequence can be matched to a specific chromosome. An important aspect that needs mention here is that it is not the change in sequencing that is detected but the amount of DNA of a particular sequence which is more or less than expected of a particular fetus. Hence, fetal DNA from all chromosomes are sequenced to determine if more sequence from seen from one chromosome than the others. This technique of massive parallel sequencing does not differentiate maternal DNA from the fetal DNA, and the total amount of DNA in the plasma is sequenced and sorted to determine if there is more or less than the expected amount

G. N. Allahbadia et al. (eds.), *Textbook of Assisted Reproduction*, https://doi.org/10.1007/978-981-15-2377-9_68

of certain fragments. Essentially, this is a quantitative test rather than a qualitative method.

Also, for this test DNA fragments (12–15 × 10^6 mapped sequences) are required in sufficient amounts to detect the difference between aneuploid and euploid fetuses.

68.2.3.2 Targeted Sequencing

In this method, only the region/chromosome of interest is sequenced, making it more efficient in terms of time and the cost as compared to the whole genome sequencing. The regions from chromosome 21, 13, and 18 are selectively amplified followed by NGS. The amount of sequencing required is significantly less than the whole genome sequencing.

68.2.3.3 Single Nucleotide Pleomorphism (SNP)-Based Tests

SNPs are specific parts of DNA that are unique to each person. They occur in 1/300 base pairs and are useful markers in clinical medicine. In this technique, the maternal blood is divided into the plasma, which contains both maternal and fetal cfDNA, and the buffy coat preparation, which is predominantly the maternal DNA. Using SNP sequencing, the maternal genotype is determined. The fetal genotype can be deduced by comparing with the combination of maternal and fetal cfDNA sequences [9].

There are drawbacks of each method. The SNP-based method is not feasible in egg donation, surrogacy, consanguinity, maternal transplant, and multiple gestation samples. The assay failure rates are also higher. However, they can be useful in cases of monosomy X and vanishing twins. The MPS-based tests are limited by inconsistent amplification and also have lower efficacy for 13, X, and Y abnormalities.

68.2.4 Steps in cfDNA Testing by Massive Parallel Sequencing

1. DNA from the maternal plasma is first extracted using the DNA extraction kit.
2. A PCR is then run to amplify the DNA fragments.
3. The DNA fragments are then sequenced and aligned to a reference human genome. Each fragment of DNA has a specific sequence of nucleotides that is specific to a chromosome, and based on these read sequences, the fragments are allotted to a chromosome during the counting.
4. Counting: A computer-generated algorithm then sorts each of these fragments into a chromosome, and the total amount of DNA distribution of the sample is generally representative of the reference human genome distribution. Any variation from this distribution, e.g., more or less of a sequence pertaining to a particular chromosome, is indicative of a trisomy or a monosomy.

68.3 Evidence for Performance of NIPT

Studies have consistently reported a very high detection rates for aneuploidies using NIPT [10–23]. A detection rate (DR) and false-positive rate (FPR) of 99% and 0.07% for Trisomy 21, 96.8% and 0.15 for Trisomy 18, and 92.1% and 0.19% for Trisomy 13, respectively, were seen in a meta-analysis by Gil et al. [24]. Thus the DR for trisomies 13 and 18 is lower than for Trisomy 21, which may be due to a lower prevalence of these aneuploidies and guanine-cytosine (GC) content of these chromosomes.

68.4 Factors Affecting Performance of NIPT

68.4.1 Rationale for Cell-Free DNA Test Failures

The test is a failure when it is reported as no result. The combined test failure rates have been reported as 1–5% for autosomal trisomies based on the technique being used. These rates are higher for X and Y chromosome abnormalities (4–7%) [25–27]. The common reasons for test failure are as follows.

68.4.1.1 Low Fetal Fraction

The absolute amount of fetal DNA with respect to the amount of maternal DNA is an important determinant of the test result. A fetal fraction of at least 4% is required for a definitive result. Up to 50% of the failures may be attributable to low fetal fraction. There could be a number of reasons for a low fetal fraction like:

- Early gestation age: Fetal fraction is less before 10 weeks of gestation and gradually increases with increasing gestational age till term [28].
- Obesity: Obese women have a lower fetal fraction due to an increase in the relative proportion of maternal as compared to fetal DNA [29].
- Fetal aneuploidies: Fetal aneuploidies may result in a lower fetal fraction leading to an increased rate of test report failures [30].

68.4.1.2 Prioritizing Performance

The failure rates of a test also vary accordingly to the acceptable false-positive and false-negative rates with an inverse correlation between the two. If the test has been reported as no result, the options are either to repeat the test, which would again be a screening test or go for a diagnostic invasive option.

68.4.2 Reasons for Test Result Inaccuracies

False positives occur when the test has falsely labelled a fetus with normal karyotype as abnormal, and false negatives occur when the test has failed to detect a fetus with abnormal karyotype.

68.4.2.1 Reasons for False-Positive Results [31]

Confined Placental Mosaicism

- The cfDNA being analyzed in maternal blood is primarily of placental origin. In conditions of placental mosaicism, the aneuploidy detected is discordant to the fetal karyotype, which can be confirmed on invasive testing.

Vanishing Twin

- Sometimes early twin demise may not be recognized if it occurs very early in gestation, and the pregnancy is considered as a singleton pregnancy. However, if the demised twin had aneuploidy, it can give a false-positive result on cfDNA testing [32].

Maternal Mosaicism

- With increasing maternal age, occasionally there is a loss of one X chromosome which can be falsely diagnosed on cfDNA testing as fetal monosomy X [33]. Sometimes, Turner's mosaic mothers can become pregnant, and in these mothers cfDNA tests can be falsely positive.

Maternal Cancer

- Tumor DNA can be aneuploid and may manifest more than one type of aneuploidy. The presence of multiple aneuploidies is an indicator of occult malignancy [34].

68.4.2.2 Reasons for False-Negative Results

Placental Mosaicism

- As with false positivity, placental mosaicism may lead to a false-negative result, as the placental karyotype may be normal in an aneuploid fetus.

Borderline Low Fetal Fraction

- A low fetal fraction precludes sequencing of adequate number of fragments and falsely leads to a screen negative result.

Technical Issues

- The guaninecytosine content of chromosome 13 is low, consequent to which the PCR becomes less reliable and decreases the detection rate for aneuploidies.

68.5 Interpretation of Test Results

The optimal utilization of any laboratory investigation depends on its clinical relevance and the ability to change practice. cfDNA indeed is a revolutionary concept which has become a fall back.

68.5.1 Reporting

The test result is reported as low-risk or high-risk for aneuploidy; positive or negative; and aneuploidy detected or not detected.

68.5.2 Implications of a Negative Test

If the NIPT report is negative, the probability of an aneuploid fetus is very remote and counselling has to be done accordingly. The routine fetal morphology scan should however be offered at 18–20 weeks, despite a negative report. cfDNA is a test to rule out only aneuploidy in the fetus. Any other genetic testing, if indicated (e.g., for raised NT or congenital malformations, etc.), must proceed as planned.

68.5.3 Implications of a Positive Test

In case of a positive test, a prompt posttest counselling should be done to convey that firstly, NIPT is only a screening test. Secondly, the possibility of a certain amount of false positivity due to the reasons mentioned above should be explained. Given these reasons, abnormal test results on NIPT should not mandate definitive management decisions. Before considering termination of pregnancy, confirmatory tests like amniocentesis or chorion villus sampling should be done.

68.5.4 No Yield

If the test reports a no yield, the options that can be given to the couple include repeat testing or definitive testing. While both options are viable, the decision should be taken keeping in mind the gestational age, as the repeat test would take 7–10 days, and a positive result would eventually require further confirmatory tests. Another point of contention would be that aneuploidies could have a low fetal fraction resulting in test failure. So the further plan should be decided after a detailed discussion.

68.6 Overall Positioning of NIPT in Aneuploidy Screening

NIPT offers additional alternatives in aneuploidy screening. The overall positioning of NIPT in the screening algorithm however is not clear. NIPT can be placed:

1. As a secondary screen
2. As a contingent screen
3. As a primary screen

68.6.1 As a Secondary Screen

This model works on offering NIPT to women who are at a high risk of aneuploidy based on their personal or family history [35], e.g.,

- Maternal age at delivery 35 years or more
- Fetal ultrasonographic findings indicating an increased risk of aneuploidy
- Personal or family history of prior pregnancy with a trisomy
- Positive first or second trimester screening test result for aneuploidy
- Parental balanced Robertsonian translocation with increased risk of T21 or T13

Positioning of NIPT here makes it an alternative to an otherwise direct invasive testing.

68.6.2 As a Contingent Screening

In this model, the population screening is done by conventional methods, which include first trimester biochemistry (beta HCG and PAPP-A) and nuchal translucency screening. Following this a risk stratification is done in which the results are divided into high, intermediate, or low risk. The risk cutoff may vary depending on the threshold for invasive testing. Generally a cutoff of 1:50–1:150 is taken as high risk and offered invasive testing directly or NIPT as a secondary screen as mentioned above. This would constitute about 3–5% of the entire population screened.

Women with risk of more than 1:1000 are generally categorized as low risk and advised routine antenatal care. This is seen in around 85% of the population.

It is the intermediate risk group, with a risk between 1:250 to 1:1000, which needs further evaluation. This group constitutes about 8–10% of the population. Traditionally, a battery of tests has been suggested to further stratify this group before offering invasive testing. After an intermediate risk in first trimester screening, a quadruple test or genetic sonogram has been used as contingent screening. NIPT can be offered in this position as a contingent screening. This makes use of the high sensitivity and specificity to screen the population further.

68.6.3 As a Primary Screen

The use of NIPT as a primary population screening test has been considered in place of serum screening. Although the detection rate is very high as compared to serum screening [36], there are certain issues that need to be considered:

1. The cost of NIPT is a constraint especially if proper pre- and posttest counselling is not built into the testing process. It leads to testing without proper interpretation and follow-up action.
2. NIPT is now considered as the most sensitive screening test for traditionally screened aneuploidies. However, even within these aneuploidies, it is more sensitive for trisomy 21 as compared to 18, 13, and sex chromosomes.
3. Using NIPT as a primary screen does not preclude the need to perform the $11–13^{+6}$ week scan as this scan encompasses more than just looking for aneuploidy, i.e., dating and structural malformations.

Therefore, at present NIPT is not recommended as a primary screening test.

68.7 Role of NIPT in Twins

Preliminary data suggest that NIPT is a feasible test option for twin gestations [37, 38]. Due to the paucity of reported studies in multiple gestations, more studies are required before establishing it in practice.

68.8 NIPT for Other Indications

68.8.1 Determination of Fetal Sex

cfDNA was used for the first time clinically for determining the fetal sex in women at risk of carrying fetuses with severe X-linked genetic disorders conditions like Duchenne muscular dystrophy. The presence of Y chromosome-specific sequences SRY or DYS14 confirms a male fetus. This removes the need for invasive testing for these conditions [39].

68.8.2 Management of RhD-Negative Pregnancies

NIPT has been used to detect the fetal RhD status in an Rh-negative mother [40–42]. Its role in the management of RhD negative mothers could be twofold.

68.8.2.1 To Guide Requirement for Monitoring

In an Rh-isoimmunized mother (indirect Coombs' test positive), determination of RhD status of the fetus can guide the monitoring as an Rh-negative fetus need not be monitored for fetal anemia by fetal Doppler, while an Rh-positive fetus needs it.

68.8.2.2 To Guide Administration of Anti-D Administration

Rh-negative mothers with partners who are heterozygous for RhD can carry either RhD-negative or positive fetus. Anti-D is administered to all women who are not isoimmunized irrespective of the fetal RhD status. With the availability of NIPT, it is possible to know the RhD status of the fetus so that anti-D administration will be administered more selectively only in those women with an Rh-positive fetus. However, at the present time, the economic feasibility of testing versus administration is not very clear.

68.8.3 Fetal or Neonatal Alloimmune Thrombocytopenia (FNAIT)

Detection of the HPA-1a gene in the maternal blood can diagnose a fetal affection of this disorder which occurs due to maternal alloantibodies against paternally inherited antigens [43, 44].

68.8.4 Monogenic Disorders

The use of cfDNA in monogenic disorders is more challenging as compared to detection of fetal sex or RhD status. If the mother is a carrier, then the detection becomes very difficult, as it requires a qualitative differentiation between the fetal and maternal mutant allele [7].

Currently NIPT can be used for detection of mutant alleles that are inherited from the father [45] or have arisen de novo [46]. One of the disorders for which clinical use of NIPT has been approved is achondroplasia [46] and its differentiation from thanatophoric dysplasia [47] and other autosomal recessive skeletal dysplasias.

68.8.5 Microdeletion Syndromes

NIPT is available commercially now for a few selected microdeletion syndromes including Di George (22q-), Wolf–Hirschhorn (4p-), Cri-du-Chat (5p-), Prader–Willi, Angelman, and 1p36 [48, 49]. Although validation data for these tests are now increasingly available, it is prudent to confine its use to situations where there is a strong possibility of such conditions rather than a blanket testing for microdeletions, as this will only increase false positives and again increasing the invasive testing rates.

68.9 Case Scenarios

1. A 36-year-old lady has had a positive quadruple test for Down syndrome at about 17 weeks gestation. Is NIPT a good option for her?

   Ans. NIPT is a good option for her as a negative test result would be reassuring and avoid an invasive procedure. In the event of a positive test a confirmatory invasive test would be in order and there would be adequate time to consider a termination of pregnancy.

2. A 40-year-old G1 woman is about 9 weeks' gestation. She has conceived by IVF and wants to know her options for aneuploidy screening. Is NIPT a good option?

   Ans. NIPT is a good option because she is at a high risk for aneuploidies because of her age. This has a better detection rate than the conventional first trimester screen (serum screening with NT scan). NIPT can be offered at an earlier gestation (any time after 10 weeks) so that pregnancy can be managed accordingly.

3. A 29-year-old patient had an NT of 4.4 mm at 12^{+5} weeks' gestation. Is NIPT a good option for her?

   Ans. Increased NT is not just a marker of aneuploidy but also for other genetic disorders or cardiac abnormalities. NIPT in such cases is not adequate for workup, and the patient should be offered a more comprehensive genetic workup with a chromosomal microarray, detailed anomaly scan, and a fetal echocardiography.

68.10 Summary

- NIPT is a highly sensitive and specific screening test for prenatal detection of fetal aneuploidies.
- It is most effective for Trisomy 21 followed by 18, 13, and sex chromosomes.
- Presently it is a screening test and definitive management decisions should not be taken based only on the result of NIPT.
- With improvement in genetic techniques, NIPY is increasingly becoming available for indications other than aneuploidies, e.g., microdeletion syndromes.

References

1. Schmorl G. Pathologische-anatomische Untersuchungen uber Puerperal-Eklampsie. Leipzig: Vogel; 1893.
2. Saiki RK, Gelfand DH, Stoffel S, et al. Primer-directed enzymatic amplification of DNA with a thermostable DNA polymerase. Science. 1988;239:487–91.
3. Lo YMD. Presence of fetal DNA in maternal plasma and serum. Lancet. 2007;350(9076):485–7.
4. Alberry M, Maddocks D, Jones M, et al. Free fetal DNA in maternal plasma in anembryonic pregnancies: confirmation that the origin is the trophoblast. Prenat Diagn. 2007;27(5):415–8.
5. Guibert J, Benachi A, Grebille AG, et al. Kinetics of SRY gene appearance in maternal serum: detection by real time PCR in early pregnancy after assisted reproductive technique. Hum Reprod. 2003;18:1733.

6. Lo YM, Zhang J, Leung TN, et al. Rapid clearance of fetal DNA from maternal plasma. Am J Hum Genet. 1999;64:218.
7. Nygren AO, Dean J, Jensen TJ, et al. Quantification of fetal DNA by use of methylation-based DNA discrimination. Clin Chem. 2010;56:1627–36.
8. Chiu RW, Akolekar R, Zheng YW, et al. Non-invasive prenatal assessment of trisomy 21 by multiplexed maternal plasma DNA sequencing: large scale validation study. Brit Med J. 2011;342:c7401.
9. Zimmermann B, Hill M, Gemelos G, et al. Noninvasive prenatal aneuploidy testing of chromosomes 13, 18, 21, X, and Y, using targeted sequencing of polymorphic loci. Prenat Diagn. 2012;32:1233–41.
10. Nicolaides KH, Syngelaki A, Gil M, et al. Validation of targeted sequencing of single-nucleotide polymorphisms for non-invasive prenatal detection of aneuploidy of chromosomes 13, 18, 21, X, and Y. Prenat Diagn. 2013;33:575–9.
11. Pergament E, Cuckle H, Zimmermann B, et al. Single-nucleotide polymorphism-based noninvasive prenatal screening in a high-risk and low-risk cohort. Obstet Gynecol. 2014;124:210–8.
12. Ehrich M, Deciu C, Zwiefelhofer T, et al. Noninvasive detection of fetal trisomy 21 by sequencing of DNA in maternal blood: a study in a clinical setting. Am J Obstet Gynecol. 2011;204:205.e1–e11.
13. Chiu R, Akolekar R, Zheng YWL, et al. Non-invasive pre-natal assessment of trisomy 21 by multiplexed maternal plasma DNA sequencing: large scale validity study. BMJ. 2011;342:c7401.
14. Palomaki GE, Kloza EM, Lambert-Messerlian GM, et al. DNA sequencing of maternal plasma to detect down syndrome: an international clinical validation study. Genet Med Off J Am Coll Med Genet. 2011;13:913–20.
15. Sparks AB, Struble CA, Wang ET, et al. Non-invasive prenatal detection and selective analysis of cell-free DNA obtained from maternal blood: evaluation for trisomy 21 and trisomy 18. Am J Obstet Gynecol. 2012;206:322.e1–5.
16. Ashoor G, Syngelaki A, Wagner M, et al. Chromosome-selective sequencing of maternal plasma cell-free DNA for first-trimester detection of trisomy 21 and trisomy 18. Am J Obstet Gynecol. 2012;206:322.e1–5.
17. Manegold-Brauer G, Lapaire O. Clinical implementation of next-generation sequencing in the field of prenatal diagnostics. https://doi.org/10.5772/61799
18. Norton ME, Brar H, Weiss J, et al. Non-invasive chromosomal evaluation (NICE) study: results of a multicenter prospective cohort study for detection of fetal trisomy 21 and trisomy 18. Am J Obstet Gynecol. 2012;207:137.e1–8.
19. Bianchi DW, Parker RL, Wentworth J, et al. DNA sequencing versus standard prenatal aneuploidy screening. N Engl J Med. 2014;370:799–808.
20. Liang D, Lv W, Wang H, et al. Non-invasive prenatal testing of fetal whole chromosome aneuploidy by massively parallel sequencing. Prenat Diagn. 2013;33:409–15.
21. Song Y, Liu C, Qi H, et al. Noninvasive prenatal testing of fetal aneuploidies by massively parallel sequencing in a prospective Chinese population. Prenat Diagn. 2013;33:700–6.
22. Stumm M, Entezami M, Haug K, et al. Diagnostic accuracy of random massively parallel sequencing for non-invasive prenatal detection of common autosomal aneuploidies: a collaborative study in Europe. Prenat Diagn. 2014;34:185–91.
23. Fairbrother G, Johnson S, Musci TJ, Song K. Clinical experience of noninvasive prenatal testing with cell-free DNA for fetal trisomies 21, 18, and 13, in a general screening population. Prenat Diagn. 2013;33:580–3.
24. Gil MM, Quezada MS, Revello R, et al. Analysis of cellfree DNA in maternal blood in screening for fetal aneuploidies: updated meta-analysis. Ultrasound Obstet Gynecol. 2015;45:249.
25. Mazloom AR, Džakula Ž, Oeth P, et al. Noninvasive prenatal detection of sex chromosomal aneuploidies by sequencing circulating cellfree DNA from maternal plasma. Prenat Diagn. 2013;33:591.
26. Samango Sprouse C, Banjevic M, Ryan A, et al. SNPbased noninvasive prenatal testing detects sex chromosome aneuploidies with high accuracy. Prenat Diagn. 2013;33:643.
27. Hooks J, Wolfberg AJ, Wang ET, et al. Noninvasive risk assessment of fetal sex chromosome aneuploidy through directed analysis and incorporation of fetal fraction. Prenat Diagn. 2014;34:496.
28. Lo YM, Tein MS, Lau TK, et al. Quantitative analysis of fetal DNA in maternal plasma and serum: implications for noninvasive prenatal diagnosis. Am J Hum Genet. 1998;62:768.
29. Canick JA, Palomaki GE, Kloza EM, et al. The impact of maternal plasma DNA fetal fraction on next generation sequencing tests for common fetal aneuploidies. Prenat Diagn. 2013;33:667.
30. Palomaki GE, Kloza EM, Lambert Messerlian GM, et al. Circulating cell free DNA testing: are some test failures informative? Prenat Diagn. 2015;35:289.
31. Hartwig TS, Ambye L, Sørensen S, Jørgensen FS. Discordant non-invasive prenatal testing (NIPT) a systematic review. Prenat Diagn. 2017;37:527.
32. Curnow KJ, Wilkins Haug L, Ryan A, et al. Detection of triploid, molar, and vanishing twin pregnancies by a single nucleotide polymorphismbased noninvasive prenatal test. Am J Obstet Gynecol. 2015;212:79.e1.
33. Wang Y, Chen Y, Tian F, et al. Maternal mosaicism is a significant contributor to discordant sex chromosomal aneuploidies associated with noninvasive prenatal testing. Clin Chem. 2014;60:251.
34. Bianchi DW, Chudova D, Sehnert AJ, et al. Noninvasive prenatal testing and incidental detection of occult maternal malignancies. JAMA. 2015;314:162.
35. American College of Obstetricians and Gynecologists Committee on Genetics. Committee opinion no. 545: noninvasive prenatal testing for fetal aneuploidy. Obstet Gynecol. 2012;120:1532.
36. Gregg AR, Skotko BG, Judith L, et al. Noninvasive prenatal screening for fetal aneuploidy, 2016 update: a position statement of the American College of Medical Genetics and Genomics. Genet Med. 2016;18:1056–65.
37. del Mar GM, Quezada MS, Bregant B, et al. Cell-free DNA analysis for trisomy risk assessment in first-trimester twin pregnancies. Fetal Diagn Ther. 2014;35:204–11.
38. Bevilacqua E, Gil MM, Nicolaides KH, et al. Performance of screening for aneuploidies by cell-free DNA analysis of maternal blood in twin pregnancies. Ultrasound Obstet Gynecol. 2015;45:61–6.
39. Hill M, Finning K, Martin P, et al. Non-invasive prenatal determination of fetal sex: translating research into clinical practice. Clin Genet. 2011;80:68–75.
40. Finning KM, Martin PG, Soothill PW, Avent ND. Prediction of fetal D status from maternal plasma: introduction of a new non-invasive fetal RHD genotyping service. Transfusion. 2002;42:1079–85.
41. Finning K, Martin P, Daniels G. A clinical service in the UK to predict fetal Rh (Rhesus) D blood group using free fetal DNA in maternal plasma. Ann N Y Acad Sci. 2004;1022:119–23.
42. Scheffer PG, van der Schoot CE, Page-Christiaens GC, de Haas M. Non-invasive fetal blood group genotyping of rhesus D, c, E and of K in alloimmunised pregnant women: evaluation of a 7-year clinical experience. BJOG. 2011;118:1340–8.
43. Scheffer PG, Ait Soussan A, Verhagen OJ, et al. Non-invasive fetal genotyping of human platelet antigen-1a. BJOG. 2011;118:1392–5.
44. Le Toriellec E, Chenet C, Kaplan C. Safe fetal platelet genotyping: new developments. Transfusion. 2013;53:1755–62.
45. Lench N, Barrett A, Fielding S, et al. The clinical implementation of non-invasive prenatal diagnosis for single gene disorders: challenges and progress made. Prenat Diagn. 2013;33:555–62.

46. Chitty LS, Griffin DR, Meaney C, et al. New aids for the non-invasive prenatal diagnosis of achondroplasia: dysmorphic features, charts of fetal size and molecular confirmation using cell-free fetal DNA in maternal plasma. Ultrasound Obstet Gynecol. 2011;37:283–9.
47. Chitty LS, Khalil A, Barrett AN, et al. Safer, accurate prenatal diagnosis of thanatophoric dysplasia using ultrasound and cell free fetal DNA. Prenat Diagn. 2013;33:416–23.
48. Lo K, Boustred C, McKay F, et al. Detection of "sub-chromosomal" pathogenic changes by sequencing cfDNA in maternal plasma: feasibility and implementation strategies. Prenat Diagn. 2014;34(Suppl 1):10.
49. Chen S, Lau TK, Zhang C, et al. A method for non-invasive detection of fetal large deletions/duplications by low coverage massively parallel sequencing. Prenat Diagn. 2013;33:584–90.

Reproductive Genetics for the Clinician

69

Stephen Brown and Jennifer Dundee

Clinical genetics, more than most other fields, is driven by technology, and the tools available for the clinical evaluation of genetic problems have expanded dramatically over the past 50 years, with each decade bringing a new revolution in methods. The first human karyotypes and the chromosomal basis of Down syndrome appeared about 1960. By the 1970s, chromosome banding techniques were developed, allowing the detection and characterization of sub-chromosomal deletions, duplications, and translocations. This led to the description of many segmental deletion syndromes. During the 1980s, it became practical to actually work with DNA and DNA level polymorphisms such as "restriction fragment length polymorphisms" or RFLPs, thus opening the door to linkage studies for gene discovery. The discovery of gene for Huntington's disease using linkage studies in 1993 was a major milestone. The 1990s saw the invention of PCR, the automation of DNA sequencing, and other technologies critical for the ultimate goal of sequencing the human genome, which was actually accomplished in 2003. The early 2000s also brought us microarray technology, vastly expanding the resolution at which genomic deletions and duplications can be visualized. Most recently, beginning in 2011, various technologies for extremely high throughput or "next-gen" DNA sequencing began to appear, initiating yet another (and arguably the biggest ever) revolution in genetic knowledge.

As each of these technologies has emerged from the research lab, they have been introduced immediately into the clinical arena, and nowhere has the impact of this technical innovation been more important than in reproductive medicine. Today, infertility specialists use conventional cytogenetics, microarray, Sanger sequencing, and next-gen sequencing to evaluate adult patients, fetuses, and preimplantation embryos. The clinical reproductive endocrinologist is confronted with genetic questions and problems every day, while at the same time, the technical knowledge and sophistication of patients and the questions they ask increase. The goal of this chapter is to provide clinicians with an up-to-date approach to genetic questions that arise in everyday practice.

S. Brown (✉) · J. Dundee
Department of Obstetrics, Gynecology and Reproductive Sciences, University of Vermont, Lerner College of Medicine, Burlington, VT, USA
e-mail: sabrown@uvm.edu

69.1 Meiosis and Aneuploidy

Meiosis, the process by which diploid germ cell precursors produce haploid gametes, is central to reproduction. In fact, the shuffling of the two parental genomes that occurs during meiosis is widely regarded as being the primary evolutionary goal of sexual reproduction. Despite its obvious evolutionary importance, reproduction in humans is surprisingly inefficient. It is estimated that, of all conceptions, about 30% of conceptions fail to implant, another 30% end as preclinical ("biochemical") losses, and another 10–15% end as first trimester miscarriages (Fig. 69.1). Ironically, in humans, errors in the segregation of chromosomes during meiosis are the leading impediment to obtaining successful pregnancies. Classic studies in the 1960s showed that about 0.3% of liveborn babies were affected with aneuploidy, but this turned out to be the tip of the iceberg. Subsequent studies in the 1970s and 1980s showed that about 50% of spontaneous miscarriages were associated with chromosome abnormalities. Given the frequency of miscarriage, this finding implied that up to 5 or 6% of all clinically recognized pregnancies are affected with aneuploidy. Follow-up studies using chromosomal polymorphisms and DNA polymorphisms to determine

G. N. Allahbadia et al. (eds.), *Textbook of Assisted Reproduction*, https://doi.org/10.1007/978-981-15-2377-9_69

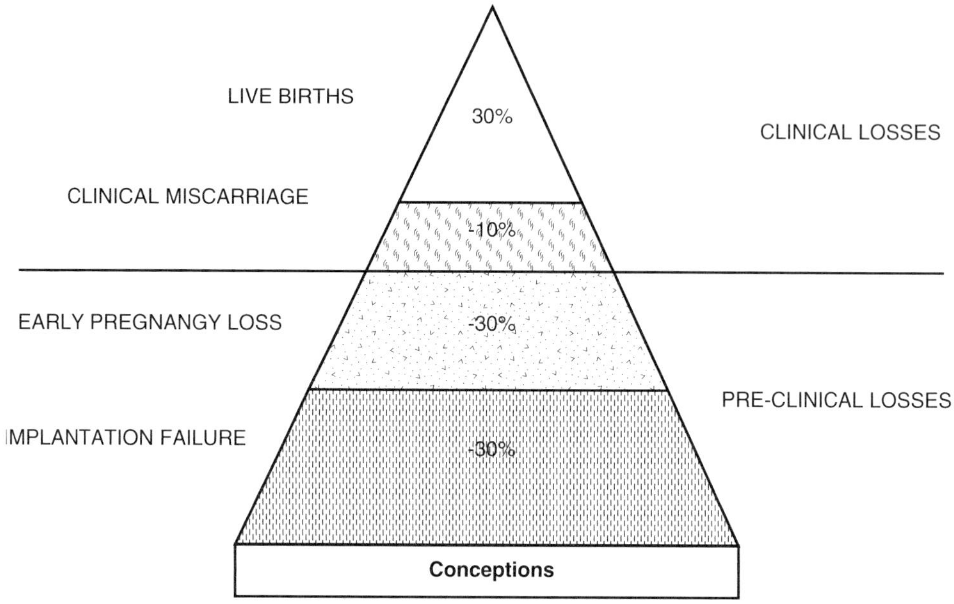

Fig. 69.1 Conceptual representation of the fate of human conceptions, showing that the majority are never clinically recognized and that the minority become successful pregnancies. (Adapted from Chard T. Frequency of implantation and early pregnancy loss in natural cycles Baillieres Clin Obstet Gynaecol 1991;Mar, 5(1):179–89, with permission)

the parental origin of chromosomes showed that the majority of fetal chromosome abnormalities arise during female meiosis, indicating that meiosis is somewhat different in males and females and that it is more error-prone in females. This finding is in good agreement with epidemiologic data showing that fetal aneuploidy risk increases with increasing maternal age but not with paternal age [1].

Over the past 25 years, a variety of studies of preimplantation embryos have appeared, with new technology driving an ever-improved ability to assess for aneuploidy. Modern studies, utilizing chromosome microarray for the assessment of all 24 chromosomes, have shown that, even in young women, about 30% of embryos are aneuploidy. By age 40, up to 70% are chromosomally abnormal [2] (Fig. 69.2). Thus, aneuploidy due to meiotic error is a major issue in human reproduction.

The development of methods for the assessment of aneuploidy in preimplantation embryos has been driven by the goal of improving the efficiency of IVF by selecting against embryos that are destined to fail due to chromosome abnormality. Early efforts to accomplish preimplantation genetic screening (PGS) using FISH technology applied to single-cell biopsies from day 3 embryos were initially said to improve the chances for success with IVF. However, when subjected to randomized trials, it became clear that, at least with FISH-based embryo screening, the overall chances of success were not significantly improved and, in at least one study, were actually reduced [3]. One proposed reason for the failure of this approach is that FISH is error-prone and limited by the fact that it only allows the assessment of a few chromosomes. More modern efforts to accomplish the goal of screening embryos for aneuploidy have made use of a series of important technological advancements, including new methods for whole genome DNA amplification in conjunction with microarray technology that allows the assessment of all 24 chromosomes. In addition, the development of methods for efficient freezing of blastocyst stage embryos now allows for multicell trophectoderm biopsies of day 5 embryos. Most recently, next-gen DNA sequencing for the assessment of aneuploidy is rapidly replacing microarray as the preferred method for aneuploidy assessment. A number of publications have claimed improvements in IVF success with the use of PGS, and there seems to be little doubt that implantation failure and early miscarriage are both reduced by selecting chromosomally normal embryos [4]. Nonetheless, there is significant controversy about whether overall success is improved [5, 6]. Resolution of the controversies surrounding the use of PGS and the establishment of guidelines for appropriate use of PGS is a pressing issue for the global REI community. Hopefully, appropriately designed randomized trials will soon clarify the circumstances in which PGS is clearly indicated.

69.2 Balanced Chromosome Translocations

About 1:500 phenotypically normal individuals is a carrier of a balanced chromosome rearrangement [7]; however, in couples with a history of miscarriage, the probability that one or the other parent is a translocation carrier is substantially increased. This is because carriers of balanced rearrangements can produce chromosomally unbalanced gametes that lead to nonviable embryos, as well as viable but developmentally abnormal offspring. Classic studies show that the incidence of translocation carrier status is 2.2% after one

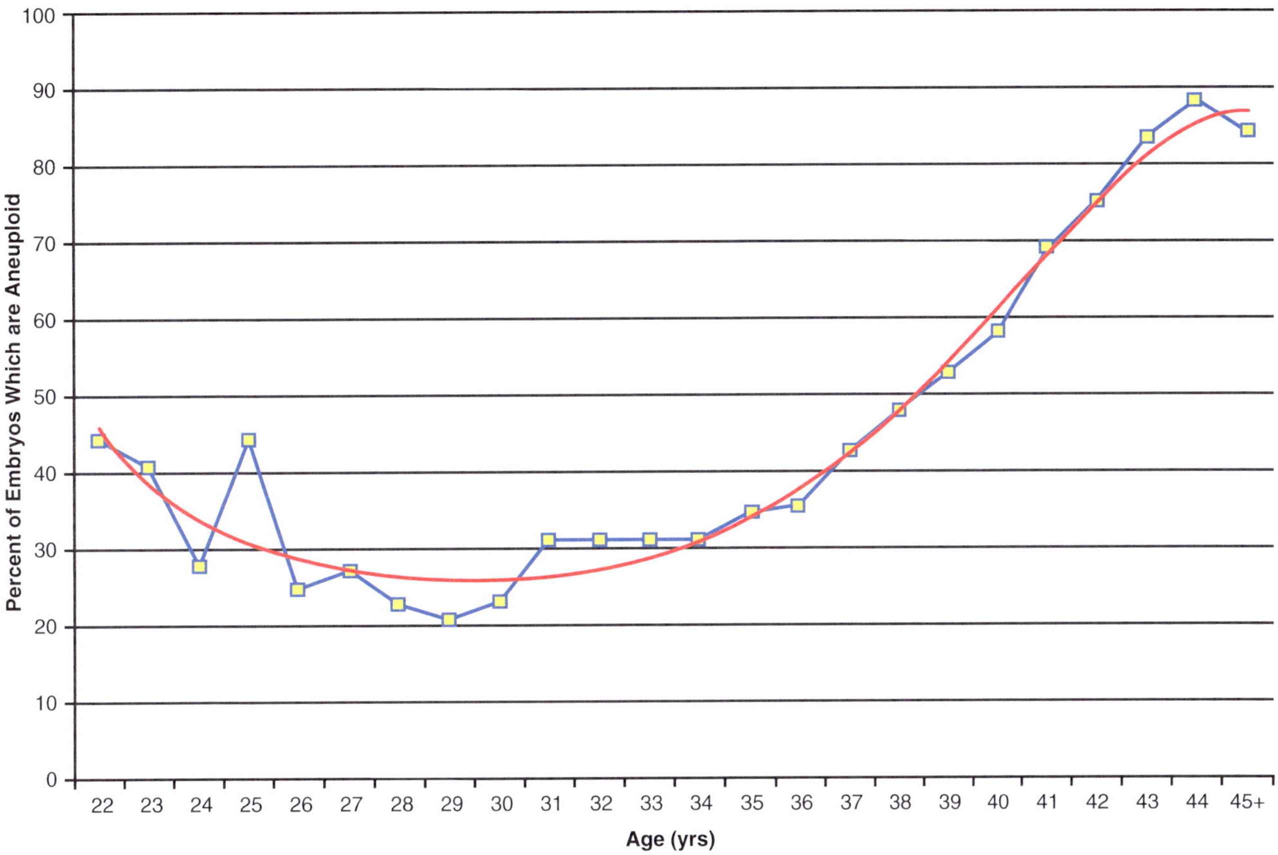

Fig. 69.2 Summary of data from PGS performed on over 15,000 trophectoderm biopsies. The overall incidence of aneuploidy is approximately 40%. (From Franasiak JM, Forman EJ, Hong KH, Werner MD, Upham KM, Treff NR, et al. The nature of aneuploidy with increasing age of the female partner: a review of 15,169 consecutive trophectoderm biopsies evaluated with comprehensive chromosomal screening. Fertil Steril. 2014;101(3):656–63 e1, with permission)

miscarriage, 4.8% after two miscarriages, and 5.2% after three [8]. This has led to the general idea that couples with recurrent loss should be evaluated for chromosome translocations; however, there is no general consensus about who should undergo such testing. For instance, the Royal College of Obstetricians and Gynaecologists recommends testing after three consecutive miscarriages, and other organizations, such as the American College of Obstetricians and Gynecologists, recommend chromosome evaluation after two. It is likely that the risk of miscarriage based on maternal age is an important factor in determining the probability of identifying a translocation carrier couple. In fact, this relationship has been documented: In couples under the age of 23 with two miscarriages, the incidence of translocation carrier was 10%, whereas it was less than 1% in couples where the female partner was over 39 [9]. Thus, chromosome analysis is more important to consider in younger couples with multiple miscarriages.

Despite the clear increase in the likelihood of miscarriage in translocation carrier couples, there is little consensus about the overall reproductive impact of balanced translocations. A large case-control study indicated that translocation carriers identified by a history of miscarriage had a very low chance to have viable unbalanced pregnancies and an overall chance to have a healthy child that was nearly equal to controls [10]. Studies of this type have led some authors to question the value of chromosome analysis in the setting of recurrent miscarriage [11, 12]. Despite the data showing a high probability of good outcome in balanced translocation carrier couples, anecdotal experience suggests that, while some translocations are unlikely to cause reproductive problems, others are associated with a high incidence of problems, including abnormal offspring and recurrent miscarriage. Consistent with this, several older studies have shown that the risk of unbalanced progeny varies dramatically, according to the particular translocation [13]. Of course, it would be very convenient to know which translocations are associated with a high risk of poor outcome and which are not; however, efforts to predict whether a given translocation will result in unbalanced progeny have not been terribly successful. Some more recent studies have attempted to use the location of breakpoints of reciprocal translocations to predict the probability of identifying usable embryos in the setting of PGD. Such studies have shown that the most asymmetrical translocations (where the size difference between the translocated segments is the largest) have the highest probability to produce unbalanced embryos; however, such predictions did not prove to be clinically useful [14]. In the end, the best indication of the reproductive significance of a balanced translocation is the couple's own history.

For an infertility specialist confronted with a couple with recurrent miscarriage and a balanced translocation, assessing the role of preimplantation genetic diagnosis (PGD) is important. The concept of using PGD to select euploid embryos is intellectually compelling, and a large number of publications have reported the successful use of PGD in this setting of a parental balanced translocation. However, systematic studies of the use of PGD in translocation couples have not been encouraging. One literature review concluded that there was insufficient data to support the use of PGD in fertile couples with a balanced chromosome translocation [15]. A more recent case-control study concluded that for fertile couples with chromosome translocation, natural conception was likely to yield a live birth faster than pregnancy achieved with PGD [16]. On the other hand, couples that have experienced recurrent miscarriage or a prior viable pregnancy with an unbalanced karyotype may have a very strong preference for IVF/PGD. Infertile couples with a balanced translocation are good candidates for PGD as well. Clearly, the role for PGD in couples with balanced translocations needs to be assessed on a case-by-case basis.

69.3 Genetics of Male Infertility

69.3.1 Cytogenetics

Male factor contributes to infertility in 50% of couples seeking treatment, so that questions relating to genetic evaluation of infertile men occur daily in an infertility practice. The first and most important type of abnormality to consider in the evaluation of male infertility is cytogenetic. Large studies indicate that the probability to identify a chromosome abnormality is inversely proportional to sperm count [17]. Men with very low sperm counts (<5 million sperm per ml) have about a 5% chance to have a recognizable chromosome abnormality, whereas those with azoospermia have up to a 15% chance to harbor a chromosome abnormality. In the setting of azoospermia, the most common finding is sex chromosome aneuploidy, typically 47 XXY or mosaic 46XY/47XXY. Men with severe oligospermia are more likely to have structural rearrangements such as balanced translocations, Robertsonian translocations, and inversions. Given the high probability to identify an important abnormality, it seems clear that men with a sperm count <5 million should have a chromosome analysis as part of their evaluation. Several authors have suggested that all men whose sperm count is low enough to require ICSI should have chromosome analysis [18, 19].

69.3.2 Translocation Carriers and Interchromosomal Effect

A number of studies utilizing FISH on single sperm from men with Robertsonian translocations have shown an increased incidence of sperm with chromosome abnormalities of chromosomes that were NOT involved in the translocation, a phenomenon known as "interchromosomal effect" [20]. Studies of embryos from couples in which the father was a Robertsonian translocation carrier have shown an increased incidence of aneuploidy of chromosomes not involved in the translocation, thus corroborating the single-sperm studies [21]. This effect may contribute to the miscarriage rate and may also lead to abnormal ongoing pregnancies, adding to the list of issues that Robertsonian translocation carriers should discuss with a geneticist.

69.3.3 Y Chromosome Microdeletions

Microdeletion of the azoospermia factor region (AZF) of the Y chromosome long arm is another potential cause of failed spermatogenesis, as is evidenced by the fact that 5% of men with oligospermia and 10% of men with azoospermia harbor such deletions [22, 23]. A number of studies have attempted to divide the AZF region into subregions (AZFa, AZFb, and AZFc) and to correlate the precise position and extent of deletion, with the severity of the defect in spermatogenesis [24]. However, this level of genetic detail is unlikely to be relevant to the clinician. Much more important is that couples understand that, if a Yq microdeletion is transmitted to a son through IVF/ICSI, defective spermatogenesis in the child is expected. Interestingly, most couples do not seem to be troubled by this possibility. Clinical experience suggests that men with oligospermia are actually relieved by the identification of a Y chromosome microdeletion.

69.3.4 CF Mutations and Congenital Bilateral Absence of the Vas Deferens

One of the mildest manifestations of loss of function of the cystic fibrosis transmembrane regulator (CFTR) is congenital bilateral absence of the vas deferens (CBAVD). In the typical CBAVD scenario, the affected individual has two different mutations in their two CFTR alleles. One mutation is severe and knocks out gene function completely, whereas the other mutation is milder. The combination results in severely reduced gene function. Because of the association between CBAVD and CF mutations, the evaluation of men with azoospermia normal testicular size and normal endocrine parameters should include testing for mutations in CFTR. Some authors have stressed that clinical evaluation for the absence of the vas deferens is unreliable, making it important to test for CFTR mutations in all men that might have obstructive azoospermia [25]. Clearly, the identification of CFTR mutation(s) in the male partner allows for appropriate testing and counseling in the female partner.

69.3.5 Advanced Paternal Age

Although advanced paternal age is not a cause of male infertility, many couples seeking infertility treatment are quite concerned about the genetic effects of increasing paternal age. Indeed, evidence accumulated over many years indicates that several types of abnormal pregnancy outcome become more frequent when the father is older. Disorders that are known to arise from single-gene mutations, such as achondroplasia and Apert syndrome as well as others, show a clear paternal age effect [26]. Molecular analysis now indicates that in those cases where a paternal age effect is present, the underlying mutations are point mutations as opposed to gene deletions or duplications [27]. In addition to these types of studies, epidemiologic studies show that autism spectrum disorder, schizophrenia, malformations, infant death, and other conditions also become more common as the father ages, although the effect size is rather small [28].

For many years, it has been hypothesized that the reason that older men produce sperm with more mutations is that their germ cells have undergone more cycles of division than younger men. It is estimated that, after puberty, a man's germ cells undergo division every 23 days. By age 20, 150 divisions are expected, and by age 50, the expected number is 840 [27]. This increase in the number of cell divisions clearly increases the chance that mutations have accumulated, but until recently, this was theoretical. With the advent of next-gen DNA sequencing, we now have solid supporting data to support this hypothesis. The number of de novo mutations appears to approximately double approximately every 16 years, so that a man who is 52 is expected to have offspring with four-fold more mutations than a 20-year-old father [29].

While these observations may be alarming to couples where the father is older, in terms of risk mitigation, there is little to offer. The overall chances of a new-onset dominant condition are still quite low, even for a father who is 55. Gene testing is impractical, since one would have to sequence the entire fetal genome. While this is technically possible, it would be ill advised, since it would result in a deluge of genetic variants of unknown significance. Likewise, prenatal ultrasound is of limited value, since most relevant conditions would not have ultrasound findings.

69.3.6 Summary

In summary, men with sperm counts less than 5 million per ml should have chromosome analysis. Those that do not have a conventional chromosome abnormality evident on routine analysis may benefit from a molecular evaluation for Y microdeletions. Men with evidence of obstructive azoospermia should be evaluated for CFTR mutations. Any man with a chromosome abnormality or a gene mutation should consult with a geneticist. Despite appropriate evaluation, a genetic cause for severe oligospermia/azoospermia is not identified in the majority of affected men.

69.4 Genetics of Premature Ovarian Insufficiency

Premature ovarian insufficiency (POI) is characterized by primary or secondary amenorrhea for at least 4 months in women under the age of 40 in conjunction with serum FSH levels above 40 IU/l (obtained twice, at least 1 month apart) and low estradiol levels (below 50 pg/ml). Classic studies indicate that (POI) affects 1:10,000 women below the age of 20 and about 1% of women by the time they reach 40 [30]. The clinician confronted with a patient with POI needs to consider several possible causes, including autoimmune disease, environmental factors, and iatrogenic and genetic factors.

69.4.1 Aneuploidy

Two functional X chromosomes are necessary for normal ovarian function, and one common cause of POI is sex chromosome aneuploidy, which is identified in about 10% of affected women [31]. Among the aneuploidies associated with POI, the most common are numerical abnormalities such as 45X and/or 46XX/45X mosaicism. Cytogenetic studies of women with POI have also identified structural abnormalities of the X chromosome, such as deletions and translocations. Review of deletion cases indicates that there are at least two regions of the X chromosome long arm where the presence of both copies is necessary for normal ovulatory function, indicating that the X chromosome is likely to contain several specific genes that are relevant to follicular survival [32]. Given that cytogenetically visible deletions of the X chromosome are known to cause POI, it is not surprising that microdeletions and duplications of the X chromosome occur as well. Microarray technology has shown that microdeletions are likely to be the cause of POI in a significant number of cases [33, 34]. This raises the question of whether microarray should be performed on women being evaluated for POI. At present there is no general consensus, but such studies may be important in select cases. The identification of a micro abnormality of the X chromosome raises the possibility that the abnormal X chromosome could be the cause of developmental abnormality when inherited by a son.

The finding of cytogenetic abnormality can have major implications for patients. Therefore, a chromosome analysis should be considered on all women being evaluated for POI. In practice, the likelihood of finding a karyotypic abnormality is much more likely in young women.

69.4.2 Fragile X Premutations

The FMR1 (fragile X mental retardation) gene, which is located on the distal X chromosome long arm, contains a CGG triplet repeat polymorphism, which normally varies between 11 and 42 repeats. Women with repeat sizes in the premutation range (greater than 55 and less than 200 repeats) are at a 13–26% risk of POI. Some studies have indicated that women with fragile X premutations who do not have overt POI have an increased incidence of ovulatory dysfunction [35]. In addition to the increased risk of POI, premutation carrier women can also have other health consequences, such as depression/anxiety. Most importantly women with premutations are at risk of having children affected with fragile X mental retardation syndrome, which occurs when premutations expand to full mutations during female meiosis. Women who are identified as permutation carriers also need to understand that boys who inherit an intact premutation are apparently at increased risk of autism [36]. For all of these reasons, women with POI should be offered fragile X testing, and those with premutations should have genetic consultation.

69.4.3 Other Single-Gene Disorders

A number of other genes where mutations can result in abnormal ovarian function have been identified and/or proposed (reviewed in [37]). While investigations into individual genes (other than FMR1) are not part of routine clinical evaluation, commercial laboratories offer next-generation sequencing panels for the evaluation of POI. Such panels may include some or all of the following genes, all of which have been implicated in POI: BMP15, CYP17A1, CYP19A1, FIGLA, FMR1, FSHR, GDF9, LHCGR, NOBOX, NR5A1, POR, PSMC3IP, and may be of benefit in select patients.

69.5 Recessive Disease Carrier Screening in Infertile Couples

Although recessive genetic conditions are individually rare, collectively they occur with surprising frequency. Estimates based on screening data suggest that about 1/500 children (depending on ethnicity) will be affected by a serious recessive condition, making it important for infertility specialists to address this issue with patients. For many years, carrier screening has been based on a combination of ethnicity and family history, with testing directed for specific conditions in selected patients. This approach is well summarized in the 2017 ACOG practice bulletin, which endorses the idea that all women/couples contemplating pregnancy should be offered screening for cystic fibrosis (CF) and spinal muscular atrophy (SMA) [38]. Hemoglobinopathies should be screened for in at-risk populations, such as people of African, Mediterranean, Middle Eastern, or South East Asian descent. Fragile X syndrome should be screened for in women with a suggestive family history of intellectual disability, and people of Ashkenazi Jewish background should be offered an appropriate panel that could include up to 20 conditions known to have increased frequency in this ethnic group.

Although this approach to carrier screening has been the standard for many years, it will fail to identify the majority of couples that are at risk for recessive or X-linked illness. With the advent of next-generation sequencing technology, the above-described screening paradigm is rapidly changing. Several commercial vendors now offer "expanded carrier screening," which can identify mutations in up to 175 recessive disease genes simultaneously. Over the next several years, such tests are expected to become cheaper and even more comprehensive. The advantages of expanded carrier screening are clear: Couples with a 25% chance to have a child, severely affected with a recessive illness, will be identified, and this will allow appropriate prenatal or preimplantation testing. Because mutation screening is done by sequencing, as opposed to mutation panels, these benefits apply to all ethnic groups [39]. However, there are clear downsides to such testing. From 30 to 50% of people tested will be identified as carriers of at least one recessive condition, making it likely that both members of a couple will need to be tested. This adds to expense, while discussions with patients about residual risks use valuable counseling resources. Some patients who are identified as carriers will very anxious about their carrier status. In addition, sequencing-based tests may reveal variants of unknown significance, potentially adding to patient anxiety.

Patient attitudes toward expanded carrier screening are likely to vary according to the situation. For the couple preparing for IVF, carrier screening may make more sense than for the couple that already has an ongoing pregnancy. In the absence of clear guidelines for the use of expanded carrier screening, it seems reasonable for infertility practices to at least make patients aware of the availability of expanded carrier screening.

69.6 Preimplantation Genetic Diagnosis for Mendelian Illness

A surprising number of couples present to infertility clinics with the desire to pursue preimplantation genetic diagnosis (PGD) for recessive, dominant, and X-linked conditions. Some couples have been identified through carrier testing, others by having already had an affected child, while others are, themselves, actually affected by dominant conditions such as polycystic kidney disease, Huntington's disease, and others. As the use of genetic technology such as extended carrier screening increases, the number of affected couples is likely to increase as well. Many such couples have turned to IVF/PGD because they do not want affected children but are unwilling or unable to risk the possibility of a decision to terminate an ongoing but affected pregnancy. In order to provide appropriate direction to such patients, infertility specialists need to have a basic technical understanding of PGD for single-gene disorders.

First, in order for PGD to be possible, the definitive causative gene mutation(s) in a patient or couple must have already been identified. In many instances, establishing what gene mutations are involved may require coordination with a geneticist. Once gene mutations have been identified, an appropriate PGD testing laboratory can be consulted about establishing a custom assay, specific for that patient or couple. In general, such an assay involves the design of PCR primers that amplify relevant genomic segments. PCR products can then be sequenced. In the simplest and earliest efforts at PGD, a single cell was removed from a day 3 embryo, and DNA prepared from it would serve as template for PCR amplification and sequencing of the relevant gene segments. While this approach was conceptually simple, it was both limited and prone to errors. When performing PCR on very small quantities of DNA, one of the two alleles of a given gene may fail to amplify, a phenomenon known as "allele dropout" or ADO. When this occurs, the sequence analysis shows the presence of only one allele. If it is the mutant allele that failed to amplify, the sequence data is easily misinterpreted as homozygous normal (false negative). In order to address this issue, most laboratories begin by performing whole genome amplification of DNA from 4 to 6 cell trophectoderm biopsies from blastocyst stage embryos. The biopsied embryos are then frozen, and the amplified DNA is used to run a single-nucleotide polymorphism (SNP) array, to genotype a large number of SNPs throughout the genome. Using family information, one can determine the SNP haplotype of the genomic region(s) surrounding the mutation(s). Then, the SNP haplotype is used to determine whether a given embryo has inherited the mutation, in a robust and highly accurate way (Fig. 69.3). Direct mutation analysis by PCR followed by sequencing is generally performed as well, providing additional analytic confidence. In addition, the amplified DNA can be used to perform comprehensive chromosome abnormality screening. This allows the selection of embryos that are chromosomally normal as well as being unaffected by a genetic illness. While PGD for single-gene genetic disease coupled with comprehensive chromosome analysis is intellectually appealing, it is sobering to consider the probability that a given embryo is normal. In the setting of a dominantly inherited condition such as polycystic kidney disease (ADPKD), 50% of embryos are expected to be affected. In a 35-year-old patient, 35% of embryos are expected to be aneuploid (Fig. 69.2), meaning that only about 33% of embryos in a 35-year-old couple ADPKD will be usable. In a cycle in which five embryos are biopsied, each of which has a 67% chance to be abnormal, there is a 15% chance that there will be no usable embryos. Patients should understand these probabilities prior to embarking on the process of IVF with PGD.

69.7 Overall Summary

Genetic problems and genetic testing both play major roles in reproductive medicine, and over the next decade, this is likely to increase dramatically. In particular, preimplantation testing for chromosome abnormalities and single-gene abnormalities is likely to become more the norm than the exception. In addition, a growing proportion of infertility patients will elect to have expanded carrier screening and will be identified as being at risk of genetic disorders. Reproductive medicine providers will be increasingly called upon to address genetic issues.

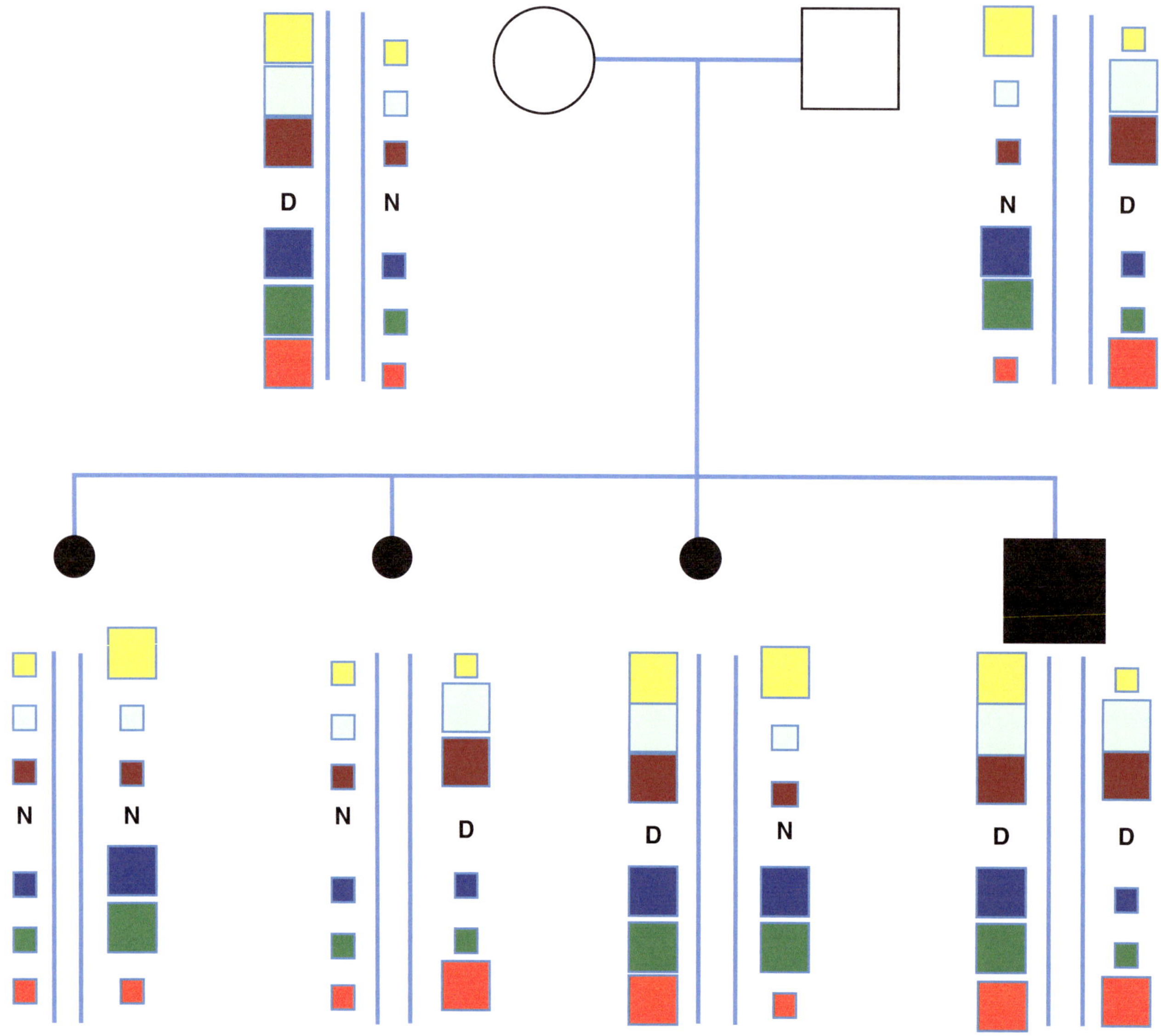

Fig. 69.3 Illustration of SNP linkage for PGD. Each colored square represents a SNP that flanks a recessive genetic disease locus, which is indicated by "D" for disease and "N" for normal. By determining the SNP genotypes in the parents and the affected son, one can deduce which SNP genotypes are associated with unaffected preimplantation embryos (depicted by small circles)

References

1. Hassold T, Hall H, Hunt P. The origin of human aneuploidy: where we have been, where we are going. Hum Mol Genet. 2007;16(2):R203–8.
2. Franasiak JM, Forman EJ, Hong KH, Werner MD, Upham KM, Treff NR, et al. The nature of aneuploidy with increasing age of the female partner: a review of 15,169 consecutive trophectoderm biopsies evaluated with comprehensive chromosomal screening. Fertil Steril. 2014;101(3):656–63.
3. Mastenbroek S, Twisk M, van der Veen F, Repping S. Preimplantation genetic screening: a systematic review and meta-analysis of RCTs. Hum Reprod Update. 2011;17(4):454–66.
4. Lee E, Illingworth P, Wilton L, Chambers GM. The clinical effectiveness of preimplantation genetic diagnosis for aneuploidy in all 24 chromosomes (PGD-A): systematic review. Hum Reprod. 2015;30(2):473–83.
5. Gleicher N, Orvieto R. Is the hypothesis of preimplantation genetic screening (PGS) still supportable? A review. J Ovarian Res. 2017;10(1):21.
6. Rubio C, Bellver J, Rodrigo L, Castillon G, Guillen A, Vidal C, et al. In vitro fertilization with preimplantation genetic diagnosis for aneuploidies in advanced maternal age: a randomized, controlled study. Fertil Steril. 2017;107(5):1122–9.
7. Jacobs PA, Frackiewicz A, Law P. Incidence and mutation rates of structural rearrangements of the autosomes in man. Ann Hum Genet. 1972;35(3):301–19.
8. De Braekeleer M, Dao TN. Cytogenetic studies in couples experiencing repeated pregnancy losses. Hum Reprod. 1990;5(5):519–28.
9. Franssen MT, Korevaar JC, Leschot NJ, Bossuyt PM, Knegt AC, Gerssen-Schoorl KB, et al. Selective chromosome analysis in couples with two or more miscarriages: case-control study. BMJ. 2005;331(7509):137–41.
10. Franssen MT, Korevaar JC, van der Veen F, Leschot NJ, Bossuyt PM, Goddijn M. Reproductive outcome after chromosome analysis

in couples with two or more miscarriages: index [corrected]-control study. BMJ. 2006;332(7544):759–63.
11. Barber JC, Cockwell AE, Grant E, Williams S, Dunn R, Ogilvie CM. Is karyotyping couples experiencing recurrent miscarriage worth the cost? BJOG. 2010;117(7):885–8.
12. van Leeuwen M, Vansenne F, Korevaar JC, van der Veen F, Goddijn M, Mol BW. Economic analysis of chromosome testing in couples with recurrent miscarriage to prevent handicapped offspring. Hum Reprod. 2013;28(7):1737–42.
13. Daniel A, Hook EB, Wulf G. Risks of unbalanced progeny at amniocentesis to carriers of chromosome rearrangements: data from United States and Canadian laboratories. Am J Med Genet. 1989;33(1):14–53.
14. Dul E, van Echten-Arends J, Groen H, Kastrop P, Wissen LA, Engelen J, et al. Can characteristics of reciprocal translocations predict the chance of transferable embryos in PGD cycles? J Clin Med. 2014;3(2):348–58.
15. Franssen MT, Musters AM, van der Veen F, Repping S, Leschot NJ, Bossuyt PM, et al. Reproductive outcome after PGD in couples with recurrent miscarriage carrying a structural chromosome abnormality: a systematic review. Hum Reprod Update. 2011;17(4):467–75.
16. Scriven PN, Flinter FA, Khalaf Y, Lashwood A, Mackie OC. Benefits and drawbacks of preimplantation genetic diagnosis (PGD) for reciprocal translocations: lessons from a prospective cohort study. Eur J Hum Genet. 2013;21(10):1035–41.
17. Mau-Holzmann UA. Somatic chromosomal abnormalities in infertile men and women. Cytogenet Genome Res. 2005;111(3–4):317–36.
18. Bonduelle M, Van Assche E, Joris H, Keymolen K, Devroey P, Van Steirteghem A, et al. Prenatal testing in ICSI pregnancies: incidence of chromosomal anomalies in 1586 karyotypes and relation to sperm parameters. Hum Reprod. 2002;17(10):2600–14.
19. Morel F, Douet-Guilbert N, Le Bris MJ, Amice V, Le Martelot MT, Roche S, et al. Chromosomal abnormalities in couples undergoing intracytoplasmic sperm injection. A study of 370 couples and review of the literature. Int J Androl. 2004;27(3):178–82.
20. Anton E, Vidal F, Blanco J. Interchromosomal effect analyses by sperm FISH: incidence and distribution among reorganization carriers. Syst Biol Reprod Med. 2011;57(6):268–78.
21. Alfarawati S, Fragouli E, Colls P, Wells D. Embryos of Robertsonian translocation carriers exhibit a mitotic interchromosomal effect that enhances genetic instability during early development. PLoS Genet. 2012;8(10):e1003025.
22. Vogt PH, Edelmann A, Kirsch S, Henegariu O, Hirschmann P, Kiesewetter F, et al. Human Y chromosome azoospermia factors (AZF) mapped to different subregions in Yq11. Hum Mol Genet. 1996;5(7):933–43.
23. Sadeghi-Nejad H, Farrokhi F. Genetics of azoospermia: current knowledge, clinical implications, and future directions. Part II: Y chromosome microdeletions. Urol J. 2007;4(4):192–206.
24. Flannigan R, Schlegel PN. Genetic diagnostics of male infertility in clinical practice. Best Pract Res Clin Obstet Gynaecol. 2017;44:26–37.
25. Dohle GR, Halley DJ, Van Hemel JO, van den Ouwel AM, Pieters MH, Weber RF, et al. Genetic risk factors in infertile men with severe oligozoospermia and azoospermia. Hum Reprod. 2002;17(1):13–6.
26. Risch N, Reich EW, Wishnick MM, McCarthy JG. Spontaneous mutation and parental age in humans. Am J Hum Genet. 1987;41(2):218–48.
27. Crow JF. The origins, patterns and implications of human spontaneous mutation. Nat Rev Genet. 2000;1(1):40–7.
28. Nybo Andersen AM, Urhoj SK. Is advanced paternal age a health risk for the offspring? Fertil Steril. 2017;107(2):312–8.
29. Kong A, Frigge ML, Masson G, Besenbacher S, Sulem P, Magnusson G, et al. Rate of de novo mutations and the importance of father's age to disease risk. Nature. 2012;488(7412):471–5.
30. Coulam CB, Adamson SC, Annegers JF. Incidence of premature ovarian failure. Obstet Gynecol. 1986;67(4):604–6.
31. Baronchelli S, Conconi D, Panzeri E, Bentivegna A, Redaelli S, Lissoni S, et al. Cytogenetics of premature ovarian failure: an investigation on 269 affected women. J Biomed Biotechnol. 2011;2011:370195.
32. Portnoi MF, Aboura A, Tachdjian G, Bouchard P, Dewailly D, Bourcigaux N, et al. Molecular cytogenetic studies of Xq critical regions in premature ovarian failure patients. Hum Reprod. 2006;21(9):2329–34.
33. Jaillard S, Akloul L, Beaumont M, Hamdi-Roze H, Dubourg C, Odent S, et al. Array-CGH diagnosis in ovarian failure: identification of new molecular actors for ovarian physiology. J Ovarian Res. 2016;9(1):63.
34. McGuire MM, Bowden W, Engel NJ, Ahn HW, Kovanci E, Rajkovic A. Genomic analysis using high-resolution single-nucleotide polymorphism arrays reveals novel microdeletions associated with premature ovarian failure. Fertil Steril. 2011;95(5):1595–600.
35. Tsafrir A, Altarescu G, Margalioth E, Brooks B, Renbaum P, Levy-Lahad E, et al. PGD for fragile X syndrome: ovarian function is the main determinant of success. Hum Reprod. 2010;25(10):2629–36.
36. Farzin F, Perry H, Hessl D, Loesch D, Cohen J, Bacalman S, et al. Autism spectrum disorders and attention-deficit/hyperactivity disorder in boys with the fragile X premutation. J Dev Behav Pediatr. 2006;27(2 Suppl):S137–44
37. Fortuno C, Labarta E. Genetics of primary ovarian insufficiency: a review. J Assist Reprod Genet. 2014;31(12):1573–85.
38. Committee on G. Committee opinion no. 691. carrier screening for genetic conditions. Obstet Gynecol. 2017;129(3):e41–55.
39. Haque IS, Lazarin GA, Kang HP, Evans EA, Goldberg JD, Wapner RJ. Modeled fetal risk of genetic diseases identified by expanded carrier screening. JAMA. 2016;316(7):734–42.

IVF Lite 2020 (ACCU-VIT + PGT-A)

70

Gautam Nand Allahbadia, Goral Gandhi,
Akanksha Allahbadia Gupta, and A. H. Maham

70.1 Introduction

Traditional stimulation protocols for medically assisted reproduction are designed to achieve high egg numbers. Consequently this increases patient discomfort, risk of OHSS, and expenses. In the past few years, milder protocols have grown in popularity. These protocols typically use either tablets given orally or low-dose gonadotropins (≤150 IU/day), shorter duration of gonadotropins, or both, compared with traditional protocols, with the aim of getting less than ten eggs per retrieval cycle. The fresh transfer pregnancy rates are lower in these mild protocols as compared to traditional protocols; however, the cumulative pregnancy rate seems to be comparable between the approaches [1]. Milder stimulation consists of a gentle controlled ovarian stimulation that aims to produce a maximum of five to six eggs. There is a false notion that IVF Lite severely decreases pregnancy and live birth rates. IVF Lite stimulation protocols with agonist trigger and freeze-all embryo protocols along with a remote single embryo transfer after genetic testing for aneuploidy (PGT-A) produce acceptable clinical pregnancy as well as live birth rates in both normal and poor responders. Moreover, IVF Lite offers many advantages such as less office visits, less number of injections and scans, and reduction in the incidence of OHSS. IVF Lite 2020 is emerging as a frontline therapy especially for patients requiring multiple egg harvesting cycles.

70.2 Why More Is Less and Less Is More?

We know that the use of high gonadotropin doses do not improve the final outcome of medically assisted reproduction [2]. IVF Lite stimulation protocols are based on the principle of better utilization of available oocytes/embryos and endometrial receptivity principles. We have growing evidence that the pregnancy rates with IVF Lite protocols are comparable to those with traditional IVF; the cumulative pregnancy rates being no different, despite having less numbers of eggs or embryos available with IVF Lite stimulation [3]. In addition to being as effective, IVF Lite is associated with a better safety profile ranking, in terms of the incidence of thromboembolic events and OHSS. Patient acceptability is better and this approach is less expensive. Newer evidence may lead to global acceptance of mini-IVF, by both patients and physicians to make IVF more accessible to couples worldwide [2, 3].

Blumenfeld surveyed literature pertaining to milder forms of stimulation for medically assisted reproduction and compared papers of "mild" or "soft" stimulation versus traditional stimulation for medically assisted reproduction [4]. He explained the paradox of "less is more" with the following explanations:

(i) In mild stimulation or natural cycles, the best follicles are selected by the principle of "quality for quantity"; (ii) increased female hormone estradiol (E2) in the late follicular part of the cycle significantly correlated with increased incidence of small for gestational age (SGA) and low-birth-weight (LBW) babies; (iii) intrafollicular estradiol, luteinizing hormone, serum testosterone, and anti-Mullerian hormone (AMH) are significantly higher in natural cycle (NC) medically assisted reproduction than in traditionally stimulated IVF cycles, suggesting an intrafollicular metabolic disruption in traditionally stimulated

G. N. Allahbadia (✉)
Consultant Reproductive Endocrinology & IVF,
Millennium Medical Center MMC IVF, Dubai Health Care City, Dubai, UAE

Bourn Hall Fertility Clinic, Jumeira, Dubai, UAE

G. Gandhi
Indo Nippon IVF, Mumbai, India

ISRME, Mumbai, India

A. A. Gupta
Indira IVF, New Delhi, India

A. H. Maham
Millennium Medical Center MMC IVF, Dubai, UAE

G. N. Allahbadia et al. (eds.), *Textbook of Assisted Reproduction*, https://doi.org/10.1007/978-981-15-2377-9_70

cycles; and (iv) very high estradiol (E2) levels increase the growth hormone-binding protein (GH-BP) and bio-neutralizing growth hormone and decrease the insulin-like growth factor (IGF) levels, which is required for optimal synergy with follicle-stimulating hormone (FSH). Blumenfeld suggested to limit retrieval of around eight to ten oocytes [4]. Milder stimulation protocols should be the way to go forward. In patients producing more than ten oocytes or where very high estradiol levels peak, either intentionally or unintentionally, a mandatory "freeze-all policy" can be instituted and remote embryo transfer (rET) can be planned in a deferred cycle [4].

Baker et al. published a retrospective study examining total gonadotropin dose in IU and live birth rates [5]. Totally 658,519 fresh IVF cycles were reported to SART between 2004 and 2012. Calculating with regression models for live birth rates comparing values for IU of FSH dose and egg number obtained was the scope of this study. Detailed additional analyses were performed on good prognosis patients (<35 years of age, body mass index <30 kg/m [2] with no DOR, no endometriosis, and no ovulatory disorders) and including days of gonadotropin injections used. With increasing FSH dose, the live birth rates decreased irrespective of the oocyte number [5]. The statistically significant findings of decrease in live birth rates with increasing gonadotropin doses were true for patients with good prognosis irrespective of female age, excluding women over 35 years who produced between 1 and 5 oocytes. The study suggested moving away from high doses of gonadotropins (FSH) [5].

IVF results over the years showed inverse relationship between oocyte efficiency and ovarian response. Zhang et al. [6] studied metaphase II (MII) oocyte efficiency according to oocyte yield in mild stimulation IVF (mIVF) and assessed whether the oocyte yield affected live birth rates. 264 infertile normo-responders ($n = 264$) less than 39 years old who underwent mIVF were included. All participants had identical ovarian stimulation protocols. All patients had a freeze-all cycle with vitrification of their blastocysts. Subsequently a single embryo (day 5) was transferred to patients in remote cycles over a 6-month duration. MII oocyte yield (low, 1–2; intermediate, 3–6; and high, ≥ 7 MII oocytes) defined the ovarian response. MII oocyte utilization rate was derived by the formula including the number of live births divided by the total number of MII oocytes produced after a single egg retrieval and subsequent remote transfers of vitrified-thawed blastocysts. The cumulative LBR over a 6-month period was the main outcome measure. Out of 1173 total retrieved oocytes (4.4 ± 0.2 per patient), there were 1019 (3.9 ± 0.2 per patient) MII or mature oocytes with a CPR of 48.1% as well as a LBR of 41.2%. The oocyte utilization rate was 30.3% in the "low" vs. 9.3% in the "intermediate" vs. 4.3% in the "high" oocyte yield groups ($p < 0.05$) which means it was inversely related to ovarian response. The implantation rate fell as the total number of mature oocytes increased and was highest in the "low" oocyte yield group ($p < 0.0001$). The cumulative LBR was almost identical in "low," "intermediate," and "high" oocyte yield groups ($p > 0.05$). The number of mature oocytes had a poor sensitivity and specificity prediction for live birth rates. These data strengthen the hypothesis of oocyte efficiency comparing conventional IVF protocols to mild stimulation protocols [6].

70.3 IVF Lite in Countries Where Embryo Freezing Is Not Allowed

In the UAE for the last decade, IVF clinics were allowed to cryopreserve only gametes and not embryos. This law has changed in 2018, and the clinics can now take individual patient permissions to freeze embryos from the Ministry of Health, UAE. Over the past decade in contradiction to the world, IVF laboratories were vitrifying oocytes and accumulating them in cases of poor responders and older women. IVF Lite in the country was done using oocyte accumulation and segmented IVF with or without genetic screening. When the requisite number was collected over multiple egg retrievals, the oocytes were thawed and injected, and the generated embryos were either transferred directly or subjected to PGT-A and then screened euploid embryos transferred. The efficiency of a good vitrification system continued giving the UAE clinics results comparable to embryo vitrification over the last decade. The rate-limiting step was the method used for vitrification and the training and experience of the Laboratory staff. From 2014, we were using published data [7, 8] to counsel our patients about the non-inferiority status of oocyte vitrification at the time of recruiting them for IVF Lite.

Herero et al. compared variable embryological and pregnancy outcomes between vitrified oocytes versus situations using vitrified embryos in patients at risk for OHSS [6]. Oocyte vitrification (Group 1) versus embryo vitrification (Group 2) was performed in a total of 96 patients. Patients had identical baseline characteristics, and no differences were observed in laboratory and clinical outcomes considering the timing of vitrification. Embryo and oocyte vitrification achieved the same live birth rates [7].

An American study reported their oocyte freezing experience in older women (over 40 years) [8]. Minimal ovarian stimulation IVF was performed in 158 women (mean age 43.9 ± 0.2). Clomiphene citrate (50 mg/day) or letrozole (2.5 mg/day) with or without low-dose gonadotropins (initiated at 75 IU/day and titrated as need be to 150 IU/day) was used in the protocols. 532 mature MII oocytes out of a total of 584 oocytes (2.1 ± 0.15 per patient) were frozen. A post-thaw ICSI was done, and a total of 344 embryos (1.9 ± 0.1 per patient) were produced. 57 good embryos were slotted for ETs and gave rise to three live births (5.3% per ET), one chemical pregnancy and three spontaneous abortions. We can use this data in counseling older women who desire autologous egg freezing [8].

70.4 Why Do Segmented IVF?

The rationale of a deferred embryo transfer whether following a conventional stimulation or a minimal stimulation is the same. Fresh embryo transfer (ET) and frozen-thawed ET (the "freeze-all" policy) was compared by Roque et al. [9], with fresh transfers performed only in cases where progesterone (P) elevation was absent. Controlled ovarian stimulation (COS) with a gonadotropin-releasing hormone antagonist protocol was performed on 530 patients with day 3 embryo transfers in all. The fresh ET group (when P levels were ≤ 1.5 ng/mL on the trigger day) included 351 patients with 179 cycles in the freeze-all group (ET performed after endometrial priming with estradiol valerate, at 6 mg/day). The implantation rate was 19.9% in the fresh ET group versus 26.5% in the freeze-all group whereas the clinical pregnancy rate was 35.9% and 46.4% while the ongoing pregnancy rate was 31.1% and 39.7% respectively. The freeze-all group had better IVF outcomes compared with the fresh ET group [8]. Endometrial receptivity may have been impaired by COS even in a select group of patients that underwent fresh ET (P levels ≤1.5 ng/mL), and outcomes may be improved recruiting patients for the freeze-all protocol [9].

70.5 Modified Natural Cycle IVF

The Steptoe-Edwards IVF miracle in 1978 was in a natural cycle. Ovarian stimulation was added to IVF protocols to achieve a greater margin for error in oocyte retrieval, fertilization, and, thus, overall pregnancy success in the early days of IVF. As laboratory technology improved, the quest to reduce the incidence of OHSS started the cycle of new research using mild IVF without hard gonadotropin stimulation protocols. An ovulation trigger using hCG and later GnRH agonist was added to the mild IVF protocols for accurate scheduling of egg retrievals and to increase oocyte yields. Later in evolution came GnRH antagonists to prevent premature ovulation. This class of protocol was labelled as the "modified natural cycle" (MNC-IVF). The modified natural IVF cycles are less expensive and give comparable pregnancy rates, and they are especially useful for patients who have an increased risk of OHSS or the patients labelled as poor responders and those wishing to avoid supernumerary embryos for freezing [10]. Here spontaneous ovulation is prevented with a small amount of hormones, and monofollicular growth is the norm. Consequently, there is no risk of OHSS, and the risk of multiples is low. On an average there is a 9.1% chance of a pregnancy after a single MNC cycle, and the cumulative pregnancy rate with a maximum of six MNC-IVF cycles is 33.4% [11]. The cumulative results of a six MNC-IVF cycles can be compared to the first COS-IVF cycle including transfer of cryopreserved embryos (33.4% versus 37.7%) [11]. Risk of a multiple pregnancy following MNC-IVF is only 0.1% and 18.3% following COS-IVF, which translates that MNC-IVF is a very good alternative option for COS-IVF [11].

The effectiveness of mild stimulation using recombinant human FSH (rhFSH) and GnRH antagonist was compared with traditional stimulation with GnRH antagonist in a multiple-dose protocol (MDP) in poor responders undergoing medically assisted reproduction (IVF/ICSI) [12]. Mild stimulation cycles give similar pregnancy rates to GnRH antagonist MDP cycles with lesser injections of rhFSH used and lesser days of injections. This can be a viable cost-effective alternate protocol as a last ditch effort before egg donation in poor responders [12].

70.6 Oral Drugs: Clomiphene Citrate or Letrozole

In routine IVF cycles, researchers have been setting up stimulation protocol studies using clomiphene citrate (CC) and letrozole with gonadotropins especially for low responders with an aim to decrease the total amount of gonadotropins used and in normo-responders to reduce the incidence of the dreaded complication of OHSS. With mild stimulation strategies in normo-responders with the use of CC and gonadotropins, the number of oocytes retrieved was on an average lesser than conventional protocols but yet gave comparable pregnancy rates. In most studies between 2000 and 2010 the cumulative pregnancy rates were lower in clomiphene cycles in fresh embryo transfers compared with conventional ovarian stimulation when frozen embryo transfers were considered [13]. Letrozole was combined with gonadotropins initially in patients with breast cancer to prevent the spikes of serum estradiol which was the norm with the use of standard controlled ovarian hyperstimulation [13]. CC and letrozole were both used with gonadotropins in poor responders and showed reduction in the amount of total gonadotropins used without affecting the pregnancy rates. The hypothesis was that letrozole used with gonadotropins may increase endometrial receptivity by optimizing integrin expression in the endometrium and by decreasing E2 levels to more physiologic bands [13].

Rose et al.'s study compared the use of clomiphene citrate and letrozole in IVF to produce only one or two embryos [14]. Either letrozole or clomiphene citrate were used with gonadotropins without using GnRH antagonists. Sixty-two patients received either letrozole or clomiphene citrate with low-dose gonadotropins in 128 treatment cycles. The hCG trigger was administered at follicle diameter of 17 mm. The oocyte retrieval was performed after 34 h followed by ICSI. The study found no statistically significant differences in the number of large follicles produced, oocytes fertilized, endometrial thickness, clinical pregnancy rates, or delivery rates in patients using clomiphene citrate versus letrozole. The peak E2 levels during treatment, which averaged 516 pg/mL with letrozole and 797 pg/mL with clomiphene citrate ($p = 0.005$), was statistically different. The premature LH surge cancellation rate was 5%. In this study an average of 2.8 mature oocytes were retrieved, 2.1 were oocytes fertilized, and 1.6 embryos were transferred into the uterus. The clinical pregnancy rate per transfer reached 25%, and the live birth rate per transfer was 19.2%. There were no clinically significant differences when letrozole or clomiphene citrate was used for mild ovarian stimulation for IVF other than peak estradiol levels [14].

Ochin et al. published a retrospective study of 65 infertile women who underwent 130 cycles in China from January 2011 to December 2014. They evaluated the low-dose clomiphene citrate plus low-dose gonadotropins on predicted normal responder patients who had an unsuspected poor IVF result, following an initial stimulation with the long GnRH agonist protocol [15]. The long agonist protocol group (Group 1) was treated with long GnRH-a protocol along with a high dose of gonadotropin injections (≥150 IU/day), compared with a second IVF cycle (Group 2) that had low-dose clomiphene citrate plus low-dose gonadotropin injections (75–112.5 IU/day). The cumulative pregnancy rate/started cycle (9.2% [6/65] vs. 51% [33/65]; $P < 0001$) was significantly better in the clomiphene citrate stimulatory protocol than the long protocol. Surprisingly the number of oocytes retrieved was also higher in the clomiphene protocol compared to the long GnRH agonist protocol (7.26 ± 1.95 vs. 5.98 ± 1.31; $P = 0.03$). There was a higher number of eggs retrieved after using a lower total dose of recombinant FSH in the CC protocol. The cumulative pregnancy rate in the low-dose CC-based protocol was much better. Thus, the clomiphene citrate plus low-dose rFSH should be the alternative viable option for similar patients in their second cycle instead of just repeating the long agonist protocol [15].

The effectiveness of clomiphene citrate (CC) versus letrozole (L) plus human menopausal gonadotropin (hMG) in gonadotropin-releasing hormone (GnRH) antagonist protocols in low responder patients with previous failed ovarian stimulation undergoing ICSI was reported recently [16]. This publication included cycles with clomiphene citrate and letrozole plus hMG using GnRH antagonist protocols in 32 low responder patients who had poor results in at least for two previous medically assisted reproduction cycles using a microdose flare protocol or GnRH antagonist protocol. 42 cycles of 32 low responders were studied. The total gonadotropin usage was significantly lower (1491 ± 873 vs. 2808 ± 1581 IU, $P = 0.005$), and mean estradiol levels on day of hCG trigger were significantly higher in the clomiphene group compared to the letrozole group (443.3 ± 255.2 vs. 255.4 ± 285.2 pg/mL, $P = 0.03$). The endometrial thickness as well as the cumulative pregnancy and live birth rates per cycle were significantly higher in the clomiphene group compared to the letrozole group (27.2 vs. 15%, 13.6 vs. 0% and 4.5 vs. 0%, respectively, $P < 0.05$). Severe low responders who had previously failed to respond to the microdose flare, or the GnRH antagonist protocols may benefit from a clomid plus hMG/GnRH antagonist protocol [16].

A study investigated IVF outcomes between patients with diminished ovarian response patients (DOR) who received three different gonadotropin doses in stimulation protocols with or without the addition of letrozole [17]. 95 patients who fulfilled two of the three Bologna criteria were included in the study. 31 patients were treated with 450 IU gonadotropins, whereas in the second group, 31 patients were treated with 300 IU. 33 patients comprised the third group and were treated with 150 IU gonadotropins along with letrozole. Their results indicated a similar number of retrieved mature and fertilized oocytes, identical fertilization rates, similar number of transferred embryos, implantation, cancellation, chemical, clinical, and ongoing pregnancy rates with no essential differences, irrespective of the doses of hMG and rFSH in POR patients. Increasing the dose of gonadotropins during stimulation is the usual approach in a poor responder but does not improve the reproductive outcomes [17]. The study summarized that letrozole in combination with low-dose gonadotropins was as effective as pure stimulation with higher doses of gonadotropins in DOR patients [17].

Song et al.'s study evaluated the efficacy of mild stimulation with clomiphene citrate on ovarian response and pregnancy rates in poor responders undergoing medically assisted reproduction [18]. This was a meta-analysis on comparing mild and traditional stimulation protocols and pregnancy outcomes. The meta-analysis on four RCTs indicated that there was no significant difference in live birth rates (OR: 0.71, 95% CI 0.22–2.29, $P = 0.57$) and clinical pregnancy rates (OR: 1.11, 95% CI 0.80–1.55, $P = 0.52$) for both these types of stimulation protocols. This study suggested that mild stimulation with clomid may be comparable with conventional COH protocols [18].

70.7 Minimal Dose Stimulation Versus Conventional Stimulation for IVF

Lazer et al. studied whether minimum-dose stimulation (MS) protocols enhance clinical pregnancy rates when compared to high-dose conventional stimulation (HS) protocols in patients with diminished ovarian reserve [19]. Inclusion criteria meant only patients with an anti-Müllerian hormone (AMH) ≤8 pmol/L and/or antral follicle count (AFC) ≤5 were included. Patients recruited in 2008 exclusively had a HS protocol, while patients recruited in 2010 were on a MS protocol. The minimum-dose protocol includes letrozole at 2.5 mg starting from day 2–6, overlapping with gonadotropins from day 3 onwards at 150 IU daily. GnRH antagonist was added at leading follicle size at a minimum of 14 mm. The high-dose group had only gonadotropins (≥300 IU/day) in their antagonist protocol. The clinical pregnancy rate and live birth rate was significantly better in the minimum-dose stimulation group when compared to the high-dose group ($P = 0.007$) [14]. The authors concluded that the MS protocol is less expensive because of the lower gonadotropin usage and gave a better clinical pregnancy rate and live birth rate than the high-dose protocol for patients with DOR [19].

Zhang et al.'s randomized non-inferiority study compared 1 cycle of mini-IVF with single embryo transfer (SET) with a cycle of conventional IVF with double embryo transfer [20]. The primary outcome was cumulative live birth rate per woman over a 6-month period. The study group included 564 patients (<39 years old) who were undergoing their first IVF cycle, and they were randomly slotted to either mini-IVF or conventional IVF. Secondary outcomes included gonadotropin use, OHSS, and multiple pregnancy rates. The cumulative live birth rate was 49% (140/285) for mini-IVF and 63% (176/279) for conventional IVF [20]. There was no OHSS in the mini-IVF group compared with 16 moderate/severe ovarian hyperstimulation syndrome cases (5.7%) in the traditional IVF group. The multiple pregnancy rates were 32% in the traditional IVF group versus 6.4% in the mini-IVF group. Use of gonadotropins was significantly less in the mini-IVF group compared with traditional IVF group (459 ± 131 vs 2079 + 389 IU; $P < 0.0001$). Compared with traditional IVF group with double embryo transfer, the mini-IVF group with single embryo transfer has a little lower live birth rate and zero OHSS cases, reduces multiple pregnancy rates, and decreases gonadotropin usage [20].

Borges et al. studied the effect of exogenous FSH on ICSI outcomes compared to the age of patient [21]. Patients undergoing COH for ICSI were split into different age groups: ≤35 y.o. ($n = 1523$), >35 and ≤ 38 y.o. ($n = 652$), >38 and ≤ 40 y.o. ($n = 332$), and > 40 y.o. ($n = 370$). Linear regression models outlined the effect of gonadotropin dose on COH, clinical, and laboratory outcomes. The authors observed that lower the age, the lower was the FSH dose needed per oocyte. In patients ≤38 y.o., there was a negative effect of the gonadotropin dose on the embryo quality and blast formation, leading to increased cycle cancellation rate. In patients more than 39 years old, there were no effects of the gonadotropin dose on the analyzed variables. They summarized that high-dose stimulation is avoidable in younger women (≤38 y.o.) based on their findings of poorer embryo quality and increased cycle cancellation rate. Mild ovarian stimulation protocols should be preferred in these cases [21].

70.8 Diminished Ovarian Reserve (DOR)

A comparison of pregnancy outcomes achieved by in vitro fertilization (IVF) minimal stimulation and conventional antagonist protocols in patients with diminished ovarian reserve (DOR) was published by Pilehvari et al. [22]. Out of 77 DOR patients undergoing IVF, 42 were included in the minimal stimulation group ($n = 42$) who received 100 mg/day clomid on day 2 of the cycle for 5 days that was followed by 150 IU/day gonadotropins (hMG) on day 5 of the cycle. The control was the conventional group ($n = 35$) who received at least 300 IU/day gonadotropin from day 2. The flexible antagonist protocol was applied for both groups. There was no difference in the number of oocytes and pregnancy rates (2.79 ± 1.96 vs. 2.20 ± 1.71 and 5.6% vs. 4.1%; $p > 0.05$). The gonadotropin usage in the minimal stimulation group was much lower than the control group (1046 ± 596 vs. 2806 ± 583). The authors stressed that mild stimulation is likely to be considered as a very patient-friendly and economical substitute for DORs [22].

In a recent publication [23], 60 DOR patients were randomized to receive either letrozole/antagonist (mild stimulation) ($n = 30$) or the agonist microdose flare protocol ($n = 30$). Both groups were identical in background and other variable characteristics. Clinical pregnancy rate was similar in both groups (13.3 vs. 16.6%). In the letrozole/antagonist protocol, the gonadotropin usage and the number of stimulation days were significantly lower. Other variables like peak E2 level on the day of hCG trigger, endometrial thickness, the retrieved oocytes, the number of fertilized oocytes, the number of transferred embryos, and the cycle cancellation rate were statistically similar. The mild protocol was cost-effective and patient-friendly and should be used in DOR patients undergoing medically assisted reproduction [23].

A prospective comparative study on 165 patients in 271 consecutive mild IVF cycles assessed the reproductive competence of oocytes obtained by follicular flushing in DOR patients [24]. Egg retrieval was scheduled 34 h after hCG trigger, and oocytes were divided into two groups: eggs obtained in the first follicular aspiration (FA, $n = 127$) and eggs obtained in the subsequent follicular flushing (FF, $n = 102$). The patient characteristics, oocyte fertilization rate, and clinical pregnancy rate per oocyte were similar in both groups. Embryo morphology (41 versus 59%, $P < 0.01$) and implantation rates (20.4 versus 34.8%, $P < 0.04$) were better in the FF group. An optimal reproductive competence was observed in oocytes retrieved after follicular flushing in mild IVF in DOR patients [24].

Progesterone during ovarian stimulation blocks the luteinizing hormone (LH) surge in normo-responders, but its role has not been defined in low responders. Chen et al. recruited a total of 204 infertile women with low ovarian reserve into the medroxyprogesterone acetate (MPA) group or the natural cycle control group alternatingly [25]. Medroxyprogesterone acetate (10 mg) was administered daily beginning from the early follicular phase, and a small amount of hMG was added in the late follicular phase if the serum FSH level was lower than 8.0 mIU/mL. As soon as a dominant follicle reached appropriate diameter, triptorelin 100 μg and hCG 1000 IU were used as ovulation triggers, and eggs were retrieved after 34–36 h. Embryos generated were cryopreserved for subsequent FET. The natural cycle IVF group was used as controls. The MPA group exhibited a larger preovulatory follicle (18.7 ± 1.8 mm vs 17.2 ± 2.2 mm), a longer follicular phase (13.6 ± 3.6 days vs 12.3 ± 3.2 days), and higher peak estradiol values (403.88 ± 167.16 vs 265.26 ± 122.16 pg/mL) while maintaining lower LH values ($P < 0.05$). Incidence of spontaneous LH surge and premature ovulation reduced significantly. A higher number of eggs and viable embryos were generated from the MPA group compared to the natural cycle group ($P < 0.05$). Also, in the MPA group the clinical pregnancy rate was slightly higher than in the natural cycle group, but the difference was not statistically significant. Progesterone-primed mild stimulation achieved optimal control of the growing dominant follicle and did not adversely affect the quality of eggs in DORs [25]. Consequently, progesterone priming is a good way to overcome premature ovulation in mild stimulation in DORs.

Three protocols for IVF/ICSI stimulation in DOR patients treatment were compared by Yu et al. [26]. The DOR patients were randomly divided into three groups: a modified gonadotropin-releasing hormone (GnRH) agonist protocol (group A), (ii) a mild stimulation protocol (group B), or (iii) an antagonist protocol (group C). Clinical variables, demographic characteristics, and pregnancy outcomes were compared between these groups. Group B (32.69%) had a higher cycle cancellation rate compared with groups A (11.11%) and C (16.67%). The early abortion rate of group C (44.44%) was higher than group A (12.50%), but not significantly different from group B (16.67%). There were no statistically significant differences in the clinical pregnancy rates and live birth rates amongst the groups. The mild stimulation protocol gave a comparable pregnancy rate as compared to the other traditional protocols [26].

70.9 Older Women

A rare case report of a 49-year-old patient who delivered twins after ICSI using her own eggs with mild ovarian stimulation was recently published [27]. The couple had both a tubal and male factor infertility. Clomid and low-dose FSH were used in the cycle followed by ICSI, where 5 2-day embryos were transferred. The babies were delivered by elective LSCS at 37 weeks for obstetric reasons including moderate PIH.

In older women with raised FSH levels, traditional ovarian stimulation is expensive and does not give good results. Mild stimulation has now come into its own and gives better-quality eggs (albeit a lesser number) as compared to the high-dose traditional stimulation [28]. Milder forms of stimulation decrease the number of days of stimulation, decrease the gonadotropin usage, and also decrease the mean number of eggs per cycle. The ratio of top-quality euploid embryos seems to be much better in mild cycles as compared with traditional protocols, while the pregnancy rates per ET are comparable. Additionally, the lesser costs, the better patient compliance, and the decreased time to complete an ART cycle make these milder approaches demographically and economically better suited. Low numbers of embryos available for transfer are always the dreaded outcome in treating of older women with IVF. A solution to this problem is to create a pool of embryos with vitrification and accumulation (ACCU-VIT) of top-grade embryos over more than one mild stimulation and modified natural IVF attempts [29]. When you reach the desired number of vitrified embryos, they can be biopsied and sent for preimplantation genetic testing (PGT-A) using next-generation sequencing (NGS), and we will then have the storage pool with only euploid embryos with maximal chances of success [28]. This would make the implantation potential for older women almost identical to normo-responders. This strategy, however, is unthinkable unless the IVF center has an excellent vitrification strategy in place. The strategy of accumulating vitrified embryos (ACCU-VIT) will become the norm in the 2020s.

70.10 Minimal Stimulation and Single Embryo Transfer (SET) with Segmented IVF

In a landmark publication, patients were not denied treatment based on their baseline FSH levels nor ovarian reserve [30]. Yet Zhang achieved wonderful pregnancy rates (20% for fresh ETs and 41% for FETs). Results such as these strengthen the case for a mild stimulation IVF protocol and remote embryo transfer of vitrified-thawed embryos as a viable alternative to traditional IVF stimulation strategies [30].

A recent study analyzed the embryological and clinical results of a single embryo transfer (SET) program vis a vis patient age (lower or equal 29, 30–34, 35–39, 40–44, and equal or higher 45 years) [31]. 7244 infertile patients underwent 20,244 cycles with a clomid-based mild stimulation protocol or alternatively using a or natural cycle protocol. A total of 10,401 fresh or frozen SET procedures were performed involving day 3 or day 5 embryos. Optimal egg retrieval rate (78.0%) showed no age-dependent loss until 45 years of age. While the fertilization (80.3%) and cleavage (91.1%) rates were not significantly different, the blastocyst formation (70.1% to 22.8%) and overall live birth rates (35.9% to 2%) showed an age-dependent decrease. Day 5/6 FET cycles gave the highest chance of a live birth per ET (41.3% to 6.1%). Although a high fertilization and cleavage rate was obtained irrespective of age, the blastocyst formation and live birth rates showed an age-dependent decreasing trend [31]. In infertile patients up until their mid-forties, an elective SET program based on a mild stimulation protocol gives acceptable live birth rates per ET. But in very advanced age group infertile patients (equal or higher than 45 years old), the success rates fall to less than 1% [31].

In unselected infertile patients following minimal ovarian stimulation/natural cycle IVF, the authors set about to determine the cumulative live birth rates (LBR) per egg retrieval [32]. Natural cycle IVF or clomiphene-based minimal ovarian stimulation was coupled with single embryo transfer in a total of 727 consecutive infertile patients who underwent 2876 (median 4) cycles with increasing use of remote frozen-thawed blastocyst transfers. The crude cumulative LBR were 65%, 60%, 39%, 15%, and 5% in patients aged 26–34, 35–37, 38–40, 41–42, and 43–44 years, respectively. No live births occurred in patients aged over 45 years in this series. The dropout rates per attempted cycle were between 13 and 25%. Success rates slowly reached a plateau, with only very few additional live births after six attempts. Majority of expected successful cases were reached within 6 months with almost maximal rates within 15 months of the first egg retrieval. This study showed us that acceptable live birth rates can be achieved with an exclusive mild stimulation/single embryo transfer program not only in patients aged <38 years but also in older patients (38–40 years) [32].

70.11 Mild Stimulation Using Corifollitropin Alfa (CFA)

A recent publication proposed mild stimulation followed by egg retrieval under local anesthesia (LA) for increased patient acceptability. The paper suggested that clomiphene citrate (CC), followed by CFA, may provide adequate stimulatory response to complete the cycle [33]. This new clomiphene citrate/CFA (CC/CFA) protocol was compared to women undergoing standard rFSH protocol (good prognosis comparative cohort: GPCC) in a 1:2 study design. The pilot study of 25 patients examined the effectiveness of clomid (100 mg from day 2–6) followed by CFA in a GnRH antagonist protocol. All egg retrievals were conducted under local block. The softer protocol saw less number of oocytes retrieved when compared to the GPCC (6.4 ± 0.7 vs. 10.7 ± 0.9, $p < 0.001$), consequently leading to a reduced number of good-quality embryos for ET or vitrification (3.7 ± 0.6 vs. 5.7 ± 0.5, $p = 0.01$). Even as the embryo quality was similar between the two groups, the endometrial thickness was significantly lower in the study group that received CC/CFA. The pregnancy rates were significantly lower in the CC/CFA group when compared to the GPCC (31.8 vs. 57.1%, $p = 0.04$), and 44% of CC/CFA patients required additional doses of rFSH to reach the hCG trigger criteria. The authors concluded that this sequential clomiphene CFA protocol did not appear to be an optimal strategy for mild IVF since it did not give adequate stimulatory effect from a single CFA injection and produced lower fresh ET pregnancy rates and lesser number of embryos for vitrification [33].

70.12 Neonatal Outcome After Minimal Stimulation

Neonatal outcome between children born after vitrified versus fresh single embryo transfer (SET) of 6623 delivered singletons following 29,944 single embryo transfers was published recently [34]. Mild IVF/natural cycle IVF followed by SET of either fresh or vitrified-thawed cleavage stage embryos or blastocysts was performed. Gestational age (38.6 ± 2 versus 38.7) and preterm delivery rate (6.9% versus 6.9%) in singletons born after the transfer of vitrified-thawed embryos were comparable to those born after fresh embryo transfers. Children born subsequent to transfers of vitrified-thawed embryos had a higher birth weight (3028 ± 465 versus 2943 ± 470 g) and lower LBW (8.5% versus 11.9%) and SGA (3.6% versus 7.6%) rates. The total birth defect rates (including minor anomalies) (2.4% versus 1.9%) and perinatal mortality rates (0.6% versus 0.5%) were similar between the two groups. The vitrification-thawing embryo transfer protocol did not increase the incidence of adverse neonatal outcomes nor birth defects following SET [34].

70.13 Preimplantation Genetic Testing for Aneuploidy (PGT-A)

The frequency of aneuploidies of the PB-I and PB-II of oocytes was reported by a Russian group [35]. FISH was performed in 238 PB-I and PB-II biopsy specimens. After COS for IVF as compared to a natural cycle, the frequency of aneuploidies in oocytes was higher. The aneuploidy rate was also higher after COH in infertile patients with female factors compared to women stimulated for IVF because of male infertility or egg donors [35]. They also surmised that oocyte aneuploidies after COS are more common in older patients after 35 years [35].

In two IVF stimulation protocols, fertilization and aneuploidy rates were compared [36]. Clomiphene citrate (CC) and human menopausal gonadotropin (hMG) were used in 349 treatment cycles and hMG after treatment with an agonist in two other study groups (long protocol), viz., Goserelin (n = 73) and Buserelin (n = 43). A cytogenetic examination was done on non-fertilized eggs in both the groups. The fertilization rates were significantly higher in the agonist/hMG group compared to the clomid/hMG group, but the cleavage rates as well as the embryo quality were not dissimilar. Out of the 736 oocytes studied via cytogenetic analysis, 256 were karyotyped, and 172 were found to be euploid, whereas 84 were found to be aneuploid. Comparatively more oocytes were aneuploid in the GnRH-a/hMG group than in the clomid/hMG group, and this finding was statistically significant [36].

32 young oocyte donors with a high response to ovarian stimulation were included in a study to test the influence of gonadotropin doses on embryo aneuploidy rates [37]. Consecutive stimulation treatments were performed for each egg donor: a standard dose protocol with a 225 IU starting dose of recombinant FSH (rFSH) and, thereafter, a reduced dose cycle with a starting dose of 150 IU recombinant FSH. In both cycles, agonist downregulation co-treatment was used. A total of 22 egg donors completed both treatment cycles with different gonadotropin doses, whereas the remaining 10 patient's cycles were cancelled due to a poor ovarian response. Significant increases in rates of fertilization and chromosomally normal blastocysts were observed in the reduced dose cycle. There were no statistically significant differences in pregnancy and implantation rates in recipients who received eggs from standard or reduced dose groups. The study suggested that in all high responder patients, one must decrease the gonadotropin dose to improve fertilization as well as quality of embryos [37].

PGS of embryos was employed in a prospective, randomized controlled study, comparing two ovarian stimulation regimens with main study characteristics being chromosome segregation behavior during meiosis and early embryo development [38]. Patients under 38 years were randomly assigned to either a mild stimulation protocol with GnRH antagonist co-treatment (67 patients) or a traditional high-dose long protocol (44 patients). On day 3, embryos were biopsied, and the copy number of 10 chromosomes was studied. They terminated the study prematurely after an unplanned interim analysis (which included 61% of the planned number of patients) found a lower embryo aneuploidy rate in the mild stimulation group. Although with mild stimulation, significantly fewer eggs and embryos were obtained following, both groups generated a similar number (1.8) of euploid embryos. The study suggested that all future ovarian stimulation protocols should avoid increasing the number of oocytes per retrieval and instead aim at generating a sufficient number of euploid embryos with a milder form of stimulation [38].

70.14 Double Stimulation in the Follicular and Luteal Phase

Antral follicles in the luteal phase enabling ovarian stimulation has been amply proved a prior. The efficiency of double stimulation, both during the follicular and luteal phases in DOR patients, was studied [39]. A total of 38 patients started with mild stimulation. After the first egg retrieval, letrozole and hMG were given in the study cycle. The double stimulation protocol yielded 167 oocytes, and a total of 26 patients (68.4%) were successful in generating one to six viable embryos which were then vitrified. Twenty-one patients were posted for a total of 23 vitrified-thawed ETs, which resulted in 13 clinical pregnancies. Double ovarian stimulation in the same menstrual cycle provides better chances for collecting oocytes in the DOR patients. This type of stimulation protocol can have a luteal phase start resulting in pooling more oocytes in shortest time. This new strategy can benefit both women with DOR and freshly diagnosed cancer patients requiring fertility preservation [39].

An Iranian study evaluated the results of double stimulations during the follicular and luteal phases in 121 DOR women. Letrozole, clomid, hMG, and GnRH agonist were used in these double stimulation cycles in the follicular and luteal phases. A total of 104 (85.9%) patients completed the study, and the initial analysis revealed that the number of retrieved eggs after the first and second stimulations were similar. The fertilization rate and the number of vitrified embryos after the conventional stimulation were significantly higher. The mean number of MII oocytes and the fertilization rate after the Shanghai protocol were higher than the standard antagonist protocol which was the control group [40].

A recent study aimed to investigate the efficacy of double stimulations during the follicular and luteal phases (duo-stim) in older women [41]. One hundred and sixteen women aged ≥38 years who received double ovarian stimulation were included, with 103 patients subdivided into 4 groups according to follicular phase stimulation strategies, including agonist short protocol (n = 27), flexible antagonist protocol (n = 32), soft stimulation protocol (n = 21), and medroxyprogesterone acetate (MPA) protocol (n = 23). The egg number and available embryos after duo-stim were twice as much as after follicular phase stimulation alone. The cycle cancellation rate decreased from 37.07% to 18.10%. 48 patients underwent 50 FETs, with a 22.00% CPR, and the implantation rate (10.53% versus 10.67%) was similar between the embryos derived from both stimulation groups. These results suggest that duo-stim could increase the PRs by accumulating more eggs or embryos in the shortest possible time which might be a more cost-effective strategy for patients in the older age groups [41].

A total of 131 patients with DORs were included in this study [42]. Thirty-three patients in the early luteal phase and 98 in the early follicular phase started ovarian stimulation with 100 mg/d clomid and 75 to 150 IU/day hMG. There were more eggs (2.8 ± 2.0 versus 2.0 ± 1.2, $p < 0.05$), more embryos (1.8 ± 1.4 versus 1.3 ± 1.1, $p < 0.05$), and more top-quality embryos (0.9 ± 0.9 versus 0.4 ± 0.6, $p < 0.05$) with a reduced cycle cancellation rate (12.1% versus 30.6%, $p < 0.05$) in the luteal stimulation group. The clinical pregnancy (17.7%, 20.0% and 41.2%) and live birth rates (10.78%, 20.0% and 29.4%) were similar ($p > 0.05$). Luteal phase stimulation can be a very good option in DORs because of increasing chances of getting top-quality embryos and by reducing the cancellation rate [42].

70.15 Advances

Do we need luteal phase progesterone support is in mild stimulation IVF protocols using Clomid and low dose FSH? [43]. The inclusion group had 15 good prognosis patients (defined as ≤38 years old with normal ovarian reserve and normo-responders, BMI <29 kg/m^2, no previous IVF cycles, no history of severe endometriosis, no history of recurrent miscarriages, no endocrine or autoimmune diseases, and no surgical semen retrievals from their partners) undergoing IVF with soft stimulation. They were monitored during the luteal phase with serial serum progesterone and LH tests. The luteal support was started only if necessary. No patient needed luteal progestogenic support since the resultant steroid environment was quite different from those in the conventional stimulation protocols. The live birth rate was 40% (6/15), the implantation rate 30% (6/20), and there were myriad advantages of the mild protocol, which included enhanced endometrial receptivity, lower expenses, and more patient compliance and acceptability. The paper suggested that the mild stimulation protocols will confer an additional benefit during the luteal phase by eliminating the necessity of luteal phase support [43].

The future trend in medically assisted reproduction (MAR) will be to decrease the intensity of ovarian stimulation protocols and to restrict the number of embryos to a single embryo transfer (SET). Contemporary literature suggests that the intensity of ovarian stimulation affects the ratio of euploid embryos [28]. Ovarian stimulation seems to have a deleterious effect on oocyte quality and embryo aneuploidy in a dose-dependent manner. We are moving to a global era of single embryo transfers, and now it becomes more important than ever before to ensure that this single embryo has the highest implantation potential. Strategies should be adopted and implemented to improve the accuracy for selecting an euploid, viable embryo with the highest implantation potential for transfer [44].

An extended refinement of morphological criteria for improving prediction of implantation potential by considering pronuclei disposition, nucleolar organization, and identification of the fastest dividing embryos with only mononucleated blastomeres as well as amalgamating morphokinetics with cytogenetics will be the future [28]. We routinely use preimplantation genetic testing (PGT-A) wherein a day 5 biopsy is tested for aneuploidy using NGS. In older patients lower oocyte yields may represent a more physiologic response to ovarian stimulation, allowing the most competent follicles and eggs to develop normally and thereby reducing the incidence of embryo aneuploidy. IVF Lite plus ACCU-VIT (accumulation of vitrified embryos) by repeated mild stimulation cycles with subsequent vitrification of blastocysts, combined with preimplantation genetic testing (PGT-A) and a remote single embryo transfer of a euploid embryo, is a promising new approach for poor responders as well as women of advanced maternal age [45, 46].

70.16 Conclusions

Traditional IVF stimulation in older women with high FSH often results in an expensive and not so successful IVF procedure with a low success rate. It is well established now that with softer stimulation, there is a greater chance of good-quality eggs (albeit a smaller number) than with higher-dose hard stimulation [2]. Milder protocols decrease the mean number of stimulation days, total dose of gonadotropins, and the mean number of eggs retrieved. But the ratio of top-quality and euploid embryos seems to be significantly higher compared with conventional hard protocols, and the pregnancy rate per embryo transfer is comparable. Additionally, the reduced costs, the better patient compliance, and the lesser days to complete an IVF cycle make these mild protocols clinically successful as well as cost-efficient over a finite period of time. The lower number of embryos generated for embryo transfer always poses a great challenge in the management of older women in MAR. We suggest building up a sufficient pool of embryos by accumulating vitrified good-grade embryos (ACCU-VIT) over several mild stimulation and natural cycles. Remember to biopsy these pooled embryos on day 5 before vitrification and freeze the biopsy separately. At the end of this accumulation process, when you have reached the requisite numbers of embryos for a particular patient, the biopsies can be subjected to a preimplantation genetic testing (PGT-A) using next-generation sequencing (NGS), and then you will carry on long-term storage of only the euploid embryos with maximum chances of implantation. This strategy works best for older women attempting to get pregnant, and now transferring a single PGT-A embryo makes the chances of success for older women similar to normal responders.

References

1. Alper MM, Fauser BC. Ovarian stimulation protocols for IVF: is more better than less? Reprod Biomed Online. 2017 Apr;34(4):345–53. https://doi.org/10.1016/j.rbmo.2017.01.010.
2. Allahbadia GN. Getting older women pregnant: contemporary thoughts. J Obstet Gynaecol India. 2016 Oct;66(5):305–9. https://doi.org/10.1007/s13224-015-0804-8.
3. Nargund G, Datta AK, Fauser BCJM. Mild stimulation for in vitro fertilization. Fertil Steril. 2017 Oct;108(4):558–67. https://doi.org/10.1016/j.fertnstert.2017.08.022.
4. Blumenfeld Z. Why more is less and less is more when it comes to ovarian stimulation. J Assist Reprod Genet. 2015 Dec;32(12):1713–9. https://doi.org/10.1007/s10815-015-0599-7.
5. Baker VL, Brown MB, Luke B, Smith GW, Ireland JJ. Gonadotropin dose is negatively correlated with live birth rate: analysis of more than 650,000 assisted reproductive technology cycles. Fertil Steril. 2015 Nov;104(5):1145–52. https://doi.org/10.1016/j.fertnstert.2015.07.1151.
6. Zhang JJ, Yang M, Merhi Z. Efficiency of metaphase II oocytes following minimal/mild ovarian stimulation in vitro fertilization. Fertil Res Pract. 2016 Sep 1;2:2. https://doi.org/10.1186/s40738-016-0025-6.
7. Herrero L, Pareja S, Aragonés M, Cobo A, Bronet F, Garcia-Velasco JA. Oocyte versus embryo vitrification for delayed embryo transfer: an observational study. Reprod Biomed Online. 2014 Nov;29(5):567–72. https://doi.org/10.1016/j.rbmo.2014.07.016.
8. Zhang JJ, Choo S, Yang M. Autologous oocyte cryopreservation in women aged 40 and older using minimal stimulation IVF. Reprod Biol Endocrinol. 2015 Oct 6;13:112. https://doi.org/10.1186/s12958-015-0110-4.
9. Roque M, Valle M, Guimarães F, Sampaio M, Geber S. Freeze-all policy: fresh vs. frozen-thawed embryo transfer. Fertil Steril. 2015 May;103(5):1190–3. https://doi.org/10.1016/j.fertnstert.2015.01.045.
10. Ho JR, Paulson RJ. Modified natural cycle in in vitro fertilization. Fertil Steril. 2017 Oct;108(4):572–6. https://doi.org/10.1016/j.fertnstert.2017.08.021.
11. Bos AM, Pelinck MJ, Dumoulin JC, Arts EG, van Echten-Arends J, Simons AH. IVF in a modified natural cycle. Ned Tijdschr Geneeskd. 2010;154(45):A2519.
12. Kim CH, Kim SR, Cheon YP, Kim SH, Chae HD, Kang BM. Minimal stimulation using gonadotropin-releasing hormone (GnRH) antagonist and recombinant human follicle-stimulating hormone versus GnRH antagonist multiple-dose protocol in low responders undergoing in vitro fertilization/intracytoplasmic sperm injection. Fertil Steril. 2009 Dec;92(6):2082–4. https://doi.org/10.1016/j.fertnstert.2009.06.005.
13. Haas J, Casper RF. In vitro fertilization treatments with the use of clomiphene citrate or letrozole. Fertil Steril. 2017 Oct;108(4):568–71. https://doi.org/10.1016/j.fertnstert.2017.08.017.
14. Rose BI, Laky DC, Rose SD. A comparison of the use of clomiphene citrate and letrozole in patients undergoing IVF with the objective of producing only one or two embryos. Facts Views Vis Obgyn. 2015;7(2):119–26.
15. Ochin H, Ma X, Wang L, Li X, Song J, Meng Y, Shen J, Cui YG, Liu J. Low dose clomiphene citrate as a mild stimulation protocol in women with unsuspected poor in vitro fertilization result can generate more oocytes with optimal cumulative pregnancy rate. J Ovarian Res. 2018 May 4;11(1):37. https://doi.org/10.1186/s13048-018-0408-x.
16. Oktem M, Guler I, Erdem M, Erdem A, Bozkurt N, Karabacak O. Comparison of the effectiveness of clomiphene citrate versus letrozole in mild IVF in poor prognosis subfertile women with failed IVF cycles. Int J Fertil Steril. 2015 Oct-Dec;9(3):285–91.
17. Bastu E, Buyru F, Ozsurmeli M, Demiral I, Dogan M, Yeh J. A randomized, single-blind, prospective trial comparing three different gonadotropin doses with or without addition of letrozole during ovulation stimulation in patients with poor ovarian response. Eur J Obstet Gynecol Reprod Biol. 2016 Aug;203:30–4. https://doi.org/10.1016/j.ejogrb.2016.05.027.
18. Song D, Shi Y, Zhong Y, Meng Q, Hou S, Li H. Efficiency of mild ovarian stimulation with clomiphene on poor ovarian responders during IVF\ICSI procedures: a meta-analysis. Eur J Obstet Gynecol Reprod Biol. 2016 Sep;204:36–43. https://doi.org/10.1016/j.ejogrb.2016.07.498.
19. Lazer T, Dar S, Shlush E, Al Kudmani BS, Quach K, Sojecki A, Glass K, Sharma P, Baratz A, Librach CL. Comparison of IVF outcomes between minimal stimulation and high-dose stimulation for patients with poor ovarian reserve. Int J Reprod Med. 2014;2014:581451. https://doi.org/10.1155/2014/581451.
20. Zhang JJ, Merhi Z, Yang M, Bodri D, Chavez-Badiola A, Repping S, van Wely M. Minimal stimulation IVF vs conventional IVF: a randomized controlled trial. Am J Obstet Gynecol. 2016 Jan;214(1):96.e1–8. https://doi.org/10.1016/j.ajog.2015.08.009.
21. Borges E Jr, Zanetti BF, Setti AS, Braga DP, Figueira RCS, Iaconelli A Jr. FSH dose to stimulate different patient' ages: when less is more. JBRA Assist Reprod. 2017 Dec 1;21(4):336–42. https://doi.org/10.5935/1518-0557.20170058.
22. Pilehvari S, Shahrokh Tehraninejad E, Hosseinrashidi B, Keikhah F, Haghollahi F, Aziminekoo E. Comparison pregnancy outcomes between minimal stimulation protocol and conventional GnRH antagonist protocols in poor ovarian responders. J Family Reprod Health. 2016 Mar;10(1):35–42.
23. Mohsen IA, El Din RE. Minimal stimulation protocol using letrozole versus microdose flare up GnRH agonist protocol in women with poor ovarian response undergoing ICSI. Gynecol Endocrinol. 2013 Feb;29(2):105–8. https://doi.org/10.3109/09513590.2012.730569.
24. Mendez Lozano DH, Brum Scheffer J, Frydman N, Fay S, Fanchin R, Frydman R. Optimal reproductive competence of oocytes retrieved through follicular flushing in minimal stimulation IVF. Reprod Biomed Online. 2008 Jan;16(1):119–23.
25. Chen Q, Wang Y, Sun L, Zhang S, Chai W, Hong Q, Long H, Wang L, Lyu Q, Kuang Y. Controlled ovulation of the dominant follicle using progestin in minimal stimulation in poor responders. Reprod Biol Endocrinol. 2017 Sep 5;15(1):71. https://doi.org/10.1186/s12958-017-0291-0.
26. Yu R, Jin H, Huang X, Lin J, Wang P. Comparison of modified agonist, mild-stimulation and antagonist protocols for in vitro fertilization in patients with diminished ovarian reserve. J Int Med Res. 2018 Jun;46:2327–37. https://doi.org/10.1177/0300060518770346.
27. Yan G, Xie X, Wang Y, Shi L, Zhou W, Liu Y, Tong X, Ji Y. Twin pregnancy after intracytoplasmic sperm injection in woman aged 49 using autologous oocytes by mild ovarian stimulation: a case report. Int J Clin Exp Med. 2015 Nov 15;8(11):21707–9.
28. Allahbadia GN. Stimulation and aneuploidy: why are milder stimulation protocols better? IVF Lite. 2016;3:41–5.
29. Allahbadia GN. Have we finally written the obituary for conventional IVF? IVF Lite. 2014;1:1–5.

30. Zhang J, Chang L, Sone Y, Silber S. Minimal ovarian stimulation (mini-IVF) for IVF utilizing vitrification and cryopreserved embryo transfer. Reprod Biomed Online. 2010 Oct;21(4):485–95. https://doi.org/10.1016/j.rbmo.2010.06.033.Epub.
31. Kato K, Takehara Y, Segawa T, Kawachiya S, Okuno T, Kobayashi T, Bodri D, Kato O. Minimal ovarian stimulation combined with elective single embryo transfer policy: age-specific results of a large, single-Centre, Japanese cohort. Reprod Biol Endocrinol. 2012 Apr 27;10:35. https://doi.org/10.1186/1477-7827-10-35.
32. Bodri D, Kawachiya S, De Brucker M, Tournaye H, Kondo M, Kato R, Matsumoto T. Cumulative success rates following mild IVF in unselected infertile patients: a 3-year, single-Centre cohort study. Reprod Biomed Online. 2014 May;28(5):572–81. https://doi.org/10.1016/j.rbmo.2014.01.002.
33. Zander-Fox D, Lane M, Hamilton H, Tremellen K. Sequential clomiphene/corifollitrophin alpha as a technique for mild controlled ovarian hyperstimulation in IVF: a proof of concept study. J Assist Reprod Genet. 2018 Apr 10;35:1047. https://doi.org/10.1007/s10815-018-1172-y.
34. Kato O, Kawasaki N, Bodri D, Kuroda T, Kawachiya S, Kato K, Takehara Y. Neonatal outcome and birth defects in 6623 singletons born following minimal ovarian stimulation and vitrified versus fresh single embryo transfer. Eur J Obstet Gynecol Reprod Biol. 2012 Mar;161(1):46–50. https://doi.org/10.1016/j.ejogrb.2011.12.005.
35. Grabar VV, Stefanovich AV. Aneuploidies in oocytes used in IVF programs. Georgian Med News. 2014;23:7–12.
36. De Sutter P, Dhont M, Vandekerckhove D. Hormonal stimulation for in vitro fertilization: a comparison of fertilization rates and cytogenetic findings in unfertilized oocytes. J Assist Reprod Genet. 1992;9:254–8.
37. Rubio C, Mercader A, Alamá P, Lizán C, Rodrigo L, Labarta E, et al. Prospective cohort study in high responder oocyte donors using two hormonal stimulation protocols: impact on embryo aneuploidy and development. Hum Reprod. 2010;25:2290–7.
38. Baart EB, Martini E, Eijkemans MJ, Van Opstal D, Beckers NG, Verhoeff A, et al. Milder ovarian stimulation for in-vitro fertilization reduces aneuploidy in the human preimplantation embryo: a randomized controlled trial. Hum Reprod. 2007;22:980–8.
39. Kuang Y, Chen Q, Hong Q, Lyu Q, Ai A, Fu Y, Shoham Z. Double stimulations during the follicular and luteal phases of poor responders in IVF/ICSI programmes (Shanghai protocol). Reprod Biomed Online. 2014 Dec;29(6):684–91. https://doi.org/10.1016/j.rbmo.2014.08.009.
40. Madani T, Hemat M, Arabipoor A, Khodabakhshi SH, Zolfaghari Z. Double mild stimulation and egg collection in the same cycle for management of poor ovarian responders. J Gynecol Obstet Hum Reprod. 2018 Dec 12;S2468–7847(18):30379. https://doi.org/10.1016/j.jogoh.2018.12.004.
41. Liu C, Jiang H, Zhang W, Yin H. Double ovarian stimulation during the follicular and luteal phase in women ≥38 years: a retrospective case-control study. Reprod Biomed Online. 2017 Dec;35(6):678–84. https://doi.org/10.1016/j.rbmo.2017.08.019.
42. Li Y, Yang W, Chen X, Li L, Zhang Q, Yang D. Comparison between follicular stimulation and luteal stimulation protocols with clomiphene and HMG in women with poor ovarian response. Gynecol Endocrinol. 2016;32(1):74–7. https://doi.org/10.3109/09513590.2015.1081683.
43. Ferraretti AP, Devroey P, Magli MC, Gianaroli L. No need for luteal phase support in IVF cycles after mild stimulation: proof-of-concept study. Reprod Biomed Online. 2017 Feb;34(2):162–5. https://doi.org/10.1016/j.rbmo.2016.10.006.
44. Allahbadia GN. IVF lite: is this the future of assisted reproduction? J Obstet Gynecol India. 2013;63:1–4.
45. Gandhi GN, Allahbadia GN, Kagalwala S, Khatoon A, Hinduja R, Allahbadia A. IVF lite - a new strategy for managing poor ovarian responders. IVF Lite. 2014;1:22–8.
46. Gandhi G, Allahbadia G, Kagalwala S, Allahbadia A, Ramesh S, Patel K, et al. ACCU-VIT: a new strategy for managing poor responders. Hum Reprod. 2013;28:i149–206.

Relevance of Embryo Aneuploidy in Medically Assisted Reproduction

71

Esther Velilla and Carmen Morales

71.1 Background

The prevalence of primary and secondary infertility has been estimated in 1.9% and 10.5%, respectively, in women of 20–44 years of age from 190 countries according published data in 2010 [1]. Aneuploidy is the main genetic factor that influences human reproductive success [2]. As it has been published, aneuploid embryos account for at least 10% of human pregnancies, and the incidence could exceed 50% for women over 35 years of age [3, 4]. Most aneuploidies compromise the implantation of the conceptuses that perish in utero, and those that implant may result in an early miscarriage or cause congenital birth defects.

Medically assisted reproduction (MAR) allows for the treatment of most infertile couples with the aim of securing a healthy birth. Therefore, in vitro fertilization (IVF) laboratories are challenged to reduce the risk associated with multiple pregnancy. For that, most of the IVF clinics have moved to the strategy of a single embryo transfer, diagnosed as chromosomally normal, since selecting just the morphologically normal ones to transfer is not enough to guarantee its success. Morphology of an embryo is weakly correlated with its viability and, hence, with its chromosome constitution. All type of uniform aneuploidies can survive to the blastocyst stage [3, 5–13]. Moreover, 40–50% blastocysts with optimal morphology can be chromosomally abnormal [14, 15], and euploid embryos do not always demonstrate better morphology than chaotic mosaics [16]. On the other hand, there is a correlation between aneuploidy and maternal age due to an increase of premature sister chromatids separation and meiotic nondisjunction of homologous chromosomes [17]. As an example, aneuploidy increases from 40% in fertile egg donors to 80% in patients of 41–42 years old [18].

However, Harton et al. in 2013 [19] demonstrated that if a chromosomally normal embryo is transferred to the uterus, the chance to implant is independent of maternal age. The transfer of abnormal embryos in an IVF cycle is related to higher rates of implantation failure and miscarriage. Although there is a direct correlation between embryo aneuploidy and maternal age, there is also positive correlation with other factors such as sperm chromosome abnormalities, altered male meiosis, or nongenetic male factor [20, 21].

Preimplantation genetic testing (PGT) has been used since the 1990s to diagnose genetically abnormal embryos for selecting, with some certainty, those genetically normal embryo(s) to be transferred to the uterus with the maximum guarantees to implant and to reach term. PGT has been incorporated into IVF laboratories to improve the efficiency of ART, increasing implantation rates while lowering pregnancy loss rate [22–29]. The success of PGT for aneuploidy screening (PGT-AS) is not limited to the technique itself but depends on different factors: (1) the optimization of the PGT-AS technique; (2) the proper selection of patients for PGT-AS; (3) the number of analyzed chromosomes (limited or comprehensive chromosome screening, CCS); and (4) the protocols of ovarian stimulation, in vitro embryo culture, and embryo(s) transfer. Focusing on PGT-AS technique, over the past years, different methodologies have been optimized to overcome many of the technical limitations intrinsic to the analysis of a single cell or a few number of them. Fluorescence in situ hybridization (FISH) on fixed nuclei from biopsied blastomeres was the technique of choice over the past two decades. However, the classic FISH technique analysis was limited to a restricted number of chromosomes [30] restricting the improvement of IVF outcomes with PGT-AS, as reported by several authors [31–38] and advised by the ESHRE PGD Consortium [39]. Therefore, the natural evolution of the PGT-AS has driven to the development, clinical validation, and application of the new emerging CCSs methodologies. Currently, the available CCS techniques developed and clinical validated for PGT-AS are array comparative genomic hybridization (aCGH) [5, 11, 15, 40], 24-chromosome FISH

E. Velilla · C. Morales (✉)
The PGD Laboratory, Jabriya Medical Center, Kuwait City, Kuwait
e-mail: esther.velilla@pgdlabs.com; carmen.morales@pgdlabs.com

G. N. Allahbadia et al. (eds.), *Textbook of Assisted Reproduction*, https://doi.org/10.1007/978-981-15-2377-9_71

(FISH-24) [41], single nucleotide polymorphism (SNP) microarray [42], quantitative real-time polymerase chain reaction (qPCR)-based CCS [43], and more recently next-generation sequencing (NGS) [44–50]. The application of CCS techniques also produces a change in the protocol of biopsy, moving from day 3 to day 5 of embryo development in order to have more quantity and quality of DNA for amplification and to overcome the high rate of mosaicism detected on cell stage embryos that can lead to misdiagnosis. Among these technologies, NGS seems to detect with higher accuracy for segmental imbalances [51, 52] and chromosomal mosaicism [51, 53–55]. Recently after three randomized control trials (RCT) testing day 5 blastocyst biopsies in good prognosis patients, there appear to be significant improvements in ongoing pregnancy rates [26, 27, 56], encouraging physicians to recommend PGT-AS on trophectoderm samples.

71.2 Is There an Optimal PGT-AS and Embryo Transfer Program?

One of the more recent discussions about PGT-AS using the new CCS platforms is which is the most efficient operating way in terms of maximizing pregnancy rates. When PGT-AS by FISH was established, most centers did the biopsy on day 3, and euploid embryos were transferred in day 5 in a fresh cycle, but pregnancy rates were not as good as expected. In the last few years, there is published evidence showing that transferring cryopreserved embryos in a non-stimulated cycle increases clinical implantation rates [57–63] and decreases low birth weight and preterm delivery rate [64, 65]. Coates et al. in 2017 [66] published a RCT comparing both approaches: to perform day 5 biopsy and vitrify all embryos while waiting for the PGT-AS results and to carry out the euploid embryo transfer in a non-stimulated cycle versus biopsing embryos at day 5 and transferring the euploid embryos on day 6 in a fresh cycle. Embryos showing slow development were biopsied on day 6 and kept frozen for a future non-stimulated transfer, in case of failed outcomes. The study was performed in a US institute with a long standing experience in embryo vitrification, embryo culture, and biopsy procedures, and the results showed, in terms of ongoing pregnancy rates and live birth rates, a trend in favor of a freeze all strategy and transference of the euploid embryos in non-stimulated cycles. Another RCT published by Rubio et al. [67] compared the effectiveness of clinical outcome with and without PGT-AS in women with advanced maternal age (from 38 to 41 years old) after embryo analysis by aCGH. They published a higher delivery rate per transfer after the first transfer attempt (52.9% vs 24.2%) and higher delivery rate per patient (36.0% vs. 21.9%) in the group that performed PGD aneuploidy screening compared to the group that did not perform PGD.

The main issue when applying the freeze all strategy is that the laboratory must optimize its culture conditions to achieve the highest rates of blastocyst formation. Moreover, vitrification and thawing protocols must be optimized in order to achieve the highest post-warming survival and cleavage development rate. Unfortunately, not all IVF laboratories around the world have standardized protocols, and, even among those following the highest quality standards, results may drastically differ from one center to another. This suggests that although publications are in favor of a specific strategy, each center should analyze its own laboratory efficiency and which strategy is the best for them. For one laboratory that does not have a good established blastocyst vitrification protocol and presents a high incidence of lysed cells and low development rate post-warming, the best approach would be to perform day 5 biopsy and transfer in a fresh cycle and only keep vitrified the D6 biopsied blastocyst for a second transfer. Another scenario may be a laboratory that presents a poor embryo culture conditions. In that way, the best approach should be to biopsy on day 3 and transfer in day 3/4 in a fresh cycle to avoid losing embryo potential.

71.3 Mosaicism

Transferring high morphological quality euploid embryos has increased pregnancy rates, but we are still faced with the challenge that some euploid embryos with a good morphology fail to implant. In this scenario, many programs have started to utilize time-lapse PGD-AS studies to correlate morphokinetics parameters and the type of aneuploidy in an attempt to identify which embryos have better competence to implant, but that said, efficiency is still not 100%. This can mainly be due to two factors: mosaicism and technical limitations.

Embryo mosaicism is one of the main sources of error when performing PGT-AS [68–76]. To establish the rate of mosaicism in preimplantation embryos is a complex task since it varies according to the embryo stage, the technology used for the diagnosis, and the skills of the genetic laboratory for the interpretation. In cleavage-stage embryos, the estimated levels of mosaicism vary from 15 to 75% while in blastocyst have been estimated in 3–24%, according to a published review [77]. The great variability on reported data can also be influenced by different factors other than PGT-AS procedure itself, including the etiology of infertility, female's age, or even in vitro culture and environmental conditions. All these elements can also impact the abnormal chromosome segregation leading to embryonic mosaicism. However, it appears that there is a general agreement for the observation that a gradual decrease in aneuploidy takes place during embryo development most probably due to self-correction mechanisms and preferential development of euploid cells.

Mosaicism occurs during mitotic division of the embryo, giving rise to chromosomally different cell lines. When analyzing one cell from the embryo, it is assumed that the result is representative of the whole embryo. In order to avoid mosaicism misdiagnosis when performing PGT-AS, two different strategies have been proposed. The first is to perform polar body 1 and 2 analysis. Using this strategy, only chromosomal abnormalities of maternal meiotic origin are analyzed, while paternal meiotic abnormalities and abnormal chromosomal mitotic segregations are not evaluated. The second is to perform trophectoderm biopsy at blastocyst stage, analyzing more than one embryonic cell in in a developmental stage with a lower rate of mosaicism compared to day 3 embryos. This strategy can be used only if a good system for day 5 embryo culture is available and if a high number of embryos is achieved. However, although mosaicism rate is lower, it can be present so there is still a risk of misdiagnosis. At the blastocyst stage, different types of mosaics have been described [78]: mosaicism that affect both trophectoderm (TFE) and inner cell mass (ICM), when the abnormal cells are confined to the TFE or ICM exclusively or when the ICM is normal TFE is abnormal (or vice versa). Depending on the type of mosaicism we are facing and the TFE cells we are biopsing by chance will condition PGT-AS misdiagnosis rate on blastocyst stage. Some studies have tried to estimate this correlation between ICM and TFE cell lines by biopsing two or three different groups of cells of the same embryo. They observed a diagnosis correlation of 95–100%, and the discordance between ICM and TFE cell lines was estimated to be around 3–4% [79, 80].

Another strategy to avoid misdiagnosis due to mosaicism on the PGT-AS results has been to perform two cells biopsy on day 3. However, this strategy has been demonstrated to be detrimental for embryo developmental competence and has not been recommended any longer.

New CCS platforms for PGT-AS such as NGS can detect low levels of diploid/aneuploid mosaicism with high accuracy (lower than 20%). Mosaic or potentially mosaic embryos have become a new category to classify embryos [81]. According PGDIS recommendations [82], embryos with a mosaicism rate lower than 20% can be considered as euploid (and then transferable), while embryos with more than 80% of abnormal cells are classified as aneuploid. The remaining ones (20–80%) can be classified as mosaics. However, to establish the thresholds between which the embryos can be considered transferable or not is a controversial issue. Simon et al. recently suggested [81] that one consider above 50% of mosaicism embryo to be classified as aneuploid and non-transferable. According to a worldwide survey from 32 countries, <10% of the analyzed embryos are classified as mosaics [81]. These embryos have a theoretically decreased implantation rate and increased risk of miscarriage, pregnancy complications, and clinically affected life births [81, 82]. Transferring embryos categorized as mosaic, although can raise some ethical considerations, is generally accepted when the couple does not have any euploid embryos [82, 83]. Different factors should be taken into consideration such as the methodology used for testing, the involved chromosomes, or the reproductive medical history of the couple [81–83]. Regarding this matter, PGDIS consortium published a suggested guideline to prioritize mosaic embryos for transfer. Patients may consider transferring a mosaic embryo only after a proper genetic counselling about the risks of miscarriage and adverse outcomes they can face.

71.4 Conclusion

One of the most important challenges for the embryologist is to discern which is the most competent embryo to transfer. Many efforts to find the magical wand have been made in studying the cytoplasmic and nuclear competence, the morphology, and morphokinetics during embryo development or in developing the most paramount technique to detect all chromosome aneuploidies. Yet still, just when we thought that we had the most comprehensive technology that permits us to screen all chromosomes, some new question arises and makes us go back in time and question all we know. Is embryo mosaicism an indicator of euploidy? Do we have to discard mosaic embryos?

References

1. Mascarenhas MN, Flaxman SR, Boerma T, Vanderpoel S, Stevens GA. National, regional, and global trends in infertility prevalence since 1990: a systematic analysis of 277 health surveys. PLoS Med. 2012;9(12):e1001356.
2. Hassold T, Hunt P. To err (meiotically) is human: the genesis of human aneuploidy. Nature Rev Genet. 2001;2:280–91.
3. Franasiak JM, Forman EJ, Hong KH, Werner MD, Upham KM, Treff NR, Scott RT. Aneuploidy across individual chromosomes at the embryonic level in trophectoderm biopsies: changes with patient age and chromosome structure. J Assist Reprod Genet. 2014 Nov;31(11):1501–9.
4. Nagaoka SI, Hassold TJ, Hunt PA. Human aneuploidy: mechanisms and new insights into an age-old problem. Nat Rev Genet. 2012;13:493–504.
5. Fragouli E, Alfarawati S, Daphnis DD, Goodall N, Mania A, Griffiths T, Wells D. Cytogenetic analysis of human blastocysts with the use of FISH, CGH and aCGH: scientific data and technical evaluation. Hum Reprod. 2011;26(2):480–90.
6. Evsikov S, Verlinsky Y. Mosaicism in the inner cell mass of human blastocysts. Hum Reprod. 1998;13(11):3151–5.
7. Magli MC, Jones GM, Gras L, Gianaroli L, Korman I, Trounson O. Chromosome mosaicism in day 3 aneuploid embryos that develop to morphologically normal blastocysts in vitro. Hum Reprod. 2000;15(8):1781–6.
8. Sandalinas M, Sadowy S, Alikani M, Calderon G, Cohen J, Munné S. Developmental ability of chromosomally abnormal

human embryos to develop to the blastocyst stage. Hum Reprod. 2001;16(9):1954–8.
9. Bielanska M, Tan SL, Ao A. High rate of mixoploidy among human blastocysts cultured in vitro. Fertil Steril. 2002;78(6):1248–53.
10. Coonen E, Derhaag JG, Dumoulin JC, et al. Anaphase lagging mainly explains chromosomal mosaicism in human preimplantation embryos. Hum Reprod. 2004;19(2):316–24.
11. Fragouli E, Katz-Jaffe M, Schoolcraft WB, Ross R, Munne S, Wells D. Comprehensive cytogenetic analysis of the human blastocyst stage. Fertil Steril. 2008;90(11):S36.
12. Santos MA, Teklenburg G, Macklon NS, Van Opstal D, Schuring-Blom GH, Krijtenburg PJ, de Vreeden-Elbertse J, Fauser BC, Baart EB. The fate of the mosaic embryo: chromosomal constitution and development of day 4, 5 and 8 human embryos. Hum Reprod. 2010;25(8):1916–26.
13. Fragouli E, Alfarawati S, Spath K, Wells D. Morphological and cytogenetic assessment of cleavage and blastocyst stage embryos. Mol Hum Reprod. 2014;20(2):117–26.
14. Wells D, Alfarawati S, Fragouli E. Use of comprehensive chromosomal screening for embryo assessment: microarrays and CGH. Mol Hum Reprod. 2008;14(12):703–10.
15. Capalbo A, Rienzi L, Cimadomo D, Maggiulli R, Elliott T, Wright G, Ubaldi FM. Correlation between standard blastocyst morphology, euploidy and implantation: an observational study in two centers involving 956 screened blastocysts. Hum Reprod. 2014;29(6):1173–81.
16. Johnson DS, Cinnioglu C, Ross R, Filby A, Gemelos G, Hill M, Ryan A, Smotrich D, Rabinowitz M, Murray MJ. Comprehensive analysis of karyotypic mosaicism between trophectoderm and inner cell mass. Mol Hum Reprod. 2010;16(12):944–9.
17. Van Steirteghem A, Liu J, Nagy Z, Joris H, Tournaye H, Liebaers I, Devroey P. Use of assisted fertilization. Hum Reprod. 1993 Nov;8(11):1784–5.
18. Ata B, Kaplan B, Danzer H, Glassner M, Opsahl M, Tan SL, Munné S. Array CGH analysis shows that aneuploidy is not related to the number of embryos generated. Reprod Biomed Online. 2012 Jun;24(6):614–20.
19. Harton GL, Munné S, Surrey M, Grifo J, Kaplan B, McCulloh DH, Griffin DK, Wells D, PGD Practitioners Group. Diminished effect of maternal age on implantation after preimplantation genetic diagnosis with array comparative genomic hybridization. Fertil Steril. 2013 Dec;100(6):1695–703.
20. Sánchez-Castro M, Jiménez-Macedo AR, Sandalinas M, Blanco J. Prognostic value of sperm fluorescence in situ hybridization analysis over PGD. Hum Reprod. 2009;24(6):1516–21.
21. Sarrate Z, Vidal F, Blanco J. Role of sperm fluorescent in situ hybridization studies in infertile patients: indications, study approach, and clinical relevance. Fertil Steril. 2010;93(6):1892–902.
22. Gianaroli L, Magli MC, Ferraretti AP, Munné S. Preimplantation diagnosis for aneuploidies in patients undergoing in vitro fertilization with a poor prognosis: identification of the categories for which it should be proposed. Fertil Steril. 1999;72(5):837–44.
23. Munné S, Magli C, Cohen J, Morton P, Sadowy S, Gianaroli L, Tucker M, Márquez C, Sable D, Ferraretti AP, Massey JB, Scott R. Positive outcome after preimplantation diagnosis of aneuploidy in human embryos. Hum Reprod. 1999;14:2191–9.
24. Munné S, Sandalinas M, Escudero T, Velilla E, Walmsley R, Sadowy S, Cohen J, Sable D. Improved implantation after preimplantation genetic diagnosis of aneuploidy. Reprod Biomed Online. 2003;7(1):91–7.
25. Munné S, Chen S, Fischer J, Colls P, Zheng X, Stevens J, Escudero T, Oter M, Schoolcraft B, Simpson JL, Cohen J. Preimplantation genetic diagnosis reduces pregnancy loss in women aged 35 years and older with a history of recurrent miscarriages. Fertil Steril. 2005;84(2):331–5.
26. Scott RT Jr, Upham KM, Forman EJ, Hong KH, Scott KL, Taylor D, Tao X, Treff NR. Blastocyst biopsy with comprehensive chromosome screening and fresh embryo transfer significantly increases in vitro fertilization implantation and delivery rates: a randomized controlled trial. Fertil Steril. 2013;100(3):697–703.
27. Yang Z, Liu J, Collins GS, Salem SA, Liu X, Lyle SS, Peck AC, Sills ES, Salem RD. Selection of single blastocysts for fresh transfer via standard morphology assessment alone and with array CGH for good prognosis IVF patients: results from a randomized pilot study. Mol Cytogenet. 2012;5(1):24.
28. Rubio C, Bellver J, Rodrigo L, Bosch E, Mercader A, Vidal C, De los Santos MJ, Giles J, Labarta E, Domingo J, Crespo J, Remohí J, Pellicer A, Simón C. Preimplantation genetic screening using fluorescence in situ hybridization in patients with repetitive implantation failure and advanced maternal age: two randomized trials. Fertil Steril. 2013;99(5):1400–7.
29. Forman EJ, Hong KH, Franasiak JM, Scott RT. Obstetrical and neonatal outcomes from the BEST trial: single embryo transfer with aneuploidy screening improves outcomes after in vitro fertilization without compromising delivery rates. Am J Obstet Gynecol. 2014;210(2):157.e1–6.
30. Munne S, Marquez C, Magli C, Morton P, Morrison L. Scoring criteria for preimplantation genetic diagnosis of numerical abnormalities for chromosomes X, Y, 13, 16, 18 and 21. Mol Hum Reprod. 1998;4:863–70.
31. Staessen C, Platteau P, Van Assche E, Michiels A, Tournaye H, Camus M, Devroey P, Liebaers I, Van Steirteghem A. Comparison of blastocyst transfer with or without preimplantation genetic diagnosis for aneuploidy screening in couples with advanced maternal age: a prospective randomized controlled trial. Hum Reprod. 2004;19(12):2849–58.
32. Mastenbroek S, Twisk M, van Echten-Arends J, Sikkema-Raddatz B, Korevaar JC, Verhoeve HR, et al. In vitro fertilization with preimplantation genetic screening. N Engl J Med. 2007;357(1):9–17.
33. Fritz MA. Perspectives on the efficacy and indications for preimplantation genetic screening: where are we now? Hum Reprod. 2008;23(12):2617–21.
34. Hardarson T, Hanson C, Lundin K, Hillensjö T, Nilsson L, Stevic J, Reismer E, Borg K, Wikland M, Bergh C. Preimplantation genetic screening in women of advanced maternal age caused a decrease in clinical pregnancy rate: a randomized controlled trial. Hum Reprod. 2008;23(12):2806–12.
35. Staessen C, Verpoest W, Donoso P, Haentjens P, Van der Elst J, Liebaers I, Devroey P. Preimplantation genetic screening does not improve delivery rate in women under the age of 36 following single-embryo transfer. Hum Reprod. 2008;23(12):2818–25.
36. Twisk M, Mastenbroek S, Hoek A, Heineman MJ, van der Veen F, Bossuyt PM, Repping S, Korevaar JC. No beneficial effect of preimplantation genètic screening in women of advanced maternal age with a high risk for embryonic aneuploidy. Hum Reprod. 2008;23(12):2813–7.
37. Schoolcraft WB, Katz-Jaffe MG, Stevens J, Rawlins M, Munne S. Preimplantation aneuploidy testing for infertile patients of advanced maternal age: a randomized prospective trial. Fertil Steril. 2009;92(1):157–62.
38. Harper JC, Harton G. The use of arrays in preimplantation genetic diagnosis and screening. Fertil Steril. 2010;94(4):1173–7.
39. Harper J, Coonen E, De Rycke M, Fiorentino F, Geraedts J, Goossens V, et al. What next for preimplantation genetic screening (PGS)? A position statement from the ESHRE PGD consortium steering committee. Hum Reprod. 2010;25(4):821–3.
40. Gutiérrez-Mateo C, Colls P, Sánchez-García J, Escudero T, Prates R, Ketterson K, Wells D, Munné S. Validation of microarray comparative genomic hybridization for comprehensive chromosome analysis of embryos. Fertil Steril. 2011;95(3):953–8.

41. Fernández S, Toro E, Colomar A, López-Teijón M, Velilla E. A 24-chromosome FISH technique in preimplantation genetic diagnosis: validation of the method. Syst Biol Reprod Med. 2015;61(3):171–7. https://doi.org/10.3109/19396368.2014.1002869.
42. Treff NR, Su J, Tao X, Levy B, Scott RT. Accurate single cell 24 chromosome aneuploidy screening using whole genome amplification and single nucleotide polymorphism microarrays. Fertil Steril. 2010;94(6):2017–21.
43. Treff NR, Tao X, Ferry KM, Su J, Taylor D, Scott RT. Development and validation of an accurate quantitative real-time polymerase chain reaction-based assay for human blastocyst comprehensive chromosomal aneuploidy screening. Fertil Steril. 2012;97(4):819–24.
44. Wells D, Kaur K, Grifo J, Glassner M, Taylor JC, Fragouli E, Munne S. Clinical utilisation of a rapid low-pass whole genome sequencing technique for the diagnosis of aneuploidy in human embryos prior to implantation. J Med Genet. 2014;51(8):553–62.
45. Fiorentino F, Biricik A, Bono S, Spizzichino L, Cotroneo E, Cottone G, Michel CE. Development and validation of a next-generation sequencing-based protocol for 24-chromosome aneuploidy screening of embryos. Fertil Steril. 2014;101(5):1375–82.
46. Fiorentino F, Bono S, Biricik A, Nuccitelli A, Cotroneo E, Cottone G, Greco E. Application of next-generation sequencing technology for comprehensive aneuploidy screening of blastocysts in clinical preimplantation genetic screening cycles. Hum Reprod. 2014;29(12):2802–13.
47. Tan Y, Yin X, Zhang S, Jiang H, Tan K, Li J, Xiong B, Gong F, Zhang C, Pan X, Chen F, Chen S, Gong C, Lu C, Luo K, Gu Y, Zhang X, Wang W, Xu X, Vajta G, Bolund L, Yang H, Lu G, Du Y, Lin G. Clinical outcome of preimplantation genetic diagnosis and screening using next generation sequencing. Gigascience. 2014;3(1):30.
48. Zheng H, Jin H, Liu L, Liu J, Wang WH. Application of next-generation sequencing for 24-chromosome aneuploidy screening of human preimplantation embryos. Mol Cytogenet. 2015;8:38.
49. Yang Z, Lin J, Zhang J, Fong WI, Li P, Zhao R, Liu X, Podevin W, Kuang Y, Liu J. Randomized comparison of next-generation sequencing and array comparative genomic hybridization for preimplantation genetic screening: a pilot study. BMC Med Genet. 2015;8:30.
50. Kung A, Munné S, Bankowski B, Coates A, Wells D. Validation of next-generation sequencing for comprehensive chromosome screening of embryos. Reprod Biomed Online. 2014;31(6):760–9.
51. Lai H-H, Chuang T-H, Wong L K, Lee M-J, Hsieh C-L, Wang H-L, Chen S-U. Identification of mosaic and segmental aneuploidies by next-generation sequencing in preimplantation genetic screening can improve clinical outcomes compared to array-comparative genomic hybridization. Mol Cytogenet. 2017;10:14. https://doi.org/10.1186/s13039-017-0315-7.
52. Bauckman K, Ribustello L, Escudero T, Armenti E, Capaldi R, Munne S. Validation of next generation sequencing (NGS) for PGD of structural chromosome abnormalities (ESHRE Abstract). Hum Reprod. 2016;31:i410.
53. Fragouli E, Alfarawati S, Spath K, Tarozzi N, Borini A, Wells D. The developmental potential of mosaic embryos (ASRM Abstract). Fertil Steril. 2015;104:e96.
54. Grifo J, Colls P, Ribustello L, Escudero T, Liu E, Munne S. Why do array-CGH(ACGH) euploid embryos miscarry? Reanalysis by NGS reveals undetected abnormalities which would have prevented 56% of the miscarriages. Fertil Steril. 2015:104e14.
55. Liu E, Escudero T, Ribustello L, Bauckman K, Colls P, Munne S. Chromosome abnormalities detected by array comparative genomic hybridization and next-generacion sequencing: results on >38000 embryos (ESHRE abstracts). Hua Reprod. 2016;31:i388.
56. Forman EJ, Li X, Ferry KM, Scott K, Treff NR, Scott RT Jr. Oocyte vitrification does not increase the risk of embryonic aneuploidy or diminish the implantation potential of blastocysts created after intracytoplasmic sperm injection: a novel, paired randomized controlled trial using DNA fingerprinting. Fertil Steril. 2012 Sep;98(3):644–9.
57. Chattacharya S. Maternal and perinatal outcomes after fresh versus frozen embryo transfer- what is the risk-benefit ratio? Fertil Steril. 2016;106:241–3.
58. Ozgur K, Berkkanoglu M, Bulut H, Humaidan P, Coetzee K. Perinatal outcomes after fresh versus vitrified–warmed blastocyst transfer: retrospective analysis. Fertil Steril. 2015;104:899–907.
59. Shapiro BS, Daneshmand ST, Garner FC, Aguieer M, Hudson C. Clinical rationale for cryopreservation of entire embryo cohorts in lieu of fresh transfer. Fertil Steril. 2014;102:3–9.
60. Shapiro BS, Daneshmand ST, Garner FC, Aguirre M, Hudson C, Thomas S. Evidence of impaired endometrial receptivity after ovarian stimulation for in vitro fertilization: a prospective randomized trial comparing fresh and frozen–thawed embryo transfer in normal responders. Fertil Steril. 2011;96:344–8.
61. Roque M, Valle M, Guimaraes F, Sampaio M, Geber S. Freeze-all policy: fresh versus frozen–thawed embryo transfer. Fertil Steril. 2015;103:1190–3.
62. Goma H, Baydoum R, Sachak S, Lapana I, Soliman S. Elective single embryo transfer: Is frozen better than fresh. JBRA Assist Reprod. 2016;20:3–7.
63. Shi Y, Wei D, Liang X, Sun Y, Liu J, Cao Y, et al. Live birth after fresh embryo transfer in women with polycistic ovary syndrome undergoing IVF /FreFro-PCOS: study protocol for a multicenter, prospective, randomized controlled trial. Trials. 2014;15:154.
64. Wennerholm UB, Henningsen AK, Romundstad LB, Bergh C, Pinborg A, Skajaerven E, et al. Perinatal outcomes of children born after frozen-thawed embryo transfer: a Nordic cohort study from CoNARTaS group. Hum Reprod. 2013;28:2545–53.
65. Maheshwari A, Battachanya S. Ellective frozen replacement cycles for all: ready for prime time? Hum Reprod. 2013;28:6–9.
66. Coates A, Kung A, Mounts E, Hesla J, Bankowski B, Barbieri E, Ata B, Cohen J, Munné S. Optimal euploid embryo transfer strategy, fresh versus frozen, after preimplantation genetic screening with next generation sequencing: a randomized controlled trial. Fertil Steril. 2017 Mar;107(3):723–30.
67. Rubio C, Bellver J, Rodrigo L, Castillón G, Guillén A, Vidal C, Giles J, Ferrando M, Cabanillas S, Remohí J, Pellicer A, Simón C. In vitro fertilization with preimplantation genetic diagnosis for aneuploidies in advanced maternal age: a randomized, controlled study. Fertil Steril. 2017 May;107(5):1122–9.
68. Los FJ, van Opstal D, van den Berg C, Braat AP, Verhoef S, Wesby-van Swaay E, van den Ouweland AM, Halley DJ. Uniparental disomy with and without confined placental mosaicism: a model for trisomic zygote rescue. Prenat Diagn. 1998 Jul;18(7):659–68.
69. Los FJ, Van Opstal D, van den Berg C. The development of cytogenetically normal, abnormal and mosaic embryos: a theoretical model. Hum Reprod Update. 2004 Jan–Feb;10(1):79–94.
70. Baart EB, Van Opstal D, Los FJ, Fauser BC, Martini E. Fluorescence in situ hybridization analysis of two blastomeres from day 3 frozen-thawed embryos followed by analysis of the remaining embryo on day 5. Hum Reprod. 2004 Mar;19(3):685–93.
71. Baart EB, Martini E, van den Berg I, Macklon NS, Galjaard RJ, Fauser BC, Van Opstal D. Preimplantation genetic screening reveals a high incidence of aneuploidy and mosaicism in embryos from young women undergoing IVF. Hum Reprod. 2006 Jan;21(1):223–33.
72. Bielanska M, Jin S, Bernier M, Tan SL, Ao A. Diploid-aneuploid mosaicism in human embryos cultured to the blastocyst stage. Fertil Steril. 2005 Aug;84(2):336–42.
73. Barbash-Hazan S, Frumkin T, Malcov M, Yaron Y, Cohen T, Azem F, Amit A, Ben-Yosef D. Preimplantation aneuploid embryos undergo self-correction in correlation with their developmental potential. Fertil Steril. 2009 Sep;92(3):890–6.

74. Daphnis DD, Fragouli E, Economou K, Jerkovic S, Craft IL, Delhanty JD, Harper JC. Analysis of the evolution of chromosome abnormalities in human embryos from Day 3 to 5 using CGH and FISH. Mol Hum Reprod. 2008 Feb;14(2):117–25.
75. Frumkin T, Malcov M, Yaron Y, Ben-Yosef D. Elucidating the origin of chromosomal aberrations in IVF embryos by preimplantation genetic analysis. Mol Cell Endocrinol. 2008 Jan 30;282(1–2):112–9.
76. Munné S, Sandalinas M, Escudero T, Márquez C, Cohen J. Chromosome mosaicism in cleavage-stage human embryos: evidence of a maternal age effect. Reprod Biomed Online. 2002 May–Jun;4(3):223–32.
77. Harton GL, Cinnioglu C, Fiorentino F. Current experience concerning mosaic embryos diagnosed during preimplantation genetic screening. Fertil Steril. 2017 May;107(5):1113–9.
78. Liu J, Wang W, Sun X, Liu L, Jin H, Li M, Witz C, Williams D, Griffith J, Skorupski J, Haddad G, Gill J. DNA microarray reveals that high proportions of human blastocysts from women of advanced maternal age are aneuploid and mosaic. Biol Reprod. 2012 Dec 27;87(6):148.
79. Johnson DS, Cinnioglu C, Ross R, Filby A, Gemelos G, Hill M, Ryan A, Smotrich D, Rabinowitz M, Murray MJ. Comprehensive analysis of karyotypic mosaicism between trophectoderm and inner cell mass. Mol Hum Reprod. 2010 Dec;16(12):944–9.
80. Capalbo A, Wright G, Elliott T, Ubaldi FM, Rienzi L, Nagy ZP. FISH reanalysis of inner cell mass and trophectoderm samples of previously array-CGH screened blastocysts shows high accuracy of diagnosis and no major diagnostic impact of mosaicism at the blastocyst stage. Hum Reprod. 2013 Aug;28(8):2298–307.
81. Simon C. Introduction: to transfer or not transfer…a mosaic embryo, that is the question. Fertil Steril. 2017 May;107(5):1083–4.
82. PGDIS Newsletter. PGDIS position statement on chromosome mosaicism and preimplantation aneuploidy testing at the blastocyst stage. Chicago: PGDIS Newsletter; 2016.
83. Sachdev NM, Maxwell SM, Besser AG, Grifo JA. Diagnosis and clinical management of embryonic mosaicism diagnosis and clinical management of embryonic mosaicism. Fertil Steril. 2017 Jan;107(1):6–11. https://doi.org/10.1016/j.fertnstert.2016.10.006.

PGT-M for Couples with a Single-Gene Disorder

72

Lawrence C. Layman

72.1 Genetic History

For all patients considering fertility, a detailed family history should be ascertained from the patient and partner (if there is a partner). Ideally, this would be a full pedigree of family members up to three generations from the individual. This entails getting the medical history of parents and sibs (first degree); aunts, uncles, and grandparents (second degree); and first cousins (third degree). This may be best done by a genetic counselor, geneticist, a nurse, or extended provider trained in performing pedigrees. It is important to ascertain the symptoms, specific diagnosis, and age of diagnosis of the disorder. Only knowing there is a history of muscular dystrophy, for example, is not sufficient to perform genetic testing. There are many different types of muscular dystrophy, so it cannot be assumed that Duchenne muscular dystrophy is present—it must be confirmed. Medical records with precise genetic testing results are required if there is to be any genetic testing of embryos. If there is a history of cancer, the age at diagnosis is more important than the age of death with regard to familial cancer, which is more likely under the age of 50 at diagnosis.

Since there are thousands of genetic diseases, it is incredibly unlikely that a clinician can be familiar with all genetic diseases. Consultation with online resources such as OMIM (Online Mendelian Inheritance in Man) will provide a clinical synopsis as well as a detailed description of the disorder and its inheritance, natural history, and involved gene(s) if known. This can be easily consulted while the patient is in the office so that preliminary genetic counseling may be performed. The inheritance of autosomal dominant, autosomal recessive, X-linked dominant, X-linked recessive, or, rarely, mitochondrial disease should be determined prior to considering any type of preconception or prenatal diagnosis (Table 72.1).

Table 72.1 Inheritance patterns of genetic disease

Inheritance	# Affected alleles to cause disease	Risk to embryo	Potential issues
Autosomal recessive	2	25% for carrier parents	Consanguinity
Autosomal dominant	1	50% if parent affected	Penetrance; variable expressivity; anticipation
X-linked recessive	1 (males) 2 (females, but rare)	50% males affected if carrier mother; 50% females carriers if carrier mother	Phenotype in females affected by non-random X-inactivation
X-linked dominant	1	50% risk if parent affected	Penetrance
Mitochondrial	Homoplasmy vs. heteroplasmy	Transmitted via females to all offspring	Phenotype worse if homoplasmy than heteroplasmy

It must be emphasized that expanded carrier screening is not a substitute for taking a family history of genetic disease. Expanded carrier screening tests for genetic diseases that are predominantly autosomal recessive in individuals without a family history of the disease. If there is a family history of a genetic disorder, the particular disease should be diagnosed in the best possible manner—not by a carrier screening method. Excellent overviews of the genetic basis for many human diseases may be found at Genereviews.org.

L. C. Layman (✉)
Section of Reproductive Endocrinology, Infertility, & Genetics, Department of Obstetrics & Gynecology, Department of Neuroscience & Regenerative Medicine, Department of Physiology, Medical College of Georgia, Augusta University, Augusta, GA, USA
e-mail: LALAYMAN@augusta.edu

G. N. Allahbadia et al. (eds.), *Textbook of Assisted Reproduction*, https://doi.org/10.1007/978-981-15-2377-9_72

72.2 Preimplantation Genetic Testing-Mutation (PGT-M)

Preimplantation genetic diagnosis (PGD) has now been renamed preimplantation genetic testing (PGT) [1]. PGT-M refers to diagnosis of monogenic/single-gene defect prior to conception. This is in contrast to PGT-A (aneuploidy), formerly known as preimplantation genetic screening, which is used to test for chromosomal abnormalities. PGT done for structural rearrangements is known as PGT-SR [1]. PGT was initiated to test at-risk embryos for genetic disease, so that a couple's risk of transmission to their offspring could ideally be eliminated. However, when looking at large numbers of cases being done, PGT-A is the most common indication for PGT, rather than PGT-M for single-gene disorders (see below). In this chapter, we will confine our topic to PGT-M of single-gene disorders.

72.3 Methods of PGT-M

72.3.1 Cell Types Used for PGT-M

To perform PGT, one or several cells must be obtained from oocytes or embryos and subjected to DNA analysis. Polar body biopsy of the first and/or second polar bodies may be performed; however, diagnosis is only useful to evaluate the maternal genome [2]. If the female patient is heterozygous for a causative mutation, the findings from the first polar biopsy should either reveal a normal genotype (which would indicate the embryo will carry the mutation) or have the mutation (which should indicate that the embryo will be normal). Biopsy of the second polar biopsy is recommended for confirmation. However, with meiosis I, crossover will occur, and if it affects the gene in question, misdiagnosis may result. For these reasons and the fact that embryos may be reproducibly cultured to day 5 blastocysts, polar body diagnosis has fallen out of favor for PGT-M in most circumstances. PGT-M has been used extensively in the literature to biopsy one cell in cleavage-stage embryos on day 3. In this case 12.5% of the embryo (one of eight cells) has been removed. Currently, the standard is to biopsy blastocyst-stage embryos by penetrating the zona with removal of 3–5 trophectoderm cells.

72.3.2 Clinical Use of PGT-M

Handyside et al. [3] had previously used polymerase chain reaction (PCR) to amplify Y-specific repeated sequence DNA from the long arm of the Y chromosome (Yq) to sex embryos for X-linked diseases to avoid transferring an affected male. Subsequently they described the first case of PGT-M for single-gene diagnosis of cystic fibrosis, an autosomal recessive disorder [4]. Both parents were heterozygous for the common ΔF508 mutation (a 3 bp deletion), now annotated as c.1521_1523delCTT (p.Phe508del). In that publication, the authors used a method called nested PCR to obtain enough DNA for diagnosis (Fig. 72.1). With this method, PCR is performed, and a small aliquot of the PCR product is reamplified by PCR using primers inside (or nested) the first primer pair. This technique allows for enrichment of the desired PCR product for analysis. They obtained a total of 16 blastomeres from 3 different carrier couples; DNA from 12 of 16 (75%) cells were successfully amplified. Two patients had suitable embryos (one noncarrier and one carrier embryo), and two embryos were transferred in both patients. One of them conceived and delivered an unaffected

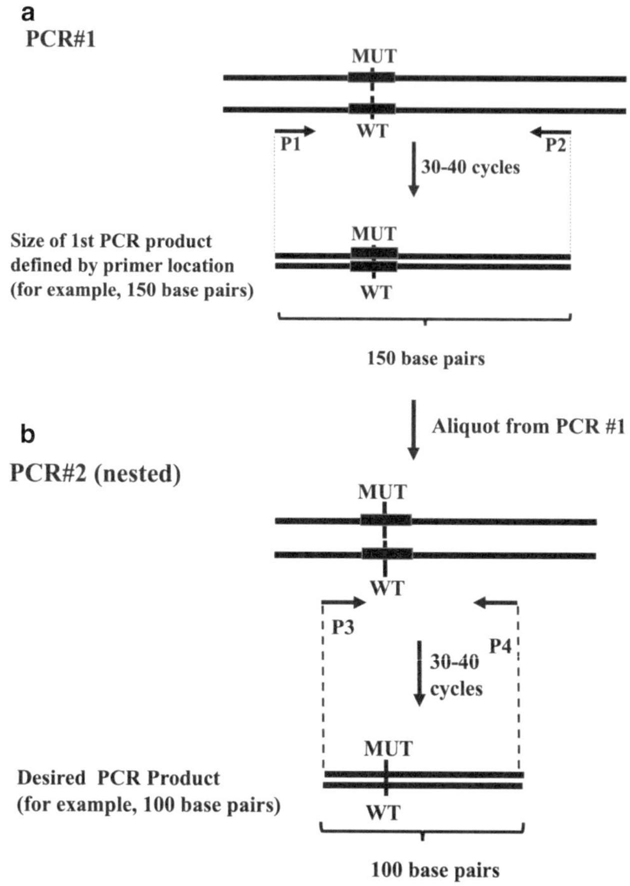

Fig. 72.1 (**a**) Polymerase chain reaction (PCR) consists of multiple cycles of denaturation of the template, followed by primer annealing and extension by the polymerase. (**b**) Nested PCR is a two-step PCR in which an aliquot of the initial PCR is reamplified using primers that are both internal to the original primers such that the resulting product is smaller, but more precise. *MUT* mutant allele, *WT* wild type (normal sequence) allele

Table 72.2 The most common genetic disorders utilized for PGT by the ESHRE PGD Consortium

Genetic disorder	Inheritance	Causative gene(s)	Considerations
Cystic fibrosis	AR	CFTR	Most point mutations; deletions also found
Myotonic dystrophy type 1	AD	*DMPK*	Triplet repeat
Huntington disease	AD	*HTT*	Triplet repeat
Sickle cell anemia/β-thalassemia	AR	*HBB*	Point mutations
Fragile X syndrome	XLD	*FMR1*	Triplet repeat
Spinal muscular atrophy	AR	*SMN1*	Deletions; nearby pseudogene
Sickle cell anemia and human leukocyte antigen	AR	*HBB/HLA* genes	Point mutations
Duchenne muscular dystrophy	XLR	*DMD*	Deletions common; large gene
Neurofibromatosis type 1	AD	*NF1*	Nearby pseudogene
Hemophilia A	XLR	*F8*	Large intronic insertion is common
Human leukocyte antigen (HLA) for acquired diseases	AR	*HLA*	Point mutations
Familial adenomatous polyposis	AD	*APC*	Point mutations and deletions
Charcot-Marie-Tooth disease type 1	AD	*PMP22, MPZ*	Point mutations and deletions
Familial amyloidotic polyneuropathy (amyloidosis, hereditary, transthyretin-related)	AD	*TTR*	Point mutations and deletions; mutations also cause familial amyloid cardiomyopathy
Marfan syndrome	AD	*FBN1*	Point mutations and deletions
Tuberous sclerosis	AD	*TSC1, TSC2*	Point mutations and deletions
Von Hippel-Lindau	AD	*VHL*	Point mutations and deletions

The most commonly tested is listed first, and they are listed in decreasing number utilized by PGT
AR autosomal recessive, *AD* autosomal dominant, *XLD* X-linked dominant, *XLR* X-linked recessive

child, but the other did not. The third patient had only one affected embryo, and one non-amplified cell, so she did not have an embryo transfer. Since this time, PGT-M has now been used for many different Mendelian disorders (Table 72.2). This first case of PGT-M exemplifies both the immense power and the concerning limitations of the PGT technique.

72.3.3 Specific DNA Methods for PGT-M

Although PCR methods have been well established for many years, the small amount of DNA in one or a few cells dramatically complicates the process, as demonstrated above by Handyside et al. [4]. When PCR is done for genetic disease in genomic DNA from adults (as in preconception diagnosis or cancer testing), 50–100 ng of DNA for 30–40 cycles of amplification are typically used. For a single diploid cell, however, there are only ~6 picograms of DNA. Therefore, for PCR, an increased number of cycles (35–60) or nested PCR, as mentioned above, is necessary. Alternatively, fluorescently labeled primers may be used, which will increase the detection of smaller amounts of the PCR product [5].

Since the amount of starting material is so small, a number of techniques have been used to amplify the entire genome. Techniques of whole genome amplification (WGA) are not new, but the procedures have improved. The principle of these techniques is to randomly amplify the entire genome such that there are enough copies of the gene of interest and enough DNA to repeat the analysis. Some are PCR-based, such as primer extension preamplification (PEP) and degenerate oligonucleotide-primed PCR (DOP). A more commonly used technique is multiple displacement amplification (MDA), which does not require PCR. In MDA, DNA is incubated with a Φ29 DNA polymerase at 30 °C and exonuclease-resistant random hexamer primers. The template is copied by a hyperbranching method, in which there is displacement of the completed strand while the polymerase begins to synthesize another one. Fragments up to 70 kb may be copied, and a 10^4–10^6 amplification may be accomplished.

A method termed multiple annealing and looping-based amplification cycles (MALBAC) amplifies DNA that forms loops, so that each strand is only amplified once [6]. In the MALBAC method, primers randomly anneal to the DNA template. The polymerase has displacement activity at higher temperatures and amplifies the template, creating so-called semi-amplicons. When the process is repeated, the semi-amplicons are amplified into full amplicons that contain complementary 3′ and 5′ ends, which then hybridize to form a looped structure. This looped structure is not able to serve as a template anymore, but the semi-amplicons and genomic DNA can be amplified. MALBAC has been reported to decrease amplification bias, require less starting DNA, and provide more in-depth coverage. The interested reader is referred to a review by Huang et al. [6]; each of the methods has its own advantages and disadvantages. The use of these techniques has improved the results obtained by PCR-based PGT-M techniques.

72.3.4 Failed Amplification, Contamination, and Allele Dropout

Failed amplification may complicate PCR with only picogram amounts of DNA template, and it is important to consider that this could happen when you discuss PGT-M with the patient. Contamination is another troublesome problem when amplifying such small amounts of starting material. This is why it is extremely important (as in any PCR) to have a clean working environment and use a negative control, which contains all reagents except DNA (the negative control lane should not have a band on a gel—or a peak on electropherogram). This is one reason intracytoplasmic sperm injection (ICSI) is also done in these circumstances.

Another problem when starting with a small amount of DNA template is allele dropout (ADO), which refers to the tendency for the polymerase in the PCR to only amplify one of the two alleles. To obviate problems of ADO, failed amplification, and contamination, the technique of multiplex PCR may be performed, in which gene-specific primers are included, as well as primers that amplify nearby polymorphisms, which are benign changes in DNA sequence, but will help identify specific alleles. By selecting polymorphisms close to the affected gene, the mutated allele could be selected by linkage analysis [7]. The expected result would be products from both reactions—if one of the two DNA fragments from either allele was missing, ADO would be present. ADO is problematic for autosomal recessive disease to avoid transfer of biallelic mutations, but is particularly difficult in autosomal dominant disease, where you cannot afford to have one affected allele (or the embryo will be affected).

In more recent years, ADO has been addressed by analyzing more useful types of polymorphisms to specifically identify each allele. Initially, this was done by using restriction enzymes that give different fragment sizes of each allele by so-called restriction fragment length polymorphisms (RFLPs), but these are not always commonly located near a specific gene of interest (Fig. 72.2 and Table 72.3). Single tandem repeat (STR) polymorphisms, such as CA repeats, are highly polymorphic and enable a much higher chance to precisely identify the allele from which they come (Fig. 72.3). The use of STRs made the selection of informative polymorphisms much more facile [7].

Since the sequencing of human genome, the locations of millions of single nucleotide polymorphisms (SNPs) are known—it is estimated that all humans possess ~10 million SNPs (Fig. 72.4). Even though SNPs typically have two different alleles, if multiple nearby SNPs could be incorporated into an assay, the specificity of allele identification would be markedly increased. Karyomapping is a technique that utilizes this principle (Fig. 72.5) [7, 8]. Karyomapping utilizes a microarray platform and incorporates ~300,000 SNPs

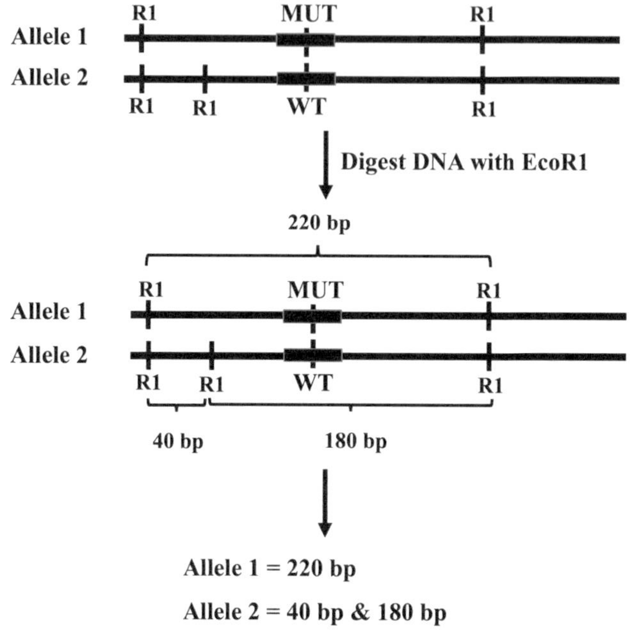

Fig. 72.2 A restriction fragment length polymorphism (RFLP) is shown. As an example, the restriction enzyme EcoRI was used to digest the PCR product. Note that allele 1 has two EcoRI (indicated as R1) cut sites while allele 2 has three EcoRI cut sites. This RFLP is heterozygous and could be used for PGT. *bp* base pairs

Table 72.3 Types of polymorphisms

Type of polymorphism	Description
Restriction fragment length polymorphism (RFLP)	Polymorphism that alters the cut site by a restriction enzyme (examples: HindIII, EcoR1); not used much for PGT because they are less frequent and may have low heterozygosity index
Short tandem repeat (STR)	Repeats of usually 2–5 bases such as CACACA, GAAGAAGAA, etc.; highly polymorphic; higher degree of heterozygosity so more valuable for PGT
Microsatellite	Another name for STR
Single nucleotide polymorphism (SNP)	Biallelic polymorphisms; degree of heterozygosity not as great as for STR, but there are many SNPs across the genome

The heterozygosity index refers to the degree to which the polymorphism is heterozygous (which then makes it useful for PGT). The higher the heterozygosity index, the more useful the polymorphism will be for family studies

spread across the genome. Therefore, for almost any genetic disease, there will be multiple SNPs near the gene of interest [7, 8]. The specific mutation may not need to be tested if there are sufficient SNPs in close proximity to the mutated allele. Karyomapping has several distinct advantages over family-based mutation and STR methods:

1. It does not require specific family-based assay generation—the same array can be used on all patients. This dramatically shortens the time to starting IVF.

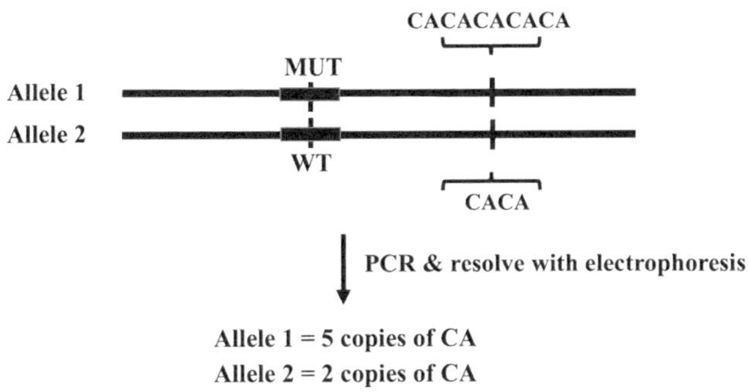

Fig. 72.3 A short tandem repeat (STR), also known as a microsatellite, is shown. Allele 1 has five copies of a CA repeat, while allele 2 has two copies. This STR is heterozygous and could be used for PGT

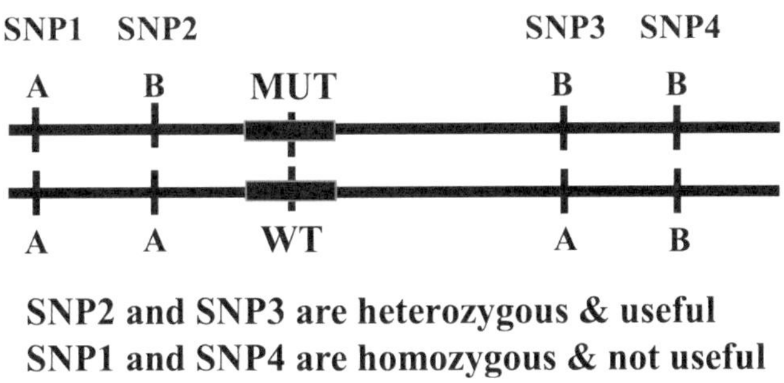

Fig. 72.4 Single nucleotide polymorphisms (SNPs) are shown. Note that of the four SNPs, each of which has an A and B allele (e.g., A could be an "A" and could be a "G"), only two are heterozygous (SNPs 2 and 3)

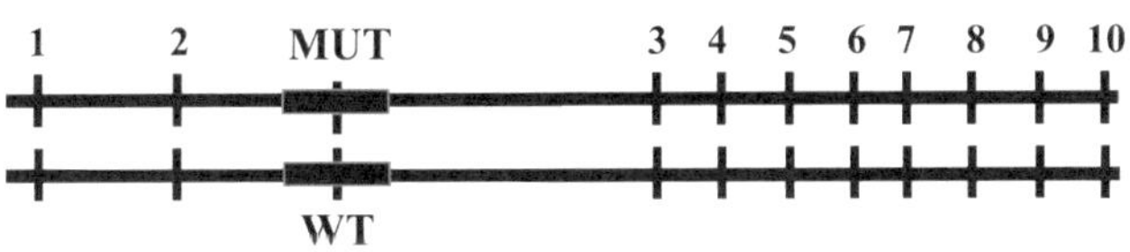

Fig. 72.5 The rationale for karyomapping is shown. Because 300,000 SNPs are present on a microarray, it is likely that there are numerous SNPs near the gene of interest (close usually means within 1,000,000 base pairs—1 megabase). Only one gene with ten different SNPs in close proximity is shown here. In reality, the 300,000 SNPs are spread throughout the genome and likely to reside close to disease-causing genes

2. The high density of SNP markers near causative genes improves diagnostic efficiency.
3. Because of the large number of SNPs, chromosome copy number can also be tested in the same assay.

Currently, PGT-A analysis typically follows PGT-M testing because it is important to avoid a deleterious allele from a Mendelian disease, but it is also prudent to avoid an aneuploid embryo [7, 8]. In fact, live births have been reported using karyomapping. Konstantinidis et al. [9] used karyomapping in 55 PGT-M cases and found that they could get a diagnosis in 99.6% vs. 96.8% of embryos using conventional PCR analysis.

Karyomapping does present some limitations. Both parents and at least one other family member are necessary for karyomapping to be informative. Karyomapping can usually be performed without the need for direct mutation detection, but occasionally this will still be necessary [7]. Next-generation DNA sequencing has also been used for PGT-M, but confirmation by Sanger sequencing is generally advisable because of errors, which, although comprising a small percent of the tested sequence, cannot afford to be missed. To date, the most common use of next-generation sequencing has been for copy number in PGT-A, but tests have been developed for spinal muscular atrophy [10] and Charcot-Marie-Tooth disease Type 1A [11], both of which are usually caused by deletions.

72.4 Testing Results: Misdiagnosis and No Diagnosis

In 2012, the ESHRE PGD Consortium collected and published 10 years of data (1997–2007) involving PGT [12]. Of 27,630 cycles, 61% were for aneuploidy screening (PGT-A), while 17% were for single-gene disorders (PGT-M), 4% for sexing for X-linked disease (relevant to PGT-M), 16% for chromosomal abnormalities, and 2% for social sexing. ICSI was used in 86% so that paternal contamination from excess sperm adherent to the zona pellucida could be excluded. Of interest, 2/3 of couples were also considered to have infertility. Laser drilling was the most common method for zona breaching, and cleavage-stage embryos were most commonly biopsied [12].

A wide variety of genetic disorders have been analyzed by PGT-M, shown in decreasing frequency in Table 72.2. In the ESHRE Consortium, cystic fibrosis was most commonly tested, followed by myotonic dystrophy type 1, Huntington disease, and hemoglobinopathies [12]. Of 4534 cycles for PGT-M, embryo transfer occurred in 3727 (82.2%), and 10/3727 (0.3%) had incorrect diagnoses for single-gene disorders. For 55 embryos, sexed because of X-linked disorders, 2/55 (3.6%) had incorrect diagnosis. The reasons for misdiagnosis include contamination, ADO, technical errors, and unknown etiologies. Clinical pregnancy rates per retrieval (22%) and per transfer (29%) are generally lower than those in recent years, probably owing to improved culture of embryos, blastocyst transfer, experience with the procedure, and PGT-A follow-up on embryos being considered for transfer [12]. Although the error rate is very low, it must be kept in mind that no embryos were available for transfer in ~18% of patients, likely due to degraded DNA, inadequate biopsy, failed amplification, and ADO.

72.4.1 Experience with PGT-M for Specific Mendelian Disorders

We have started with an overview of the methods and types of diseases that can be tested for using PGT-M, but it is important to consider how well PGT-M works for specific genetic diseases. In this section, PGT-M experience for three different genetic diseases—neurofibromatosis type 1 (autosomal dominant), fragile X syndrome (X-linked dominant), and cystic fibrosis (autosomal recessive)—will be examined. As will be seen, the lessons learned from clinical utility should be understood by the clinician ordering these tests.

72.4.2 Autosomal Dominant Disease: Neurofibromatosis Type 1 (NF1)

Much can be learned, particularly on how to counsel patients, by examining the experience of a large PGT laboratory for diagnosis of a specific Mendelian disorder [13]. Between 2004 and 2013, 77 couples had 156 PGT-M cycles for neurofibromatosis 1 (NF1), an autosomal dominant condition with complete penetrance, which has been the sixth most common Mendelian disease to have PGT-M [13]. Affected patients present with multiple benign neurofibromas; mild intellectual deficits/learning disabilities; facial, optic, skeletal, and cardiovascular abnormalities; as well as a predisposition to benign and malignant tumors. NF1 is caused by mutations in the neurofibromin (*NF1*) gene in more than 95% of patients.

Since this study occurred between 2004 and 2013, the predominant cell type analyzed was cleavage-stage biopsy of a single blastomere on day 3 [13]. Prior to 2010, PGT was done by direct PCR on the single cell using nested primers. After 2010, WGA was performed (amounting to just over half of the embryos), and enough PCR product was available so that six different flanking markers of *NF1* could be tested to be sure that recombination did not occur. PCR was then analyzed by capillary electrophoresis to get an individual genotype of each allele, which was then compared to the embryo haplotype. Some of the samples were also tested by PGT-A using a chromosomal microarray for detection of insertion/deletions (indels), also known as copy number variants (CNVs), that were 10 megabases or larger.

Demographic data was collected, including sporadic or familial transmission. NF1 is autosomal dominant, but half of new cases are new mutations, so other family members may not yet be affected (of course, the affected individual has a 50% chance of passing on to her/his offspring). Of the presenting couples, 3 of 81 (3.7%) were not able to be tested because molecular probes could not be generated, and one couple underwent IVF, but no embryos sufficient for biopsy were obtained [13]. Of 156 cycles, 1356 embryos were biopsied, and of these, 1322/1356 (97%) were able to be analyzed. However, a clear molecular diagnosis was obtained in 1060/1322 (80%) of embryos. Of the 20% that resulted in the inability to get a diagnosis, more than half had insufficient molecular data and about 40% had inconclusive results. As expected, close to half (46%) of embryos were unaffected and could be transferred. Approximately 87% of the 156 cycles produced at least one unaffected embryo (median 3). Definitive diagnoses were more likely when there was known NF1 inheritance (84%) vs. sporadic (76%) and when the center had multiple NF1 referrals. Interestingly, the success of getting a molecular diagnosis was not associated with embryo quality, academic affiliation of the medical center, or use of WGA. Overall, 27% of couples having at least one IVF/PGT-M cycle conceived and had an unaffected live birth, and the chance of pregnancy correlated with the number of unaffected embryos available.

Approximately 5% of couples with NF1 who wanted to undergo PGT-M could not do so. Molecular probes could not be designed for three couples (3.7%), most likely because of the inability to differentiate the *NF1* gene from an *NF1* pseudogene. To fully discriminate these alleles, sufficient family members must be available. Overall, about 80% of embryos were able to receive a diagnosis. This is slightly less than that for myotonic dystrophy type 1 (86.6%) and Huntington disease (87.8%) from the ESHRE Consortium [12]. Interestingly, these latter two disorders are triplet repeat diseases, which also have their own special considerations.

72.4.3 X-Linked Dominant Disease: Fragile X Syndrome

Fragile X syndrome is the most common single-gene cause of intellectual disability in humans. It is an X-linked dominant condition with reduced penetrance that presents in males with varying degrees of moderate to severe intellectual disability, hyperactivity, autism, facial abnormalities, large ears, skeletal abnormalities, cardiac valve anomalies, and macroorchidism. About half of affected females have mild intellectual disability or learning disability. More than 98% of affected males and females possess >200 copies of a CGG triplet repeat in the 5′-untranslated region of the *FMR1* gene on Xq27.3, which is termed a full mutation. Carrier females, and some males, may have 55–200 repeats, which is known as a premutation [14]. Women with the premutation are at increased risk for premature ovarian insufficiency (10–15%) by age 40, and both male and female premutation carriers are at risk for tremor/ataxia later in life. Expansion of the premutation may occur in mitosis in the embryo of a carrier female to a full mutation, and this risk of expansion and subsequent intellectual disability in males increases with the size of the triplet repeat.

PGT-M for fragile X syndrome poses some specific issues that must be considered. The triplet CGG repeat has very high GC content and is difficult to amplify by PCR, particularly in single cells. The first PGT-M for fragile X syndrome was performed in 1995 and was based exclusively on detection of nonexpanded maternal and paternal *FMR1* alleles [15]. Although not commonly known by clinicians, this method can only be offered to informative couples (meaning you can distinguish both maternal alleles and the one paternal allele). For example, if the carrier mother has 28 and 78 repeats and father has 39 repeats, the assay is informative since all three repeat sizes are different. However, if the father had the same number of repeats as the mother (28 repeats, in this example), this assay would not be able to be used for diagnosis. Perhaps somewhat surprisingly, only about 63% of all couples will have informative *FMR1* alleles [13]. As with all other diseases using small amounts of starting DNA, ADO can occur.

In 2001, the first indirect test for fragile X syndrome was reported, and the authors suggested they could offer PGT to ~90% of interested couples. An indirect test does not measure the number of CGG repeats, and if there are not informative markers and/or ADO, misdiagnosis may occur. Therefore, the best approach is to include both direct and indirect tests. Some investigators utilized MDA to amplify the genome, followed by a combination of direct and nearby (linked) STR markers. There were improvements in that successful amplification increased from 41% to 66% of cases, but there was still a high rate of no amplification [16]. When tested clinically, they reported one live-born, unaffected child [16] Other investigators also utilized MDA and analyzed the products by a combination of fluorescent PCR of the *FMR1* CGG repeats, *AMELY* (amelogenin) to identify Y sequences, and two polymorphic markers [17]. In preclinical tests, successful amplification rates of the CGG repeat and the polymorphisms DXS1215 and FRAXAC1 were 84.2%, 87.5%, and 75.0%, respectively. ADO rates, however, were still high and ranged from 31.3% for the direct test to 57.1% and 50.0% for both markers [17]. In 2 PGT cycles, they were able to successfully diagnose 20 of 30 embryos as normal (n = 10), affected (n = 4), and premutation carriers (n = 6). Although three unaffected embryos were transferred, the patients did not conceive [17]. Despite improvements, these studies demonstrate the difficulty in getting a diagnosis on every patient who comes in for PGT-M for fragile X syndrome.

More recently, others have reported methods to increase the amplification rate of both alleles and the diagnostic detection rate. Kieffer et al. [14] had traditionally used a direct test and amplification of *SRY* on the short arm of Y (Yp), but they have now reported an indirect multiplex test using four STR (microsatellite) markers combined with a Y chromosome marker. They performed this test alone or in combination with the direct test. Unfortunately, even using five polymorphic markers, just over one third of couples were not informative for CGG repeats.

These investigators sought to improve the detection rate of both indirect and direct tests. They identified five new markers that exhibited 69% to 81% heterozygosity. In their new indirect test, they tested the 5 markers along with one of the previous ones and *AMELY* in a multiplex single-round PCR test of 55 cycles. Their definition of a "direct test" was expanded to include four new markers and *AMELY* sequences in addition to testing the CGG repeats in a multiplex PCR.

They tested both the direct and indirect tests in single-cell analyses using lymphoblasts from 3 control male cell lines, 2 control female cell lines, and 1 female with 23 and 70 repeats (premutation). They obtained a PCR signal in 94% for the new indirect and 90% for the new direct test. Successful amplification exceeded 80% for each marker. The mean rate of non-informativeness was markedly reduced—26% for the new indirect and 23% for the new direct test. In combining the indirect and direct tests, 63% and 64% of cells, respectively, tested had a complete genotype for all cells tested. They were able to obtain a conclusive genotype (not with every marker, but enough to be informative) in 100% of both tests. These new tests have only preliminary use in PGT cycles, but their adopted strategy allows the potential for 96% of couples to be diagnosed.

72.4.4 Autosomal Recessive Disease: Cystic Fibrosis

Cystic fibrosis is the most common indication for genetic testing using PGT-M [18]. Cystic fibrosis is an autosomal recessive condition affecting ~1/4000 individuals of European descent. Mutations in the causative gene, cystic fibrosis transmembrane conductance regulator (*CFTR*), lead to absent or decreased chloride and bicarbonate transport across the apical membranes of secretory epithelial cells, which results in thickened secretions in the lung, pancreatic and biliary ducts, GI tract, and vas deferens. Patients with CF typically present with failure to thrive and develop progressive pulmonary disease, pancreatic insufficiency, and gastrointestinal and nutritional defects. Males may have bilateral congenital absence of the vas deferens. A clinical test of an increased sweat chloride suggests diagnosis, which is confirmed with mutations in the *CFTR* gene.

A publication from the European Society of Human Genetics (ESHG) in 2016 provides international guidelines for PGT-M for CF. Since it is an autosomal recessive disease, both parents will be carriers, and their genotype and informative genetic markers should be known prior to testing. There is not a universally accepted method, but the combination of direct and indirect tests is advised. Current recommendations advocate that at least two fully informative markers within 1 megabase (Mb) on both sides of the gene and intragenic markers should be included when they are available. Recombination within the *CFTR* gene is rarely described, so it is acceptable to perform PGT-M by an indirect method using intragenic STRs located on the same side of the variant if other markers are inconclusive or noninformative. If MDA is used, ESHG suggests using two markers on each side of the gene because of high ADO rates. Customized protocols should be validated.

72.5 Summary

As can be seen from the examples of fragile X syndrome (X-linked dominant), neurofibromatosis type 1 (autosomal dominant), and cystic fibrosis (autosomal recessive), some similar themes emerge. Comprehensive counseling should be performed when first discussing expectations with prospective PGT-M couples. Important topics to stress include:

1. Knowing the phenotype/genotype of the disorder.
2. Understanding the frequency of gene mutations in the disorder (in NF1, e.g., 95% of cases have a mutation in the *NF1* gene [not 100%]; therefore, it may not be useful to do PGT-M in 5% of people right at the outset).
3. Even when the gene is known, molecular diagnosis is not always possible prior to the start of the cycle.
4. Not all embryos will be acceptable to biopsy.
5. No DNA will be obtained on some embryos.
6. Specific diagnosis may not be possible for all available embryos.
7. Some patients may have no embryos to transfer.

Clinicians should be aware regarding the methodology used for PGT-M so they can adequately counsel or have a geneticist/genetic counselor available. Fortunately, misdiagnosis rates are very small, and with the advent of blastocyst biopsy, more cells will be available and hopefully improved methods and informative genotypes will be accomplished. Lastly, it is important, as evidenced by these three genetic diseases illustrated here (fragile X syndrome, NF1, and CF), to analyze disease-specific testing of reproductive outcomes.

References

1. Zegers-Hochschild F, Adamson GD, Dyer S, et al. The international glossary on infertility and fertility care, 2017. Hum Reprod. 2017;32:1786–801.
2. Cimadomo D, Capalbo A, Ubaldi FM, et al. The impact of biopsy on human embryo developmental potential during preimplantation genetic diagnosis. Biomed Res Int. 2016;2016:7193075.
3. Handyside AH, Kontogianni EH, Hardy K, Winston RM. Pregnancies from biopsied human preimplantation embryos sexed by Y-specific DNA amplification. Nature. 1990;344:768–70.
4. Handyside AH, Lesko JG, Tarin JJ, Winston RM, Hughes MR. Birth of a normal girl after in vitro fertilization and preimplantation diagnostic testing for cystic fibrosis. N Engl J Med. 1992;327:905–9.
5. Braude P, Pickering S, Flinter F, Ogilvie CM. Preimplantation genetic diagnosis. Nat Rev Genet. 2002;3:941–53.
6. Huang L, Ma F, Chapman A, Lu S, Xie XS. Single-cell whole-genome amplification and sequencing: methodology and applications. Annu Rev Genomics Hum Genet. 2015;16:79–102.
7. Handyside AH. Live births following karyomapping - a "key" milestone in the development of preimplantation genetic diagnosis. Reprod Biomed Online. 2015;31:307–8.
8. Thornhill AR, Handyside AH, Ottolini C, et al. Karyomapping-a comprehensive means of simultaneous monogenic and cytogenetic PGD: comparison with standard approaches in real time for Marfan syndrome. J Assist Reprod Genet. 2015;32:347–56.
9. Konstantinidis M, Prates R, Goodall NN, et al. Live births following Karyomapping of human blastocysts: experience from clinical application of the method. Reprod Biomed Online. 2015;31:394–403.
10. Ren Y, Zhi X, Zhu X, et al. Clinical applications of MARSALA for preimplantation genetic diagnosis of spinal muscular atrophy. J Genet Genomics. 2016;43:541–7.
11. Gui B, Yang P, Yao Z, et al. A new next-generation sequencing-based assay for concurrent preimplantation genetic diagnosis of Charcot-Marie-Tooth disease type 1A and aneuploidy screening. J Genet Genomics. 2016;43:155–9.
12. Harper JC, Wilton L, Traeger-Synodinos J, et al. The ESHRE PGD consortium: 10 years of data collection. Hum Reprod Update. 2012;18:234–47.
13. Merker VL, Murphy TP, Hughes JB, et al. Outcomes of preimplantation genetic diagnosis in neurofibromatosis type 1. Fertil Steril. 2015;103:761–8.
14. Kieffer E, Nicod JC, Gardes N, et al. Improving preimplantation genetic diagnosis for Fragile X syndrome: two new powerful single-round multiplex indirect and direct tests. Eur J Hum Genet. 2016;24:221–7.
15. Apessos A, Abou-Sleiman PM, Harper JC, Delhanty JD. Preimplantation genetic diagnosis of the fragile X syndrome by use of linked polymorphic markers. Prenat Diagn. 2001;21:504–11.
16. Burlet P, Frydman N, Gigarel N, et al. Multiple displacement amplification improves PGD for fragile X syndrome. Mol Hum Reprod. 2006;12:647–52.
17. Lee HS, Kim MJ, Lim CK, Cho JW, Song IO, Kang IS. Multiple displacement amplification for preimplantation genetic diagnosis of fragile X syndrome. Genet Mol Res. 2011;10:2851–9.
18. Girardet A, Viart V, Plaza S, et al. The improvement of the best practice guidelines for preimplantation genetic diagnosis of cystic fibrosis: toward an international consensus. Eur J Hum Genet. 2016;24:469–78.

Preimplantation Genetic Testing for Aneuploidies (PGT-A) in Recurrent Miscarriage

73

A. Vaiarelli, D. Cimadomo, L. Rienzi, and F. M. Ubaldi

73.1 Introduction

Human reproduction is a very inefficient process. The possibility of conceiving per menstrual cycle is as low as 20% [1]. Furthermore, early pregnancy loss, also referred to as miscarriage or spontaneous abortion, is defined as the loss of a clinical pregnancy before 20 weeks of gestation or, if the gestational age is unknown, the loss of an embryo/fetus of <400 g [2].

Recurrent miscarriage (RM) is an important issue in the field of reproductive medicine. It has been estimated it affects 2–5% of the women attempting to conceive, and about 1% of women may go through three or more miscarriages in their reproductive lifespan [1]. The definition of RM has long been debated and is different among the international societies. According to the European Society for Human Reproduction and Embryology (ESHRE) [3, 4], RM is defined as three consecutive pregnancy losses, including the non-visualized ones. On the contrary, the American Society for Reproductive Medicine (ASRM) defined RM as two or more clinical pregnancy losses documented by ultrasonography or histopathologic evaluation, but not necessarily consecutive [5]. This difference in its definition affects also how its incidence and prevalence are calculated across different countries; indeed an international consensus is eagerly needed. The international societies are instead concordant that biochemical pregnancy losses, defined as a positive pregnancy test not associated with the establishment of a pregnancy [6], should not be considered proper miscarriages.

From a clinical perspective, few cases of RM derive from a single pathogenic cause; most of them may in fact have a multifactorial background which involves the interaction of multiple genetic and environmental parameters. Therefore, the outcome for the couples with RM is not determined by a single factor, and it should be carefully tailored upon each couple's specific characteristics and clinical history.

The aim of this chapter is to summarize the current knowledge upon the causes of RM and discuss the role of preimplantation genetic testing for aneuploidies (PGT-A) and/or for structural rearrangements (PGT-SR) in patients with such indication.

73.2 Overview of the Main Factors Related to Recurrent Miscarriage

Each couple with RM has a different prognosis largely dependent upon their individual clinical history, a thorough diagnostic workup, and maternal age. Especially the latter is one of the most important elements to predict the reproductive potential of a woman [7]. Indeed, if the fertility rate decreases as the woman ages, the miscarriage rate follows an opposite trend. To this regard, Nybo Anderson and colleagues showed that the risk of miscarriage increases from 8.9% when a woman is aged 20–24 to 74.7% by the age of 44. They set 35 years as the age threshold beyond which this increase becomes more evident. Furthermore, this study also reported that the experience of a miscarriage is prognostic upon further pregnancy losses in following attempts to conceive. For instance, up to 35% and 45% of the parous and nulliparous women who have already experienced three spontaneous abortions may, respectively, undergo a further miscarriage [8].

A thorough investigation of the incidence of karyotypic imbalances in miscarriages highlights that some embryos affected by trisomies for few autosomes or sex chromosome aneuploidies may develop up to this stage of prenatal development, and collectively they account for 60–70% of the first trimester losses in humans [9, 10] (see the specific paragraph treating this topic hereafter). Nevertheless, additional factors can be associated with an increased risk for RM, such as uterine anomalies, antiphospholipid syndrome, and hormonal and metabolic disorders. Moreover, several other

A. Vaiarelli · D. Cimadomo · L. Rienzi · F. M. Ubaldi (✉)
GENERA, Center for Reproductive Medicine, Valle Giulia Clinic, Rome, Italy

G. N. Allahbadia et al. (eds.), *Textbook of Assisted Reproduction*, https://doi.org/10.1007/978-981-15-2377-9_73

etiologies, as chronic endometritis, inherited thrombophilia, luteal phase deficiency, and high sperm DNA fragmentation, have been proposed as possible causes of RM, but are still to be considered controversial [1].

In the next paragraph, we will go through the proposed strategies for a diagnostic workup in patients that experienced RM.

73.3 Proposed Workup for Patients That Experienced Repeated Miscarriage

Preconception counseling is pivotal for patients with a history of RM, who may be more concerned and require more reassurance for the future attempts. Several investigations, ranging from genetic testing to lifestyle modifications and medication, could have a positive effect on the chances of obtaining a healthy baby. A universally valid workup has not been defined yet, even because any couple has its own medical history, and tailored investigations should be conducted by considering several clinical parameters.

At first, an accurate anamnesis should be conducted for both partners aiming at defining their modifiable lifestyle habits (smoking, abuse of alcohol, diet, etc.) and their family history of infertility and miscarriage [11].

Secondly, a specific blood workup is required to examine possible factors that can affect the prognosis of the couples and the possibility for the woman to carry a pregnancy to term [1]. They may include:

(a) Prolactin (PRL) [12].
(b) Thyroid-stimulating hormone (TSH) serum levels and, in case of abnormal levels, also thyroid autoantibodies testing [13].
(c) Antiphospholipid antibody syndrome could also be investigated by testing anticardiolipin antibodies, anti-β II glycoprotein I antibodies, and lupus anticoagulant [14].
(d) Factor V Leiden, prothrombin gene mutation, protein C and protein S deficiency, antithrombin III deficiency, and hyper-homocysteine, since thrombophilia is one of the causes associated with RM [15].

Nonetheless, for what concerns, for instance, the association of the latter with RM, a meta-analysis of 9 studies including overall 1228 women with an experience of at least two previous miscarriages failed to show any positive impact of anticoagulation treatment (aspirin and low-molecular-weight heparin, or the combination of both) upon a further attempt to conceive [16]. Indeed, this is an example that more consistent data from multicenter studies are yet required to solve the current controversies upon this topic.

Thirdly, a transvaginal three-dimensional ultrasound, sonohysterography, and hysteroscopy should be performed to evaluate the uterine cavity, and pelvic magnetic resonance imaging can also be useful in complex cases of anatomic defects. In fact, uterine anomalies have been reported in up to 20% of women that experienced RM [1, 17].

Besides all the anatomic, endocrine, and immunologic evaluations we may conduct, for about half of the women affected from RM, its causes go undetected, and the main answers up to date could be generally found in the genetics [5, 11].

73.4 The Genetic Cause of Miscarriage

There is a clear association between maternal age and the incidence of aneuploidies in the embryos produced [7, 18, 19]. However, more than 90% of the chromosomally abnormal embryos, even if they may develop as fully expanded good-quality blastocysts or follow a standard morphodynamic development in vitro [20, 21], either do not implant or are spontaneously aborted. Whole chromosome copy number variations, such as trisomy, polyploidy, or sex chromosome aneuploidies (e.g., 45, X karyotype), are mostly observed in spontaneous abortions. Specifically, almost half of the products of conception after a miscarriage may carry chromosomal abnormalities, a rate that varies depending on woman age and may rise up to 70% [7, 22, 23]. This is mainly due to the meiotic impairment of oogenesis, which is a clear consequence of aging, and may follow different paths, such as meiosis I or meiosis II non-disjunction, premature separation of sister chromatids, or the recently described reverse segregation [24–26]. Oogenesis is indeed a long path: the ovarian reserve is established at birth and depleted from menarche to menopause, the oocytes arrest in the late prophase of meiosis I for decades, and, once recruited, they undergo an asymmetrical division and a fast meiosis II post-fertilization. Conversely, spermatogenesis begins with puberty, proceeds uninterrupted, and leads to symmetrical divisions. It has been in fact estimated that only a minority (1–2%) of the spermatozoa carry chromosomal impairments [9, 18], probably also caused by gender-specific differences in the meiotic silencing checkpoint. Essentially, this mechanism seems to be more stringent during sperm than during oocyte maturation processes, thus leading to the arrest of sperms that do not show a perfect matching of the chromosomes [27].

Another important genetic cause of miscarriage is structural chromosomal abnormalities. The most frequent are balanced reciprocal translocations that have an incidence in prenatal diagnosis of 1/560 fetuses and balanced Robertsonian translocations and inversions with an incidence of 1/1100–

1200 fetuses. The incidence of unbalanced structural abnormalities is instead even lower [28, 29]. These chromosomal imbalances are independent from maternal age and may equally affect both the partners. In this regard, a history of RM in young women advocates an increased risk of structural chromosome abnormality in one of the components of the couple [29]. Indeed, the incidence of balanced structural chromosome abnormalities is 0.7% in the general population, but it increases to 2.2% after one miscarriage, 4.8% after two miscarriages, and up to 5.2% after three miscarriages [30]. Yet, RM is more frequent when the abnormality is present in the maternal karyotype rather than in paternal one, and again this is probably caused by the differences in the stringency of the meiotic silencing checkpoint [27]. Possibly, as suggested in cytogenetic studies of gametes from patients with balanced structural chromosome abnormalities, such impairments in males more commonly result in a lower fertility, rather than in the production of chromosomally imbalanced sperms [31].

Segmental (or partial) aneuploidies, either copy number variations (CNVs) or microdeletions and microduplications (MMs), are another class of chromosomal imbalances apparently not related to maternal age or gender in general that may be responsible for RM [32, 33]. However, only in <1% they are inherited [34]; it is most probable for them to occur because of a de novo mutation, equally probable during either oogenesis and spermatogenesis or post-fertilization mitotic events. Their estimated prevalence in the newborn population ranges between 0.5 and 2/10000 [35, 36]. Even if their incidence is largely lower than whole chromosome aneuploidies, they may have an equally dramatic impact on reproduction if the copy number state of putative dosage sensitive genes is altered. Notably though, many segmental aneuploidies do not have a clear pathogenic definition and should be considered variants of unknown significance, whose incidence in miscarriages is 2–3%, different from the pathogenic ones which may reach up to 5% and 0.5% in spontaneous abortions and newborns, respectively [37].

Other chromosomal causes of miscarriage may be embryonic mosaicism (as we will discuss later in this chapter), ploidy impairments, or uniparental disomy. For all of them, the incidence in miscarriage is never higher than 2% [33, 38, 39]. However, they cannot be predicted or accurately diagnosed because of either biological or technical issues (or both), and there is no risk factor related to parental characteristics to predict them.

Future molecular studies on the patients who experienced RM and/or on the products of conception themselves may provide a more thorough view of the mechanisms underlying the occurrence of miscarriage and possibly novel strategies for prevention and/or treatment.

73.5 What Can We Do for Woman with RM?

Historically, chromosome analysis has been suggested for couples with RM. However, some controversy still exists upon its prognostic value. Those in favor of a routine karyotyping suggest that it should be included as part of the counseling provided to couples with RM, while the opponents claim that even in the presence of RM, only a selected population of patients may benefit from it [29]. Specifically, parental karyotyping is suggested especially in case of young women that underwent more than two pregnancy losses.

In general, though, no strategies are available to counteract the age-related increase of aneuploidies or the establishment of a pregnancy characterized by a partial or structural chromosomal abnormality. In this regard, diagnostic programs either in the preimplantation period on the embryos produced during IVF treatments or in the prenatal period (prenatal diagnosis, PND) were introduced to limit the occurrence of aneuploid pregnancies, especially for older women or with specific indications [40]. Currently, the only available options to minimize this risk are (i) fertility preservation in young women by oocyte vitrification; (ii) egg or sperm donation, where allowed by the local regulation; or (iii) PGT-A and/or PGT-SR at the blastocyst stage during IVF cycles.

PGT is a diagnostic approach aimed at identifying chromosomally normal blastocysts within a cohort of embryo produced during ART. This embryo selection strategy prevents aneuploid blastocysts from being transferred, thus reducing both the risk for implantation failure per transfer and miscarriage due to chromosomal impairments [41–43].

At first, PGT (which was previously wrongly referred to as preimplantation genetic screening, PGS) did not show any clinical value in its first version [44], which was designed as a largely ineffective, if not detrimental [45, 46], strategy based on the 9 chromosome-FISH analysis of a single blastomere retrieved from cleavage stage embryos. Conversely, now it is conducted through 24-chromosome testing techniques, namely, array comparative genome hybridization (aCGH), single nucleotide polymorphisms array (SNP-array), quantitative polymerase chain reaction (qPCR), or next-generation sequencing (NGS), on trophectoderm biopsies at the blastocyst stage, a strategy that (i) ensures reliable information; (ii) does not impact embryo reproductive potential [45, 46]; (iii) is cost-effective since the analysis is conducted only on developmentally competent embryos that developed as blastocysts; (iv) guarantees high positive and negative clinical predictive values, which are ≥50% independently from maternal age and ≥ 96%, respectively [47]; and (v) provides a more efficient IVF treatment in terms of higher implantation and lower miscarriage rates according to all the randomized controlled trials (RCTs) conducted up to now and reviewed in two recent meta-analyses [41, 42].

Nevertheless, first class data from RCTs about its efficacy on a per intention-to-treat basis, as well as an analysis of its cost-effectiveness, are still required [43]. Only one study to date showed a comparable efficacy, but lower multiple pregnancy and miscarriage rates when a euploid single blastocyst transfer policy was introduced in a single large IVF center with respect to the previous untested double embryo transfer policy, but it is limited from its retrospective and observational design [48].

At present, PGT could be considered a valid option for couples with RM to select euploid blastocysts with the highest possible developmental potential and the lowest possible risk of miscarriage. Furthermore, it allows to confidently adopt a single embryo transfer policy, thus inherently reducing the risk for multiple pregnancies and relatively negative obstetrical and perinatal outcomes [49, 50].

73.6 The Criticisms Underneath Preimplantation Genetic Testing Technology

In a recent paper, Murugappan and colleagues compared the pregnancy outcomes after IVF-PGT versus the expected management in patients with RM [51]. They claimed that the former provides similar outcomes in terms of pregnancy, live birth, and clinical miscarriage rates per intent to treat as the latter. This paper had a great impact in the scientific community, especially since it was highlighted by the editor in chief of the journal as an evidence that PGT should not be considered a valid clinical option for the treatment of RM. However, Rienzi et al. [52], besides appreciating the effort invested in performing this study due to the absence of clear evidences and an international consensus upon this issue, pointed out some methodological criticisms in its design that unequivocally undermine its reliability. Firstly, no randomization was performed, and there was a significant difference of 2 years in the maternal age between the IVF-PGT (37.1 ± 4.1) and the expected management (35.7 ± 3.9) groups; and secondly, in 20% ($n = 40/198$) of the IVF cycles, no aneuploidy testing was actually conducted because of poor blastocyst yield and/or embryo morphological quality. As expected, these standard IVF cycles resulted in 50% miscarriage rate versus 14% in the PGT group ($p = 0.003$). In other terms, the paper by Murugappan and colleagues does not represent high-quality data not using PGT in RM patients. On the contrary, it implicitly stresses the evidence that morphological criteria are very poor predictors of embryo chromosomal architecture and viability. Indeed, if few or only poor-quality blastocysts are produced during an IVF cycle, this should not be a reason to cancel aneuploidy testing, thereby exposing the patients to the consequences of an aneuploid embryo transfer. PGT is not a tool to assess embryo quality; it rather is a diagnostic test to exclude reproductively incompetent embryos from the cohort, namely, the embryos that may generate implantation failures or miscarriages.

There is also a concern about clinically recognizable false-negative errors in PGT, in other terms the risk that an aneuploid blastocyst is diagnosed as euploid and results in a miscarriage or chromosomally abnormal pregnancy. To date, two papers have been published that showed these data with two different molecular techniques: Werner et al. reported it to be as low as 0.32% per clinical pregnancy and 0.13% per ongoing pregnancy by qPCR-based trophectoderm analysis [53], while Tiegs et al. reported it to be 1.5% per clinical pregnancy and a 0.7% per ongoing pregnancy by array-CGH [54].

False-positive results are instead an issue that may result in a different consequence, namely, euploid blastocysts diagnosed as aneuploid and thereby prevented from being transferred. Only Scott and colleagues to date could provide some tremendously valuable data about the negative predictive value of PGT. In a non-selection prospective study conducted by SNP-array, where a trophectoderm biopsy was retrieved and analyzed only after embryo transfer and in a blinded fashion with respect to the clinical outcome, they reported that 4% of the embryos that would have been identified as aneuploid were instead implanted [47]. Later, the same group presented a study to the ASRM annual meeting in 2015 (Werner et al., 2015, ASRM national meeting), where the same design was applied, but a targeted-NGS molecular analysis was conducted. None of the 41 blastocysts that would have been diagnosed aneuploid were then implanted in this interim analysis.

Another important current hot topic in the international scientific and clinical community, which is closely related to the risk for both false-positive and false-negative results, is the issue of chromosomal mosaicism. It is defined as the presence of cell lines with different karyotypes within the same embryo, which may arise because of a mitotic missegregation that occurred post-fertilization. The earlier the error occurs along preimplantation development, the higher the extent of mosaicism. Importantly, aneuploid mosaicism (the presence of cells with different aneuploid chromosomal constitution) does not represent a problem for the diagnosis; only a euploid/aneuploid constitution does. From a biological perspective, an unavoidable sampling bias limits the possibility to identify and properly diagnose mosaic embryos; from a technical perspective, the current comprehensive chromosome testing molecular techniques may suggest the presence of mosaicism through an intermediate log2 ratio for a given chromosome, yet it is not possible to resolve a genuine biological variability from a possible amplification bias

[55, 56]. The most probable prevalence of mosaicism in human blastocysts, collectively reported by basic research studies that analyzed disaggregated blastocysts (inner cell mass and 2–3 fragments of trophectoderm) donated for research, is 5% [56]. Its impact in clinical pregnancies achieved from infertile women, reported on thousands of specimens in PND by Huang and colleagues, never exceeds 1.4% after either spontaneous or IVF-derived conceptions, where real mosaicism (not only confined to the placenta) accounts for about 0.5% [38]. Recently, Greco and colleagues in a paper published in the *New England Journal of Medicine* reported the clinical outcomes after the transfer of 18 allegedly mosaic euploid/aneuploid embryos according to an aCGH-based diagnosis in couples with no other transferable embryo produced during a PGT cycle [57]. They resulted in six full-term pregnancies of chromosomally normal children. This paper, especially with the implementation of novel more sensible NGS-based techniques, introduced the yet controversial transfer of allegedly mosaic embryos in the clinical practice. Clearly, a thorough counseling, which must acknowledge the biological and technical limitations of this controversial practice, should be provided to the couple.

The starting amount of DNA which is retrieved from a biopsy is not sufficient itself to conduct the downstream molecular analyses; therefore, preamplification protocols are required for PGT. Mainly whole genome amplification (WGA) or targeted amplifications strategies may be applied. The former elicits a random amplification of 40–60% of the genome, while the latter allows the sole amplification of predetermined sequences on each chromosome. In a paper published in the *European Journal of Human Genetics*, Capalbo and colleagues blindly compared WGA-based aCGH and targeted qPCR on two different trophectoderm biopsies obtained from aneuploid blastocysts and, in case of discordant results, analyzed a third biopsy by WGA-based SNP-array [58]. They reported 99.9% of concordance between the methods on a per chromosome analysis. However, if a discordant diagnosis was returned, aCGH was reported as significantly more prone to false-positive errors with respect to qPCR (7% versus 0.5%; $p < 0.01$). This is ascribable to WGA itself and to the amplification bias that may derive from it, thereby impacting the reliability of the diagnosis. Similarly, the doubt that part of the blastocysts diagnosed as "mosaic" with WGA-based methods could actually be the result of technical errors persists. There is therefore the need for a more thorough validation of the techniques used to this end, by studying multiple biopsies of the same allegedly mosaic blastocyst with different molecular approaches (preferably one of the two should be a targeted approach), before this practice could be adopted in PGT cycles.

Nevertheless, targeted approaches are limited to the diagnosis of only full chromosome aneuploidies and admit a 0.5% risk for clinically significant segmental aneuploidies to term. However, this limitation, for what concerns de novo CNVs and MMs, is shared with WGA-based technologies, which cover just a portion of the genome (40–60%) [59] and may be biased [58] by the preamplification protocol itself. On top of that, a repository database of CNVs/MMs and their consequences on preimplantation embryo development is still missing. It is therefore complex to provide a clinical interpretation of the reproductive impact of any given segmental aneuploidy detected in the preimplantation period.

73.7 Future Perspectives

Even if PGT-A is an efficient diagnostic tool, it cannot change the embryo intrinsic implantation potential or improve its reproductive competence. The scientific community is therefore investing big efforts to this end.

Firstly, by unveiling any other factor, besides female aging, which may cause aneuploidies [60], some guidelines may be provided to the community to reduce the prevalence of miscarriages and try to broaden woman reproductive lifespan. Moreover, cellular processes involved in chromosome missegregation may be targeted to prevent (or find a solution to) their occurrence. For instance, Wu et al. are investigating the effects of salubrinal in obese mice, as a tool to counteract the diet-derived metabolic stress in the endoplasmic reticulum and reestablish the oocyte maturation potential both in vivo and in vitro [61].

Secondly, by comprehensively characterizing the meiotic machinery and all its different components, we may identify putative key gene/protein targets, whose functionality must be preserved to prevent defective chromosome segregation (e.g., DNA damage response genes (for instance, [62, 63])).

Thirdly, chromosome therapy is a fascinating future perspective to perform functional correction on living cells. Up to now, two protocols have been set up in human/animal cell models: the *XIST (X-inactive specific transcript)*-driven heterochromatization of chromosome 21 [64] and the *ZSCAN4 (zinc finger and SCAN domain containing 4)* mRNA-mediated correction of trisomy 18 and 21 [65].

Lastly, several functional and molecular studies in both the academic and clinical fields are ongoing to characterize also the endometrial cells and their receptive potential [66–70]. These studies may bring about novel evidences to increase our knowledge of this topic and possibly introduce novel tools to treat this condition.

73.8 Conclusion

RM is an important reproductive topic. Various etiologies have been identified over the years, and successful treatment strategies have been implemented. A comprehensive workup can be started following two consecutive losses, especially in women aged >35 years, to identify treatable causes that include uterine abnormalities and immunological, endocrine, and genetic conditions. The modification of some lifestyle habits should also be proposed to increase the reproductive prognosis of a couple. Nevertheless, almost half of the RM cases are still unexplained and yet require future specific investigations. Whatever the cause of RM is, thorough investigations and follow-up supported by a psychological care may help many couples to obtain a successful live birth.

RM is one of the main indications for PGT. However, even if Chen and colleagues reported that the miscarriage rate is significantly lowered after euploid embryo transfer in their meta-analysis [42], some limitations exist. Specifically, data about PGT clinical efficacy per intention to treat and cost-effectiveness are yet missing, and a clear international consensus has not been reached yet. Many clinical studies are in the pipeline, and several research projects are investigating the issue of RM, especially for what concerns the non-chromosomic pregnancy losses, which will hopefully provide novel evidences in the next years.

References

1. El Hachem H, Crepaux V, May-Panloup P, Descamps P, Legendre G, Bouet PE. Recurrent pregnancy loss: current perspectives. Int J Women's Health. 2017;9:331–45.
2. Zegers-Hochschild F, Adamson GD, de Mouzon J, Ishihara O, Mansour R, Nygren K, et al. International Committee for Monitoring Assisted Reproductive Technology (ICMART) and the World Health Organization (WHO) revised glossary of ART terminology, 2009. Fertil Steril. 2009;92:1520–4.
3. Kolte AM, Bernardi LA, Christiansen OB, Quenby S, Farquharson RG, Goddijn M, et al. Terminology for pregnancy loss prior to viability: a consensus statement from the ESHRE early pregnancy special interest group. Hum Reprod. 2015;30:495–8.
4. Jauniaux E, Farquharson RG, Christiansen OB, Exalto N. Evidence-based guidelines for the investigation and medical treatment of recurrent miscarriage. Hum Reprod. 2006;21:2216–22.
5. Practice Committee of the American Society for Reproductive M. Evaluation and treatment of recurrent pregnancy loss: a committee opinion. Fertil Steril. 2012;98:1103–11.
6. Lenton EA, Hooper M, King H, Kumar A, Monks N, Verma S, et al. Normal and abnormal implantation in spontaneous in-vivo and in-vitro human pregnancies. J Reprod Fertil. 1991;92:555–65.
7. Heffner LJ. Advanced maternal age - how old is too old? N Engl J Med. 2004;351:1927–9.
8. Nybo Andersen AM, Wohlfahrt J, Christens P, Olsen J, Melbye M. Maternal age and fetal loss: population based register linkage study. BMJ. 2000;320:1708–12.
9. Hassold T, Hunt P. To err (meiotically) is human: the genesis of human aneuploidy. Nat Rev Genet. 2001;2:280–91.
10. Nagaoka SI, Hassold TJ, Hunt PA. Human aneuploidy: mechanisms and new insights into an age-old problem. Nat Rev Genet. 2012;13:493–504.
11. Kutteh WH. Novel strategies for the management of recurrent pregnancy loss. Semin Reprod Med. 2015;33:161–8.
12. Chen H, Fu J, Huang W. Dopamine agonists for preventing future miscarriage in women with idiopathic hyperprolactinemia and recurrent miscarriage history. Cochrane Database Syst Rev. 2016;7:CD008883.
13. De Carolis C, Greco E, Guarino MD, Perricone C, Dal Lago A, Giacomelli R, et al. Anti-thyroid antibodies and antiphospholipid syndrome: evidence of reduced fecundity and of poor pregnancy outcome in recurrent spontaneous aborters. Am J Reprod Immunol. 2004;52:263–6.
14. Opatrny L, David M, Kahn SR, Shrier I, Rey E. Association between antiphospholipid antibodies and recurrent fetal loss in women without autoimmune disease: a metaanalysis. J Rheumatol. 2006;33:2214–21.
15. Rey E, Kahn SR, David M, Shrier I. Thrombophilic disorders and fetal loss: a meta-analysis. Lancet. 2003;361:901–8.
16. de Jong PG, Kaandorp S, Di Nisio M, Goddijn M, Middeldorp S. Aspirin and/or heparin for women with unexplained recurrent miscarriage with or without inherited thrombophilia. Cochrane Database Syst Rev. 2014:CD004734.
17. Sugiura-Ogasawara M, Ozaki Y, Katano K, Suzumori N, Mizutani E. Uterine anomaly and recurrent pregnancy loss. Semin Reprod Med. 2011;29:514–21.
18. Hassold T, Hall H, Hunt P. The origin of human aneuploidy: where we have been, where we are going. Hum Mol Genet. 2007;16(2):R203–8.
19. Franasiak JM, Forman EJ, Hong KH, Werner MD, Upham KM, Treff NR, et al. The nature of aneuploidy with increasing age of the female partner: a review of 15,169 consecutive trophectoderm biopsies evaluated with comprehensive chromosomal screening. Fertil Steril. 2014;101:656–63.
20. Capalbo A, Rienzi L, Cimadomo D, Maggiulli R, Elliott T, Wright G, et al. Correlation between standard blastocyst morphology, euploidy and implantation: an observational study in two centers involving 956 screened blastocysts. Hum Reprod. 2014;29:1173–81.
21. Rienzi L, Capalbo A, Stoppa M, Romano S, Maggiulli R, Albricci L, et al. No evidence of association between blastocyst aneuploidy and morphokinetic assessment in a selected population of poor-prognosis patients: a longitudinal cohort study. Reprod Biomed Online. 2015;30:57–66.
22. Sugiura-Ogasawara M, Ozaki Y, Katano K, Suzumori N, Kitaori T, Mizutani E. Abnormal embryonic karyotype is the most frequent cause of recurrent miscarriage. Hum Reprod. 2012;27:2297–303.
23. Werner M, Reh A, Grifo J, Perle MA. Characteristics of chromosomal abnormalities diagnosed after spontaneous abortions in an infertile population. J Assist Reprod Genet. 2012;29:817–20.
24. Ottolini CS, Newnham LJ, Capalbo A, Natesan SA, Joshi HA, Cimadomo D, et al. Genome-wide maps of recombination and chromosome segregation in human oocytes and embryos show selection for maternal recombination rates. Nat Genet. 2015;47:727–35.
25. Capalbo A, Bono S, Spizzichino L, Biricik A, Baldi M, Colamaria S, et al. Sequential comprehensive chromosome analysis on polar bodies, blastomeres and trophoblast: insights into female meiotic errors and chromosomal segregation in the preimplantation window of embryo development. Hum Reprod. 2013;28:509–18.
26. Handyside AH, Montag M, Magli MC, Repping S, Harper J, Schmutzler A, et al. Multiple meiotic errors caused by predivision of chromatids in women of advanced maternal age undergoing in vitro fertilisation. Eur J Hum Genet. 2012;20:742–7.
27. Turner JM. Meiotic silencing in mammals. Annu Rev Genet. 2015;49:395–412.
28. Forabosco A, Percesepe A, Santucci S. Incidence of non-age-dependent chromosomal abnormalities: a population-based study on 88965 amniocenteses. Eur J Hum Genet. 2009;17:897–903.
29. Franssen MT, Korevaar JC, Leschot NJ, Bossuyt PM, Knegt AC, Gerssen-Schoorl KB, et al. Selective chromosome analysis in couples with two or more miscarriages: case-control study. BMJ. 2005;331:137–41.

30. De Braekeleer M, Dao TN. Cytogenetic studies in couples experiencing repeated pregnancy losses. Hum Reprod. 1990;5:519–28.
31. Kurahashi H, Tsutsumi M, Nishiyama S, Kogo H, Inagaki H, Ohye T. Molecular basis of maternal age-related increase in oocyte aneuploidy. Congenit Anom (Kyoto). 2012;52:8–15.
32. Ottolini CS, Capalbo A, Newnham L, Cimadomo D, Natesan SA, Hoffmann ER, et al. Generation of meiomaps of genome-wide recombination and chromosome segregation in human oocytes. Nat Protoc. 2016;11:1229–43.
33. Wang Y, Cheng Q, Meng L, Luo C, Hu H, Zhang J, et al. Clinical application of SNP array analysis in first-trimester pregnancy loss: a prospective study. Clin Genet. 2016;91(6):849–58.
34. Levy B, Sigurjonsson S, Pettersen B, Maisenbacher MK, Hall MP, Demko Z, et al. Genomic imbalance in products of conception: single-nucleotide polymorphism chromosomal microarray analysis. Obstet Gynecol. 2014;124:202–9.
35. Kort DH, Chia G, Treff NR, Tanaka AJ, Xing T, Vensand LB, et al. Human embryos commonly form abnormal nuclei during development: a mechanism of DNA damage, embryonic aneuploidy, and developmental arrest. Hum Reprod. 2016;31:312–23.
36. Vega M, Breborowicz A, Moshier EL, McGovern PG, Keltz MD. Blastulation rates decline in a linear fashion from euploid to aneuploid embryos with single versus multiple chromosomal errors. Fertil Steril. 2014;102:394–8.
37. Wapner RJ, Martin CL, Levy B, Ballif BC, Eng CM, Zachary JM, et al. Chromosomal microarray versus karyotyping for prenatal diagnosis. N Engl J Med. 2012;367:2175–84.
38. Huang A, Adusumalli J, Patel S, Liem J, Williams J 3rd, Pisarska MD. Prevalence of chromosomal mosaicism in pregnancies from couples with infertility. Fertil Steril. 2009;91:2355–60.
39. Gueye NA, Devkota B, Taylor D, Pfundt R, Scott RT Jr, Treff NR. Uniparental disomy in the human blastocyst is exceedingly rare. Fertil Steril. 2014;101:232–6.
40. Vermeesch JR, Voet T, Devriendt K. Prenatal and pre-implantation genetic diagnosis. Nat Rev Genet. 2016;17:643–56.
41. Dahdouh EM, Balayla J, Garcia-Velasco JA. Comprehensive chromosome screening improves embryo selection: a meta-analysis. Fertil Steril. 2015;104:1503–12.
42. Chen M, Wei S, Hu J, Quan S. Can comprehensive chromosome screening technology improve IVF/ICSI outcomes? A meta-analysis. PLoS One. 2015;10:e0140779.
43. Vaiarelli A, Cimadomo D, Capalbo A, Orlando G, Sapienza F, Colamaria S, et al. Pre-implantation genetic testing in ART: who will benefit and what is the evidence? J Assist Reprod Genet. 2016;33:1273–8.
44. Mastenbroek S, Twisk M, van der Veen F, Repping S. Preimplantation genetic screening: a systematic review and meta-analysis of RCTs. Hum Reprod Update. 2011;17:454–66.
45. Scott RT Jr, Upham KM, Forman EJ, Zhao T, Treff NR. Cleavage-stage biopsy significantly impairs human embryonic implantation potential while blastocyst biopsy does not: a randomized and paired clinical trial. Fertil Steril. 2013;100:624–30.
46. Cimadomo D, Capalbo A, Ubaldi FM, Scarica C, Palagiano A, Canipari R, et al. The impact of biopsy on human embryo developmental potential during preimplantation genetic diagnosis. Biomed Res Int. 2016;2016:7193075.
47. Scott RT Jr, Ferry K, Su J, Tao X, Scott K, Treff NR. Comprehensive chromosome screening is highly predictive of the reproductive potential of human embryos: a prospective, blinded, nonselection study. Fertil Steril. 2012;97:870–5.
48. Ubaldi FM, Capalbo A, Colamaria S, Ferrero S, Maggiulli R, Vajta G, et al. Reduction of multiple pregnancies in the advanced maternal age population after implementation of an elective single embryo transfer policy coupled with enhanced embryo selection: pre- and post-intervention study. Hum Reprod. 2015;30:2097–106.
49. Forman EJ, Hong KH, Ferry KM, Tao X, Taylor D, Levy B, et al. In vitro fertilization with single euploid blastocyst transfer: a randomized controlled trial. Fertil Steril. 2013;100:100–7.
50. Forman EJ, Hong KH, Franasiak JM, Scott RT Jr. Obstetrical and neonatal outcomes from the BEST Trial: single embryo transfer with aneuploidy screening improves outcomes after in vitro fertilization without compromising delivery rates. Am J Obstet Gynecol. 2014;210:157.e1–6.
51. Murugappan G, Shahine LK, Perfetto CO, Hickok LR, Lathi RB. Intent to treat analysis of in vitro fertilization and preimplantation genetic screening versus expectant management in patients with recurrent pregnancy loss. Hum Reprod. 2016;31:1668–74.
52. Rienzi L, Capalbo A, Vajta G, Ubaldi FM. PGS for recurrent pregnancy loss: still an open question. Hum Reprod. 2017;32:476–7.
53. Werner MD, Leondires MP, Schoolcraft WB, Miller BT, Copperman AB, Robins ED, et al. Clinically recognizable error rate after the transfer of comprehensive chromosomal screened euploid embryos is low. Fertil Steril. 2014;102:1613–8.
54. Tiegs AW, Hodes-Wertz B, McCulloh DH, Munne S, Grifo JA. Discrepant diagnosis rate of array comparative genomic hybridization in thawed euploid blastocysts. J Assist Reprod Genet. 2016;33:893–7.
55. Capalbo A, Rienzi L. Mosaicism between trophectoderm and inner cell mass. Fertil Steril. 2017;107:1098–106.
56. Capalbo A, Ubaldi FM, Rienzi L, Scott R, Treff N. Detecting mosaicism in trophectoderm biopsies: current challenges and future possibilities. Hum Reprod. 2016;32(3):492–8.
57. Greco E, Minasi MG, Fiorentino F. Healthy babies after intrauterine transfer of mosaic aneuploid blastocysts. N Engl J Med. 2015;373:2089–90.
58. Capalbo A, Treff NR, Cimadomo D, Tao X, Upham K, Ubaldi FM, et al. Comparison of array comparative genomic hybridization and quantitative real-time PCR-based aneuploidy screening of blastocyst biopsies. Eur J Hum Genet. 2015;23:901–6.
59. Gawad C, Koh W, Quake SR. Single-cell genome sequencing: current state of the science. Nat Rev Genet. 2016;17:175–88.
60. Hunter JE, Allen EG, Shin M, Bean LJ, Correa A, Druschel C, et al. The association of low socioeconomic status and the risk of having a child with Down syndrome: a report from the national Down syndrome project. Genet Med. 2013;15:698–705.
61. Wu LL, Russell DL, Wong SL, Chen M, Tsai TS, St John JC, et al. Mitochondrial dysfunction in oocytes of obese mothers: transmission to offspring and reversal by pharmacological endoplasmic reticulum stress inhibitors. Development. 2015;142:681–91.
62. Caburet S, Arboleda VA, Llano E, Overbeek PA, Barbero JL, Oka K, et al. Mutant cohesin in premature ovarian failure. N Engl J Med. 2014;370:943–9.
63. Hopkins J, Hwang G, Jacob J, Sapp N, Bedigian R, Oka K, et al. Meiosis-specific cohesin component, Stag3 is essential for maintaining centromere chromatid cohesion, and required for DNA repair and synapsis between homologous chromosomes. PLoS Genet. 2014;10:e1004413.
64. Jiang J, Jing Y, Cost GJ, Chiang JC, Kolpa HJ, Cotton AM, et al. Translating dosage compensation to trisomy 21. Nature. 2013;500:296–300.
65. Amano T, Jeffries E, Amano M, Ko AC, Yu H, Ko MS. Correction of Down syndrome and Edwards syndrome aneuploidies in human cell cultures. DNA Res. 2015;22:331–42.
66. Larsen EC, Christiansen OB, Kolte AM, Macklon N. New insights into mechanisms behind miscarriage. BMC Med. 2013;11:154.
67. Weimar CH, Macklon NS, Post Uiterweer ED, Brosens JJ, Gellersen B. The motile and invasive capacity of human endometrial stromal cells: implications for normal and impaired reproductive function. Hum Reprod Update. 2013;19:542–57.
68. Weimar CH, Post Uiterweer ED, Teklenburg G, Heijnen CJ, Macklon NS. In-vitro model systems for the study of human

embryo-endometrium interactions. Reprod Biomed Online. 2013;27:461–76.

69. Diaz-Gimeno P, Ruiz-Alonso M, Blesa D, Bosch N, Martinez-Conejero JA, Alama P, et al. The accuracy and reproducibility of the endometrial receptivity array is superior to histology as a diagnostic method for endometrial receptivity. Fertil Steril. 2013;99:508–17.

70. Ruiz-Alonso M, Blesa D, Diaz-Gimeno P, Gomez E, Fernandez-Sanchez M, Carranza F, et al. The endometrial receptivity array for diagnosis and personalized embryo transfer as a treatment for patients with repeated implantation failure. Fertil Steril. 2013;100:818–24.

Part IX

IVF Laboratory

74 Setting Up an IVF Laboratory

Stephen Troup

The design of an IVF laboratory needs to incorporate a number of key considerations ranging from where the laboratory is situated relative to other rooms, through to its size, configuration, the equipment it houses and even what the walls might be painted with (or not). Not only does the design of the laboratory affect the environment in which people work and their efficiency, but more importantly, it can affect the outcome of the treatments that take place therein.

This chapter seeks to describe some of the fundamental design features of the IVF laboratory with reference to the basic physiological needs of gametes and embryos cultured in vitro, together with suggestions and recommendations as to how these needs might be best met. It must be recognised, however, that there are 'many ways to skin the cat' and that the content of this chapter is a combination of scientific evidence where it is available, accepted dogma and straightforward common sense.

As a starting point, it seems prudent to consider some features of the female reproductive tract in terms of it being the 'best' environment in which gametes and embryos will thrive. In simple terms, the female reproductive provides an environment which:

1. Is at a constant 37 °C and varies very little from this
2. Is a supportive milieu for the early embryo which is at the correct pH and supplies appropriate nutrients
3. Protects the early embryo from potential damage by infective agents, physical damage, exposure to light and toxins
4. Contains biological selection mechanisms leading to embryo implantation and live birth
5. Although it seems rather obvious, ensures that the baby belongs to the mother!

In considering IVF laboratory design, it is worthwhile being mindful of these fundamental requirements.

We will discuss the design of the IVF laboratory by considering the following eight questions:

1. Where should it be ideally situated?
2. What size and shape should it be?
3. What are the regulatory requirements?
4. How do we make it clean, warm and toxin-free?
5. How do we handle and observe our embryos?
6. How do we make sure there are no mix-ups?
7. How do we monitor the facilities?
8. How do we store cryopreserved gametes and embryos?

Some of the issues discussed in this chapter relate to the design of a new laboratory, but many are principles and ideas that can also be applied to an existing laboratory set-up. Finally, it is essential that an experienced clinical embryologist is part of the design and implementation team tasked with setting up an IVF laboratory—it is all too easy to underestimate the importance of the often-overlooked idiosyncrasies associated with successful IVF, and the person best placed to advise on such things is the clinical embryologist.

74.1 Where Should an IVF Laboratory Be Situated?

There are several factors that should be considered when choosing where to site an IVF laboratory, some of which are, of course, easier to control than others. Ideally, the quality of air that enters the laboratory should be as high as possible (although this risk can be mitigated by air purification systems discussed below). As such, it makes sense to site the lab away from any form of manufacturing plant, which might, for example, release airborne toxins. Similarly, airborne pollution from traffic, railways or airports is best avoided. Many centres in recent years have moved away from a conventional

S. Troup (✉)
Reproductive Science Consultancy Ltd, Wilmslow, UK
e-mail: steve@rsc.me.uk

G. N. Allahbadia et al. (eds.), *Textbook of Assisted Reproduction*, https://doi.org/10.1007/978-981-15-2377-9_74

hospital-based site to facilities on business or science parks, with which also often come the advantages of lower costs and, crucially, easier parking for patients.

74.2 What Size and Shape Should an IVF Laboratory Be?

It is commonplace and prudent to engage the services of clean-room specialists in the design of an IVF laboratory to ensure that any specific regulatory clean-room requirements are met. The use of clean-room specialists is recommended for both new-build projects and refits alike. Such experts are familiar with how, for example, the shape of a room or the equipment therein might affect airflow and hence the sterile function of the room; the concept of air pressure cascades to ensure the IVF laboratory itself is the cleanest part of the room arrangement; and how to generate the clean air in the first place.

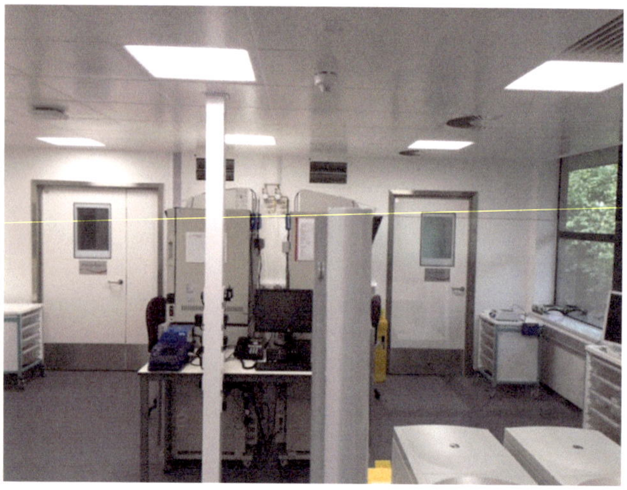

Fig. 74.1 The location of the embryology laboratory. This should be directly adjacent to the procedure rooms where oocyte collections and embryo transfers take place. (Courtesy of the Knutsford Hewitt Fertility Center, Liverpool Women's NHS Foundation Trust, Liverpool, UK)

In considering the design of an IVF laboratory, it is also extremely important to consider a number of key adjacencies. It is highly desirable to have direct access between the 'procedure' room(s) where egg collection and embryo transfer procedures take place and the laboratory itself (Fig. 74.1).

Such access can take the form of a conventional clean-room hatch arrangement or perhaps, more sensibly, door access, with the latter more readily facilitating communication between embryology and clinical teams. It is also 'good clean-room practice' that a dedicated store be situated near the laboratory, or ideally directly adjacent, with a 'materials-transfer' hatch directly into the laboratory. Similarly, hatch access between the cryostore facility and the main laboratory might be considered desirable (Fig. 74.2).

Some laboratories have also arranged to have their semen sample production facilities directly adjacent to the main IVF laboratory linked by a pass-through hatch (Fig. 74.2b). Whilst this arrangement undoubtedly lessens patient embarrassment in terms of not having to physically hand over the semen sample, consideration needs to be given to privacy within the sample collection room particularly in terms of noise and, crucially, the requirement to develop a robust chain of custody.

Unfortunately, there is no simple metric that can be applied to determine the size of an IVF laboratory other than the simple fact that I have yet to visit a laboratory that is too big. There are, however, some important considerations

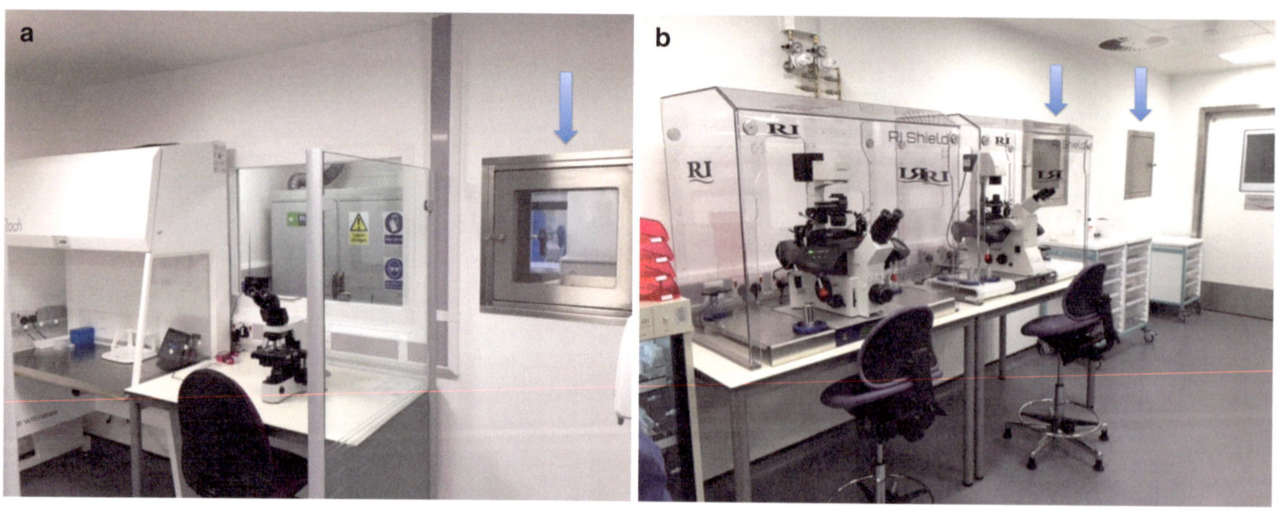

Fig. 74.2 Hatches link into the embryology lab. Hatches can be used to link to various rooms that ensure sterility and safety, such as the cryostore, or for the delivery of sterile consumables or andrology specimens. (**a**) This hatch (arrow 1) links the lab to the cryostore; (**b**) these two hatches link into the laboratory clean store (arrow 2) and the male specimen sample production room (arrow 3). (Courtesy of the Knutsford Hewitt Fertility Center, Liverpool Women's NHS Foundation Trust, Liverpool, UK)

when attempting to gauge correct laboratory size. Most importantly, consideration needs to be given to the safety of the gametes and embryos that are to be processed through the laboratory. It makes sense, therefore, to allow for wide circulation spaces to minimise the chances of accidental collision—it seems likely that embryologists will always have to carry vessels containing gametes and embryos around the laboratory. Similarly, blind corners should be avoided if at all possible.

Of course, consideration should also be given to the amount, type and positioning of equipment within the laboratory. In relation to the latter, care should be taken with the positioning of air inlet vents. The cooling effect of a flow of air, for example, over a dish on an ICSI rig should not be underestimated and although such an effect can be compensated for and dealt with, as part of the equipment validation process, the problem is far better designed out at the outset if at all possible.

The laboratory will require a considerable number of power outlets, data points and gas outlets, and a simple rule to follow in this respect is to install more than you think are needed! It is far better to have a number of redundant power outlets than to have to use extension cables (the use of which is now frowned upon or indeed prohibited in some institutions) or to have to retrospectively install additional sockets in an operational clean-room laboratory. The positioning of outlets and gas manifolds is also very important, as these are difficult to move once installed. It may, for example, make sense to position gas manifolds higher on a wall to allow equipment to be sited underneath them, or alternatively outside the laboratory.

Finally, it is rare that a laboratory remains filled with the same equipment throughout its life. Equipment is replaced and updated and new developments occur. As such, it seems sensible to design the laboratory with inherent flexibility. For example, it may be better to consider mobile, rather than fixed, benching and storage (Fig. 74.3). Similarly, mobile screens can effectively create rooms within rooms (Fig. 74.4). Incorporating 'mobility' into the laboratory also facilitates cleaning and decontamination, an essential element of an effective laboratory.

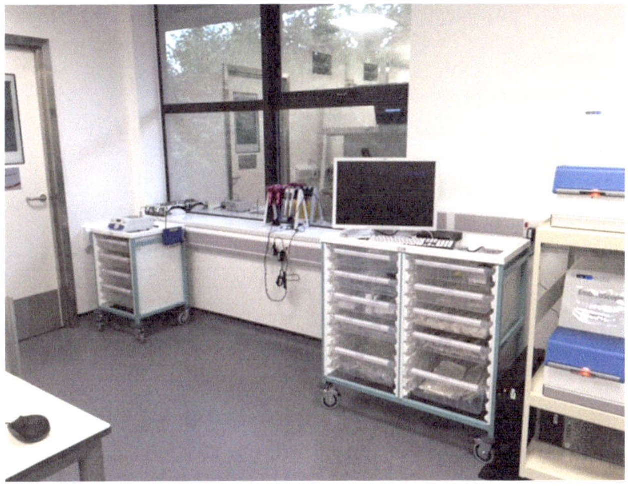

Fig. 74.3 Mobile furniture. Rather than using fixed fixtures and fittings, mobile units allow for laboratory redesign according to changing requirements. (Courtesy of the Knutsford Hewitt Fertility Center, Liverpool Women's NHS Foundation Trust, Liverpool, UK)

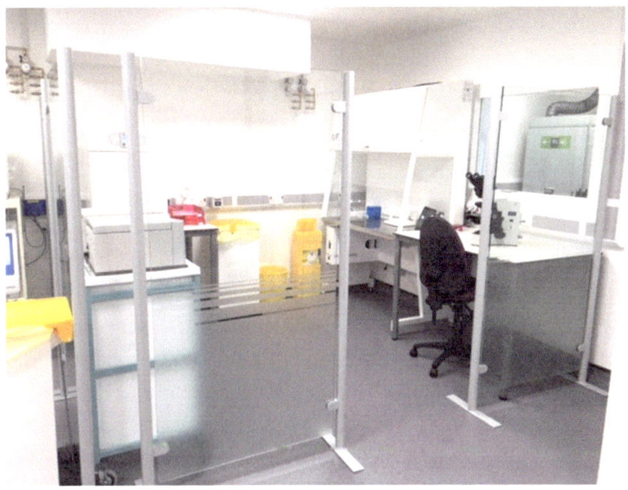

Fig. 74.4 Creating a room within a room using screens. (Courtesy of the Knutsford Hewitt Fertility Center, Liverpool Women's NHS Foundation Trust, Liverpool, UK)

74.3 What Are the Regulatory Requirements?

It would be unusual nowadays to construct an IVF laboratory that does not meet the broad requirements of 'clean-room' design, although the actual regulatory requirements are not that difficult to achieve. As a pragmatic benchmark, the EU Tissue and Cells Directive (2004/23/EC) [1] contains clauses that specify the air quality that should be achieved in a laboratory handling gametes and embryos. It is interesting to note that this EU Directive has been interpreted differently by EU member states with some choosing to ignore the Directive completely. Nevertheless, in the UK, the Human Fertilization & Embryology Authority (HFEA) were appointed as the so-called competent authority in terms of implementing the Directive. Following professional body consultation, the HFEA decided that in simple terms, gametes and embryos should be handled in Grade C air, with the quality of background air being Grade D (Table 74.1). Grade C and D specify the levels of particulate and microbial contamination permissible whilst the room is at rest and during operation. The definition of these air qualities is provided by the Medicines and Healthcare products Regulatory Agency (MHRA) [2]. Importantly, using a combination of clean-room

Table 74.1 Air grades for microbial contamination, measured as colony forming units (cfus) forming on a settle plate containing agar, after exposure to air for 4 h and air particle counts, measured as the number of 0.5 μm particles/m^3

Grade	Settle plates (diam. 90 mm) cfu/4 h	Particles (number of 0.5 μm particles/m^3)
A	<1	3500
B	10	3500
C	100	350,000
D	200	3,500,000

Table data based on MHRA—Rules and Guidance for Pharmaceutical Manufacturers and Distributors 2002; and on ISO14644

design and good practice means that operating an IVF laboratory to these levels of cleanliness is easily achievable.

74.4 How Do We Make the Environment for the Gametes and Embryos Clean, Warm and Toxin-Free?

Described above are the clean-room requirements in terms of generating an environment full of filtered high-efficiency particulate air (HEPA-filtered) that is constantly and frequently replenished. This approach usually includes the design of positive-pressure air cascades within the laboratory and adjacent rooms such that the highest air pressure is in laboratory itself, causing particles and contaminants to be 'blown' away from the room. However, such a clean-room arrangement will be entirely ineffectual without the rigorous application of rules around clothing (in particular footwear), restricted access, personal hygiene, cleaning schedules and frequent and regular environmental monitoring to ensure the clean-room status is adequately maintained.

If one accepts that the human female reproductive tract is the ideal environment in which eggs and embryos will thrive, then it makes sense to try to mimic some of its fundamental attributes in the IVF laboratory. Human eggs and embryos are particularly susceptible to damage by even slight reductions in temperature below normal body temperature [3]. There are several ways in which the dishes or tubes containing gametes and embryos can be kept as close to body temperature as possible including incubation systems, heated blocks and surfaces and heated cabinets.

However, there are two reasons why the IVF laboratory should be equipped with an air-conditioning system capable of providing not only clean air (as described above) but air at a constant temperature. Firstly, although effective procedures will limit the time gametes and embryos are not in the incubator to a minimum, short periods of exposure to ambient temperature are inevitable and, as such, an IVF laboratory that is consistently warm is highly desirable, although consideration must be given to the working environment for staff who can spend many hours within the laboratory.

Perhaps less obvious is the fact that most incubators commonly used within IVF laboratories do not have the ability to cool below the ambient temperature of the laboratory. Indeed, more often than not, as the ambient temperature of the laboratory approaches that of the temperature set point of the incubator, the incubator temperature will start to rise above its set point with obvious potential detrimental effects to gametes or embryos therein. This consideration is particularly important in warmer climates although it is easy to overlook in climates with large differences in temperatures between summer and winter.

The in vivo development of an embryo affords it a level of protection against toxic substances although the blood-placental barrier is 'leaky' and a relatively poor block to chemicals—often demonstrated by the large number of substances and foods avoided by pregnant women. Nevertheless, it is common sense to design an IVF laboratory such that exposure to potential gamete-toxic substances is minimised. Of particular concern within the IVF laboratory is presence of volatile organic compounds (VOCs).

VOCs are chemicals with a high vapour pressure at room temperature and low boiling point. VOCs have been demonstrated to be embryo-toxic [4], and there many potential sources to consider in the construction and operation of an IVF laboratory. Some of the more obvious sources of VOCs are solvent-based paints, glues and sealants. Most of these have a familiar and easily recognisable odour by virtue of the large number of VOCs being released by them. Solvent-based products should be avoided at all costs, particularly as entirely suitable water-based, odourless alternatives are now readily available.

Less obviously, VOCs are often present in new IVF laboratory equipment (e.g. incubators). It is therefore prudent to unpack and install new equipment quickly and to allow it to operate empty for as long a period of time as possible before using it for gamete or embryo culture. VOCs can be filtered out of the IVF laboratory environment, and a variety of fixed, in-line and mobile filters are commercially available for this purpose. Indeed, VOC filters are often incorporated into the design of some incubator systems.

The presence of VOCs can be readily monitored using handheld detection devices. Monitoring of VOC levels in the IVF laboratory should form part of the ongoing environmental monitoring procedures of the laboratory. However, this is particularly important following construction work or the installation of new equipment.

74.5 How Do We Handle and Observe Our Embryos?

Continuing the premise that 'the in vivo situation is ideal' allows us to consider the best ways in which to handle and observe embryos during their time in vitro. This section deals with the equipment that might be best suited for the IVF laboratory in order to at least approximate the in vivo environment, recognising that:

1. A degree of gamete and embryo manipulation remains inevitable.
2. It is necessary to observe embryo development in order to assess developmental competence and select those embryos with the highest implantation potential.

Given the above, the ideal IVF laboratory would, of course, be a laboratory-sized incubator with stable temperature and filtered gas supplies in which the embryologists would work observing and manipulating gametes and embryos at their leisure, in the knowledge that the embryo environment remained entirely stable (as is the case in vivo). Under these circumstances, stress to the embryo by changing its environment would be minimised. Clearly, however, such an arrangement is not tenable, and our challenge is to get as close to this situation as possible by designing IVF laboratories and using equipment in such a way as to minimise stress to the embryo.

In terms of being able to observe the embryo whilst maintaining a stable environment, the advent of commercially available time-lapse imaging (TLI) systems in recent years has taken us much closer to being able to achieve the desirable stable culture situation. There are now a number of commercially available TLI systems, and whilst the evidence base around the efficacy of morphokinetic embryo selection algorithms remains controversial, the stable culture conditions afforded by such incubator systems remain highly desirable. In terms of lab design, TLI incubators are space-efficient, can facilitate remote access to imaging and certainly contribute to efficient use of the embryologists' time.

74.6 How Do We Ensure There Are No Mix-Ups?

Virtually all realms of modern society would consider it a fundamental right of our existence as human beings to know with certainty who our biological parents are. Yet the Internet and media provide a rich and surprisingly persistent source of articles in which 'mix-ups' in IVF labs are (often sensationally) described. Indeed, there has been at least one reported 'serious' mix-up in IVF laboratories around the world every year for the last 20 years, and although the incidence might be considered low, the fact that mix-ups continue to occur is significant cause for concern. Furthermore, it seems reasonable to assume that the reported events are only the 'tip of the iceberg' and one wonders how many mix-ups continue to take place in IVF labs unreported—or even unnoticed!

An IVF lab should contain systems that, as far as possible, minimise the risk of mix-ups occurring. In the UK, and in response to a widely publicised incident in 2002 where a white couple gave birth to black twins following a mix-up in the IVF laboratory, the HFEA introduced requirements within IVF labs that witnessing by a suitably trained individual must take place at any point at which a mix-up could occur [5]. This requirement is now enshrined in the HFEA's Code of Practice which IVF labs in the UK are required to adhere to [6].

Although a regulatory requirement in the UK, the principle of procedure witnessing should be built into the design and operation of any IVF lab. However, asking a colleague to 'manually' witness a procedure is less than ideal as it can be distracting and time-consuming (up to 20 min could be spent simply witnessing the key laboratory procedures in an IVF cycle). Fortunately, alongside the requirement to witness key IVF laboratory procedures came the development of electronic systems capable of facilitating this element of IVF lab practice.

Two approaches to electronic witnessing have been commercially developed using either barcode or radio frequency identification (RFID) technology. There are several systems now commercially available utilising these technologies, and it is for the embryologists involved in the lab design and operation to choose the system best suited to their needs, as pros and cons exist with both barcode and RFID systems.

Reassuringly, prior to the introduction of these systems into UK IVF laboratories, the HFEA went to considerable lengths to investigate not only the systems' efficacy but also their safety [7]. In this author's opinion, it would seem foolhardy to not incorporate an electronic witnessing system into the design of any IVF laboratory.

74.7 How Do We Monitor the Facilities?

The precious nature of the gametes and embryos within an IVF laboratory requires us to ensure that all facilities and equipment are remotely monitored when the laboratory is unattended and indeed and also when the laboratory is staffed. Some countries place a regulatory requirement on the need to suitably and continuously monitor equipment. For example, in the UK the HFEA places a condition of an IVF centre's licence that states:

> where equipment or materials affect critical processing or storage parameters (e.g. temperature, pressure, particle counts, microbial contamination levels), they must be identified and be the subject of appropriate monitoring, alerts, alarms … [8].

There are many alarm monitoring systems commercially available, although most share the common features of being able to monitor critical parameters, to record data and to instigate an alarm both locally and remotely should a parameter fall out of its preset range. Increasingly, as technology has advanced, alarm monitoring systems are able to operate wirelessly and are relatively simple to install into a new or existing facility.

74.8 How Do We Store Cryopreserved Gametes and Embryos?

Perhaps the most difficult area within an IVF laboratory to design and set up effectively is the cryostore facility, principally by virtue of the significant health and safety considerations that surround the inevitable use of liquid nitrogen (LN2). Great expertise exists within the companies that manufacture and install cryostorage facilities. Furthermore, an active dialogue between the embryologist in charge of the laboratory and the supplier is of particular importance in this area.

There are principally two approaches to the provision of LN2 to a cryostore. Perhaps the most commonly used approach is to have LN2 delivered from a specialist supplier to the centre. It can then be stored for use at the centre, either in smaller pressurised storage vessels which are mobile, or in much larger 'fixed' pressurised vessels which tend to be sited externally, with the LN2 being piped into the laboratory.

The mobile storage tanks have the advantage of being more easily stored within the internal cryostorage laboratory. However, their mobility itself can cause problems as, for example, moving such a vessel between floors using an elevator requires a stringent standard operating procedure to protect those involved.

The requirement to move LN2 within a centre can be obviated by the installation of an externally sited fixed tank. Whilst this is in many ways highly desirable, it is all too easy to not consider the considerable cost involved in cooling the pipeline that delivers LN2 to the laboratory. It is important to remember that each time the LN2 tap in the laboratory is turned on, the entire length of the pipeline (in spite of it being designed for purpose and vacuum-lined) will need to cool to −196 °C before any liquid will appear in the laboratory.

In recent years, many IVF laboratories have chosen to install their own LN2 generators. These devices range in size and generating capability (producing ~20 litres LN2 per day upwards) and are often no bigger than a large filing cabinet and so can easily be located within the cryostore itself. Such machines are able to extract nitrogen gas from the atmosphere and convert it directly into LN2. Although commercial manufacturers are few and far between, the use of LN2 generators overcomes many of the difficulties described above and (depending on usage) generates LN2, which, on a 'price per litre' basis, can be significantly cheaper than commercially sourced LN2.

It is crucial when setting up a cryostore to balance the needs of the laboratory, the health and safety of staff and the costs involved in not only setting up the laboratory in the first place but also the ongoing running costs.

74.9 Summary

In conclusion, there are many elements to consider when designing an IVF laboratory, but in essence, the design of a successful IVF laboratory will follow the simple premise that form should follow function as far as possible.

In this respect, therefore, those involved in the setting up, and indeed day-to-day operation, of an IVF laboratory should also hold uppermost in their considerations the fact that an IVF laboratory should be set up to provide conditions which emulate the in vivo environment as far as possible.

Whilst compromise is inevitable perhaps as a result of configuration, regulation or financial restrictions, the design and set-up of the most successful IVF laboratories should cause the gametes and embryos therein to be minimally compromised.

References

1. Directive 2004/23/EC of the European Parliament and of the Council of March 2004 on setting standards of quality and safety for the donation, procurement, testing, processing, preservation, storage and distribution of human tissues and cells. Official Journal of the European Journal.
2. Medicines and Healthcare products Regulatory Agency. MHRA – rules and guidance for pharmaceutical manufacturers and distributors 2002.
3. Pickering SJ, Braude PR, Johnson MH, Cant A, Currie J. Transient cooling to room temperature can cause irreversible disruption of the meiotic spindle in the human oocyte. Fertil Steril. 1990;54:102–8.
4. Khoudja RY, Xu Y, Li T, Zhou C. Better IVF outcomes following improvements in laboratory air quality. J Assist Reprod Genet. 2013;30(1):69–76.
5. Dyer C. Biological father declared the legal father in IVF mix up. BMJ. 2003;326(7388):518.
6. Human Fertilisation and Embryology Authority Code of Practice, Edition 9 (2009).
7. Human Fertilisation and Embryology Authority Advisory Group on Safety and New Technologies.
8. Human Fertilisation and Embryology Authority, 2017 - Licence condition T24.

Air Quality in the IVF Laboratory

75

Normand Brais

Evidence has accumulated over the years that following the standard guidelines and codes for designing healthcare facility ventilation systems is far from being sufficient to ensure a sterile environment [1–4]. Sterility is generally defined as 99.9999% reduction of a population of microorganisms. This means that as little as one microorganism in a million is expected to survive after disinfection.

Standard traditional air filtration with HEPA (high-efficiency particulate air) filters or ULPA (ultralow penetration air) filters have been widely adopted in clinical ventilation systems to control airborne pathogens. However, multiple studies have demonstrated that despite using such filters, viral and bacterial airborne contamination are still ubiquitous in these ventilation systems [5–7].

The most common cause of filter ineffectiveness relates to the filter rack seal joints bypass, filter puncture leakage, and poor installation or maintenance. Furthermore, all filters show a significant drop in their capture efficiency for a certain range of particulate size. In this critical size range, particles are either too small to be captured by interception/impaction or too large or to be removed by diffusion/electrostasis. This is just a straightforward consequence of the fundamental principles of filtration physics [8].

HEPA filters also display a weakness at a critical particle size between 0.1 and 0.4 microns as shown in Fig. 75.1. HEPA filter efficiency drops to a minimum value of 99.95% at a critical point for particles called MPPs (most penetrating particles) which are around 0.2 microns in size.

If a HEPA filter is challenged with a concentration of one million particles per cubic meter falling within its vulnerable size range, for each cubic meter of air as much as 500 particles every hour will pass through the filter. During the course of a single day, a 1000 m^3/h "fresh air" ventilation system would allow 12 million viable particles to contaminate the aseptic zone.

It is also worth noting that in order to perform according to specifications, the air velocity facing the filters must be below a specified value. For HEPA filters, it is generally recommended not to exceed an incoming velocity of more than 1.3 m/s. Since many air handling units are often designed to operate at much higher velocities, the performance of HEPA filters may end up being substandard.

Within the filter vulnerable particle size extended range of 0.02–0.7 micron, several microorganisms (also called "viable particulates") are typically found. Many of the biocontaminants in this critical size range are highly undesirable inside a medical environment.

When challenged by one million particles, some viable microorganisms can penetrate through the filter if they are ~0.2 microns in size. Considering that sterility is defined as less than one survivor in a one million microorganism population, it is quite clear that the HEPA air disinfection process filtration is not sufficient for IVF laboratories and, as such, requires a finishing step.

Unlike filtration, ultraviolet germicidal irradiation (UVGI) does not capture or retain microorganisms, but rather, it sterilizes them by damaging their DNA/RNA strands as they pass by an intense germicidal UV light zone. Contrary to a filter that accumulates particulates until the pressure drop increases to a point where it needs replacement, UV disinfection systems have a negligible pressure drop and require comparatively very low maintenance.

75.1 Fundamentals of Ultraviolet Disinfection Process

75.1.1 UV Light Spectrum

We cannot see the UV light spectrum, which extends from 100 to 400 nm. The UV spectrum has been arbitrarily classified into four subdivisions:

N. Brais (✉)
Sanuvox Technologies, Inc., Montreal, QC, Canada
e-mail: bma@bma.ca; nbrais@bma.ca

G. N. Allahbadia et al. (eds.), *Textbook of Assisted Reproduction*, https://doi.org/10.1007/978-981-15-2377-9_75

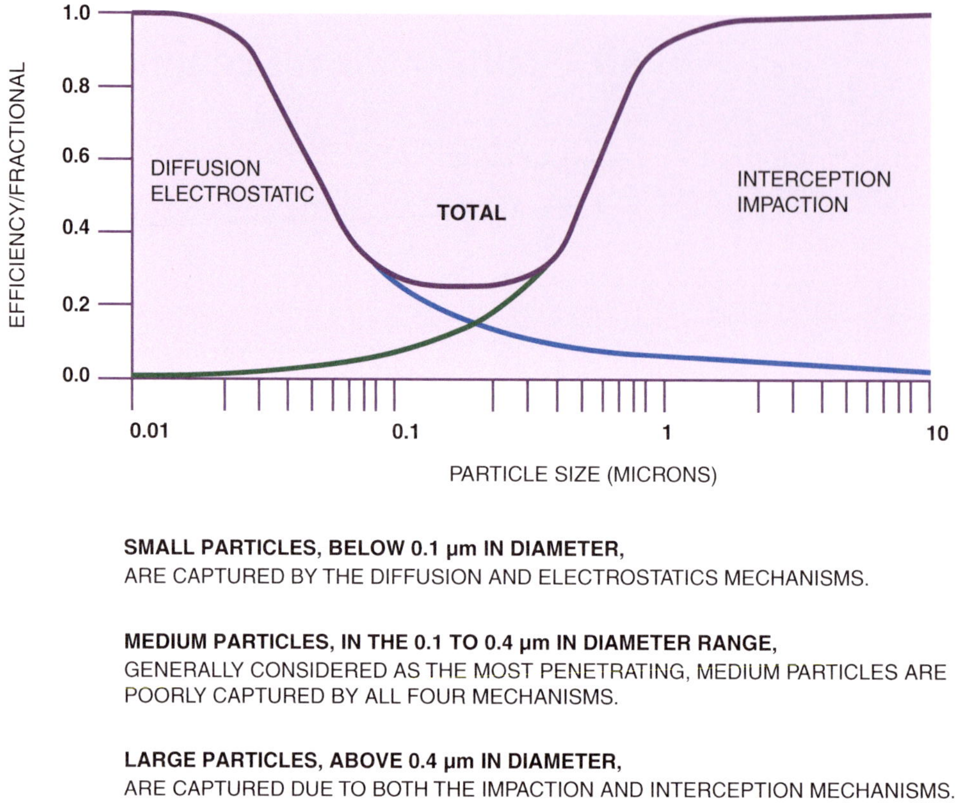

Fig. 75.1 Fundamental principles of air filtration. (From Da Roza RA, Particle size for greatest penetration of HEPA filters and their true efficiency. National Technical Information Service, U.S. Department of Commerce, 5285 Port Royal Road, Springfield, VA 22161, USA)

- UV-A band (400–315 nm)—mainly from sunlight reaching the Earth's surface, not absorbed by the ozone layer
- UV-B band (315–280 nm)—causes skin to redden, mostly absorbed by the ozone layer
- UV-C band (280–200 nm)—the most effective for germicidal effect, fully absorbed by the ozone layer
- Far or vacuum UV (200–30 nm)—ozone producing and ionizing radiation

75.1.2 UV Disruption of DNA and RNA

The discovery of microbial disinfection by UV light dates back to 1877 [9]. Then later, in 1928, F.L. Gates [10] identified the specific wavelength of UV light that was responsible for the observed germicidal effect. It was during this first half of the twentieth century that quantum mechanics helped to explain how DNA/RNA interacted with specific wavelengths.

We now know that nucleic acids have a peak absorption spectra at wavelengths of 265 nm; hence, these are most effective germicidal [11], causing the most damage to the genetic material of sterilized microbes.

UV disinfection works by causing cumulative molecular damage to the molecules in the strands of DNA and RNA. The disruption of nucleic acids by UV light has the ability to affect the complete spectrum of microorganisms, making them all sterile given a sufficient dosage and consequently making them unable to infect a host. Within the limits of experimental accuracy, the lethal action of germicidal UV appears to be independent of the nature of the organism, and, unlike antibiotics, there has been no sign of adaptive resistance after almost a century of wide usage for drinking water disinfection.

Most commercially available germicidal light sources are based on fluorescent tube technology and emit between 30 and 35% of their input power at 253.7 nanometers, a wavelength very close to the peak germicidal wavelength of 265 nm.

UVGI sterilization of microorganisms is therefore achieved in practice with the low cost and widely available wavelength of 253.7 nm. The quantum energy carried by UV-C photons is high enough to dissociate most single chemical bonds between carbon, hydrogen, oxygen, and nitrogen atoms. The molecular disruption caused by these energetic photons results in irreversible damage to the nucleic acids of a microorganism until it is no longer viable.

UV radiation damages DNA by causing cyclobutane pyrimidine dimers (CPDs) and pyrimidine-pyrimidone 6-4 photoproducts (6-4 PPs) to form [12]. While CPDs covalently bond between pyrimidines, UV-C causes the most dimers to form from thymine, the least from cytosine, with an intermediate level from mixed dimers [13].

For RNA viruses, UV irradiation causes the pyrimidine photoproducts to form from the nucleotide uracil.

Provided the UV dose is high enough to prevent any repair mechanisms, then the nucleic acid is permanently altered, with genetic replication and transcription impaired, resulting in viral death.

For more information, please see the in-depth review by Kowalski, which describes in detail how nucleic acids are damaged by UV [13].

75.1.3 UV Dose: Response Calculation

Mathematically, UVGI disinfection can be considered as an assault of photons onto a microbe. An amount of energy called a quantum E_λ is carried by each photon. Each quantum E_λ has a value linked to the light wavelength according to the Planck-Einstein equation:

$$E_\lambda = hc / \lambda \qquad (75.1)$$

where

h = Planck's constant, 6.626×10^{-34} J·s
c = speed of light in vacuum, 2.998×10^{8} m/s
λ = wavelength, m

Using this equation, each UV-C photon conveys an energy at a wavelength of 253.7 nm, equal to 7.83×10^{-19} J. Therefore, the number of photons per joule is the inverse, i.e., 1.28×10^{18} photons per joule. Given that 1 watt of power equals 1 joule of energy per second, then a UV intensity of 100 W/m^2 will result in a flow of 1.28×10^{20} photons per second per square meter.

For a virus that is 0.2-micron diameter, the target area is only 3.14×10^{-14} m^2. However, despite its small size, every second this virus will be bombarded by as much as four million photons!

If a microbe is subjected to sufficient photonic bombardment, the accumulated photochemical damage will render it dysfunctional. Realistically though, only a few of the high numbers of photons actually hit the virus. The effectiveness of UV disinfection for a specific area of a virus depends on many factors, such as the particular distribution of its DNA sequence, its protein shell, and the number of destroyed molecules relative to the number of photons absorbed by the virus. A promising and useful predictive method based on the above-described photon bombardment concept and successful hit probability has been published to predict the UV susceptibility of microorganisms as a function of their genome without using classical experimental bio-lab test procedure [14].

Given the above, the microbial response to a UV dose can also be considered, based on the rate of microbial death relative to the number of successful hits over a specific period. If successful hits are described as the product of the UV power per unit area I, the number of bio-organism N, the bio-organism effective UV inactivation cross section k, and the exposure time t, then:

$$\text{Hit rate} = dN / dt = k\,N\,I\,t \qquad (75.2)$$

Integration of Eq. (75.2) yields:

$$N(t) = N_0 e^{-kIt} \qquad (75.3)$$

where

N_0 = initial number of microorganisms
N_t = number of microorganisms surviving after any time t
k = a microorganism-dependent UV susceptibility constant (m^2/Joule)
I = the irradiance UV intensity received by the microorganism (watt/m^2)
t = the exposure time (seconds)

The fraction of microorganisms initially present, which survive at any given time, is called the survival ratio S and can be expressed as:

$$S = \frac{N_t}{N_0} \qquad (75.4)$$

The sterilized fraction is what is called the disinfection rate which is simply 1 minus the survival ratio.

$$\text{Disinfection} = 1 - S = 1 - e^{-kIt} \qquad (75.5)$$

As explained above, we can define the germicidal UV dose by the total number of UV photons emitted per unit area during a time interval, which can be written as:

$$\text{UV Dose} = I \times t \quad \text{in Joule / m}^2 \qquad (75.6)$$

By substituting Eq. (75.6) in Eq. (75.5), we finally get the well-verified germicidal UV dose-response relation:

$$\text{Disinfection} = 1 - e^{-k\,\text{UV Dose}} \qquad (75.7)$$

Equation (75.7) shows that a specific disinfection rate is provided by a specific dose, regardless of the exposure time or intensity. However, exposure time is different for surface disinfection compared to airborne disinfection. The disinfection exposure time of air in the induct depends on airflow speed and so could only be for milliseconds. This contrasts to a longer exposure time of minutes/hours for stationary surfaces such as wall, floors, or air cooling or heating coils. Thus, to be effective, airborne microbes need to be subjected to UV intensities far higher than those used to disinfect surfaces.

There is an exponential time decay relation for some microorganisms of concern under a constant UVGI intensity of 10 mW/cm^2. Significant differences exist in the exposure time required for the same level of disinfection between the most and least UV-susceptible microorganisms of concern. The one that requires the highest dosage will be the one governing the sizing of the UV system.

75.1.4 How Susceptible Are Microbes to UV Energy?

UV inactivation depends on the microbe. Fungal spores are least susceptible, followed by bacterial spores and mycobacteria, with vegetative bacteria having the highest susceptibility. However, this is a loose guide as individual species can vary in resistance, and spore-forming bacteria and fungi can have vegetative forms, which have greater susceptibility. Viruses are more problematic to categorize as they have the highest range of variation to susceptibility.

If we look at Eq. (75.5), a higher UV dose is needed to disinfect microbes with a lower k value, noting that units of k are m^2/Joule, which is the inverse of the units used in UV dose. As an example, in 1964, Jensen calculated the UV susceptibility of influenza A virus to be 0.0119 m^2/J. Given this, the UV dose needed to reach 90% disinfection of a population of influenza A virus can be calculated as:

$$D90 = \frac{\ln(10)}{k} = \frac{2.303}{k} \quad \text{in J/m}^2 \tag{75.8}$$

This gives a D90 value for influenza A virus of 19.3 J/m^2. The required UV dosage to obtain a desired disinfection level can therefore be calculated, such that a UV dose of twice/thrice the D90 should provide a 99% and 99.9% disinfection levels, respectively. The disinfection LOG value, i.e., the number of 9s, is equal to the delivered UV dose divided by the D90 value.

To reach sterility, a condition that we have previously defined as a disinfection level of 6 LOG or 99.9999%, at least six times the D90 value of the most resistant microorganism must be delivered. For further information on published UV susceptibility k values, please see the referenced work of Kowalski [13].

75.2 UVGI Dosage Required for Adequate Air Disinfection of IVF Clinics

Given the nature of the sensitive procedures performed within IVF clinics, where pre-implantation embryos are being manipulated in vitro, the target air disinfection level should be as close as possible to total sterility. To determine the required UV dose for IVF clinics, we should first examine the list of the microorganisms of concern that fall within the vulnerable size range of HEPA filters and compare their UV susceptibility k to find out the most resilient species.

The most resilient microorganism is the bacteria *Francisella tularensis*, which requires a UV dose of 25.59 mJ/cm^2 for 90% disinfection. In order to reach 6 LOG of overall disinfection after filtration, the UV system must therefore be designed to at least sterilize 499 of the 500 remaining bacteria, i.e., a disinfection rate of 499/500 = 99.8% which is just a little short of 3 LOG (99.9%). Consequently, the UV system sizing criteria consist in delivering a UVGI dose of a little less than three times 25.59 mJ/cm^2. An exact calculation shows that a dose of 75 mJ/cm^2 must be delivered to the air stream before entering the aseptic space.

This UV dosage ensures an overall disinfection of at least 6 LOG for all of the microorganisms of concern.

When filtration is used in conjunction with UVGI disinfection, a combined disinfection efficiency can be calculated using the following formula:

$$\text{Disinfection}_{\text{overall}} = 1 - (1 - \text{Filter}_{\text{eff}})(1 - \text{UV}_{\text{eff}}) \tag{75.9}$$

Therefore, to attain an overall disinfection of 99.9999%, i.e., 6 LOG of sterility equivalent, the following UV disinfection efficiency is required for a given filtration efficiency:

$$\text{UV}_{\text{eff}} = 1 - \frac{10^{-6}}{1 - \text{Filter}_{\text{eff}}} \tag{75.10}$$

According to Eq. (75.10), if the HEPA filter MPP efficiency is 99.95% for the most penetrating particle size, then the UV disinfection efficiency must be designed to be superior to 99.8% so that an overall disinfection above 99.9999% or 6 LOG is achieved.

Using Eq. (75.7) with the controlling UV susceptibility value of *Francisella tularensis*, the minimum required UV dose to reach 99.8% disinfection is computed to be 75 mJ/cm^2.

Repeating the above calculation, but with a higher-performing ULPA filter, where the MPP efficiency is equal or greater than 99.99%, then the UV dose needed to complete the disinfection and ensure air sterility drops to 50 mJ/cm^2.

75.2.1 UVGI Air Disinfection System Design Guidelines for IVF

So how much UV power does it take for a given airflow to deliver the target UV dose that will ensure sterility?

Before getting into an example of such a design, it is important to note that Eq. (75.7) does not give any indication of the distribution of UV energy as a function of x, y, and z coordinate given by set of UV lamps positioned inside an air duct.

To further complicated matters, an air duct causes microbe mobility, which can be either turbulent or stratified. Unlike turbulent air, the worst-case scenario is a stratified "laminar" air stream. The physical geometry of the duct and the fact that the light intensity decays as an inverse square law with the distance from the source are also important. Thus, the number and position of UV lamps within the duct need consideration, as these factors will affect the final delivered UV dose. A computerized program is needed to calculate the UV irradiation field inside a duct. This should also take into account the surfaces of duct wall which can reflect UV, to enhance performance.

Initial UVGI air stream disinfection systems design guidelines based the average UVGI dose on size and number of lamps and reflective surfaces [15]. However, the designs suffered had several flaws:

1. The real three-dimensional intensity field was not defined, but was evaluated based on the lamp power rating.
2. Lamps were specified without regard to lamp positioning.
3. Duct dimensions were not accounted for when correcting from reflectivity.

Even today, too many UV systems are unfortunately sized using crude rules, such as packing all ductwork with successions of lamps. Such misuse has invariably ended up with poor performances and deceived some UV system users.

Nowadays, computational power allows for adequate custom-sizing of any in-duct UV disinfection system. Proper calculations for predicting the applied UV dose must take into account the relevant input parameters: lamp characteristics, placement, and orientation, alongside geometry and surface reflectivity. The following parameters need consideration:

- Airflow rate
- Height, width, and length of duct
- % Reflectivity of inner surfaces
- Lamp UV output power (W), lamp length and diameter
- 3-D positioning coordinates of each UV lamp (x_i, y_i, z_i)
- Target microorganism susceptibility constant k (m^2/J)

Taking all these critical sizing variables into account, Kowalski [16] proposed a dimensional analysis to assess how effective the UV system would be for providing disinfection. This results in a useful simplified general scaling correlation to provide a UV dose based on airflow, UV output power, and duct length. The formula is as follows:

$$\text{UV dose} \sim P \times L / Q \qquad (75.11)$$

where

P = power output of UV source in watt
Q = airflow in m^3/s
L = UV exposure length

For upscaling or downscaling purposes, Eq. (75.11) tells us that if the flow rate is doubled in the same duct size, then the UV power or number of lamps must be doubled as well, to ensure the same disinfection performance. The same can be said about the duct UV exposure length L; if it's reduced by half to make the system more compact, then the UV output power will have to be doubled to compensate.

Applying this correlation to the previous example, where 250 watt of UV output over 2 m exposure length provided a given disinfection level to an airflow of 1000 m^3/h, we can work out how much UV output would be required to ensure the same level of disinfection for an airflow of 2000 m^3/h over the same exposure length. The answer is simply twice the UV output, i.e., 500 watt.

By observing in Eq. 75.11 that the airflow Q is the product of the duct cross-section A by the air velocity V and that the UV exposure time t is simply the ratio of the duct length L to the air velocity V, we can rewrite it as follows:

$$\text{UV dose} \sim P \times t / A \qquad (75.12)$$

This scaling relation concisely expresses the fact that the delivered UV dose is the product of UV lamps output power in watts with the exposure time in seconds divided by the duct cross-sectional area. Figure 75.2 shows an actual picture of the UVGI disinfection system described and calculated in this example.

It is worth mentioning that the inner duct wall reflectivity significantly contributes to the total UV field. Inter-reflections, caused by reflections echoing between surfaces, will help to achieve steady state at the speed of light. This converges to a finite value, which relies on the inner surface reflective properties and geometry of the duct. The physical process of inter-reflections is also taken into account by computer models. Neglecting to use highly reflective duct lining surfaces such as polished aluminum severely impairs UV system performance.

It should be noted that the reflective properties for UVC wavelength are very different compared to visible light reflectivity. Despite its reflective features for visible light,

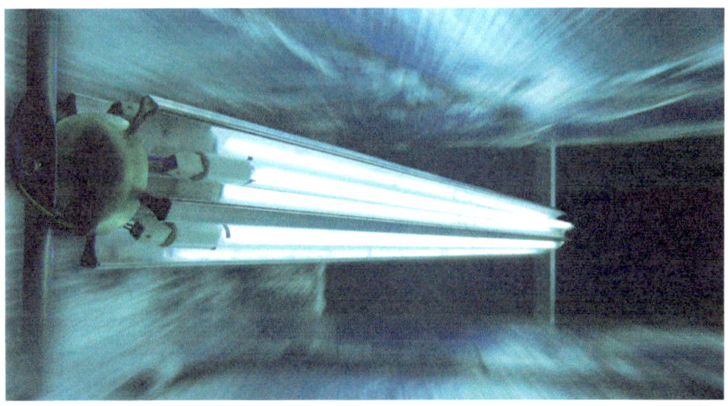

Fig. 75.2 Photo of a Biowall™ disinfection installation. (Courtesy of Sanuvox Technologies, Montreal, Canada)

stainless steel has a low UVC reflectivity of only 20%. Aluminum with a reflectivity ranging from 73 to 87% is the optimal low-cost material of choice to line an air duct to improve UV disinfection performance. UVC reflectivity data is published and must be included in a proper calculation to maximize the energy efficiency of the UV disinfection system.

75.2.2 Effect of Air Velocity, Temperature, and Lamp Aging on UV System Output

Air temperature and velocity may vary over a wide range within a ventilation system, causing significant variations in UV lamp output. As such, these factors must be adequately accounted for.

Maximum UV output requires a UV lamp surface temperature of 38–50 °C. The UV lamp temperature could become too low if the air is moving, and the UV output will then fall. To minimize the chilling effect and allow higher operating efficiency under cold airflow condition, it is preferable to install the UV lamps parallel to the flow instead of perpendicular cross-flow.

UV lamp output also decreases over time due to lamp aging, with UV lamps rated in terms of effective hours of UV emission. Toward the end of the useful life (20,000 h), the intensity of a UV lamp is estimated to be around 80% compared to the intensity of a UV lamp measured at 100 h of operation. The germicidal lifespan is reduced, even though blue light continues to be emitted. It is therefore important to consider UVGI systems designed based on intensity at "the end of effective life."

As well as aging, other factors to consider include the lamp type and the ambient conditions when used.

These can accumulate in ventilation systems to reduce the effective emission by up to 50% [17].

75.3 Ultraviolet Surface Disinfection

Pathogens can be transmitted via environmental surfaces, yet suboptimal surface disinfection in healthcare facilities has been observed to be substandard [17]. UVGI surface disinfection systems can either be mobile or fixed.

75.3.1 Mobile UVGI Surface Disinfection Units

Mobile UVGI units are momentarily placed in contaminated areas to disinfect whole room surfaces. The unit shown in Fig. 75.3 has sufficient UVGI power to provide a 6 LOG disinfection for *Clostridium difficile* spores in a square room (5 m × 5 m) on all exposed surfaces within 15 min. A mobile unit can be equipped with multiple motion sensors that will cause it to shut down if someone enters the room during the sterilization cycle. It is also equipped with a data-logger that will keep a time and location record of every disinfection cycle performed during a given period.

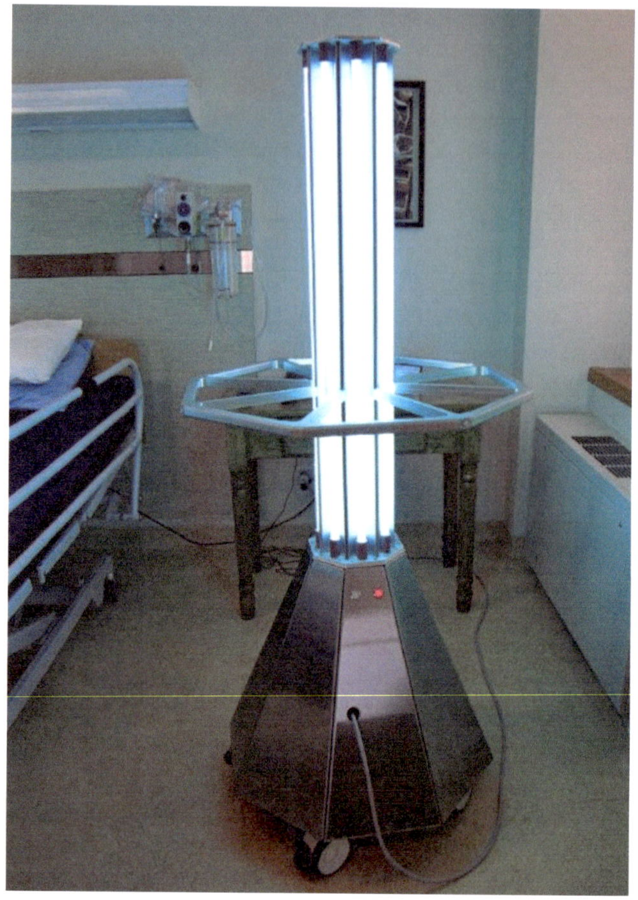

Fig. 75.3 Mobile UV unit for whole room surface disinfection. (Courtesy of Sanuvox Technologies, Montreal, Canada)

75.3.2 Fixed Automated UVGI Disinfection Units

In critical areas, such as egg collection rooms and IVF labs, permanent automatic UVGI units can be used (Fig. 75.4). These units are activated automatically when the rooms are unoccupied after each entry or use. They include a programmable logic controller with a timer, redundant motion detectors, and door switch for personnel safety.

With a properly engineered UV output relative to the size of the room that ensures a minimum UVGI intensity of 30 microwatt/cm^2 on the target surfaces, a disinfection cycle time of 5–10 min has demonstrated up to 6 LOG disinfection of the most commonly found pathogens. Table 75.1 shows typical expected disinfection results.

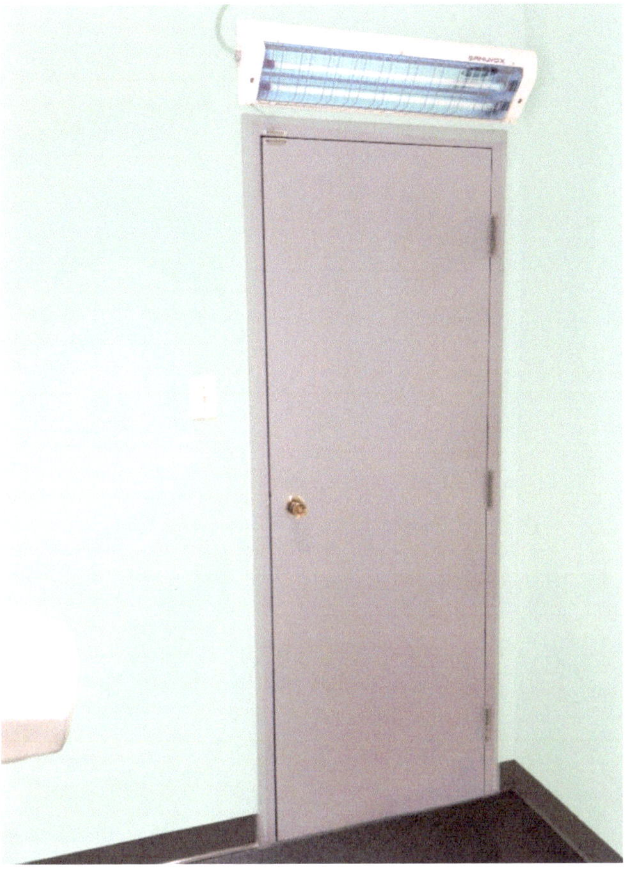

Fig. 75.4 Automatic washroom UV disinfection unit with motion sensors. (Courtesy of Sanuvox Technologies, Montreal, Canada)

Table 75.1 Typical expected disinfection with fixed UVGI units

Disinfection percent	5 min cycle	10 min cycle
	9.0 mJ/cm²	18.0 mJ/cm²
C. diff	96.872%	99.9022%
E. coli	99.9999%	100.0000%
Enterobacter cloacae	96.0766%	99.8461%
Klebsiella pneumoniae	99.2788%	99.9948%
Legionella pneumophila	100.0000%	100.0000%
Listeria monocytogenes	100.0000%	100.0000%
MRSA	99.9962%	100.0000%
Mycobacterium tuberculosis	100.0000%	100.0000%
Pseudomonas aeruginosa	99.9919%	100.0000%
Salmonella	100.0000%	100.0000%
Serratia marcescens	99.9806%	100.0000%
Staphylococcus epidermis	100.0000%	100.0000%
VRE	97.6971%	99.9470%

75.3.3 Air Conditioning Cooling Coils Disinfection

A plethora of bacterial and fungal spores can grow in the moist environment provided by heating, ventilating, and air conditioning (HVAC) systems, with the high relative humidity helping to promote germination. Microbe nutrients can be provided by dust and biofilms of environmental bacteria. Consequently, the following molds and bacteria are ubiquitous inside an HVAC: *Aspergillus*, *Penicillium*, *Mucor*, *Cladosporium*, *Fusarium*, *Alternaria*, *Pseudomonas aeruginosa*, *E.coli*, *Salmonella*, and *Legionella*.

When HVAC technicians open unit, they can encounter slimy residue of mold biofilm on the coil and drain pan. This impairs the heat transfer capacity of the system to transfer heat, leading to higher operating costs, but also causes an undesirable smell.

Regular cleaning of the coil can help, taking care not to use unsafe or flammable detergents. Acids and high-pressure washing are also discouraged as these can shorten the coil lifespan. Even with frequent cleaning, mold can regrow within a month.

Air conditioning cooling coil fins constitute a fertile wet surface area at constant temperature that ends up being a major bacteria and mold incubator and reservoir. The removal of fungal growth inside cooling coils HVAC system is a common well-known application of fixed UVGI systems. Elimination of the air conditioning reservoir of microorganisms significantly reduces airborne infections. Since biofilm-coated coils also impair heat transfer performance, the energy consumption is reduced with substantial energy saving paybacks.

Since the UV light can be operated 24 h a day every day, the disinfection of the air handling units requires little power. Figure 75.5 shows a typical installation to maintain cooling coils biologically clean along with the engineering sizing software calculation to ensure adequate UV dosage across the coil surface and between the fins.

To maintain a coil free of bio-contaminant, a constant minimum UV intensity of 0.25 mW/cm² is required on its surface. Simple petri dish contact tests performed over the last 20 years have shown that this intensity is more than sufficient to ensure that 99% of the most resilient mold *Aspergillus niger* will be rendered sterile after 3600 s of exposure. It follows that the required average UV output power per square meter of coil is only 2.5 watt and, considering the standard UV lamp efficiency of 33% and an overall uniformity compensation multiplier of 1.33, a total input power consumption of 10 watt per square meter of coil is all it takes to keep it sterile and clean at all times.

75.4 UVGI System Maintenance Guidelines

75.4.1 Lamp Replacement

UV lamps replacement should be in line with manufacturer recommendations. Although lamps can operate for up to 2 consecutive years, annual replacement (8760 h under continuous use) ensures that the correct UV dosage is always provided. It should be noted that while lamps may appear to

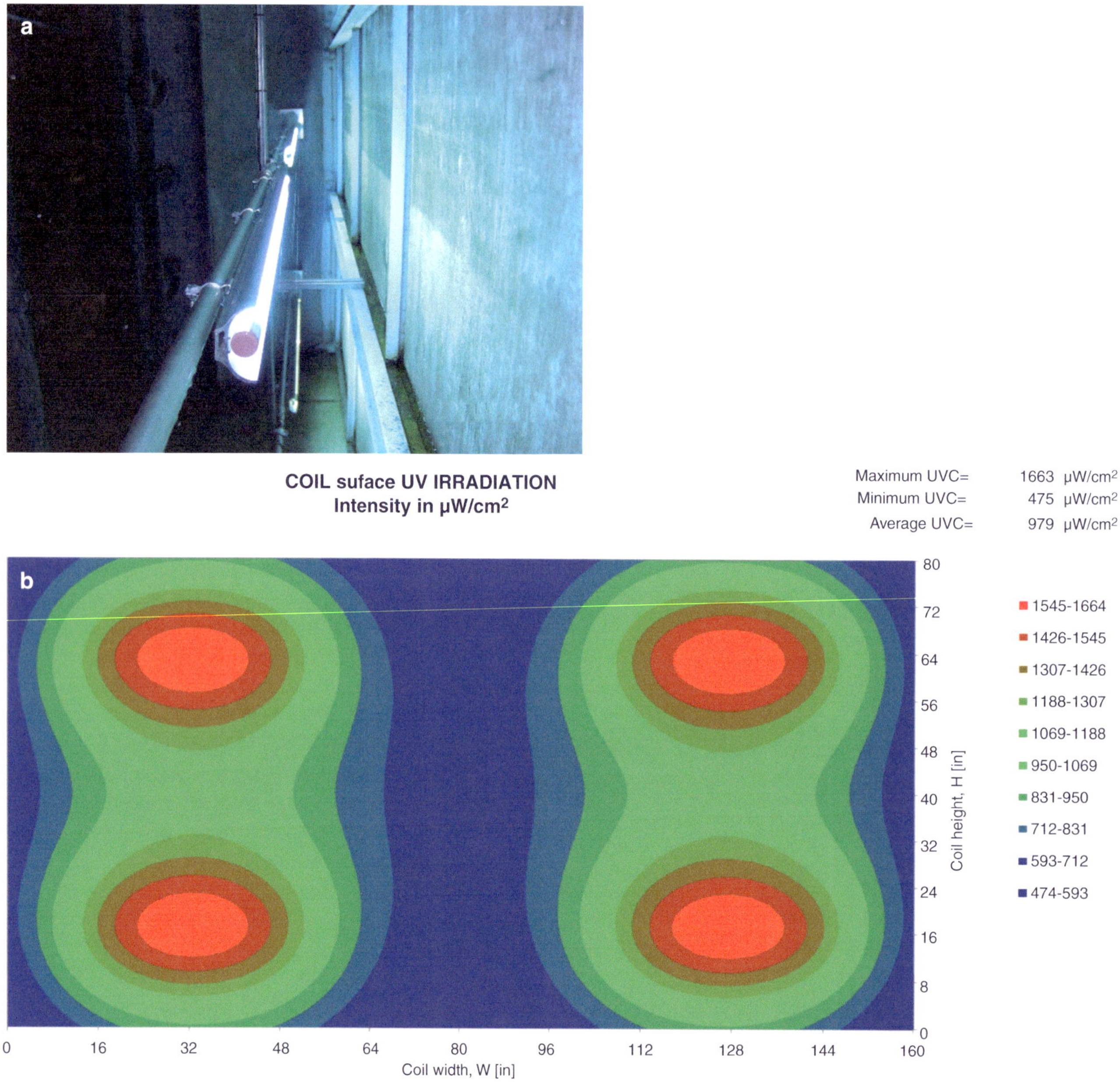

Fig. 75.5 (**a** and **b**) Air conditioning cooling coil UVGI disinfection system engineered with appropriate software. (Courtesy of Sanuvox Technologies, Montreal, Canada)

operate beyond 2 years, the germicidal UV output is reduced. Lamp failure is also promoted by frequent switching *on*/*off*.

75.4.2 Lamp Disposal

UV lamps should be treated as hazardous waste, with disposal performed in accordance with disposal guidelines for conventional commercial fluorescent bulbs, noting that they are mercury-containing devices. While some countries allow for general discarding of low-mercury bulbs, national and local jurisdictions should be consulted to confirm if these are classified as hazardous waste.

The US Environmental Protection Agency has promulgated "Universal Waste" regulations to several types of hazardous waste including mercury bulbs. Mercury lamps can be treated as regular waste for transport to a recycling facility.

75.4.3 Inspection

It is important that UVGI systems can automatically alarm if a UVC lamp fails. Any failed lamp should be replaced immediately. Dirty lamps, soiled due to inadequate pre-filtration or airborne bio-aerosols, can either be replaced or cleaned using isopropyl alcohol or a commercial glass cleaner or isopropyl alcohol and a lint-free cloth.

75.4.4 Safety Design Guidance

It is important to prevent UV light "leaking" outside of the HVAC equipment. As such, in-duct UV systems should be fully enclosed, and all access panels should carry exterior labels highlighting the potential hazard of UV exposure [18].

Positive disconnection devices, capable of being locked, should be fitted to all lamps. These should be situated next to the main access panel, external to the lamp chamber. The UV system should automatically shut down if any access panel is opened. Only authorized persons should be able to access the UV "*On/off*" switches, and they should be locked to prevent accidentally turning off. It is important not to locate the UV "*On/off*" switches next to the general room lighting switches.

75.5 Conclusion

When properly engineered, germicidal UV systems can provide extremely efficient disinfection for the IVF laboratory, including equipment, surfaces, and air supply systems. Further applications include disinfection of operating rooms, walls and floors, medical equipment, and cooling coils in HVACs. Public health agencies, such as the Centers for Disease Control in the USA, recommend the use of UVGI to disrupt the transmission of pathogens in building ventilation systems.

The current uncommonness of UV disinfection is essentially due to the false perception that HEPA air filters are sufficient to provide sterilized air. Years of cumulated field experiences have shown that filters are certainly necessary but not sufficient. When dealing with sub-micron bio-contaminants in the size range of 0.1–0.4 micron, even the best filtration technologies fail to stop them all. Unlike filters, UVGI technology does not capture the bio-contaminants, but it can effectively sterilize them when a proper dosage of ultraviolet is applied. The UVGI technology has the ability to sterilize a plethora of microbes in air streams, as well as on contaminated wall and objects.

References

1. American Institute of Architects. Guidelines for design and construction of hospital and healthcare facilities. Washington, DC: AIA; 2001.
2. American Society of Heating, Refrigerating, and Air-Conditioning Engineers. HVAC design manual for hospital and clinics. Atlanta: ASHRAE; 2003.
3. American Society of Heating, Refrigerating, and Air-Conditioning Engineers. Handbook - HVAC applications. Atlanta: ASHRAE; 2003.
4. CDC. Guidelines for environmental infection control in health-care facilities. Atlanta: U.S. Department of Health and Human Services Centers for Disease Control and Prevention; 2003.
5. Kato S, Sung M, University of Tokyo. Using UVGI to counter contaminant dispersion. IFHE Digest. 2011.
6. Menzies D, Popa J, Hanley JA, Rand T, Milton DK. Effect of ultraviolet germicidal lights installed in office ventilation systems on workers' health and well being: double-blind multiple cross-over trial. Lancet Med J. 2003;362:1785–91.
7. Menzies D, Adhikari N, Arietta M, Loo V. Efficacy of environmental measures in reducing potentially infectious bioaerosols during sputum induction. Infect Control Hosp Epidemiol. 2003;24:7.
8. Kowalski WJ, Bahnfleth W. MERV filter models for aerobiological applications. Air Media. 2002:13–7.
9. Downes A, Blunt T. Research on the effect of light upon bacteria and other organisms, vol. 26. London: Proceedings of the Royal Society; 1877. p. 488.
10. Gates, F.L. On nuclear derivatives and the lethal action of UV light. 1928.
11. Davidson JN. The biochemistry of nucleic acids. 5th ed. London: Methuen; 1965.
12. Setlow RB. Cyclobutane-type pyrimidine dimmers in polynucleotides. Science. 1966;153:379–86.
13. Kowalski W. Ultraviolet germicidal irradiation handbook. Berlin: Springer; 2009.
14. Kowalski WJ, Bahnfleth WP, Hernandez MT. A genomic model for the prediction of ultraviolet inactivation rate constants for RNA and DNA viruses.
15. Luckiesh M, Holladay LL. Designing installations of germicidal lamps for occupied rooms. Gen Elect Rev. 1942;45(6):343–9.
16. Lee B, Bahnfleth W, Auer K. Life cycle cost simulation of in-duct ultraviolet germicidal irradiation system.
17. Kowalski W. Hospital airborne infection control. Boca Raton: Taylor & Francis; 2012.
18. Engineers, American Society of Heating Refrigerating and Air Conditioning. ASHRAE handbook - chapter 16; 2008.

pH, Temperature, and Light

76

Kimball O. Pomeroy and Michael L. Reed

76.1 pH Homeostasis in Oocytes and Embryos

In clinical IVF, the incubator is a surrogate oviduct and uterus. Its purpose is to provide an ideal environment for fertilization and the growth of the developing preimplantation embryo. During this stage, the embryo normally travels through a dynamic environment from the oviduct to the uterus. Temperature, pH, osmolality, and many other environmental factors change during its journey. Current incubators and culture media are fairly static. The incubator must often provide an environment that is a compromise—suitable for sperm, oocytes, and the various stages of preimplantation embryo development. This system should not just address ideal growth but should also allow for ideal expression of embryonic genes. It should provide for the necessary chemicals, growth factors, proteins, osmolality, temperature, and pH. Almost all current culture media have been developed for mice gametes and embryos and then applied to humans. In addition, we often are not aware of the ideal conditions for human gametes and embryos.

76.1.1 pH

pH is the measurement of the concentration of the hydrogen ion (H^+) and conversely the hydroxide ion (–OH) concentration in a solution. It is the negative logarithm of the H^+ activity. Since this is a logarithmic scale, the difference in concentration from a pH 5 to 6 is tenfold, and the difference between pH 7.35 and 7.55 is a 60% increase.

K. O. Pomeroy (✉)
The World Egg Bank, Phoenix, AZ, USA

M. L. Reed
The Fertility Center of New Mexico, Albuquerque, NM, USA

76.1.2 Cell Response to pH Changes

Maintaining of a proper internal pH (pH_i) is important for the survival of all cells. The activities of many intracellular enzymes are regulated by pH. Protein synthesis [1], DNA and RNA synthesis [2], as well as contractility of myosin [3] are affected by pH. Changes in pH have even been theorized to be important in the control of the cell cycle and cell division of several cell types [4]. It is the production of proton gradients (H^+) that drives the ATP synthases to produce ATP, the "energy currency" of most cells. For these processes to occur, pH must be precisely regulated.

All animal cells that have been examined, aside from non-nucleated erythrocytes, vigorously regulate their pH_i [5]. They do this by sensing changes in pH_i and then appropriately speeding up or slowing down the activity of transporters that move acids and/or bases across the plasma membrane. The vital process of pH_i homeostasis is regulated by a delicate balance between the rate of metabolic acid generation and the activity of acid/base transporters in the plasma membrane. When an acid or base load is applied in the cell, these transporter proteins will react and maintain homeostasis by shuttling acids or bases into or out of the cell.

Three transport proteins have been identified in oocytes and embryos (Table 76.1). Two transporters function to over-

Table 76.1 A list of transport proteins used in pH homeostasis, the reproductive cells in which they function, and their protective roles

Transporter	Abbreviation	Oocyte	Embryo	Aids in recovery from
Sodium hydrogen exchanger (antiporter)	NHE		X	Acidosis
Sodium-dependent chloride-bicarbonate exchanger	NDCBE		X	Acidosis
Anion exchanger (bicarbonate-chloride exchanger)	AE	X	X	Alkalosis

G. N. Allahbadia et al. (eds.), *Textbook of Assisted Reproduction*, https://doi.org/10.1007/978-981-15-2377-9_76

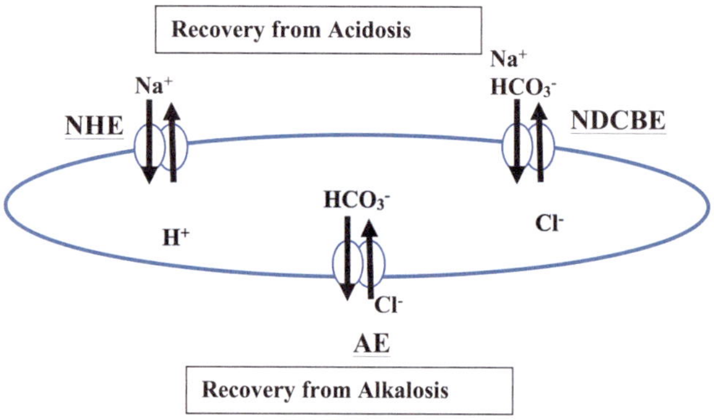

Fig. 76.1 Schematic of the function of three transporter molecules

come acid loads by increasing the pH, and the third overcomes alkaline loads by decreasing the pH (Fig. 76.1).

Na^+/H^+ antiporters (exchangers) play a major role in maintaining the pH_i from bacteria to humans. These proteins exchange Na^+ for a H^+. When intracellular pH falls (an acid load), this protein will absorb a Na^+ molecule and extrude a H^+, thus increasing the pH inside of the cell. The second protein involved in alkalizing the cytosol is the sodium-dependent chloride bicarbonate exchanger. Sodium and bicarbonate are transported into the cell in exchange for the external transport of chloride. The major transporter used to acidify the cytosol is the anion exchanger (HCO_3^-/Cl^- exchanger) which pumps out bicarbonate in exchange for pumping in chloride.

76.1.3 pH of Oviduct and Uterus/pH of Oocytes and Embryos

In trying to identify the optimal pH for culturing oocytes and embryos, the pH of the oviduct and the uterus is a good start. There are data for the sheep, cow, and mouse, but whether these really pertain to the human reproductive tract is questionable. Historically, pH of media has been designed around the pH of blood—7.35 to 7.45. Only the oviduct of the human appears to be in this range [6].

During reproduction, the oocyte, as part of a cumulus-oocyte-complex (COC), must leave the follicle where the pH is about 7.5–7.7 [7]. It must then pass into the oviduct with a pH of 7.28–7.7 [6] where it may be fertilized and then transverse to the uterus, where the embryo enters most likely as a morula [8–10] and where the pH has been measured from 7.0 to 7.2 [11]. As the embryo navigates this wide range of different external pH, it must be able to maintain the proper internal pH demanded by the intracellular environment. The pH_i of the oocyte has been measured to be about 7.0–7.1 and the pH of the cleavage embryo at 7.12 [12]. It is the role of the various transport proteins mentioned above to modulate the pH to a range that is acceptable to the cell(s). It should also be appreciated that this is not without cost. Too many fluctuations in external pH may tax the embryo's energy stores, resulting in embryo death. It has been shown in mouse embryos that raising the pH_i by 0.1–0.15 pH units can result in increased glycolysis and lowered oxidative metabolism [13, 14].

Human cleavage-stage embryos appear to be able to respond to both alkaline and acid loads and have active Na^+/H^+ antiporters, anion exchangers, and sodium-dependent chloride bicarbonate exchangers [7, 12]. In contrast, human oocytes appear to be able to regulate against alkaline loads but not acid loads. They appear to have an active anion exchanger but impaired Na^+/H^- antiporter and sodium-dependent chloride bicarbonate exchanger activity. Human oocytes thus appear to not to be able to regulate acid loads effectively.

Bicarbonate is necessary to adequately control acid loads as the Na^+/H^+ antiporter. It only kicks in below about pH 6.8. It is up to the sodium-dependent chloride bicarbonate exchanger to perform the fine pH control around the internal pH_i of the embryo, which is pH 7.1 [12]. This is one of the reasons it is important that handling media (and flushing media) should contain some bicarbonate. If handling media did not contain bicarbonate, it would rob the embryo of the ability to regulate its pH above pH 6.8. Since oocytes do not have a fully active mechanism to modify their internal pH, care must be taken to ensure that (1) bicarbonate is present in the media and (2) the external pH does not vary much from the pH_i of the oocyte, which is about pH 7.1.

As regards vitrification, it has been shown that vitrified hamster 2-cell embryos lose their ability to regulate pH_i effectively for up to 6 h after warming [14]. The pH_i of these embryos goes from 7.24 to 7.34 after warming and results in reduced activity of both the Na^+/H^+ antiporter and anion exchanger systems. Whether this occurs in other mammals, like humans, remains to be seen. However, caution should be exercised after the warming of vitrified human embryos so that the external pH is optimized. pH excursions should be avoided.

76.1.4 pH of Culture Media

A wide variety of media have been used for the successful culture of human embryos. The manufacturers of these media recommend pH targets that range from 7.2 to 7.5. The first media used for human IVF were based on media used in tissue culture. These were often simple salt solutions (like Earle's) or complex media (like Ham's F10). The pH of these media was set to the same levels as those used in the cell line from which it was borrowed. Later, more complex media were developed, based mainly on research examining the constituents of the human oviduct [15]. Still, embryologists are, for the most part, stuck with the prior tissue culture pHs, around 7.35.

Later, media were developed that attempted to imitate some aspects of the dynamic nature of the oviduct and uterus. These sequential media [16, 17] used one medium for the first 3 days of embryo culture and another for the subsequent days up to day 7. By adding amino acids, embryologists were finally able to routinely get human embryos to the blastocysts stage. Of note, these newer media were formulated first for mouse embryos and then applied to human embryos. To indicate the lack of concern with pH at this time, none of these studies even mention the pH of the culture media.

The pH of IVF media is determined mainly by the concentration of CO_2 in the incubator and the concentration of bicarbonate in the media. CO_2, provided by gas cylinders attached to the incubator, must first permeate and equilibrate with any oil overlay and then with the actual culture media. The CO_2 in solution then reacts with the bicarbonate in the medium to form carbonic acid. The amount of carbonic acid formed depends primarily on the amount of bicarbonate and CO_2 in the medium. In the laboratory, pH of the medium can be adjusted by changing the amount of CO_2 delivered to the incubator—more CO_2 results in more carbonic acid and a lower pH. Proper quality control of the incubator pH should include more than setting CO_2 and measuring its concentration.

Fyrite is an inaccurate method of measuring CO_2 [18] and is a poor substitute for actual pH measurements. To ensure the proper pH of media, one must measure it directly with a pH probe. This will especially be important when one is trying to troubleshoot culture problems. A detailed discussion of how to perform pH measurements can be found in a review by the embryologist Pool (2004) [18]. Briefly a calomel or a double junction silver/silver chloride probe, less than 1 year old, should be used. All media should contain the same concentration of protein used in culture. Calibration and test measurements should be measured at 37 °C.

The addition of proteins and the elevation (altitude) of the laboratory are two other factors that can affect the pH. This means that each laboratory will need to adjust the CO_2 of its incubators in order to produce the desired pH in the culture media. pH should be measured after protein supplementation as this can change the media pH. Figure 76.2 shows two media with protein (personal communication Jason Swain). The silver bar is for media supplemented with protein by the manufacturer (where pH is adjusted after protein supplementation). The blue bars are the same media as in the gray bars (without protein added by the manufacturer) but supplemented by the laboratory with a protein source (10% v/v SSS). Note that the pH is lower when protein is added by the laboratory by almost 0.1 pH point. Most likely this is due to simple dilution of bicarbonate by the added protein solution.

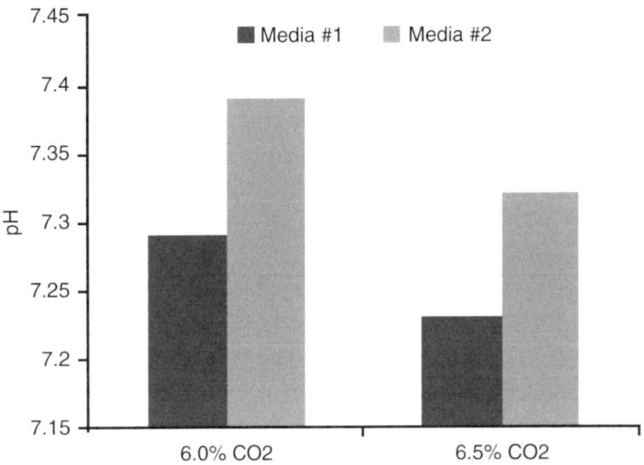

Fig. 76.2 Y-axis pH of media. #1 is media where 10% protein (SSS) was added by the laboratory and #2 is media with protein added during its manufacture. (Personal communication, Jason Swain, 2017)

Improper pH may not only affect the pH_i of the cell but may also have an indirect effect on some of the properties of the major protein found in media, albumin. An improper pH may affect the ability of albumin to act as a chelator, modifier of pH, antioxidant, carrier of fatty acids, etc. [19].

What is not often appreciated is that pH is also affected by temperature. (This is distinct from the effect of temperature on the pH probe's ability to provide an accurate pH.) The pH of pure water at 0 °C is 7.47, but at 25 °C it is 7.00 and at 100 °C it is 6.14. This is important to remember when considering use of non-CO_2-buffered media (handling or modified media) and the use of these buffers where temperature is poorly controlled for vitrification.

As mentioned previously, pH deviations should be avoided in order to increase viability of the embryo. This dictates a precise range for all media used in IVF. Retrieval media (flush media), culture media, handling media, etc. should all follow this range, and any exceptions should be based on physiology. Care should be taken that embryos and oocytes are not exposed to alkaline conditions above pH 7.45.

Currently, many embryologists use media that are closer to the pH_i of embryos (pH 7.2). This has probably slowly evolved as embryologists observed better embryo development with lower pHs than those previously recommended. It has been proposed that a constant pH close to the pH_i of the embryo will put less stress on the embryo that may result in the use of limited supplies of energy in the form of ATP [20].

76.1.5 Adjuvant Media and pH

Not only must an optimum pH be maintained in culture medium; it is also important in the use of adjuvant media—flush media, ICSI media, handling media, and vitrification media. Synthetic organic buffers, like HEPES or MOPS, are often used in IVF for the handling of gametes or embryos outside of CO_2 incubators. What may not be appreciated is that temperature can affect the pK_a of these buffers as well as the pH of the media [21]. When these buffers go from 37 °C to 25 °C, their pH can decrease by about 0.2 pH units.

The pH of media during an oocyte collection should also be examined to ensure that during routine use the proper pH is obtained. One should pay particular attention to those situations where the temperature of the medium may change. When one is making culture dishes for IVF, it is important that the dishes be allowed sufficient time to equilibrate with the incubator. One study [22], using four-well dishes with 50 μl or 500 μl of media and 500 μl of oil, indicated that a minimum of 10 h was necessary for the media to equilibrate to pH. The size of the droplet did not make a difference. If pre-equilibrated oil was used, equilibration time was decreased to less than 1 h. They also found that removal of equilibrated dishes for up to 5 min had minimal effect on the pH of the media.

Some laboratories use portable, mobile incubators (originally these units, referred to by some as isolettes, were actually modified newborn baby incubators) to aid them during retrievals or the transfer of embryos; the units house a microscope and have controllers for temperature, CO_2, and humidity. Many of these incubators use a thermal conductivity device to determine the CO_2 concentration of the gasses inside the incubator. This type of device will provide an inaccurate reading if the humidity of the chamber changes. The device may read 6.2% CO_2, while in reality, the humidity has decreased due to improper humidification or constant opening and closing of the hand ports. The embryologist may actually be working in an environment with a much lower CO_2 concentration and thus a more alkaline external pH. An infrared CO_2 controller will be more accurate in these situations.

In order to have consistent results when working with gametes and embryos, it is important to always be aware of how the external pH can be affected by what you are doing. All aspects of IVF should be characterized for pH fluctuations by first determining the goal pH for media and then assuring that the goal is met with minimal pH excursions. pH should be verified when new lots of media are added to the system, when gas cylinders are changed, or when any major change in the culture environment or methods occurs. One should empirically determine the maximum amount of time a dish can be left on the bench, by measuring pH changes in test media during mock procedures.

76.2 Temperature

The ideal temperature for human gamete and embryo handling has not been clearly defined, but most embryologists will strive to maintain 37.0 °C for all surfaces, media, and equipment to minimize "physiological and genetic stress" and other factors that could impact on in vitro development [23–26].

In 1936, embryologist Gregory Pincus [27] said:

> In obtaining both unfertilized and fertilized ova for culture in vitro, the use of a warm washing solution is preferable. This is often practically difficult and rabbit ova at least are not materially affected by handling at room temperature over a period of several hours.

During this period, Pincus was studying oocyte cooling and parthenogenetic activation.

In 1968, another embryologist, Ralph Brinster [28], wrote:

> The cultivation temperature has not been studied to a great extent, but Alliston (1965) has shown that rabbit ova cultivated at 40 °C for 6 h do not develop as well as controls cultivated at 37 °C when transferred to foster mothers. In the absence of contradictory evidence, it is generally considered that a temperature of 37°–37.5° is the best temperature in which to maintain the cultures.

The actual control temperature was 38 °C [29], but the context is correct.

It is important to realize that a lot of the information on embryo culture, including temperature, has been translated from work with other species, e.g., for mouse, rat, and rabbit [30]; as such, studies must be evaluated in context according to requirements and findings for different species.

76.2.1 In Vivo Temperatures

In vivo core temperatures for ovaries, oviducts, and the uterus during ovulation, fertilization, and development, and eventual deposition of the embryo into the uterine environment, have been discussed at length [31]. Specific to female (non-human) physiology, Hunter [32, 33] described temperature gradients across ovaries, and differential temperatures between isthmus and ampulla oviduct, and has stated that the deep rectal temperature for any species could be misleading and may not translate to in vitro conditions. Preovulatory follicles are cooler than surrounding tissue, and isthmus and ampulla temperatures differ by 0.9–1.6 °C in rabbit and 0.2–1.6 °C for the pig.

One possible explanation regarding the oviduct is the mounting evidence for mammalian sperm thermotaxis (human included). Sperm appear to be uniquely sensitive to temperature gradients [34]. El-Sheikh Ali and colleagues [35] described that in cattle, there is an increasing thermal gradient from the vagina to the deep uterine horn relative to the steroid hormone concentrations, albeit within a very narrow temperature range of less than 0.5 °C.

If human body temperature is accepted as 36.6–37.3 °C (rectal), which end of this spectrum is most appropriate for in vitro procedures, and what temperature best represents physiological reproductive temperature? Should in vitro temperature be static or dynamic according to in vivo conditions? Hunter expressed concerns about accepted, deep body and physiological temperatures in the human relevant to ART and proposed expanding research into effects of temperature on molecular aspects of reproductive processes [32].

76.2.2 In Vitro Temperature Control

In vitro, the temperatures for oocyte and embryo handling/maintenance are controlled by equipment and technique. There have been many studies and discussions on this topic. Two excellent resources are McCulloh (2012) (laboratory management and quality control [36]) and Elder et al. (2015) (detailed descriptions of temperature control and equipment management, among other topics in the book [37]).

76.2.3 Sperm

Testicles and epididymal structures for most mammals operate outside of the body cavity (human, cattle, sheep, goats) or near to the body (rabbit, rodent, pig). Sperm are generated and reside in organs slightly cooler than core body temperature. The exceptions to this include the hippopotamus, elephant, and aquatic (fresh and marine) mammals, which all have internalized testicles and storage structures.

Sperm tolerate and function at cooler-than-body temperatures; exposing germinal and storage organs (externalized) to body (and above body) temperature can be damaging to sperm, e.g., adversely impacting on in vitro acrosome function [38]. Furthermore, the adverse effect of raised temperature associated with varicoceles in the human is well recognized [39]. Sperm function (motility, capacitation, fertilization, and post-fertilization events) can be maintained and prolonged at room and colder temperatures with appropriate technique and/or extenders [40–43]. In fact, many protocols for human ART and sperm processing for insemination involve room temperature handling of human sperm.

76.2.4 Oocytes

The oocyte spindle has been studied extensively in several species and specifically in relation to temperature and oocyte competency. In a classic study, Pickering and colleagues [44] cooled a small number of human oocytes for observation of cytoskeletal changes. After warming oocytes back to 37 °C after 10 or 30 min at room temperature, not all spindle structures reformed with fidelity; the results were broadly accepted as critical to human IVF procedures. Sathananthan's team [45] cooled mouse oocytes rapidly from 37 to 15, 4, 0, and −7 °C for subsequent evaluation by light and electron microscopy. Cooling below 15 °C induced major spindle depolymerization and some reversible changes in cytoplasmic components. A detailed study by Zenzes and colleagues [46] demonstrated that human oocyte spindles shortened after 2–3 min at 0 °C, and after 10 min, spindles depolymerized completely. Yet chromosomes were not dispersed; two separate microtubule classes were discussed, and the authors concluded that depolymerization was time-dependent and tubulin reorganization could depend on the class of tubulin affected. In context, these papers represent foundation studies, evaluating extreme oocyte cooling without cryoprotective agents.

In one study, living (not fixed) spindle dynamics were evaluated using polarized light microscopy after cooling oocytes. Microtubule reassembly was delayed after warming following an exposure to 25 and 28 °C, but not 33 or 37 °C [47], and downstream metrics, e.g., fertilization rates, were higher when ICSI was performed at 37 °C [48].

Lenz and colleagues [38] demonstrated that in cows, mishandling of sperm/oocyte co-incubation or micromanipulation could impact outcomes. Acrosome function was impaired at 40 °C, but at the lower temperatures (35 and 37 °C), fertilization was impaired when compared to controls at 39 °C (with 39 °C being the body temperature of the cow). In human oocytes, a time-by-temperature interaction was observed, involving oocyte spindle and chromosome competency [49]. Sun and colleagues [50] found that at 37 °C, human oocyte spindles were stable for 20 min, but microtubules depolymerized at 39 °C (10 min) and 40 °C (1 min). Cooler temperatures were not evaluated, but it appears that human oocytes should not be exposed to temperatures ≥38 °C.

There is credible evidence (unpublished, Swain and Pool, pers. comm.) to suggest human oocytes may be cooled to room temperature during periods of micromanipulation without compromising downstream events. Data shared by Swain and Pool (Tables 76.2 and 76.3) for fertilization and developmental metrics, for a very large number of oocytes from two laboratories using similar protocols, are compelling. While no direct comparisons were performed (37 °C to room temperature ICSI), it appears oocyte competence and meiotic spindle microtubule fidelity may be more robust than imagined.

Table 76.2 Fertilization rates over a 10-year time frame for IVF and ICSI procedures

	IVF & ICSI	ICSI[a]
Main lab	12,545/18,002 (69.7%)	7076/10,124 (69.9%)
Satellite lab	6688/9172 (72.9%)	2499/3589 (69.6%)
Combined	19,233/27,174 (70.8%)	9575/13,713 (69.8%)

Swain and Pool, unpublished, with permission
[a]Room temperature

Table 76.3 Clinical outcomes following room temperature ICSI; day 3 transfer

	Patient age 23–45	Patient age ≤35
Clinical pregnancy	407/740 (55.0%)	244/389 (62.7%)
Delivery	348/740 (47.0%)	214/289 (55.0%)
Implantation rate	531/1607 (33.0%)	333/804 (41.4%)

Swain and Pool, unpublished, with permission

Yang's team [51] found that porcine oocytes could be cultured at room temperature for up to 3 days, as intact COCs, and maintain their meiotic and cytoplasmic competence upon warming and fertilization. Immature horse COCs could also be held under conditions simulating transport at room temperature in buffered culture medium, with acceptable blastocyst rates following ICSI [52].

Based on the available information, it would seem prudent to minimize temperature extremes (below or above body temperature) for prolonged periods of time during oocyte recovery, processing, and micromanipulation. Most importantly, exposing human oocytes to temperatures ≥38 °C for any length of time should be minimized.

76.2.5 Embryos

Most embryologists agree that human embryos should be maintained at a (relative) constant temperature, with minimal environmental excursions from stage to stage during culture and during routine evaluations, micromanipulation, preparation for transfer, and so on. However, for context, before cryopreservation was commonplace in ART, storage and transport of gametes and embryos of various species, laboratory and livestock, was an important topic [53].

Mouse embryos enclosed in oviducts were transported successfully at 4 °C [54], and cleavage-stage bovine embryos [55] were stored for 30 min at 0 °C. Cattle embryos could be held at 4 °C for up to 7 days, without cryopreservation, yielding 24/32 pregnancies [56]. Grau and colleagues [57] maintained human tri-pronucleate cleavage and blastocyst-stage embryos at 4 °C for 48 h and showed that development to blastocyst, or blastocyst re-expansion, was reduced after 48 h, but not after 24 h. Lastly, another study [58] demonstrated that where human blastocysts were cooled during transport to another facility for cryopreservation, after warming, clinical pregnancy and delivery rates were improved for the transported group (note that after 30 min, medium temperature dropped from 33 °C to approximately 24 °C).

Regarding in vitro culture of human embryos, Hong and colleagues [59] described a well-controlled study where sibling human oocytes were prospectively randomized to incubation at one of two temperatures, 36 °C and 37 °C; multiple incubators were utilized, and care was taken at all steps to minimize study variation. Incubator stability was 36 ± 0.07 °C and 37 ± 0.04 °C. Fertilization and embryonic aneuploidy rates were not significantly different; however, there were significantly higher cleavage-stage cell numbers, blastocyst formation rates, and "usable" blastocyst numbers with incubation at 37 °C compared to 36 °C. Interestingly, there were no differences in implantation rates per embryo transferred.

Higher-than-body temperatures were not addressed by Hong's team, but in vivo and in vitro heat stress does elicit concern [60–63]. McCulloh, in his chapter on laboratory quality control [36], described an experience where fertilization, poly-pronuclear rate, and subsequent embryo cleavage were adversely affected due to an incubator operating "out of control"—an inaccurate thermometer reported 37 °C, when the actual temperature was 41 °C.

Choi and colleagues [64] exposed one-cell mouse zygotes to elevated temperatures (37 °C, 39 °C, 40 °C, and 41 °C) for short- (8 h) and long-term (96 h) intervals. Severe, short-term heat stress compromised early cleavage, while trophectoderm cell number and quality was diminished with long-term heat stress, despite formation of blastocyst-stage embryos. Gene expression was also altered, as were post-transfer fetal metrics. Youssef and colleagues [65] examined the ideal culture temperature for mouse embryos (where body temperature is 37 °C). They found variable blastocyst and hatching blastocyst conversion rates with culture at 36, 37, 37.5, 38, and 39 °C; blastocyst hatching was highest at 37.5 °C, but combined blastocyst and blastocyst hatching rate was higher at 37 °C.

Following fertilization, oocytes appear to be more tolerant of cooler temperatures than pre-fertilization oocytes, especially when later-stage embryos form. In the human IVF laboratory, this may be comforting, regarding (1) planned events (e.g., evaluations on various days (without time-lapse), assisted hatching, transfer, biopsy, or cryopreservation), or (2) unplanned events (e.g., power loss, embryo transfers that take longer than usual).

In conclusion, oocyte cytoskeletal and cytoplasmic components appear to be sensitive to cooler-than-body temperature, particularly when there are excursions below 33 °C for longer periods of time (unless bolstered by cryoprotective agents). COCs may be more tolerant of cooling than exposed oocytes.

Human oocytes and embryos are sensitive to temperatures above accepted body temperature. In vitro temperature excursions (unplanned) can be largely avoided by having a series of defined and dedicated equipment and technique protocols in place.

Considering that human culture media and products are performance-validated at 37 °C, bioassays, and human IVF procedures alike, might not perform as expected at different temperatures (which are conditions unlikely to be validated by the manufacturers).

Quality management is tied directly to regulatory compliance and medical/legal concerns, no matter the biological (outcomes) performance of a laboratory. As such, acceptable temperature targets for each phase of the human IVF process should be selected, and steps should be taken to maintain and monitor those targets.

76.3 The Effect of Light on Embryos and Embryo Culture

In order to work with embryos in the laboratory, they must be examined at various stages, and this requires their exposure to light. The longest and most intense exposure to light is when they are examined under a microscope to perform ICSI or to grade. They are also exposed briefly to the ambient light in the room as they are moved from incubators to benches and back. Normally, during in vivo culture, they are not exposed to light. Embryos then may not have developed via evolution protective measures to protect them from light. Light exposure occurs during retrieval of oocytes, during gamete processing, during manipulations and grading of embryos, during fertilization checks, and during embryo transfer.

Pioneering embryologist Sir Robert Edwards was concerned about the effect of light on embryos:

> Light has also been one of my major concerns ever since IVF began. We were aware of the many papers on mammals published by embryologists on the evolution of reactive oxygen species in response to light exposure, and its deleterious effects on embryo growth. We could not afford any risks with human embryos to be replaced into the mother, so we used green filters routinely to remove some of the light radiation, lower the light intensity and produce a more acceptable colour for the eye by modifying the harsh artificial light from the microscope. The potential effects of light concerned me in another way. During transfer, gynaecologists often used an intense operating theatre light to shine on the cervical os. Yet this was where the embryo is passed during the transfer process. At the last moment, after hormone stimulation, oocyte collection, fertilization and cleavage in vitro, these precious embryos could be exposed to an intense light which might impair their ongoing development. We therefore dimmed this light during transfer to avoid any damage to the embryos in the last stage of their ex-utero existence. Several investigators have disparaged my attitude, and they may even be right when they claim that human embryos can tolerate this degree of intense light exposure. But I have never seen any evidence on this point from these investigators, and it is surely better to be safe than sorry. So I still use many of these precautions [66].

As far as we are aware, no well-designed studies to investigate the effect of light on human gametes and embryos have been performed. The information that we have regarding the type of lighting, duration of exposure, or exposure to specific wavelengths has only been performed on animal models like rabbits, hamsters, and mice.

The most important variables to examine when measuring light are duration of exposure, intensity of exposure, and, finally, the wavelength of light. Light intensity is often measured in lux, but this measurement is the intensity as measured by the human eye and is not useful for non-visible wavelengths. Lux also does not take into account the length of exposure. A better measure of intensity is irradiance (w/m^2). As a measurement of power, it includes the duration of the exposure. Most of the studies on the influence of light on cells do not include this measurement of irradiance. This makes it difficult to even determine the exposure of the cells to light.

Light might affect a reproductive cell in several ways. There may be a direct effect—light stresses the cell and activates stress genes. Light could directly damage DNA via ionization. Light could also indirectly affect cells—oxidizing components of the media or oil or even changing a component into a toxicant. This indirect process can occur via photooxidation—a chemical reaction between light and components of culture medium and oil. Light has been implicated in the oxidation of oil used in the culture of human embryos [67]. This same photooxidation could also produce changes in the lipid membranes of sperm and oocytes, inhibiting the process of fertilization. Production of hydrogen peroxide, a toxic substance, can also take place when media containing HEPES and riboflavin are exposed to light [68–72].

One of the first observations pointing to light's damaging effects on cells was the observation that light exposure killed protozoans placed in an acridine dye solution [68]. Light modified the acridine, causing decreased photosynthesis and inhibition of replication and growth. This effect, where light modifies media components into toxicants, has been shown by others [69, 70, 72].

Light has been shown to damage the gametes or embryos of rabbits [73], hamster [74–77], and mouse [78]. Even though bovine embryos show no negative growth effects from light exposure, they do show higher levels of the inducible stress protein, HSP70 [79].

The spectrum of light that appears to be most damaging is the visible blue to ultraviolet light (range of 445–500 nm, Fig. 76.3). No studies to date have examined the wavelengths that might damage DNA in human gametes or embryos, but UVB radiation (290–300 nm) has been shown to damage the

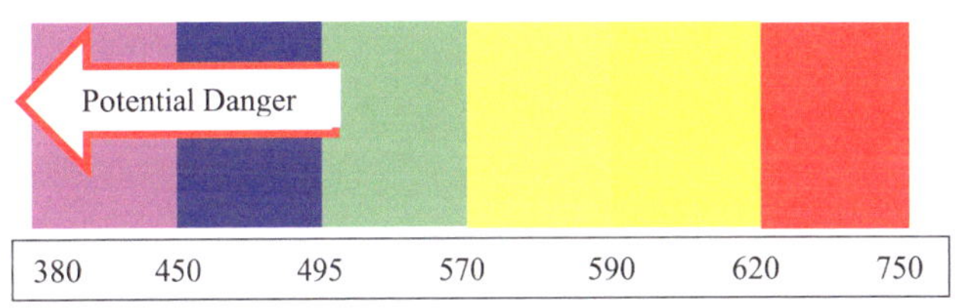

Fig. 76.3 The visible light wavelength (nm)

DNA of sea urchin embryos [80] and damage proteins and membrane lipids [81]. A cascade reaction of peroxides can be initiated by exposure to light and/or heat, resulting in the production of water-soluble toxicants in culture droplets [82–84].

76.4 Conclusion

While there is substantial evidence that light can be harmful to non-primate mammalian gametes and embryos, there is little conclusive evidence that light is harmful to human gametes or embryos. Light can affect the quality of oil and culture media, by modifying oil and media components, including buffers such as HEPES. The most damaging spectrum of light appears to be in the blue visible and ultraviolet spectrum (<500 nm). By including antioxidants or by excluding photooxidative media components, it may be possible to reduce the effects of light on embryos. Reducing the amount of harmful wavelengths in IVF laboratories via limited exposure to any light, use of ambient light filters, and avoidance of fluorescent lighting may also minimize these negative effects of light.

When constructing an embryology laboratory, care should be taken to avoid direct sunlight. This may necessitate the covering of any exterior windows with reflecting film. Hood lights, ambient lights, headlamps, and microscope lamps should be used sparingly. A green bypass filter might be useful to minimize potential damage from microscope lights. Recent developments in time-lapse imaging mean that it is now even more important to understand the role light might play in growing human embryos in vitro.

References

1. Winkler M. Regulation of protein synthesis in sea urchin eggs by intracellular pH. Kroc Found Ser. 1982;15:325–40.
2. Gerson DF. Intracellular pH: its measurement, regulation and utilization in cellular functions. New York: Alan R. Liss; 1982. p. 375–83.
3. Condeelis JS, Taylor DL. The contractile basis of amoeboid movement: the control of gelation, solation, and contraction in extracts from dictyostelium discoideum. J Cell Biol. 1977 Sep 1;74(3):901–27.
4. Gillies RJ, Deamer DW. Intracellular pH changes during the cell cycle in Tetrahymena. J Cell Physiol. 1979 Jul 1;100(1):23–31.
5. Roos A, Boron WF. Intracellular pH. Physiol Rev. 1981 Apr;61(2):296–434.
6. David A, Serr DM, Czernobilsky B. Chemical composition of human oviduct fluid. Fertil Steril. 1973 Jun;24(6):435–9.
7. Dale B, Menezo Y, Cohen J, DiMatteo L, Wilding M. Intracellular pH regulation in the human oocyte. Hum Reprod. 1998 Apr;13(4):964–70.
8. Buster JE, Bustillo M, Rodi A, Cohen S, Hamiltion M, Simon J, et al. Biologic and morphologic development of donated human ova recovered by nonsurgical uterine lavage. Am J Obstet Gynecol. 1985;153(2):211–7.
9. Carson SA, Smith A, Scoggan J, Buster JE. Superovulation fails to increase blastocyst yield after uterine lavage. Prenat Diagn. 1991;11(8):513–22.
10. Formigli L, Roccio C, Stangalini A, Coglitore M, Formigli G. Non-surgical flushing of the uterus for pre-embryo recovery: possible clinical applications. Hum Reprod. 1990;5(3):329–35.
11. Yedwab GA, Paz G, Homonnai TZ, David MP, Kraicer PF. The temperature, pH, and partial pressure of oxygen in the cervix and uterus of women and uterus of rats during the cycle. Fertil Steril. 1976 Mar;27(3):304–9.
12. Phillips KP, Leveille M-C, Claman P, Baltz JM. Intracellular pH regulation in human preimplantation embryos. Hum Reprod. 2000;15(4):896–904.
13. Edwards LJ, Williams DA, Gardner DK. Intracellular pH of the mouse preimplantation embryo: amino acids act as buffers of intracellular pH. Hum Reprod. 1998 Dec;13(12):3441–8.
14. Lane M, Lyons EA, Bavister BD. Cryopreservation reduces the ability of hamster 2-cell embryos to regulate intracellular pH. Hum Reprod. 2000 Feb;15(2):389–94.
15. Quinn P, Kerin JF, Warnes GM. Improved pregnancy rate in human in vitro fertilization with the use of a medium based on the composition of human tubal fluid. Fertil Steril. 1985 Oct 1;44(4):493–8.
16. Gardner DK. Mammalian embryo culture in the absence of serum or somatic cell support. Cell Biol Int. 1994 Dec;18(12):1163–79.
17. Gardner DK, Lane M. Alleviation of the "2-cell block" and development to the blastocyst of CF1 mouse embryos: role of amino acids, EDTA and physical parameters. Hum Reprod. 1996 Dec;11(12):2703–12.
18. Pool TB. Optimizing pH in clinical IVF. Clin Embryol. 2004;7:1–7.
19. Francis GL. Albumin and mammalian cell culture: implications for biotechnology applications. Cytotechnology. 2010 Jan;62(1):1–16.
20. Lane M. Mechanisms for managing cellular and homeostatic stress in vitro. Theriogenology. 2001;93(5):225–36.
21. Swain JE, Pool TB. New pH-buffering system for media utilized during gamete and embryo manipulations for assisted reproduction. Reprod Biomed Online. 2009;18(6):799–810.
22. Steel T, Conaghan J. pH equilibration dynamics of culture medium under oil. Fertil Steril. 2008 Apr 1;89(4):S27.
23. Leese HL. Metabolism of the preimplantation embryo: 40 years on. Reproduction. 2012;143:417–27.
24. Leese HL, Baumann CG, Brison D, McEvoy TG, Sturmey RG. Metabolism of the viable embryo: quietness revisited. Mol Hum Reprod. 2008;14(12):667–72.
25. Menezo Y, Lichtblau I, Elder K. New insights into human preimplantation metabolism in vivo and in vitro. J Assist Reprod Genet. 2013;30:293–303.
26. Wale PL, Gardner DK. The effects of chemical and physical factors on mammalian embryo culture and their importance for the practice of assisted human reproduction. Hum Reprod Update. 2016;22(1):2–22.
27. Pincus GG. The eggs of mammals. New York: The Macmillan Company; 1936. p. 159.
28. Brinster RL. In vitro culture of mammalian embryos. J Anim Sci. 1968:1–14.
29. Alliston C, Howarth B, Ulberg L. Embryonic mortality following culture in vitro for one- and wo-cell rabbit eggs at elevated temperatures. J Reprod Fertil. 1965;9:337–41.
30. Vogel B, Wagner H, Gmoser J, Worner A, Loschberger A, Peters L, et al. Touch-free measurement of body temperature using close-up thermography of the ocular surface. MethodsX. 2016;3:407–16.
31. Ng KYB, Mingels R, Morgan H, Macklon N, Cheong Y. In vivo oxygen, temperature and pH dynamics in the female reproductive tract and their importance in human conception: a systematic review. Hum Reprod Update. 2018;24(1):15–34.
32. Hunter R. Temperature gradients in female reproductive tissues. Reprod Biomed Online. 2012;24:377–80.

33. Hunter R. Temperature gradients in female reproductive tissues and their potential significance. Anim Reprod. 2009;6(1):7–15.
34. Perez-Cerezales S, Boryshpolets S, Afanzar O, Brandis A, Nevo R, Kiss V, et al. Involvement of opsins in mammalian sperm thermotaxis. Sci Rep. 2015;5:16146.
35. El-Sheikh Ali H, Kitahara G, Tamura Y, Kobayashi I, Hammi K, Torisu S, et al. Presence of a temperature gradient among genital tract portions and the thermal changes within these portions over the estrous cycle in beef cows. J Assist Reprod Dev. 2013;59(1):59–65.
36. McCulloh D. Quality control: maintaining stability in the laboratory. In: Textbook of assisted reproductive techniques, volume one: laboratory perspectives. London: Informa Healthcare; 2012. p. 9–30.
37. Elder K, Van den Bergh M, Woodward B. Temperature control in the IVF laboratory. In: Troubleshooting and problem-solving in the IVF laboratory. Cambridge: Cambridge University Press; 2015. p. 79–103.
38. Lenz R, Ball G, Leibfried M, Ax R, First N. In vitro maturation and fertilization of bovine oocytes are temperature-dependent processes. Biol Reprod. 1983;29:173–9.
39. The Handbook of Andrology. Second. Lawrence, Kansas: Allen Press; 2010.
40. Foote RH. The history of artificial insemination: selected notes and notables. J Anim Sci. 2002;80:1–10.
41. Rehman RU, Zhao C, Shah MA, Qureshi MS, Wang X. Semen extenders and artificial insemination in ruminants. Veterinaria. 2013;1(1):1–8.
42. Riel JM, Yamauchi Y, Huang TT, Grove J, Ward MA. Short-term storage of human spermatozoa in electrolyte-free medium without freezing maintains sperm chromatin integrity better than cryopreservation. Biol Reprod. 2011;85(3):536–47.
43. Said A-H, Reed ML. Increased count, motility, and total motile sperm cells collected across three consecutive ejaculations within 24 h of oocyte retrieval: implications for management of men presenting with low numbers of motile sperm for assisted reproduction. J Assist Reprod Genet. 2015;32(7):1049–55.
44. Pickering SJ, Braude PR, Johnson MH, Cant A, Currie J. Transient cooling to room temperature can cause irreversible disruption of the meiotic spindle in the human oocyte. Fertil Steril. 1990;54(1):102–8.
45. Sathananthan AH, Kirby C, Trounson A, Philopatos D, Shaw J. The effects of cooling mouse oocytes. J Assist Reprod Dev. 1992;9:139–48.
46. Zenzes MT, Bielecki R, Casper RF, Leibo S. Effects of chilling to 0C on the morphology of meiotic spindles in the human metaphase II oocyte. Fertil Steril. 2001;75(4):769–77.
47. Wang W-H, Meng L, Hackett RJ, Odenbourg R, Keefe DL. Limited recovery of meiotic spindles in living human oocytes after cooling-rewarming observed using polarized light microscopy. Hum Reprod Update. 2001;16(11):2374–8.
48. Wang W-H, Meng L, Hackett RJ, Odenbourg R, Keefe DL. Rigorous thermal control during intracytoplasmic sperm injection stabilizes the meiotic spindle and improves fertilization and pregnancy rates. Fertil Steril. 2002;77(6):1274–7.
49. Almeida P, Bolton V. The effect of temperature fluctuations on the cytoskeletal organization and chromosomal constitution of the human oocyte. Zygote. 1995;3(4):357–65.
50. Sun X-F, Wang W-H, Keefe DL. Overheating is detrimental to meiotic spindles within in vitro matured human oocytes. Zygote. 2004;12(1):65–70.
51. Yang C-R, Miao D-Q, Zhang Q-H, Guo L, Tong J-S, Wei Y, et al. Short-term preservation of porcine oocytes in ambient temperature: novel approaches. PLoS One. 2010;5(12):e14242.
52. Foss R, Ortis H, Hinrichs K. Effect of potential oocyte transport protocols on blastocyst rates after intracytoplasmic sperm injection in the horse. Equine Vet J. 2013;45:39–43.
53. Maurer RR. Storage of mammalian oocytes and embryos: a review. Can J Anim Sci. 1976;56:131–45.
54. Kamimura E, Nakashima T, Ogawa M, Ohwada K, Nakagata N. Study of low-temperature (4C) transport of mouse two-cell embryos enclosed in oviducts. Comp Med. 2003;53(4):393–6.
55. Balasubramanian S, Rho G-J. Effect of chilling on the development of in vitro produced bovine embryos at various cleavage stages. J Assit Reprod Genet. 2006;23(2):55–61.
56. Ideta A, Aoyagi Y, Tsuchiya K, Kamijima T, Nishimiya Y, Tsuda S. A simple medium enables bovine embryos to be held for seven days at 4C. Sci Rep. 2013;3:1173.
57. Grau N, Aparicio B, Escrich L, Mercader A, Delgado A, Remohi J, et al. Short-term storage of tripronucleated human embryos. J Assist Reprod Genet. 2013;30:1043–7.
58. Bareh G, Robinson R, Knudtson J, Retzloff M, Neal G, Pool T. Frozen embryo transfer outcomes between embryos from a satellite facility transported to the central facility prior to cryopreservation versus those from the central lab immediately cryopreserved. Fertil Steril. 2013;100(3):S175.
59. Hong KH, Lee H, Forman EJ, Upham KM, Scott RJ. Examining the temperature of embryo culture in in vitro fertilization: a randomized controlled trial comparing traditional core temperature (37C) to a more physiologic, cooler temperature (36C). Fertil Steril. 2014;102:767–73.
60. Hansen PJ. Effects of heat stress on mammalian reproduction. Philos Trans R Soc B. 2009;364:3341–50.
61. Lavy G, Diamond MP, Pellicer A, Vaughn WK, DeCherney AH. The effect of the incubation temperature on the cleavage rate of mouse embryos in vitro. J In Vitro Fert Embryo Transf. 1988;5(3):167–70.
62. Sakatani M. Effects of heat stress on bovine preimplantation embryos produced in vitro. J Assist Reprod Dev. 2017;63(4):347–52.
63. Sakatani M, Bonilla L, Dobbs KB, Block J, Ozawa M, Shanker S, et al. Changes in the transcriptome of morula-stage bovine embryos caused by heat shock: relationship to developmental acquisition of thermotolerance. Reprod Biol Endocrinol. 2013;11:3.
64. Choi I, Dasari A, Kim N-H, Campbell KH. Effects of prolonged exposure of mouse embryos to elevated temperatures on embryonic developmental competence. Reprod Biomed Online. 2015;31:171–9.
65. Youssef A, Kandil M, Makhlouf A, Habib D, Mesiano S, Liu J, et al. Impact of incubation temperature on mouse embryo development. Fertil Steril. 2016;105(2):e45.
66. Edwards RG. New concepts in embryonic growth and implantation. Hum Reprod. 1998;13(Suppl 3):271–82.
67. Otsuki J, Nagai Y, Chiba K. Damage of embryo development caused by peroxidized mineral oil and its association with albumin in culture. Fertil Steril. 2009 May;91(5):1745–9.
68. Hill R Jr, Bensch K, King DW. Photosensitization of nucleic acids and proteins: the photodynamic action of acridine orange on living cells in culture. Exp Cell Res. 1960;21:106–17.
69. Stoien J, Wang R. Effect of near-ultraviolet and visible light on mammalian cells in culture II. Formation of toxic photoproducts in tissue culture medium by black light. PNAS. 1974;71:3961–5.
70. Wang R. Lethal effect of "daylight" fluorescent light on human cells in tissue-culture medium. Photochem Photobiol. 1975;21:373–5.
71. Wang R, Nixon B. Identification of hydrogen peroxide as a photoproduct toxic to human cells in tissue-culture medium irradiated with "daylight" fluorescent light. In Vitro. 1978;14:715–22.
72. Zigler J, Lepe-Zuniga J, Vistica B, Gery I. Analysis of the cytotoxic effects of light-exposed hepes-containing culture medium. In Vitro Cell Dev Biol Plant. 1985;1:282–7.
73. Daniel J. Cleavage of mammalian ova inhibited by visible light. Nature. 1964;201:316–7.
74. Yamauchi Y, Yanagimachi R, Horiuchi T. Full-term development of golden hamster oocytes following intracytoplasmic sperm injection. Biol Reprod. 2002;67:534–9.

75. Hirao Y, Yanagimachi R. Detrimental effect of visible light on meiosis of mammalian eggs in vitro. J Exp Zool. 1978;206:365–9.
76. Umaoka Y, Noda Y, Nakayama T, Narimoto K, Mori T, Iritani A. Effect of visual light on in vitro embryonic development in the hamster. Theriogenology. 1992;38:1043–4.
77. Oh S, Gong S, Lee S, Lee E, Lim J. Light intensity and wavelength during embryo manipulation are important factors for maintaining viability of preimplantation embryos in vitro. Fertil Steril. 2007;88:1150–7.
78. Takenaka M, Horiuchi T, Yanagimachi R. Effects of light on development of mammalian zygotes. PNAS. 2007;104:14289–93.
79. Korhonen K, Sjovall S, Viitanen J, Ketoja E, Makarevich A, Peippo J. Viability of bovine embryos following exposure to the green filtered or wider bandwidth light during in vitro embryo production. Hum Reprod. 2009;24:308–14.
80. Lesser M, Kruse V, Barry T. Exposure to ultraviolet radiation causes apoptosis in developing sea urchin embryos. J Exp Biol. 2003;206:4097–103.
81. Halliwell B. Reactive oxygen species antioxidants. Redox biology is a fundamental theme of aerobic life. Plant Physiol. 2006;141:312–22.
82. Otsuki J, Nagai Y, Chiba K. Damage of embryo development caused by peroxidized mineral oil and its association with albumin in culture. Fertil Steril. 2009;91:1745–9.
83. Otsuki J, Nagai Y, Chiba K. Peroxidation of mineral oil used in droplet culture is detrimental to fertilization and embryo development. Fertil Steril. 2007;88:741–3.
84. Provo M, Herr C. Washed paraffin oil becomes toxic to mouse embryos upon exposure to sunlight. Theriogenology. 1998;49:214.

77 A Comparison of Embryo Culture Incubators for the IVF Laboratory

Jason E. Swain

77.1 Introduction

Minimizing environmental stressors and reducing variability during embryo culture are required to achieve optimal embryo development and maximize assisted reproductive technology (ART) outcomes. Key environmental variables to consider include carbon dioxide levels/pH of the culture medium, temperature stability, oxygen concentration, media evaporation/osmolality, and air quality. Importantly, all of these potential environmental stressors and others can be impacted or regulated by the laboratory incubator, which house gametes/embryos for the majority of their time in vitro. As a result, incubators are likely the most important pieces of equipment within the IVF laboratory, maintaining environmental stability within the culture system. As a result, incubator selection and proper use/management are critical for success of an IVF program.

With advances in manufacturing and technology, several incubator models now exist with varying capacities and capabilities and differing methods of controlling their internal environment (Table 77.1). This results in an increasing complexity when attempting to select an appropriate culture incubator for the IVF laboratory.

77.2 Incubator Function

The primary function of an incubator within the IVF laboratory is to provide a stable environment to hold gametes and embryos during their culture and development in vitro. To achieve this goal, an incubator must regulate several environmental variables, including gas concentrations (oxygen and carbon dioxide), temperature, and humidity. This must be done in a clean environment free of contamination and volatile organic compounds (VOCs), which can impair development. Importantly, a variety of methods are utilized by different incubators to maintain this stability. Additionally, considerations exist before selection and implementation of an incubator into the IVF laboratory.

77.2.1 Gas Atmosphere and Sensors

A primary function of a laboratory incubator is to consistently and reliably provide the appropriate gas atmosphere. Specifically, regulation of the concentration of carbon dioxide (CO_2) is of paramount importance, as this gas helps regulate the pH of the culture medium. The pH of media is an important variable that can significantly impact gamete function and embryo development [1–4].

Modern embryo culture incubators must also be able to provide an environment with a reduced concentration of oxygen (O_2). While atmospheric O_2 concentration is ~21%, it has long been shown that a reduced incubator oxygen concentration of ~5% during preimplantation embryo development is beneficial for embryo development and live birth in a variety of animal species, as well as human [5–7], most notably when used throughout the entire culture period to the blastocyst stage [8–10]. Reduced O_2 concentration is most commonly achieved by supplying a balance of nitrogen gas to displace atmospheric O_2 to achieve the desired O_2 concentration within the incubator. Whether a further reduction in O_2 concentration <5% is beneficial for human embryos is unknown but an active area of ongoing research [11, 12].

Rapid and accurate measurement of CO_2 and O_2 concentrations by the incubator is required to achieve target set points in a timely fashion and ensure appropriate growth conditions are maintained. Paramount to this essential function is the type of sensor installed. The two primary methods used in IVF incubators to monitor CO_2 concentration include thermal conductivity (TC) or infrared (IR) sensors (Fig. 77.1).

TC sensors operate via measurement of resistance between two thermistors, with one enclosed within an impermeable chamber and the other exposed to the incubator

J. E. Swain (✉)
CCRM IVF Network, Lone Tree, CO, USA
e-mail: jswain@ccrmivf.com

G. N. Allahbadia et al. (eds.), *Textbook of Assisted Reproduction*, https://doi.org/10.1007/978-981-15-2377-9_77

Table 77.1 Incubator technology variables that should be considered when evaluating and selecting a unit for the laboratory

	Gas type	CO_2 sensor	O_2 sensor	Temperature	Volume[a,b]	Humidity	Contamination control[d,e]	Other
Options	– CO_2-only – Low O_2 mixer – Low O_2 premixed cylinder	– IR – TC	–Zirconium – Galvanic (Fuel cell)	– Air jacket – Water jacket – Direct heat	– Benchtop 2-chamber Multichamber Other (i.e., timelapse) – Small-box – Large-box	– Yes[c] – No	– Heat – Internal UV – H_2O_2 – Copper alloy – External/internal HEPA – External/Internal VOC filter	– Data logging – Cost – Patient capacity – Service – Technology integration (dynamic culture, time-lapse cameras, alarm connectivity, real-time pH sensors, etc.)

[a]Actual volumes will vary from unit to unit
[b]Other novel designs exist, but these are general terms to refer to the most commonly used incubators in the IVF lab
[c]Some units bubble gas through a water pan to expedite re-humidification
[d]Ease of removing inner parts and/or wiping interior also is important to consider
[e]Presence/absence of an internal fan or other features may influence

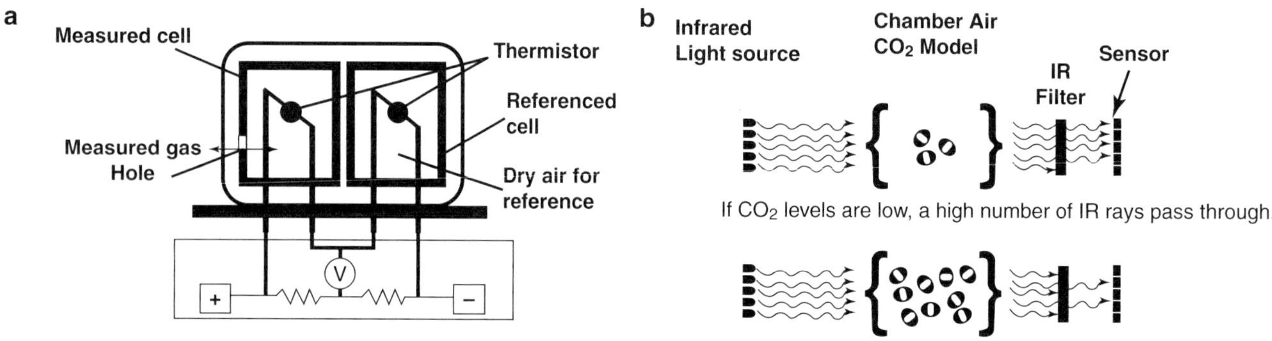

Fig. 77.1 Types of CO_2 sensors commonly used in culture incubators. (**a**) TC and (**b**) IR sensors

chamber [13]. The presence of CO_2 in the incubator chamber changes the resistance between the two thermistors and permits measurement of gas concentrations. Importantly, temperature and humidity impact the resistance of TC sensors and impact their measurements.

In contrast to TC sensor, IR sensors are largely independent of both humidity and temperature. IR sensors emit light and utilize specialized optics to detect IR light absorbance, which is relative to the levels of CO_2 inside the incubator chamber [14]. Thus, compared to IR sensors, incubators utilizing TC sensors tend to take a longer period of time to measure and therefore stabilize CO_2 levels following door openings since the gas concentrations cannot be fully determined and subsequently adjusted until both temperature and humidity stabilize. Due to reduction in cost and improvements to IR sensor lifespan, many embryo specific/modern IVF laboratory incubators utilize IR sensors and have become the preferred option for use.

Similar to incubator CO_2 sensors, two primary types of gas sensor are used to assess incubator O_2 concentration. These two types of O_2 sensors are galvanic/fuel cell or zirconium sensors [15] (Fig. 77.2). Though modern galvanic sensors have improved the rapidness of their responsiveness, they still tend to have slower response times compared to zirconium sensors. Additionally, compared to zirconium sensors, galvanic sensors tend to require more frequent replacement to ensure proper function.

Importantly, for both incubator O_2 and CO_2 readings, external incubator digital displays should not be solely relied upon to indicate rapidness of atmospheric recovery times during re-equilibration. Some incubator models are programmed to display their programmed set points prior to achieving re-equilibration of internal gas concentrations. If trying to assess environmental stability or speed of atmospheric recovery in IVF incubator chambers, the use of an independent measuring device placed within the incubator chamber is recommended for a more accurate assessment or comparison. These independent measuring devices may include independent gas sensors like fyrite or as part of an alarm system. Additionally, real-time pH meters may offer accurate assessment of CO_2 gas recovery (Fig. 77.3).

It should also be mentioned that accurate gas levels can be achieved in the absence of gas sensors or without gas mixers inside the incubator through use of cylinders of medical grade premixed gas. These premixed gases can be supplied directly to an incubator or to a sealed modular chamber placed inside the incubator, rather than requiring the incubator to have an internal gas mixer to adjust the gases into the proper ratios. Using this premixed gas approach, appropriate CO_2/O_2 concentrations are quickly achieved as soon as the

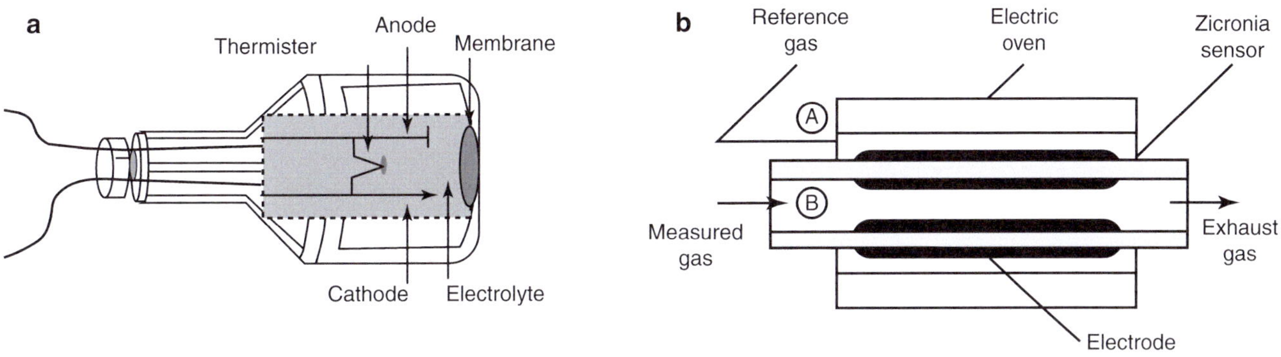

Fig. 77.2 Types of O_2 sensors commonly used in culture incubators. (**a**) Galvanic/fuel cells and (**b**) zirconium

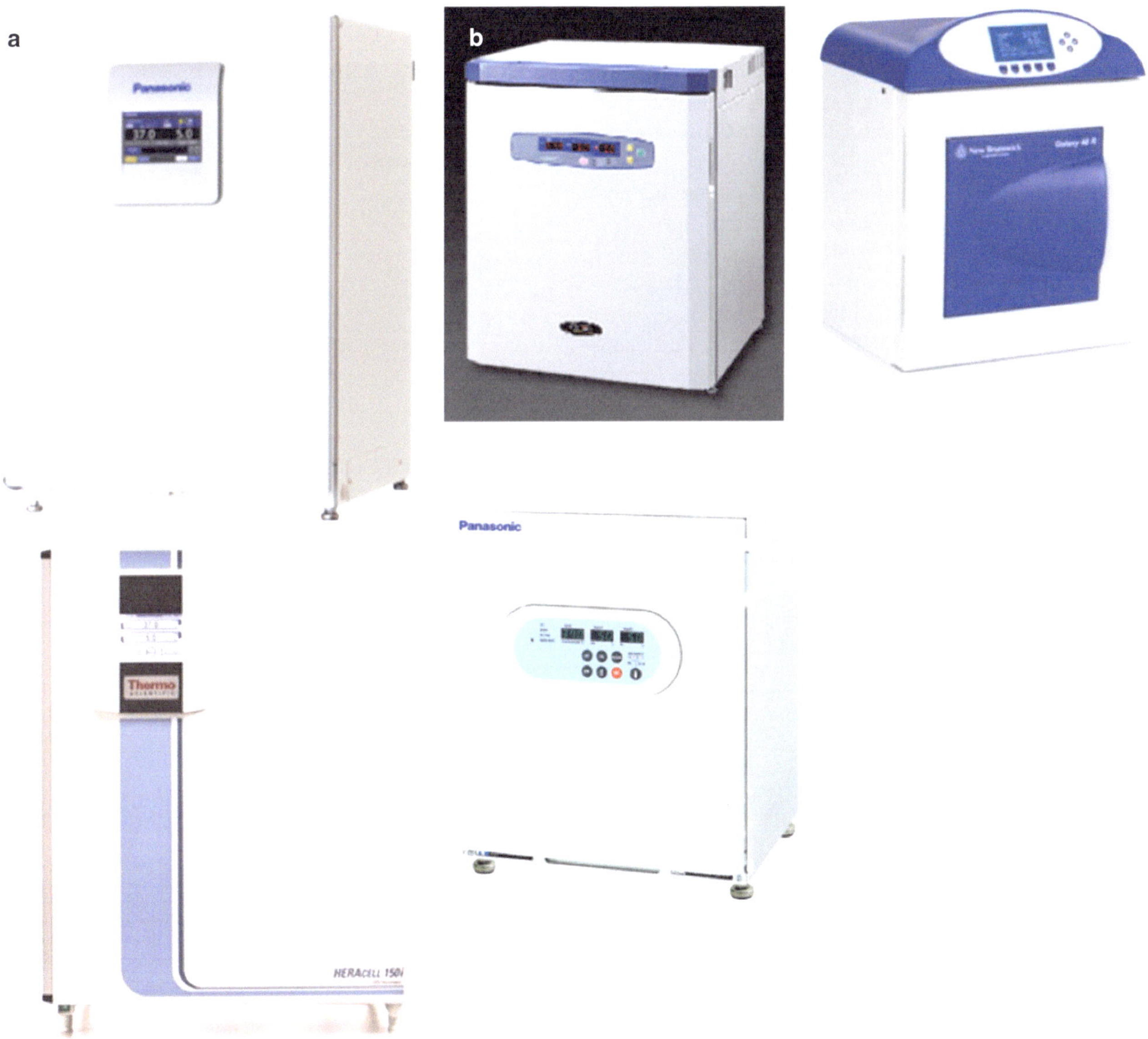

Fig. 77.3 Type of incubators commonly found in IVF laboratories. (**a**) Large-box incubators can vary in size but are generally ~150 L. (**b**) Small-box incubators generally range in size from around 30–55 L

incubator volume has been filled with the premixed gas. Importantly, implementation of proper quality control is essential to ensure that the premixed gas concentrations/ratios inside the gas cylinder yield the appropriate/desired pH and growth conditions in the culture medium required by the particular laboratory. Factors such as the media used, protein type and concentration, and laboratory elevation above sea level will dictate what CO_2 concentration is required to obtain the desired media pH.

77.2.2 Incubator Chamber Size and Number

Chamber volume and the number of chambers are important factors to consider for incubator function and selection. Regardless of the gas sensor used or method of gas supply, incubator chamber volume influences gas equilibration and recovery timing. With door openings, traditional "large-box" incubators (~150–200 L) may require an extended time to refill with CO_2 and/or nitrogen gases. "Small-box" incubators (~14–50 L) have received increased use in IVF laboratories. Depending on the laboratory workflow, these smaller incubators may help improve gas recovery and reduce environmental stress, leading to improved outcomes compared to large-box incubators [16]. In cases of "box-type" incubators, often one patient is placed per shelf, and these units are useful for equilibration of media and holding test tubes for process like sperm preparation.

New incubators now being commonly used include benchtop/top load units of varying sizes/configurations. These incubators are designed specifically for clinical IVF and have extremely small chambers (~0.3–0.5 L), further improving atmospheric/environmental recovery time (Table 77.2). These modern benchtop incubators often provide several individual chambers for single patient use (Fig. 77.4).

Table 77.2 Types of modern benchtop IVF incubators and humidity options

Make/model	Type	Controlled humidity
K-systems G210	Multichamber	No
K-systems G185	Multichamber	No
Astec EC-6S	Multichamber	No
Astec EC-9	Multichamber	No
ESCO Miri Multiroom	Multichamber	No
IKS DS-1	Multichamber	Option yes
Synvivo CNC-I091	Multichamber	No
ESCO Miri TL	Timelapse	No
Vitrolife Embryoscope	Timelapase	No
Vitrolife Embryoscope plus	Timelapse	No
Genea Biomedx Geri	Timelapse	Option yes
Cook K-MINC	Dual chamber	Yes
Planer BT-37/INC-A20	Dual chamber	Yes
Labotect Labo C-Top	Dual chamber	Yes
Astec IVF Cube	Multichamber removeable	Yes
Planer CT37stax	Multichamber removeable	Yes

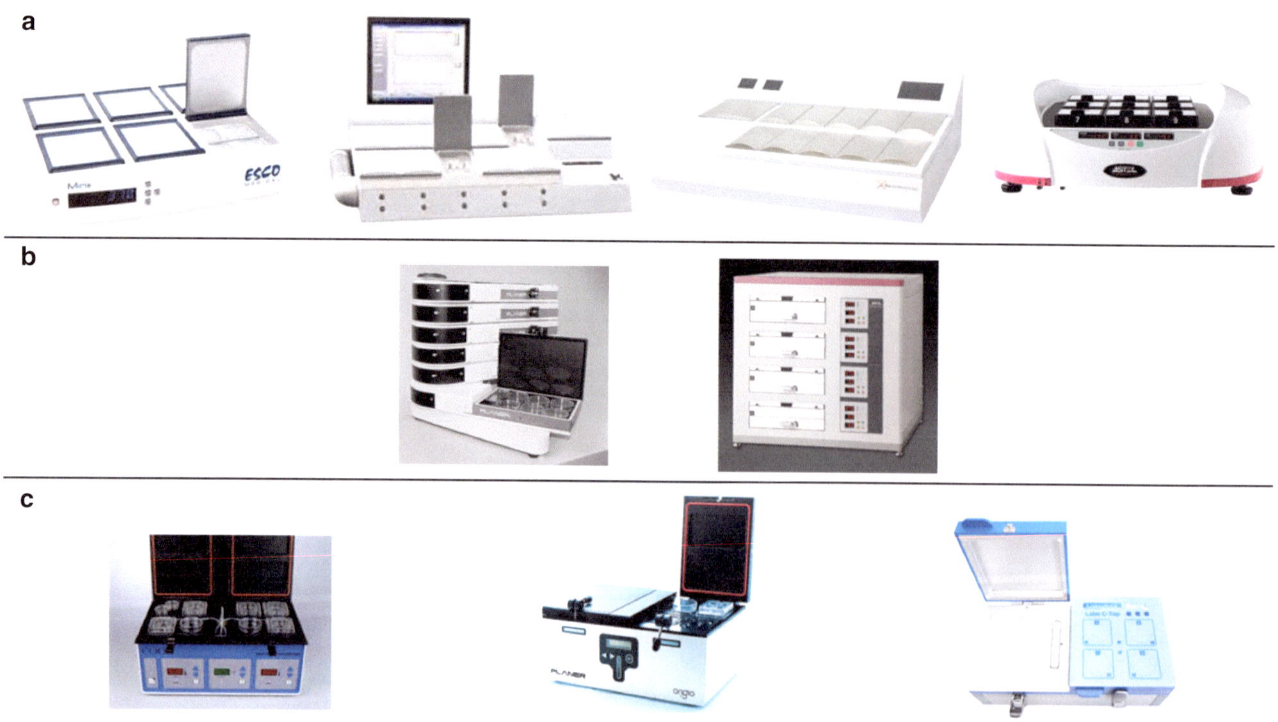

Fig. 77.4 A variety of modern benchtop incubators commercially available for use in IVF laboratories. Size, number of chambers, and various accessories vary between systems. (**a**) multichamber systems, (**b**) multichamber systems with removable incubator boxes, and (**c**) dual-chamber systems

A mixture of incubator types is often useful within the IVF laboratory, and, as will be discussed, incubator management is a key component for optimized incubator function regardless of chamber number or size.

77.2.3 Air Filtration and Quality

Another variable relevant to incubator gas atmosphere that impacts functional capability is air quality. Air quality, specifically the presence and amount of volatile organic compounds (VOCs), may negatively impact preimplantation embryo development [17–20], though relevant levels of VOCs are still unknown. As a result, most laboratories have dedicated air handling systems to filter out particulates, as well as VOCs, and various studies indicate a benefit to embryo development and/or outcomes once air quality is improved [20, 21]. However, while air quality inside the main IVF laboratory is important, the quality of the air/atmosphere inside the incubator chamber itself is of greater concern.

Background laboratory air quality will impact on the atmospheric quality within the incubator, especially in CO_2-only incubators, which carry a balance of ~94% room air. However, the quality of gas from the supply tanks must also be considered, especially in low O_2 incubators, which flood their interiors with nitrogen from these tanks to reduce O_2 levels to ~5%. VOCs have been detected in gas supply tanks used for IVF incubators [18]. In these cases, filtering the supply gases through inline filters prior to incubator entry may be an effective approach to improving incubator atmosphere. These inline filters contain HEPA (high-efficiency particulate air) filtration to reduce particle counts. Furthermore, additional filter methods to reduce VOCs include activated charcoal or potassium permanganate. At least one preliminary study showed improvement in embryo development following implementation of inline gas VOC filters [22].

Placement of specialized VOC filtration units inside incubators may also improve air quality and outcomes [19, 23, 24], though this is not always the case [25–27]. Their effectiveness depends on their size, and fitting into smaller incubators may be problematic. An emerging approach to improve air quality that is now being added to some incubators includes recirculating atmosphere via an ultraviolet light source to reduce possible microbials and to photocatalytically breakdown VOCs [28, 29].

It should be mentioned that incubators that utilize cylinders of premixed gas have the ability to filter the entirety of the gas supply prior to entering the incubator chamber. By contrast, incubators that mix the gases themselves, such as either CO_2-only or low O_2 incubators, have at least some portion of room air present, though if room air is of high quality this likely poses little problem. Also, it is important to note that the plasticware or internal incubator components may "off-gas" inside the elevated temperatures of the incubator chamber [17]. Thus, despite having acceptable outside air quality or a prefiltered gas supply, VOCs may still be present inside an incubator. In these cases, proper initial cleaning of incubators and off-gassing of devices and supplies may help address concerns. Additionally, placement of modular VOC filter units in the incubator chamber or recirculation of chamber atmosphere through external filters may also be effective.

77.2.4 Temperature Regulation and Stability

It is well-known that temperature can impact various aspects of gamete and embryo function, most notably meiotic spindle stability in the oocyte [30–32], possibly embryo metabolism [33] and mitotic cell division timings [34]. However, data indicate that temperature gradients may exist in the female reproductive tract [35–37]. Thus, while the optimal target temperature for IVF incubators that contain varying cell types and embryos at different developmental stages is still unknown [27, 38], maintaining a controlled/stable temperature inside the incubator while cells are inside is mandatory for reducing harmful environmental stress.

Three primary methods of heating are utilized in IVF incubators. Two methods, used primarily in box-type incubators, include a water jacket or air jacket, both of which warm the air in the incubator chamber and may or may not include an internal fan to circulate. The third heating method used by primarily newer IVF-specific benchtop/top load units entails contact of the warmed incubator surface and direct heat transfer to the culture dish and enclosed medium. Some incubators may warm the base of the chamber, while others may warm the tops and bases. Importantly, each of the three warming methods utilized in culture incubators has benefits and limitations.

Water-jacketed incubators retain heat for longer during incubator openings or power failure. However, these units are heavy, tend to have a higher power consumption, and may burden emergency power supplies. There are also concerns that contamination may originate from inside the water jacket. Conversely, air-jacketed incubators warm up quickly but do not retain heat for long periods with interrupted power supply. The third heating approach, utilizing direct heat/contact, results in very rapid heat recovery following opening of the incubator, but similar to air-jacketed units, maintaining this temperature for any period of time during power interruption can be problematic.

Importantly, temperature gradients can exist inside any type of incubator, regardless of the type of warming approach employed. Such gradients are most common in box-type incubators utilizing water or air jackets. A preliminary report indicated slight temperature variations when culture dishes were placed in various locations within a large-box water-jacketed incubator, with measurements varying between 36.97, 37.17, and 37.23 °C [39]. Whether such minor fluctuations are detrimental is unknown, but independent temperature measurement between shelves on box-type units, known as temperature-mapping, is recommended. Furthermore, verifying the temperature between individual culture chambers or across warmed surfaces of various benchtop/top load unit configurations can give critical information on temperature accuracy and stability that could impact gamete and embryo development and function.

77.2.5 Humidity and Evaporation

Many incubators provide an elevated humidity in order to reduce media evaporation from the higher incubation temperature during culture. This helps avoid detrimental rises in medium osmolality that can compromise preimplantation embryo development [40, 41]. Humidification inside the incubator is usually achieved in a passive fashion, via evaporation or bubbling inlet gases through a water reservoir placed in the bottom of the incubator chamber. Importantly, the presence of a water reservoir for humidity is also a potential source of contamination and should be monitored with and water exchanged/replaced regularly.

It should be noted that humidity inside the incubator is not necessarily required to culture embryos. Many new IVF-specific benchtop incubators do not provide humidification (Table 77.2). If sufficient amounts of oil overlay are used and media is exchanged/replenished appropriately, high-quality embryo development in a non-humidified incubator is achievable. Importantly, evaporation of media can occur despite use of mineral oil overlay in non-humidified incubators [42]. Thus, variables such as volume of media and amount of oil and number of days of continuous culture should be considered and osmolality measured to confirm appropriateness of culture conditions. This is likely even more important with the increased use of single-step culture media and uninterrupted culture, where evaporation is more likely to occur over time.

Interestingly, a recent study indicated that humidification of a dry benchtop incubator resulted in improved embryo development compared to the totally dry incubator [43]. While evaporation of media was not assessed in this study, an increase in osmolality, or possibly even media pH, was assumed to be a possible cause. However, placement of water into a normally dry incubator can be problematic, due to condensation within the chamber and possible issues with internal electrical components that were not developed for use in a humidified environment.

77.2.6 Other Considerations

Other considerations for incubator selection include approaches available for cleaning and sterilization to reduce chances of contamination. Various incubators are constructed with copper-containing alloys, as copper can act as an antimicrobial and antifungal agent [44, 45]. However, at least one study suggested that oxidized copper particles from incubator walls may have detrimental effects on bovine embryo development [16], though the experimental design utilized prevented any conclusive correlation and several copper-containing incubators are used successfully for human embryo culture.

As an alternative for contamination control, some air-jacketed incubators feature heat decontamination cycling capability. Other incubator types can be outfitted with hydrogen peroxide sterilization capability by the manufacturer. Ultraviolet light treatment of water pans is also available to reduce incidence of contamination on some units, though this feature is often turned off to avoid possible damage to cells cultured inside the incubator. Most incubators can be sanitized and/or cleaned by removing inner pieces for autoclaving and wiping down the interior of the unit with embryo-safe products, such as hydrogen peroxide or other commercial IVF cleaning solutions, preferably with low VOC content. Incubators with fewer removable parts or lacking internal circulation fans are easier to clean and may help reduce the risk of contamination.

Daily monitoring for quality control/assurance is another consideration when selecting a laboratory incubator. When dealing with multiple chambers in a benchtop incubator, daily measurement of gas levels or temperatures in each chamber can be time-consuming. However, newer technologies are starting to address these issues, with the availability of small real-time temperature sensors for each chamber [46] or real-time pH sensors.

Incubator selection criteria include other practical items as well. These include the space occupied, the manner in which chamber doors open and close and latch, how gas concentrations may be measured, ability for incubators or chambers to be connected to the current alarm system, and availability of preventative maintenance and service. It is recommended that "demo" units of incubators be trialed or careful examination of units at exhibit halls or in other laboratories be conducted, prior to purchasing and clinical implementation.

77.3 Comparative Studies and Clinical Outcomes

Very few comparative studies examining environmental stability and recovery of particular incubator units exist in the peer reviewed literature, and even fewer studies exist comparing outcomes of embryo development or assisted reproductive outcomes. Furthermore, careful examination of the existing literature is required to understand why any reported differences may exist, and this scrutiny often points out limitations in study design that need to be considered when interpreting results.

A comparison of a small two chamber benchtop/top load units (~0.43 L) using direct heat versus a large-box (~170 L) incubator using a water jacket and no inner doors demonstrated a significantly faster recovery of temperature in the benchtop/top load, direct heat unit [47]. Temperature in the benchtop/top load unit recovered to 37 °C within 5.5–6.5 minutes, dependent upon the volume of medium tested, while the large-box incubator failed to reach the set point following a 20-min recovery (36.2 and 36.7 °C). Whether the same would hold true with an air-jacketed box-type incubator, small- or large-sized, or with units using sealed inner doors is unknown. Interestingly, the use of milled aluminum blocks to hold culture dishes within box-type incubators was able to help maintain stable temperature within the culture dish [47]. These data demonstrate the importance of proper incubator management in optimizing incubator stability and performance. Whether this would translate to differences in embryo development or clinical outcomes is unknown.

When comparing a small benchtop incubator unit with two top load chambers (~0.43 L) and a small-box incubator (~32 L), it was found that after a 5 s opening that the benchtop/top load unit had improved temperature recovery (5 min vs. 30 min) and O_2 recovery (3 min vs. 8 min), improved "good" early embryo development (40% vs. 38%), and improved "good" blastocyst formation (15% vs. 8%) [48]. Interestingly, this study measured O_2 recovery rather than CO_2 recovery. While O_2 and CO_2 will recover at the same rate in the benchtop unit due to using a premixed gas supply, O_2 will recover much more slowly than CO_2 in the box unit that uses separate gas supplies due to the larger amount of nitrogen needed in the larger volume. It is unknown if such large differences would exist if measuring CO_2, which is likely more important. Furthermore, in this case, the small-box unit was outfitted with outdated technology and utilized a TC CO_2 sensor and was water-jacketed. Whether the same differences would be apparent if using the faster IR CO_2 sensor and air-jacket heated unit is unknown. Importantly, no oil overlay was used in this study, and overall blastocyst conversion rates in both incubators were low. It is possible that the use of oil overlay would have stabilized pH and temperature and perhaps improved the suboptimal growth conditions. Thus, while the benchtop/top load unit likely recovered atmosphere and temperature more rapidly, a more thorough examination of the study design reveals that the discrepancies between the two incubators may not be as pronounced if using more modern/optimized approaches.

In another study, a box-type incubator and a small two-chambered benchtop/top load units were compared, examining the recovery of temperature, CO_2, and humidity. In addition, fertilization rate, embryo quality, clinical pregnancy, and implantation rates were compared between the incubator types [49]. Following a 10-s incubator opening, it was found that there was a significant difference in temperature recovery (1 min vs. 180 min), CO_2 recovery (8 min vs. 120 min), and humidity recovery (12 min vs. 180 min), with faster recovery occurring in the benchtop/top load unit. Of note, the large-box incubator was outfitted with non-airtight inner doors which may not provide a stable gas environment as newer incubator units which employ this stabilization measure. Additionally, large-box incubators used in the study utilized the slower TC sensor and were water-jacketed. Finally, the benchtop/top load unit utilized low O_2 culture via premixed gas, while the large-box incubator used CO_2 only. As previously mentioned, low O_2 appears to produce improved preimplantation embryo development and clinical outcomes compared to high oxygen culture [5–7]. Furthermore, the use of premixed medical gas in the benchtop/top load unit may provide improved air quality over use of ~94% room air in the large-box incubator. Support for this theory can be found in a preliminary study that compared the same type of large-box and a small benchtop/top load incubator. In this study, results indicated that indeed air quality/gas composition may be partially responsible for improved mouse blastocyst development observed in two out of five different culture media in the benchtop unit compared to the large-box incubator. Interestingly, it is unknown why the benefit was not observed in the all the media types, although other culture system variables may have existed between the incubators [50]. These same confounding variables in the culture system exist in another study that compared the same type of large-box and benchtop unit [51] and make it impossible to precisely assess the impact of the incubator as the sole factor. Despite the differences in the culture parameters and suboptimal culture conditions provided in the large box incubators in these studies, there were no reports of significant difference in human embryo development, clinical pregnancy, or implantation rates [49].

In a comparative study examining culture incubators using human donor oocytes, clinical outcomes between a benchtop/time-lapse incubator and a large-box incubator were assessed (large-box incubator size confirmed via personnel communication M. Cruz). Despite significant differences in embryo handling approaches, including an uninterrupted embryo culture paradigm in the benchtop incubator while handling/removing embryos at least twice from the large-box incubator, as well as use of low O_2 in the benchtop unit but high O_2 the large-box, no difference in blastocyst formation, blastocyst score/quality, or ongoing clinical pregnancy was reported [52]. Additionally, embryos were cultured individually in microdrops in the large-box incubator while being placed into individual microwells for the benchtop (pers. comm. M. Cruz). This difference in culture dishes is important to note because the type of culture

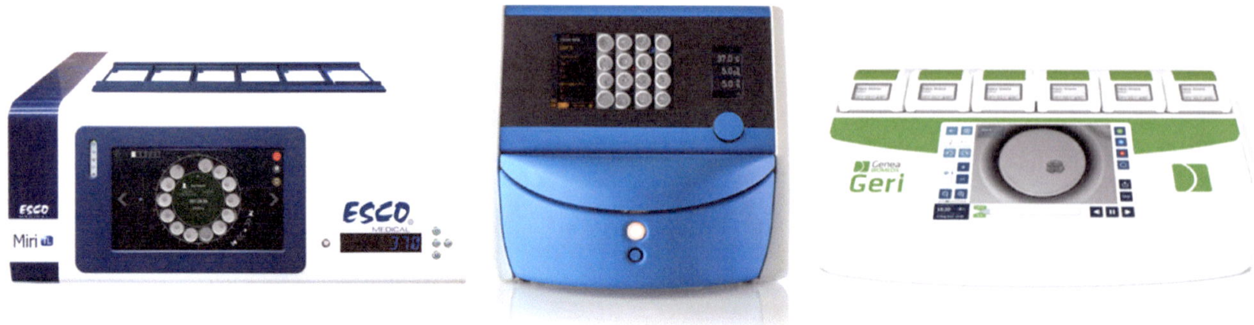

Fig. 77.5 Three modern incubators incorporating time-lapse imaging (TLI) that utilize individual chambers for each patient to provide environmental stability. Patient capacity and accessories available vary between systems

platform used can create unique microenvironments and differentially impact embryo development [53]. While no significant difference between the numbers of day 3 or day 5 transfers based on a particular incubator was reported (benchtop/time-lapse vs. box incubator) [52], upon reanalysis of the reported data using different statistical software, it appears that more day 5 transfers were performed from the larger box-incubator (34/58) compared to the smaller time-lapse incubator (19/50). It is a common practice for day 5 transfer to be dictated by superior quality or quantity of available embryos though no differences in clinical outcomes were reported. Thus, the use of smaller benchtop incubators does not necessarily equate to better embryo quality, as several other culture system variables are can impact development (Fig. 77.5).

Another published report compared a benchtop/time-lapse incubator versus a standard large-box unit (large-box incubator size confirmed via pers. comm. J. Hindkjær) using the key performance indicators of embryo development, clinical pregnancy, and implantation rates. Even with several confounding variables between the two incubator treatments, such as the use of different culture dishes (Embryoslide™ vs. Nunc 4-well) and embryo culture density (single vs. group), no statistically significant differences in any examined endpoint were noted [54]. While neither incubator used low O_2 (pers.comm. K. Kirkegaard), other conditions used in the incubators, such as humidity or pH similarities/differences, were not reported. Failure to properly control all these sort of impactful culture system variables between incubators makes it impossible to truly determine "superiority" of a particular incubator over another. Thus, while these published reports help demonstrate safety of time-lapse imaging (TLI) systems for embryos, the use of a smaller model incubator does not guarantee superior clinical outcomes. The same data could be used to defend an alternate viewpoint and to demonstrate that a large-box incubator, with proper management, can yield similar outcomes to a TLI benchtop unit.

A more recent retrospective observational multicenter cohort study compared clinical pregnancies following transfer of embryos cultured in a TLI incubator compared to a large-box CO_2 incubator with a TC sensor. The study demonstrated a 20.1% increase in clinical pregnancy per oocyte retrieval or 15.7% per embryo transfer [55]. However, as pointed out in the paper, this could be due to a variety of factors including, but not limited to, improved embryo selection via TLI and from the uninterrupted culture approach utilized in the TLI unit. Importantly, the medical gas supply of the TLI incubator was extensively filtered via HEPA, active carbon, and UV, while the large-box incubator was not. An improved approach to isolate the impact of the incubators may include comparison of outcomes using TLI inside a large-box incubator with similar air quality to those from a benchtop TLI incubator.

An additional retrospective matched-pair analysis of a TLI system to a large-box incubator was performed [56]. Approximately half of the patients cultured in the large-box incubator used high O_2 culture, while the TLI incubator utilized low O_2 culture. Using four-well dishes in the box incubator compared to a culture slide in the TLI incubator, clinical outcomes were compared. There was no comparison of preimplantation embryo development. Higher clinical pregnancy, implantation, and live birth rates were associated with the TLI system compared to the large-box incubator. Importantly, several variables in the culture system differed between incubator treatments due to the retrospective nature of the study (method of embryo selection, lot numbers of various culture items, oxygen tension, etc.). Thus, it is difficult to determine if one incubator was truly more efficient than another in terms of improved embryo quality or if the culture system as a whole was primarily responsible for reported differences

A prospective study using patient randomization examined outcomes following culture of embryos in a TLI incubator after 2 days to that of embryos cultured in a standard box incubator [57]. Both systems utilized low O_2 and the same media. The box incubator had embryos cultured in 20 μL microdrops, while the TLI system utilized the proprietary TLI culture slide. Embryos cultured in the TLI system were not disturbed, while those cultured in the box incubator were removed for observations at three time points. No difference in the number of good quality embryos between the incubators was observed on day 2. No differences in pregnancy or implantation were noted, but patients with transfers from embryos cultured in the TLI system had higher rates of miscarriage. Whether similar results would be observed following extended culture to the blastocyst stage is unknown.

Another prospective comparison of a box incubator to a TLI system was performed using a poor prognosis patient population. Using 20 μL drops in a standard petri dish in a box incubator or use of 25 μL of media in a conical culture slide in a TLI incubator, patients were randomized and outcomes compared after 3 days of culture [58]. Both incubator systems utilized low O_2 and the same media. Embryos in the box incubator were removed and examined three times, while those in the TLI incubator were left undisturbed and imaged using the TLI monitoring system. Looking at 16 patients (44 zygotes) in the TLI incubator and 15 patients (42 zygotes) in the box incubator, no differences in embryos quality were noted on day 3, and no differences in pregnancy rates were identified (18.8 vs. 20.0%). The authors noted significantly that more time was required to utilize the TLI incubator compared to the standard culture system. Seven oocyte donors were also randomly assigned to the two culture systems. It was noted that with 36 embryos cultured in the TLI system, lower levels of Grade A embryos were available, though no differences in Grade A+B embryos were noted between the two systems. Low numbers and lack of blastocyst culture should be noted.

To illustrate the importance of other factors regulating embryo development other than the actual incubator type or chamber size, a comparison of two identical ten-chamber benchtop units was performed, creating humidity in one incubator through addition of a water dish while leaving the other incubator non-humidified. Patient randomization was utilized, and no differences between patient populations were noted. All other conditions were similar. The authors reported that embryos cultured in the non-humidified incubator had impaired development on day 3 and day 5, and transfers yielded lower pregnancy rates [43].

While new incubator technology should be beneficial, it should be noted that "more physiologic" approaches, which are less technologically advance, can also potentially lend themselves to improved embryo development. A comparison between a vaginal culture capsule and a box-type low $O_{2\ \text{incubator}}$ was performed following patient randomization [59]. While more cleaved embryos (88 vs. 69%) and more overall blastocysts >2BB (51 vs. 31%) were present in the box incubator, the authors noted no difference in the number of high-quality blastocysts available for transfer, and only the in vivo cultured embryos yielded fully hatched blastocysts. No differences in pregnancy or implantation were observed following transfer. Thus, while preimplantation embryos would never normally see the vagina and variations may exist between patients in terms of the environmental conditions present during vaginal culture, this approach does appear to be able to provide good quality embryos for use. Whether the same findings would hold if compared to a modern benchtop incubator is unknown.

In summary, examination of comparative studies on embryo culture incubators indicates some differences are apparent between units in endpoints like environmental recovery, including gas atmosphere and temperature. These environmental recovery differences depend largely on the size of the incubator and the technology utilized in the unit, such as gas sensor type or temperature control approach. Importantly, careful attention must be paid to the use of optimal available technology/approaches for each incubator type to better assess comparisons between units. Many of the existing reports compare newer smaller benchtop units or TLI units to older outdated large-box incubators. While this reflects many real-world system changes, comparison of new smaller units to an "optimized" large-box or small-box unit might be more insightful into impact of the incubator itself.

Additionally, it becomes apparent in examining prospective studies that while smaller incubator units recover gas atmosphere and temperature more rapidly, which undoubtedly reduces environmental stress, this may not necessarily equate to better clinical outcomes. Furthermore, published comparative studies fail to properly control confounding variables, such as gas environment, type of dish used, and embryo selection methods. This makes it very difficult to determine potential impact and or superiority of a particular incubator type.

77.4 Incubator Management

A critical review of existing comparative incubator studies makes it clear that it is not possible to determine the "best" incubator. Superiority of an incubator will vary for each laboratory based on particular use and needs. As previously mentioned, results can vary between incubators types for a variety of reasons [16, 27]. This reinforces the need for strict quality control as well as proper management of laboratory IVF incubators to optimize function and outcomes [27]. Insight into specific incubator units, both benchtop/top load and standard box-type, their functioning and potential drawbacks can be found elsewhere [60]. Regardless of the specific model of incubator utilized within the laboratory, without proper incubator management, environmental stability and embryo development can be compromised in even the most cutting-edge unit employing the newest technology.

Proper incubator management involves steps aimed at maintaining environmental stability inside the unit. A critical approach to achieve this includes distribution of patient samples and proper workflow to avoid overuse of specific incubators. Not taking these measures results in "overcrowding" and an inability to maintain a stable culture environment due to repeated door openings/closing. Thus, incubator management requires a sufficient number of units based not only on total cycle volume but also on the time frame of when these cycles are performed. For example, an IVF laboratory that performs 300 cycles spread over a 12-month period will have a different requirement for number of incubators than an IVF laboratory that performs the same 300 cycles batched at intervals throughout the year. The number of incubators needed will also differ for laboratories that perform blastocyst culture compared to those that do not.

In addition to considering the number of incubators required, the use or workflow between incubators must also be considered. Preferential use of a particular unit over others as a result of a more convenient location/proximity can compromise the environmental stability of the individual incubator due to increased openings/closing. It was demonstrated that reducing door opening from six to four times over a 6-day period on a small-box incubator utilizing a water jacket with TC CO_2 and galvanic O_2 sensors resulted in significant improved human blastocyst formation (53 vs. 43%) and "good" quality blastocysts (60% vs. 51%), though no differences in day 3 embryo quality, implantation, or clinical pregnancy rates were noted [61]. Further supporting the benefit of reduced incubator door openings and improved embryo development, the use of a gas-sealed modular chamber placed inside the incubator to stabilize gas atmosphere resulted in significantly improved mouse blastocyst development and increased cell number compared to embryos cultured in a standard box incubator opened approximately 11 times per day [62]. Similar improvements in mouse embryo development and clinical outcomes were observed with use of a large enclosed isolator-based culture system, likely due, in part, to improved environmental stability [63]. Thus, IVF cases should be distributed as evenly as possible between all available incubators to avoid overuse or excessive door openings, regardless of the size or format of the unit.

Another method to reduce incubator door opening includes the use of "holding" incubators that can be used for transient procedures, such as dish equilibration, sperm swim-up/capacitation, or even brief culture of thawed embryos prior to same-day/immediate transfer. Using older "outdated" incubators, like many large-box units, for these purposes may help reduce excessive use of incubators used primarily for extended embryo culture.

Finally, the use of various commercially available incubator adjuncts can help with incubator management and improve environmental stability. These approaches include use of gas or air filters to improve air quality. Additionally, the use of inner doors on box-type incubators can aid in reducing gas loss. Desiccator jars or modular chambers can maintain gas atmosphere within box-type incubators during repeated openings/closings, and specialized milled aluminum blocks designed to hold culture dishes can help maintain a stable temperature.

77.5 Incorporating New Technology and Future Directions

Another important consideration for incubator selection entails the ability to implement new technology. The field has already seen an increase in new incubators incorporating TLI with small individual chambers for each patient. These incubators often require fewer door openings and provide a more stable growth environment. However, future improvements may be achievable.

Recent advances in dynamic embryo culture include motorized tilting devices, vibrating platforms, or even piezo-actuated pin systems [53, 64, 65], all which require standard box-type (large or small) incubators for placement. While with proper management, these innovations are aimed at improving embryo development and/or selection and may be performed in a similar fashion as benchtop units. Indeed, perhaps novel dynamic culture devices can be scaled down to permit incorporation into small benchtop/top load incubators (Fig. 77.6).

For example, emerging TLI devices could potentially be modified to incorporate dynamic vibrational culture. One could envision a small vibrating motor, similar to those used to vibrate cellular phones, attached to the area housing the embryo dish to provide gentle mechanical stimulation for brief periods between image capture. Prior studies indicate that 5 s of vibration at 44 Hz or other similar brief intervals improved embryo development and outcomes [66–69], though rates of control samples are often poor and there is disagreement that the beneficial effects exist [70].

Furthermore, microfluidic capabilities could be incorporated to help with media exchange or novel dishware utilized where lyophilized media would be reconstituted automatically inside the incubator with an automated water pipetting system and equilibrated at the appropriate time. The embryos could then be moved along a microfluidic pathway to this new media, thereby achieving uninterrupted embryo culture but not being confined to using a single-step media while alleviating potential concerns about ammonia buildup. Additionally, more insightful noninvasive imaging technology could be implemented to supplement the normal

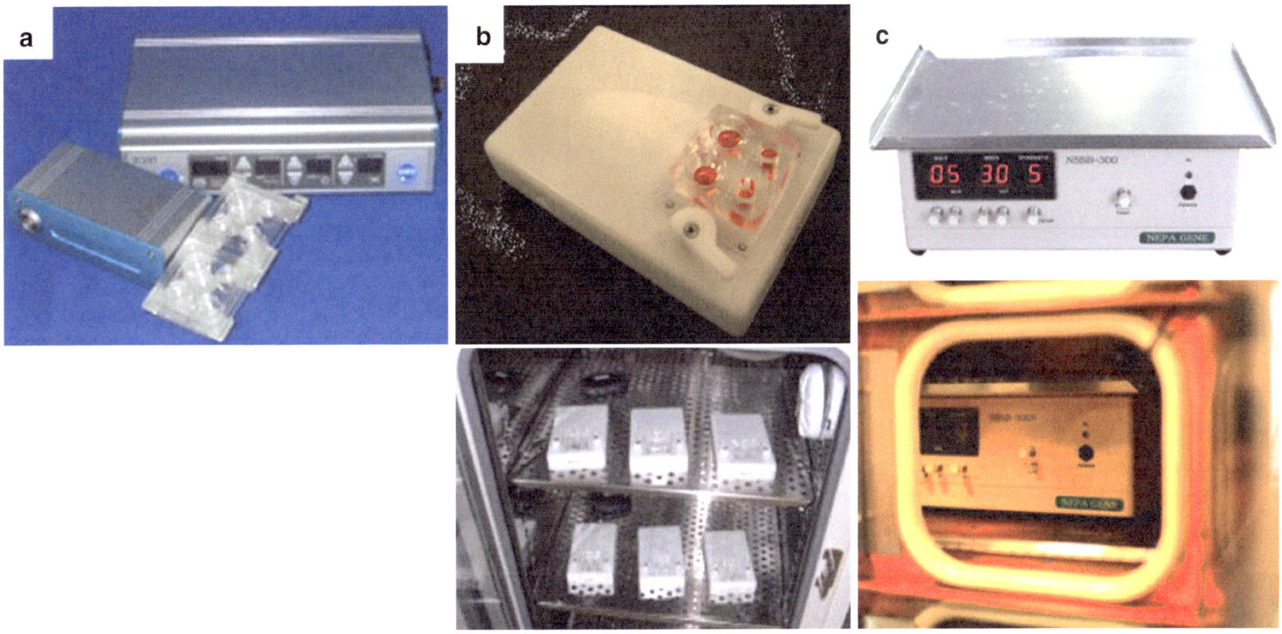

Fig. 77.6 Examples of novel, dynamic embryo culture platforms that may require specific incubator/space requirements for clinical use. (**a**) Motorized tilting device, (**b**) piezo-actuated microfluidic platform, and (**c**) vibrating platforms

dark field or bright field images commonly used currently [71].

77.6 Conclusion

Incubator selection is perhaps one of the most important decisions for an IVF laboratory, as these pieces of equipment control the growth environment of the preimplantation embryo via regulation of several environmental variables. While newer and more novel culture approaches may reduce the need for traditional incubators [63, 72–81], for the time being, these laboratory workhorses remain a central part of a modern IVF laboratory. Functional aspects of the incubator, such as gas capability and sensor type, as well as temperature control and size/patient capacity, are important considerations. Smaller incubator units, especially benchtop/top load devices, result in faster temperature and gas recovery. However, no published studies have demonstrated a clear benefit of any particular incubator type in terms of human preimplantation embryo development or clinical outcomes. Regardless of the incubator type, low O_2 capability should be utilized, and an IR CO_2 sensor is preferable for those units that mix the gases internally to permit the quickest gas recovery. Practical issues, such as cost and space requirements, must also be considered. The appropriate number and type of incubators are needed to adequately support the patient caseload, and this requirement must be determined on a lab-by-lab basis based on workflow. A combination of different incubator types, including large and small-box as well as benchtop/top load within a lab, helps cover multiple scenarios and offers several options for utilization, including implementation of emerging technologies.

Importantly, to improve incubator function and help optimize performance, proper incubator management is essential. Regardless of the size of the incubator or the technology incorporated/utilized, failure to implement proper management of case workflow or failure to perform proper daily quality assurance/control can compromise the culture conditions provided by any incubator. Proper incubator management should consider the daily caseload, rather than annual cycle number to avoid unnecessarily high incubator door openings/closings and maintain a stable internal growth environment. As technology continues to advance and new culture platforms and embryo selection technologies become available, incubators will undoubtedly need to continue to evolve to meet the changing needs of the field.

References

1. Swain JE. Is there an optimal pH for culture media used in clinical IVF? Hum Reprod Update. 2012;18(3):333–9. PubMed PMID: 22311857. Epub 2012/02/09.eng
2. Swain JE. Optimizing the culture environment in the IVF laboratory: impact of pH and buffer capacity on gamete and embryo quality. Reprod Biomed Online. 2010;21(1):6–16. PubMed PMID: 20570214. Epub 2010/06/24.eng
3. Swain JE. Media composition: pH and buffers. Methods Mol Biol. 2012;912:161–75. PubMed PMID: 22829374
4. Swain JE, Pool TB. New pH-buffering system for media utilized during gamete and embryo manipulations for assisted reproduction.

Reprod Biomed Online. 2009;18(6):799–810. PubMed PMID: 19490784. Epub 2009/06/06.eng
5. Bavister B. Oxygen concentration and preimplantation development. Reprod Biomed Online. 2004;9(5):484–6. PubMed PMID: 15588462. Epub 2004/12/14.eng
6. Bontekoe S, Mantikou E, van Wely M, Seshadri S, Repping S, Mastenbroek S. Low oxygen concentrations for embryo culture in assisted reproductive technologies. Cochrane Database Syst Rev. 2012;7:CD008950. PubMed PMID: 22786519. Epub 2012/07/13. eng
7. Mantikou E, Bontekoe S, van Wely M, Seshadri S, Repping S, Mastenbroek S. Low oxygen concentrations for embryo culture in assisted reproductive technologies. Hum Reprod Update 2013;19(3):209. PubMed PMID: 23377864. Epub 2013/02/05.eng.
8. Kovacic B, Vlaisavljevic V. Influence of atmospheric versus reduced oxygen concentration on development of human blastocysts in vitro: a prospective study on sibling oocytes. Reprod Biomed Online. 2008;17(2):229–36. PubMed PMID: 18681997. Epub 2008/08/07.eng
9. Meintjes M, Chantilis SJ, Douglas JD, Rodriguez AJ, Guerami AR, Bookout DM, et al. A controlled randomized trial evaluating the effect of lowered incubator oxygen tension on live births in a predominantly blastocyst transfer program. Hum Reprod. 2009;24(2):300–7. PubMed PMID: 18927130. Epub 2008/10/18. eng.
10. Waldenstrom U, Engstrom AB, Hellberg D, Nilsson S. Low-oxygen compared with high-oxygen atmosphere in blastocyst culture, a prospective randomized study. Fertil Steril. 2009;91(6):2461–5. PubMed PMID: 18554591. Epub 2008/06/17.eng
11. Morin SJ. Oxygen tension in embryo culture: does a shift to 2% O2 in extended culture represent the most physiologic system? Journal of assisted reproduction and genetics. 2017;34(3):309–14. PubMed PMID: 28181051. Pubmed Central PMCID: 5360691.
12. Bolnick A, Awonuga AO, Yang Y, Abdulhasan M, Xie Y, Zhou S, et al. Using stem cell oxygen physiology to optimize blastocyst culture while minimizing hypoxic stress. J Assist Reprod Genet. 2017; 34(10):1251–9. PubMed PMID: 28647787.
13. Chou J. Electrochemical sensors. Hazardous gas monitors: a practical guide to selection, operation and applications. New York: McGraw Hill; 1999. p. 27–35.
14. Chou J. Infrared sensors. Hazardous gas monitors: a practical guide to selection, operation and applications. New York: McGraw Hill; 1999. p. 55–72.
15. Instruments H. Oxygen sensors: theory and application. http://www.hitech-instcouk/pdfs/technical/oxygen_sensorspdf [Internet].
16. Avery B, Greve T. Impact of incubator type on the yield of in vitro produced bovine blastocysts. Acta Vet Scand. 1992;33(4):341–8. PubMed PMID: 1488949. Epub 1992/01/01.eng
17. Cohen J, Gilligan A, Esposito W, Schimmel T, Dale B. Ambient air and its potential effects on conception in vitro. Hum Reprod. 1997;12(8):1742–9. PubMed PMID: 9308805. Epub 1997/08/01. eng
18. Hall J, Gilligan A, Schimmel T, Cecchi M, Cohen J. The origin, effects and control of air pollution in laboratories used for human embryo culture. Human reproduction. 1998; 13(Suppl 4):146–55 PubMed PMID: 10091065. Epub 1999/03/26.eng.
19. Merton JS, Vermeulen ZL, Otter T, Mullaart E, de Ruigh L, Hasler JF. Carbon-activated gas filtration during in vitro culture increased pregnancy rate following transfer of in vitro-produced bovine embryos. Theriogenology 2007;67(7):1233-1238. PubMed PMID: 17331571. Epub 2007/03/03.eng.
20. Khoudja RY, Xu Y, Li T, Zhou C. Better IVF outcomes following improvements in laboratory air quality. J Assist Reprod Genet. 2013; 30(1):69–76. PubMed PMID: 23242648. Pubmed Central PMCID: 3553352. Epub 2012/12/18.eng.
21. Boone WR, Johnson JE, Locke AJ, Crane MM, Price TM. Control of air quality in an assisted reproductive technology laboratory. Fertil Steril. 1999;71(1):150–4. PubMed PMID: 9935133. Epub 1999/02/06.eng
22. Esteves SC, Gomes AP, Verza Jr S. Control of air pollution in assisted reproductive technology laboratory and adjacent areas improves embryo formation, cleavage and pregnancy rates and decreases abortion rate: comparison between a class 100 (ISO 5) and a class 1.000 (ISO 6) cleanroom for micromanipulation and embryo culture. Fertil Steril 2004;82(Suppl 2):S259–S260.
23. Schimmel T, Gilligan A, Garrisi G, Espositi B, Cecchi M, Dale B, et al. Removal of volatile organic compounds from incbuators used for gamete and embryo culture. Fertil Steril. 1997;68(Suppl 1):s165.
24. Mayer J, Nechchiri F, Weedon V, Jones E, Kalin H, Ochniger S, et al. Prospective randomized crossover analysis of the impact of an IVF incubator air filtration system (coda, genx) on clinical pregnancy rates. Fertil Steril. 1999;72(Suppl 1):s42.
25. McLellan S, Panagoulopoulos C, Dickinson K, Wright D, Toght T, Lanzendorf S. Effect of incubator air filtration system on IVF outcomes. Fertil Steril. 2001;76(Suppl 1):s103.
26. Battaglia D, Khabani A, Rainer C, Moore D. Prospective randomized trial of incubator CODA filtration unites revealed no effect on outcome. Fertil Steril. 2001;75(Suppl 1):s6.
27. Higdon HL 3rd, Blackhurst DW, Boone WR. Incubator management in an assisted reproductive technology laboratory. Fertil Steril. 2008;89(3):703–10. PubMed PMID: 17524397. Epub 2007/05/26. eng
28. Chapuis Y, Klvana D, Guy C, Kirchnerova J. Photocatalytic oxidation of volatile organic compounds using fluorescent visible light. J Air Waste Manag Assoc. 2002;52(7):845–54. PubMed PMID: 12139349. Epub 2002/07/26.eng
29. Sharmin R, Ray MB. Application of ultraviolet light-emitting diode photocatalysis to remove volatile organic compounds from indoor air. J Air Waste Manag Assoc. 2012;62(9):1032–9. PubMed PMID: 23019817. Epub 2012/10/02.eng
30. Wang WH, Meng L, Hackett RJ, Oldenbourg R, Keefe DL. Rigorous thermal control during intracytoplasmic sperm injection stabilizes the meiotic spindle and improves fertilization and pregnancy rates. Fertil Steril. 2002;77(6):1274–7. PubMed PMID: 12057740. Epub 2002/06/12.eng
31. Wang WH, Meng L, Hackett RJ, Odenbourg R, Keefe DL. Limited recovery of meiotic spindles in living human oocytes after cooling-rewarming observed using polarized light microscopy. Hum Reprod. 2001;16(11):2374–8. PubMed PMID: 11679523. Epub 2001/10/27.eng
32. Sun XF, Wang WH, Keefe DL. Overheating is detrimental to meiotic spindles within in vitro matured human oocytes. Zygote. 2004;12(1):65–70. PubMed PMID: 15214582. Epub 2004/06/25. eng
33. Leese HJ, Baumann CG, Brison DR, McEvoy TG, Sturmey RG. Metabolism of the viable mammalian embryo: quietness revisited. Mol Hum Reprod. 2008;14(12):667–72. PubMed PMID: 19019836. Pubmed Central PMCID: 2639445. Epub 2008/11/21.eng.
34. Walters EA, Brown JL, Krisher R, Voelkel S, Swain JE. Impact of a controlled culture temperature gradient on mouse embryo development and morphokinetics. Reprod Biomed Online. 2020; 40(4):494–9. PubMed PMID: 32171708.
35. Hunter RH, Einer-Jensen N. Pre-ovulatory temperature gradients within mammalian ovaries: a review. J Anim Physiol Anim Nutr (Berl). 2005;89(7-8):240–3. PubMed PMID: 15972073. Epub 2005/06/24.eng
36. Hunter RH, Einer-Jensen N, Greve T. Presence and significance of temperature gradients among different ovarian tissues. Microsc Res Tech. 2006;69(6):501–7. PubMed PMID: 16703612. Epub 2006/05/17.eng

37. Hunter RH. Temperature gradients in female reproductive tissues. Reprod Biomed Online. 2012;24(4):377–80. PubMed PMID: 22369989. Epub 2012/03/01.eng
38. Hong K, Forman E, Lee H, Ferry K, Treff N, Scott R. Optimizing the temperature for embryo culture in IVF: a randomized controlled trial (RCT) comparing standard culture temperature of 37C to the reduced more physiologic temperature of 36C. Fertil Steril. 2012;98(3):s167.
39. Stoddart N, Rho H, Maisel H, Zhao T, Tarantino S, Fleming S. Influence of the position of the culture dish within the incubator chamber and temperature of culture media on clinical outcome following Assisted Reproductive Technology (ART) treatment. Fertil Steril. 2003;80.(suppl(3):s164–5.
40. Swain JE, Cabrera L, Xu X, Smith GD. Microdrop preparation factors influence culture-media osmolality, which can impair mouse embryo preimplantation development. Reprod Biomed Online. 2012;24(2):142–7. PubMed PMID: 22197605. Epub 2011/12/27. eng
41. Lane M, Mitchell M, Cashman KS, Feil D, Wakefield S, Zander-Fox DL. To QC or not to QC: the key to a consistent laboratory? Reprod Fertil Dev. 2008;20(1):23–32. PubMed PMID: 18154695. Epub 2007/12/25.eng
42. Swain J, Schoolcraft W, Bossert N, Batcheller A. Media osmolality changes over 7 days following culture in a non-humidified benchtop incubator. Fertil Steril 2016;106(3):e362.
43. Fawzy M, AbdelRahman MY, Zidan MH, Abdel Hafez FF, Abdelghafar H, Al-Inany H, et al. Humid versus dry incubator: a prospective, randomized, controlled trial. Fertil Steril. 2017; 108(2):277–83. PubMed PMID: 28651960.
44. Borkow G, Gabbay J. Putting copper into action: copper-impregnated products with potent biocidal activities. FASEB J. 2004;18(14):1728–30. PubMed PMID: 15345689. Epub 2004/09/04.eng
45. Grass G, Rensing C, Solioz M. Metallic copper as an antimicrobial surface. Appl Environ Microbiol. 2011;77(5):1541–7. PubMed PMID: 21193661. Pubmed Central PMCID: 3067274. Epub 2011/01/05.eng.
46. Jarmuz P, Barrett D, Sakkas D. Continual temperature and humidity measurement allows more efficient and accurate monitoring of incubator performance. Fertil Steril. 2014;102(35 suppl):e133.
47. Cooke S, Tyler JP, Driscoll G. Objective assessments of temperature maintenance using in vitro culture techniques. J Assist Reprod Genet. 2002;19(8):368–75. PubMed PMID: 12182443. Pubmed Central PMCID: 3455576. Epub 2002/08/17.eng.
48. Fujiwara M, Takahashi K, Izuno M, Duan YR, Kazono M, Kimura F, et al. Effect of micro-environment maintenance on embryo culture after in-vitro fertilization: comparison of top-load mini incubator and conventional front-load incubator. J Assist Reprod Genet. 2007;24(1):5–9. PubMed PMID: 17160731. Pubmed Central PMCID: 3455086. Epub 2006/12/13.eng.
49. Lee M, Grazi R, Seifer D. Incorporation of the Cook K-Minc incubator and media system into the IVF lab: the future of IVF. J Clin Embryol. 2013;13(3):21–32.
50. Morbeck D, Fredrickson J, Walker D, Daftary G. Culture in a benchtop incubator reduces in vitro stress in a sensitive mouse embryo QC assay: potential role of air quality. Fertil Steril. 2011;96(3):s249.
51. Mortimer S, Fluker M, Yuzpe A. Effect of culture system upon fertilization rate and embryo development for patients 40 years and older. Hum Reprod. 2003;80(suppl 3):s168.
52. Cruz M, Gadea B, Garrido N, Pedersen KS, Martinez M, Perez-Cano I, et al. Embryo quality, blastocyst and ongoing pregnancy rates in oocyte donation patients whose embryos were monitored by time-lapse imaging. J Assist Reprod Genet. 2011;28(7):569–73. PubMed PMID: 21394522. Pubmed Central PMCID: 3162049. Epub 2011/03/12.eng.
53. Swain JE, Smith GD. Advances in embryo culture platforms: novel approaches to improve preimplantation embryo development through modifications of the microenvironment. Hum Reprod Update. 2011;17(4):541–57. PubMed PMID: 21454356. Epub 2011/04/02.eng
54. Kirkegaard K, Hindkjaer JJ, Grondahl ML, Kesmodel US, Ingerslev HJ. A randomized clinical trial comparing embryo culture in a conventional incubator with a time-lapse incubator. J Assist Reprod Genet. 2012;29(6):565–72. PubMed PMID: 22460082. Pubmed Central PMCID: 3370049. Epub 2012/03/31.eng.
55. Meseguer M, Rubio I, Cruz M, Basile N, Marcos J, Requena A. Embryo incubation and selection in a time-lapse monitoring system improves pregnancy outcome compared with a standard incubator: a retrospective cohort study. Fertil Steril. 2012;98(6):1481–9. e10. PubMed PMID: 22975113
56. Barrie A, Homburg R, McDowell G, Brown J, Kingsland C, Troup S. Embryos cultured in a time-lapse system result in superior treatment outcomes: a strict matched pair analysis. Hum Fertil. 2017;20(3):179–85. PubMed PMID: 27884061
57. Park H, Bergh C, Selleskog U, Thurin-Kjellberg A, Lundin K. No benefit of culturing embryos in a closed system compared with a conventional incubator in terms of number of good quality embryos: results from an RCT. Hum Reprod. 2015;30(2):268–75. PubMed PMID: 25432920
58. Wu L, Han W, Wang J, Zhang X, Liu W, Xiong S, et al. Embryo culture using a time-lapse monitoring system improves live birth rates compared with a conventional culture system: a prospective cohort study. Hum Fertil. 2017;09:1–8. PubMed PMID: 28597711
59. Doody KJ, Broome EJ, Doody KM. Comparing blastocyst quality and live birth rates of intravaginal culture using INVOcell to traditional in vitro incubation in a randomized open-label prospective controlled trial. J Assist Reprod Genet. 2016;33(4):495–500. PubMed PMID: 26843390. Pubmed Central PMCID: 4818641.
60. Meintjes M. CO2 and Low-O2 Incubators. In: Nagy Z, Varghese A, Agarwal A, editors. Practical manual of in vitro fertilization. New York: Springer; 2012. p. 61–70.
61. Zhang JQ, Li XL, Peng Y, Guo X, Heng BC, Tong GQ. Reduction in exposure of human embryos outside the incubator enhances embryo quality and blastulation rate. Reprod Biomed Online. 2010;20(4):510–5. PubMed PMID: 20129824. Epub 2010/02/05. eng
62. Gardner DK, Lane M. Alleviation of the '2-cell block' and development to the blastocyst of CF1 mouse embryos: role of amino acids, EDTA and physical parameters. Hum Reprod. 1996;11(12):2703–12. PubMed PMID: 9021376
63. Hyslop L, Prathalingam N, Nowak L, Fenwick J, Harbottle S, Byerley S, et al. A novel isolator-based system promotes viability of human embryos during laboratory processing. PLoS One. 2012;7(2):e31010. PubMed PMID: 22393356. Pubmed Central PMCID: 3290619. Epub 2012/03/07.eng.
64. Smith GD, Takayama S, Swain JE. Rethinking in vitro embryo culture: new developments in culture platforms and potential to improve assisted reproductive technologies. Biol Reprod. 2012;86(3):62. PubMed PMID: 21998170. Pubmed Central PMCID: 3316262. Epub 2011/10/15.eng.
65. Swain JE, Lai D, Takayama S, Smith GD. Thinking big by thinking small: application of microfluidic technology to improve ART. Lab Chip. 2013;13(7):1213–24. PubMed PMID: 23400523. Epub 2013/02/13.eng
66. Isachenko E, Maettner R, Isachenko V, Roth S, Kreienberg R, Sterzik K. Mechanical agitation during the in vitro culture of human pre-implantation embryos drastically increases the pregnancy rate. Clin Lab. 2010;56(11–12):569–76. PubMed PMID: 21141442. Epub 2010/12/15.eng
67. Isachenko V, Maettner R, Sterzik K, Strehler E, Kreinberg R, Hancke K, et al. In-vitro culture of human embryos with mechanical micro-

vibration increases implantation rates. Reprod Biomed Online. 2011;22(6):536–44.
68. Hur YS, Park JH, Ryu EK, Park SJ, Lee JH, Lee SH, et al. Effect of micro-vibration culture system on embryo development. J Assist Reprod Genet. 2013;30(6):835–41. PubMed PMID: 23657828. Pubmed Central PMCID: 3696450. Epub 2013/05/10.eng.
69. Isachenko V, Sterzik K, Maettner R, Isachenko E, Todorov P, Rahimi G, et al. In vitro microvibration increases implantation rate after embryonic cell transplantation. Cell Transplant. 2017;26(5):789–94. PubMed PMID: 27725062
70. Juneau CR, Franasiak JM, Morin SJ, Werner MD, Upham KM, Scott RT. EnMotion: embryos natural motion. blastulation is not different between static and dynamic culture systems. Fertil Steril. 2016;106(3):e358–9.
71. Jasensky J, Swain JE. Peering beneath the surface: novel imaging techniques to noninvasively select gametes and embryos for ART. Biol Reprod. 2013;89(4):105. PubMed PMID: 24068105
72. Ranoux C, Aubriot FX, Dubuisson JB, Cardone V, Foulot H, Poirot C, et al. A new in vitro fertilization technique: intravaginal culture. Fertility and sterility. 1988;49(4):654–7. PubMed PMID: 3350160. Epub 1988/04/01.eng.
73. Ranoux C, Seibel MM. New techniques in fertilization: intravaginal culture and microvolume straw. J In Vitro Fert Embryo Transf. 1990;7(1):6–8. PubMed PMID: 2187040. Epub 1990/02/01.eng
74. Taymor ML, Ranoux CJ, Gross GL. Natural oocyte retrieval with intravaginal fertilization: a simplified approach to in vitro fertilization. Obstet Gynecol. 1992;80(5):888–91. PubMed PMID: 1407935. Epub 1992/11/01.eng
75. Vajta G, Holm P, Greve T, Callesen H. The submarine incubation system, a new tool for in vitro embryo culture: a technique report. Theriogenology. 1997;48(8):1379–85.
76. Suzuki T, Sumantri C, Khan NH, Murakami M, Saha S. Development of a simple, portable carbon dioxide incubator for in vitro production of bovine embryos. Anim Reprod Sci. 1999;54(3):149–57. PubMed PMID: 10066102. Epub 1999/03/05.eng
77. Varisanga MD, Dong YJ, Mtango NR, Fahrudin M, Ni Wayan KK, Suzuki T. Bovine blastocysts obtained from reconstructed cytoplast and karyoplasts using a simple portable CO2 incubator. Cloning. 2000;2(4):167–73. PubMed PMID: 16218853. Epub 2005/10/13.eng
78. Vajta G, Bartels P, Joubert J, de la Rey M, Treadwell R, Callesen H. Production of a healthy calf by somatic cell nuclear transfer without micromanipulators and carbon dioxide incubators using the Handmade Cloning (HMC) and the Submarine Incubation System (SIS). Theriogenology. 2004;62(8):1465–72. PubMed PMID: 15451255. Epub 2004/09/29.eng
79. Blockeel C, Mock P, Verheyen G, Bouche N, Le Goff P, Heyman Y, et al. An in vivo culture system for human embryos using an encapsulation technology: a pilot study. Hum Reprod. 2009;24(4):790–6. PubMed PMID: 19273881. Pubmed Central PMCID: 2656929. Epub 2009/03/11.eng
80. Swain JE. A self-contained culture platform using carbon dioxide produced from a chemical reaction supports mouse blastocyst development in vitro. J Reprod Dev. 2011;57(4):551–5. PubMed PMID: 21532256. Epub 2011/05/03.eng
81. Itoi F, Tokoro M, Terashita Y, Yamagata K, Fukunaga N, Asada Y, et al. Offspring from mouse embryos developed using a simple incubator-free culture system with a deoxidizing agent. PLoS One. 2012;7(10):e47512. PubMed PMID: 23056643. Pubmed Central PMCID: 3467247. Epub 2012/10/12.eng.

Quality Management Systems

78

Linsey White and Bryan J. Woodward

A successful fertility clinic requires a strong quality management system (QMS) to deliver a desired level of excellence. The QMS should include quality policies, quality assurance and quality control. Maintaining quality is a continuous process which should be regularly risk assessed and audited to ensure the highest expectations are met for patients and staff. Furthermore, quality should be embedded within the organization with full managerial supervision and support. This enables troubleshooting via a cycle of continuous improvement, which enhances quality, leading to increased patient satisfaction, alongside improved satisfaction of investors and staff. A fertility clinic with a well-established and functioning QMS implements effective quality management on a daily basis. All areas can be evaluated and audited with the highest standard of results achieved.

An iterative four-step quality management tool of "*plan-do-check-act*", known as the Deming Cycle, is used across many industries for the control and continuous improvement of processes and procedures [1] (Fig. 78.1). The "*plan*" phase involves assessing and deciding on which process needs to be improved, with a clear goal to reach. The "*do*" phase allows the action plan to be implemented and data to be gathered to look at the effectiveness of the change or new process. At the "*check*" phase, the data is evaluated alongside the plan and desired outcome, forming a gap analysis or appraisal. Finally, the "*act*" phase demonstrates the new and improved process can become the baseline, provided the desired outcome has been met. When put together, the Deming Cycle is continuous, with numerous processes seven completing the cycle several times to continuously refine the process.

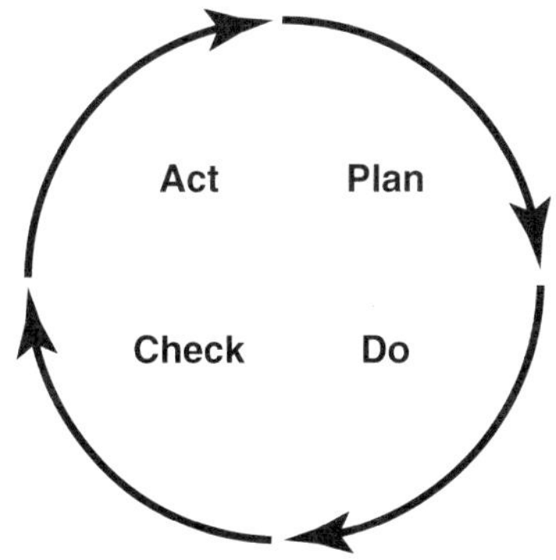

Fig. 78.1 The Deming Cycle, whereby a four-step quality management tool of "*plan-do-check-act*" is used to control and continuously improve procedures

78.1 Establishing a Quality Management System

In the UK, the Human Fertilization and Embryology Authority (HFEA) requires all licensed fertility clinics to have a QMS [2], stating:

> The centre must put in place a QMS and implement this system to continually improve the quality and effectiveness of the service provided in accordance with the conditions of this licence and the guidance on good practice as set out in the HFEA's Code of Practice.
>
> (Guidance Note T32, HFEA Code of Practice, 2019)

The HFEA provides its own definition of a QMS as:

> The organisational structure, defined responsibilities, procedures, processes and resources for implementing quality management (i.e. the co-ordinated activities to direct and control an organisation with regard to quality), including all activities which contribute to quality, directly or indirectly
>
> (Section 23.1, HFEA Code of Practice, 2019)

L. White
Assisted Conception Service, NHS Greater Glasgow and Clyde, Glasgow, UK

B. J. Woodward (✉)
X&Y Fertility, Leicester, UK

G. N. Allahbadia et al. (eds.), *Textbook of Assisted Reproduction*, https://doi.org/10.1007/978-981-15-2377-9_78

All HFEA-licensed fertility clinics have had to align their QMSs to account for the HFEA's interpretation of the European Union (EU) Tissue and Cells Directive 2004/23/EC [3]. This Directive affected all EU Member States, accepting that interpretation of the Directive differed according to the country. An effective QMS requires regular review regardless of the geographical location but may need to adapt to new local legislation as it changes.

78.1.1 External Standards

Many fertility clinics consult external standards to supplement their QMS, such as the International Organization for Standardization (ISO; www.iso.org), which provides sets of standards for a specific level of quality.

ISO standards that relate to assisted conception include:

- ISO 9000:2000. Quality Management Systems: Fundamental and vocabulary
- ISO 9001:2008. Quality Management Systems: Requirements
- ISO 15189:2012. Medical laboratories: Requirements for quality and competence

Other approaches to QMS development, such as "Lean & 5S" and "Six Sigma" have their roots in successful car manufacturing companies. For example, "Lean & 5S" is an operating philosophy originally developed by Toyota to help reduce costs and turnover time. Similarly, Motorola developed "Six Sigma", a philosophy that reduces "variability" to help solve problems. "Six Sigma" solves all problem using a five-step DMAIC process: *define, measure, analyse, improve and control.*

> A systematic approach to identify and eliminate waste through continuous improvement by flowing the product only when the customer needs it in pursuit of perfection
> (US Department of Commerce's National Institute of Standards & Technology Manufacturing Extension Partnership)

External standards tend to be short documents with wide-ranging statements to allow interpretation by different industries. The requirements of specific organizations may also need to be considered by fertility clinics, e.g. in the UK, clinics need to consider the HFEA, the Care Quality Commission, the National Health Service (NHS) Litigation Agency and the UK Accreditation Service.

If external standards are implemented, a high-level quality can be consistently maintained within the fertility unit. This ensures patients receive an agreed standard of care throughout their treatment, whilst the clinic can also work continuously to improve the service delivered. Thus, the QMS provides a management framework to monitor and enhance performance.

78.1.2 The Quality Manual

The quality manual should describe the clinic in its entirety and all activities taking place. It should also be a fluid document that all staff can input into, with regular reviews and updates as processes evolve and improve. As such, the quality manual is a vital component of the QMS.

The quality manual should consist of guidance on the processes and procedures imperative to running the clinic, such as management of staff, non-conformances, corrective and preventive procedures, document control, internal auditing and records. Each section should be written in such a way that it is easily understood by all staff. When the benefits of quality are appreciated by all team members, then quality manual becomes an essential document for management of the fertility clinic, In the UK, the importance sits alongside the HFEA Code of Practice, with both working in synergy.

78.2 Organizational Structure, Management and Responsibility

Fertility clinics should designate one person to have overall responsibility for all activity taking place. In the UK, this person is called the "Person Responsible" or "PR". With support from the senior management team (usually represented by senior staff from the medical, nursing, scientific and administration teams), the PR directs the organizational structure by assigning clear roles, job descriptions and responsibilities to all staff and ensuring they have skills required to fulfil these roles.

An organizational chart should be included in the quality manual to show that the clinic has the correct number of staff of sufficient grade, skills and experience, to perform the treatments to a require level of quality. It also defines accountability and reporting relationships (Fig. 78.2).

Each position within the organization should be clearly defined by a job description specifying the requirements, e.g. appropriate education, skills, training and experience. Job descriptions can be used as part of the hiring process but also to ensure staff are sufficiently skilled and aware of their responsibilities to meet the clinic's objectives throughout their service. All staff should possess the desired key skills, and these should be developed throughout their employment with an appraisal system implemented to monitor and evaluate each individual's service. Appraisals or regular staff reviews should highlight training needs, with individuals having a personal training file including evaluation of performance and competence and an appraisal report containing recommendations for improvements to benefit the clinic. Staff engagement is imperative for the clinic to deliver high standards of patient care. When quality is present, individu-

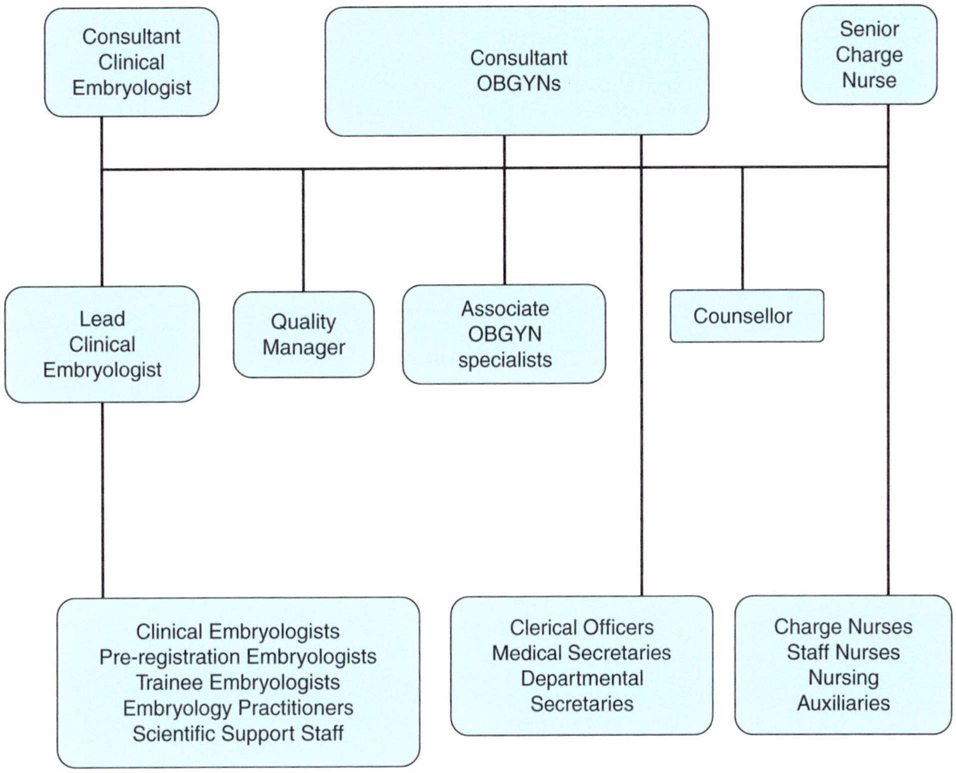

Fig. 78.2 A typical organizational chart for a fertility clinic

als should competently perform their designated tasks in line with the SOPs and remain engaged in the clinic objections and quality policy.

The organizational chart (Fig. 78.2) requires timely reviews to ensure its effectiveness in supporting the ever-changing clinic needs. For example, fluctuations in cycle numbers may warrant a change in the number of certain types of staff, which should be regularly reviewed throughout management and quality review and auditing.

All staff should comply with ethical conduct, which is usually covered by the codes of conduct from respective professional bodies, e.g. in the UK there are codes from the Royal College of Nursing (RCN), the Royal College of Obstetrians and Gynecologists (RCOG) and the Royal College of Pathologists (RCPath), whilst laboratory staff additionally sign up to codes from the Health and Care Professions Council (HCPC) and the Association of Reproductive and Clinical Scientists (ARCS).

78.2.1 The Quality Manager

The quality manager must have a deep understanding of all aspects of the QMS and the requirements of the internal and external standards to be achieved. Often the quality manager may have other responsibilities within the clinic, although the importance of quality should not be sacrificed with QMS implementation treated as priority.

The quality manager's role includes:

(i) Ensuring Code of Practice requirements are met and communicating with the national regulatory body as required
(ii) Ensuring resources are available to implement and maintain the QMS and that staff are aware of the associated tasks
(iii) Monitoring training compliance to ensure that employee skills are of the required standard and offer additional support and retraining where necessary
(iv) Completing audits and identifying the need for changes and opportunities for improvement
(v) Establishing the quality policy and objectives
(vi) Monitoring key performance indicators (KPIs) and implementing data-driven improvements

78.2.2 Quality Policy and Objectives

The quality policy is a statement showing the clinic's intention to work towards key areas, e.g. achieving patient satisfaction, training staff and working with suppliers to achieve the best outcomes for patient treatment.

In the UK, the HFEA defines a Quality Policy as:

> the overall intentions and direction of an organisation related to quality as formally expressed by centre management. A quality policy statement defines or describes an organisation's

> intentions and commitment to quality and provides a framework for setting quality objectives and planning.
>
> (Section 23.6, HFEA Code of Practice, 2019)

The approved quality policy should be displayed in the clinic, for both staff and patients to see. To ensure the quality objectives meet patient needs, they should be measurable and regularly reviewed such that the objectives are reached and maintained.

78.3 Control of Equipment

78.3.1 Validation

Validation or verification should be completed on all critical equipment and processes to verify that they are performing to the specifications required and thereby give confidence in the system.

Typically validation documents include:

- The validation master plan (VMP). This document defines the scope, planning and management of complete validation process. The VMP summarizes details of the equipment and the strategy for the whole validation process. This should be completed and circulated to all senior members of staff to ensure the correct variables are being verified.
- The user requirement specification (URS). This document demonstrates the need and purpose of the equipment or process. This document ensures that equipment and processes have all the necessary requirements to ensure they are fit for purpose.
- The qualifications. These are documents supporting the installation, operation and processing of equipment or processes, and include the:
  - Installation qualification (IQ)—to verify that installation of an item of equipment or a process is correct and ensures the equipment is functioning as per manufacturer's guidance
  - Operation qualification (OQ)—to demonstrate the ability of the equipment or process to operate as specified in the URS
  - Process qualification (PQ)—to show satisfactory completion of the OQ, demonstrating outputs of a process meets all specifications
- The validation report (VR). This document pulls together all documents and verifies all requirements of the VMP have been met. The VR gives recommendations for improvement and risk mitigation. The VR also specifies the timelines for maintenance, calibration and revalidation.

78.3.2 Calibration and Maintenance

Calibration is performed by checking and comparing the equipment to a known standard. This process may require adjustment of the instrument to bring it to the standard and reset values. The majority of equipment requires some kind of maintenance and calibration, with the frequency usually defined by manufacturer specifications or quality manual, depending of importance of equipment to the process. An evaluation should be carried out to assess frequency of usage, importance of equipment, and how often the equipment malfunctions or drifts from the desired levels and therefore requires servicing and calibration. Records of unplanned maintenance and breakdowns should be recorded as this could highlight suboptimal equipment. Suboptimal performing equipment should be segregated and not used until calibration and revalidation has taken place.

78.3.3 Third-Party Agreements

Third-party agreements (TPAs) are contracts between fertility clinics and suppliers of equipment, consumables and services. TPAs cover the conditions to be met by both parties to deliver the desired service. This allows approval and monitoring of the suppliers to ensure needs and expectations of the clinic are met. TPAs are sometimes referred to as service-level agreements (SLAs), more often for services rather than products between departments within the same organization.

In the UK, the HFEA Code of Practice defines a TPA as:

> an agreement in writing between a person who holds a licence and another person which is made in accordance with any licence conditions imposed by the Authority for the purpose of securing compliance with the requirements of Article 24 of the first Directive (relations between tissue establishments and third parties) and under which the other person -
>
> (a) procures, tests or processes gametes or embryos (or both), on behalf of the holder of the licence, or
> (b) supplies to the holder of the licence any goods or services (including distribution services) which may affect the quality or safety of gametes or embryos
>
> (Mandatory Requirement 2A, HFEA Code of Practice, 2019)

78.3.4 Traceability and Identification

In fertility clinics, high-level identification and traceability are needed to allow verification of all equipment and consumables. This allows investigation and segregation should non-conforming material and retrospective investigation. All consumables should be batch controlled by documenting the product identifier, batch number and expiry date. Traceability can be useful for investigations if trends in changes to performance are observed or a safety field notice is issued from the manufacturer.

All equipment and consumables should be identified as "approved for use" such that they comply with all legislative requirements. These items should be checked to ensure there was not deterioration to quality during shipping from the supplier to the clinic. TPAs with companies supplying culture media should stipulate that the "cold chain" (temperature from the factory, throughout transit to the clinic) is not compromised. This can be monitored by data loggers that measure temperature throughout transit to confirm that the quality of the media will be optimal for clinic use. If there is a change to the transport method without prior agreement from the clinic, then the TPA has not been adhered too and the media should not be used clinically.

In Europe, incoming consumables should be approved by supplier by CE (Conformite Europeene) marking of the product. A CE mark is the manufacturer's declaration that the product complies with the essential requirements of the relevant European health, safety and environmental protection legislation. The CE mark often indicates the product has been placed legally on the market and there is free movement of the product within complying counties within the EU. However, CE marking is not always available, in which case in-house testing should be undertaken.

The HFEA Code of Practice states:

> The centre should use only media and consumables that have been CE-marked at a classification suitable for their intended purpose. Modifying existing devices (for example, adding calcium ionophore to culture medium) or using them 'off label' for purposes not intended by the manufacturer (for example, using a medium for a different purpose from that specified) has safety implications. It may also count as manufacture of a new device under the Medical Devices Regulations.
>
> (section 26.4, HFEA Code of Practice, 2019)

78.4 Document Control and Record Keeping

Documentation control within a fertility clinic is imperative to ensure consistency exists throughout all procedures. Documents are often controlled electronically via quality management software designed to monitor all documents and ensure training, review and regular audits as stipulated by the quality manual.

Good document control ensures that all staff perform standard operating procedures (SOPs) in the same way, using the same recording methods (e.g. forms or worksheets) to minimize inter-operator variation (Fig. 78.3). Only current and approved versions of documents, forms and any other paperwork should be available. When documents are reviewed and changed, all staff should have access to up-to-date versions to ensure all processes are carried out as per the changes. Adherence to older uncontrolled versions of SOPs could impact on the safety of patients, their gametes and/or embryos and also on staff.

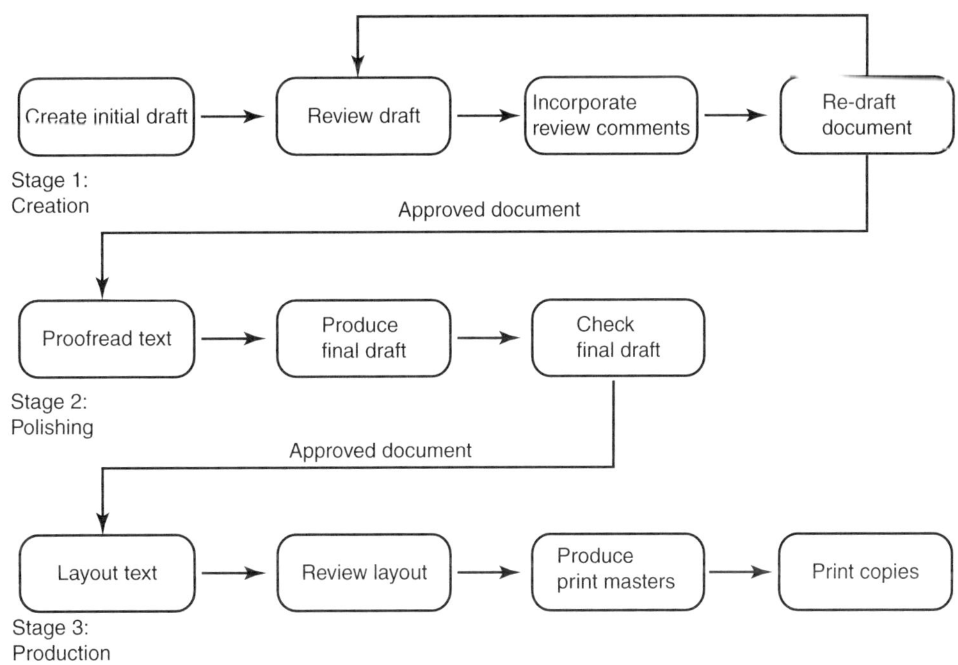

Fig. 78.3 The process of document control

Any deviation from an agreed process should be logged as a non-conformance (NC) to ensure traceability of all events. Staff should be allowed the opportunity to justify deviations and update appropriate SOPs if required. Although a deviation is a NC, it may lead to an improvement and could therefore contribute to the quality feedback improvement loop.

Recommendations for document management:

- Allocate each document:
  - A code to allow them to be controlled and tracked, e.g. SOP-XXX, FORM-YYY
  - A numerical or alphabetical revision which should be updated each time the document is reviewed and changed. With previous versions archived for reference only, access should be restricted to prevent adherence to previous documents.
- Document changes should be carried out by someone with expertise of the process. All changes should then be peer reviewed before approval for use.
- For traceability, a full justification of why changes were made should be recorded, assessing the possible impact of the change, including any changes to risk level and validation documented.
- Documents should be available at all times to operators in the format that cannot be amended, e.g. a PDF version.
- Documents should follow the same templates to allow consistency and ease of use throughout.
- Referencing should be made to other documents where applicable, e.g. references or links to related worksheets.
- Documents should be appropriately filed to allow traceability with a recommended retention of files for a specific period of time if not electronic.

78.5 Audits and Quality Improvements

Quality indicators, also known as key performance indicators (KPIs), should be continuously monitored to allow evaluation and outcome of clinic procedures. Data trends should drive improvement; therefore, it is important to record data accurately for statistical analysis.

The HFEA Code of Practice states:

> Required standards of quality and safety, in the form of quality indicators for all activities authorised by this licence and other activities carried out in the course of providing treatment services that do not require a licence, must be established.
> (Guidance note T35, HFEA Code of Practice, 2019)

Examples of KPIs include the percentages of eggs collected relative to the number of follicles, oocytes fertilized relative to the number of oocytes collected and live births relative to the number of embryo transfers performed.

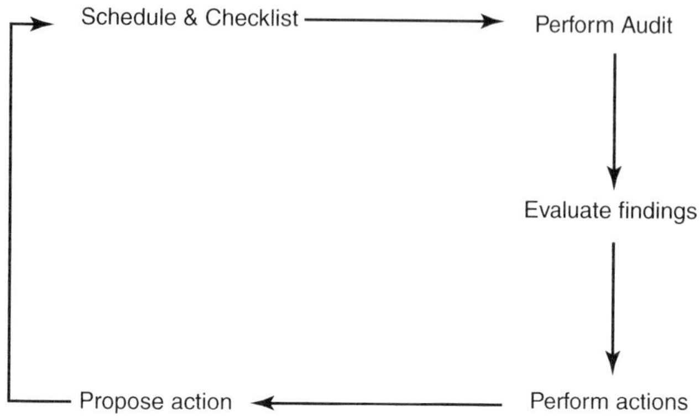

Fig. 78.4 The continuous audit loop

Audits are used to monitor the output of documented processes and provide an objective evaluation to determine whether the process is being carried out as per the clinic requirement. This is managed via an audit schedule to look at as many areas as possible, concentrating on processes that have been recently introduced or changed. An audit schedule usually runs over a reasonable period of time, such as 2 years (Fig. 78.4). Unscheduled audits may also be undertaken at any point, particularly if there are concerns about a process.

Audits establish whether all activities that affect quality are being carried out correctly and effectively by staff. Audits should be carried out by a trained auditor, and it is recommended the auditor does not work directly on the process being evaluated to enable them to look at processes objectively. Audits can be performed internally (within the organization by a trained member of staff) and externally (via external assessment, e.g. from the HFEA or supplier audits). Audits should be welcomed, as they introduce continuous improvement and give patients and staff a further degree of confidence in the clinic.

Following an audit, a report should be completed with any NCs or observations discussed and actioned by department senior staff, as necessary. They can be used to measure compliance with policies, procedures or requirements (e.g. the HFEA Code of Practice).

The HFEA Code of Practice states that:

> ...audits must be performed at least every two years, by trained and competent staff and in an independent way. Findings and corrective actions must be documented and implemented.
> (Guidance Note T36, HFEA Code of Practice, 2019)

Audit findings should be investigated with an action plan put in place to resolve and correct any issues. The period of time required to resolve findings varies, according to the number of changes required. It is important a full investigation takes place before a corrective action is implemented to ensure the root cause of the issue is resolved.

78.6 Non-conformance Reporting, Corrective Action and Preventive Action

When reporting NCs, a document should be generated to ensure the root cause is identified and resolved. Immediate remedial action should be implemented, to allow the operator/process to continue. This should be followed up with an investigation and implementation of appropriate actions to resolve the issue, in a timely manner.

Corrective action preventive action (CAPA) is often used to resolve NCs and mitigate the risk of them occurring again in the future. Corrective action (CA) is proposed and implemented after an initial investigation of a NC. A problem-solving method of investigation, such as the "*5 whys*" may be used. "*5 whys*" solves problems by asking "*why*" no fewer than five times to drill down to the root cause.

Preventive actions (PA) are often more difficult to put in place as they require action to be put in place before any NC occurs. This takes into account that it is often difficult to foresee issues with processes without trialling them first. PAs may be identified at routine audits as observations for improvement.

78.7 Risk Management

Risk management is the process of identifying and mitigating all potential risks to the fertility service in order to minimize their impact. These could be risks to patients and their gametes or embryos or risks to staff by any process. All major processes should be risk assessed within the clinic when they are introduced or significant changes take place, to ensure safety and fit for purpose.

Failure Mode Effects Analysis (FMEA) is an approach often used to assess risk. This is a step-by-step approach used to numerically analyse risks, whereby each risk is discussed in turn and scored according to the likelihood of occurrence and severity. These individual scores are then ranked by a traffic light system, with red risks requiring an immediate and effective action to be implemented, orange risks requiring a corrective action to be put in place to reduce risk and a green risk should also have a corrective action implemented although not as crucial. See FMEA's website for the criticality matrix.

Risk management should be integrated into all processes throughout the QMS to mitigate risk as much as possible. Identifying all the potential hazards at an early stage allows appropriate controls to be identified and incorporated into the service development (Fig. 78.5). This is a proactive process, and all staff should be engaged in risk management and encouraged to identify potential risks.

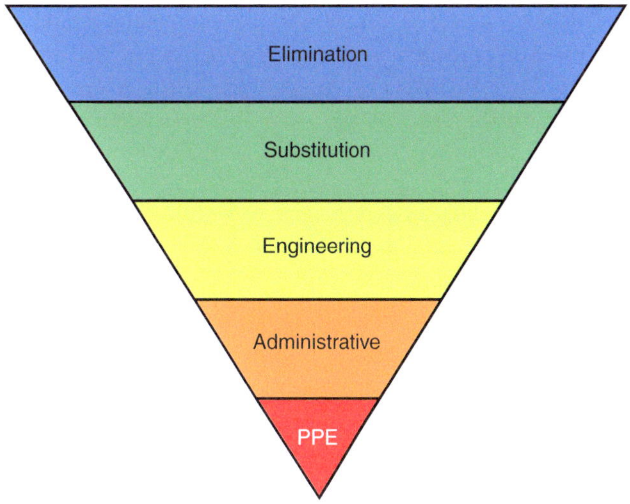

Fig. 78.5 Risk assessment guide. Blue, physically remove the hazard; green, replace the hazard; yellow, isolate people from the hazard; orange, change the way people work; red, protect the worker with personal protection equipment (PPE)

78.8 Patient Satisfaction and Complaints

Clinics should monitor patient satisfaction to identify, assess and react to emerging issues and to identify opportunities for the continuous improvement of service. This allows the clinics to make improvements and deliver care to a high standard.

Clinics should have a clear complaints procedure as, unfortunately, complaints are inevitable. Patient complaints allow the opportunity for a clinic to provide feedback before, throughout and after their treatment. Complaints should be fully investigated and evaluated, with a suitable CAPA put in place, if appropriate. Complaints should not be ignored and an action plan with a follow-up for each case should take place. Complaints should also be reviewed annually to allow any trends to be observed, so that quality can be improved.

78.9 The Management Review Meeting

The management team should formally meet at least annually to evaluate the effectiveness of the QMS and general organization of the fertility clinic. This meeting provides an opportunity for the team to examine if the expected results are achieved and the functions meet expectation. The capability of the organization and requirements for the future can then be considered.

The management review meeting (MRM) is an opportunity to get a group of senior decision-makers together to review the organizations quality and to make improvements and changes where necessary. NCs and complaints should be reviewed and preventive measures put in place where possible for future occurrences. As such, the MRM is one of the most important meetings that a fertility clinic undertakes.

78.10 Conclusion

The objective of this chapter was to demonstrate some of the key aspects of a successful QMS for a fertility clinic. Managing quality is crucial to all services and businesses. Quality helps to maintain patient satisfaction and reduce risk, making good business sense. It is hoped that, with correct guidance, everyone will realize why it is imperative to have quality embedded into all aspects of a clinic, as the benefits of bringing quality deliver improved outcomes for both patients and staff.

References

1. Wang LR, Wang Y, Lou Y, Li Y, Zhang XG. The role of quality control circles in sustained improvement of medical quality. Springerplus. 2013;2(1):141.
2. European Union. Commission Directive 2004/23/EC of the European Parliament and of the Council of 31 March 2004 on setting standards of quality and safety for the donation, procurement, testing, processing, preservation, storage and distribution of human tissues and cells. Offic J Eur Union. L102/48.
3. Human Fertilisation and Embryology Authority. Code of practice. 9th ed; 2019.

Risk Management in Medically Assisted Reproduction

79

Ajibike Oyewumi

Healthcare, by its very nature, deals with risk. To tackle the disease or challenge that the patient presents with, some kind of remedy that invades or alters the body or the body's responses has to be instituted. The anticipated benefit makes it justifiable to take these actions. However, the remedies or remedial actions may have some harmful consequences. The potential harmful consequences of the beneficial remedies are what constitute the risks. The overall objective of all healthcare organisations is to deliver the best quality of care possible, without error or harm to the patient, the staff, the organisation and the society.

Modern healthcare, including assisted reproductive technology (ART), is immensely complex. Kenneth Kizer, a former head of the US Veterans Affairs Health System, stated that modern healthcare has turned in the most complex enterprises ever tackled by humans [1]. Causes of complexity in healthcare include the use of highly complicated technologies, the use of many potent drugs, differing education and training of providers, often confused lines of authority, highly shifting physical settings and multiple providers looking after various aspects of the patients and needing multiple hand-offs. Furthermore, there may be communication barriers, patients who are medically diverse, a large variety of care processes and the time-pressured surroundings in which the providers work. All of this complexity brings with it risks and makes the system error-prone [1, 2].

Risks and adverse events have been studied more in other aspects of healthcare than in ART. The World Health Organisation (WHO) estimated that about one in ten patients are harmed while receiving healthcare worldwide [3]. This number is an estimated average and will vary by region and by care delivered. A research scan published in 2011 by the Health Foundation included more than 100 studies and reviews, predominantly from the USA, Australasia, Europe and the UK. This more recent research suggested that levels of harm ranged from 3 to 25% in acute care. Half to one third of these events were thought to be preventable [4].

ART treatment programmes are complicated due to the use of high-tech equipment and procedures in the clinical laboratory, including gamete and embryo micromanipulation and cryopreservation and pre-implantation genetic testing, in addition to the reasons stated above. The patient population being treated is also broadening and often involves patients with pre-existing conditions and multiple parties, including the future parents, gamete donors or gestational surrogates [5]. In addition, ART requires the integration of multiple disciplines, as in many, if not most, aspects of healthcare. It has been suggested that this multidisciplinary nature, which necessitates multiple hand-off of patients and patient materials, could mean that the risk of incidents could even be higher than in other areas of clinical practice [6].

A study from the Netherlands published in 2011 found that the overall death rate in IVF pregnancies was 42 per 100,000 women, compared with 6 deaths per 100,000 in all pregnancies [7]. In a 10 year study performed by Boston IVF Andrology and Embryology laboratories in the USA, the overall rates of moderate and significant errors ("Moderate: a problem negatively affecting a cycle but not to the extent that it is lost; Significant: loss of a cycle due to loss/mishandling of gametes or embryos; and Major: systemic problems affecting multiple patients") per procedure and per cycle were 0.05% and 0.18%, respectively. These rates, when compared to rates of 2.7–12% that result from laboratory errors in other areas of medicine, were very favourable [5]. In the UK, the Human Embryology and Fertilization Authority (HFFEA) reported an average 500–600 incidents per year out of more than 60,000 cycles of IVF treatment [8].

All these data point to the fact that though quite low, there is a risk of adverse events associated with ART that cannot be ignored. These adverse outcomes also increase the risk of lawsuits and claims against the organisation in charge of the ART.

A. Oyewumi (✉)
Lagoon Hospital, Ikoyi, Lagos, Nigeria

G. N. Allahbadia et al. (eds.), *Textbook of Assisted Reproduction*, https://doi.org/10.1007/978-981-15-2377-9_79

Risk management in healthcare can be traced back in history to Ignaz Semmelweis and Florence Nightingale. Semmelweis required that doctors and students clean their hands in chlorinated lime water before entering the labour ward especially when coming in from the autopsy room. However, risk management only really started to be appreciated after World War II, with sources citing modern risk management beginning around 1955–1964 [9–11].

Risk management in healthcare in its present form emerged in the mid-1970s, when healthcare institutions experienced a rapid rise in lawsuits and claims costs [9, 10]. At this time, the corporate world found a means of addressing the management of risk through the purchase of insurance. As malpractice verdicts and settlements continued to rise, a more proactive approach to managing risk began to evolve and develop resulting in risk management in healthcare [10, 11].

79.1 Hazards, Risks and Their Consequences

It is important to know the difference between two closely related yet distinct concepts: hazard and risk. Hazard can be defined as a source of potential harm or a situation with a potential to cause loss. It is an intrinsic property which is an immutable condition of a given situation or activity. This implies that hazards cannot be altered.

Risk is the chance that something unwelcome or unpleasant could lead to injury or loss. Risk in healthcare may be clinical or non-clinical. Non-clinical risks generally encompass areas of administration, finance, technology, environment, human resources, staff safety and health and safety, all of which might influence public opinion and reputation. Clinical risks arise from clinical processes relating to the patient, either directly and indirectly. The consequences of clinical risks have been termed "adverse events". Adverse events can be preventable or non-preventable. When the events have catastrophic, irreversible impacts, like disability or death, they have been termed sentinel events. Thankfully these are rare.

In the UK, the HFEA defines an adverse incident as:

> "any event, circumstance, activity or action which has caused, or has been identified as potentially causing harm, loss or damage to patients, their embryos and/or gametes, or to staff of a licensed centre." These include incidents which are clinical, laboratory-based or administrative [8].

Risks to be considered in the ART setting are related to the clinical, laboratory and administrative aspects. Others are financial, legal and ethical. These are important to consider as there could be issues arising in relation to accessing treatment and the possible impact on the health of the staff, the public and future generations [6]. Adverse events which occur in fertility practice can be classified as:

- Clinical (such as hospital admissions due to ovarian hyperstimulation syndrome)
- Laboratory-based (such as loss of sperm, eggs or embryos and IVF mix-ups)
- Administrative errors (such as breaches of confidentiality and record keeping errors) [8]

The consequences of known risks in medical practice and ART should be prevented by having a proactive approach to managing the risks.

Risk management (RM) is the process by which the risk can be measured or estimated, and then strategies can be developed to prevent or manage it.

As RM evolved, the focus shifted from managing solely professional liabilities to managing patient safety and loss prevention [12]. However, RM principles are applicable across all areas of healthcare strategy and operations, and this has led to the promotion of a broader, comprehensive organisation-wide approach of enterprise risk management (ERM) approach [13, 14].

- "RM is an integral part of all organizational processes" [15].
- "It is not a stand-alone activity that is separate from the main activities and processes of the organisation. RM is part of the responsibilities of management and an integral part of all organisational processes, including strategic planning and all project and change management processes" [16].

Notwithstanding the approach used in RM in an organisation, the primary goal should be to reduce harm and improve patients' quality of life.

79.2 Risk Management and Quality Management

RM and quality improvement should be considered as integrated rather than separate streams when determining all areas of operation. These include clinical practice, equipment procurement and design, capital development, management of contractors and the workforce, workplace health and safety, information technology and financial planning [15, 16].

79.3 Aims of Risk Management

RM helps to highlight situations that are error-prone and to implement systems that help to prevent the errors from happening; to address errors before they cause harm or loss or to mitigate harm from errors before they impact on patients, staff or the organisation. Other goals of RM include enhancing patient outcomes, effective management of resources, supporting legislative and regulatory compliance and safeguarding financial security and continued viability of the organisation [15, 16].

The benefits of RM are often very clear to those involved in RM, quality and patient safety. However, staff who are overworked might perceive it as just another task or burden [6].

The consequences of not pursuing RM include [17]:

- The organisation will be always reactive to risk and make decisions based on inadequate information and knowledge of future risks and consequences.
- Scarce resources will be expended to correct problems that could have been avoided.
- Catastrophic problems will occur without warning, and the organisation may be unable to respond rapidly to such events.
- Recovery thereafter may be very difficult and/or costly or even impossible.

79.4 Risk Categories

79.4.1 Scope of the Risk Management Programme

Developing a comprehensive RM programme involves looking beyond the clinical- and patient-related risk. To be truly comprehensive, a RM programme should include the following categories or domains of risk shown in Table 79.1 [17–19].

79.5 Risk Management Strategies

The ultimate goal of RM is to identify appropriate strategies that can be used to avoid or eliminate the identified risk when possible. If, however, a risk cannot be eliminated, then it must be managed.

Table 79.1 Risk categories

Patient care	Facilities
Financial	Property related
Strategic	Operational
Legal/regulatory	Medical products and technology
Human resources—medical and non-medical	Natural hazards

79.5.1 Key Components of Risk Management

When developing a RM strategy, three key components need to be in place: organisational commitment, integration and stakeholder engagement.

79.5.2 Organisational Commitment

Organisational commitment [17, 18] involves the leadership team at all levels, including the board, who should clearly and unequivocally demonstrate its commitment to RM and safety, to all staff. This can be performed by providing approval support and active participation in the programme when required. It also involves developing accountability systems and assignment of responsibility with support for the various roles within the system. The importance of safety should be clearly stated in the institution's policies, and it should involve all aspects of organisational life.

79.5.3 Integration

The RM programme should be integrated with other systems, initiatives and aspects of the organisational culture and strategy, particularly regarding quality and safety (see section above). Efforts should be made to create operational links and avoid duplication of efforts. Access should be provided to all levels of the organisation, with defined accountabilities and identification of resources.

79.5.4 Stakeholder Engagement

All stakeholders should be made aware of safety and its importance. It is necessary to incorporate safety in the daily operations of the organisation. The RM policy and its challenges should be explained to all stakeholders. Input from clinical staff should be sought throughout the process and included into the RM programme. Efforts should be made to seek the commitment of the clinical staff and to encourage ownership of the programme by all staff.

79.5.5 Risk Management Process

The RM process (clinical and non-clinical) involves a number of steps. These steps have been labelled differently by various authors, organisations and entities. In general, they follow the same principles of identifying the risk; assessing the risk; responding to the risk and evaluation of the RM process and the programme [16–20].

The ISO 31000:2009 [16–18] which is largely based on the AS/NZS 4360:2004 process identifies the five steps in the RM process as:

- Risk identification
- Risk analysis
- Risk evaluation and prioritisation
- Risk response or treatment
- Review evaluation and monitoring.

It also includes some other components: establishing the context in which risk is to be managed; communication and consultation with all stakeholders and the monitoring and review of the RM programme in the process.

Though the process is depicted as stepwise, in reality it is most often iterative between the steps. As well as considerable iteration between the steps, consideration must be given to involve continuous application to the elements of "Communication and Consultation" and "Monitoring and Review". These two additional processes flow across the five steps of the RM process. Both are vital to effective RM and need to be implemented simultaneously at each level of the RM process.

79.5.6 Establish the Context

It is important to establish the context of the RM process quite clearly at the beginning of the process. This step defines the parameters within which risks will be managed and clarifies the goals, objectives and the scope of the process, taking into account the internal and external environment.

Establishing the context includes getting a comprehensive appreciation of all the factors that may have an impact on the ability of the organisation to achieve its intended outcomes. A set of key risk criteria must then be defined for structuring identification and response to the identified risk. Such criteria may be based on clinical, regulatory operational, technical, financial, legal, social and humanitarian factors.

79.5.6.1 External Context

In defining the external context, it is important to consider who the external stakeholders are and their relationship with the organisation. ART centres should be considered within the context of government regulations, professional guidelines, licensing and accreditation requirements. Furthermore, they should be considered within the context of the competition in the industry (generating referrals, outcomes, pricing, etc.). Some countries have established comprehensive legislation and regulations that govern most aspects of ART such as the UK, Japan, the European Union and a number of Australian states. However, others, such as the USA, are not as regulated and rely on professional clinical and ethical guidelines and the general regulation of medical practice to govern this area [21, 22].

79.5.6.2 Internal Context

Understanding the internal context involves consideration of the internal stakeholders and the environment. ART centres exist in different settings. Some are part of a larger multi-speciality organisation, while others exist as mono-speciality units. Those that exist as part of a larger organisation will be influenced by the culture, structure, policies and processes of the corporate body [16, 17].

79.5.7 Risk Identification

Risk identification is the use of a well-structured systematic process to find, recognise and describe risks in the healthcare environment or process that constitutes potential loss exposures for the institution. Risk identification is not a one-time process but should be ongoing and dynamic. Over time, all significant risks to the organisation need to be identified, assessed, treated and monitored. However, because it is not possible to deal with all the risks at the same time, risks that may pose an internal or external threat should be identified and prioritised.

To identify risks, the exposure in the risk categories in Table 79.1 should be considered. The following components should be understood:

- What are the issues that may arise, the possible locations and timing and under what circumstances?
- How is this likely to occur?
- Who are the persons that may be involved?
- How will the information about the identified risks be gathered?
- How reliable is/are the source(s) of information?
- Have all the right stakeholders been engaged in the process of identifying the risk?

Possible sources of information for identifying risks are shown in Table 79.2.

There are a variety of methodologies, processes and tools available to assist in risk identification. Tools can be retrospective or prospective [17, 18, 22].

The following are a few of the various tools available:

- Root cause analysis (RCA)
- Failure Mode and Effects Analysis (FMEA)
- Event tree analysis (ETA) and hazard identification
- Questionnaires
- Brainstorming

Table 79.2 Sources of information for risk identification

Sentinel event reports	Previous risk registers
Satisfaction surveys	Brainstorming
Patient feedback	Strategic and business plans
Complaint data	SWOT analysis (to identify the Strengths, Weaknesses, Opportunities and Threats of a possible event) and environmental scans
Clinical audits; morbidity and mortality reviews	Flow charting, system design review
Interview/focus group discussion	Systems engineering
Quality/performance improvement data	Work breakdown structure analysis
Medico-legal data	Operational modelling
Audits or physical inspections	Decision trees
Licensing or accreditation reports	Personal experience or past organisational experience

- Focus groups
- Interviews
- Patient satisfaction surveys

It is critical to perform a thorough and comprehensive risk identification, because a risk that is not identified will not be included in the risk analysis. On the other hand, it is important to limit the number of risks identified, as it will be difficult to operationalise a list of many risks. The number of risks can be limited by focusing on only the most significant ones. The criteria for determining "significance" may differ depending on the organisation. One method that may be used is to consider those risks that might require the attention of senior leadership [23].

Key risks areas in ART identified by the HFEA in the UK [24] and by the European Society of Human Reproduction and Embryology (ESHRE) [25, 26] are based on findings from reported incidents over time. These include risks related to the gamete or embryo (such as incorrect identification, cross-infection, damage or loss) and to the patient (including failure of the consenting process, multiple pregnancy, cross-infection and errors in the donor information).

79.5.8 Risk Analysis

Risk analysis is the process used to understand the nature, sources and causes of risk identified. It also involves the evaluation of the information collected during the risk identification process to determine the probability that the consequence of the risk will occur (likelihood) and the potential severity of harm or loss associated with an identified risk [16, 18, 19]. Risk analysis should take into account existing controls.

79.5.8.1 Types of Analysis

There are three types of methodologies for risk analysis:

- **Quantitative methods**—These are the most accurate, provided the data is available. Examples include Probabilistic Analysis, Life-Cycle Cos Analysis, Influence Diagrams, etc.
- **Qualitative methods**—These depend on the experience and judgement of the assessors. It should therefore be performed by those who have a good grasp of the processes or situations and the organisational context. Examples include brainstorming and expert judgement.
- **Semi-Qualitative methods**—These involve the allocation of numbers or letters to qualitative rankings, e.g. A, B, C or 1, 2, 3 to represent high, medium or low. Care should be taken to ensure that the rankings are understood as approximations only, since they are not precise.

Ranking of risks is undertaken using the Likelihood Categories Table (Table 79.3), Consequence Categories Table (Table 79.4) and Risk Assessment Matrix (Fig. 79.1). The tables and matrix are to be used as guides to grading, and each incident should be considered in the context of all the available information.

Organisations can choose to adapt or adopt one of the many tables developed by other institutions, or they can develop one that meets their needs.

The tables below are provided by the HFEA to guide the mandatory reporting system in the UK [24]. For tables that include all aspects of the organisation, you can refer to the Clinical Risk Management Guidelines for the Western Australian Health System [15]

- Incidents are graded A if they fall in the red zone (the most serious), B if the fall in the yellow zone and C if the fall in the green zone.
- The red zone is the most serious, while the green zone is called as a "near miss", taking into account the severity of the outcome, or potential outcome, and the likelihood of a reoccurrence (Likelihood × Severity) [8, 24].

Table 79.3 Likelihood table

Likelihood level	Descriptor of risk likelihood	Definition
5	Almost certain	Likely to occur on many occasions
4	Likely	Probable but not persistent
3	Possible	May occur occasionally
2	Unlikely	Not expected to happen again but possible
1	Rare	Difficult to believe it could happen again

From the HFEA: Adverse incidents in fertility clinics: lessons to learn, 2010–2012 report [8]

Table 79.4 Consequences table

Severity level	Descriptor	Actual or potential impact on individual	Actual or potential impact on organisation	Numbers affected	Potential for complaint or litigation
5	Severe	Death of patient/staff, loss of all samples for many patients	Multi-agency investigation, adverse publicity, prosecution, loss of HFEA licence	One (e.g. death) or many (e.g. major cryostorage tank failure)	Litigation expected/ certain. Possible prosecution
4	Major	Major harm, professional misconduct, loss of all samples for a few patients, recurrent significant breach of HFEA Code of Practice (COP)	Costs, reputation damage, negative impact on staff morale, disciplinary hearings, loss of HFEA licence or conditions on practice	Smaller numbers 2–5	Litigation expected/ certain. Action taken by professional organisations, e.g. Health and Safety Executive (HSE), MHRA* or the General Medical Council (GMC)
3	Moderate	Semi-permanent harm, loss of all samples for one or loss of most samples for some patients, significant breach of COP	RIDDOR± or MHRA* reportable, compensation costs (e.g. provision of a complimentary treatment cycle)	1–2	Litigation possible but not certain. High potential for complaint
2	Minor	Short-term injury, minor breach of HFEA COP, avoidable risk, loss of one of many samples for a patient	Minimal risk to organisation	1	Complaint possible, litigation unlikely
1	Insignificant	No injury or adverse outcome	No risk to the organisation	1	Complaint and litigation unlikely

From the HFEA: Adverse incidents in fertility clinics: lessons to learn, 2010–2012 report [8].
*RIDDOR = Reporting of Injuries, Diseases and Dangerous Occurrences Regulations; MHRA = Medicines and Healthcare products Regulatory Agency)

Fig. 79.1 Risk level estimator (matrix) (from The HFEA website www.hfea.gov.uk)

Likelihood → / Severity ↓	Almost certain 5	Likely 4	Possible 3	Unlikely 2	Rare 1
Severe 5	25	20	15	10	5
Major 4	20	16	12	8	4
Moderate 3	15	12	9	6	3
Minor 2	10	8	6	4	2
Insignificant 1	5	4	3	2	1

79.5.9 Evaluate and Prioritise the Risk

At this stage, the organisation should review the risks identified against the criteria established at the onset while establishing the context for the RM process. The purpose is to determine which of the risks are acceptable or unacceptable, develop a prioritised list and determine which risks require treatment, the mode of treatment and at which level of the organisation they should be managed.

79.5.10 Treatment or Response to Risk

There are a number of options available to treat or respond to risks which may or may not be appropriate in a particular circumstance (Fig. 79.2).

79.5.10.1 Risk Acceptance

This is a conscious decision made to live with the consequences of a risk. It is important to note that acceptance does

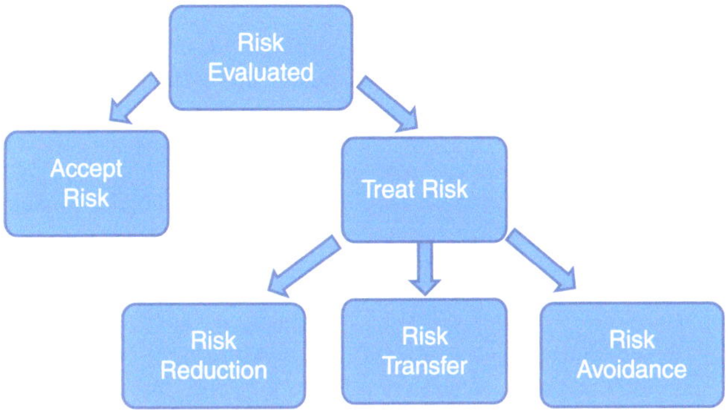

Fig. 79.2 Options for responding to risks

not indicate that the risk is insignificant. Neither does it mean that the risk will be ignored.

Some of the reasons why risks may be considered acceptable include:

- If the potential benefits of the situation outweigh the potential consequences
- If the risk is out of the control of the organisation and therefore there is no control or treatment available
- If the risk ranks low enough as to make committing resources to manage it inefficient

If the risk is found to be unacceptable, then it has to be treated. An example is accepting the risk of earthquakes and its consequences on the clinic and laboratory in earthquake prone regions.

Risk treatment options include risk avoidance, reduction and transfer.

79.5.10.2 Risk Avoidance

Risk can be avoided by choosing:

- Not to become involved in activities that can generate the risk
- An alternative activity that has less risk for the organisation
- An alternative method, pathway or process that is less risky to complete the desired activity or removing the hazard

Examples include prohibiting the use of fragrances and the wearing of perfumes in the IVF laboratory or referral of seropositive patients to centres that are better equipped to manage them so as to avoid the risk of cross-contamination.

79.5.10.3 Risk Reduction

This involves taking appropriate measures to reduce the possibility of an adverse event, its consequences or both. The establishment of identification or witnessing protocols is an example of risk reduction techniques. Witnessing provides assurance that all gametes or embryos are identifiable at all stages of the laboratory and treatment process, thereby preventing any gamete or embryo mismatches [28]. The practice of elective single embryo transfer (eSET) in patients that have high chances of multiple pregnancy, establishment of early warning or detection systems, e.g. fitting alarms to cryotanks to indicate a low level and/or high temperature alarm, is another example of RM in IVF clinics and laboratories [25]

79.5.10.4 Risk Transfer

This describes the shifting of the burden of the risk to another party that can better manage or control the risks. The most common method is insurance. Other methods of risk transfer are by legislation, contracts and administrative processes.

Setting up a quality management system (QMS) in the fertility clinic and laboratory is one of the ways of managing or responding to risk in ART. Some jurisdictions have made the establishment of a QMS mandatory for fertility clinics as a pre-condition for licensing, e.g. the HFEA in the UK [26].

Having a QMS involves control of documents and records; control of nonconformities; instituting corrective and preventive action; human resource management and the monitoring and measurement of quality [27, 28]. These are areas that have been linked with documented risks and adverse outcomes in ART.

79.5.11 Review and Monitor

Overall, it is the responsibility of the leadership to monitor and evaluate all aspects of the organisation's RM programme. Mechanisms should be developed to evaluate the outcomes and impact of RM systems and processes at all levels of the organisation. Key performance indicators (KPIs) should be developed to monitor and demonstrate the effectiveness of the programme. These KPIs should be reported to stakeholders regularly, so that areas that need attention and action are swiftly identified. This action should also be shared with colleagues, particularly those that have responsibility for quality improvement and patient safety, as they are opportunities for improvement.

The progress of the programme should also be evaluated against:

- Expected benefits such as improvement in allocation of resources
- Improved organisational preparedness for crises
- Identification of risks in areas that could have been missed [23]

The risks within an organisation are not static, and changes in risks identified and risk ratings can also be tracked over time [23].

79.6 Documentation of Risk Management Activities and Outcomes

The findings and results from the risk assessment activity should be documented in a Risk Register, which is the central repository of all documentation pertaining to an organisation's management of identified risks [16, 17, 23]. The Risk Register provides a way to compare and evaluate different types of risks. Furthermore, the list of significant risks can then be ranked in order of priority.

The Risk Register is considered a living document subject to review at regular intervals and as new information about risks comes to light. It will form the basis for reporting about the RM programme to senior leadership.

The Risk Register is also a valuable resource for setting organisational priorities and should be integrated into the organisation's strategic planning process.

79.7 Conclusion

An increasing number of people seeking to get pregnant are opting for the use of ART. Though the numbers of adverse events recorded are very low, ART patients have been shown to be at a higher risk of adverse events than the general population [2, 5, 27]. These incidents can put the patients, their gametes and embryos, the staff and the organisation in jeopardy. It is therefore imperative to develop a comprehensive and effective strategy to reduce the risks. Identification of the risk (clinical and non-clinical) areas is the first step in the approach to develop a risk-free IVF programme.

Essential elements in the development of a successful RM programme include demonstrable leadership commitment to the programme, integration of the risk program with the organisation's strategy objectives and with the quality and patient safety and adequate stakeholder engagement and involvement. Instituting a QMS in the clinic and laboratory is a good way to help manage risk. It is, however, important to note that it is not the documentation of the QMS but the spirit that makes the difference.

References

1. Kizer KW. Patient centre care: essential but probably not sufficient. Qual Saf Health Care. 2002;11:117–8.
2. de Ziegler D, Gambone JC, Meldrum DR, Chapron C. Risk and safety management in infertility and assisted reproductive technology (ART): from the doctor's office to the ART procedure. Fert Steril. 2013;100(6):1509–17.
3. World Health Organisation. Patient safety. Magnitude. Accessed 2 Mar 2017. http://www.who.int/patientsafety/en/
4. The Health Foundation. Research scan: evidence of harm. London, UK. November 2011
5. Sakkas D, Pool TB, Barrett CB. Analyzing IVF laboratory error rates: highlight or hide? RBM Online. 2015;31:447–8.
6. Kennedy CR, Mortimer D. Risk management in IVF. Best Pract Res Clin Obstet Gynaecol. 2007;21(4):691–712.
7. Bewley S, Foo L, Braude P. Adverse outcomes from IVF. BMJ. 2011;342:d436.
8. Human Fertilization and Embryology Authority. Adverse incidents in fertility clinics: lessons to learn. United Kingdom. 2010–2012.
9. Messano GA, De Bono V, Di Folco F, Marsella LT. Past and present of risk management in healthcare Ig. Sanità Pubbl. 2014;(70): 421–7.
10. Crockford GN. The bibliography and history of risk management: some preliminary observations. Geneva Pap Risk Insur. 1982;7:169–79.
11. Kuhn AM, Youngberg BJ. The need for risk management to evolve to assure a culture of safety. Qual Saf Health Care. 2002;(11):158–62.
12. Card AJ, Klein VR. A new frontier in healthcare risk management: working to reduce avoidable patient suffering. J Healthcare Risk Manag. 2015;35(3):31–7.
13. Van Seaton H. Enterprise risk management: COSO, New COSO, ISO 31000. Presentation to Council of Standards Australia on Nov. 6, 2009 and the Council of Standards New Zealand on Oct. 16, 2009.
14. The Australian Council on Healthcare Standards (ACHS) Risk Management and Quality Improvement Handbook. EQuIPNational. July 2013.
15. Carroll RL, Hoppes M, Hagg-Rickert S, Youngberg BJ. Enterprise risk management: a framework for success. American Society for Healthcare Risk Management; 2014.
16. Clinical Risk Management Guidelines for the Western Australian Health System Information series no. 8. Department of Health. East Perth, Western Australia.
17. Mortimer ST, Mortimer D. Quality and risk management in the IVF laboratory. 2nd ed. Cambridge, UK: Cambridge University Press; 2015.
18. McCaffrey JJ, Hagg-Rickert S. Development of a risk management program. In: Carroll RL, editor. Risk management handbook for health care organizations, student ed.; Hoboken, NJ, Wiley; 2009.
19. Kavaler F, Alexander RS. Risk management in healthcare institutions: limiting liability and enhancing care. 3rd ed. Burlington, MA: Jones and Bartlett; 2014.
20. Frith L, Blyth E. Assisted reproductive technology in the USA: is more regulation needed? RBM Online. 2014;29(4):516–23.
21. European Union. Commission Directive 2006/17/EC implementing Directive 2004/23/EC of the European Parliament and of the Council as regards certain technical requirements for the donation, procurement and testing of human tissues and cells. Offic J Eur Union. L38/40:9.2.2006.
22. https://healthit.ahrq.gov/health-it-tools-and-resources/workflow-assessment-health-it-toolkit/all-workflow-tools/risk
23. Integrated risk management for healthcare organizations. Risk Resource Guide Healthcare Insurance Reciprocal of Canada (HIROC). October 2014.
24. Human Fertilisation and Embryology Authority. HFEA risk tool. Accessed on the HFEA website on 26 Mar 2017. http://www.hfea.gov.uk/6674.html

25. Land JA, Evers JL. Risks and complications in assisted reproduction techniques: report of an ESHRE consensus meeting. Hum Reprod. 2003;18:455–7.
26. Human Fertilisation and Embryology Authority HFEA Code of Practice. 8th ed. United Kingdom; 2016.
27. Jain K. How safe is your IVF program? Fertil Sci Res. 2014;1:63–6.
28. Alper MM. Experience with ISO quality control in assisted reproductive technology. Fertil Steril. 2013;100:1503–8.

Screening for Infections Prior to Medically Assisted Reproduction

80

Ciara Hughes, Tim Dineen, and Bryan J. Woodward

Clinics offering assisted reproductive services should aim to provide couples or individuals the opportunity to have a healthy child in the safest possible manner. An aspect of particular concern for reproductive specialists is the risk of viral cross-contamination and infection during treatment.

If isolation of gametes or embryos during incubation, processing and cryostorage is compromised, there is an infection risk which can have either a vertical or horizontal mode of transmission, occurring from partner-to-partner, female-to-foetus, donor-to-recipient and patient-to-patient. Many infections have the potential to result in serious and life-threatening illnesses. Clinics have a responsibility to ensure that they have adequate screening policies and appropriate procedures in place. Furthermore, clinics who treat people who test positive for a blood-borne virus (BBV) or other sexually transmitted infection (STI) should have the necessary protocols (clinical and laboratory), facility infrastructure and equipment. This is needed to ensure safety for those individuals, their partner or recipients, other patients and the healthcare staff providing the treatment.

In 2004, the European Union (EU) issued a Parent Directive to all countries in the European Economic Area (EEA), known as the European Tissue and Cells Directive (EUTCD) (2004/23/EC) [1]. This was followed by two further Technical Directives (2006/17/EC) [2], (2006/86/EC) [3]. These Directives aimed to harmonize the regulatory approach across Europe, by setting standards of quality and safety for the donation, procurement, testing, processing, preservation, storage and distribution of human tissues and cells.

One area of the Directives that was highly debated related to the timing and frequency of the screening for assisted reproductive treatment (ART) or medically assisted reproduction (MAR) [4]. This discussion led to another Directive being issued in (2012/39/EU) [5], which amended further the requirements for screening specifically for ART.

This chapter reviews the current screening guidelines in Europe: who should be screened, when should they be screened, and what should they be screened for?

80.1 Why Is Screening Necessary?

From an individual's perspective, screening is important from a medical, ethical and legal viewpoint, as measures, such as referral to an appropriate physician for information about their condition, prognosis and treatment, can be taken in the event of a positive result. They can also be counselled about their reproductive options [4].

80.1.1 Legal and Regulatory Requirements

In 1995, the European Society of Human Reproduction and Embryology (ESHRE) recommended screening for both partners for hepatitis B (HBV), hepatitis C (HCV) and human immunodeficiency virus (HIV) prior to undergoing ART [6]. For all EEA countries, this became a legal requirement on 7 April 2004, with incorporation into their national laws required by 7 April 2006. The debate that followed related mainly to the timing and frequency of testing, with different countries adopting different interpretations of 'time of donation' [7].

In 2015, ESHRE revised their guidelines for good practice in IVF laboratories, stating that '*patients must be screened for infectious diseases according to national and international regulations*' [8].

C. Hughes (✉)
Embryology Department, Beacon Care Fertility, Dublin, Ireland

T. Dineen
Waterstone Clinic, Tivoli, Cork, Ireland

B. J. Woodward
X&Y Fertility, Leicester, UK

G. N. Allahbadia et al. (eds.), *Textbook of Assisted Reproduction*, https://doi.org/10.1007/978-981-15-2377-9_80

In 2008, the American Society of Reproductive Medicine (ASRM) published recommendations to reduce the risk of viral transmission during ART [9]. These guidelines were updated in 2013 and the title was amended to reflect that the document related specifically to the use of autologous gametes and that 'sexually intimate partners are excluded from United States Food and Drug Administration (FDA) mandated screening and testing for viral infections' [10]. Screening of gamete or embryo donors however is mandatory under federal law, with each state and local municipality having its own standards.

There has always been a concern regarding the risks of contamination and infection transmission in ART [11], since males have transmitted HIV, HBV or HCV to their partners via their infected semen [12, 13]. HCV contamination during fertility treatment has also been reported, although this was not traced directly to laboratory procedures [14].

The risk of cross-contamination during cryostorage was highlighted by HBV transmission from cryostored bone marrow [15]; yet the overall number of cross-contamination incidents reported in ART is still relatively low. However, cross-contamination can cause chronic lifelong infections and every effort should be taken to keep minimize risk.

80.1.2 Advantages and Disadvantages of Screening

From a clinical perspective, biological screening prior to donation is advantageous since it helps to prevent:

(i) Infection of viruses and other organisms from the donor to:
   (a) A recipient (in the case of a sexual partner)
   (b) A non-partner (in the case of gamete or embryo donation or a mix-up of gametes or embryos)
(ii) Cross-contamination in the ART facility, which could cause infection of:
   (a) Other patients
   (b) Members of staff
(iii) Viral transmission from the donor to the embryo
(iv) Cross-contamination between samples in the cryobanks

Disadvantages of screening primarily relate to cost and inconvenience. If people seeking ART don't receive state funding, they may face significant financial costs. Even if they have budgeted for the main cost of IVF or ICSI treatment, they may not have factored in costs of additional screening tests, investigations, travel, accommodation, medication and other 'add-ons' [16]. It is also time-consuming for both the clinic and the couple to attend appointments for repeat screening and may cause additional stress for the couple.

80.2 Who Should Be Screened and Do Some People Require More Specific Screening?

80.2.1 Couples Seeking Fertility Treatment with Their Own Gametes

There is a significant difference in the screening requirements for cohabiting couples who are seeking fertility treatment compared to individuals or couples who are donating gametes or embryos. In most cases, couples trying to conceive are sexually active without barrier contraception. Therefore, it is highly likely that if one partner has an STI, this will be passed on [17]. In cases where one partner is known to be BBV-positive, then ART treatment may reduce the risk of horizontal transmission [18–20].

Basic semen analysis clients, attending for diagnostic purposes only, do not require screening if the samples are examined in a laboratory dedicated to such assessments or in a designated space within the main laboratory with the appropriate operator precautions [7].

For couples undergoing a cycle of IVF or ICSI treatment using their own gametes, it is now accepted standard practice that both partners should be screened prior to commencing ART. For couples undergoing intrauterine insemination (IUI), it has been debated as to whether it is necessary to screen both partners, just the male or neither. Annex III of EU 2006/17/EC 2.2 states:

> In the case of sperm processed for IUI and not to be stored, if the tissue establishment can demonstrate that the risk of cross-contamination and staff exposure has been addressed through the use of validated processes, biological testing may not be required.

Most ART laboratories may process semen for IUI using the same equipment and area as for processing semen for IVF and ICSI. This increases the risk of cross-contamination even if equipment is decontaminated after every procedure. As a result, many clinics reduce this risk by routinely screening the male as for IVF or ICSI.

However, there is no requirement found in any legislation or regulation reviewed that dictates that the female needs to be screened. Clinics may opt to screen the female voluntarily as good clinical practice to establish viral screen status prior to attempting to achieve a pregnancy. Ultimately, the risk to the female of infection is reduced by sperm washing (when compared to natural intercourse) [18–20]. As a result of the costs and time frames involved, many clinics opt not to carry out screening for females undergoing IUI.

80.2.2 Individuals Who Are Donating Their Gametes or Embryos to a Third Party

At the turn of the century in the UK, the British Andrology Society published sperm donor screening guidelines [21] and the British Fertility Society published egg and embryo donor screening guidelines [22]. In 2008, these UK guidelines were collated and updated into a single document to reflect the introduction of the EUTCD and legal changes to sperm donation [23]. Screening not only covered BBVs and STIs but also age, history (genetic, medical and surgical and reproductive and sexual) and karyotyping.

Understandably, there are additional requirements for donor screening to reduce any infection risk to the recipient. In 2013, the ASRM practice committee published updated recommendations for gamete and embryo donation that outlines very specific screening requirements for gamete and embryo donation [24].

80.2.3 The Female Recipient and Male Partner in Third Party Donations

From the literature to date, there is no legal requirement outlining compulsory testing of the female recipient of donor material or of the male partner that is not biologically involved in the treatment. The 2013 ASRM guidelines recognized that donor screening is not a federal requirement but made very specific recommendations for screening of both the female recipient of the donor material and also of the male partner [24].

Most obstetricians will perform biological screening as part of good clinical practice for the female during pregnancy irrespective of the method of conception [25]. However, it could be argued that male screening is excessive and costly, when he has no involvement in a biological sense. The ASRM makes the argument that screening both partners will address any potential medical and legal issues that could arise should the partner seroconvert during or after donor use. If the male partner were found to be positive, it would also allow the clinical team the opportunity to ensure that he is referred for appropriate treatment and given advice on preventing transmission [24]. A similar argument can be made for screening the female partner in a same-sex couple having donor insemination treatment.

80.2.4 Healthcare Professionals in ART

Healthcare professionals are exposed to an infection risk from either blood sampling or handling of gametes and embryos from BBV-positive patients. To date, as far as we are aware, no case has been reported of infections from samples to the clinic staff [26].

Many clinics worldwide choose not to treat BBV-positive patients and refer them elsewhere. If clinics don't have the additional training, isolation equipment or separate cryostorage facilities, then this could be the safest approach. Whilst this reduces the risk of staff infection, universal precautions should always be adhered to minimize risk.

Conversely, although it has not been reported to date, it is theoretically possible that a BBV-positive healthcare staff member could infect a patient or their gametes and embryos. However, healthcare staff screening can be controversial, due to the possible impact on their employment role and duties if they were to test BBV-positive.

Legally, employees do not have to disclose if they have been tested for BBVs or their status [27], accepting that different countries and healthcare institutions have different staff screening policies. In both the UK and Ireland, under the relevant Health and Safety at Work Acts, employers have a legal duty to protect their employees and anyone else who might possibly be at risk of infection and have issued guidelines which outline the appropriate risk assessments and immunization advice for healthcare workers. The ESHRE 2015 guidelines for good laboratory practice made recommendations for personnel specifically in the ART setting [8] (Table 80.1).

Table 80.1 Recommendations for personnel working in ART

Recommendations for personnel working in ART
• Staff should be: – Vaccinated against HBV (and other viruses should vaccinations become available) – Informed when a viral-positive patient is to be treated so that they can take measures when handling potentially infectious biological material • Standard operating procedures should cover eventualities where infection might take place, e.g. needle stick injuries • Treatment of viral-positive patients should only be performed in IVF laboratories with dedicated areas or equipment or alternatively to specific time slots with subsequent decontamination of allocated areas and equipment

80.3 When to Screen and How Often?

When the EUTCD was implemented, there was no coherent approach across the EU community to either the interpretation of the 'time of donation' for testing nor the frequency of retesting for ART patients [7]. An ESHRE task force reported that within 19 countries that responded to a questionnaire, the variation of screening interval ranged from 3 to 24 months, with the most common being every 12 months [28].

80.3.1 Time of Initial Testing

The EU Directive 2006/17/EC Annex III stated that for partner donation 'biological screening must be carried out at the time of donation'. In Ireland at that time, it was agreed, following much debate with the Ireland competent authority that this could be extended to within 30 days of treatment for every cycle, but this still remained costly and time-consuming, particularly if cycles were cancelled or delayed. Other countries had interpreted time of donation differently [7] (Table 80.2).

In the USA, gamete donation is regulated by the FDA, with the minimal requirements for screening and applying only to those individuals or couples acting as a third-party donor [29]. Testing originally had to be at the 'time of donation' which was the same as for the EUTCD. However, an amendment following input from various stakeholders instigated a change in the ruling, stipulating that oocyte donors must be screened within 30 days prior to procurement. This allowed for proper donor eligibility assessment which would not be possible if taken on day of oocyte retrieval. Sperm donors were to be assessed at time of donation or within 7 days prior.

As screening was not required for couples in an intimate relationship who may then have embryos that they wished to donate to other couples, it became evident that these embryos could not be donated as the original screening criteria had not been met. Given the reduced availability of embryo donations, the FDA issued a ruling to allow embryo donation without the need for screening results at the time of donation.

Ideally, the donation could proceed if the appropriate tests were performed at the time when the decision was made to donate the embryos, with the couple being counselled accordingly. However, in the absence of any screening, a recipient couple could proceed with treatment using donor embryos following informed consent, knowing that the embryos had been labelled with 'not evaluated for infectious substances' and having been advised of the communicable disease risk [30].

Table 80.2 Initial variation in interpretation of the 'time of donation' for partner-partner donation in different European Countries

Country	Time of donation
Ireland	Within 30 days
Italy	Within 90 days
Germany, Greece, Belgium	At time of treatment
France and Spain	6 months prior to treatment
Netherlands and Norway	Maximum 12 months prior to treatment

From Dineen T, Woodward BJ. Chapter 10—Other factors to consider with sperm preparation for treatment. From "Male infertility: sperm diagnosis, management and delivery". Publishers Jaypee, India. ISBN 678-1-907816-46-8, with permission

80.3.2 Screening Frequency

Screening frequency for ART became a highly debated aspect of the EUTCD, particularly with regard to cohabiting couples. Several papers were published following EUTCD implementation showing no reported cases of HIV, HBV or HCV seroconversion in cohabiting couples and that the original screening frequency was excessive [17, 31–33].

In 2010, the European Commission issued a request to the European Centre for Disease Prevention and Control (ECDC), for their assistance to investigate the health risks of a potential change of EU legislation on tissue and cells. This followed many member states arguing that the testing requirements in the parent EUTCD did not improve the safety of the process compared to periodic screening of partners donating reproductive cells [34]. This report suggested that the commission should change the testing requirements to once per year, provided the clinic could demonstrate that the risks of staff exposure, cross-contamination and potential gamete mix-ups had been minimized through the use of validated quality and safety processes.

Recommendations were also made to centralise reporting of BBV testing via a standard protocol within the EU as part of quality assurance for tissue and cell donation establishments. It further recommended reviewing the chance of infecting embryos with BBVs and the risks of BBV transmission in cryostorage, as well as the possible risk of gamete mix-ups. To date, neither these recommendations have been realised.

In 2012, the EU Directive 2006/17/EC provided an updated testing frequency specific to ART from 'at the time of donation' to 'blood samples must be obtained within 3 months before the first donation'. If additional partner donations were made by the same donor, then more blood draws were needed, with frequency set by national legislation, but being within at least 24 months from previous sampling [5]. This was transposed into law in Ireland and the UK in 2012. Most clinics now operate the 3-month pre-treatment initial screen. Many clinics that already had a policy in place for screening once per year chose to remain with this time frame based on the demographics and prevalence in the clinics specific area.

Although the risk of seroconversion in cohabiting couples has been assessed and considered low when using their own gametes, there still remains a theoretical risk that seroconversion could occur.

80.4 What Biological Screening Tests Should Be Performed?

A survey was conducted in 2013 by the European Commission of all the member states regarding testing of donors of reproductive tissues and cells with data reported from 2011 [35].

Most of the reporting countries complied with the requirements in Annex III of 2006/17/EC with the exception of Lithuania and Poland due to an inappropriate transposition of the Directives for the ART sector. Three member states (Austria, Belgium and Finland) were reported to have more stringent requirements than outlined in the Directive in that they required mandatory nucleic acid testing (NAT) for HIV, HBV and HCV [35]. Table 80.3 indicates the testing performed in 2011 for of each member state.

Many of the guidelines or codes of practice published have statements such as '*Patients must be screened for infectious diseases according to national and international regulation*' [8]. Others have incorporated the requirements from the EUTCD directly [36, 37]. In addition to the well-known BBVs (HIV, HBV and HCV), clinics are now required to keep up-to-date with the increase in the incidence of new viruses that may pose a risk to health such as the West Nile virus (WNV) and the Zika virus.

ART clinics in Ireland and UK benefit from regular updates by the Health Products Regulatory Authority (HPRA) and the Human Fertilization and Embryology Authority (HFEA) respectively. For those countries that may not have notification processes in place, the ECDC [38], the Centres for Disease Control and Prevention (CDC) [39] and the World Health Organisation (WHO) [40] websites can be consulted regularly in order to keep abreast of disease outbreaks and testing advice.

The EUTCD has a significant difference in the screening tests required for partner and non-partner donation. Guidelines for specific tests should be assessed and adapted according to geographic region and prevalence of disease in that specific region [41]. Routine screening for genital infections, i.e. syphilis, gonorrhoea, chlamydia, herpes simplex, human papillomavirus and vaginal infection should be assessed alongside a full medical history/physical examination of both partners and the disease prevalence [41]. Risk assessment questionnaires should be designed based on this information and should request information on recent travel history to examine the possibility of infections such as the WNV, Zika, COVID-19, etc. Recent potential exposure to risk such as recent surgery, blood transfusion or body piercing should also be assessed. These risk assessments are often similar to the questionnaires used by the local blood transfusion organizations and these could be considered as a template on which to base the reproductive screening questionnaire.

Screening for every known virus or infection is impractical and costly. However, if a virus or infection is not detected and a cross-contamination occurs, the outcome can be very serious resulting in a chronic long-term health issue for the recipient or offspring.

80.4.1 Partner Donation

The minimal biological screening requirement of the EUTCD for all individuals or couples, as updated in 2012, is for HIV, HBV and HCV. These are legal requirements for all countries in the EEA [2].

Global variation remains regarding screening recommendations for couples using their own gametes but most countries perform the tests for HIV, HBC and HCV voluntarily as good clinical practice.

The European Commission in 2012, in addition to changing the time of screening, also updated the 2006/17/EC Directive regarding human T-cell lymphotropic viruses I–II (HTLV I-II) testing. The original Directive had requested testing to be performed in areas of high incidence. However, it had proven difficult to determine what exactly 'an area of high incidence' was and therefore screening policies had not been uniformly implemented across Europe [5]. The term 'incidence' measures the frequency of new disease cases, whilst 'prevalence' is the population percentage that is affected by a particular disease at a specific time. As prevalence data is more available, the 2012/39/EU Directive update reflected this change.

Regarding additional screening for partner donation, a risk assessment questionnaire should be completed with the couple. After reviewing this information, a decision can then be taken as to whether further testing is required or if treatment needs to be deferred.

80.4.2 Non-partner Donations

Whilst several guidelines give recommendations for genetic testing, blood typing and rhesus status, [2, 23, 24], only those proposed for BBVs and other STIs will be considered here. In 2013, the ASRM practice committee guidelines for gamete and embryo donation outlined specific screening requirements for both the female recipient and male partner, even in cases of sperm donation (Table 80.4).

In the UK, joint professional body guidelines for donor screening were issued [23]. These aimed to safeguard recipients of donor gametes and embryos from infection passed from a donor, whilst safeguarding donor-conceived offspring from picking up an infection or serious heritable disorder. Screening for HTLV and transmissible spongiform encephalopathies (TSE) such as Creutzfeldt-Jakob disease (CJD) were recommended. Even though validated testing was not available to confirm pre-mortem CJD, it was suggested that the donor should be rejected if they had 'been diagnosed with a prion-related disease or have first degree family members similarly diagnosed; undergone an invasive neurosurgi-

Table 80.3 Testing of donors of reproductive tissues and cells performed by EU member states (2011 data)

Tests for donors of reproductive tissues and cells/ country	Anti HIV 1Ab	Anti-HIV 2Ab	HIV ag	Nat HIV 1	HB sAg	AntiBc Ab	NAT HBV	Anti HCV Ab	NAT HCV	NAT chlamydia	*T. pallidum*	HTLV 1	Nat HTLV 1
Austria	Y	Y		Y	Y	Y	Y		Y	Y	Y		
Belgium	Y	Y		Y	Y	Y	Y	Y	Y	Y	Y		
Bulgaria	Y	Y			Y	Y		Y		Y	Y		
Cyprus	Y	Y			Y	Y		Y		Y	Y		
Czech Republic	Y	Y	Y		Y	Y		Y		Y	Y		
Germany	Y	Y			Y	Y		Y		Y	Y		
Denmark	Y	Y			Y	Y		Y		Y	Y		
Estonia	Y	Y		Y	Y	Y		Y	Y	Y	Y		
Spain	Y	Y	Y	Y	Y	Y	Y	Y	Y	Y	Y	Y	Y
Finland	Y	Y	Y	Y	Y	Y	Y	Y	Y	Y	Y		
France	Y	Y	Y		Y	Y		Y		Y	Y		
Croatia	Y	Y	Y		Y	Y		Y		Y	Y		
Hungary	Y	Y			Y	Y		Y			Y		
Ireland	Y	Y			Y	Y		Y			Y		
Italy	Y	Y			Y	Y		Y			Y		
Liech-tenstein	Y	Y			Y	Y		Y					
Lithuania	Y	Y									Y		
Luxem-bourg	Y	Y			Y	Y		Y			Y	Y	
Latvia	Y	Y			Y	Y		Y		Y	Y		
Malta	Y	Y			Y	Y		Y			Y		
Nether-lands	Y	Y			Y	Y		Y		Y	Y		
Norway	Y	Y			Y	Y		Y		Y	Y	Y	
Poland	Y	Y			Y	Y					Y		
Portugal	Y	Y			Y	Y		Y		Y	Y	Y	
Romania	Y	Y	Y		Y	Y		Y			Y	Y	Y
Sweden	Y	Y	Y		Y	Y		Y			Y	Y	
Slovenia	Y	Y	Y		Y	Y		Y			Y		
Slovakia	Y	Y			Y	Y		Y			Y		
UK	Y	Y			Y	Y		Y			Y	Y	

Table 80.4 Outline of the guidelines published in 2013 by the ASRM for the biological screening recommended for gamete and embryo donor, female recipients and male partners

	ASRM Sperm donation			ASRM Oocyte donation			ASRM Embryo donation At least 180 days after cryopreservation[a]	
Biological test	Donor	Female recipient	Male partner	Donor	Female recipient	Male partner	Female (donor)	Male (donor)
Human immunodeficiency virus (HIV 1 NAT testing & HIV 2 Ab) HIV Group 0 antibodies	Recommended	Recommended	Recommended	Recommended	Recommended	Recommended	Recommended	Recommended
Hepatitis B (HBsAg and AntiHBc IgG, IgM)	Recommended	Recommended	Recommended	Recommended	Recommended	Recommended	Recommended	Recommended
Hepatitis C (HCV) Antibody and NAT	Recommended	Recommended	Recommended	Recommended	Recommended	Recommended	Recommended	Recommended
Human T-lymphotropic virus (HTLV-I)	Recommended	Request at clinician's discretion	Request at clinician's discretion					Recommended
Cytomegalovirus (CMV IgG, IgM)	Recommended	Recommended						Recommended
Chlamydia (*Chlamydia trachomatis*)	Recommended	Recommended	Recommended	Recommended	Recommended		Recommended	Recommended
Syphilis (*Treponema pallidum*)	Recommended	Recommended	Recommended	Recommended	Recommended	Recommended	Recommended	Recommended
Gonorrhoea (*Neisseria Gonorrhoeae*)	Recommended	Recommended	Recommended	Recommended	Recommended		Recommended	Recommended
West Nile virus (WNV)	Not requested for but if any history or symptoms, defer for 120 days			Not requested for but if any history or symptoms, defer for 120 days				
Transmissible spongiform encephalopathies *Creutzfeldt-Jakob disease (CJD)*	Not requested but reject if any diagnosis has been made			Not requested for but reject if any diagnosis has been made				
Quarantine—180 days	Not discussed			Considered not practical for eggs but should be considered for resulting embryos				

[a]ASRM recommends that the recipients submit to the same blood tests for infectious disease as for donors for sperm donation

cal procedure; or received invasive pituitary-derived growth hormone, cornea, sclera or dura mater'.

Considerable research has since been undertaken to address the lack of validated blood tests for routine screening for asymptomatic donors of CJD. Whilst some research shows promise [42, 43], no test has been confirmed as validated. Table 80.5 shows a comparison of recommended test for donors between the EUTCD, HFEA, Joint UK Professional Bodies and the Irish Legislation, including those for CJD.

Table 80.5 Recommended biological screening for donors other than partners

Biological test	EUTCD As stipulated by section 2 of Annex III of the European Union Tissues and Cells Directive 2006	HFE Act and 9th Code of Practice	UK Joint Association Guidelines[a]	IRISH Statutory Instruments 158/2006 209/2014
Human immunodeficiency virus (HIV 1 & 2)	Legal requirement	Legal requirement	Recommended	Legal requirement
Hepatitis B (HBsAg and AntiHBc)	Legal requirement	Legal requirement	Recommended	Legal requirement
Hepatitis C (HCV)	Legal requirement	Legal requirement	Recommended	Legal requirement
Human T-lymphotropic virus (HTLV-I)	Legal requirement but only if donors/sexual partner living in or originating from high prevalence area	Legal requirement but only if donors / sexual partner living in or originating from high prevalence area	Recommended	Legal requirement but only if donors/sexual partner living in or originating from high prevalence area
Cytomegalovirus (CMV IgG, IgM)	Not specifically requested May be requested under general STI investigation following medical/ physical assessment	Not specifically requested May be requested under general STI investigation following medical/ physical assessment	Recommended	Not specifically requested May be requested under general STI investigation following medical/ physical assessment
Chlamydia (*Chlamydia trachomatis*)	Legal requirement NAT testing	Legal requirement NAT testing for sperm donors only	Recommended	Legal requirement NAT testing for sperm donors only
Syphilis (*Treponema pallidum*)	Legal requirement	Legal requirement	Recommended	Legal requirement
Gonorrhoea (*Neisseria gonorrhoeae*)	Not specifically requested May be requested under general STI investigation following medical/ physical assessment	Not specifically requested May be requested under general STI investigation following medical/ physical assessment	Recommended	Not specifically requested May be requested under general STI investigation following medical/ physical assessment
Human papillomavirus (HPV)	Not specifically requested May be requested under general STI investigation following medical/ physical assessment	Not specifically requested May be requested under general STI investigation following medical/ physical assessment	Physical examination—defer if necessary	Not specifically requested May be requested under general STI investigation following medical/ physical assessment
Herpes simplex virus (HSV)	Not specifically requested May be requested under general STI investigation following medical/ physical assessment	Not specifically requested May be requested under general STI investigation following medical/ physical assessment	Physical examination—defer if necessary	Not specifically requested May be requested under general STI investigation following medical/ physical assessment
Epstein-Barr virus (EBV)	Not specifically requested May be requested under general STI investigation following medical/ physical assessment	Not specifically requested May be requested under general STI investigation following medical/ physical assessment	Not requested	Not specifically requested May be requested under general STI investigation following medical/ physical assessment
West Nile virus (WNV)	Request test based on demographics and medical and recent travel history	Request test based on demographics and medical and recent travel history	Not requested	Request test based on demographics and medical and recent travel history
Zika virus	Request test based on demographics and medical and recent travel history	Request test based on demographics and medical and recent travel history	Not requested	Request test based on demographics and medical and recent travel history

Table 80.5 (continued)

Biological test	EUTCD As stipulated by section 2 of Annex III of the European Union Tissues and Cells Directive 2006	HFE Act and 9th Code of Practice	UK Joint Association Guidelines[a]	IRISH Statutory Instruments 158/2006 209/2014
Ebola	Request test based on demographics and medical and recent travel history	Request test based on demographics and medical and recent travel history	Not requested	Request test based on demographics and medical and recent travel history
Malaria	Request test based on demographics and medical and recent travel history	Request test based on demographics and medical and recent travel history	Not requested	Request test based on demographics and medical and recent travel history
T. cruzi	Request test based on demographics and medical and recent travel history	Request test based on demographics and medical and recent travel history	Not requested	Request test based on demographics and medical and recent travel history
Quarantine 180 day period with retest recommended	Legal requirement unless nucleic acid amplification technique (NAT) or validated virus inactivation step has been carried out	Legal requirement unless nucleic acid amplification technique (NAT) or validated virus inactivation step has been carried out	Sperm Recommended Oocytes—not recommended—recipients to be warned of risks Embryo—where possible screen retrospectively	Legal requirement unless nucleic acid amplification technique (NAT) or validated virus inactivation step has been carried out
Transmissible spongiform encephalopathies *Creutzfeldt-Jakob disease (CJD)*	Not requested	Not requested	Recommended. Currently no test available but exclusion criteria applied	Not requested

Comparing EUTCD as stipulated by section 2 of Annex III of the European Union Tissues and Cells Directive 2006, HFEA, UK Joint guidelines
[a]ABA/ACE/BAS and BFS guidelines and the Irish legislation

80.5 Should Screening for Cytomegalovirus Be Routine?

80.5.1 The Background to CMV

Historically, rubella was the most prevalent infectious cause of embryo fetopathy worldwide. However, a systemic vaccination and screening program reduced its prevalence significantly, and it has now been replaced by cytomegalovirus (CMV) [44]. According to the EUTCD [2], the need for CMV screening relates to where the donors have recently travelled to and their likelihood of exposure.

In Europe, an estimated 0.5–0.9% of children are born with congenital CMV infection [44], with ~11% of these infants being symptomatic [45]. There is a 30–40% risk of vertical transmission with primary maternal CMV infection in pregnancy, of these ~10–20% will have evidence of infection at birth [46]. Primary infection during the first trimester of pregnancy can result in impaired vision, progressive sensorineural hearing loss and mental retardation for the offspring [44]. Given the viral prevalence and the potential adverse fetal impact, the question is whether or not to routinely screen for CMV in pregnancy [47–49], or more specifically prior to ART [44].

80.5.2 CMV: Who Should Be Screened and When?

Women who are either contemplating pregnancy or who have already conceived should at least consider CMV screening. A review of the literature indicates that there is no clear policy for screening couples for CMV who intend to use their own gametes, unless the clinician identifies a risk in the medical history that would warrant such screening. Some might argue that it would be a waste of resources to universally screen women who are already pregnant or who are contemplating pregnancy. However, if there were a proven intervention that could help treat the infection, then universal screening would be preferred and considered the most cost-effective strategy [47]. This approach is still under debate.

80.5.3 Laboratory Testing for CMV

CMV infection can be detected by testing for CMV-specific IgG and IgM antibodies. IgM antibodies are first exposed early in the primary infection and IgG antibodies are produced within a few weeks of initial infection but will generally remain throughout life as a constant indication of previous infection. However, CMV antibody response is inconsistent particularly with IgM, with antibodies persisting for months following primary infection and even increasing in concentration during reactivation of viral replication [50, 51]. In addition, discordance has been reported among the commercial CMV IgM tests, together with results that were false-positive [52]. This uncertainty has given rise to concerns about the interpretation of these results.

The Centre for the Disease Control and the UK National Screening Committee do not recommend systematic population screening for CMV in pregnancy [53, 54]. The Institute of Medicine in the USA identified vaccine development for CMV as a major public health priority back in 1999 [55], but a review of the literature would suggest that a robust vaccination for CMV still requires more research and safety validation before it could be implemented.

The authors believe that until safe and successful CMV vaccination programs exist, routine screening for all couples (using own gametes) undergoing ART is not currently warranted. However, all people contemplating pregnancy should be given advice regarding the spread of CMV particularly in terms of hygiene.

80.5.4 CMV Testing Using Donors Other Than Partners

The EUTCD states that the CMV screening should be carried out only if there is a recent travel or exposure history. In an ideal situation, only negative donors should be recruited but, with an acute shortage of donors, there has been much debate as to whether this is a reasonable approach [56].

There is little data available to confirm if CMV can be transmitted through the donation of eggs or embryos, but it is agreed that it is likely to be considerably lower than with sperm donation. The joint UK guidelines recommend recruitment of CMV-negative donors and if sufficient in numbers, then recruitment of positive donors should be avoided [23]. CMV-positive donors should only be used with CMV-positive recipients. Anyone who seroconverts or who is positive with CMV IgM should defer donation. These guidelines apply to all sperm, egg and embryo donors.

The ASRM guidelines concur with this strategy for sperm donation, whilst for egg donors, there is no requirement for CMV testing and for embryo donors there is only a requirement for the male to be tested for CMV.

80.6 Conclusion

A report from the European Commission indicated that EUTCD implementation has been considered 'adequate', with all Member States now having appointed competent authorities [35]. However, some Member States had differing approaches in the implementation which has restricted the ever-increasing demand to transfer gametes and embryos between countries. Safe distribution requires clinics to establish standardised screening methods.

The EUTCD states:

> The availability of human tissues and cells used for therapeutic purposes is dependent on community citizens who are prepared to donate them. In order to safe guard public health and to prevent the transmission of infectious diseases by these tissues and cells, all safety measures need to be taken during their donation, procurement, testing, processing, preservation, storage, distribution and use [1].

This legislation forces clinics in Europe to do their utmost to minimise cross-contamination risks. In summary, each clinic should develop a robust system for assessing individuals medically and physically to identify additional risks. Screening policies should comply with local and national legislation and consider local demographics and prevalence of BBV and other STIs. Quality management systems should underpin the running of a clinic to ensure that protocols are in place for training, procedures, screening and quarantine.

There should also be a mechanism to ensure that when new risks are identified, e.g. the Zika virus, that the information can be effectively communicated to staff so that they are aware of the additional precautions that may need to be taken. The laboratory must have either isolation facilities (including cryostorage), for known positive cases. If the facilities don't permit this, they should have dedicated time allocations for the handling of these cases with validated decontamination protocols. Universal precautions should apply in all cases where potentially infectious materials are handled, but additional training should be provided for known positive cases as they may require additional processing steps.

ART clinics may need to revisit their screening programmes to allow the treatment of BBV-positive individuals, to minimize transmission risk between the couple and to others attending and working in the clinic. Preventing access to ART may no longer be the solution, especially given the advances in treatment for such infections that have been made and the improved life expectancy [57].

References

1. European Union. Commission Directive 2004/23/EC of the European Parliament and of the Council of 31 March 2004 on setting standards of quality and safety for the donation, procurement, testing, processing, preservation, storage and distribution of human tissues and cells. Offic J Eur Union. L102/48.
2. European Union. Commission Directive 2006/17/EC of 8 February 2006 implementing Directive 2004/23/EC of the European Parliament and of the Council as regards certain technical requirements for the donation, procurement and testing of human tissues and cells. Offic J Eur Union. L38/40.

3. European Union. Commission Directive 2006/86/EC of 24 October 2006 implementing Directive 2004/23/EC of the European Parliament and of the Council as regards traceability requirements, notification of serious adverse reactions and events and certain technical requirements for the coding, processing, preservation, storage and distribution of human tissues and cells. Offic J Eur Union. L294/32.
4. Engelert Y, Lesage B, Liesnard C, Van den Bergh M. Design of a high security assisted reproduction technology laboratory for hepatitis B, C and HIV positive patients. Hum Reprod. 2002;17:393.
5. European Union. Commission Directive 2012/39/EC of 26 November 2012 amending Directive 2006/17/EC as regards certain technical requirements for the testing of human tissues and cells Offic J Eur Union. L327/24.
6. Van den Eede B. Investigation and treatment of infertile couples. ESHRE guidelines for good clinical and laboratory practice. European Society of Human Reproduction and Embryology. Hum Reprod. 1995;10:1246–71.
7. Dineen TM, Woodward B. Other factors to consider with sperm preparation for treatment. In: Mehta J, Woodward B, editors. Male infertility: sperm diagnosis, management and delivery. London: JP Medical; 2014. p. 71–80.
8. De los Santos MJ, Apter S, Coticchio G, Debrock S, Lundin K, Plancha CE, Prados F, Rienzi L, Verheyen G, Woodward B, Vermeulen N. ESHRE Revised guidelines for good practice in IVF laboratories (2015). Hum Reprod. 2016;31(4):685–6.
9. Practice Committee of the American Society for Reproductive Medicine. Recommendations for reducing the risk of viral transmission. Fertil Steril. 2006; 86(5): S11–S1.
10. Practice Committee of the American Society for Reproductive Medicine. Recommendations for reducing the risk of viral transmission during fertility treatment with the use of autologous gametes: a committee opinion. Fertil Steril. 2013;99(2):340–6.
11. Steyaert SR, Leroux-Roels GG, Dhont M. Infections in IVF : review and guidelines. Hum Reprod Update. 2000;5(6):432–41.
12. Englert Y, Lesage B, Van Vooren JP, Liesnard C, Place I, Vannin AS, Emiliani S, Delbaere A. Medically assisted reproduction in the presence of chronic viral diseases. Hum Reprod Update. 2004;10:149–62.
13. Sauer MV. Sperm washing techniques address the fertility need of HIV seropositive men: a clinical review. Reprod Biomed Online. 2005;10:135–40.
14. Lesourd F, Izopet J, Mervan C, Payen JL, Sandres K, Monrozies X, Parinaud J. Transmissions of hepatitis C virus during the ancillary procedures for assisted conception. Hum Reprod. 2000;15:1083–5.
15. Tedder RS, Zuckerman MA, Goldstone AH, Hawkins AE, Fielding A, Briggs EM, et al. Hepatitis B transmission from contaminated cryopreservation tank. Lancet. 1995;346:137–40.
16. Kelly J, Hughes C, Harrison RF. The hidden costs of IVF. Ir Med J. 2006;99(5):142–3.
17. Wingfield M, Cottell E. Viral screening of couples undergoing partner donation in assisted reproduction with regard to EU Directives 2004/23/EC, 2006/17/EC and 2006/86/EC: what is the evidence for repeated screening? Hum Reprod. 2010;25(12):3058–65.
18. Abou-Setta AM. Transmission risk of hepatitis C virus via semen during assisted reproduction: how real is it? Hum Reprod. 2004;(12):2711–7.
19. Gilling-Smith C, Emiliani S, Almeida P, Liesnard C, Englert Y. Laboratory safety during assisted reproduction in patients with blood borne viruses. Hum Repod. 2005;20:1433–8.
20. Allahbadia GN. Viral hepatitis and assisted reproduction. J Obstet Gynecol India. 2015;66(6):397–403.
21. British Andrology Society. Guidelines for the screening of semen donors for donor insemination. Hum Reprod. 1999;14:1823–6.
22. Aird I, Barratt C, Murdoch A. and BFS Committee. BFS recommendations for good practice on screening of egg and embryo donors. Hum Fertil. 2000;3:162–5.
23. Association of Biomedical Andrologists, Association of Clinical Embryologists, British Andrology Society, British Fertility Society & Royal College of Obstetricians and Gynaecologists. UK guidelines for the medical and laboratory screening of sperm, egg and embryo donors. Hum Fertil. 2008; 11(4):201–210.
24. Practice Committee of the American Society for Reproductive Medicine. Recommendation for gamete and embryo donation: a committee opinion. Fertil Steril. 2013;99(1):47–62.
25. National Health Service (NHS) UK. Infectious diseases in pregnancy screening (IDPS): programme overview. Available from: https://www.gov.uk/guidance/infectious-diseases-in-pregnancy-screening-programme-overview.
26. Magli C, Van den Abbeel E, Lundin K, Royere D, Vander Elst J, Gianaroli L. Committee of the Special interest group on Embryology. Revised guidelines for good practice in IVF laboratories. Hum Reprod. 2008;23:1523–262.
27. Health and safety Executive UK. Blood-borne viruses in the workplace. Guidance for employers and employees. Available from http://www.hse.gov.uk/pubns/indg342.pdf
28. Mocanu E. O-244 EU Tissues and cells directive—State of the art. Hum Reprod. 2010; 25.
29. Food and Drug Administration. Code of Federal Regulations 21 Available from: https://www.accessdata.fda.gov/scripts/cdrh/cfdocs/cfcfr/CFRSearch.cfm?fr=1271.90
30. Food and Drug Administration. Human cells, tissues, and cellular and tissue-based products; donor screening and testing; and related labelling. Available from: http://www.fda.gov/BiologicsBloodVaccines/TissueTissueProducts/QuestionsaboutTissues/ucm136397.htm
31. Pepas L, MacMahon Eel Youkhy T, Khalaf Y, Brause P. Viral screening before each cycle of assisted conception treatment is expensive and unnecessary: a survey of result from a UK inner city clinic. Hum Fertil (Camb). 2011;14:224–9.
32. Hughes C, Grundy K, Emerson G, Mocanu E. Viral screening at the time of each donation in ART patient: is it justified? Hum Reprod. 2011;26(11):3169–72.
33. Mocanu EV. Facts and myths in serological screening of ART couples. Facts Views Vis Obgyn. 2012;4(3):198–202.
34. European Centre for Disease prevention and Control. Technical report. Risk assessment on change of testing requirements for partner donation of reproductive cells. Available from: http://ec.europa.eu/health//sites/health/files/sti_prevention/docs/ecdc_ra_donation_reproductive_cells.pdf.
35. European Commission. Commission staff working document on the implementation of Directives 2004/23/EC, 2006/17/EC and 2006/86/EC on setting standards of quality and safety for the donation, procurement, testing, processing, preservation, storage and distribution of human tissues and cells. *Accompanying the document.* Report from the Commission to the European Parliament, the Council, The European Economic and Social Committee and the Committee of the Regions on the Implementation of Directives 2004/23/EC, 2006/17/EC and 2006/86/EC setting standards of quality and safety for human tissues and cells. Available from: http://eur-lex.europa.eu/legal-content/EN/TXT/?uri=CELEX%3A52016SC0127
36. Human Fertilisation and Embryology Authority. 9th Code of Practice, UK. Available from: https://www.hfea.gov.uk/media/2565/hfea-draft-code-of-practice-9th-edition-consultation-version.pdf
37. European Communities (Quality and Safety of Human Tissues and Cells) Regulations 2006. S.I. No. 158/2006. Available from: http://www.irishstatutebook.ie/eli/2006/si/158/made/en/print#article1
38. http://ecdc.europa.eu/en/Pages/home.aspx
39. https://www.cdc.gov/
40. www.who.int/
41. Elder K, Baker, D, Ribes J. Prevention: patient screening and the use of donor gametes. In: Infections, infertility and assisted reproduction. New York: Cambridge University Press; 2011. p 353–64.

42. Jackson GS, Burk-Rafel J, Edgeworth JA, Sicilia A, Abdilahi S, Korteweg J, Mackey J, Thomas C, Wang G, Schott JM, Mummery C, Chinnery PF, Mead S, Collinge J. Population screening for variant Creutzfeldt-Jakob disease using a novel blood test: diagnostic accuracy and feasibility study. JAMA Neurol. 2014;71(4):421–8.
43. Concha-Marambio L, Pritzkow S, Moda F, Tagliavini F, Ironside JW, Schulz PE, Soto C. Detection of prions in blood from patients with variant Creutzfeldt-Jakob disease. Sci Transl Med. 2016;8(370):370ra183.
44. Kling C, Kabelitz D. Congenital HCMV and assisted reproduction: why not use the chance for primary screening? Arch Gynecol Obstet. 2015; 291:1205–11.
45. Kenneson A, Canoon MJ. Review and meta-analysis of the epidemiology of congenital cytomegalovirus (CMV) infection. Rev Med Virol. 2007;17(4):253–76.
46. Bhide A, Papageorghiou AT. Managing primary CMV infection in pregnancy. BJOG. 2008;115:805–7.
47. Cahill AG, Odibo AO, Stamilio DM, Macones GA. Screening and treating for primary cytomegalovirus infection in pregnancy: where do we stand? A decision analytic and economic analysis. Am J Obstet Gynecol. 2009;201:466.e1–7.
48. Carlson A, Norwitz ER, Stiller RJ. Cytomegalovirus infection in pregnancy: should all women be screened? Rev Obstet Gynecol. 2010;4(3):172–9.
49. Walker SP, Palma-Dias R, Wood EM, Shekleton P, Giles ML. Cytomegalovirus in pregnancy: to screen or not to screen. BMC Pregnancy Childbirth. 2013;13:96.
50. Nyholm JL, Schleiss MR. Prevention of maternal cytomegalovirus infection: current status and future prospects. Int J Womens Health. 2010;(2):23–35.
51. Elder K, Baker D, Ribes J. Cytomegalovirus and blood-borne viruses. In: Infections, infertility and assisted reproduction. New York: Cambridge University Press; 2011. p. 262–9.
52. Lazzarotto T, Brojanac S, Maine GT, Landini MP. Search for cytomegalovirus-specific immunoglobulin M: comparison between a new western blot, conventional western blot, and nine commercially available assays. Clin Diagn Lab Immunol. 1997;4(4):483–6.
53. Centres for Disease Control and Prevention (CDCP). Cytomegalovirus (CMV) and Congenital CMV infection. Available from: https://www.cdc.gov/cmv/clinical/features.html.
54. UK National Screening Committee. Current UK NSC recommendations. Available from: https://legacyscreening.phe.org.uk/screening-recommendations.php.
55. Stratton K, Durch J, Lawrence R. Vaccines for the 21st century: a tool for decision making. Washington, DC: National Academy Press; 2001.
56. Liesnard CA, Revelard P. Englert. Screening standards in assisted reproductive technologies. Is the British Andrology Society recommendation to recruit cytomegalovirus negative semen donors only, a reasonable one? Hum Reprod. 2001;16:1789–91.
57. Savasi V, Ferrazzi E, Fiore S. Reproductive assistance for infected couples with blood-borne viruses. Placenta. 2008:S160–5.

Treating Patients with Blood-Borne Viruses

81

Michael Bright Yakass, Bryan J. Woodward, and Osbourne Quaye

81.1 Learning Objectives

At the end of this chapter, the reader will appreciate:

- The basic pathobiology of viruses of reproductive health importance
- How to handle samples from patients with blood-borne viruses
- The basic laboratory setup to handle these samples
- The biosafety controls to be instituted

Viral infections are a public health concern in people of reproductive age globally, with prevalence varying according to location and exposure to risk factors (Table 81.1). About 37 million people are estimated to be infected by the human immunodeficiency virus (HIV), with about 50–60% of them in their reproductive ages [1]. Viral coinfections in an individual are common, with about three million HIV-infected persons also infected with the Hepatitis B virus (HBV) [2]. With the improvement and efficacy in highly activated antiretroviral therapy (HAART), public awareness, and healthy diets, HIV-infected persons are living longer than they used to a decade or two ago, and many of them wish to fulfill their human right to produce a family of their own [3]. To accomplish this safely, many people are resorting to medically assisted reproduction to minimize the risk of infecting their partners and/or their prospective children.

In order not to deny virus-infected people fertility treatment, laboratories should put in place safety measures to prevent or avoid contamination and infection of the laboratory personnel and patients receiving treatment.

The European Society of Human Reproduction and Embryology (ESHRE) [4] and the American Society for Reproductive Medicine (ASRM) [5] have both issued guidelines on risk reduction when handling gametes of virus-infected patients.

81.2 Basic Biology of Viruses

Viruses are obligate intracellular parasites, meaning that they need a living host to propagate and infect new host cells. Most viruses are in sizes ranging from 30 to 500 nm and can only be observed with an electron microscope. The naming of viruses has been somewhat haphazard: sometimes named after the person who first isolated the virus (e.g., Epstein-Barr virus, named after British scientists M.A. Epstein and Y.M. Barr), from whom the virus was first isolated (e.g., Asibi strain of yellow fever virus, named after a Ghanaian patient), or the town/city the virus was first isolated in (e.g., Zika virus, after the Zika Forest in Uganda). Viruses have been reclassified into families, genus, and species according to their genetic material (RNA or DNA), sizes, and shapes.

Most viruses go through a common life cycle of attachment, entry, uncoating, replication, protein synthesis, assembly, and egress/budding out to infect other cells. One thing is common to most viruses: they seize the host transcription and translation apparatus to propagate more viruses. Like other pathogens, viruses tend to preferentially infect certain kinds of cells. For example, HBV mainly infects hepatocytes, whereas HIV infects CD4+ T-helper cells.

M. B. Yakass (✉)
Virology Laboratory, West African Centre for Cell Biology of Infectious Pathogens, Department of Biochemistry, Cell & Molecular Biology, University of Ghana, Accra, Ghana

Assisted Conception Unit, Lister Hospital & Fertility Centre, Accra, Ghana

B. J. Woodward
X&Y Fertility, Leicester, UK

O. Quaye
Virology Laboratory, West African Centre for Cell Biology of Infectious Pathogens, Department of Biochemistry, Cell & Molecular Biology, University of Ghana, Accra, Ghana

G. N. Allahbadia et al. (eds.), *Textbook of Assisted Reproduction*, https://doi.org/10.1007/978-981-15-2377-9_81

81.2.1 Viral Genomes and Replication

A virus may have DNA or RNA as the genetic material. There are seven different viral genomes: double-stranded DNA (dsDNA), gapped dsDNA, single-stranded DNA (ssDNA), dsRNA, plus (+) strand ssRNA, minus (–) strand ssRNA, and (+) strand ssRNA with DNA intermediate. Since a virus lacks translation apparatus, all viral genomes must make mRNA to be read and translated by host ribosomes.

Depending on the viral genome and associated proteins, some viruses may integrate into host DNA or remain as non-integrants in the nucleus or cytoplasm of infected cells. Some RNA viruses, called retroviruses (e.g., HIV), contain an enzyme called reverse transcriptase, which makes a complementary DNA strand that is then inserted into host DNA before transcription and translation of viral proteins can occur (Fig. 81.1).

Table 81.1 Risk factors for viral infections

HIV/Hepatitis B and C
Unsafe sex—vaginal or anal intercourse with infected person
Injections—recreational drug use
Vertical transmission—mother-to-child
Blood transfusion
Occupational—healthworkers
Multiple sex partners
Migration—travelling to endemic countries

81.3 Viruses of Reproductive Health Importance

A number of viruses have been noted to be of reproductive health importance mainly because they are transmitted sexually, in utero or in perinatal stages. For the purposes of this chapter, a few well-researched viruses of reproductive health importance will be discussed. It should be noted other viruses may also impact on reproductive health, but they are less researched, such as West Nile virus which was detected in patients in France and Slovenia in 2018.

81.3.1 Human Immunodeficiency Virus (HIV)

HIV is a *retrovirus* infecting mainly the immune cell CD4+ T-helper. The RNA genome is reverse transcribed by a reverse transcriptase enzyme into a double-stranded DNA, which is integrated into the host DNA using the viral integrase enzyme. HIV-1 is prevalent worldwide, whereas HIV-2 is mostly found in West Africa. Currently there are no vaccines for HIV, and affected individuals can be treated via antiretroviral therapy. Shedding of the virus has been detected in seminal [6] and follicular fluids [7]; however, semen is the main route of transmission.

HIV-infected males generally have reduced sperm quality (concentration and motility) [8]. A proteomic analysis of semen produced by HIV-infected males on antiretroviral

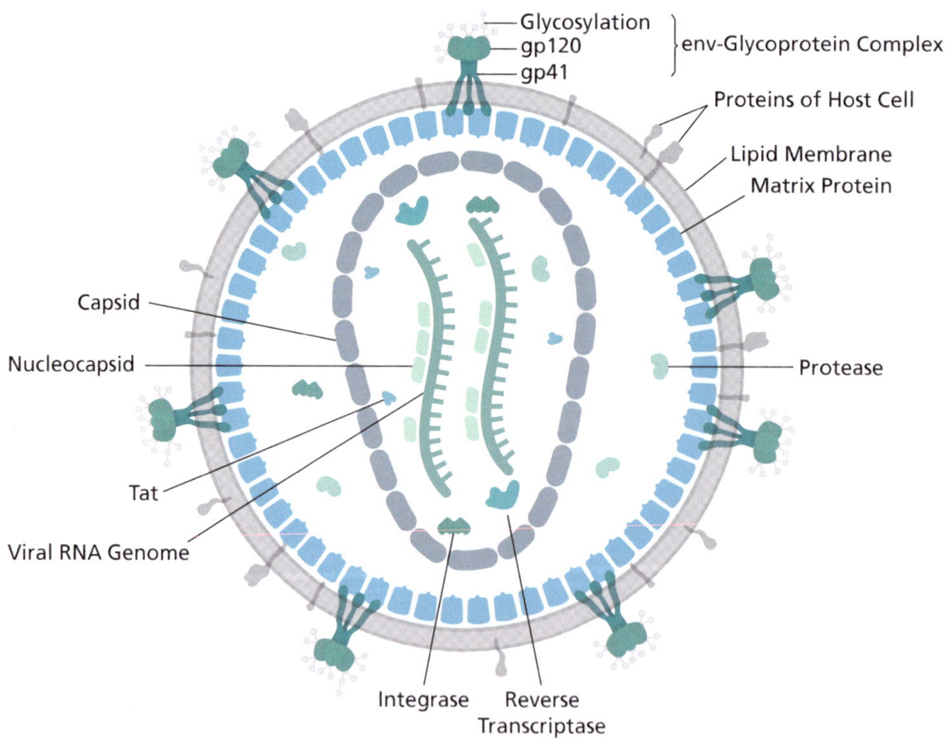

Fig. 81.1 A diagrammatic illustration of a typical virus (HIV). The diagram shows the typical structure of a virus, with the nucleic acid material encapsulated in a nucleocapsid (a capsid of a virus with the enclosed nucleic acid) (from Thomas Splettstoesser (www.scistyle.com), https://en.wikipedia.org/wiki/Structure_and_genome_of_HIV)

therapy revealed reduced expression of 14 proteins involved in sperm motility [8]. HIV in ART has been well-researched and hence has been used as an example extensively in this chapter.

81.3.2 Hepatitis B Virus (HBV)

HBV is a DNA virus belonging to the *Hepadnaviridae* family with the main routes of transmission being sexual intercourse and sharing needles for injection drug use. Since HBV vaccines are available, it is recommended that all patients are vaccinated and all healthcare personnel are also vaccinated against prior to working in ART.

HBV has been detected in semen of infected men [9]. In a case-control study, HBV-infected males and their uninfected partners undergoing in vitro fertilization/intracytoplasmic sperm injection (IVF/ICSI) treatment had significantly reduced semen parameters (sperm count and motility), fertilization rate, embryo quality, implantation, and clinical pregnancy rates compared to matched uninfected controls [10].

81.3.3 Hepatitis C Virus (HCV)

HCV is a single-stranded RNA virus belonging to the *Flaviviridae* family and is transmitted via body fluids of infected persons. Currently there is no licensed vaccine against HCV, but highly effective antiviral therapy is available. HCV has been detected in blood, saliva, follicular fluid, semen, and culture medium of embryos resulting from fertilization using sperm prepared from HCV-infected semen. However, HCV was not detected in culture medium at the time of embryo transfer, following the intervention of serial rinsing in multiple droplets of culture media on a daily basis [11, 12].

81.3.4 Zika Virus (ZIKV)

ZIKV is a positive-sense single-stranded RNA virus belonging to the *Flaviviridae* family and transmitted via the bites of infected *Aedes* mosquitoes. At present, there is no licensed vaccine against ZIKV. ZIKV-infected adults are mostly asymptomatic, but with outbreaks of ZIKV in South America and the spread across many countries in Europe and North America, there have been many reports of congenital abnormalities (microcephaly) in children born to ZIKV-infected parents. ZIKV has been associated with reduced sperm count and can be detected by reverse transcriptase polymerase chain reaction (RT-PCR) in semen after density-gradient centrifugation (DGC) washing protocols [13] and even 6 months after onset of symptoms [14].

Table 81.2 Viruses of reproductive health importance

Virus	Detected in semen? (REF)	Detected in FF (REF)
Human immunodeficiency virus (HIV)	+ [6]	+ [7]
Hepatitis B virus (HBV)	+ [9]	+ [16]
Hepatitis C virus (HCV)	+ [11]	+ [12]
Hepatitis D virus (HDV)	+ [17]	+ [17]
Zika virus (ZIKV)	+ [14]	ND
Ebola virus (EBOV)	+ [15]	ND
Human herpes virus (HHV)	+ [18]	ND
Herpes simplex virus (HSV)	+ [19]	+ [20]
Cytomegalovirus (CMV)	+ [21]	+ [20]
Epstein-Barr virus (EBV)	+ [19]	ND
Human papilloma virus (HPV)	+ [18]	ND

FF follicular fluid, *ND* plausible but no data

81.3.5 Ebola Virus (EBOV)

EBOV is a negative-sense RNA virus belonging to the family *Filoviridae* and transmitted via body fluids of infected persons. Currently, there is no licensed vaccine against EBOV. The 2013–2016 EBOV outbreaks in West Africa took several lives, but many thousands survived the hemorrhagic disease, and the virus may still remain dormant in them for many months or years, which poses risk to themselves and/or their sexual partners. EBOV RNA is detectable by RT-PCR in semen 12 months after recovery [15] (Table 81.2).

81.4 Blood Testing

Individuals seeking ART should be tested for viruses according to national and international guidelines. Considering the emotional trauma associated with receiving news of viral positivity, it is important that patients are given the necessary education and awareness and their consents taken before performing such tests. Some consider that counselling should be provided before having such screening tests, although this may not be practical.

All patients seeking ART should undergo testing for HIV, HBV, and HCV. Gamete donors may be additionally required to have screening for *Cytomegalovirus* (CMV), but this has not gained widespread acceptance in the fertility clinics for autologous gamete usage. Some countries also required screening for human T-cell lymphotropic virus (HTLV-1 antibody) if the patients live in or originate from high prevalence areas.

Due to viral latency (the period of one contracting a virus and the time it is actually detected by laboratory diagnosis), some clinics prefer individuals to be tested at least 3 months prior to gamete retrieval and fertilization. That way, a repeated virus testing could be performed after 3 months to confirm absence of virus in patients' samples.

81.5 Laboratory Setup for Treating Patients with Blood-Borne Viruses

Most of the blood-borne viruses (BBVs) of reproductive health importance (HIV, HBV, and HCV) can be handled in a biosafety level 2 (BSL-2) environment. The IVF laboratory that treats BBV-infected patients must be set up to minimize the risk of infection to clinic personnel (horizontal transmission), the gametes and embryos of the infected couple (vertical transmission), gametes and embryos of other patients being treated in the same laboratory (nosocomial infection), and other nonclinical staff that may interact with the laboratory.

Such a lab should have the practices and components in place to address issues relating personnel, primary barriers, and relevant procedures.

81.5.1 Personnel

- A laboratory manager who is knowledgeable in viruses of reproductive health importance should lead the laboratory.
- All staff should be fully trained on effective handling of infectious agents.
- There should be regular competence checks of staff on the institutional biosafety manual, and all staff should be updated whenever changes or relevant updates are made.
- All personnel should receive the needed immunizations (e.g., against HBV), and the laboratory manager should ensure this is adhered to.
- A comprehensive biosafety manual should be prepared, made available in the laboratory, and all personnel should read this prior to undertaking any treatment. This manual should describe the kind of infectious agents to be handled in the laboratory, who is permitted to process such samples, a step-by-step protocol on handling infectious gametes and embryos, measures to prevent infections, and efficient waste disposal practices.
- There should be a clear procedure to follow if personnel suspect they have been exposed to any infectious samples via an accident such as a needlestick injury.

81.5.2 Primary Barriers

- A separate containment IVF laboratory with specifications befitting a BSL-2 should be created to treat virus-infected patients. In situations where this physical separation is not possible, procure separate laboratory equipment such as centrifuge and biological safety cabinet (BSC) class II for the specific handling of samples from virus-infected patients or separate patients "in-time" by scheduling treatment on different days for virus-infected patients. If treating both virus-infected and uninfected patients on the same day, also separate them "in-time" by putting all infected patients last on the procedure list so that effective decontamination of the laboratory and equipment can be performed after cases.
- The laboratory should be designed such that it makes it easy to clean—from walls to floors whenever necessary.
- There should be a dedicated incubator for handling gametes and embryos from virus-infected patients, which should be regularly cleaned with appropriate embryo-tested detergents and the incubator-specific decontamination cycles performed after cleaning.
- A portable size autoclave should be made available in the laboratory or adjoining sterilization room for autoclaving biological waste before disposal at the incinerator.
- All needles and sharps should be safely disposed of in sharps containers.
- Disposable gowns/aprons, facemasks, head covers, gloves, and other personal protective equipment should be worn during treatment.
- Separate dewars for storing gametes and embryos from virus-infected patients should be provided, and access should be appropriately secured.

81.5.3 Relevant Procedures

- Work surfaces including biosafety cabinets should be completely decontaminated with 70% alcohol or other embryo-tested disinfectant followed with two changes of distilled water immediately after processing gametes and embryos. **Note that processed semen, oocytes, and embryos should be safely stored away in incubators before applying disinfectants.**
- At the close of workday, the dedicated centrifuge for virus samples should be completely decontaminated with embryo-tested detergent followed with two changes of distilled water. Weights (filled centrifuge tubes) that are used as balance in virus-dedicated centrifuge should be discarded at the close of workday.
- All procedures such as centrifugation, oocyte retrievals, and handling should be carefully performed to minimize aerosol formation.
- All infectious waste including tubes, culture dishes with media, follicular fluid, and semen should be disposed of safely into autoclavable plastic bags. All sealed bags **must** be autoclaved in the laboratory or adjoining sterilization room before disposing off the waste at the incinerator.

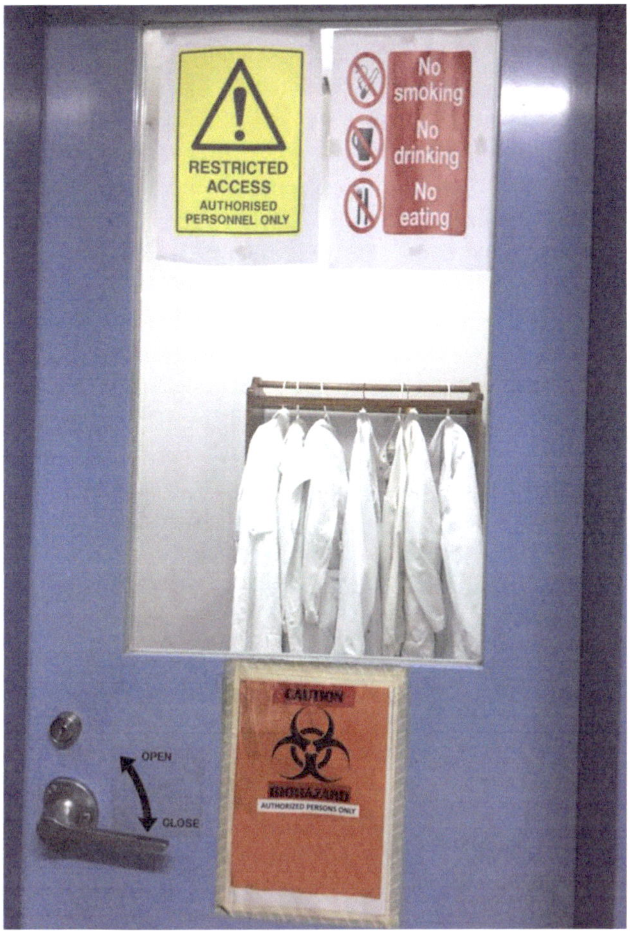

Fig. 81.2 Entrance to an IVF lab that treats virus-infected patients

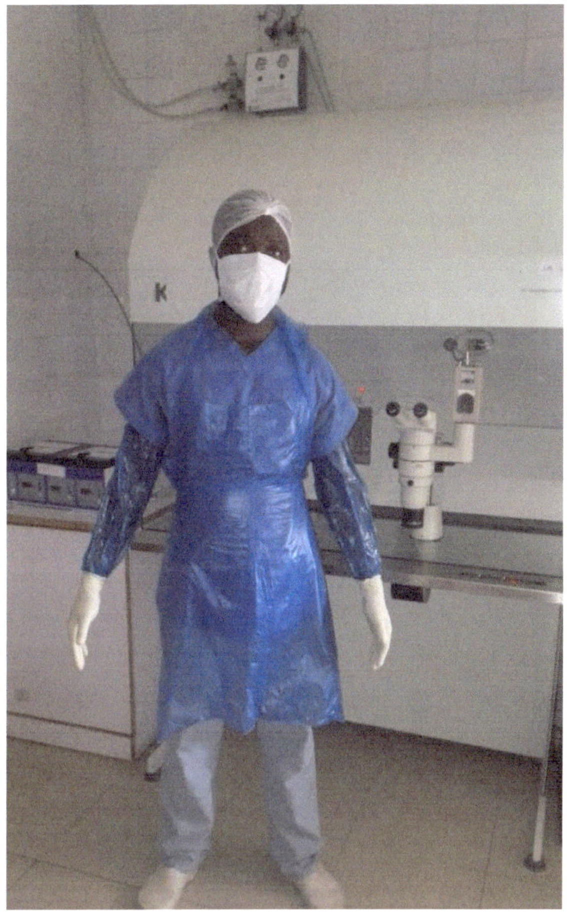

Fig. 81.3 A laboratory personnel appropriately gowned to work on virus-infected samples

- Access to the IVF laboratory treating BBV-positive patients should be completely restricted to laboratory personnel only. The door to the laboratory should be marked as "Out of Bounds" and with the biohazard sign (Fig. 81.2).
- As per standard practice, needles and syringes must never be recapped.
- When treating BBV-positive patients, the use of glassware and needles should be minimized. Glassware should be replaced with plasticware whenever possible.
- Facemasks and goggles should be worn especially when performing procedures that may cause splashes of infectious fluids, e.g., follicular fluids during oocyte retrievals.
- Disposable gowns/aprons and double pair of gloves should be worn whenever working on infected samples (Fig. 81.3). Stained gloves should be changed—the technique is to wear double gloves (two pairs), so when you need to change the gloves, you can easily remove the second layer/pair of gloves without exposing your bare hands unnecessarily when handling infected samples. Double gloving also adds an additional barrier against needlestick injuries.
- Broken glass Pasteur pipettes should never be handled even with gloved hands. Such broken items should be swept using a brush and dustpan and appropriately discarded in puncture-proof sharps container.
- Any excessive spillages, needlesticks, and events that pose infection risk to personnel must be immediately reported to the laboratory manager and records of treatment and/or monitoring of symptoms of such exposures duly recorded [22].

81.6 Treating Serodiscordant Couples

Serodiscordant couples seeking ART should first be referred to an infectious disease specialist/virologist who can check the disease status and advise on an appropriate drug regimen (if this is not already in place). It is recommended that the uninfected partner in serodiscordant couples start pre-exposure prophylaxis (PrEP) treatment before seeking ART [23].

81.6.1 Seropositive Female

In the case of a virus-infected female partner of a serodiscordant couple, semen from the uninfected male can be processed for self-insemination, intrauterine insemination (IUI), IVF, or ICSI, which completely eliminates the risk of infecting the uninfected male. The risk of mother-to-child (vertical) transmission has been reduced to <2% in mothers on the highly active antiretroviral therapy (HAART) [24].

It is thought that with oocytes, the surrounding cumulus or granulosa cells harbor the viruses [25]; hence it is recommended that retrieved oocytes from virus-infected females should be denuded almost immediately and processed for ICSI rather than proceed with conventional IVF to minimize contact of oocytes and granulosa cells [25].

Adhering to the following precautions when handling oocytes from virus-infected females will prevent contamination and infection:

- All procedures should be performed in a biosafety class II cabinet while wearing appropriate personal protective equipment (PPE).
- Oocytes should be rinsed in a minimum of two changes of warmed media, and perform denudation as soon as practicable.
- Embryos from virus-infected females should be cultured in a separate and dedicated incubator.
- Since the risk of vertical transmission may be increased with multiple pregnancies, consider replacing fewer embryos at transfer. An elective single-embryo transfer (eSET) is recommended [25]. Culture to the blastocyst stage may be helpful for embryo selection for eSET.

81.6.2 Seropositive Male

There are four possible approaches to treating a couple with a seropositive male and a seronegative female:

1. Couples can engage in unprotected intercourse, but only around the time of ovulation. This is the riskiest approach as it exposes the uninfected woman to infection unnecessarily. In one report, 4 out of 92 uninfected women with HIV-infected males seroconverted to HIV; 2 after 7 months of follow-up and 2 after delivery [26]. The seroconversion rate of HIV-negative women having unprotected intercourse with their HIV-positive male partners has been reported to vary depending on the disease severity and stage of the infected male. In a prospective longitudinal study, the rate of seroconversion was reported to be in the range from 0.7 to 5 per 1000 episodes of unprotected intercourse [27]. However, the risk of transmission of viruses through unprotected intercourse is real and cannot be overemphasized.
2. Performing a modified DGC technique and inseminating the washed semen into the uterus of the unaffected female via IUI. In a meta-analysis of 8212 seronegative females who had IUIs with washed semen from HIV-seropositive males, none seroconverted [28]. As a smaller insemination volume is used in IVF (usually 10–20 μl) as compared to IUI (usually 0.3–0.5 ml), it could be thought that the risk of transmission of HIV to uninfected females might be higher in IUI than in IVF, but there is no empirical data to support this. When semen washing was performed, neither IUI nor IVF resulted in HIV transmission to uninfected females and their newborns even 6 months after delivery [29].
3. Performing IVF/ICSI with the washed semen sample. This is the method of choice especially in cases of poor semen quality in the seropositive male and or blocked tubes in the seronegative female. Considering the risk of infection and/or contamination, ICSI has been indicated as the preferred technique for fertilizing oocytes over conventional IVF [30].
4. Avoid use of sperm from the BBV-positive partner altogether. While sperm washing of BB-positive sperm is effective, this technique may not definitely eliminate the virus. Therefore, an alternative option is to use donated sperm. In HIV-discordant couples with an infected male, accepting donated sperm will eliminate the possible risk of infecting the mother and the prospective child(ren). However, in our experience, most infected males prefer to have their own genetically related children, especially when they have good sperm parameters, so use of donor sperm is rarely chosen. Other options could also be adoption or to remain childless.

81.6.2.1 Modified DGC Protocol

A slightly modified DGC protocol as described below is used to process semen from virus-infected males, but it is recommended that every laboratory should establish a working protocol according to national and regional guidelines.

- To ensure efficient removal of infected leucocytes and cellular debris, it is advisable to use 1 ml each of three layers gradient—90/70/40 % for the DGC.
- Use a disposable Pasteur pipette to transfer semen from the specimen container onto the upper layer of the gradients. Centrifuge for 300 g for 10 min.
- After centrifugation, carefully aspirate the supernatant (with a Pasteur pipette) to prevent mixing, and discard.
- Carefully aspirate the pellet using a fresh Pasteur pipette into a fresh tube containing sperm washing medium. Centrifuge for 200 g for 10 min.

- Aspirate and discard the supernatant as before. Now, use the swim-up technique. Overlay pellet with warmed fertilization/sperm processing medium, and keep at a 45° slanted position. Motile sperms should migrate into the overlaid medium. Carefully aspirate the upper portion of the medium, containing migrated sperms, gently to prevent mixing, and use for downstream procedures such as for IUI, IVF/ICSI.
- Use disposable counting chamber to assess the sperm concentration and motility.

There are conflicting reports on the success of DGC eliminating viruses in semen. For example, after DGC, there was complete removal of HIV in 741 semen samples [31] and human herpes virus (HHV 6/7) [32], whereas removal of herpes simplex virus (HSV) and *Cytomegalovirus* (CMV) failed significantly [32].

81.6.2.2 Double-Layer Tube Technique

The double-layered tube device, ProInsert (Nidacon, Sweden), is designed to minimize the risk of recontaminating the sediment or washed sperm when processing virus-infected semen using DGC. With this tube, the sperm pellet could be aspirated without touching the upper layers of semen and gradient expected to contain trapped cellular debris, leucocytes, and viruses. In one study using the ProInsert tube of the 103 HIV-infected semen that was processed, viral DNA was detected in only 2 of the processed samples by PCR [33].

81.7 Virus Testing in Post-sperm Wash Sample

A quality control system that includes viral testing in a post-sperm wash sample is essential in the treatment of IVF patients with blood-borne viral infections, since the wash process may not yield guaranteed virus-free sample. A basic lateral flow assay simply detecting the presence or absence of viral proteins is not an ideal quality control instrument, as this assay requires very high viral protein thresholds for detection (low sensitivity). PCR offers a better specificity and sensitivity, able to detect very minute quantities of viral nucleic acids and therefore recommended for quality control testing of post-sperm wash samples. For example, the AMPLICOR HIV-1 MONITOR (Roche), a PCR-based assay, has been reported to give 100% sensitivity in detecting 7.5 copies/reaction of HIV-1 RNA/DNA [34].

Since PCR-based assays can be performed within a few hours, the washed semen could be stored at room temperature for the meantime or cryopreserved and thawed for IUI or ICSI if the PCR indicates no amplification of viral RNA/DNA. When the post-wash semen has residual viral RNA/DNA, fresh semen can be obtained from the man for another wash procedure, or a donor semen can be used, or the post-wash semen containing the residual viral nucleic acid can be used, with all the recommended options being at the consent of the couple.

Nucleic acid testing (NAT), which is based on the principle of PCR to amplify specific targeted sequences of viruses, has been extensively used in screening donated blood prior to transfusions. NAT is a highly sensitive and specific molecular biology tool and is able to detect minute titers of viruses in the sample. NAT could be performed on pooled samples, and hence clinics handling many or batched BBV-infected males can perform this assay simultaneously to be efficient at time and resource use [35].

81.8 Cryopreserving Gametes and Embryos

Several studies have investigated the possibility of viral contamination between gametes and embryos that are stored in liquid nitrogen (LN2). However, to date there has been no report of viral transmission from frozen semen used for inseminations or IVF/ICSI in clinical IVF applications [36]. No viral nucleic acid has been detected in sampled LN2 and LN2 storage tanks containing embryos from HIV-, HCV-, and HBV-infected couples [37]. However, in experimental settings, the risk of viral transmission or cross contamination from infected LN2 to bovine embryos has been demonstrated [38]. Since there is a risk, the closed system of cryopreservation has been recommended over open systems especially when cryopreserving gametes and embryos from virus-infected couples. Several clinics in Europe currently use the heat-sealed CryoBiosystem (CBS) straws in cryopreserving gametes and embryos to minimize or prevent the risk of viral contamination from liquid phase LN2.

Semen, especially from donors, should be quarantined until the donor repeats serum virus testing for HIV, HBV, and HCV before samples are moved into appropriate LN2 dewars. Dewars meant for quarantine should be decontaminated after it was used to quarantine virus-infected gamete or embryos.

81.9 Effects of Viral Infections on Outcomes of ART

The impact viral infections may have on ART outcome has been studied with varying results. In a case-controlled study, HIV-seropositive women <35 years of age had similar pregnancy and live birth rates compared to their age-matched seronegative controls, whereas live birth rates were significantly reduced in older (>35 years) HIV-seropositive women

[39]. In another case-controlled study, HIV-infected women had significantly reduced implantation and live birth rates compared to matched controls [40]. Such reduced outcomes have been attributed in part to mitochondrial DNA depletion in oocytes of virus-infected women on HAART [41]. Obstetric outcomes (premature delivery, birth weights, miscarriage) are generally favorable for serodiscordant couples [42], but it is recommended that all infants perinatally exposed to HIV should be placed on antiretroviral therapy for at least 6 weeks after delivery [43].

81.10 Controversies on Virus-Infected Gametes

The role of sperm cells as vectors for the transmission of HIV to oocytes and embryos has been suggested. While sperm cell surfaces are devoid of the CD4+ receptor, which is required on HIV target cells, the human mannose receptor (hMR) is abundant on the surface of sperm cells. hMR on sperm surface has been demonstrated to bind to HIV and hence can lead to the internalization of HIV in sperm cells [44, 45]. It has been demonstrated that HIV provirus is integrated in the genome of sperm cells, and such sperms could achieve fertilization as unaffected sperm cells. HIV gag and pol DNA were also detected by fluorescent in situ hybridization (FISH) in two-cell embryos resulting from fertilization with sperm cells containing integrated HIV provirus [46].

In another study of serodiscordant couples, eight HBV-infected males, their uninfected partners, and their aborted fetuses were screened by nested PCR to amplify the C gene of HBV. All the eight women tested negative for all markers of HBV infection, but the PCR of aborted fetuses amplified the HBV C gene. The authors report that sequences of HBV C gene amplified in father/fetus pair showed great similarity with some specific point mutations at same nucleotide position in father and fetus [47] suggesting a possible father-to-child vertical transmission through infected sperm cells.

81.11 Conclusion

Viral infections play a critical role in the safety and outcomes of ART, and hence people seeking such procedures should be tested for viruses according to national and international guidelines. Establishing and enforcing institutional biosafety protocols will assist in limiting the risk of infection of gametes, patients, and personnel working in a facility treating BBV-infected couples.

References

1. UNAIDS. Global AIDS Update. 2016.
2. Kourtis AP, Bulterys M, Hu DJ, Jamieson DJ. HIV–HBV coinfection — a global challenge. N Engl J Med. 2012;366(19):1749–52.
3. Oladapo OT, Daniel OJ, Odusoga OL. Ayoola-Sotubo O. Fertility desires and intentions of HIV-positive patients at a suburban specialist center. J Natl Med Assoc. 2005;97(12):1672–81.
4. De los Santos MJ, Apter S, Coticchio G, Debrock S, Lundin K, Plancha CE, et al. Revised guidelines for good practice in IVF laboratories (2015). Hum Reprod. 2016;31(4):685–6.
5. ASRM. Recommendations for reducing the risk of viral transmission during fertility treatment with the use of autologous gametes: a committee opinion. Fertil Steril. 2013;99(2):340–6.
6. Houzet L, Matusali G, Dejucq-Rainsford N. Origins of HIV-infected leukocytes and virions in semen. J Infect Dis. 2014;210(suppl 3):S622–30.
7. Bertrand E, Zissis G, Marissens D, Gerard M, Rozenberg S, Barlow P, et al. Presence of HIV-1 in follicular fluids, flushes and cumulus oophorus cells of HIV-1-seropositive women during assisted-reproduction technology. Aids. 2004;18(5):823–5.
8. Pilatz A, Discher T, Lochnit G, Wolf J, Schuppe HC, Schuttler CG, et al. Semen quality in HIV patients under stable antiretroviral therapy is impaired compared to WHO 2010 reference values and on sperm proteome level. Aids. 2014;28(6):875–80.
9. Jenison SA, Lemon SM, Baker LN, Newbold JE. Quantitative analysis of hepatitis B virus DNA in saliva and semen of chronically infected homosexual men. J Infect Dis. 1987;156(2):299–307.
10. Zhou XP, Hu XL, Zhu YM, Qu F, Sun SJ, Qian YL. Comparison of semen quality and outcome of assisted reproductive techniques in Chinese men with and without hepatitis B. Asian J Androl. 2011;13(3):465–9.
11. Leruez-Ville M, Kunstmann JM, De Almeida M, Rouzioux C, Chaix ML. Detection of hepatitis C virus in the semen of infected men. Lancet. 2000;356(9223):42–3.
12. Devaux A, Soula V, Sifer C, Branger M, Naouri M, Porcher R, et al. Hepatitis C virus detection in follicular fluid and culture media from HCV+ women, and viral risk during IVF procedures. Hum Reprod. 2003;18(11):2342–9.
13. Joguet G, Mansuy JM, Matusali G, Hamdi S, Walschaerts M, Pavili L, et al. Effect of acute Zika virus infection on sperm and virus clearance in body fluids: a prospective observational study. Lancet Infect Dis. 2017;17(11):1200–8.
14. Nicastri E, Castilletti C, Liuzzi G, Iannetta M, Capobianchi MR, Ippolito G. Persistent detection of Zika virus RNA in semen for six months after symptom onset in a traveller returning from Haiti to Italy, February 2016. Euro Surveill. 2016;21(32)
15. Deen GF, Broutet N, Xu W, Knust B, Sesay FR, McDonald SLR, et al. Ebola RNA persistence in semen of Ebola virus disease survivors—final report. N Engl J Med. 2017;377(15):1428–37.
16. Taylor PJ, Gill MJ, Mahadevan M, Pattinson HA. Hepatitis B virus in human follicular fluid. Fertil Steril. 1987;48(3):514.
17. Mansour W, Lemoine M, Neri Pinto F, Llabador de Royer MA, Le Gal F, Yazbeck C, et al. Markers of hepatitis delta virus infection can be detected in follicular fluid and semen. J Clin Virol. 2014;61(2):279–81.
18. Kaspersen MD, Bungum M, Fedder J, Bonde J, Larsen PB, Ingerslev HJ, et al. No increased sperm DNA fragmentation index in semen containing human papillomavirus or herpesvirus. Andrology. 2013;1(3):361–4.

19. Kapranos N, Petrakou E, Anastasiadou C, Kotronias D. Detection of herpes simplex virus, cytomegalovirus, and Epstein-Barr virus in the semen of men attending an infertility clinic. Fertil Steril. 2003;79(Suppl 3):1566–70.
20. Ardizzoni A, Manca L, Capodanno F, Baschieri MC, Rondini I, Peppoloni S, et al. Detection of follicular fluid and serum antibodies by protein microarrays in women undergoing in vitro fertilization treatment. J Reprod Immunol. 2011;89(1):62–9.
21. Lupton J, Vernamonti J, McCabe C, Noble J, Yin HZ, Eyre RC, et al. Cytomegalovirus and human immunodeficiency virus in semen of homosexual men. Fertil Steril. 2014;101(2):350–8.
22. Centers fDCaP. Biosafety in microbiological and biomedical laboratories. 5th ed. 2009.
23. WHO. Guideline on when to start antiretroviral therapy and on pre-exposure prophylaxis for HIV. Geneva; 2015.
24. Siegfried N, van der Merwe L, Brocklehurst P, Sint TT. Antiretrovirals for reducing the risk of mother-to-child transmission of HIV infection. Cochrane Database Syst Rev. 2011;(7):CD003510.
25. Jindal SK, Rawlins RG, Muller CH, Drobnis EZ. Guidelines for risk reduction when handling gametes from infectious patients seeking assisted reproductive technologies. Reprod Biomed Online. 2016;33(2):121–30.
26. Mandelbrot L, Heard I, Henrion-Geant E, Henrion R. Natural conception in HIV-negative women with HIV-infected partners. Lancet. 1997;349(9055):850–1.
27. de Vincenzi I. A longitudinal study of human immunodeficiency virus transmission by heterosexual partners. European Study Group on Heterosexual Transmission of HIV. N Engl J Med. 1994;331(6):341–6.
28. Barnes A, Riche D, Mena L, Sison T, Barry L, Reddy R, et al. Efficacy and safety of intrauterine insemination and assisted reproductive technology in populations serodiscordant for human immunodeficiency virus: a systematic review and meta-analysis. Fertil Steril. 2014;102(2):424–34.
29. Vitorino RL, Grinsztejn BG, de Andrade CA, Hokerberg YH, de Souza CT, Friedman RK, et al. Systematic review of the effectiveness and safety of assisted reproduction techniques in couples serodiscordant for human immunodeficiency virus where the man is positive. Fertil Steril. 2011;95(5):1684–90.
30. Palermo GD, Neri QV, Rosenwaks Z. To ICSI or not to ICSI. Semin Reprod Med. 2015;33(2):92–102.
31. Savasi V, Ferrazzi E, Lanzani C, Oneta M, Parrilla B, Persico T. Safety of sperm washing and ART outcome in 741 HIV-1-serodiscordant couples. Hum Reprod. 2007;22(3):772–7.
32. Michou V, Liarmakopoulou S, Thomas D, Tsimaratou K, Makarounis K, Constantoulakis P, et al. Herpes virus infected spermatozoa following density gradient centrifugation for IVF purposes. Andrologia. 2012;44(3):174–80.
33. Fourie JM, Loskutoff N, Huyser C. Semen decontamination for the elimination of seminal HIV-1. Reprod Biomed Online. 2015;30(3):296–302.
34. Zamora MJ, Obradors A, Woodward B, Vernaeve V, Vassena R. Semen residual viral load and reproductive outcomes in HIV-infected men undergoing ICSI after extended semen preparation. Reprod Biomed Online. 2016;32(6):584–90.
35. Hans R, Marwaha N. Nucleic acid testing-benefits and constraints. Asian J Transfus Sci. 2014;8(1):2–3.
36. Pomeroy KO, Harris S, Conaghan J, Papadakis M, Centola G, Basuray R, et al. Storage of cryopreserved reproductive tissues: evidence that cross-contamination of infectious agents is a negligible risk. Fertil Steril. 2010;94(4):1181–8.
37. Cobo A, Bellver J, de los Santos MJ, Remohi J. Viral screening of spent culture media and liquid nitrogen samples of oocytes and embryos from hepatitis B, hepatitis C, and human immunodeficiency virus chronically infected women undergoing in vitro fertilization cycles. Fertil Steril. 2012;97(1):74–8.
38. Bielanski A, Nadin-Davis S, Sapp T, Lutze-Wallace C. Viral contamination of embryos cryopreserved in liquid nitrogen. Cryobiology. 2000;40(2):110–6.
39. Nurudeen SK, Grossman LC, Bourne L, Guarnaccia MM, Sauer MV, Douglas NC. Reproductive outcomes of HIV seropositive women treated by assisted reproduction. J Womens Health (2002). 2013;22(3):243–9.
40. Stora C, Epelboin S, Devouche E, Matheron S, Epelboin L, Yazbeck C, et al. Women infected with human immunodeficiency virus type 1 have poorer assisted reproduction outcomes: a case-control study. Fertil Steril. 2016;105(5):1193–201.
41. Lopez S, Coll O, Durban M, Hernandez S, Vidal R, Suy A, et al. Mitochondrial DNA depletion in oocytes of HIV-infected antiretroviral-treated infertile women. Antivir Ther. 2008;13(6):833–8.
42. Cleary-Goldman J, Pena JE, Thornton MH 2nd, Robinson JN, D'Alton ME, Sauer MV. Obstetric outcomes of human immunodeficiency virus-1-serodiscordant couples following in vitro fertilization with intracytoplasmic sperm injection. Am J Perinatol. 2003;20(6):305–11.
43. Chappell CA, Cohn SE. Prevention of perinatal transmission of human immunodeficiency virus. Infect Dis Clin North Am. 2014;28(4):529–47.
44. Cardona-Maya W, Lopez-Herrera A, Velilla-Hernandez P, Rugeles MT, Cadavid AP. The role of mannose receptor on HIV-1 entry into human spermatozoa. Am J Reprod Immunol. 2006;55(4):241–5.
45. Fanibunda SE, Velhal SM, Raghavan VP, Bandivdekar AH. CD4 independent binding of HIV gp120 to mannose receptor on human spermatozoa. J Acquir Immune Defic Syndr (1999). 2008;48(4):389–97.
46. Wang D, Li LB, Hou ZW, Kang XJ, Xie QD, Yu XJ, et al. The integrated HIV-1 provirus in patient sperm chromosome and its transfer into the early embryo by fertilization. PLoS One. 2011;6(12):e28586.
47. Wang S, Peng G, Li M, Xiao H, Jiang P, Zeng N, et al. Identification of hepatitis B virus vertical transmission from father to fetus by direct sequencing. Southeast Asian J Trop Med Public Health. 2003;34(1):106–13.

Laboratory Aspects of In Vitro Maturation Cycles

82

Weon-Young Son, Sara Henderson, and Jin-Tae Chung

82.1 Introduction

Infertile women with polycystic ovaries have comprised the majority of patients undergoing IVM to avoid ovarian hyperstimulation syndrome (OHSS) caused by exogenous gonadotropins stimulation. However, indications for IVM are widened to include various reasons of infertility, especially for poor ovarian reserve [1, 2] and fertility preservation [3]. The research for improvements in IVM is continuing, and improved pregnancy rates have recently been established by a number of centers [4, 5]. Nonetheless, the reduced pregnancy rates per cycle compared to conventional IVF represent a major obstacle that needs to be overcome for widespread uptake of IVM. This lower efficiency manifests at multiple levels: particularly lower metaphase II (M-II) rates (typically 40–60%) but also lower subsequent embryo development rates [6] and, in some centers, higher miscarriage rates.

Therefore, understanding oocyte maturation process and the details of human IVM is crucial to improve results. We will review oocyte maturation mechanisms and the laboratory aspects in IVM cycles.

82.2 Oocyte Maturation

An in-depth understanding of oocyte maturation process is required to develop "high-quality oocytes" in vitro. Oocyte maturation refers to both nuclear and cytoplasmic maturation. The nuclear maturation in the oocyte implies the resumption of the first meiotic division and progression to metaphase II (M-II). Cytoplasmic maturation involves metabolic and structural changes in the organelles, which are required for fertilization and early embryo development.

W.-Y. Son (✉) · S. Henderson · J.-T Chung
MUHC Reproductive Centre, Department of Obstetrics and Gynecology, McGill University Health Center (MUHC), McGill University, Montreal, QC, Canada
e-mail: weon-young.son@muhc.mcgill.ca

Oocytes inside follicles are arrested in prophase I (germinal vesicle (GV) stage) until luteinizing hormone (LH) surge even though chromatin configuration and transcriptional activity are different between growing follicles. It is well established that this meiotic arrest is maintained by high cyclic adenosine 3′,5′-monophosphate (cAMP) levels within the oocyte. Gap junctions between oocytes and cumulus cells (CCs), as well as between cumulus cells themselves, regulate cAMP levels. Regulatory molecules for meiotic arrest as well as nutrients and metabolites are bi-directionally transferred through the gap junction. High cAMP levels within the oocyte before the LH surge are maintained by three mechanisms. Firstly, cAMP enters the oocyte from CCs through the gap junctions [7], and it is also produced by the oocyte itself via G protein-coupled receptors in the oocyte membrane [8]. Finally, guanosine 3′,5′-cyclic monophosphate (cGMP), an inhibitor of phosphodiesterase 3A (PDE3A: oocyte-specific phosphodiesterase), crosses through gap junctions into the oocyte [9], where it prevents hydrolysis of cAMP by PDE3A. The high intra-ovarian cAMP concentration inactivates the meiosis-promoting factor (MPF) and blocks meiotic progression.

After the LH surge, the preovulatory follicle rapidly increases in volume, and the CCs in cumulus oocyte complex (COC) are expanded physiologically. Hyaluronan (HA) is mainly involved in the cumulus cell expansion and is synthesized in the plasma membrane of the CCs [10]. The cumulus expansion disrupts the Cx43 gap junction in the COCs which inhibits the transport of cAMP from cumulus cells into oocytes leading to the activation of MPF and meiotic resumption of oocytes [11]. It has been suggested that the secretion of a soluble factor from oocytes is involved in HAS2 (hyaluronan synthase 2) mRNA expression, HA synthesis, and cumulus expansion in vitro. Probable oocyte-secreted factors include growth differentiation factor-9 (GDF-9), bone morphogenetic protein 15 (BMP-15), and BMP-6 [12].

G. N. Allahbadia et al. (eds.), *Textbook of Assisted Reproduction*, https://doi.org/10.1007/978-981-15-2377-9_82

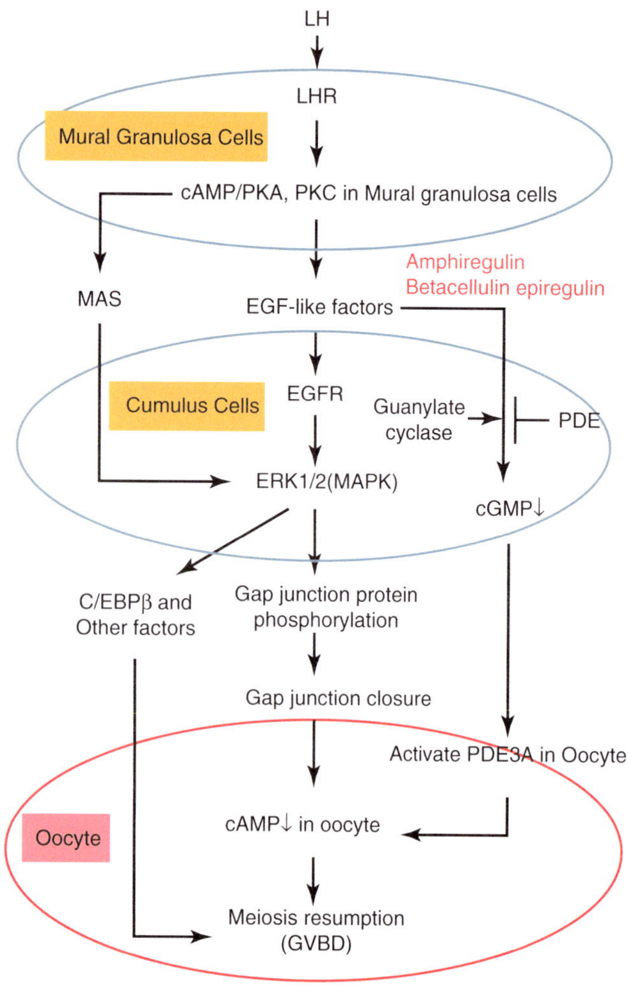

Fig. 82.1 Signal transduction in follicular somatic cells and oocyte regulating oocyte meiosis after LH surge. CAAT-enhancer-binding protein (C/EBPβ)

Figure 82.1 illustrates the signaling pathways involved in oocyte maturation in vivo. LH receptor (LHR) expression is much higher in mural granulosa layers than in CCs. Mural granulosa cell (GCs) activation by LH induces the expression of EGF-like growth factors, amphiregulin, betacellulin, and epiregulin, as second signals [13]. CCs are the main target for EGF-induced meiotic resumption. The LH surge leads to a drop in follicular and oocyte cGMP levels [14]. Mitogen-activated protein kinase (MAPK) in CCs is immediately activated following EGF administration. Increased activation of MAPK in follicular somatic cells may lead to resumption of meiosis by inducing the synthesis of downstream meiosis resumption-inducing factor(s), as well as phosphorylation of gap junction proteins. Altogether, cAMP-mediated meiotic arrest is lifted, and oocyte maturation is induced. Therefore, both the oocyte itself and the GCs play a role in the regulation of oocyte maturation and development [12].

82.3 Clinical Application of Human Immature Oocyte Maturation Program

In vivo oocyte maturation is a complex process orchestrated by hormonal signals, surrounding somatic cells, and transcription factors. However, immature oocytes retrieved from antral follicles start hormone-independent, spontaneous meiotic maturation in vitro. In vitro maturation is associated with premature disruption of oocyte-cumulus cell gap junctions, preventing the crossing of beneficial factors, such as nucleotides and nutrients from CCs to the oocyte. This may impair the composition of oocyte cytoplasm.

Cyclic AMP analogues, kinase, or PDE inhibitors have been used to delay spontaneous IVM, by mimicking in vivo mechanisms [15, 16]. However, the effect was not significant, especially in humans. Recently, an Australian group suggested an IVM system called "Simulated physiological oocyte maturation (SPOM)," and they reported improved outcomes in mouse and bovine models [17]. Whether it would be applicable in human IVM system or not remains to be determined.

Gonadotropin stimulation of ovaries is widely employed to improve the quality and quantity of oocytes in human IVM programs [18].

82.4 Laboratory Procedure of IVM

82.4.1 Oocyte Retrieval

The follicular aspirate is collected in collection tubes containing flushing media with 2 U heparin to prevent the formation of blood clots during retrieval. Multiple snap needle punctures are needed because follicles are small (2–13 mm) and bloody aspirates may block the thin needle lumen with lower aspiration pressure. As in direct aspiration of immature oocytes from ex vivo ovarian tissues or ovaries during the cesarean section, the tissues/ovaries are held with one hand, and direct aspiration of small follicles containing immature oocytes is performed using a simple 5 or 10 mL syringe (containing HEPES-buffered IVF media with proteins) and 22-gauge needle.

82.4.2 Oocyte Identification

The follicular aspirate is first examined under a stereomicroscope to identify COC. Since the COCs aspirated from IVM cycles have a small amount of cells compared to those from controlled ovarian hyperstimulation (COH) cycles, they can be easily overlooked by embryologists. Therefore, the bottom portion of the tube holds a small volume of follicular

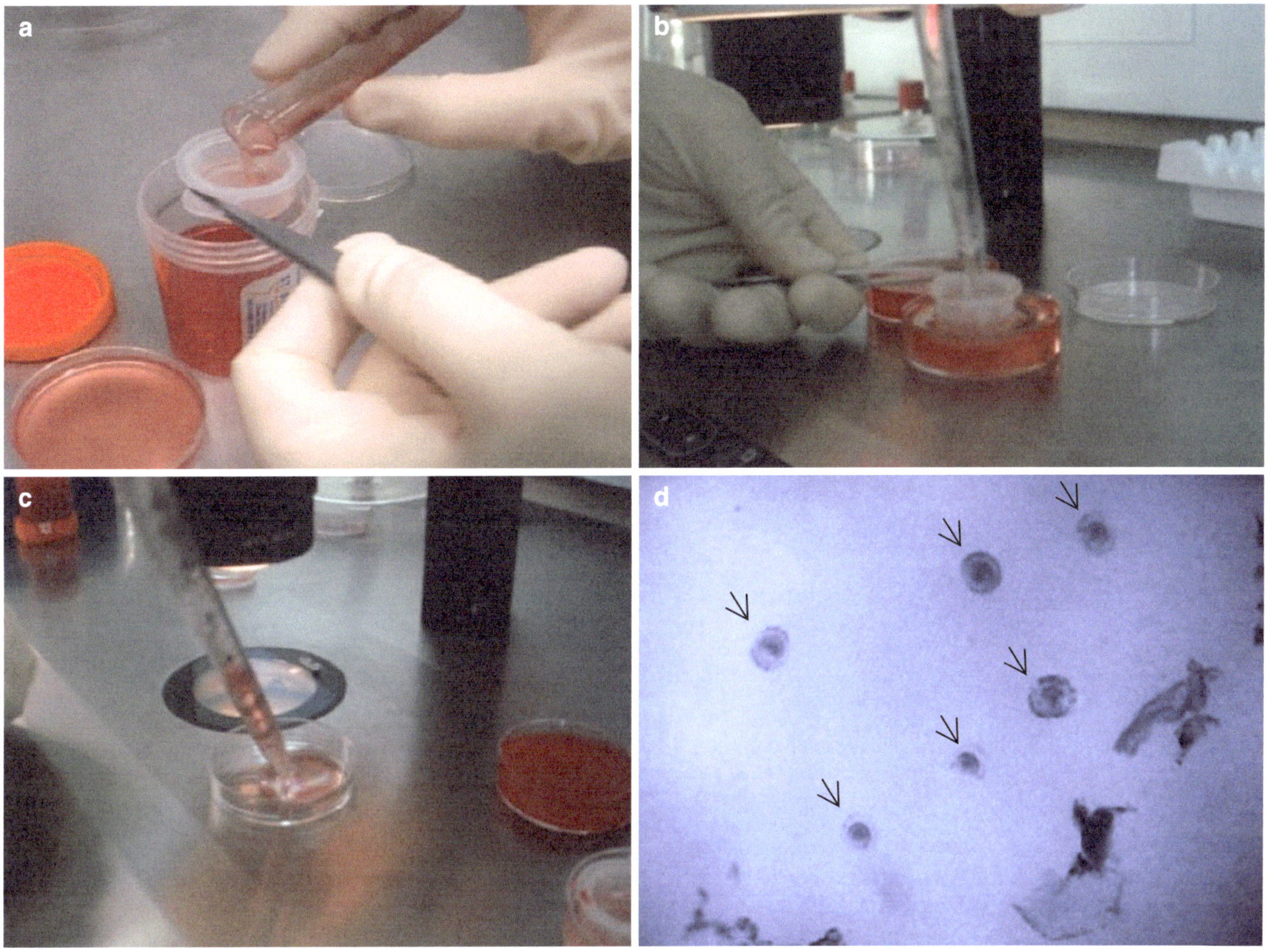

Fig. 82.2 Filter method. (**a**) Filtering of follicular aspirates, (**b**) washing the filtrate with fresh media, (**c**) transfer washed filtrates to a new Petri dish, (**d**) cumulus oocyte complexes in the Petri dish (arrow)

aspirate to facilitate the identification of oocytes since they most likely will sink to the bottom of the tube. In hCG-primed IVM cycles, the CCs of some of the COCs have already started expansion in vivo and thus facilitate detachment from the follicles. It makes oocyte retrieval and COC identification for both clinician and embryologist easier than non-hCG-primed IVM cycles. This method allows for more efficient and timely communicates between clinician and embryologist regarding the number and morphology of oocytes retrieved during the process.

The other method is to use a cell strainer device made of a nylon mesh of 70-μm pores (Fig. 82.2) [19]. The follicular aspirates in collection tubes are filtered with the cell strainer. After filtering all follicular aspirates, the collected aspirates are washed with fresh medium (containing HEPES-buffered IVF media with proteins) to remove red blood cells and small cells. They are then transferred to a new Petri dish to search for COC under a stereomicroscope. This method is mainly performed in the IVM cycles without hCG-priming such as non-, FSH-primed IVM cycles or follicle aspirates from ovarian tissue, since COCs show similar color to mural GCs without CCs expansion (Fig. 82.3A).

In order to avoid the expanded COCs block in pores of the filter, once oocytes with expanded CCs are identified directly under stereomicroscope, only the remaining aspirates are filtered through a cell strainer to facilitate identification of those oocytes with a small amount or a compact CCs.

82.4.3 Cumulus Oocyte Morphology in Relation to hCG Exposure

COC morphology varies in cycles with and without hCG priming [20] (Fig. 82.3). Oocytes with dispersed CC are only found in hCG-primed-IVM cycles (Fig. 82.3B). In the non-hCG-primed IVM cycles, immature oocytes surrounded by multiple layers of CCs had higher embryo developmental potential than oocytes without multilayer CCs [21]. In hCG-primed IVM cycles, the oocytes with dispersed CCs had higher rate of in vitro maturation and

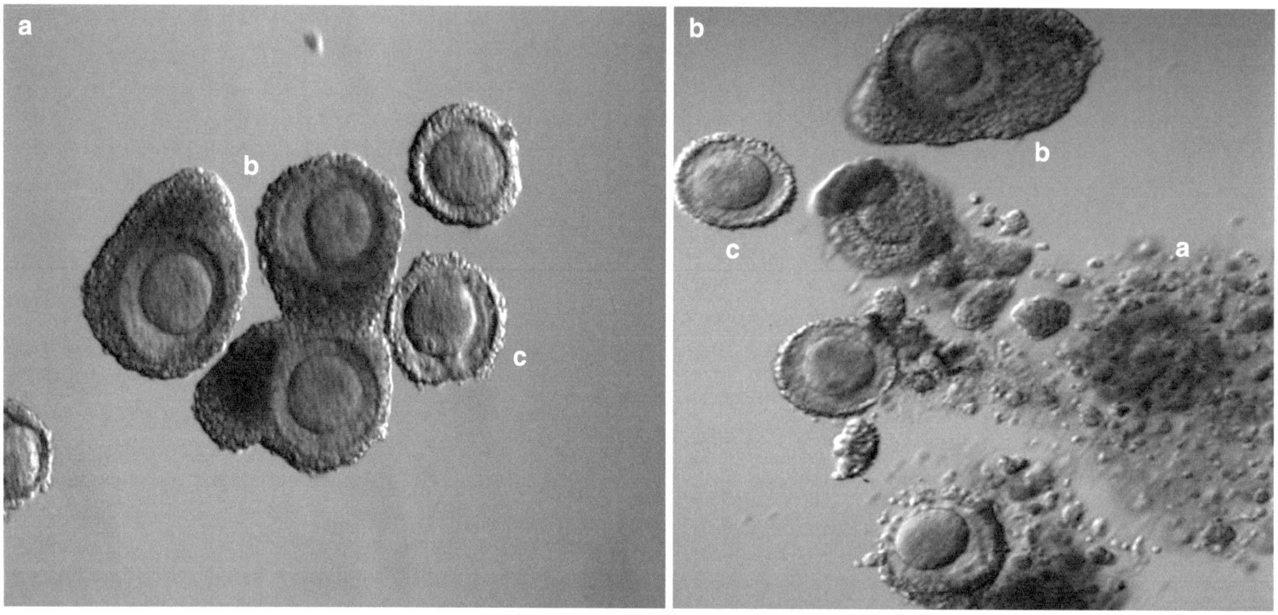

Fig. 82.3 Cumulus oocyte complex (COC) just after oocyte retrieval (**A**) from non-hCG-primed IVM cycles. (**B**) From hCG-primed IVM cycles. (**a**) Oocyte with dispersed cumulus cells (CCs), (**b**) oocyte with compacted CCs, (**c**) oocytes with sparse CCs

matured faster than oocytes without dispersed CCs [22]. Immature oocytes collected in COH cycles had similar results [15]. Actually, most of immature oocytes obtained from COH cycles have expanded CCs, and more than 80% reach in vitro maturation if the CCs are attached and cultured for 24 h (personal experience). In general, oocytes that reach maturation faster can produce better developmental potential and less aneuploidy rate than those reaching maturation late in IVM cycles [23–26]. Therefore, higher pregnancy rate can be obtained in the IVM cycles that had transferred embryos derived from faster in vitro matured oocytes than late ones [27].

82.4.4 In Vivo Matured Oocytes in hCG-Primed IVM Cycles

In vivo matured oocytes can be collected alongside immature oocytes in hCG-primed IVM cycles. All the oocytes with an extruded polar body (PB) have expanded CCs. This implies that a few of them have already resumed meiosis and/or extruded PB [20, 24, 27, 28]. The number of good quality at cleavage or at blastocysts produced from in vivo matured oocytes was significantly higher than that of in vitro matured oocytes [20, 25], resulting in higher clinical pregnancy rate in the cycles where transferred embryos were derived from in vivo matured oocytes [24, 29]. Sometimes in vivo matured oocytes can be collected from follicles measuring <10 mm at the time of retrieval. Multiple in vivo matured oocytes can usually be retrieved in hCG-primed IVM cycles [28]. Recently, Jeppesen et al. [30] showed that in humans LHR expression was maximal in GCs from preovulatory follicles and a majority of antral follicles with a diameter of 3–10 mm expressed LHR at approximately 10% of the maximum. This report could explain the reason for retrieving mature oocytes even from small diameter antral follicles in hCG-primed IVM cycles.

To evaluate oocyte maturity in IVM cycles associated with hCG priming, spreading method can be used easily: after identifying expanded COC, they are removed from the Petri dish, and follicular aspirates in the Petri dish are discarded while keeping a small amount of fluid in the dish. The COCs are spread into the Petri dish to observe oocyte cytoplasm under the dissecting microscope (Fig. 82.4). This procedure should be performed quickly before the follicular fluid dries out on the Petri dish. It would be difficult to identify oocytes with the first PB but easy to separate oocytes with and without GV in cytoplasm with this method. When GV is not observed in the cytoplasm, CCs are removed to assess maturity. If M-II oocytes are overlooked at the time of retrieval, they will be aged by the time of CC removal (24 h later), and their developmental competence might be compensated. Therefore, identification of in vivo matured oocytes is very important in hCG-primed IVM cycles. Some IVF clinics are removing expanded CCs 6 h after egg retrieval to evaluate precise oocyte maturity [31].

82.4.5 IVM Culture Medium and Supplements

Most human IVM media composition is informed by experiences in other mammalian species. Recently, commercial IVM media (SAGE or Medi-Cult) became available.

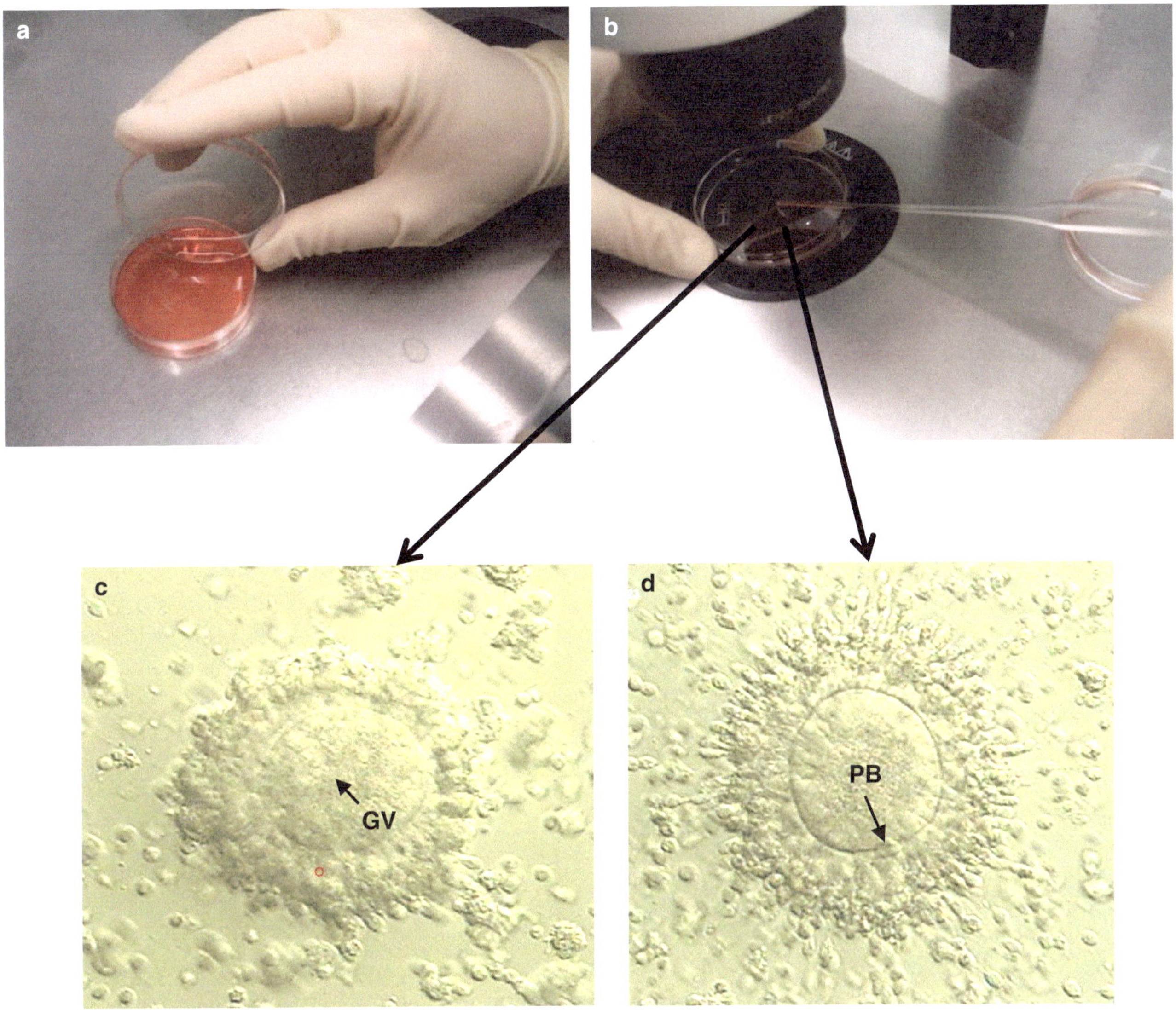

Fig. 82.4 The process to assess oocyte maturity with spreading method. (**a**) Removing most of follicular fluid (**b**) put the identified COC with dispersed CCs on the Petri dish. (**c**) A GV-stage oocyte with expanded cumulus cells, (**d**) metaphase II (M-II)-stage oocyte with dispersed cumulus cells. GV, germinal vesicle; PB, 1st polar body

However, IVM, fertilization, embryo development, and pregnancy rates are found to be similar with TCM 199-based and Medi-Cult commercial IVM media [32, 33] or between SAGE commercial IVM media and blastocyst IVF media [34]. Therefore, despite the availability of commercial human IVM culture media, the developmental competency of immature oocytes is not improved over complex culture medium or regular IVF media. Optimal culture medium for human immature oocytes is still to be developed. Regular IVF blastocyst culture medium may be a good choice, especially for clinics where IVM cycles are not routinely done.

Currently, most IVM protocols involve supplement serum, FSH, or other additives such as LH/hCG and/or EGF into IVM culture medium based on their physiological role in oocyte maturation in vivo. Since serum sources from other patients or from animals have potential sources of infectious agents, the patient's own serum, human serum albumin (HSA), or synthetic serum substitutes have been used as protein supplementation in IVM media.

FSH is normally added to the culture medium since FSH is involved in the development of preovulatory follicles in vivo [35], for induction of LH receptors and for inducing EGF-like growth factors. FSH and LH have been reported to improve human oocyte maturation and embryo cleavage [36, 37]. hCG and LH are reported to be equally effective in promoting oocyte maturation in vitro [38]. However, hCG in the culture medium was not found to improve IVM and embryonic development in one study [39]. Therefore, the role of gonadotropin and their optimal concentration in culture medium still need to be studied. Gonadotropins may not have the same role in oocyte maturation in vitro due to the absence of mural cells, which respond to LH/hCG signals involved in upregulation of EGF-like growth factors in vivo. EGF itself could help in vitro maturation of oocytes. Indeed, EGF supplementation of IVM medium is reported to improve nuclear maturation of cumulus-denuded human GV-stage oocytes and increase fertilization rate of n cumulus-intact immature oocytes [40].

82.4.6 Culture Time for Assessing In Vitro Maturation of Immature Oocytes

Separating M-II stage oocytes with extruded first PB from the germinal vesicle breakdown (GVBD)-stage oocytes is pretty hard without CCs denudation due to variable orientation of the first PB on the Petri dish. The GVBD oocytes could become M-II and be inseminated on the same day after removing CCs. Oocyte maturity would be evaluated again early in the morning of day 1, and ICSI would be performed immediately if there are any M-II oocytes. By the end of day 1, the presence of zygotes would be evaluated since aged oocytes could show earlier fertilization sign than usual and separated from the other oocytes that had been injected at the same time but show no sign of fertilization. When zygotes are not observed, signs of fertilization would be checked again the next morning.

The maturity status of GV-stage oocytes does not require re-assessment on the same day in hCG-primed IVM cycles. In the non-hCG-primed IVM cycles, COCs retrieved from antral follicles usually have a compact mass of CCs with oocytes at GV-stage and therefore do not need to assess oocyte maturity on the collection day.

Some of the GV-stage oocytes at collection can reach M-II stage oocytes after 24 h of maturation in both hCG-primed and unprimed IVM cycles [20, 33, 39]. Most studies reported 40–60 % rate of in vitro maturation after day 1 culture (24–30 h) in IVM cycles [20, 39]. However, oocytes were inseminated 48 or 56 h after assessing maturation in non-primed IVM cycles, and oocyte maturity was not even assessed on day 1 in earlier studies [41, 42]. Therefore, many oocytes must have been arrested at the M-II stage for 24–30 h before insemination. This places them well past the optimal fertilization time and was the one of the main reasons for poor clinical outcomes for the first several years after starting human IVM program.

It would not be suggested to use M-II oocytes matured after day 2 culture unless there are not enough mature oocytes on day 1 since the embryos produced from late matured ones (day 2) had poor developmental potential and had higher aneuploidy rate.

Since time-lapse incubator system (TLS) has been developed, the time period of oocyte IVM from GV-stage oocytes could be observed, although most of CCs at GV-stages are removed to see the first PB extrusion in the TLS which may act differently than oocytes with intact CC. In the GV-stage oocytes retrieved from FSH-hCG-stimulated IVM cycles, the average time from GV- to GVBD-stage was 3.3 h (±2.3, range: 0.5–9.3 h) and GBVD- to M-II-stage was 12. 5 h (±1.5, range: 7.7–15.6 h) after beginning culture in IVM media [43].

Therefore, oocyte maturity should be assessed after day 1 culture in the entire IVM program.

82.4.7 Insemination of Mature Oocytes Produced from IVM Cycles

ICSI has been used to increase the chances of fertilization whether or not a male factor has been detected as a result of the theoretical concern of zona pellucida hardening during the in vitro culture of the immature oocytes [44]. ICSI resulted in a higher fertilization rate than IVF insemination in several studies [33, 45]. However, Walls et al. [46] recently reported similar fertilization rate between IVF and ICSI insemination in IVM oocytes. Therefore, whether ICSI is beneficial or absolutely necessary to effectively inseminate IVM oocytes in the absence of sperm factors is still controversial. Nevertheless, ICSI is the commonly used method of insemination to increase fertilization in the majority of IVM studies.

82.4.8 ICSI Timing

Asynchronous maturation of the immature oocytes is typical of human IVM cycles. Therefore, optimal ICSI timing is important to ensure maximal fertilization and embryo development.

Balakier et al. [47] suggested that the IVM oocytes obtained from COH cycles needed at least 3 h before insemination after extruding the 1st PB to obtain reasonable fertilization rates. Meanwhile, developmental potential would be negatively affected if IVM oocytes were post-maturation aging. Thus, the optimal interval between extrusion of the first PB and ICSI is crucial in human IVM. Hyun et al. [48] reported that human oocytes matured in vitro needed at least 1 h after the first PB extrusion to complete nuclear maturation, and better quality embryos were produced when ICSI was done 3 h after 1st PB in hCG-primed IVM cycles. Recently, using TLS in FSH-hCG-primed IVM cycles, Gunasheela et al. [49] reported that ICSI 3–6 h after the 1st PB extrusion was associated with higher fertilization rate (83.1%) than < 3 h (40%) or > 6 h (64 %). Likewise, no good quality morula/blastocysts were developed when ICSI was performed < 3 h after the 1st PB extrusion.

It is important to note that the time for completing nuclear/cytoplasmic maturation after the first PB extrusion depends on the source of immature oocytes (from COH cycles or IVM cycles) as well as on IVM culture system. Practically, however, it would be easier to remove CCs in the afternoon of day 1 after culturing for and perform ICSI 3 h after observing the first PB, in order to avoid several ICSI times for an IVM cycle.

82.4.9 Culture of IVM Embryos

Once zygotes are formed, the remaining embryology work is the same as IVF cycles such as embryo culture and transfer and embryo cryopreservation.

82.5 Cryopreservation of Oocytes Obtained from IVM Cycles

Based on the success of "oocyte vitrification," the American Society for Reproductive Medicine (ASRM) has endorsed oocyte cryopreservation as a fertility preservation strategy for women with cancer and other conditions which require gonadotoxic treatments [50]. However, COH for IVF is contraindicated for women with hormone-dependent cancers. Moreover, chemo- or radiation-therapy cannot be delayed to do an IVF cycle in many cases. Immature oocyte collection can be an alternative under these conditions [51]. A few live births have been reported after IVM oocyte cryopreservation [52–56], yet live birth using cryopreserved IVM oocytes for fertility preservation was not reported at the time of writing. Some live births have been reported using vitrified/warmed IVM embryos produced from immature oocytes retrieved from ex vivo ovarian tissue [57–59].

Immature oocytes can be cryopreserved at the GV-stage (before IVM) of after reaching maturation (after IVM). Vitrification after reaching M-II-stage seems better than vitrification at the GV-stage in terms of survival rate and embryo developmental potential after warming [60, 61].

Therefore, IVM- or cryo-technology still needs to be advanced for optimal cryopreservation of smaller GV-stage oocytes. The results can be improved by (i) improving the quality of in vitro produced oocytes by optimizing in vitro conditions and/or (ii) adapting cryopreservation methods to the cellular properties of oocytes before/after in vitro maturation.

82.6 Conclusion

Manipulation of oocytes collected from IVM cycles is more technically demanding and time consuming as compared to stimulated IVF cycles. Embryologists should be adequately trained by an experienced supervisor before embarking on IVM cycles [19]. Laboratory procedure requires optimization as well [19]. Recently, 3-D culture systems [62–64], addition of EGF-like growth factors (amphiregulin and epiregulin) [65] or oocyte secreting factors (GDF-9 and BMP-15) [66, 67] to culture medium have been tried to improve human IVM culture systems. However, they are still suboptimal to support IVM of human immature oocytes and further research is required to develop the optimal human IVM culture medium. It is not only culture media that is important but also the physical aspect of culture such as a 3-D culture system with proper pressure in order to mimic the inside of a follicle. It is also important for the IVM culture media/system to be simple to manage to facilitate handling by the embryologist in the embryology laboratory.

References

1. Hyman JH, Sokal-Arnon T, Son WY, Tan SL, Dahan MH. Live birth of twins after performing early hCG administration as a modification of natural cycle in vitro fertilization, in a women with decreased ovarian reserve. Arch Gynecol Obstet. 2015;291:219–22.
2. Nayot D, Chung JT, Son WY, Ao A, Hughes M, Dahan MH. Live birth following serial vitrification of embryos and PGD for fragile X syndrome in a patient with the premutation and decreased ovarian reserve. J Assist Reprod Genet. 2013;30:1439–44.
3. Creux H, Monnier P, Son WY, Tulandi T, Buckett W. Immature oocyte retrieval and in vitro oocyte maturation at different phases of the menstrual cycle in women with cancer who require urgent gonadotoxic treatment. Fertil Steril. 2017;107:198–204.
4. Das M, Son WY, Buckett W, Tulandi T, Holzer H. In-vitro maturation versus IVF with GnRH antagonist for women with polycystic ovary syndrome: treatment outcome and rates of ovarian hyperstimulation syndrome. Reprod Biomed Online. 2014;29:545–51.
5. Junk SM, Yeap D. Improved implantation and ongoing pregnancy rates after single-embryo transfer with an optimized protocol for in vitro oocyte maturation in women with polycystic ovaries and polycystic ovary syndrome. Fertil Steril. 2012;98:888–92.
6. Walls ML, Ryan JP, Keelan JA, Hart R. In vitro maturation is associated with increased early embryo arrest without impairing morphokinetic development of useable embryos progressing to blastocysts. Hum Reprod. 2015;30:1842–9.
7. Anderson E, Albertini DF. Gap junctions between the oocyte and companion follicle cells in the mammalian ovary. J Cell Biol. 1976;71:680–6.
8. Mehlmann LM, Jones TL, Jaffe LA. Meiotic arrest in the mouse follicle maintained by a Gs protein in the oocyte. Science. 2002;297:1343–5.
9. Hubbard CJ, Terranova PF. Inhibitory action of cyclic guanosine 5′-phosphoric acid (GMP) on oocyte maturation: dependence on an intact cumulus. Biol Reprod. 1982;26:628–32.
10. Salustri A, Yanagishita M, Hascall VC. Synthesis and accumulation of hyaluronic acid and proteoglycans in the mouse cumulus cell-oocyte complex during follicle-stimulating hormone-induced mucification. J Biol Chem. 1989;264:13840–7.
11. Norris RP, Freudzon M, Mehlmann LM, Cowan AE, Simon AM, Paul DL, et al. Luteinizing hormone causes MAP kinase-dependent phosphorylation and closure of connexin 43 gap junctions in mouse ovarian follicles: one of two paths to meiotic resumption. Development. 2008;135:3229–38.

12. Gilchrist RB, Lane M, Thompson JG. Oocyte-secreted factors: regulators of cumulus cell function and oocyte quality. Hum Reprod Update. 2008;14:159–77.
13. Park JY, Su YQ, Ariga M, Law E, Jin SL, Conti M. EGF-like growth factors as mediators of LH action in the ovulatory follicle. Science. 2004;303:682–4.
14. Norris RP, Ratzan WJ, Freudzon M, Mehlmann LM, Krall J, Movsesian MA, et al. Cyclic GMP from the surrounding somatic cells regulates cyclic AMP and meiosis in the mouse oocyte. Development. 2009;136:1869–78.
15. Nogueira D, Ron-El R, Friedler S, Schachter M, Raziel A, Cortvrindt R, et al. Meiotic arrest in vitro by phosphodiesterase 3-inhibitor enhances maturation capacity of human oocytes and allows subsequent embryonic development. Biol Reprod. 2006;74:177–84.
16. Shu YM, Zeng HT, Ren Z, Zhuang GL, Liang XY, Shen HW, et al. Effects of cilostamide and forskolin on the meiotic resumption and embryonic development of immature human oocytes. Hum Reprod. 2008;23:504–13.
17. Albuz FK, Sasseville M, Lane M, Armstrong DT, Thompson JG, Gilchrist RB. Simulated physiological oocyte maturation (SPOM): a novel in vitro maturation system that substantially improves embryo yield and pregnancy outcomes. Hum Reprod. 2010;25:2999–3011.
18. Dahan MH, Tan SL, Chung J, Son WY. Clinical definition paper on in vitro maturation of human oocytes. Hum Reprod. 2016;31:1383–6.
19. Son WY, Tan SL. Laboratory and embryological aspects of hCG-primed in vitro maturation cycles for patients with polycystic ovaries. Hum Reprod Update. 2010;16:675–89.
20. Son WY, Yoon SH, Lim JH. Effect of gonadotrophin priming on in-vitro maturation of oocytes collected from women at risk of OHSS. RBM Online. 2006;13:340–8.
21. Russell JB. Immature oocytes retrieval combined with in-vitro oocyte maturation. Hum Reprod. 1998;13(Suppl 3):63–70.
22. Yang SH, Son WY, Yoon SH, Ko Y, Lim JH. Correlation between in vitro maturation and expression of LH receptor in cumulus cells of the oocytes collected from PCOS patients in HCG-primed IVM cycles. Hum Reprod. 2005;20:2097–103.
23. Smitz J, Picton HM, Platteau P, Rutherford A, Cortvrindt R, Clyde J, et al. Principal findings from a multicenter trial investigating the safety of follicular-fluid meiosis-activating sterol for in vitro maturation of human cumulus-enclosed oocytes. Fertil Steril. 2007;87:949–64.
24. Son WY, Chung JT, Demirtas E, Holzer H, Sylvestre C, Buckett W, et al. Comparison of cycles programmed for IVM with and without in vivo matured oocytes retrieved. RBM Online. 2008;17:59–67.
25. Son WY, Lee SY, Lim JH. Fertilization, cleavage and blastocyst development according to the maturation timing of oocytes in in vitro maturation cycles. Hum Reprod. 2005;20:3204–7.
26. Zhang XY, Ata B, Son WY, Buckett WM, Tan SL, Ao A. Chromosome abnormality rates in human embryos obtained from in-vitro maturation and IVF treatment cycles. Reprod Biomed Online. 2010;21:552–9.
27. Son WY, Chung JT, Chian RC, Herrero B, Demirtas E, Elizur S, et al. A 38-hour interval between hCG priming and oocyte retrieval increases in vivo and in vitro oocyte maturation rate in programmed IVM cycles. Hum Reprod. 2008;23:2010–6.
28. Son WY, Chung JT, Herrero B, Dean N, Demirtas E, Holzer H, et al. Selection of the optimal day for oocyte retrieval based on the diameter of the dominant follicle in hCG-primed in vitro maturation cycles. Hum Reprod. 2008;23:2680–5.
29. Fadini R, Dal Canto MB, Mignini Renzini M, Brambillasca F, Comi R, Fumagalli D, et al. Effect of different gonadotrophin priming on IVM of oocytes from women with normal ovaries: a prospective randomized study. RBM Online. 2009;19:343–51.
30. Jeppesen JV, Kristensen SG, Nielsen ME, Humaidan P, Dal Canto M, Fadini R, et al. LH-receptor gene expression in human granulosa and cumulus cells from antral and preovulatory follicles. J Clin Endocrinol Metab. 2012;97:E1524–31.
31. Fadini R, Coticchio G, Brambillasca F, Mignini Renzini M, Novara PV, Brigante C, et al. Clinical outcomes from mature oocytes derived from preovulatory and antral follicles: reflections on follicle physiology and oocyte competence. J Assist Reprod Genet. 2015;32:255–61.
32. Filali M, Hesters L, Fanchin R, Tachdjian G, Frydman R, Frydman N. Retrospective comparison of two media for in-vitro maturation of oocytes. RBM Online. 2008;16:250–6.
33. Söderström-Anttila V, Mäkinen S, Tuuri T, Suikkari AM. Favourable pregnancy results with insemination of in vitro matured oocytes from unstimulated patients. Hum Reprod. 2005;20:1534–40.
34. Pongsuthirak P, Songveeratham S, Vutyavanich T. Comparison of blastocyst and Sage media for in vitro maturation of human immature oocytes. Reprod Sci. 2015;22:343–6.
35. Abir R, Franks S, Mobberley MA, Moore PA, Margara RA, Winston RM. Mechanical isolation and *in vitro* growth of preantral and small antral human follicles. Fertil Steril. 1997;68:682–8.
36. Anderiesz C, Ferraretti A, Magli C, Fiorentino A, Fortini D, Gianaroli L, et al. Effect of recombinant human gonadotrophins on human, bovine and murine oocyte meiosis, fertilization and embryonic development *in vitro*. Hum Reprod. 2000;15:1140–8.
37. Durinzi KL, Wentz AC, Saniga EM, Johnson DE, Lanzendorf SE. Follicle stimulating hormone effects on immature human oocytes: *in vitro* maturation and hormone production. J Assist Reprod Genet. 1997;14:199–204.
38. Hreinsson J, Rosenlund B, Friden B, Levkov L, Ek I, Suikkari AM, et al. Recombinant LH is equally effective as recombinant hCG in promoting oocyte maturation in a clinical in-vitro maturation programme: a randomized study. Hum Reprod. 2003;18:2131–6.
39. Ge HS, Huang XF, Zhang W, Zhao JZ, Lin JJ, Zhou W. Exposure to human chorionic gonadotropin during in vitro maturation does not improve the maturation rate and developmental potential of immature oocytes from patients with polycystic ovary syndrome. Fertil Steril. 2008;89:98–103.
40. Goud PT, Goud AP, Qian C, Laverge H, Van der Elst J, De Sutter P, et al. In-vitro maturation of human germinal vesicle stage oocytes: role of cumulus cells and epidermal growth factor in the culture medium. Hum Reprod. 1998;13:1638–44.
41. Son WY, Park SE, Lee KA, Lee WS, Ko JJ, Yoon TK, et al. Effect of 1,2-propanediol and freezing-thawing on the in vitro developmental capacity of human immature oocytes. Fertil Steril. 1996;66:995–9.
42. Trounson AO, Wood C, Kausche A. In-vitro maturation and the fertilization and developmental competence of oocytes recovered from untreated polycystic ovarian patients. Fertil Steril. 1994;62:353–62.
43. Gunasheela D, Menon J, Amitha J, Nirmala H, Uttur G, Deepanjali G, et al. Diameter of immature oocytes collected in IVM cycles and its association with nuclear maturation timing. Hum Reprod. 2016;31(suppl_1):i211.
44. Nagy ZP, Cecile J, Liu J, Loccufier A, Devroey P, Van Steirteghem A. Pregnancy and birth after intracytoplasmic sperm injection of in vitro matured germinal-vesicle stage oocytes: case report. Fertil Steril. 1996;65:1047–50.
45. Hwang JL, Lin YH, Tsai YL. In vitro maturation and fertilization of immature oocytes: a comprehensive study of fertilization techniques. J Assist Reprod Genet. 2000;17:39–43.
46. Walls M, Junk S, Ryan JP, Hart R. IVF versus ICSI for the fertilization of in-vitro matured human oocytes. Reprod Biomed Online. 2012;25:603–7.
47. Balakier H, Sojecki A, Motamedi G, Librach C. Time-dependent capability of human oocytes for activation and pronuclear formation during metaphase II arrest. Hum Reprod. 2004;19:982–7.

48. Hyun CS, Cha JH, Son WY, Yoon SH, Kim KA, Lim JH. Optimal ICSI timing after the first polar body extrusion in in vitro matured human oocytes. Hum Reprod. 2007;22:1991–5.
49. Gunasheela D, Nirmala H, Uttur G, Deepanjali G, Son WY. The dynamic of in vitro maturation (IVM) and their optimal ICSI timing of germinal vesicle oocytes retrieved from IVM cycles. Hum Reprod. 2017;32(suppl_1):i.
50. Practice Committee of the American Society for Reproductive Medicine. ASRM Practice Committee response to Rybak and Lieman: elective self-donation of oocytes. Fertil Steril. 2009;92:1513–4.
51. Ata B, Shalom-Paz E, Chian RC, Tan SL. In vitro maturation of oocytes as a strategy for fertility preservation. Clin Obstet Gynecol. 2010;53:775–86.
52. Chen H, Lv JQ, Ge HS, Wu XM, Xi HT, Chi HH, et al. Live birth following vitrification of in vitro matured oocytes derived from sibling smaller follicles at follicle selection phase in the context of in vitro fertilization. Gynecol Endocrinol. 2014;30:624–6.
53. Chian RC, Huang JY, Gilbert L, Son WY, Holzer H, Cui SJ, et al. Obstetric outcomes following vitrification of in vitro and in vivo matured oocytes. Fertil Steril. 2009;91:2391–8.
54. El Hachem H, Poulain M, Finet A, Fanchin R, Frydman N, Grynberg MH. Live birth after frozen-thawed oocytes matured in vitro in a PCOS patient: a model for improving implantation rates in IVM cycles and objectively assessing the real potential of development of frozen oocytes matured in vitro. Gynecol Endocrinol. 2014;30:415–8.
55. Gunasheela S, Gunasheela D, Jaykumar A, Hiremath N, Son WY. Live birth after in vitro maturation and vitrification of immature oocytes retrieved from conventional IVF cycle: a case report. J Assist Reprod Genet. 2012;29:1073–6.
56. Tucker MJ, Wright G, Morton PC, Massey JB. Birth after cryopreservation of immature oocytes with subsequent in vitro maturation. Fertil Steril. 1998;70:578–9.
57. Prasath EB, Chan ML, Wong WH, Lim CJ, Tharmalingam MD, Hendricks M, et al. First pregnancy and live birth resulting from cryopreserved embryos obtained from in vitro matured oocytes after oophorectomy in an ovarian cancer patient. Hum Reprod. 2014;29:276–8.
58. Segers I, Mateizel I, Van Moer E, Smitz J, Tournaye H, Verheyen G, et al. In vitro maturation (IVM) of oocytes recovered from ovariectomy specimens in the laboratory: a promising "ex vivo" method of oocyte cryopreservation resulting in the first report of an ongoing pregnancy in Europe. J Assist Reprod Genet. 2015;32:1221–31.
59. Uzelac PS, Delaney AA, Christensen GL, Bohler HC, Nakajima ST. Live birth following in vitro maturation of oocytes retrieved from extracorporeal ovarian tissue aspiration and embryo cryopreservation for 5 years. Fertil Steril. 2015;104:1258–60.
60. Cao Y, Xing Q, Zhang ZG, Wei ZL, Zhou P, Cong L. Cryopreservation of immature and in-vitro matured human oocytes by vitrification. Reprod Biomed Online. 2009;19:369–73.
61. Fasano G, Demeestere I, Englert Y. In-vitro maturation of human oocytes: before or after vitrification? J Assist Reprod Genet. 2012;29:507–12.
62. Combelles CM, Fissore RA, Albertini DF, Racowsky C. In vitro maturation of human oocytes and cumulus cells using a co-culture three-dimensional collagen gel system. Hum Reprod. 2005;20:1349–58.
63. Vanhoutte L, Nogueira D, De Sutter P. Prematuration of human denuded oocytes in a three-dimensional co-culture system: effects on meiosis progression and developmental competence. Hum Reprod. 2009;24:658–69.
64. Vanhoutte L, Nogueira D, Dumortier F, De Sutter P. Assessment of a new in vitro maturation system for mouse and human cumulus-enclosed oocytes: three-dimensional prematuration culture in the presence of a phosphodiesterase 3-inhibitor. Hum Reprod. 2009;24:1946–59.
65. Ben-Ami I, Komsky A, Bern O, Kasterstein E, Komarovsky D, et al. In vitro maturation of human germinal vesicle-stage oocytes: role of epidermal growth factor-like growth factors in the culture medium. Hum Reprod. 2011;26:76–81.
66. Hussein TS, Thompson JG, Gilchrist RB. Oocyte-secreted factors enhance oocyte developmental competence. Dev Biol. 2006;296:514–21.
67. Yeo CX, Gilchrist RB, Thompson JG, Lane M. Exogenous growth differentiation factor 9 in oocyte maturation media enhances subsequent embryo development and fetal viability in mice. Hum Reprod. 2008;23:67–73.

Complications of Oocyte Retrieval

83

Funda Gode, Suleyman Akarsu, and Ahmet Zeki Isik

Oocyte pick-up is one of the cornerstones of the in vitro fertilization (IVF) cycle. The first oocyte was obtained by laparotomy, resulting in the first IVF human pregnancy, in 1973 [1]. The laparoscopic approach was typically applied until transvaginal ultrasound-guided oocyte pick-up, which was first described in 1985 [2–4]. This procedure became the preferred method worldwide, as it has many advantages over the laparoscopic approach, such as ease of learning and application, good safety and effectiveness, and a more practical daily procedure for clinicians [5].

Although ultrasound-guided oocyte pick-up is a simple procedure, some serious complications can occur, including hemorrhage, infection, and injury to adjacent pelvic structures. Furthermore, certain rare complications, including ureteral obstruction, ureterovaginal fistula, and vertebral osteomyelitis have been observed in some case reports [6–8]. Anesthetic complications can also occur, as the procedure is often performed under local or general anesthesia. In this chapter, we discuss both common and rare complications of oocyte pick-up and propose some recommendations for making the procedure safer.

83.1 Hemorrhage

Minimal bleeding, which stops spontaneously, is common during the transvaginal oocyte retrieval procedure. An estimated 230 ml blood loss within 24 h after a non-complicated oocyte retrieval is considered normal [9]. However, bleeding can be serious if the aspiration needle directly injures a blood vessel in a pelvic organ (uterus, bladder, or ovary) or an iliac vessel.

The most common form of bleeding is from the vaginal vault, which has been reported to occur in 1.4–18.4% of all punctures [10]. Fortunately, this type of bleeding often stops spontaneously or can be controlled by local pressure and topical hemostatic agents [11]. A speculum should not be used, as it may stretch the vaginal walls and prolong bleeding [12, 13]. However, suturing of the lesion is necessary in cases of serious bleeding. Therefore, optimal vaginal exploration is helpful for appropriate management in these cases [14].

Intra-abdominal bleeding is most often associated with damage to the fine vascular network of blood vessels on the ovarian surface and theca internal layer and tends to result in varying degrees of blood loss [15]. Bleeding related to damaged pelvic organs or pelvic blood vessels might be more serious. Severe intra-abdominal bleeding is rare, occurring in 0–1.3% of oocyte retrieval procedures [12–16]. Most cases are diagnosed several hours after oocyte pick-up, with a reported interval between oocyte pick-up and surgical intervention ranging from 3 to 18 h [16–18]. Vital signs, symptoms, and blood hemoglobin levels should be evaluated immediately in cases of suspected intraperitoneal bleeding. Ultrasound may be helpful to determine the extent of bleeding and the intra-abdominal fluid level. A prompt drop in hemoglobin, hemodynamic instability, or a massive volume of fluid in the abdominal cavity requires emergent management via blood transfusion and procedures such as laparoscopy or laparotomy [14]. Alternatively, pelvic arterial embolization can be performed in hemodynamically stable patients if facilities for interventional vascular radiology are available. Kart et al. reported life-threatening intra-abdominal bleeding after oocyte retrieval that was successfully managed with bilateral uterine artery embolization. The authors mentioned that empiric embolization of the anterior division of the internal iliac arteries can be performed if the exact source of the bleeding cannot be identified [15].

The most important factor for preventing intraperitoneal bleeding is careful performance of the procedure with good technique. Ultrasonographic visualization of the ovaries by pressing the ultrasonographic probe firmly against the vaginal wall will decrease the distance between the needle and ovary. An assistant can help by applying pressure against the

F. Gode (✉) · S. Akarsu · A. Z. Isik
In Vitro Fertilization Unit, Izmir Medicalpark Hospital, Karsiyaka, Izmir, Turkey

G. N. Allahbadia et al. (eds.), *Textbook of Assisted Reproduction*, https://doi.org/10.1007/978-981-15-2377-9_83

abdomen to fix mobile and abnormally located ovaries. One needle puncture and sequential aspiration of the follicles with the same puncture decreases the bleeding risk. Additionally, visualization of all round structures, in both the longitudinal and transverse axes, and detection of the iliac vessels are important for a safe procedure [13]. Misidentifying the iliac vessels as ovarian follicles can lead to serious complications. Color Doppler ultrasound is also recommended to distinguish major and minor blood vessels and to minimize hemorrhage during follicular aspiration [17]. At the end of the procedure, excessive collection of fluid or blood in the pelvis should be checked [13].

Needle size can also be a factor, where the smaller size of newly designed needles has been associated with less vaginal bleeding in recent reports [18, 19]. Follicular flushing with solutions containing heparin is related to bleeding from the small intrafollicular blood vessels and can cause a hemoperitoneum [16]. Therefore, aspirating the follicles quickly without flushing might be helpful to avoid excessive bleeding from follicles.

Retroperitoneal bleeding can be catastrophic, as the bleeding may not be detected by ultrasonography after the procedure and symptoms can occur later. Azem et al. reported massive retroperitoneal bleeding resulting from injury to the midsacral vein. The bleeding was controlled with a metal clip [20]. A life-threatening hemorrhage from a pseudoaneurysm of the obturator artery has also been reported, successfully managed with a covered stent under computed tomography angiography guidance. The authors mentioned that a retroperitoneal bleed is usually concealed and requires specific management [21].

Management of patients with coagulation disorders undergoing transvaginal oocyte retrieval is also important. The overall risk of complications for patients with bleeding disorders is unknown; however, severe intra-abdominal hemorrhage has been reported in patients with von Willebrand disease, essential thrombocytopenia, and factor XI deficiency [22–24]. Peavey et al. reported successful prophylaxis of a hemorrhage by using fresh frozen plasma, recombinant factor, intravenous immunoglobulin, and desmopressin in patients with von Willebrand disease and in hemophilia carriers before oocyte retrieval [25]. Specific attention should be paid to patients with a family history of unusual bleeding so that known bleeding abnormalities can be corrected prior to transvaginal oocyte retrieval, which can minimize bleeding in this population. However, up to 534 coagulation tests may be needed to detect a single coagulation disorder. Therefore, screening for coagulation disorders in all patients undergoing transvaginal oocyte retrieval is useless for prediction [26].

It may be necessary to pass the aspiration needle through the myometrium and endometrium to retrieve oocytes in some patients due to anatomical variations, which can increase bleeding and infection risk. Fixing the uterus with a tenaculum is recommended in such cases to stabilize the ovaries and ensure easier oocyte retrieval [13].

83.2 Pelvic Infection

Infection is another important complication after transvaginal oocyte retrieval. The general incidence of pelvic infections after transvaginal oocyte retrieval is <1%, with more severe pelvic abscesses or tubo-ovarian abscesses occurring in <0.3% of cases [27–30]. The severity of infection ranges from a minor infection with pyrexia, leukocytosis, and abdominal pain to a major medical event, such as a pelvic abscess [12, 31]. The potential risk factors for pelvic infection after transvaginal oocyte retrieval are endometriosis, history of pelvic inflammatory disease (PID), pelvic surgery, and pelvic adhesions [12, 16, 30].

The microorganisms isolated from pelvic abscesses are commonly detected in the vagina [12, 13]. As pelvic infections have not previously been reported after laparoscopic or abdominal oocyte retrieval, direct inoculation of vaginal microorganisms has been suggested as the potential cause of pelvic infections. Therefore, minimizing the number of vaginal penetrations is generally recommended for decreasing the risk of infection [12]. Other preventive strategies include disinfecting the probe between use, sterilizing the needle guides, using sterile covers on the ultrasound probe and machine, and applying sterile drapes to cover the patient's legs and perigenital area [13, 32]. There is no consensus on vaginal preparation before oocyte retrieval. Different solutions, including povidone-iodine and chlorhexidine, have been used as a preventive strategy. Van Os et al. reported that pregnancy rates are lower when iodine-containing solutions are used [33]. In contrast, Tsai et al. reported that vaginal douching with aqueous povidone-iodine, followed by irrigation with normal saline immediately before oocyte retrieval, is effective in preventing a pelvic infection without compromising the outcome of IVF treatment [34]. The authors suggested that the potential detrimental effects of iodine on oocytes can be prevented by irrigating with saline to flush away the iodine.

The role of antibiotic prophylaxis for preventing a pelvic infection is also controversial. Use of antibiotics does not seem to affect pelvic infection rates. The incidence of pelvic infection in a study that included 2670 procedures was 0.6% without antibiotic prophylaxis [12]. Pelvic infection in donor cycles dropped from 0.4% to 0% with the use of prophylactic antibiotics; however, the sample size was not large enough to detect statistical significance [31]. Tureck et al. reported a 1.3% infection rate even though patients received prophylactic antibiotics [10]. Although there is no standard guideline for using antibiotics, antibiotic prophylaxis is generally recommended for patients with risk factors such as history of endometriosis, PID, pelvic adhesions, or pelvic surgery [35].

Endometriosis is a significant risk factor by providing culture medium for bacteria following oocyte retrieval. Moini et al. reported 10 cases of acute PID (0.12%) among 5958 transvaginal oocyte retrievals. Endometriosis was detected in eight of the ten patients, which supports a role of endometriosis in increasing pelvic infection rate [36]. No pelvic infections were reported in a recent series of 214 IVF cycles performed in women with endometriomas. In that study, a 4-day prophylaxis plus ceftriaxone regimen was systematically prescribed, and the endometrial puncture rate was 3%. Avoiding aspiration of the endometrioma was recommended during the procedure [35].

Management of a pelvic infection following oocyte retrieval depends on the severity of the condition. Abdominal pain, fever, and leukocytosis should be evaluated. Hospitalization and intravenous antibiotics might be sufficient in mild PID. However, accurate diagnosis and prompt intervention of ovarian abscesses are extremely important, as the clinical condition of the patient can deteriorate very quickly. Medical treatment alone is successful in only 34–87.5% of patients with a pelvic abscess [34]. Surgical intervention via laparoscopy or laparotomy should be performed when medical therapy is unsuccessful within 72 h. Ultrasound-guided drainage of the abscess is another alternative to surgery, but a 6.6% incidence of residual abscess has been reported in these cases [37].

Another important issue in pelvic infection cases is reduced implantation rates. PID at the critical time of implantation results in failed conception [38]. The potential explanations for thaws are endotoxemia, prolonged release of prostaglandins, local inflammatory reaction, and an increase in body temperature that affects implantation and the conceptus [14]. Therefore, embryo cryopreservation and embryo transfer are recommended for subsequent cycles in cases of pelvic infection.

83.3 Pelvic Injury

The pelvic anatomical structures, including the bowel, ureters, and blood vessels, can be inadvertently injured by the aspiration needle during transvaginal oocyte retrieval. The risk of bowel injury appears to be very low, as no cases were reported in large series [12, 39]. However, some case reports have presented perforated appendicitis following transvaginal oocyte retrieval [27, 40]. Previous surgery and history of a pelvic infection, endometriosis, and adhesions might be predisposing factors.

Ureteral injury, ureterovaginal fistula, and obstruction have also been reported in the literature [7, 41, 42]. The anatomic position of the ureters anterolateral to the upper fornices of the vagina, changes in anatomical structure due to endometriosis or pelvic surgery, mechanical pressure of the vaginal probe, and difficulties identifying the ureters during oocyte retrieval are potential predisposing factors for ureteral injury [41]. Doppler ultrasound and maintenance of the needle guide in a lateral position before puncture are recommended to prevent injury to anterior structures [43]. Patients might present with fever, nausea, vomiting, lower abdominal and flank pain, suprapubic pain, and irritative urinary symptoms [7]. These general symptoms are nonspecific to distinguish a pelvic injury from oophoritis or ovarian hyperstimulation. Therefore, renal ultrasonography and abdominal imaging are helpful for an accurate diagnosis. Ureteral injury can be viewed as a result of direct needle trauma or secondary to necrosis induced by fluid collection and obstruction, which might lead to serious sequelae, such as ureterovaginal fistula or renal dysfunction. Therefore, persistent fever and vaginal leakage should raise suspicion. Most cases can be managed by conservative treatment with ureteral stenting or a nephrostomy tube, but two cases underwent ureterovesical reimplantation. Prompt evaluation and early suspicion are helpful for less invasive modalities.

Oocyte retrieval can also result in bladder injury. However, formation of a vesicovaginal fistula is extremely rare. Al-Shaikh et al. reported a vesicovaginal fistula after oocyte retrieval. The patient presented with a watery vaginal discharge after embryo transfer. Conservative management in the form of bladder catheterization for 3 weeks was initiated. The authors stated that early intervention with a Foley catheter cured the condition without long-term morbidity [44].

Some very uncommon complications have been reported in the literature. Almog et al. described a case of vertebral osteomyelitis treated by antibiotics [45]. Bentov et al. reported two cases of periumbilical hematoma as a result of retroperitoneal bleeding [46]. In addition, a pseudoaneurysm with massive hematuria was described following transvaginal oocyte retrieval [47].

83.4 Conclusion

Transvaginal oocyte retrieval is a frequently used procedure during IVF cycles. Vaginal and intraperitoneal bleeding, pelvic infection and abscesses, and injury to pelvic structures are the most likely complications following the procedure. Although these complications are reportedly rare, they can lead to life-threatening conditions. Therefore, preventive strategies should be seriously considered, including sterilization and adequate equipment. Proper training of staff is also extremely important. Patients should be informed in detail about the incidence of complications and informed consent should be obtained before the procedure.

References

1. De Kretzer D, Dennis P, Hudson B, et al. Transfer of a human zygote. Lancet. 1973;2:728–9.
2. Berger MJ, Smith DM, Taymor ML, Thompson RS. Laparoscopic recovery of mature human oocytes. Fertil Steril. 1975;26:513–22.
3. Steptoe PC, Edwards RG. Laparoscopic recovery of preovulatory human oocytes after priming of ovaries with gonadotropins. Lancet. 1970;1:683–9.
4. Wickland M, Lennart E, Hamberger L. Transvesical and transvaginal approaches for the aspiration of follicles by the use of ultrasound. Ann NY Acad Sci. 1985;442:184–6.
5. Kovacs GT, King C, Cameron I, et al. A comparison of vaginal ultrasonic-guided and laparoscopic retrieval of oocytes for in vitro fertilization. Asia Ocenia J Obstet Gynaecol. 1990;16:39–43.
6. Miller PB, Price T, Nichols JE Jr, Hill L. Acute ureteral obstruction following transvaginal oocyte retrieval-a case report. Hum Reprod. 2002;17:137–8.
7. Von Eye Corleta H, Moretto M, DÀvila AM, Berger M. Immediate ureterovaginal fistula secondary to oocyte retrieval-a case report. Fertil Steril. 2008;90:2006.e1–3.
8. Almog B, Rimon E, Yovel I, et al. Vertebral osteomyelitis: a rare complication of transvaginal ultrasound-guided oocyte retrieval. Fertil Steril. 2000;73:1250–2.
9. Dessole S, Rubattu G, Ambrosini G, Miele M, Nardelli GB, Cherci PL. Blood loss following non-complicated transvaginal oocyte retrieval for IVF. Fertil Steril. 2001;76:205–6.
10. Tureck RW, Garcia C, Blasco L, Mastroianni L. Perioperative complications arising after transvaginal oocyte retrieval. Obstet Gynecol. 1993;81:590–3.
11. Lenz S, Leeton J, Renou P. Transvaginal recovery of oocytes for in vitro fertilization using vaginal ultrasound. J In Vitro Fert Embryo Transf. 1987;4:51–5.
12. Benett SJ, Waterstone JJ, Cheng WC, Parsons J. Complications of transvaginal ultrasound–directed follicle aspiration: a review of 2670 consecutive procedures. J Assist Reprod Genet. 1993;10:772–8.
13. El-Shawarby SA, Margara RA, Trew GH, Lavery SA. A review of complications following transvaginal oocyte retrieval for in-vitro fertilization. Hum Fertil. 2004;7(2):127–33.
14. Gardner DK, Weissman A, Howles CM, Shoham Z. Textbook of assisted reproductive techniques. Bleeding, severe pelvic infection and ectopic pregnancy. 4th edition. Volume 2: Clinical perspectives; 2012, 62, p. 374–81.
15. Kart C, Guven S, Aran T, Dinc H. Life threatening intraabdominal bleeding after oocyte retrieval successfully managed with angiographic embolization. Fertil Steril. 2011;96:e99–e102.
16. Dicker D, Ashkenazi J, Feldberg D, et al. Severe abdominal complications after transvaginal ultrasonographically guided retrieval of oocytes for in vitro fertilization and embryo transfer. Fertil Steril. 1993;59:1313–5.
17. Shalev J, Orvieto R, Meizner I. Use of color Doppler sonography during follicular aspiration in patients undergoing in vitro fertilization may reduce the risk of blood vessel injury. Fertil Steril. 2004;81:1408–10.
18. Nakagawa K, Nishi Y, Kaneyama M, Sugiyama R, Motoyama H, Sugiyama R. The effect of a newly designed needle on the pain and bleeding of patients during oocyte retrieval of a single follicle. J Reprod Infertil. 2015;16(4):207–11.
19. Wikland M, Blad S, Bungum L, Hillensjö T, Karlström PO, Nilsson S. A randomized controlled study comparing pain experience between a newly designed needle with a thin tip and a standard needle for oocyte aspiration. Hum Reprod. 2011;26(6):1377–83.
20. Azem F, Wolf Y, Botchan A, Amit A, Lessing JB, Kluger Y. Massive retroperitoneal bleeding : a complication of transvaginal ultrasonography guided oocyte retrieval for IVF-ET. Fertil Steril. 2000;74:405–6.
21. Bolster F, Mocanu E, Geoghegan LL. Transvaginal oocyte retrieval complicated by life-threatening obturator artery haemorrhage and managed by a vessel-preserving technique. Ulster Med J. 2014;83(3):146–8.
22. Moayeri SE, Coutre SE, Ramirez EJ, Westphal LM. Von Willebrand disease presenting as recurrent hemorrhage after transvaginal oocyte retrieval. Am J Obstet Gynecol. 2007;196:e10–1.
23. El-Shawarby SA, Margara RA, Trew GH, Laffan MA, Lavery SA. Thrombocythemia and hemoperitoneum after transvaginal oocyte retrieval for in vitro fertilization. Fertil Steril. 2004;82: 735–7.
24. Battaglia C, Regnani G, Giulini S, Madgar L, Genazzani AD, Volpe A. Severe intraabdominal bleeding after transvaginal oocyte retrieval for IVF-ET and coagulation factor XI deficiency: a case report. J Assist Reprod Genet. 2001;18:178–81.
25. Peavey M, Steward R, Paulyson-Nunez K, James A. Succesful prophylactic regimens for transvaginal oocyte retrieval in women with bleeding diatheses. Haemophila. 2013;19:174–92.
26. Revel A, Schejter-Dinur Y, Yahalomi SZ, et al. Is routine screening needed for coagulation abnormalities before oocyte retrieval? Fertil Steril. 2011;95:1182–4.
27. Roest J, Mous HV, Zeilmaker GH, Verhoeff A. The incidence of major clinical complications in a Dutch transport IVF programme. Hum Reprod Update. 1996;4:345–53.
28. Bodri D, Guillen JJ, Polo A, Trullenque M, Esteve C, Coll O. Complications related to ovarian stimulation and oocyte retrieval in 4052 oocyte donor cycles. Reprod Biomed Online. 2008;2:237–43.
29. Ludwig AK, Glawatz M, Griesinger G, Diedritch K, Ludwig M. Perioperative and postoperative complications of transvaginal ultrasound-guided oocyte retrieval: prospective study of >1000 oocyte retrievals. Hum Reprod. 2006;12:3235–40.
30. Asemota OA, Girda E, Duenas O, Neal-Perry G, Pollack S. Actinomycosis pelvic abscess after in vitro fertilization. Fertil Steril. 2013;100:408–11.
31. Hignett M, Claman P. High rates of perforation are found in endovaginal ultrasound probe covers before and after oocyte retrieval for IVF-ET. J Assist Reprod Genet. 2008;7:341–3.
32. Van Os HC, Roozenburg BJ, Janssen-Caspers HA, Leerentveld RA, Scholtes MC, Zeilmaker GH, et al. Vaginal disinfection with povidon iodine and the outcome of in-vitro fertilization. Hum Reprod. 1992;7:349–50.
33. Tsai YC, Lin MYS, Chen SH, Chung MT, Loo TC, Huang KF, Lin LY. Vaginal disinfection with povidone iodine immediately before oocyte retrieval is effective in preventing pelvic abscess formation without compromising the outcome of IVF-ET. J Assist Reprod Genet. 2005;22(4):173–5.
34. Kelada E, Ghani R. Bilateral ovarian abscesses following transvaginal oocyte retrieval for IVF: a case report and review of literature. J Assist Reprod Genet. 2007;24:143–5.
35. Benaglia L, Somigliana E, Iemello R, Colpi E, Nicolosi AE, Ragni G. Endometrioma and oocyte retrieval-induced pelvic abscess: a clinical concern or an exceptional complication. Fertil Steril. 2008;89(5):1263–6.
36. Moini A, Riazi K, Amid V, Ashrafi M, Tehraninejad E, Madani T, Owj M. Endometriosis may contribute to oocyte retrieval-induced pelvic inflammatory disease: report of eight cases. J Assist Reprod Genet. 2005;22(7):307–9.
37. Gjelland K, Ekerhovd E, Granberg S. Transvaginal ultrasound-guided aspiration for treatment of tubo-ovarian abscess: a study of 302 cases. Am J Obstet Gynecol. 2005;193:1323–30.
38. Ashkenazi J, Farhi J, Dicker D, et al. Acute pelvic inflammatory disease after oocyte retrieval: adverse effects on the results of implantation. Fertil Steril. 1994;61:526–8.

39. Aragona C, Mohamed M, Espinola MS, Linari A, Pecorini F, Micara G, Sbracia M. Clinical complications after transvaginal oocyte retrieval in 7098 IVF cycles. Fertil Steril. 2011;95:293–4.
40. Akman MA, Katz E, Damewood M, Ramzy AI, Garcia JE. Perforated appendicitis and ectopic pregnancy following IVF. Hum Reprod. 1995;10:3325–6.
41. Grynberg M, Berwanger AL, Toledano M, Frydman R, Deffieux X, Fanchin R. Ureteral injury after transvaginal ultrasound-guided oocyte retrieval: a complication of in vitro fertilization-embryo transfer that may lurk undetected in women presenting with severe ovarian hyperstimulation syndrome. Fertil Steril. 2011;96(4):869–71.
42. Mongiu AK, Helfand BT, Kielb SJ. Ureterovaginal fistula formation after oocyte retrieval. Urology. 2009;73(2):444.e1–3.
43. Miller PB, Price T, Nichols JE, Hill L. Acute ureteral obstruction following transvaginal oocyte retrieval for IVF. Hum Reprod. 2002;17:137–8.
44. Al-Shaikh G, Abotalib Z. Vesicovaginal fistula formation after oocyte retrieval. Taiwan J Obstet Gynecol. 2013;52:597–8.
45. Almog B, Rimon E, Yovel I, et al. Vertebral osteomyelitis: a rare complication of transvaginal oocyte retrieval. Fertil Steril. 2000;73:1250–2.
46. Bentov Y, Levitas E, Silberstein T, Potashnik G. Cullen's sign following ultrasound guided transvaginal oocyte retrieval. Fertil Steril. 2006;85:227.
47. Jayakrishnan K, Raman VK, Vijayalakshmi VK, Baheti S, Nambiar D. Massive hematuria with hemodynamic instability-complication of oocyte retrieval. Fertil Steril. 2011;96:e22–4.

Follicular Flushing at Oocyte Retrieval in Medically Assisted Reproduction

84

Pinar Caglar Aytac and Bulent Haydardedeoglu

Throughout the 1970s oocyte retrieval has been performed via laparoscopy. In the mid-1980s after ultrasound was introduced for oocyte retrieval (OR), initially transvesical OR was performed under abdominal ultrasound guidance. All these efforts were expensive and prone to many complications. However, development of transvaginal ultrasonography in the late 1980s and 1990s let us retrieve oocytes in an easier and more convenient way. Consequently, OR became an outpatient procedure. With advances in technology, transvaginal probes provided better resolution, enabling us to visualize and collect oocytes from ovaries located further in the pelvis, due to adhesions after pelvic infections or surgeries.

After the introduction of double-lumen catheters, some non-randomized studies suggested that follicle flushing had promising results that could increase the numbers of collected oocyte [1–3]. Bagtharia and Haloob suggested that flushing follicles up to six times can increase oocyte yield up to 97% compared to aspiration only for which oocyte yield was 40% [3]. Oocyte retrieval is the harvest of all efforts ovarian hyperstimulation in assisted reproductive technologies or medically assisted reproduction (MAR). Live birth rate, which is the end point of in vitro fertilization (IVF), is correlated with the number of oocytes and is optimal around 15 oocytes [4]. A survey showed that more than 50% of IVF clinics in Australia used follicular flushing to prevent oocyte retention in the aspirated follicles in MAR [5]. Similarly, many IVF clinics began to flush follicles to obtain more oocytes with double-lumen catheters despite the controversies.

Nevertheless prospective controlled studies and Cochrane analysis were performed which showed that follicular flushing had no benefit compared to standard single-lumen catheters [6–10]. Among these, the only study to report live birth rate (LBR), which also had the largest study population, showed that flushing follicles did not yield more oocytes during OPU and resulted in similar LBRs in IVF [6]. Later, two review and meta-analyses reported that follicular flushing had no effect in collected number of oocytes and live birth rates over traditional single aspiration; moreover, this procedure increased OR procedure time and the cost of IVF by increasing flushing medium utilization [11, 12].

P. C. Aytac · B. Haydardedeoglu (✉)
Faculty of Medicine, Department of Obstetrics and Gynecology, Division of Reproductive Endocrinology and IVF Unit, Baskent University, Adana, Turkey

84.1 Oocyte Retrieval in Poor Responders

Most of the studies investigating the efficacy of flushing involved women with unexplained infertility. However, women with poor ovarian reserve or poor response to ovarian stimulation have lower oocyte yield, therefore maximizing the retrieval of the developed oocytes is even more crucial in these populations. The first randomized controlled study in poor responders showed no difference in the number of oocytes retrieved, implantation rate and ongoing pregnancy rates between the flushing and the control groups [8]. Of note, this study had a small sample size with 15 patients in each group. It was calculated that at least 162 poor responders should be randomized to show an improvement of one oocyte retrieved via flushing [13]. Other RCTs failed to show superiority of flushing over aspirating only in poor responders, with regard to number of oocytes retrieved [14–16].

In a study by Von Horn K et al., a modified double-lumen needle (17G, Gynetics®) with another double-lumen needle (17G, Steiner-Tan Needle®) were compared for flushing oocytes in poor responders, but no difference was shown in retrieved numbers of oocytes [16]. However, Mok-Lin E et al. demonstrated that quality of oocytes, implantation rate, and clinical pregnancy rate were lower in the cycle that had follicular flushing with double-lumen needle [14]. They speculated that increased intrafollicular pressure during

G. N. Allahbadia et al. (eds.), *Textbook of Assisted Reproduction*, https://doi.org/10.1007/978-981-15-2377-9_84

flushing, increased anesthesia time or aspirating all granulosa cells might impair oocyte quality and pregnancy rate. Other RCTs did not demonstrate detrimental effect of flushing on oocyte quality or live birth rate in poor responders [15, 16]. Flushing oocytes in natural cycle IVF did not impair the length of luteal phase or progesterone and estradiol concentrationts in von Wollf et al.'s study [17]. Thus, it can be thought that flushing of granulosa cells does not impair implantation and pregnancy rates in natural cycle IVF. In conclusion, the available studies show that follicular flushing in poor responders does not increase oocyte yield, implantation rate, or live birth rates.

84.2 In Vitro Maturation

Oocyte retrieval in vitro maturation (IVM) cycles, in which oocytes that are smaller than 14 mm in diamater are retrieved, may be impaired because of problematic detachment of immature oocytes from compact granulocytes. However, there is only one abstract involving only four women, reporting 100% oocyte retrieval rate in 3 women and 71% in one woman. They also reported decreased number of vaginal punctures to achieve these rates [18]. Still, there is not enough data on the role of flushing in IVM.

84.3 Natural Cycles and Milder Stimulation IVF

In a study by von Wolff M, flushing follicles resulted in an increase in oocyte retrieval rate from 44.5% up to 80.5% after three times flushing in monofollicular natural IVF cycles. Accordingly, number of transferred embryos increased as well [19]. In the another study on milder stimulation in IVF, follicular flushing resulted in similar oocyte yield and clinical pregnancy rate, whereas oocyte quality and implantation rates were improved [20]. These were not RCTs, and in both, flushing was performed when no oocyte was detected in the initial aspiration. However, this method does not rule out the possibility that the oocyte was in the lumen of the needle or the tube in the first place. Therefore, well-designed and larger trials are required to show if there is any benefit from flushing in natural, semi-natural or mild IVF cycles.

84.4 Reproductive Outcomes

Another question regarding flushing is wheher it has a detrimental effect on IVF outcomes due to possible damage to oocytes or any other impact due to the procedure. In von Wolff et al.'s study, luteal phase length or estrogen or progesteron levels in the luteal phase did not change after flushing in natural IVF cycles [17]. Lozono Mendez DH et al. [20] suggested that follicular flushing increased oocyte quality and implantation rates, where as a study by contrary to the study of Mok-Lin E et al. denied these findings [14]. Most of the RCTs on the subject demonstrated no decrease in oocyte quality or pregnancy or live birth rates [6, 7, 15, 16].

84.5 Preparation for Oocyte Retrieval

Generally, OR is performed under sedation anesthesia under of transvaginal ultrasonography guidance. First, vagina is cleansed with saline. If iodine is used for vaginal preparation in selected patients, it should be followed by a thorough application of saline to remove any left over, to prevent toxic effects of iodine to oocytes [21, 22]. In our clinic, we rinse the vagina with warm saline and clean the cervical secretions with gauze. In patients with endometrioma, 2 g cephazoline sodium is administered intravenously before ½ h of OR. Routinely oral antibiotic azithromycin 500 mg is also given after ORU procedure daily for 3 days for suspected infection prevention in our clinic.

84.6 Aspiration Techniques

The technique of OR is universally similar in most IVF centers. Patients are placed in lithotomy position under anesthesia. The vaginal probe of ultrasound is completely draped with sterile plastic bag. The needle guide is attached over the plastic bag on the designated place securely. The needle guide can be disposable or reusable. The aspiration needle is connected to sterile tubes, which are placed in an incubator to maintain a temperature similar to that of the abdominal cavity. The tubes are plugged and have to outlets, one from the plastic tuba connected to the aspiration needle, and the other connected to the suction device. Suction device is controlled by the clinician, using a pedal.

We prefer suction pressure to be around 80–100 mmHg in our clinic. Higher pressures can be used for removing plugs in the aspiration needles. In the single-lumen needle, there is one plastic lumen that connects the tube and the needle. In the double lumen catheter, there are two plastic lumens, one for aspirating and the other for irrigating the follicle. The irrigation line is attached to an injector containing follicular flushing medium (Quinn's Advantage, Medium with HEPES; USA).

Placing the probe so that there is minimal distance between the ovary and the lateral fornix reduces complications. Then, the needle is placed into the guide and inserted in the nearest follicle. Follicle is aspirated until it is totally collapsed. If using a double-lumen needle for flushing, then 2 ml medium at 37 C is injected into each follicle manually while the needle is kept in place. The injection-aspiration process is repeated three times. Aspiration pressure is strictly maintained between 80 and 100 mmHg [15].

In a study by Sasamoto Y et al. rotating the single-lumen needle while in the follicle was shown to improve retrieval of retained cumulus complex and oocytes in the cattle [23]. In our clinic we use 17G (gauge) single-lumen needle (Cook, Ireland) and 16.5G double-lumen needle (Vitrolife, Sweden).

While the preferred pressure for aspiration may vary, it is generally between 80–220 mmHg. One study showed that oocytes were not affected by aspiration pressure 140 mmHg compared to 120 mmHg [24].

Two animal studies showed that while oocyte recovery rate was improved by increasing aspiration pressure, oocytes retrieved in higher pressures were more likely to be denuded of cumulus cells [25, 26].

84.7 Conclusion

In MAR, follicular flushing has no advantage over aspirating only in OR. Specific populations, such as poor responders or patients undergoing natural IVF, do not benefit from flushing either. Moreover, it is prolongs the procedure time and costs more due to increased use of medium and prolonged anesthesia.

References

1. Waterstone JJ, Parsons JH. A prospective-study to investigate the value of flushing follicles during transvaginal ultrasound-directed follicle aspiration. Fertil Steril. 1992;57:221–3.
2. Elhussein E, Balen AH, Tan SL. A prospective-study comparing the outcome of oocytes retrieved in the aspirate with those retrieved in the flush during transvaginal ultrasound directed oocyte recovery for in vitro fertilization. Br J Obstet Gynaecol. 1992;99:841–4.
3. Bagtharia S, Haloob ARK. Is there a benefit from routine follicular flushing for oocyte retrieval? J Obstet Gynaecol. 2005;25:374–6.
4. Sunkara SK, Rittenberg V, Raine-Fenning N, Bhattacharya S, Zamora J, Coomarasamy A. Association between the number of eggs and live birth in IVF treatment: an analysis of 400 135 treatment cycles. Hum Reprod. 2011;26(7):1768–74.
5. Knight DC, Tyler JP, Driscoll GL. Follicular flushing at oocyte retrieval: a reappraisal. Aust NZ J Obstet Gynaecol. 2001;41(2):210–3.
6. Haydardedeoglu B, Cok T, Kilicdag EB, Parlakgumus AH, Simsek E, Bagis T. In vitro fertilization-intracytoplasmic sperm injection outcomes in single- versus double-lumen oocyte retrieval needles in normally responding patients: a randomized trial. Fertil Steril. 2011;95(2):812–4.
7. Tan SL, Waterstone J, Wren M, Parsons J. A prospective randomized study comparing aspiration only with aspiration and flushing for transvaginal ultrasound-directed oocyte recovery. Fertil Steril. 1992;58:356–60.
8. Levens ED, Whitcomb BW, Payson MD, Larsen FW. Ovarian follicular flushing among low-responding patients undergoing assisted reproductive technology. Fertil Steril. 2009;91(Suppl 4):1381–4.
9. Kara M, Aydin T, Turktekin N. Is follicular flushing really effective? A clinical study. Arch Gynecol Obstet. 2012;286(4):1061–4.
10. Wongtra-Ngan S, Vutyavanich T, Brown J. Follicular flushing during oocyte retrieval in assisted reproductive techniques. Cochrane Database Syst Rev. 2010;9:CD004634.
11. Levy G, Hill MJ, Ramirez CI, Correa L, Ryan ME, DeCherney AH, Levens ED, Whitcomb BW. The use of follicle flushing during oocyte retrieval in assisted reproductive technologies: a systematic review and meta-analysis. Hum Reprod. 2012;27(8):2373–9.
12. Roque M, Sampaio M, Geber S. Follicular flushing during oocyte retrieval: a systematic review and meta-analysis. J Assist Reprod Genet. 2012;29(11):1249–54.
13. Hill MJ, Levens ED. Is there a benefit in follicular flushing in assisted reproductive technology? Curr Opin Obstet Gynecol. 2010;22(3):208–12.
14. Mok-Lin E, Brauer AA, Schattman G, Zaninovic N, Rosenwaks Z, Spandorfer S. Follicular flushing and in vitro fertilization outcomes in the poorest responders: a randomized controlled trial. Hum Reprod. 2013;28(11):2990–5.
15. Haydardedeoglu B, Gjemalaj F, Aytac PC, Kilicdag EB. Direct aspiration versus follicular flushing in poor responders undergoing intracytoplasmic sperm injection: a randomised controlled trial. BJOG. 2017;124(8):1190–6.
16. Von Horn K, Depenbusch M, Schultze-Mosgau A, Griesinger G. Randomized, open trial comparing a modified double-lumen needle follicular flushing system with a single-lumen aspiration needle in IVF patients with poor ovarian response. Hum Reprod. 2017;32(4):832–5.
17. von Wolff M, Kohl Schwartz A, Stute P, Fäh M, Otti G, Schürch R, Rohner S. Follicular flushing in natural cycle IVF does not affect the luteal phase – a prospective controlled study. Reprod Biomed Online. 2017;35(1):37–41.
18. Uzelac PS, Christensen GL, Nakajima ST. Follicular flushing avoids multiple vaginal punctures and may aid in oocyte recovery in in vitro maturation (IVM). Fertil Steril. 2009;91:S5.
19. von Wolff M, Hua YZ, Santi A, Ocon E, Weiss B. Follicle flushing in monofollicular in vitro fertilization almost doubles the number of transferable embryos. Acta Obstet Gynecol Scand. 2013 Mar;92(3):346–8.
20. Mendez Lozano DH, Brum Scheffer J, Frydman N, Fay S, Fanchin R, Frydman R. Optimal reproductive competence of oocytes retrieved through follicular flushing in minimal stimulation IVF. Reprod Biomed Online. 2008;16(1):119–23.
21. Hannoun A, Awwad J, Zreik T, Ghaziri G, Abu-Musa A. Effect of betadine vaginal preparation during oocyte aspiration in in vitro fertilization cycles on pregnancy outcome. Gynecol Obstet Investig. 2008;66(4):274–8.
22. Tsai YC, Lin MY, Chen SH, Chung MT, Loo TC, Huang KF, Lin LY. Vaginal disinfection with povidone-iodine immediately before oocyte retrieval is effective in preventing pelvic abscess formation without compromising the outcome of IVF-ET. J Assist Reprod Genet. 2005;22(4):173–5.
23. Sasamoto Y, Sakaguchi M, Katagiri S, Yamada Y, Takahashi Y. The effects of twisting and type of aspiration needle on the efficiency of transvaginal ultrasound-guided ovum pick-up in cattle. J Vet Med Sci. 2003;65:1083–6.
24. Kumaran A, Narayan PK, Pai PJ, Ramachandran A, Mathews B, Adiga SK. Oocyte retrieval at 140-mmHg negative aspiration pressure: a promising alternative to flushing and aspiration in assisted reproduction in women with low ovarian reserve. J Hum Reprod Sci. 2015;8(2):98–102.
25. Bols PE, Van Soom A, Ysebaert MT, Vandenheede JM, de Kruif A. Effects of aspiration vacuum and needle diameter on cumulus oocyte complex morphology and developmental capacity of bovine oocytes. Theriogenology. 1996;45:1001–14.
26. Fry RC, Niall EM, Simpson TL, Squires TJ, Reynolds J. The collection of oocytes from bovine ovaries. Theriogenology. 1997;47:977–87.

85 Handling Unhealthy or Poor-Quality Sperm Samples in a Medically Assisted Reproduction Laboratory

Sheryl Homa

A significant proportion of men attending for medically assisted reproduction (MAR) have poor-quality sperm. Although many of the factors contributing to poor sperm quality may be addressed through medical intervention and lifestyle modifications, there will inevitably be men who continue to demonstrate poor semen parameters and will need MAR to achieve a family.

The aim of any sperm handling procedure in the MAR laboratory is to select the most motile, genetically healthy, and functionally active sperm from a given sample, as these are the most likely to result in a healthy ongoing pregnancy. Routine protocols may have to be adjusted for "difficult" samples, and specific protocols implemented to obtain sperm from a retrograde ejaculate or a surgically retrieved testicular sample.

While there are many step-by-step guides to routine handling and processing of sperm samples [1, 2], this chapter focuses on the variety and adaptations of sperm handling techniques available for optimizing sperm quality for MAR.

85.1 Handling Samples with Abnormal Semen Parameters

The processing of difficult samples relies predominantly on variations of the standard discontinuous density gradient centrifugation (DGC) technique. However, removal of seminal plasma and the mechanical shearing force of extensive centrifugation at speeds of 600 g and above can cause an increase in oxidative stress and sperm DNA damage [3], so it is important to minimize these steps as much as possible. A minimum speed (g force) and length of time of centrifugation are recommended, as well as a reduction to the number of repetitive centrifugation steps.

85.1.1 Increased Viscosity

Viscous samples significantly hamper recovery of sperm from semen. There are several procedures that may be attempted to reduce viscosity, including:

1. Incubating the semen for 30 min at 36 ± 1 °C to encourage liquefaction and reduce viscosity.
2. Diluting the semen 1:1 v/v with culture medium. This process involves mixing by gently inverting or by drawing the sample up and down with a sterile Pasteur pipette. The diluted semen can then be layered directly onto a discontinuous density gradient before centrifugation. This should always be the method of choice as it is the least harmful to sperm.
3. Treating the semen with proteolytic enzymes such as bromelain, α-chymotrypsin, trypsin, or α-amylase to improve sample handling [2, 4]. Proteases effectively reduce semen viscosity without affecting sperm motility; however, there is a risk that sperm may be damaged, and there is a paucity of evidence to confirm they can be used safely in MAR. Although proteases may be helpful in the diagnostic andrology laboratory for semen analysis, only compounds that have been thoroughly tested should be used in MAR. In Europe, this includes CE-marking for clinical use.
4. Increasing centrifugal force and or time of centrifugation may improve the yield of sperm. However, samples should not be centrifuged for more than 500 g for 20 min (see above).

Please note, mechanical manipulation with a needle and syringe should never be used to decrease viscosity due to the increased risk of structural and DNA damage to the sperm.

S. Homa (✉)
Andrology Solutions, London, UK
e-mail: s.homa@andrologysolutions.co.uk

G. N. Allahbadia et al. (eds.), *Textbook of Assisted Reproduction*, https://doi.org/10.1007/978-981-15-2377-9_85

85.1.2 Extensive Debris

If a sample has macromolecular debris, including cellular or acellular aggregates or gel bodies, it is recommended to allow the sample to settle in a 15 ml centrifuge tube for a short period of time. The supernatant can then be layered onto the gradient, leaving large aggregates and gel bodies behind.

Semen with significant debris leads to "raft" formation at the interface between density gradients, preventing sperm from moving through and resulting in negligible pellet formation after centrifugation.

To mitigate these effects, the following procedure is recommended:

- Gently mix the semen with a small amount of "upper layer" before centrifuging.
- Layer smaller volumes of semen over the gradient, e.g., no more than 1 ml to be layered over a 1 ml 40/45%:1 ml 80/90% two-step colloid layer (Fig. 85.1b).
- Include an intermediate layer of 60% colloid in the DGC (Fig. 85.1c).
- Increase the volume of each gradient layer, e.g., up to 2 ml (Fig. 85.1d). Longer column lengths or additional density layers can help to prevent raft formation, increasing sperm yield.

85.1.3 Poor Motility (Asthenozoospermia) and Vitality (Necrozoospermia)

Astheno- or necrozoospermia often results from a toxic environment in the epididymis due to male accessory gland infection, epididymal dysfunction or partial obstruction, or seminal fluid stasis from a lack of sexual activity or spinal cord injury (SCI).

As a result, a population of aging, apoptotic sperm accumulate in the epididymis and vas deferens. Ejaculates are often characterized by alterations in seminal plasma pH with increased debris, polymorphonuclear leukocytes (PMNs), and oxidative stress.

Repetitive ejaculation depletes epididymal stores of senescent sperm and improves motility and vitality [5, 6]. Therefore, asking the patient to ejaculate twice a day for several days beforehand will encourage clearance of residual older sperm, enhancing the proportion of newly formed sperm in the ejaculate. Additionally, providing a second sample within 3 h minimizes exposure of newly produced sperm to a hostile epididymal environment, increasing motility and vitality [5, 6] and reducing reactive oxygen species (ROS) and DNA damage [5, 7]. This technique can help even when there is complete asthenozoospermia or necrozoospermia. If the patient finds it difficult to maintain this intense frequency of ejaculation, a

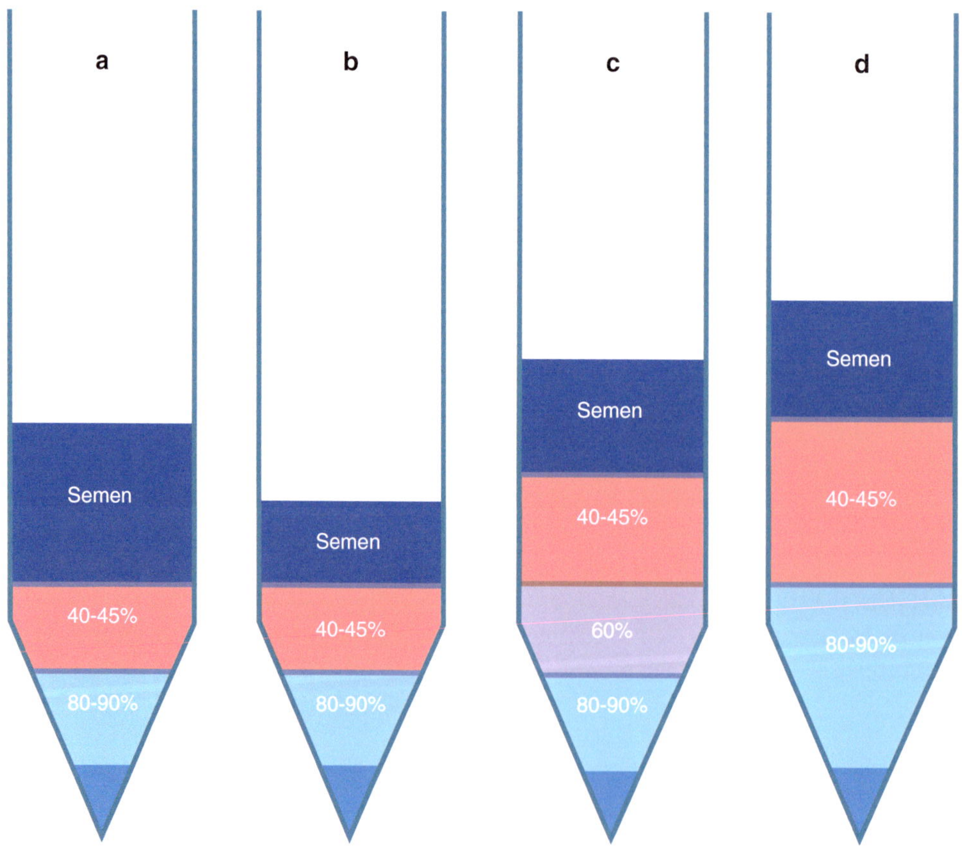

Fig. 85.1 Sperm preparation from samples with extensive debris. (**a**) Routine density gradient for samples with insignificant debris. Layer up to 2 ml semen over 1 ml upper layer and 1 ml lower layer. (**b**) Reducing semen volume. (**c**) Additional density layer. (**d**) Increased volume of density layers

second sample produced an hour later on the day of treatment should suffice.

Asthenozoospermic samples should be prepared by DGC as for sperm with normal motility. Occasionally, asthenozoospermia is associated with structural defects. Adjusting the lower density layer by diluting it 9:1 v/v with culture medium may improve the yield but will most likely reduce motility. Alternatively, if immotility is due to antisperm antibodies, then ejaculation into culture medium should be advised.

Separation of apoptotic from non-apoptotic sperm can be achieved by magnetic-activated cell sorting (MACS) (Fig. 85.2). This process involves washing the sperm through an affinity column packed with superparamagnetic microspheres coated with Annexin V antibodies. Following exposure to a magnetic field, the Annexin V binds to phosphatidylserine residues that are exposed on the sperm plasma membrane surface during apoptosis. MACS is a relatively safe method that has been shown to improve motility and vitality of the sample, especially when used in conjunction with DGC [8], although swim-up after DGC may be more effective. However, there is conflicting data regarding improvement in clinical outcome using this technique [9].

For samples with negligible motility, the hypo-osmotic swelling (HOS) test can be used to select viable sperm for ICSI treatment [10] (Fig. 85.3). Sperm selection by this method may improve both fertilization and pregnancy rates. However, caution should be taken when using the HOS test as it cannot distinguish between dead sperm that already have coiled tails.

An alternative method for stimulating sperm motility is to add a nonspecific inhibitor of cAMP phosphodiesterase (PDE) such as pentoxifylline to the washed sample. PDE inhibitors increase both total and progressive motility and cervical mucus penetration [4, 10]. However, they may interfere with capacitation and induce premature acrosome reaction [11]. As the safety of these compounds for use in the clinic has yet to be fully validated, PDE inhibitors should only be used when absolutely necessary for ICSI treatment. It is not advisable to use these compounds for IVF or intrauterine insemination (IUI) treatment or prior to sperm storage.

If sperm remain immotile after all attempts to improve motility have failed, a diagnostic vitality test using eosin Y or eosin-nigrosin can be performed on a small aliquot of the sample that is going to be used for treatment. This will provide a measure of the extent of vital sperm if the decision is made to continue with the ICSI. This may be more acceptable to the patient than using a sperm donor at the outset. However, oocyte cryopreservation should also be considered in such extreme instances.

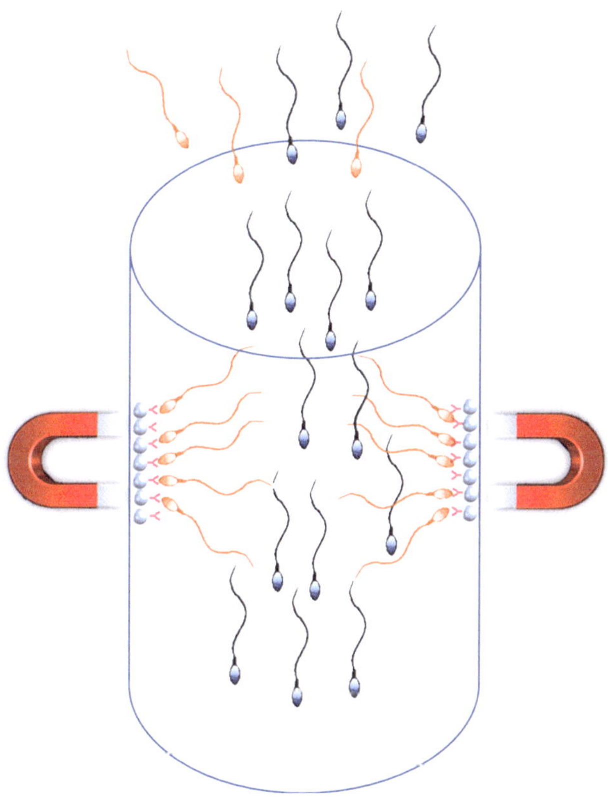

Fig. 85.2 Magnetic-activated cell sorting (MACS). Sperm are passed through a column containing colloidal superparamagnetic microspheres conjugated with Annexin V antibodies. Apoptotic sperm (red) bind to the Annexin V whilst healthy viable sperm (blue) pass through the gradient

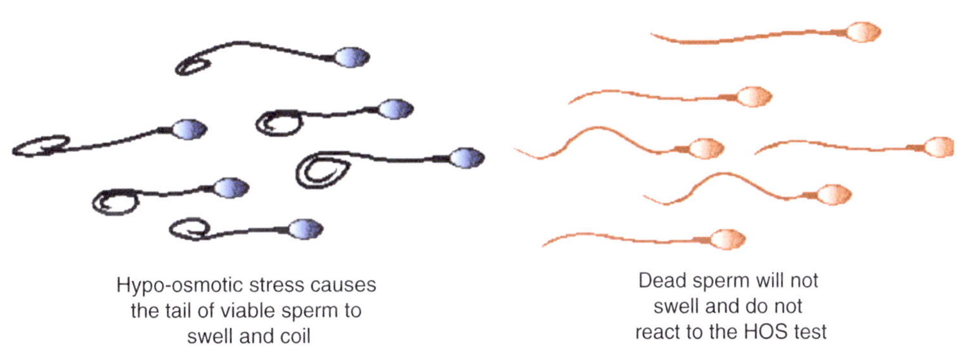

Fig. 85.3 Hypo-osmotic swelling test (HOS) to determine viability. Sperm with coiled tails (blue) are viable

85.1.4 Low Count (Oligozoospermia)

Oligozoospermic samples require processing for ICSI treatment. As long as there are enough sperm for ICSI treatment, normal DGC methods are recommended. Sperm reach their isopycnic (buoyant density) points following centrifugation at 300 g after 20 min [1, 12], so any increase in centrifugation speed or time past this point may be superfluous to increasing yield.

Alternatively, a number of adjustments can be made to routine protocols to enhance the recovery of very low numbers of sperm for MAR, such as:

- Requesting a 5 days abstinence instead of 2–3, as each day may extend the numbers of sperm
- Requesting production of two samples to boost numbers of sperm prepared for treatment
- Diluting the lower layer (9:1 v/v with culture medium) to encourage recovery of a larger number of sperm. This risks reducing the percentage motility in the final preparation and recovering a higher proportion of abnormal sperm
- Reducing the volume of the gradient layers to decrease the distance that the sperm travel to increase the motile sperm yield
- Layering the sample over a single layer density colloid (40%) instead of the standard two-step gradient (if the count is very low)
- Only performing one wash of the pellet retrieved from DGC

Glass filtration is an alternative method for preparing oligoasthenozoospermic samples [4]. This technique separates sperm according to the filtration effect of the glass wool and the ability of the sperm to self-propel through it. It requires a subsequent centrifugation step to remove the seminal fluid. Yields have been reported to be high, and the recovered sperm have improved DNA integrity [13]; however, glass wool is expensive and may fragment during the washing process.

The most difficult cases are inevitably cryptozoospermic samples. In such cases, sperm are so scarce that preparation through standard DGC risks losing all of the sperm. One option is to resort to direct centrifugation of the whole semen sample. However, this method is not recommended as healthy sperm will become concentrated in the pellet alongside damaged sperm and polymorphonuclear leukocytes (PMNs). This may cause irreversible damage to the healthy sperm, detrimentally affecting the ability to fertilize, particularly in samples from men diagnosed with infertility [10]. Accepting this risk, in cases where sperm numbers are extremely low, may be the only option for finding sufficient sperm for treatment.

85.1.5 Poor Morphology (Teratozoospermia)

Morphology (Fig. 85.4) has probably the weakest correlation to fertility of all the major parameters that are measured in semen. With the exception of monomorphic abnormalities such as macrocephaly and globozoospermia, there is no direct correlation between teratozoospermia and genetic anomalies [14].

DGC is reported to be the optimal technique for enriching sperm with normal morphology, utilizing the principle that abnormal sperm tend to have a lower density and are less likely to pellet.

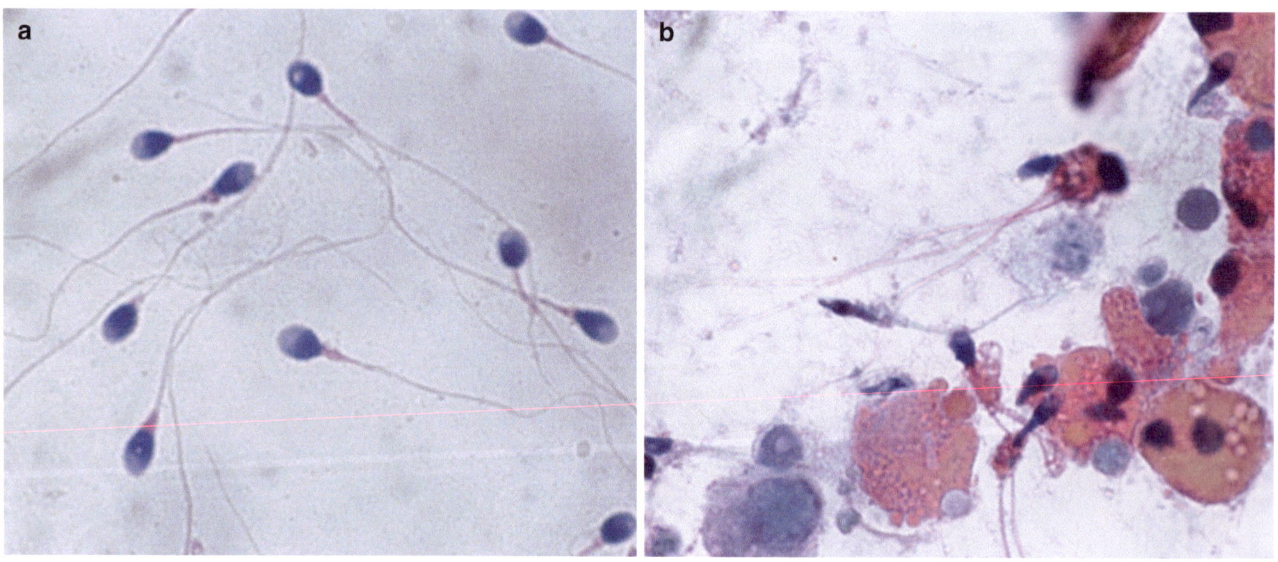

Fig. 85.4 Normal (**a**) versus abnormal (**b**) sperm samples. Semen samples were stained using Papanicolaou stain

The development of MSOME (motile sperm organelle morphology examination) implements real-time high-resolution differential interference contrast optics with computer-assisted magnification to evaluate nuclear morphology of motile sperm [15]. Sperm are selected at ×6000 magnification according to the presence of vacuoles present on the sperm head. These vacuoles were thought to represent abnormal morphology, although this has been disputed [16].

Early studies were encouraging [15], reporting improved pregnancy rates and reduced miscarriage rates using MSOME in conjunction with ICSI (IMSI—intracytoplasmic morphologically selected sperm injection). However, more recent studies show conflicting evidence for the benefits of IMSI [17, 18]. Furthermore, the technique may compromise sperm safety, since sperm can be exposed for up to 5 h during the selection process, risking DNA damage and oxidative stress.

85.1.6 Cellular Contamination

Polymorphonuclear leukocytes (PMNs) (Fig. 85.5) are a significant risk to sperm quality as they are a major source of ROS. High ROS are not only the main cause of sperm DNA damage but also impair semen parameters and fertilization and adversely affect blastocyst development and IVF pregnancy rates [19]. All efforts to reduce PMN contamination must be implemented before the sperm are used for MAR. Typical causes of PMN are infection, inflammation (e.g., prostatitis), varicocele, smoking, etc.

If PMNs remain following clinical intervention, it is recommended to process the semen by DGC centrifugation to remove them. Addition of glass wool filtration prior to centrifugation has been shown to remove up to 90% seminal leukocytes [4]. Direct swim-up may also be used; however the sperm yield will most likely be much lower than with DGC.

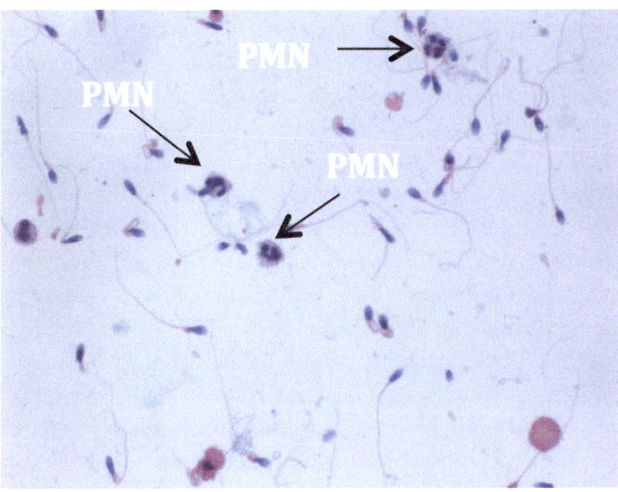

Fig. 85.5 Semen sample containing more than 1 million per ml polymorphonuclear leukocytes (PMN). Sample stained with Papanicolaou stain

85.1.7 Poor Genetic Integrity

Infertile men contain a significantly higher proportion of sperm with damaged DNA [20] or aneuploidy [21]. This has been linked to poor embryo development, reduced implantation and pregnancy rates, and increased miscarriage [22].

Preparing sperm using DGC at 300 g results in an enrichment of a fraction of sperm with improved DNA integrity and morphology [23]. Further enrichment of sperm with good chromatin quality may be obtained using DGC in conjunction with MACS [8]. However, the use of MSOME to select sperm with reduced DNA damage remains controversial [17].

Novel methods have recently been introduced to separate highly motile, morphologically normal sperm with minimal DNA fragmentation using microfluidic sorting [9]. The platform consists of a microchip with two channels separated by a membrane composed of a meshwork of micropores (Fig. 85.6). The membrane permits migration of functionally competent motile sperm while preventing compromised sperm from penetrating, mimicking the natural selection process for sperm in the female tract. Semen is layered in the lower channel beneath the membrane, and culture medium is layered in the channel above the membrane. The platform is then incubated at 37 °C for 30 min. The motile sperm that migrate through the membrane are collected from the top layer and are ready for use in MAR. This technique obviates the need for DGC and minimizes preparation time, both of which may induce exposure to oxidative stress and sperm DNA fragmentation. Preliminary results are encouraging, demonstrating good recovery rates with sperm that have significantly higher motility and reduced DNA damage compared to those prepared by other methods [9, 24]. However, it is yet to be established whether the technique is more efficient in improving clinical outcome.

A technique that uses petri dishes coated in hyaluronic acid to bind to mature sperm (PICSI) has been used with some success to increase the selection of both euploid sperm [25] and sperm with reduced sperm DNA fragmentation [26]. The principle behind this technique is that immature sperm are more likely to be aneuploid with fragmented DNA than their mature counterparts and only mature sperm express receptors for hyaluronic acid. ICSI is therefore carried out using only sperm bound to the dish. While early results for PICSI were promising, two large multicenter randomized controlled studies showed no increase in the rates of implantation, clinical pregnancy [27], or live birth [28] compared to standard ICSI. However, importantly, there was a significant reduction in the incidence of miscarriage [27, 28] indicating that this technique may be beneficial for cou-

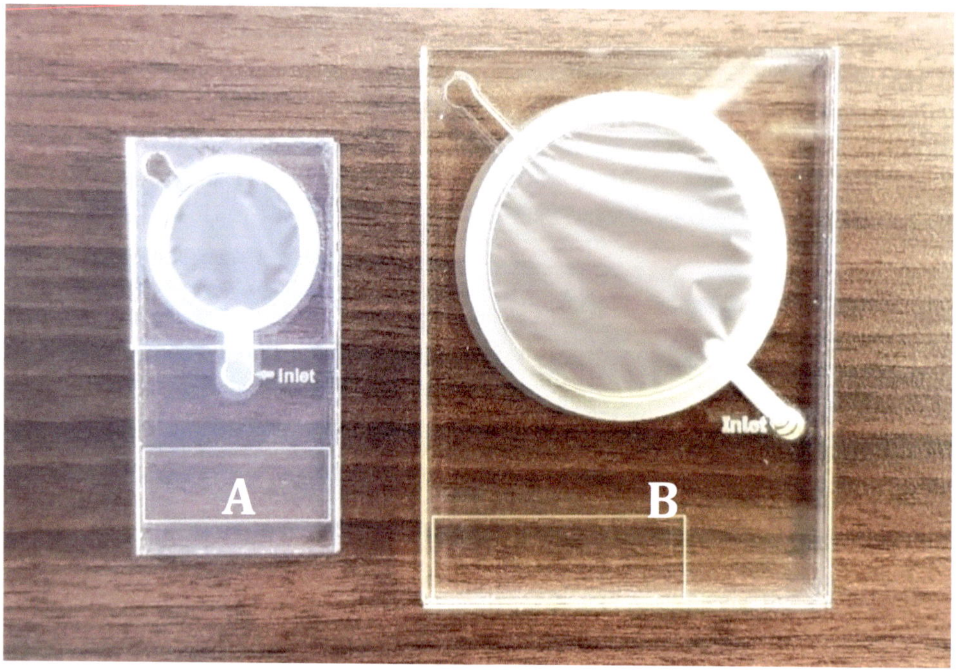

Fig. 85.6 Microfluidic sorting chip. Chambers are available in two sizes to accommodate small volumes up to 0.85 ml (**a**) or up to 3 ml (**b**)

ples experiencing recurrent pregnancy loss. Clearly more studies are required to confirm clinical benefit.

Finally, for sperm samples that are known to have high levels of DNA fragmentation, a novel approach is to ask the patient to have only 1-day abstinence and then prepare sperm for ICSI treatment from a second ejaculate produced within 3 h of the first, count permitting. This technique should reduce levels of DNA damage in the resultant sperm preparation (see Sect. 85.1.3).

85.2 Handling Compromised Semen

85.2.1 Semen Samples with Infectious Disease

For discordant couples attending for fertility treatment where the male partner has infectious disease, there is the risk of transferring virus to the partner or any unborn child. Although this risk is always present between such partners trying to conceive naturally, it is advantageous to minimize the risk of viral transmission during MAR. Patients that should be vaccinated against their partner's infection where possible and must continue with protected intercourse. As a virus is more likely to be present in the seminal fluid rather than adhered to sperm, sperm from infected males are subjected to extensive washing and swim-up following DGC to try to remove all trace of seminal fluid prior to use [29, 30]. Viral load in the fresh semen and subsequent sperm wash should be assessed by PCR to determine the efficacy of the procedure. The prepared sample can be cryopreserved for later use, and only the virus-free sample used for ICSI. While this protocol may limit the transmission of bacterial or viral infection, there is no guarantee that the sample will be completely free of infective agents. However, to date there are no reported cases of HIV transmission to female partners or any resulting child using this technique.

85.2.2 Semen Samples from Men with Spinal Cord Injury

Spinal cord injury (SCI) often results in neurogenic reproductive dysfunction, manifested by erectile dysfunction, an inability to ejaculate and compromised semen quality, specifically asthenozoospermia accompanied by necrozoospermia [31]. Although spermatogenesis may be affected by SCI, sperm count is usually unaffected. Stagnation in the epididymis due to prolonged periods of sexual abstinence and an abnormal testicular milieu is thought to be contributing factors to poor semen quality in SCI men primarily due to seminal plasma factors, including ROS arising from residual PMNs [31]. SCI patients exhibit a decrease in sperm mitochondrial activity and an increase in sperm DNA fragmentation [32]. Furthermore, SCI patients may develop bladder infections from catheterization that could affect sperm quality.

Ejaculates from SCI men may be obtained using penile vibration (PV) or electroejaculation (EEJ) for subsequent use with MAR [32]. The quality of ejaculated sperm collected from men with SCI is usually insufficient for IUI treatment although there are reports of successful outcome using this procedure [33].

Semen quality becomes impaired within 2 weeks of a sustained injury. Hence, if possible, semen should be collected and stored within this time frame to ensure maximum quality. Semen should be processed as soon as it is collected as the quality of the sperm will rapidly deteriorate the longer they remain in the ejaculate.

Sperm quality collected by PV is considered to be superior to that collected by EEJ. However, if EEJ is to be used, the bladder should be washed with HEPES buffer beforehand, just in case there is no antegrade ejaculate. The bladder can then be catheterized and flushed with additional HEPES buffer to collect any retrograde semen.

Depending on the severity of the SCI, an ejaculate may not be obtained. In such instances, surgical testicular sperm retrieval can be considered.

85.2.3 Retrograde Semen Samples

A major cause of anejaculation or aspermia is retrograde ejaculation (RE), rendering the patient infertile. This occurs when there is incomplete closure of the bladder sphincter muscle at ejaculation, resulting in transport of the ejaculate into the bladder. RE results from peripheral nerve injury, e.g., diabetes mellitus, or following lumbar spine surgery, as well as central nervous system damage following SCI and myelodysplasia.

Certain medications are associated with RE, e.g., α-blockers, antidepressants, antipsychotics, and antihypertensives. Interestingly, pseudoephedrine (Sudafed) has been found to be an effective treatment for many men with RE [34]. This can be incorporated into the protocol for sperm collection as described in the box below.

Recommended Protocol for Retrograde Sample Collection

1. On the day prior to sample production the man should:
   (a) Take one tablespoon of sodium bicarbonate dissolved in water in the morning and in the evening. A urinary alkalizer available from a pharmacy may be suitable for use.
   (b) Take 60 mg of pseudoephedrine every 6 h.
2. On the day of sample production, he should:
   (a) Take two 60 mg doses of pseudoephedrine and one tablespoon of bicarbonate, followed by breakfast. He may drink a glass of milk with breakfast and pass urine.
3. Upon arrival at the laboratory, he should:
   (a) Wait until he feels the need to urinate again before producing his sample.
   (b) Try to ejaculate and collect any semen produced. He should then proceed to collect a urine sample into a separate container immediately afterward. It is important that he collects the entire urine sample.
4. In the lab, centrifuge the urine as quickly as possible. Resuspend the combined pellets into culture medium and wash before layering over density gradients as usual (see 1).

RE may be either partial or complete, depending on whether there is any antegrade ejaculate. After ejaculation, there will always be residual sperm in the post-ejaculatory urine washed out from the urethra. As much as 15% of the total sperm may occur in the urine following normal ejaculation [35]. If the percentage in the urine is increased, this is evidence for RE.

If there are sufficient sperm in the antegrade ejaculate for use in MAR, then the amount of sperm in the bladder is irrelevant. However, if there are insufficient sperm in the antegrade ejaculate or if there is complete RE, then sperm should be prepared from the post-ejaculatory urine for use in treatment.

RE sperm can be used successfully with IUI and ICSI treatment [36, 37] with live births reported at around 14% [36] and 28% [37], respectively. Prepared RE samples tend to have poor recovery rates post-thawing, so it is always preferable to prepare a fresh sample on the day of treatment if possible.

There are two essential components to handling sperm collected from urine:

- Exposure to urine will potentially harm the sperm as many of the components in urine are toxic. The pH is acidic which is also deleterious to sperm, so the bladder must be neutralized prior to sperm entry.
- Exposure time to urine must be minimized to prevent the sperm from dying. The sperm must be retrieved from the urine and transferred into culture medium as quickly as possible. For practical purposes, it may be helpful to have two andrologists processing the sample together.

85.3 Handling Testicular Sperm

85.3.1 PESA Samples

Sperm aspirated from the epididymis are relatively motile and usually not contaminated with other cells. However, they do tend to lose their motility quite quickly once removed from their physiological environment. It is important therefore to process these sperm as soon as possible following aspiration. Since the samples should be relatively clean, they can be washed by a simple centrifugation and resuspension step without risking considerable oxidative stress. Alternatively, centrifuge the aspirate through a single layer density gradient using 40% colloid.

85.3.2 Testicular Biopsies

Testicular biopsy samples are notoriously difficult to handle. All processing must occur in a buffered medium to protect the sample while working in theatre or in a class II cabinet.

Performing an initial testicular sperm extraction (TESE) procedure on the day of egg collection is not recommended due to the physical demands, high cost, and emotional toll on a couple of finding no sperm on the day. This should only be performed if there are facilities for oocyte cryopreservation.

Surgeons may elect to perform a TESE in advance of treatment, especially when there is no guarantee of finding sperm. These samples may then be frozen for later use. There is no significant difference in ICSI outcome using fresh or frozen testicular sperm [38]. However, if the number of sperm is extremely low, there is no guarantee that viable sperm will be found upon thawing. Under these circumstances, patients should be counselled that they may require synchronous TESE arranged for the day of egg collection.

Alternatively, a repeat sperm retrieval may be performed a day or two in advance of egg collection and the samples cultured prior to use for ICSI [38]. An advantage of this approach is that it may relieve the difficulties encountered with coordinating synchronous sperm retrievals. However, culturing sperm in medium for any length of time may increase the risk of sperm DNA damage [31], although prolonged testicular sperm culture does not appear to affect ICSI outcome [39]. On the other hand, sperm viability and pregnancy rates are significantly reduced if the sperm are exposed to prolonged culture prior to cryopreservation [40].

Tips for Performing and Processing Testicular Sperm

- Surgical sperm retrievals may be performed in an alternative location to the MAR laboratory. Samples should be transported in an appropriate buffered culture medium in a temperature-controlled incubator without compromising sperm quality [41].
- Testicular temperature ranges between 32 and 34 °C. Ideally incubators and warm plates should be set at this temperature for handling this sperm. If this is not possible, ambient temperature is preferable [42].
- It is essential to tease out sperm from the seminiferous tubules into a minimal amount of culture medium. If sperm numbers are small, teasing into large volumes of fluid will dilute the sperm so that it may be impossible to find them.
- Always remember to keep the tissue and cell suspensions moist. Working with small volumes of fluid exposed to air risks drying out the sample, resulting in increased pH and osmolarity due to solute concentration as the fluid evaporates, causing irreparable damage to sperm. Ensure samples are always replaced in closed test tubes or into a humidified incubator while teasing the remaining tissue or checking for sperm on slides.
- MicroTESE samples should be teased in a shallow petri dish, preferably the lid, as this allows a shallower angle to work with, affording optimal handling conditions with the teasing instruments.
- Tease the seminiferous tubules with a sterile small gauge needle and use a sterile blunt instrument, e.g., the blunt side of a stitch removal blade, moving the edge over the tubules to tease out the sperm (Fig. 85.7).
- Microscope cover slips are not recommended for testicular tissue processing as hands are too close to the petri dish, risking contamination. The coverslips are fragile and prone to breaking, becoming a safety hazard.
- Enzymatic digestion of the tissue with collagenase or mechanical tissue homogenization should never be used as these methods stimulate the production of ROS, seriously compromising sperm quality and DNA integrity.

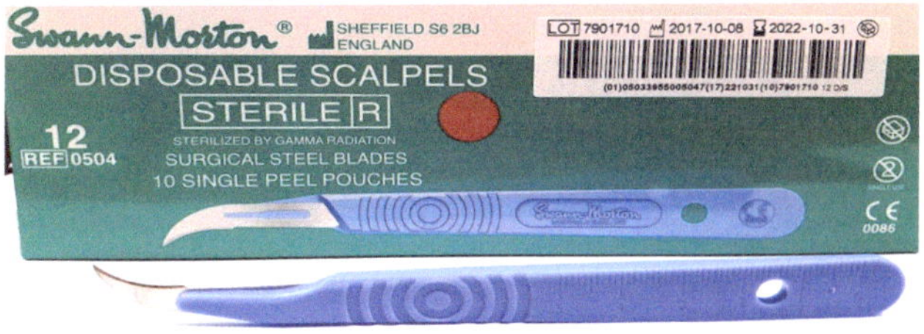

Fig. 85.7 The blunt edge of disposable scalpels can be used to break the seminferous tubules to tease out the sperm

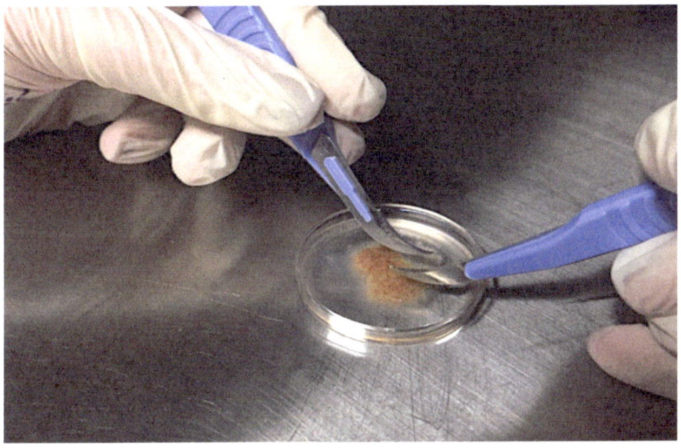

Fig. 85.8 Searching for testicular sperm takes a considerable amount of time and it may be preferable for one andrologist to process the tissue while another microscopically examines the cell suspension for sperm

85.3.3 Searching for Testicular Sperm

When searching biopsied tissue, it is essential to carry out a thorough examination of the dish or the slide to look for sperm. This involves scanning from the corner position upward and then moves across one field of view and scans downward to the bottom of the coverslip or dish, so that everything has been scanned. This process takes a considerable amount of time, and it may be preferable for one andrologist to process the tissue, while another microscopically examines the cell suspension for sperm (Fig. 85.8). The presence of sperm should be confirmed with a colleague if possible.

If sperm numbers are very low, it may take several hours to thoroughly search for sperm. If no sperm are found, it may be useful to cryopreserve the cell suspension and request a histology report to confirm the findings.

In cases of complete azoospermia, it is extremely important to remember that a man's life can be completely changed by how the embryologist relates this information. Telling a man that he has no usable sperm for treatment is devastating, so it is essential to take all the time necessary to ensure no stone is left unturned in the quest for finding usable sperm.

Care needs to be taken when identifying vital sperm for use in ICSI. Clearly, motile sperm are ideal, but testicular sperm do not fully acquire the ability to move until they arrive in the epididymis, so most are immotile. Motile sperm may only exhibit occasional twitching, and, if the slide is scanned too quickly, it is easy to miss. If no motile sperm are seen, vital sperm may be identified by using the HOS test [10] or pentoxifylline [4, 10] to encourage motility as described above. Alternatively, TESE samples may be cultured for up to 72 h to improve motility (see Sect. 85.3.1).

85.4 Cryopreservation of Poor-Quality Samples

The choice of cryoprotecting agent (CPA) and the method of freezing and thawing are essential to good sperm recovery. It is crucial to add the CPA very slowly, drop by drop, to prevent osmotic shock. Freezing in TEST-yolk buffer (TYB) may be more efficient at protecting sperm motility, vitality, and morphology than use of glycerol as the only CPA [43], possibly because TYB protects sperm membrane fluidity and integrity during the freezing process and protects during the thawing process.

However, as egg yolk is derived from birds, there is concern that TYB may harbor viruses or other organisms. For this reason, clinics tend to favor CPAs without egg yolk, using TYB only when sperm quality is particularly poor and there is a risk of very poor post-thaw recovery. If TYB is used, it should be derived from certified virus-free flocks, heat-inactivated at 56 °C, endotoxin-tested and approved for clinical use.

85.4.1 Cryopreservation of Poor-Quality Semen

A difficulty with freezing unprocessed cryptozoospermic samples is that they require an extended length of time to locate the sperm, if at all, following thawing. For such samples, it may be advantageous to cryopreserve individual sperm in a variety of cryopreservation vehicles, e.g., plastic microbeads. However, the safety of this technique is questionable [44]. Alternatively, follow the recommendations in 1.4 above to concentrate sperm numbers prior to cryopreservation.

Men with pathology of the male accessory glands, partial RE, or hypogonadism often have severely low volumes. An option is to ask the patient to ejaculate into a specimen container primed with 1–2 ml buffered culture medium to extend the sample, so it can be frozen in multiple straws or vials.

As the seminal fluid from an infertile man may contain apoptotic sperm, bacteria, and leukocytes (which are a major source of ROS), it may be advantageous to perform a sperm preparation prior to cryopreservation to remove the seminal fluid, thereby protecting the sperm DNA from damage [45].

85.4.2 Cryopreservation of Testicular Sperm

Epididymal sperm are devoid of all proteins, lipids, carbohydrates, as well as antioxidants to protect against ROS-induced damage. Therefore, these sperm should be frozen in a CPA that will offer maximum protection, such as TYB [46]. Using this cryopreservation method has shown no significant difference between fertilization and pregnancy rates using fresh versus frozen epididymal sperm.

When freezing surgically retrieved testicular sperm, where possible, it helps to maximize the numbers of straws stored, to minimize the necessity of a repeat surgical procedure. Sufficient numbers of sperm should be provided in each vial/straw to provide a good chance of finding sperm following thawing.

It is recommended that a "test thaw" is performed on cryopreserved samples, if there are sufficient sperm to do so. This provides essential information for the clinician and the MAR lab regarding patient management. It helps to determine if sperm will be found in the thawed sample on the day of egg collection and also whether donor sperm should be offered as back up.

85.4.3 Cryopreservation of Sperm from Men with Cancer

Men diagnosed with cancer may be referred urgently for fertility preservation prior to imminent surgery and or radio- or chemotherapy that may make them sterile. Often these patients have very limited time to attend the clinic for sperm storage and may not be compliant with regard to sample production.

There are several ways in which handling of such samples can be maximized for subsequent use. The volume of the sample per straw can be reduced to allow more straws to be frozen. Furthermore, if the patient if able, he can be asked to produce more than one sample when he attends: the second sample may have a lower count but may still be sufficient for ICSI.

On the day of ICSI treatment, another option is to refreeze the remainder of the sample for subsequent use [47]. While sperm continue to lose motility with each successive round of freezing and thawing, sufficient viable sperm may remain for subsequent use in another ICSI treatment cycle (Royle and Homa, unpublished results). However, it is not known whether DNA damage would be increased to a clinically significant level in such samples.

85.5 Conclusion

There are a plethora of methods available for improving the yield of actively motile sperm from poor-quality samples. However, it is very important to ensure that the methods are safe to use and do not affect the genetic integrity or the functional capability of the sperm. The method of choice should always be the least invasive, with minimal exposure to mechanical manipulation. In addition, the time for processing the sperm should be kept to a minimum. Methods to improve handling of poor-quality samples may only involve simple changes to established protocols. On the other hand, the implementation of novel methods may involve exposure of sperm to additional biochemicals that must be verified for safety. Furthermore, they may require expensive equipment which will increase the cost. It is therefore essential that there is a clear evidence base for the safety and clinical outcome of these technologically advanced methods in order to justify their use in MAR.

Acknowledgments The author would like to thank Nadia Graham for the illustrations.

References

1. Bjorndhal L, Mortimer D, Barratt C, Castilla J, Menkveld R, Kvist U, et al. A practical guide to basic laboratory andrology. Cambridge: Cambridge University Press; 2010.
2. World Health Organization, editor. WHO laboratory manual for the examination and processing of human semen. 5th ed. Geneva: World Health Organization; 2010.
3. Aitken RJ, Clarkson JS. Significance of reactive oxygen species and antioxidants in defining the efficacy of sperm preparation techniques. J Androl. 1988;9:367–76.
4. Henkel RR, Schill WB. Sperm preparation for ART. Reprod Biol Endocrinol. 2003;1:108.
5. Correa-Perez JR, Fernandez-Pelegrina R, Aslanis P, Zavos PM. Clinical management of men producing ejaculates characterized by high levels of dead sperm and altered seminal plasma factors consistent with epididymal necrospermia. Fertil Steril. 2004;81:148–50.
6. Alipour H, Van Der Horst G, Christiansen OB, Dardmeh F, Jorgensen N, Nielsen HI, et al. Improved sperm kinematics in semen samples collected after 2 h versus 4-7 days of ejaculation abstinence. Hum Reprod. 2017;32:1364–72.
7. Agarwal A, Gupta S, Du Plessis S, Sharma R, Esteves SC, Cirenza C, et al. Abstinence time and its impact on basic and advanced semen parameters. Urology. 2016;94: 102–10.
8. Manuel TJ, José MM, María CA, Carlos Z, Estela MP. Use of Annexin V based sperm selection in assisted reproduction. Andrology (Los Angel). 2017;6:1000182.
9. Vaughan DA, Sakkas D. Sperm selection methods in the 21st century. Biol Reprod. 2019. pii: ioz032.
10. Nordhoff V. How to select immotile but viable spermatozoa on the day of intracytoplasmic sperm injection? An embryologist's view. Andrology. 2015;3:156–62.

11. Glenn DR, McVicar CM, McClure N, Lewis SE. Sildenafil citrate improves sperm motility but causes a premature acrosome reaction in vitro. Fertil Steril. 2007;87(5):1064–70.
12. Mortimer D. Sperm preparation methods. J Androl. 2000;21:357–66.
13. Larson KL, Brannian JD, Timm BK, Jost LK, Evenson DP. Density gradient centrifugation and glass wool filtration of semen remove spermatozoa with damaged chromatin structure. Hum Reprod. 1999;14(8):2015–9.
14. Sun F, Ko E, Martin RH. Is there a relationship between sperm chromosome abnormalities and sperm morphology? Reprod Biol Endocrinol. 2006;4:1.
15. Berkovitz A, Eltes F, Lederman H, Peer S, Ellenbogen A, Feldberg B, et al. How to improve IVF-ICSI outcome by sperm selection. Reprod Biomed Online. 2006;12:634–8.
16. Fortunato A, Boni R, Leo R, Nacchia G, Liquori F, Casale S, et al. Vacuoles in sperm head are not associated with head morphology, DNA damage and reproductive success. Reprod Biomed Online. 2016;32:154–61.
17. Setti AS, Paes de Almeida Ferreira Braga D, Iaconelli A Jr, Aoki T, Borges E Jr. Twelve years of MSOME and IMSI: a review. Reprod Biomed Online. 2013;27:338–52.
18. Teixeira DM, Barbosa MA, Ferriani RA, Navarro PA, Raine-Fenning N, Nastri CO, et al. Regular (ICSI) versus ultra-high magnification (IMSI) sperm selection for assisted reproduction. Cochrane Database Syst Rev. 2013;7:CD010167.
19. Aitken RJ, Smith TB, Jobling MS, Baker MA, De Iuliis GN. Oxidative stress and male reproductive health. Asian J Androl. 2014;16:31–8.
20. Santi D, Spaggiari G, Simoni M. Sperm DNA fragmentation index as a promising predictive tool for male infertility diagnosis and treatment management-meta-analyses. Reprod Biomed Online. 2018;37(3):315–26.
21. Harton GL, Tempest HG. Chromosomal disorders and male infertility. Asian J Androl. 2012;14(1):32–9.
22. Simon L, Emery BR, Carrell DT. Review: diagnosis and impact of sperm DNA alterations in assisted reproduction. Best Pract Res Clin Obstet Gynaecol. 2017;44:38–56.
23. Tomlinson MJ, Moffatt O, Manicardi GC, Bizzaro D, Afnan M, Sakkas D. Interrelationships between seminal parameters and sperm nuclear DNA damage before and after density gradient centrifugation: implications for assisted conception. Hum Reprod. 2001,16:2160–5.
24. Quinn MM, Jalalian L, Ribeiro S, Ona K, Demirci U, Cedars MI, Rosen MP. Microfluidic sorting selects sperm for clinical use with reduced DNA damage compared to density gradient centrifugation with swim-up in split semen samples. Hum Reprod. 2018;33:1388. https://doi.org/10.1093/humrep/dey239.
25. Huszar G, Jakab A, Sakkas D, Ozenci CC, Cayli S, Delpiano E, Ozkavukcu S. Fertility testing and ICSI sperm selection by hyaluronic acid binding: clinical and genetic aspects. Reprod Biomed Online. 2007;14:650–63.
26. Parmegiani L, Cognigni GE, Bernardi S, Troilo E, Ciampaglia W, Filicori M. "Physiologic ICSI": hyaluronic acid (HA) favors selection of spermatozoa without DNA fragmentation and with normal nucleus, resulting in improvement of embryo quality. Fertil Steril. 2010;93:598–604.
27. Worrilow KC, Eid S, Woodhouse D, Perloe M, Smith S, Witmyer J, Ivani K, Khoury C, Ball GD, Elliot T, Lieberman J. Use of hyaluronan in the selection of sperm for intracytoplasmic sperm injection (ICSI): significant improvement in clinical outcomes-multicenter, double-blinded and randomized controlled trial. Hum Reprod. 2013;28:306–14.
28. Miller D, Pavitt S, Sharma V, Forbes G, Hooper R, Bhattacharya S, Kirkman-Brown J, Coomarasamy A, Lewis S, Cutting R, Brison D, Pacey A, et al. Physiological, hyaluronanselected intracytoplasmic sperm injection for infertility treatment (HABSelect): a parallel, two-group, randomised trial. Lancet. 2019;393:416–22.
29. Nicopoullos JD, Almeida P, Vourliotis M, Goulding R, Gilling-Smith C. A decade of the sperm-washing programme: where are we now? Hum Fertil. 2010;13:90–7.
30. Pfeifer S, Goldberg J, McClure R, Lobo R, Thomas M, Widra E, et al. Recommendations for reducing the risk of viral transmission during fertility treatment with the use of autologous gametes: a committee opinion. Practice Committee of American Society for Reproductive Medicine. Fertil Steril. 2013;99:340–6.
31. Patki P, Woodhouse J, Hamid R, Craggs M, Shah J. Effect of spinal cord injury on semen parameters. J Spinal Cord Med. 2008;31:27–32.
32. DeForge D, Blackmer J, Garritty C, Yazdi F, Cronin V, Barrowman N, et al. Fertility following spinal cord injury: a systematic review. Spinal Cord. 2005;43:693–703.
33. Kafetsoulis A, Brackett NL, Ibrahim E, Attia GR, Lynne CM. Current trends in the treatment of infertility in men with spinal cord injury. Fertil Steril. 2006;86(4):781–9.
34. Shoshany O, Abhyankar N, Elyaguov J, Niederberger C. Efficacy of treatment with pseudoephedrine in men with retrograde ejaculation. Andrology. 2017;5:744–8.
35. Sigman M, Boyle K, Jarow JP. Prevalence of sperm in the post-ejaculatory urine of fertile and subfertile men. Urology. 2008;71:110–2.
36. Jefferys A, Siassakos D, Wardle P. The management of retrograde ejaculation: a systematic review and update. Fertil Steril. 2012;97:306–12.
37. Philippon M, Karsenty G, Bernuz B, Courbiere B, Brue T, Saïas-Magnan J, et al. Successful pregnancies and healthy live births using frozen-thawed sperm retrieved by a new modified Hotchkiss procedure in males with retrograde ejaculation: first case series. Basic Clin Androl. 2015;25:5.
38. Karacan M, Alwaeely F, Erkan S, Çebi Z, Berberoğlugil M, Batukan M, et al. Outcome of intracytoplasmic sperm injection cycles with fresh testicular spermatozoa obtained on the day of or the day before oocyte collection and with cryopreserved testicular sperm in patients with azoospermia. Fertil Steril. 2013;100:975–80.
39. Nabi A, Khalili MA, Halvaei I, et al. Prolonged incubation of processed human spermatozoa will increase DNA fragmentation. Andrologia. 2014;46:374–9.
40. Desch L, Bruno C, Herbemont C, Michel F, Bechoua S, Girod S, et al. Impact on ICSI outcomes of adding 24 h of in vitro culture before testicular sperm freezing: a retrospective study. Basic Clin Androl. 2015;25:6.
41. Omurtag K, Cooper A, Bullock A, Naughton C, Ratts V, Odem R, Lanzendorf SE. Sperm recovery and IVF after testicular sperm extraction (TESE): effect of male diagnosis and use of off-site surgical centers on sperm recovery and IVF. PLoS One. 2013;8(7):e69838.
42. Thijssen A, Klerkx E, Huyser C, Bosmans E, Campo R, Ombelet W. Influence of temperature and sperm preparation on the quality of spermatozoa. Reprod Biomed Online. 2014;28:436–42.
43. Stanic P, Tandara M, Sonicki Z, Simunic V, Radakovic B, Suchanek E. Comparison of protective media and freezing techniques for cryopreservation of human semen. Eur J Obstet Gynecol Reprod Biol. 2000;91:65–70.
44. Di Santo M, Tarozzi N, Nadalini M, Borini A. Human sperm cryopreservation: update on techniques, effect on DNA integrity, and implications for ART. Adv Urol. 2012;2012:854837.
45. Petyim S, Neungton C, Thanaboonyawat I, Laokirkkiat P, Choavaratana R. Sperm preparation before freezing improves sperm motility and reduces apoptosis in post-freezing-thawing sperm compared with post-thawing sperm preparation. J Assist Reprod Genet. 2014;31:1673–80.
46. Patrizio P. Cryopreservation of epididymal sperm. Mol Cell Endocrinol. 2000;169:11–4.
47. Ofeim O, Brown TA, Gilbert BR. Effects of serial thaw-refreeze cycles on human sperm motility and viability. Fertil Steril. 2001;2001(75):1242–3.

Conventional IVF

86

Cornelia G. A. Meyer

Nowadays, IVF is a well-established and effective treatment option to help infertile couples throughout the world. The clinical technique of conventional IVF (cIVF) was developed by the British physiologist Robert Edwards and his colleagues, Patrick Steptoe and Jean Purdy. Edwards had the vision that a human oocyte could be fertilized in vitro and that the resulting embryo could enable a pregnancy to ensue, after transfer to the uterus. In 1978, his vision was realized with the birth of the world's first cIVF baby, Louise Brown. It took a further three decades to pass before Edwards was finally awarded the Nobel Prize in Medicine for his outstanding work.

> The most important thing in life is having a child.
> Nothing is more special than a child. (Robert Edwards)

In 1992, another milestone was reached for medically assisted reproduction (MAR), when the technique of intracytoplasmic sperm injection (ICSI) was introduced to enable a man to father a child, even if he has a very low number of poor-quality sperm. In the years since, there has been a trend to overuse the ICSI technique to treat all types of infertility, even though evidence of the benefit of this approach is questionable [1]. This is cause for concern, and many consider that the method of fertilization should be chosen based on a precise indication, rather than an "ICSI for all" approach.

86.1 Indications for IVF

It was in the eighteenth century that the German physician and anatomist Martin Naboth recognized the association between tubal blockage and infertility, publishing his findings in 1707 in "De Sterilitate Mulierum" (On Sterility in Woman). cIVF was originally developed to help women who suffered infertility due to problems with their fallopian tubes. Tubal infertility is estimated to account for around a third of all subfertility cases, and the frequency may be even higher in populations where sexually transmitted infections (STIs) are more prevalent [2]. Impaired tubal function and patency may result from acquiring STIs or surgical damage. Apart from helping with peritubal adhesions, tubal surgery usually is considered to be less effective for aiding conception than cIVF [2].

In contrast to tubal infertility, a standard infertility evaluation may fail to reveal any obvious cause. This occurs for 15–30% of all infertile couples and is referred to as "unexplained" or idiopathic infertility [3]. cIVF may not be the most cost-effective therapy for unexplained infertility but can be the treatment of choice, particularly if less costly therapies, such as intrauterine insemination (IUI), have failed [4].

Endometriosis is another common cause of infertility, affecting around 10–15% women during their reproductive lifetime [5]. The condition can be detrimental to multiple aspects of the reproductive cycle, having adverse effects on all stages, from the developing follicle and the resulting quality of the oocyte, due to embryo quality and the lining of the endometrium which might prevent implantation of a hatching blastocyst [6]. Compared to ICSI, performing cIVF for severe cases of endometriosis-associated infertility may result in either complete fertilization failure (12.7 vs. 1.8%) or an inability to activate the block to polyspermy leading to higher rates of triploidy (3.9 vs. 0.9%) [7]. A similar situation has been reported for infertility patients diagnosed with polycystic ovarian syndrome (PCOS), which has led some fertility teams to promote the use of ICSI over cIVF if a zona pellucida malfunction is suspected [8].

For many couples diagnosed with moderate male factor infertility in which the husband's sperm function is not severely deficient but shows moderate oligoasthenoteratozoospermia, cIVF can be an option. Tournaye and colleagues showed that cases with moderate male subfertility can be effectively treated with cIVF [9]. When using a high insemination concentration (HIC), the fertilization results did not significantly differ from those obtained with microinjected

C. G. A. Meyer (✉)
Cryos International, Aarhus, Denmark
e-mail: cgam@cryosinternational.com

G. N. Allahbadia et al. (eds.), *Textbook of Assisted Reproduction*, https://doi.org/10.1007/978-981-15-2377-9_86

sibling oocytes (HIC of 800,000 motile sperm/mL compared to standard insemination concentration of 200,000 motile sperm/mL) [9].

For male patients with borderline semen quality, it is not easy to determine the optimal treatment. The overall aim is to maximize the chance of fertilization without resorting to ICSI. In such situations, if several oocytes are collected, a more cautious approach could be to allocate half of the oocytes to cIVF and half to ICSI [10].

Severe deficits in semen quality are a clear contraindication for cIVF. Thus, ICSI would be the preferred insemination method in situations where the original sperm morphology is considered suboptimal [11], there are high titers of antisperm antibodies [12], or the concentration of progressively motile sperm is <1 million/ml after preparation of the semen sample [13].

86.2 Cases Where cIVF Versus ICSI Needs Consideration

Studies on sibling oocytes have shown that patients with increased oocyte immaturity may benefit from cIVF [14]. Conventional insemination allows unrestricted oocyte-sperm interaction, such that the maturation processes can be completed whilst the oocytes remain enclosed within the cumulus-oocyte-complex (COC), thus optimizing the timing for fertilization.

Whilst ICSI may be advised in cases where the number of COCs collected is low, it has been demonstrated that the rates of fertilization, pregnancy, and miscarriage are no better than if cIVF had been used [15].

Oocytes collected from women over 35 years of age have shown similar fertilization results to those of younger women when undergoing cIVF [16]. Suspected structural defects in these "older" oocytes that might have led to impaired fertilization rates have proven false, and thus advanced maternal age is not an acceptable contraindication for cIVF.

With regard to fertilization outcome of cryopreserved-thawed/warmed oocytes, the results in the literature are contradictory, although ICSI seems to be the preferred method of fertilization. Cryopreservation may lead to the zona becoming hardened, due to the cortical granules being released prematurely, and this can deter sperm entry with cIVF [17, 18]. However, these findings might depend on the cryopreservation protocol and on the composition of the cryopreservation medium, rather than on the cryopreservation method itself [19]. High fertilization rates after vitrification have been reported, but this was influenced by how intact the corona radiata was [20]. For oocytes that have undergone slow freezing followed by thawing, good fertilization and pregnancy rates have been reported after cIVF, on a par with those reported after ICSI [21].

Zona hardening has also been postulated for oocytes that have been exposed to longer culture periods associated with being matured in vitro, and this was thought to negatively impact the fertilization outcome with cIVF. However, a different study on sibling in vitro-matured oocytes from PCOS patients showed that the fertilization rate was not significantly affected by use of cIVF over ICSI [22].

A notable exception, where conventionally inseminated oocytes should be avoided, is for ART cycles including preimplantation genetic diagnosis (PGD). This is because cIVF increased the risk of sample contamination of the biopsied cells, due to the extra sperm that are often attached to the zona.

86.3 Factors Predicting cIVF Success

The likelihood of success of cIVF treatment is affected by the cause of the infertility [23]. This is influenced by the period of time that a couple has endured infertility, since the duration of infertility has been shown to be inversely correlated to pregnancy rates for couples undergoing cIVF treatment [24]. Female age also impacts on cIVF success, as oocyte quality decreases drastically when women reach their mid-30s. How a woman responds to ovarian stimulation should also be considered, as higher pregnancy rates have been linked to treatments where high numbers of COCs are collected [24]. Beside the various infertility indications, another factor that impacts on the cIVF outcome is the number of previous unsuccessful IVF attempts, since an inverse relationship with cIVF success has been noted [23].

86.4 Conventional IVF Procedure: Bringing Sperm and Eggs Together

86.4.1 Options for Semen Sample Preparation

Several factors have a major impact on the fertilization outcome when conventional insemination is being used. Obtaining an adequate number of selected functional sperm is one of them. To do this, various sperm preparation techniques have been established, such as simple washing procedures with subsequent resuspension of sperm, swim-up migration, density gradient centrifugation, or microfluidic sperm sorting ([25, 26]; Figs. 86.1 and 86.2).

All of these techniques have been developed in order to purify viable sperm away from the seminal plasma, non-motile or damaged sperm, sperm fragments, leukocytes, bacteria, and other decapacitating factors. The overall aim is to protect and improve sperm function and prevent damage. At the same time, sperm preparation techniques aim to reduce the percentage of dysfunctional sperm and reduce the detrimental effects from sperm that may be producing reactive

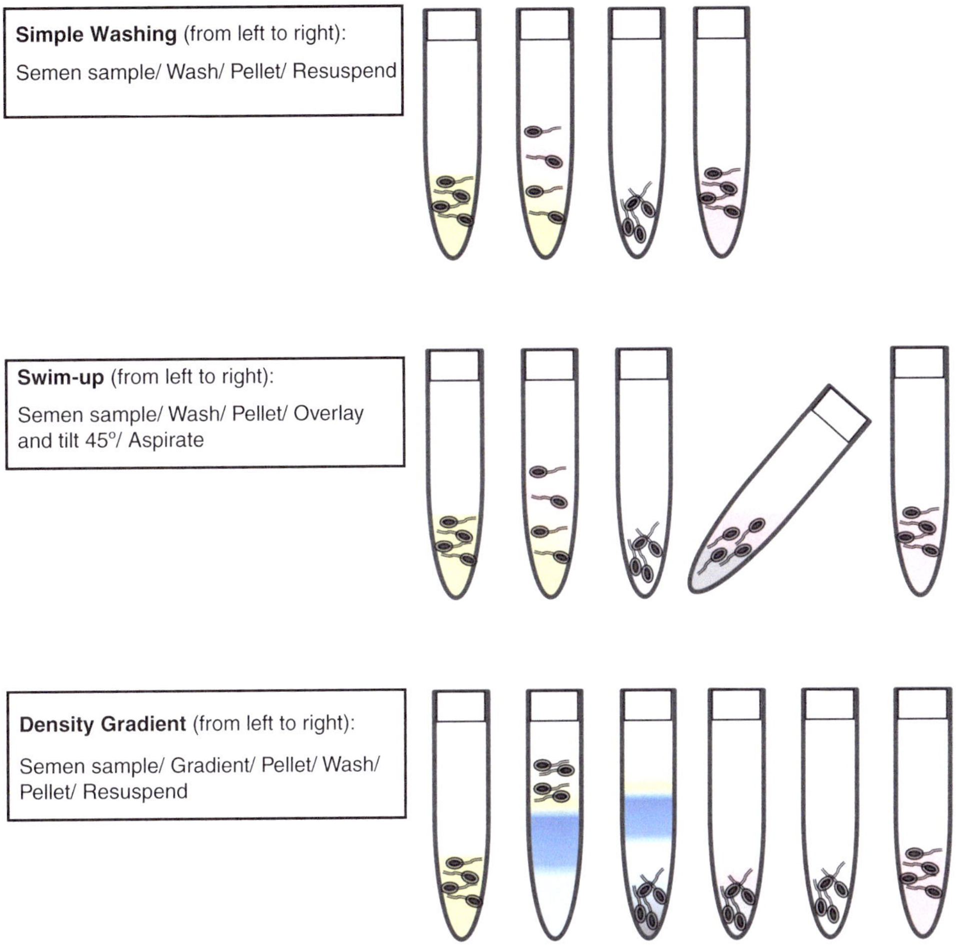

Fig. 86.1 Frequently used sperm preparation techniques and their characteristic purification steps

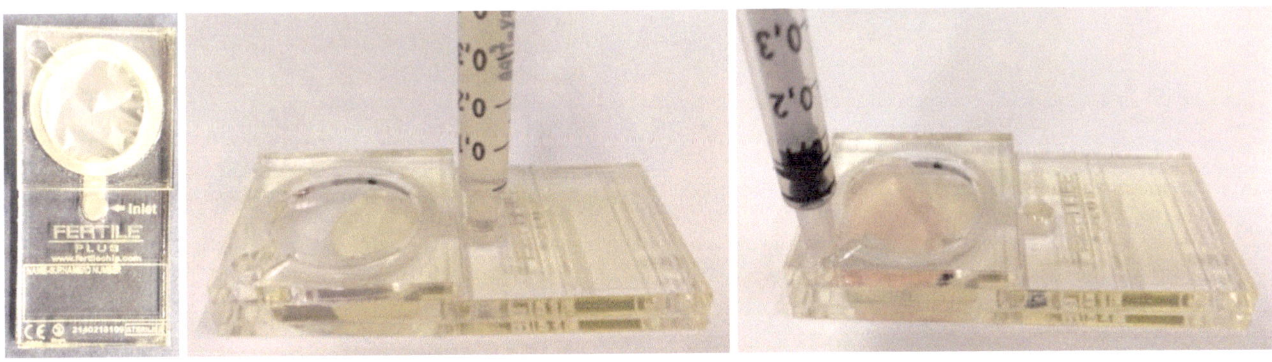

Fig. 86.2 Microfluidic sperm sorting; Fertile Plus® sperm sorting chip (left); application of semen sample (middle); subsequent overlaying with sperm preparation medium (right)

oxygen species (ROS). Each method of sperm preparation varies in efficiency, depending on the semen sample quality. Thus, technique selection requires a careful and specific choice in every individual case. Prior to treatment, it is advisable to perform a test sperm preparation in order to propose the most adequate preparation technique "on the day."

To avoid prolonged sperm exposure to seminal plasma, the semen analysis and preparation should be initiated within 60 min of production. In general, for a semen sample with initial normal semen parameters, the final prepared sample should ideally have a high proportion of sperm that are the optimal shape with >1 million motile sperm per ml [11]. Typically, a total motile count ranging between 0.2 and 0.5×10^6/ml is used [9, 27]. The final sperm suspension should provide sufficient progressively motile sperm to optimize the chance of normal fertilization. At present, no reliable cut-off values are available that allow a precise prediction of the fertilization outcome.

Prior to insemination, the purified and concentrated motile sperm should be transferred to a special fertilization medium, which needs to be compatible with oocyte culture in terms of buffering system and pH.

86.4.2 Grading Oocyte Maturity

Oocytes at various stages of meiotic maturity can be obtained during follicle aspiration, as they are retrieved prior to ovulation [28]. Oocyte maturation is a complex process whereby contemporaneous changes to the cytoplasm and genome must take place. However, in superovulation cycles for cIVF treatment, cytoplasmic maturity is sometimes asynchronous with nuclear maturity [29]. To allow oocytes to complete their maturation process after follicle aspiration, in order to reach the maximum fertilization potential, a preincubation prior to cIVF has been recommended [30–32].

Following COC retrieval, oocyte maturity is initially evaluated from the visual characteristics of the COC, incorporating assessment of the oocyte (if visible), the corona radiata, and the cumulus oophorus (Table 86.1). Microscopic COC assessment may provide valuable information about when to perform the insemination and also about the likelihood of fertilization outcome (Fig. 86.3). For example, a dense corona radiata layer has been correlated with a decreased oocyte maturity [33, 34]. In such instances, in order to optimize the likelihood of fertilization of mature oocytes, it may be worth considering a delay to the time of insemination.

As well as cumulus maturation and expansion, other morphological anomalies may provide useful information regarding the developmental potential of oocytes. For example, a lower rate of fertilization and development to the blastocyst stage has been linked to oocytes originating from COCs where blood clots were observed within the original cumulus matrix

Table 86.1 Predicted oocyte maturity grading based on morphological characteristics in terms of the cumulus-oocyte-complex

Morphological characteristics	Grade 1 Mature or preovulatory	Grade 2 Approximately mature	Grade 3 Immature	Grade 4 Postmature	Grade 5 Atretic
Cumulus mass	Very expanded	Expanded	Dense and compact	Very expanded; often having clumps	Rarely present
Corona radiata	Very radiant, revealing a distinct zona pellucida	Slightly compact	If present: Very adherent, compact layer of corona cells	Radiant; yet often clumped and irregular or incomplete; zona pellucida visible	If present: Clumped and very irregular; zona pellucida very visible
Ooplasm	Clear		If visible: Revealing the presence of the germinal vesicle	Either slightly granular or dark	Dark and frequently misshapen
Detached membrane granulosa cells	Expanded and well aggregated	Expanded and well aggregated	Compact and non-aggregated	Small and relatively non-aggregated	Very small clumps of cells

Adapted from Lin YC, Chang SY, Lan KC, Huang HW, Chang CY, Tsai MY, et al. Human oocyte maturity in vivo determines the outcome of blastocyst development in vitro. J Assist Reprod Genet. 2003; 20: 506–12, with permission
The grading takes into account the cumulus compactness, corona density, and cytoplasm granularity of the oocyte if visible

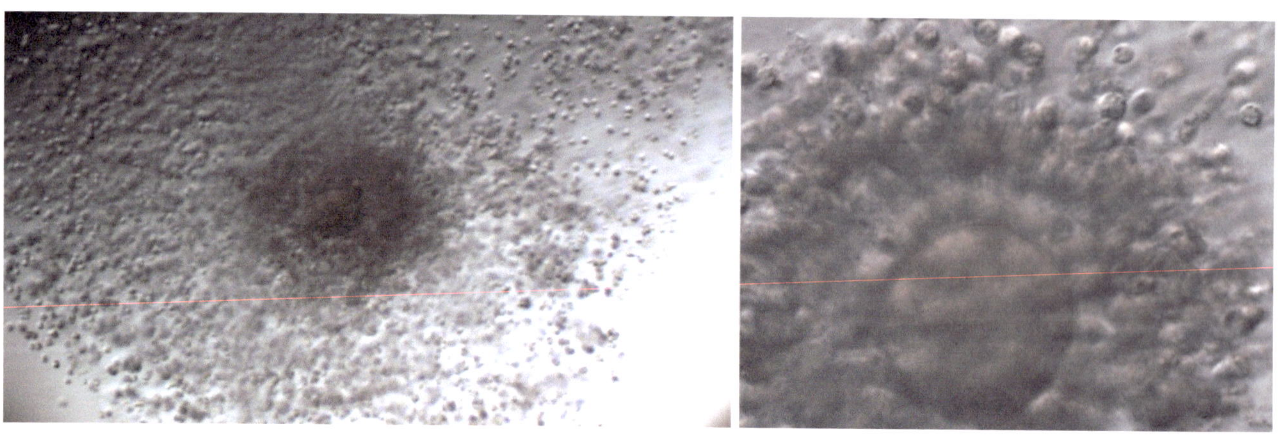

Fig. 86.3 Expanded cumulus-oocyte-complex (left); MII oocyte with radiant corona radiata and distinct zona pellucida (right)

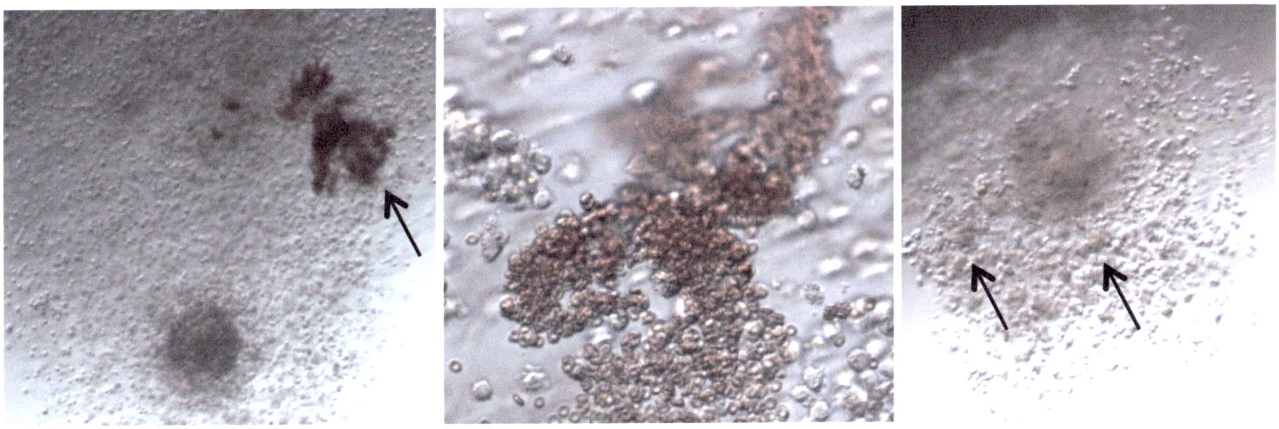

Fig. 86.4 Cumulus-oocyte-complexes with blood inclusions (left and middle); COC with postmature oocyte and amorphous clumps (right)

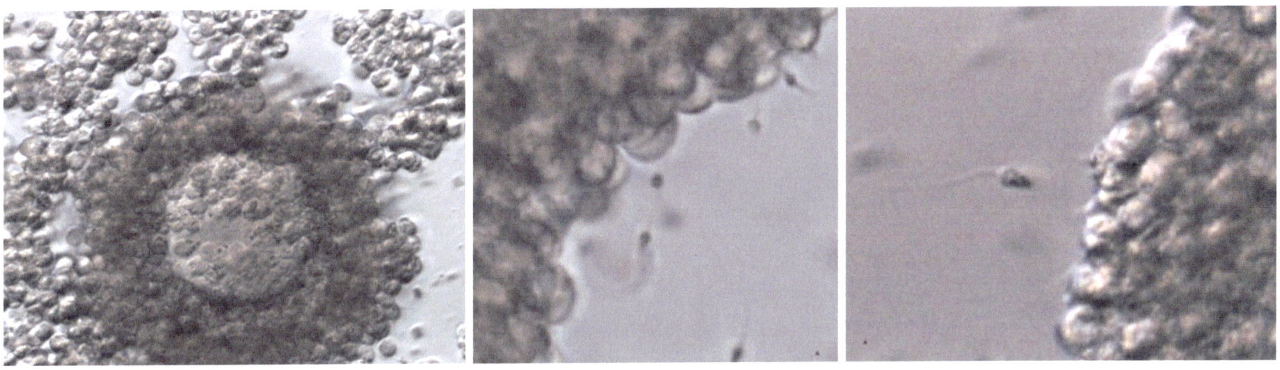

Fig. 86.5 Cumulus-oocyte-complex (left); cumulus cells-spermatozoa interaction (middle and right)

(Fig. 86.4) [33]. Whilst it could be useful to dissect blood clots from COCs, this may not actually improve the oocyte quality, as the COCs may simply have originated from poor-quality follicles and be adversely affected as a result. However, for cIVF it is still advisable to dissect away any blood inclusions, in order to remove any potential source of ROS.

86.4.3 Oocyte Insemination

The insemination time depends on the timing of the ovulation induction (e.g., the trigger injection) and follicle aspiration. An incubation period for freshly collected COCs of 2–6 h in vitro prior to cIVF has been recommended to optimize fertilization and pregnancy outcome [31].

After this time, a defined volume of the prepared sperm is added to the droplet that already contains the COCs, using a sterile pipette (Fig. 86.5). The actual final concentration of motile sperm may depend on several factors such as whether the COCs are cultured in droplets overlaid with oil or in open culture without oil. The number of COCs in each droplet is also worth considering. The final sperm concentration in the media with the COCs should be around 100,000 progressively motile sperm/ml. However, the insemination concentration can be reduced, for example, if a previous cycle with cIVF resulted in a high rate of polyspermy.

For conventional insemination, typically a fertilization medium is used, since this contains a higher concentration of glucose than normal culture medium in order to optimize the sperm motility and movement characteristics.

86.5 Co-incubation Period

In standard cIVF insemination protocols, uninterrupted co-culture of sperm and COCs is performed up to the time of the fertilization check the following morning. However, it has been suggested that exposing the COCs to sperm for this long period of time could potentially may be harmful to the oocytes [35]. An extended co-incubation time may lead to suboptimal culture conditions, since sperm metabolic waste products may accumulate, e.g., ROS. Satisfactory fertilization results have been reported following a shorter co-incubation time of just 2 h [35], whilst some even consider a very brief exposure of 30 s to be sufficient [36]. Before a change to standard protocols takes place, further studies are needed to ascertain how relevant the co-incubation period is, in terms of final outcomes such as the rates of miscarriage and live birth.

86.6 Assessing Fertilization

After completion of the insemination procedure, the COCs are carefully dissected to observe the oocytes in detail. This process usually takes place 16–18 h after the insemination and involves denudation of any cumulus cells, prior to transfer of the oocytes from the fertilization medium to fresh embryo culture medium (Fig. 86.6). Each oocyte must be microscopically examined to confirm if the cytoplasm contains two pronuclei (PN) and if the perivitelline space contains two polar bodies (PBs). If so, it is accepted that the oocyte has been successfully fertilized by a single sperm. If only one PN is observed, a second evaluation of the PN status is recommended to be performed 4 h later, in case a second PN develops.

86.6.1 Total Fertilization Failure

cIVF is a well-established technique and in general achieves high fertilization rates of around 67%, within a competency value of ≥60% for the "normal IVF fertilization rate" [37]. However, fertilization failure can still take place for couples undergoing both cIVF and ICSI (cIVF 5–10% vs. ICSI 2–3%, [38]).

The possible etiologies of total fertilization failure (TFF) are complex, but it is accepted that for the majority of cases, the oocyte has failed to be penetrated by the sperm. Analysis of failed fertilized oocytes revealed that the majority of these oocytes contained no sperm tail and chromatin after conventional insemination [39]. Despite these sperm-related factors, a defect in the PN formation or oocyte activation might be another cause for fertilization failure [38] as well as an inability of the chromatin to undergo the required changes within the cytoplasm [39].

Additionally, cycle-specific parameters have to be considered. This occasionally contributes to unexpected TFF after cIVF in a second treatment cycle, even though fertilization may have been achieved in a first treatment cycle.

Semen quality is usually assessed in line with the procedures and lower reference limits described by the World Health Organization [40]. This assessment can help fertility specialists to predict the likelihood of fertilization with cIVF, accepting that some men may be infertile due to defects in sperm function that cannot be ascertained from a basic semen analysis [41].

Depending on the infertility indication, the risk of TFF after cIVF has been estimated to be around 13% in cases where the man has normal semen parameters and tubal factor infertility and around 17% if there is unexplained infertility. However, if there are problems with sperm progressive motility, then the TFF risk can be up to 50% [42–44]. Elucidating the etiology of TFF is necessary in order to optimize patient counseling and future treatment outcomes.

For couples with unexplained infertility, the incidence of TFF with cIVF may be higher. Although the precise etiology for these incidences is not fully understood, the most likely explanations are an inability of the sperm to enter the oocyte and defective sperm chromatin [45]. Whilst ICSI can decrease the risk of TFF, there remains an inability to foresee which couples may benefit most from having ICSI rather than cIVF. When considering which insemination technique to undertake, it is important to consider the possible improvement ICSI can offer against the procedural

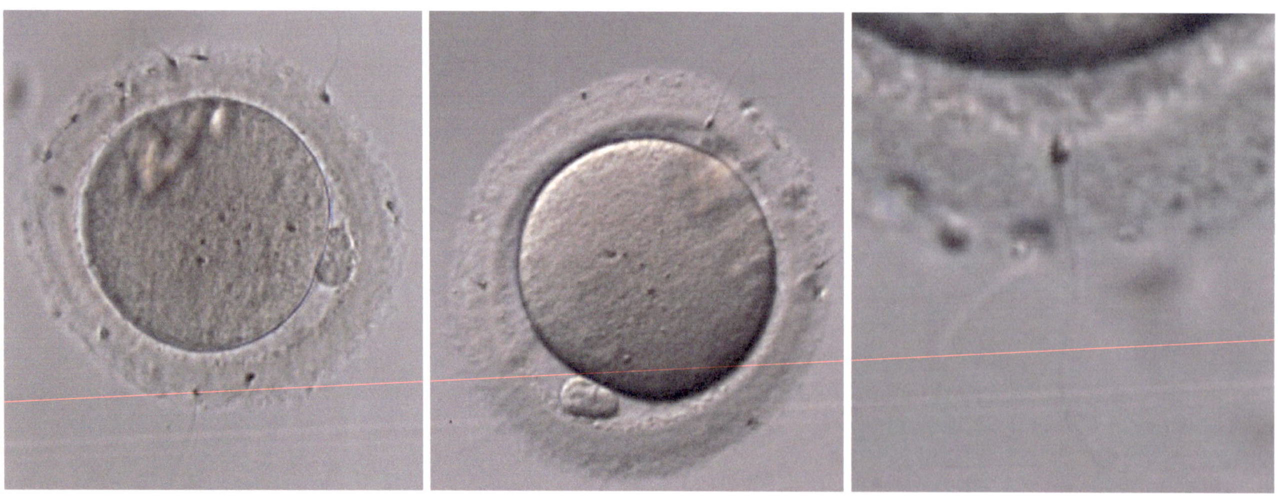

Fig. 86.6 Denuded MII oocyte post-insemination showing good (left) and fair (middle) sperm interaction with the zona pellucida; sperm reaching the perivitelline space (right)

hazards and additional costs that may come with micromanipulation.

86.7 Half Conventional cIVF: Half ICSI

To avoid making the choice in favor of cIVF or ICSI, there is an alternative approach referred to as "split" or "half-half" cIVF-ICSI. Using this practice, half of the cohort of COCs is allocated to cIVF, whilst the remaining COCs are denuded and subjected to ICSI. The strategy of split cIVF-ICSI may also be a possible policy in cases where a mild male factor is suspected and may prevent TFF in one out of four cycles [46].

86.8 The Future

This chapter has considered various aspects linked to cIVF. Whilst advances have taken place in the way cIVF is performed, the process continues to be suboptimal compared to in vivo fertilization. Further improvements are therefore needed. For example, it may be useful to include techniques such as microfluidics that mimic more closely the natural sperm selection processes in the tubal-uterine environment [47].

A take-home message from this chapter is that rather than succumbing to the temptation of performing 100% ICSI for all cycles to avoid the risk of TFF, it is worth considering cIVF as a treatment option where this more natural method of fertilization could be possible. cIVF should continue to have a prominent role in ART, and future developments in the cIVF laboratory can only improve success rates further.

References

1. Dyer S, Chambers GM, de Mouzon J, Nygren KG, Zegers-Hochschild F, Mansour R, et al. International Committee for monitoring assisted reproductive technologies world report: assisted reproductive technology 2008, 2009 and 2010. Hum Reprod. 2016;0:1–22.
2. Khalaf Y. Tubal subfertility. BMJ. 2003;327(7415):610–3.
3. Practice committee of American Society for Reproductive Medicine. Effectiveness and treatment for unexplained infertility. Fertil Steril. 2006;86:111–4.
4. Centers for Disease Control and Prevention, American Society for Reproductive Medicine, Society for Assisted Reproductive Technology. 2006 Assisted Reproductive Technology Success Rates: National Summary and Fertility Clinic Reports, Atlanta: U.S. Department of Health and Human Services, Centers for Disease Control and Prevention; 2008.
5. Hemmings R, Rivard M, Olive DL, Poliquin-Fleury J, Gagne D, Hugo P, et al. Evaluation of risk factors associated with endometriosis. Fertil Steril. 2004;81:1513–21.
6. Barnhart K, Dunsmoor-Su R, Coutifaris C. Effect of endometriosis on in vitro fertilization. Fertil Steril. 2002;77:1148–55.
7. Komsky-Elbaz A, Raziel A, Friedler S, Strassburger D, Kasterstein E, Komarovsky D, Ron-El R, Ben-Ami I. Conventional IVF versus ICSI in sibling oocytes from couples with endometriosis and normozoospermic semen. J Assist Reprod Genet. 2013;30:251–7.
8. Hwang JL, Seow KM, Lin YH, Hsieh BC, Huang LW, Chen HJ, et al. IVF versus ICSI in sibling oocytes from patients with polycystic ovarian syndrome: a randomized controlled trial. Hum Reprod. 2005;20:1261–5.
9. Tournaye H, Verheyen G, Albano C, Camus M, Van Landuyt L, Devroey P, et al. Intracytoplasmic sperm injection versus in vitro fertilization: a randomized controlled trial and a meta-analysis of the literature. Fertil Steril. 2002;78:1030–7.
10. Van der Westerlaken L, Naaktgeboren N, Verburg H, Dieben S, Helmerhorst FM. Conventional in vitro fertilization versus intracytoplasmic sperm injection in patients with borderline semen: a randomized study using sibling oocytes. Fertil Steril. 2006;85:395–400.
11. Coetzee K, Kruger T, Lombard C. Predictive value of normal sperm morphology: a structured literature review. Hum Reprod Update. 1998;4:73–82.
12. The ESHRE Capri Workshop Group. Intracytoplasmic sperm injection (ICSI) in 2006: evidence and evolution. Hum Reprod Update. 2007;13:515–26.
13. Rhemrev JPT, Lens JW, McDonnell J, Schoemaker J, Vermeiden JPW. The postwash total progressively motile sperm cell count is a reliable predictor of total fertilization failure during in vitro fertilization treatment. Fertil Steril. 2001;76:884–91.
14. Taylor TH, Wright G, Jones-Colon S, Mitchell-Leef D, Kort HI, Nagy ZP. Comparison of ICSI and conventional IVF in patients with increased oocyte immaturity. Reprod Biomed Online. 2008;17:46–52.
15. The Practice Committees of the American Society for Reproductive Medicine and Society for Assisted Reproductive Technology. Intracytoplasmic sperm injection (ICSI) for non-male factor infertility: a committee opinion. Fertil Steril. 2012;98:1395–9.
16. Kim HH, Bundorf MK, Behr B, McCallum SW. Use and outcome of intracytoplasmic sperm injection for non-male factor infertility. Fertil Steril. 2007;88:622–8.
17. Vincent C, Pickering SJ, Johnson MH. The hardening effect of dimethylsulphoxide on the mouse zona pellucida requires the presence of an oocyte and is associated with reduction in the number of cortical granules present. J Reprod Fertil. 1990;89:253–9.
18. George MA, Johnson MH, Vincent C. Use of fetal bovine serum to protect against zona hardening during preparation of mouse oocytes for cryopreservation. Hum Reprod. 1992;7:408–12.
19. Larman MG, Sheehan CB, Gardner DK. Calcium-free vitrification reduces cryoprotectant-induced zona pellucida hardening and increases fertilization rates in mouse oocytes. Reprod. 2006;131:53–61.
20. Tong X-H, Wu L-M, Jin R-T, Luo L-H, Luan H-B, Liu Y-S. Fertilization rates are improved after IVF if the corona radiate is left intact in vitrified-warmed human oocytes. Hum Reprod. 2012;27:3208–14.
21. Li X-H, Chen S-U, Zhang X, Tang M, Kui Y-R, Wu X, et al. Cryopreserved oocytes of infertile couples undergoing assisted reproductive technology could be an important source of oocyte donation: a clinical report of successful pregnancies. Hum Reprod. 2005;20:3390–4.
22. Walls M, Junk S, Ryan JP, Hart R. IVF versus ICSI of in-vitro matured human oocytes. Reprod Biomed Online. 2012;25:603–7.
23. Nelson SM, Lawler DA. Predicting live birth, preterm delivery, and low birth weight in infants born from in vitro fertilisation: a prospective study of 144,018 treatment cycles. PLoS. 2011;8:e1000386.
24. Van Loendersloot LL, van Wely M, Limpens J, Bossuyt PM, Repping S, van der Veen F. Predictive factors in in vitro fertiliza-

tion (IVF): a systematic review and meta-analysis. Hum Reprod Update. 2010;16:577–89.
25. Henkel RR, Schill W-B. Sperm preparation for ART. Reprod Biol Endocrinol. 2003;1:108–42.
26. Quinn MM, Jalalian L, Ribeiro S, Ona K, Demirci U, Cedars MI, Rosen MP. Microfluidic sorting selects sperm for clinical use with reduced DNA damage compared to density gradient centrifugation with swim-up in split semen samples. Hum Reprod. 2018;33:1–6.
27. Payne D, Matthews CD. Intracytoplasmic sperm injection – clinical results from the reproductive medicine unit. Adelaide Reprod Fertil Dev. 1995;7:219–27.
28. Balakier H, Sojecki A, Motamedi G, Librach C. Time-dependent capability of human oocytes for activation and pronuclear formation during metaphase II arrest. Hum Reprod. 2004;19:982–7.
29. Sundstrom P, Nilsson BO. Meiotic and cytoplasmic maturation of oocytes collected in stimulated cycles is asynchronous. Hum Reprod. 1988;3:613–9.
30. Trounson AO, Mohr LR, Wood C, Leeton JF. Effect of delayed insemination on in vitro fertilization, culture and transfer of human embryos. J Reprod Fertil. 1982;64:285–94.
31. Harrison KL, Wilson LM, Breen TM, Pope AK, Cummins JM, Hennessey JF. Fertilization of human oocytes in relation to varying delay before insemination. Fertil Steril. 1988;50:294–7.
32. Khan I, Staessen C, van den Abbeel E, Camus M, Wisanto A, Smitz J, Devroey P, van Steirteghem AC. Time of insemination and its effect on in-vitro fertilization, cleavage and pregnancy rates in GnRH agonist/HMG-stimulated cycles. Hum Reprod. 1989;4:921–6.
33. Ebner T, Moser M, Shebl O, Sommergruber M, Yaman C, Tews G. Blood clots in the cumulus-oocyte-complex predict poor oocyte quality and post-fertilization development. Reprod Biomed Online. 2008;16:801–7.
34. Lin YC, Chang SY, Lan KC, Huang HW, Chang CY, Tsai MY, et al. Human oocyte maturity in vivo determines the outcome of blastocyst development in vitro. J Assist Reprod Genet. 2003;20:506–12.
35. Kattera S, Chen C. Short coincubation of gametes in in vitro fertilization improves implantation and pregnancy rates: a prospective, randomized, controlled study. Fertil Steril. 2003;80:1017–21.
36. Bungum M, Bungum L, Humaidan P. A prospective study, using sibling oocytes, examining the effect of 30 seconds versus 90 minutes gamete co-incubation in IVF. Hum Reprod. 2006;21:518–23.
37. European Society for Human Reproduction and Embryology (ESHRE) Special Interest Group of Embryology and Alpha Scientists in Reproductive Medicine. The Vienna consensus: report of an expert meeting on the development of ART laboratory performance indicators. RBMOnline. 2017;1–17.
38. Mahutte NG, Arici A. Failed fertilization: is it predictable? Curr Opin Obstet Gynecol Rev. 2003;15:211–8.
39. Rawe VY, Brugo Olmedo S, Nodar FN, Doncel GD, Acosta AA, Vitullo AD. Cytoskeletal organization defects and abortive activation in human oocytes after IVF and ICSI failure. Mol Hum Reprod. 2000;6:510–6.
40. World Health Organization. WHO Laboratory Manual for the examination and processing of human semen. 5th ed. Geneva: World Health Organization; 2010.
41. Ergur AR, Dokras A, Giraldo JL, Habana A, Kovanci E, Huszar G. Sperm maturity and treatment choice of in vitro fertilization (IVF) or intracytoplasmic sperm injection: diminished sperm HspA2 chaperone levels predict IVF failure. Fertil Steril. 2002;77:910–8.
42. Staessen C, Camus M, Clasen K, De Vos A, van Steirteghem A. Conventional in-vitro fertilization versus intracytoplasmic sperm injection in sibling oocytes from couples with tubal infertility and normozoospermic semen. Hum Reprod. 1999;14:2474–9.
43. Hershlag A, Paine T, Kvapil G, Feng H, Napolitano B. In vitro fertilization-intracytoplasmic sperm injection split: an insemination method to prevent fertilization failure. Fertil Steril. 2002;77:229–32.
44. Verheyen G, Tournaye H, Staessen C, De Vos A, Vandervorst M, Van Steirteghem A. Controlled comparison of in-vitro fertilization and intracytoplasmic sperm injection in patients with asthenozoospermia. Hum Reprod. 1999;14:2313–9.
45. Finch KA, Fonseka KG, Abogrein A, Ioannou D, Handyside AH, Thornhill AR, et al. Nuclear organization in human sperm: preliminary evidence for altered sex chromosome centromere position in infertile males. Hum Reprod. 2008;23:1263–70.
46. Van der Westerlaken L, Helmerhorst F, Dieben S, Naaktgeboren N. Intracytoplasmic sperm injection as a treatment for unexplained total fertilization failure or low fertilization after conventional *in vitro* fertilization. Fertil Steril. 2005;83:612–7.
47. Wheeler MB, Rubessa M. Integration of microfluidics in animal in vitro embryo production. Mol Hum Reprod. 2017;23(4):269.

ICSI: Yesterday, Today, and Tomorrow

87

Henry E. Malter

Intracytoplasmic sperm injection (ICSI) is a cumbersome name for a seemingly simple technique that has remained a major pillar of human-assisted reproductive medicine practice for over 20 years. Is there anything further to write about ICSI? Embarking on this chapter, I'm not really sure. However, it is always worthwhile to take stock and not accept a potentially erroneous or even detrimental status quo. I will do my best to present a current and up-to-date review of ICSI and its proper place within assisted reproductive technology (ART). Hopefully this will be of some immediate value and also utility as we move forward into the fourth decade of assisting patients in achieving their goal of realizing the birth of healthy offspring. We will begin with a historical discussion of the work leading up to ICSI and then examine the current clinical situation and the expansion of the use of ICSI beyond male factor patients. We will briefly go over the history and current status of follow-up and criticism of ICSI followed by a look at the potential future for the technique. Figure 87.1 provides a visual summary on some of the topics under discussion.

87.1 Historical Perspective

The interaction between egg and sperm was always a tantalizing biological scenario to examine, and the specifics of this process still remain to be fully elucidated. It is also of primary importance in both human and agricultural/research animal reproduction.

Sperm-egg fusion leading to subsequent fertilization is a highly complex biological process involving unique cell–cell interaction, recognition, signal transmission, membrane fusion, activation, chromatin remodeling, and other molecular components. It culminates the long journey of the spermatozoa from its site of production in the testes, through the male reproductive tract, through the female tract, and then through the outer cellular investments of the mature egg. The idea of circumventing all of this complexity and simply forcibly inserting a sperm cell into an egg seems questionable but has been a perennial developmental biology and animal research activity.

The first reported instance of successfully injecting a sperm cell into a mammalian egg was reported by Lin in the mouse [1]. Later this work was repeated and expanded in the golden hamster in the laboratory of Ryuzo Yanagimachi in 1976 [2]. Their experiments established that apparently normal sperm decondensation and pronuclear (PN) formation could occur following injection into the cytoplasm. This was quite a surprising landmark result considering that apparently normal fertilization occurred with testicular hamster and even freeze-dried human sperm via a physical scenario that circumvented most aspects of the normal fertilization process.

The first mammalian offspring from ICSI occurred in the rabbit reported in essentially simultaneous publications by Carol Keefer in the USA and Iritani and Hosoi in Japan [3, 4]. Their work was actually concurrent with the first human report of direct sperm injection leading to PN formation by Susan Lanzendorf and colleagues [5]. Unfortunately the results of that study were not promising causing a dampening of interest in direct injection.

In human clinical ART, male factor fertility due to low sperm number and low motility had been a recognized issue going back to the first days of IVF [6]. Early attempts involved various techniques to isolate motile sperm and concentrate them in the vicinity of the egg in microdrop culture. Considering the complex and difficult animal injection protocols and disappointing direct injection human results, alternative concepts for promoting sperm-egg fusion were proposed and had a modest clinical vogue.

Simply opening the zona pellucida or injecting sperm under the zona and adjacent to the oolemma provided minor improvements in mild male factor cases [7–12]. However, the clinical application of these techniques did forever

H. E. Malter (✉)
Fertility Center of the Carolinas, University of South Carolina School of Medicine, Greenville, SC, USA
e-mail: henry.malter@prismahealth.org

G. N. Allahbadia et al. (eds.), *Textbook of Assisted Reproduction*, https://doi.org/10.1007/978-981-15-2377-9_87

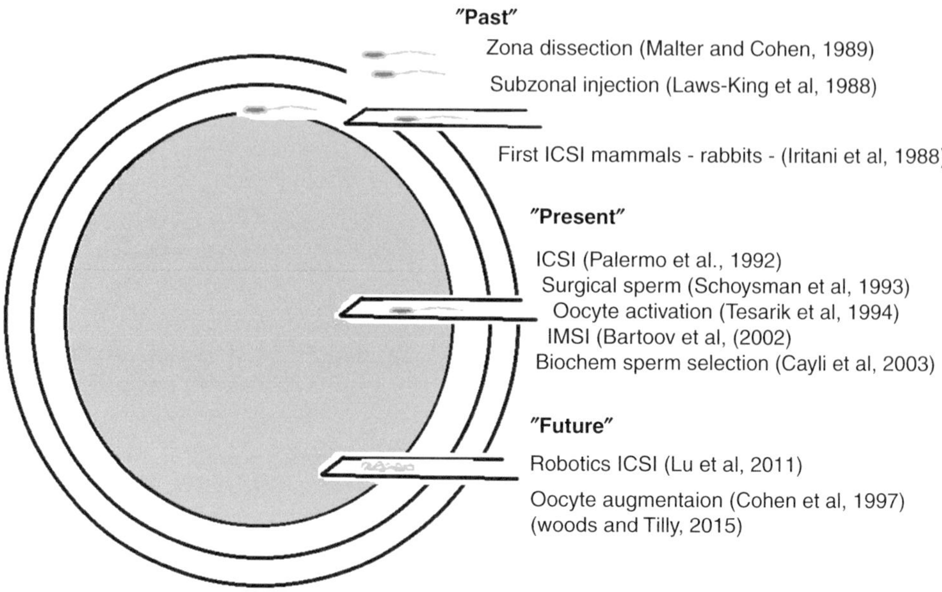

Fig. 87.1 A limited schematic representation of the past, present, and future of ICSI

change the human ART lab by proving that the micromanipulation of human eggs and embryos was compatible with good outcome and the birth of healthy children [13].

Zona opening protocols also demonstrated some interesting aspects of the human fertilization process in that polyspermy (not observed when the mouse zona is opened) was a major issue and made those techniques essentially unusable [14]. Embryonic zona opening has of course continued to be an important technique in promoting hatching and biopsy [15, 16].

Zona opening and subzonal sperm insertion continued for a brief period, but in the early 1990s, Gianpiero Palermo and coworkers in Brussels fortuitously observed successful viable fertilization when the plasma membrane of human eggs was apparently pierced during attempts at subzonal injection [17]. The Brussels team pursued and refined the technique to create a working direct injection protocol that led to the first human births. They somewhat ponderously termed the technique intracytoplasmic sperm injection (ICSI) to delineate it from the subzonal injection procedure [18].

Using direct injection of single sperm, excellent rates of fertilization and embryo development were achieved making even the most severe male factor cases clinically treatable. Using ICSI, almost all manifestations of male factor infertility can be addressed down to a female to male gamete ratio of 1:1.

87.2 Current Laboratory Aspects

In surveys of ICSI, wide variation in sperm and egg quality do not seem to result in much variation in outcome [19, 20]. There are some critical factors including proper sperm cell immobilization and confirmation of oocyte membrane breakage resulting in true intracytoplasmic injection.

ICSI, by design, can obviously achieve fertilization with individual viable spermatozoa, and so even severely compromised ejaculates from extreme male factor patients can be used with good success. Very quickly the technique was also used with success in the most challenging azoospermic cases where very limited epididymal or testicular sperm were obtained via surgery and biopsy [21, 22]. Even in cases where fully mature spermatozoa are not available, surgically obtained immature spermatids can be injected and result in terms of development though at a greatly reduced rate of success [23, 24].

One obvious characteristic of ICSI is that the embryologist becomes the sperm selector bypassing millions of years of coevolution between the sperm and female reproductive tract. In the original procedure, sperm were observed at approximately 200 to 400× magnification on a standard inverted microscope. Sperm with overtly normal morphology and motility were chosen for injection. Results using this level of "selection" were quite good, and fertilization/development could be achieved with highly compromised samples including those with zero normal forms on a standard semen analysis. However, over the years, a variety of potential improvements to the sperm selection process have been proposed.

A first question concerns sperm viability. Motile sperm are preferably chosen, but in some cases, particularly surgically retrieved samples, such cells may be few and far between or apparently absent. Initially immotile viable sperm can be stimulated into motility via administering various pharmacological agents affecting cellular energy metabolism such as methylxanthines (phosphodiesterase inhibitors), intracellular Ca modulators, or ATP itself [25–27]. It should be noted that all of these agents have potentially serious negative effects on the oocyte and subsequent development so that care must be taken [28].

Immotile viable sperm can apparently be identified simply by gentle probing with the injection needle to confirm tail flexibility and vitality [29]. Probably the most common technique is hypoosmotic treatment using diluted 50% media which delineates cells with intact viable membranes by their characteristic swelling behavior. A more modern alternative challenges individual cells with a "shot" of laser energy directed at the terminal portion of the sperm tail [30].

Of course, sperm motility itself makes ICSI somewhat of a challenge were it not reduced via the use of viscous media. The large majority of ICSI is performed using commercial media containing polyvinylpyrrolidone (PVP). However, there is some evidence of toxicity and detrimental effects in both sperm and embryos [31, 32]. An alternative is to use a media containing hyaluronic acid as the viscosity increasing agent which would seem to provide a more physiological option [33].

Among viable sperm, it would be desirable to select cells which would have the greatest chance of achieving fertilization and normal term development. A variety of schemes have been proposed in this area although a complete understanding of what constitutes such a "perfect" or at least developmentally competent sperm cell is certainly still lacking.

Obviously the selection process itself must be benign to subsequent sperm function. One idea is to simply "look" more carefully at each sperm cell to identify morphological abnormalities that might be associated with function or downstream developmental issues. High magnification (6000×) sperm observation using a complicated and expensive video microscopy setup forms the basis of several clinical techniques originally described as motile sperm organelle morphology examination (MSOME) or intracytoplasmic morphologically selected sperm injection (IMSI) by Bartoov and colleagues [34, 35]. Several individual morphological aspects have been connected with sperm dysfunction. Defects in the head/neck piece area have been associated with subsequent centriolar dysfunction and early developmental abnormalities although high magnification observation is not necessarily required [36].

The presence of sperm head vacuoles is another morphological indicator associated with downstream developmental issues [37]. Sperm head abnormalities (head geometry and vacuoles) revealed by high magnification observation and image analysis have been correlated with DNA fragmentation [38]. Clinically, high magnification sperm selection against such abnormalities has been reported to increase implantation rates [39]. While other studies have failed to demonstrate any real positive effect, a recent meta-analysis did support improved implantation and pregnancy rates and reduced miscarriage rates in the treatment of male factor couples [37, 40, 41]. The very high cost in both equipment and time has kept this promising technique in limited clinical use.

Biochemical selection of sperm for ICSI has been suggested based on a determination of the presence of the HspA2 hyaluronic acid receptor protein on the sperm surface. The presence of this protein is associated with sperm maturity, while its deficit is associated with maturation arrest and chromosomal abnormality [42, 43]. This concept has been incorporated into clinical tests for HA binding activity as well as a selection device for identifying motile sperm for injection that will bind HA. However, a major 2016 meta-analysis of this concept demonstrated that its clinical application yielded no improvement in fertilization or pregnancy rates with some evidence of improvement in embryo development and concluded that further study was warranted [44].

Another biochemical sperm selection technique involves identifying sperm that bind to annexin V—a marker of membrane phosphatidyl serine and apoptosis [45]. However, it is unclear that this cumbersome technique involving magnetic-activated cell sorting of live sperm provides benefit over standard sperm preparation techniques [46, 47].

As discussed below, oocyte activation defects arising from obvious sperm deficits such as 100% globozoospermia can be successfully proactively addressed via ICSI followed by artificial egg activation protocols [48]. An excellent review addressing sperm-specific issues involving ICSI is provided by Neri and coauthors [26].

87.3 Clinical Aspects of ICSI: Moving Beyond Male Factor Patients

Over the past 20 years, ICSI has clearly expanded out from this initial indication of male factor infertility. According to the 2014 Centers for Disease Control summary of over 200,000 ART cycles in the USA, male factor issues played a role in perhaps 50% of cycles, while ICSI was used in 69% of cycles. This preponderance of ICSI cycles above the level of male factor infertility is observed to greater and lesser degrees elsewhere around the world [49].

Considerable debate has occurred over whether there are non-male factor reasons to apply ICSI though many clinics, including in full disclosure, the author's, currently perform ICSI on essentially all cycles [50]. Anecdotally, some very large clinics operate in highly regimented fashion in terms of staff and resources, and ICSI seems to logistically allow for tighter control over the flow and timing of daily operations. One obvious reason is to avoid fertilization failure which is known to occur spontaneously in between 5 and 15% of ART cycles but also in 3–5% of initial ICSI cycles [51, 52].

Some data backs up the idea that ICSI will consistently result in a spontaneous reduction of such failed cycles. For example, in one study on cycles following a complete fertilization failure insemination cycle, ICSI did provide a significant increase in subsequent fertilization of 48% per retrieved oocyte compared with 11% for subsequent insemination [53]. Idiopathic fertilization failure would be particularly troublesome in poor-responding patients with few mature oocytes available.

However, in a randomized trial involving non-male factor cycles with fewer than six eggs, embryo yield, implantation, and pregnancy rate was no different between ICSI and insemination [54]. In couples with idiopathic infertility (another potential ICSI indication), a meta-analysis demonstrated that ICSI did result in higher fertilization with an established higher risk of fertilization failure in insemination cycles [55].

One aspect of ART failure that ICSI has revealed, and perhaps provides a partial solution to, is the failure of oocyte activation which could theoretically occur from either sperm or egg deficits. This has no doubt been a ubiquitous, though fortunately rare, occurrence in all treatment cycles, but particularly revealed by ICSI when the introduction of a viable sperm cell into a mature egg can be strictly confirmed.

Various strategies have been proposed to artificially activate eggs following ICSI, usually in a subsequent cycle following fertilization failure from suspected activation failure. These include mechanical, electrical, and direct chemical stimulation to trigger intracellular Ca^{2+} oscillations [56–58]. Many pregnancies and healthy term deliveries have been achieved by these invasive protocols, and follow-up studies on the resulting offspring are reassuring [53, 59].

The American Society of Reproductive Medicine (ASRM) produced an excellent practice committee opinion on the use of ICSI in non-male factor infertility in 2012 [60].

87.4 Follow-Up and Criticism

Considering its invasive nature, ICSI has properly been the subject of analysis, follow-up on the resulting offspring, and associated criticism. The technique was adopted quickly based on proven clinical success and some early follow-up studies. However, ICSI obviously bypasses many cellular aspects of the fertilization process which could potentially result in cryptic aberrations and downstream effects on development.

Follow-up basic research in captive nonhuman primates demonstrated several differences in sperm decondensation behavior and timing between injected sperm and natural sperm-egg fusion-mediated fertilization [61]. While demonstrating that spindle formation was essentially identical to that observed in inseminated oocytes, various sperm cell components are abnormally present and persistent inside the egg including the tail, acrosomal contents, and the perinuclear theca. Despite these early distinctions, at 20 h postfertilization, ICSI and inseminated macaque oocytes are ultrastructurally indistinguishable [62]. Obviously the non-vital microscopy required to fully elucidate post-ICSI ultrastructure is highly problematic in human clinical material.

In a minor study on the ultrastructure of human in vitro mature oocytes post-ICSI, some injection-associated plasma membrane damage and possible unique events such as the acrosome reaction occurring within the ooplasm were observed. However, sperm components did not obviously persist in the cytoplasm, and sperm DNA decondensation and pronuclear formation appeared relatively normal. In general, the timing of early post-ICSI development in the human seems unremarkable.

It is worth noting that despite these observed ultrastructural aspects, healthy offspring (with some follow-up work) have been produced from ART using ICSI in both rhesus macaques and baboons [63, 64]. It must also be noted that human eggs and embryos are developmentally distinct from other model systems in often profound ways. From the author's personal experience in research and large animal reproduction, compared with other mammalian species, cytoplasmic sperm injection does seem to be a much more straightforward and "forgiving" technique in the human.

A basic question obviously concerns the possible effects of ICSI on the associated conceived offspring. A large number of well-performed follow-up studies have taken place from the first year following adoption to the present day—on young adults conceived from the first clinical applications—and only a limited subset of these can be discussed.

A 2012 meta-analysis identified 24 studies comparing over 27,000 ICSI-conceived children with over 46,000 children conceived by standard insemination and demonstrated no increased risk of birth defects when ICSI was applied [65]. Many such follow-up studies, performed essentially every few years since the inception of the technique, have demonstrated no differences or only minor differences in ICSI offspring compared with similar selected cohorts of naturally conceived children in a wide range of growth and developmental markers, chromosomal aspects, and physiological aspects [66–68].

This brings up the issue of true "controls" for such studies since the genetic background of children conceived in couples experiencing infertility issues, particularly severe male factor couples, could be quite unique from those conceived in fertile couples in the general population. This issue challenges the majority of such follow-up studies.

Nevertheless, evidence from some studies has shown unique apparent deficits in ICSI offspring. A major prospective study conducted 10 years after the first ICSI use and monitored over 3000 ICSI pregnancies beginning at 16 weeks. The rate of major malformations (8.6%) was in fact significantly increased with a relative risk of 1.25 compared with a large similar cohort of naturally conceived children [69]. A study on 300 5-year-old ICSI children (again compared with matched controls from the general population) showed no effect on growth and general health though interestingly ICSI-conceived children in this study did have higher rates of surgical and therapeutic medical interventions [70].

A specific area of concern comes directly from the basic success of ICSI in facilitating the birth of children for men with severe male factor abnormalities and potentially associated underlying genetic lesions. The incidence in sex chromosome abnormalities and general structural abnormalities does seem to be slightly increased in ICSI offspring compared again to the normal population rate [71, 72]. Also, severe male factor patients have an increased incidence of micro-deletions in the azoospermia factors region of the Y chromosome, and these can definitely be transmitted to resulting male offspring, in most cases arguably uniquely, via ICSI [73, 74].

Young men conceived from ICSI had normal pubertal development and comparable levels of most reproductive hormones in comparison to spontaneously conceived counterparts, though mild aberrations in both inhibin B and follicle stimulation hormone levels were observed [75, 76]. Very recently, the same group has reported on the semen quality of young men conceived via ICSI finding that they had lower median sperm concentrations and total motile sperm counts (both essentially halved) compared with naturally conceived controls. Interestingly, no direct correlation could be identified in semen quality between fathers and ICSI-conceived sons.

In conclusion, there have been a variety of minor differences observed in ICSI offspring but in most cases only in comparison to naturally conceived children—a questionable control. For the most part, no significant differences in a wide range of developmental metrics have been observed. The severe male factor-associated issues would seem to present more of a population-based counseling aspect than suggesting caution in application. Male factor patients deserve to have the chance to be fathers, and, in many cases, ICSI provides the only possibility of achieving this. The birth of millions of healthy ICSI babies at this point is reassuring in all regards, and no doubt further follow-up studies perhaps with more subtle metrics will be continued as the first ICSI offspring enter adulthood.

87.5 The Future

The future of ICSI can be considered both from the perspective of potential "improvements" to the technique itself and in its potential application. The basic ICSI technique has been unchanged for almost 20 years. However, it is a time-consuming activity requiring considerable training and skill.

Robotic automation of assisted reproduction laboratory aspects is no doubt on the near horizon. In fact, experimentally, an essentially automated ICSI system has already been developed which included video-guided sperm capture and immobilization, vacuum-driven positioning of multiple eggs, and successful injection using live video image-directed robotic micromanipulation units [77].

No doubt with further advancement in image analysis, microfluidics, and robotics, new systems with improved outcome and utility can be developed. Potential improvements in sperm selection for ICSI will continue to be pursued. While current variations such as high magnification or hyaluronic acid binding selection have failed to completely capture mainstream clinical capture, these or similar techniques might show clinical importance if better targeted based on a better understanding of genetic and other patient variations.

Perhaps there are ways to facilitate other sperm selection methods involving synthetic cumulus cells or zona surfaces as shown from prior experimental work [78, 79].

Ultimately, one concept I feel could be pursued is a system for the video, perhaps "artificial intelligence" driven, identification of screened sperm cells with desired "normal" physical or other selection characteristics to the injection system through microfluidics [80].

Also in ICSI's future, and in fact already being pursued, are clinical protocols using the basic ICSI technique to actually modify and theoretically "augment" patient eggs. Manipulation of ooplasm has been pursued via research attempting to alter cytoplasmic developmental determinants or manipulate the ooplasmic mitochondrial make-up [81, 82].

Based on evidence of efficacy and positive effects from ooplasmic manipulation in these and other experiments, the augmentation of human ooplasm was attempted in a clinical trial using a modified form of ICSI [83]. A small amount of cytoplasm from a healthy young donor egg was first aspirated and then injected along with the sperm cell into theoretically compromised patient eggs. In a preliminary trial in carefully selected couples exhibiting consistent total failure in prior assisted reproduction attempts, the technique resulted in considerable success [84, 85]. Unfortunately, since the ooplasmic transfer resulted in a limited instance of mitochondrial DNA transfer between individuals, it was determined to fall under the regulatory purview of the US Food and Drug Administration who requested an extensive investigative new drug protocol be performed prior to continued application. This protocol was well beyond the capability of the team involved, and further application of the technique was voluntarily terminated.

A version of the technique termed autologous germline mitochondrial energy transfer (AUGMENT) was pursued in which a proprietary preparation supposedly containing mitochondria derived from the patient's own "ovarian stem cells" was injected, essentially via ICSI, into their eggs to improve outcome during subsequent ART procedures [86, 87]. Despite promising initial clinical trial results, continued evaluation of the technique suggested that it failed to improve outcome in patients with prior failure using standard ART and was associated with a reduction in euploid embryos [88, 89]. However, the preliminary results, gathered at multiple clinics, did suggest that a practically workable solution in addressing ooplasmic deficits might still be obtained via intracytoplasmic injection. Obviously mitochondrial augmentation cannot address every possible source of potential deficits which could arise from a variety of other ooplasmic sources, and nuclear transfer experiments—providing a complete cytoplasmic exchange—have also been recently reported [90, 91]. If further, perhaps patient-specific ooplasmic deficits could be identified and proper augmentation material developed perhaps from stem cell-derived sources, direct injection via ICSI would seem to offer the least invasive and potentially most efficacious method for introduction.

87.6 Conclusion

ICSI has made a tremendous impact on the utility and success of human-assisted reproduction. Through ICSI, fertilization and subsequent healthy human offspring can be facilitated in essentially all manifestations of male gamete deficit and dysfunction. Many of these couples would never have been able to conceive healthy children without ICSI.

The technique may be providing further utility in making ART a more efficacious and successful process beyond male factor issues, but this concept will continue to be evaluated. In general, despite some identified concerns in the resulting offspring, particularly related to severe male factor patients, ICSI would seem to be fully compatible with normal human development particularly when considered with other less invasive forms of treatment required by infertile couples. Comparisons with the fertile population will always be problematic, and with proper, current counseling ICSI should remain a valid treatment option. The future of ICSI is of course the subject of speculation, but already the technique has provided utility in attempts to "improve" human oocytes, and no doubt advancements in ICSI as a male infertility treatment will also occur.

References

1. Lin TP. Microinjection of mouse eggs. Science. 1966;151:333–7.
2. Uehara T, Yanagimachi R. Microsurgical injection of spermatozoa into hamster eggs with subsequent transformation of sperm nuclei into male pronuclei. Biol Reprod. 1976;15:467–70.
3. Iritani A, Utsumi K, Miyake M, Hosoi Y, Saeki K. In vitro fertilization by a routine method and by micromanipulation. Ann NY Acad Sci. 1988;541:583–90.
4. Keefer CL. Fertilization by sperm injection in the rabbit. Gamete Res. 1989;22:59–69.
5. Lanzendorf SE, Maloney MK, Veeck LL, Slusser J, Hodgen GD, Rosenwaks Z. A preclinical evaluation of pronuclear formation by microinjection of human spermatozoa into human oocytes. Fertil Steril. 1988;49:835–42.
6. Cohen J, Edwards RG, Fehilly CB, Fishel CB, Hewitt J, Rowland G, et al. Treatment of male infertility by in vitro fertilization: factors affecting fertilization and pregnancy. Acat Eur Fertil. 1984;15:455–65.
7. Cohen J, Malter H, Fehilly C, Wright G, Elsner C, Kort H, et al. Implantation of embryos after partial opening of oocyte zona pellucida to facilitate sperm penetration. Lancet. 1988;2:162.
8. Gordon JW, Talansky BE. Assisted fertilization by zona drilling: a mouse model for correction of oligospermia. J Exp Zool. 1986;239:347–54.
9. Gordon JW, Grunfeld L, Garrisi GJ, Talansky BE, Richards C, Laufer N. Fertilization of human oocytes by sperm from infertile males after zona pellucida drilling. Fertil Steril. 1988;50:68–73.
10. Lacham O, Trounson A, Holden C, Mann J, Sathananthan H. Fertilization and development of mouse eggs injected under the zona pellucida with single spermatozoa treated to induce the acrosome reaction. Gamete Res. 1989;23:233–43.
11. Laws-King A, Trounson A, Sathananthan H, Kola I. Fertilization of human oocytes by microinjection of a single spermatozoon under the zona pellucida. Fertil Steril. 1987;48:637–42.
12. Ng SC, Bongso A, Chang SI, Sathananthan H, Ratnam S. Transfer of human sperm into the perivitelline space of human oocytes after zona-drilling or zona-puncture. Fertil Steril. 1989;52:73–8.
13. Malter HE, Cohen J. Partial zona dissection of the human oocyte: a nontraumatic method using micromanipulation to assist zona pellucida penetration. Fertil Steril. 1989;51:139–48.
14. Malter H, Talansky B, Gordon J, Cohen J. Monospermy and polyspermy after partial zona dissection of reinseminated human oocytes. Gamete Res. 1989;3:377–86.
15. Cohen J, Elsner C, Kort H, Malter H, Massey J, Mayer MP, et al. Impairment of the hatching process following IVF in the human and improvement of implantation by assisting hatching using micromanipulation. Hum Reprod. 1990;5:7–13.
16. De Boer K, McArthur S, Murray C, Jansen RPS. First live birth following blastocyst biopsy and PGD analysis. Reprod Biomed Online. 2002;4:35.
17. Palermo GD, O'Neill CL, Chow S, Cheung S, Parella N, Pereira N, Rosenwaks Z. Intracytoplasmic sperm injection: state of the art in humans. Reproduction. 2017;154:F93–F110.
18. Palermo G, Joris H, Devroey P, Van Steirteghem AC. Pregnancies after intracytoplasmic injection of single spermatozoon into an oocyte. Lancet. 1992;340:17–8.
19. Joris H, Nagy Z, Van de Velde H, De Vos A, Van Steirteghem A. Intracytoplasmic sperm injection: laboratory set-up and injection procedure. Hum Reprod. 1998;13(Suppl 1):76–86.
20. Malter HE, Cohen J. Intracytoplasmic sperm injection: technical aspects. In: Vayena E, Rowe PJ, Griffin PD, editors. Current practices and controversies in assisted reproduction. World Health Organization: Geneva; 2002. p. 126–32.
21. Devroey P, Liu J, Nagy Z, Goossens A, Tournaye H, Camus, et al. Pregnancies after testicular sperm extraction and intracytoplasmic sperm injection in non-obstructive azoospermia. Hum Reprod. 1995;10:1457–60.
22. Schoysman R, Vanderzwalmen P, Nijs M, Segal-Bertin G, van de Casseye M. Successful fertilization by testicular spermatozoa in an in vitro fertilization programme. Hum Reprod. 1993;8:1339–40.
23. Tanaka A, Nagayoshi M, Takemoto Y, Tanaka I, Kusunoki H, Watanabe S, et al. Fourteen babies born after round spermatid injection into human oocytes. PNAS. 2015;112:14629–34.
24. Vanderzwalmen P, Zech H, Birkenfeld A, Yemini M, Bertin G, Lejeune B, et al. Intracytoplasmic injection of spermatids retrieved from testicular tissue: influence of testicular pathology,

type of selected spermatids and oocyte activation. Hum Reprod. 1997;12:1203–13.
25. Carlomagno G, Nordio M, Chiu TT, Unfer V. Contribution of myo-inositol and melatonin to human reproduction. Eur J Obstet Gynecol Reprod Biol. 2011;159:267–72.
26. Neri QV, Lee B, Rosenwaks Z, Machaca K, Palermo GD. Understanding fertilization through intracytoplasmic sperm injection (ICSI). Cell Calcium. 2014;55:24–37.
27. Tarlatzis BC, Kolibianakis EM, Bontis J, Tousiou M, Lagos S, Mantalenakis S. Effect of pentoxifylline on human sperm motility and fertilizing capacity. Arch Androl. 1995;34:33–42.
28. Tournaye H, Van der Linden M, Van den Abbeel E, Devroey P, Van Steirteghem A. Effects of pentoxifylline on in-vitro development of preimplantation mouse embryos. Hum Reprod. 1993;8:1475–80.
29. Soares JB, Glina S, Antunes N Jr, Wonchockier R, Galuppo AG, Mizrahi FE. Sperm tail flexibility test: a simple test for selecting viable spermatozoa for intracytoplasmic sperm injection from semen samples without motile spermatozoa. Rev Hosp Clin Fac Med Sao Paulo. 2003;58:250–3.
30. Aktan TM, Montag M, Duman S, Gorkemli H, Rink K, Yurdakul T. Use of a laser to detect viable but immotile spermatozoa. Andrologia. 2004;36:366–9.
31. Mizuno K, Hoshi K, Huang T. Fertilization and embryo development in a mouse ICSI model using human and mouse sperm after immobilization in polyvinylpyrrolidone. Hum Reprod. 2002;17:2350–5.
32. Strehler E, Baccetti B, Sterzik K, Capitani S, Collodel G, De Santo M, et al. Detrimental effects of polyvinylpyrrolidone on the ultrastructure of spermatozoa (Notulae seminologicae 13). Hum Reprod. 1998;13:120–3.
33. Balaban B, Lundin K, Morrell JM, Tjellstrom H, Urman B, Holmes PV. An alternative to PVP for slowing sperm prior to ICSI. Hum Reprod. 2003;18:1887–9.
34. Bartoov B, Berkovitz A, Eltes F. Selection of spermatozoa with normal nuclei to improve the pregnancy rate with intracytoplasmic sperm injection. N Engl J Med. 2001;345:1067–8.
35. Bartoov B, Berkovitz A, Eltes F, Kogosowski A, Menezo Y, Barak Y. Real-time fine morphology of motile human sperm cells is associated with IVF-ICSI outcome. J Androl. 2002;23:1–8.
36. Rawe VY, Brugo Olmedo S, Nodar FN, Vitullo AD. Microtubules and parental genome organization during abnormal fertilization in humans. Zygote. 2002;10:223–8.
37. Setti AS, Braga DP, Figueira RC, Iaconelli A Jr, Borges E. Intracytoplasmic morphologically selected sperm injection results in improved clinical outcomes in couples with previous ICSI failures or male factor infertility: a meta-analysis. Eur J Obstet Gynecol Reprod Biol. 2014;183:96–103.
38. Utsuno H, Oka K, Yamamoto A, Shiozawa T. Evaluation of sperm head shape at high magnification revealed correlation of sperm DNA fragmentation with aberrant head ellipticity and angularity. Fertil Steril. 2013;99:1573–80.
39. Vanderzwalmen P, Hiemer A, Rubner P, Bach M, Neyer A, Stecher A, et al. Blastocyst development after sperm selection at high magnification is associated with size and number of nuclear vacuoles. Reprod Biomed Online. 2008;17:617–27.
40. Mauri AL, Petersen CG, Oliveira JB, Massaro FC, Baruffi RL, Franco JG Jr. Comparison of day 2 embryo quality after conventional ICSI versus intracytoplasmic morphologically selected sperm injection (IMSI) using sibling oocytes. Eur J Obstet Gynecol Reprod Biol. 2010;150:42–6.
41. Oliveira JB, Petersen CG, Massaro FC, Baruffi RL, Mauri AL, Silva LF, et al. Motile sperm organelle morphology examination (MSOME): intervariation study of normal sperm and sperm with large nuclear vacuoles. Reprod Biol Endocrinol. 2010;8:56.
42. Cayli S, Jakab A, Ovari L, Delpiano E, Celik-Ozenci C, Sakkas D, et al. Biochemical markers of sperm function: male fertility and sperm selection for ICSI. Reprod Biomed Online. 2003;7:462–8.
43. Huszar G, Jakab A, Sakkas D, Ozenci CC, Cayli S, Delpiano E, et al. Fertility testing and ICSI sperm selection by hyaluronic acid binding: clinical and genetic aspects. Reprod Biomed Online. 2007;14:650–63.
44. Beck-Fruchter R, Shalev E, Weiss A. Clinical benefit using sperm hyaluronic acid binding technique in ICSI cycles: a systematic review and meta-analysis. Reprod Biomed Online. 2016;32:286–98.
45. Vermes I, Haanen C, Steffens-Nakken H. A novel assay for apoptosis. Flow cytometric detection of phosphatidylserine expression on early apoptotic cells using fluorescein labelled Annexin V. J Immunol Methods. 1995;184:39–51.
46. Nadalini M, Tarozzi N, Di Santo M, Borini A. Annexin V magnetic-activated cell sorting versus swim-up for the selection of human sperm in ART: is the new approach better than the traditional one? J Assist Reprod Genet. 2014;31:1045–51.
47. Romany L, Garrido N, Motato Y, Aparicio B, Remohí J, Meseguer M. Removal of annexin V-positive sperm cells for intracytoplasmic sperm injection in ovum donation cycles does not improve reproductive outcome: a controlled and randomized trial in unselected males. Fertil Steril. 2014;102:1567–75.
48. Egashira A, Murakami M, Haigo K, Horiuchi T, Kuramoto T. A successful pregnancy and live birth after intracytoplasmic sperm injection with globozoospermic sperm and electrical oocyte activation. Fertil Steril. 2009;92:2035–9.
49. Dyer S, Chambers GM, De Mouzon J, Nygren KG, Zegers-Hochschild F, Mansour R, et al. International Committee for Monitoring Assisted Reproductive Technologies. World report on Assisted Reproductive Technologies: 2008, 2009 and 2010. Hum Reprod. 2016;31:1588–609.
50. Evers JL. Santa Claus in the fertility clinic. Hum Reprod. 2016;31:1381–2.
51. Molloy D, Harrison K, Breen T, Hennessey J. The predictive value of idiopathic failure to fertilize on the first in vitro fertilization attempt. Fertil Steril. 1991;56:285–9.
52. Roest J, Van Heusden AM, Zeilmaker GH, Verhoeff A. Treatment policy after poor fertilization in the first IVF cycle. J Assist Reprod Genet. 1998;15:18–21.
53. Vanden Meerschaut F, D'Haeseleer E, Roeyers H, Oostra A, Van Lierde K, De Sutter P. Neonatal and developmental outcome of children born following assisted oocyte activation (AOA). Fertil Steril. 2012;98:S16.
54. Moreno C, Ruiz A, Simón C, Pellicer A, Remohí J. Intracytoplasmic sperm injection as a routine indication in low responder patients. Hum Reprod. 1998;13:2126–9.
55. Johnson LN, Sasson IE, Sammel MD, Dokras A. Does intracytoplasmic sperm injection improve the fertilization rate and decrease the total fertilization failure rate in couples with well-defined unexplained infertility? A systematic review and meta-analysis. Fertil Steril. 2013;100:704–11.
56. Nasr-Esfahani MH, Deemeh MR, Tavalaee M. Artificial oocyte activation and intracytoplasmic sperm injection. Fertil Steril. 2010;94:520–6.
57. Tesarik J, Sousa M, Testart J. Human oocyte activation after intracytoplasmic sperm injection. Hum Reprod. 1994;9:511–8.
58. Yanagida K, Katayose H, Yazawa H, Kimura Y, Sato A, Yanagimachi H, Yanagimachi R. Successful fertilization and pregnancy following ICSI and electrical oocyte activation. Hum Reprod. 1999;14:1307–11.
59. Kyono K, Takisawa T, Nakajo Y, Doshida M, Toya M. Birth and follow-up of babies born following ICSI with oocyte activation using strontium chloride or calcium ionophore A23187. J Mamm Ova Res. 2012;29:35–40.
60. Practice Committee of the ASRM and SART. Intracytoplasmic sperm injection (ICSI) for non-male factor infertility: a committee opinion. Fertil Steril. 2012;98:1395–9.
61. Hewitson L, Simerly C, Dominko T, Schatten G. Cellular and molecular events after in vitro fertilization and intracytoplasmic sperm injection. Theriogenology. 2000;53:95–104.
62. Ramalho-Santos J, Sutovsky P, Simerly C, Oko R, Wessel GM, Hewitson L, et al. ICSI choreography: fate of sperm structures after

monospermic rhesus ICSI and first cell cycle implications. Hum Reprod. 2000;15:2610–20.
63. Sackett G, Ruppenthal G, Hewitson L, Simerly C, Schatten G. Neonatal behavior and infant cognitive development in rhesus macaques produced by assisted reproductive technologies. Dev Psychobiol. 2006;48:243–65.
64. Simerly CR, Castro CA, Jacoby E, Grund K, Turpin J, McFarland D, et al. Assisted reproductive technologies (ART) with baboons generate live offspring: a nonhuman primate model for ART and reproductive sciences. Reprod Sci. 2010;17:917–30.
65. Wen J, Jiang J, Ding C, Dai J, Liu Y, Xia Y, et al. Birth defects in children conceived by in-vitro fertilization and intracytoplasmic sperm injection: a meta-analysis. Fertil Steril. 2012;97:1331–7.
66. Belva F, Henriet S, Liebaers I, Van Steirteghem A, Celestin-Westreich S, Bonduelle M. Medical outcome of 8-year-old singleton ICSI children (born at 32 weeks' gestation) and a spontaneously conceived comparison group. Hum Reprod. 2007;22:506–15.
67. Bonduelle M, Legein J, Buysse A, Van Assche E, Wisanto A, Devroey P, et al. Prospective follow-up study of 423 children born after intracytoplasmic sperm injection. Hum Reprod. 1996;11:1558–64.
68. Bowen JR, Gibson F, Leslie GI, Saunders DM. Medical and developmental outcome at 1 year for children conceived by intracytoplasmic sperm injection. Lancet. 1998;351:1529–34.
69. Katalinic A, Rosch C, Ludwig M. Pregnancy course and outcome after intracytoplasmic sperm injection: a controlled, prospective cohort study. Fertil Steril. 2004;81:1604–16.
70. Bonduelle M, Wennerholm UB, Loft A, Tarlatzis BC, Peters C, Henriet S, et al. A multi-centre cohort study of the physical health of 5-year-old children conceived after intracytoplasmic sperm injection, in vitro fertilization and natural conception. Hum Reprod. 2005;20:413–9.
71. Bonduelle M, Aytoz A, Van Assche E, Devroey P, Liebaers I, Van Steirteghem A. Incidence of chromosomal aberrations in children born after assisted reproduction through intracytoplasmic sperm injection. Hum Reprod. 1998;13:781–2.
72. Munne S, Marquez C, Reing A, Garrisi J, Alikani M. Chromosome abnormalities in embryos obtained after conventional in vitro fertilization and intracytoplasmic sperm injection. Fertil Steril. 1998;69:904–8.
73. Girardi SK, Mielnik A, Schlegel PN. Submicroscopic deletions in the Y chromosome of infertile men. Hum Reprod. 1997;12:1635–41.
74. Kent-First MG, Kol S, Muallem A, Ofir R, Manor D, Blazer S, et al. The incidence and possible relevance of Y-linked microdeletions in babies born after intracytoplasmic sperm injection and their infertile fathers. Mol Hum Reprod. 1996;2:943–50.
75. Belva F, Bonduelle M, Painter RC, Schiettecatte J, Devroey P, De Schepper J. Serum inhibin B concentrations in pubertal boys conceived by ICSI: first results. Hum Reprod. 2010;25:2811–4.
76. Belva F, Bonduelle M, Schiettecatte J, Tournaye H, Painter RC, Devroey P, De Schepper J. Salivary testosterone concentrations in pubertal ICSI boys compared with spontaneously conceived boys. Hum Reprod. 2011;26:438–41.
77. Lu Z, Zhang X, Leung C, Esfandiari N, Casper RF, Sun Y. Robotic ICSI (intracytoplasmic sperm injection). IEEE Trans Biomed Eng. 2011;58:2102–8.
78. Black M, Liu DY, Bourne H, Baker HW. Comparison of outcomes of conventional intracytoplasmic sperm injection and intracytoplasmic sperm injection using sperm bound to the zona pellucida of immature oocytes. Fertil Steril. 2010;93:672–4.
79. Hong SJ, Chiu PC, Lee KF, Tse JM, Ho PC, Yeung WS. Establishment of a capillary-cumulus model to study the selection of sperm for fertilization by the cumulus oophorus. Hum Reprod. 2004;19:1562–9.
80. Knowlton SM, Sadasivam M, Tasoglu S. Microfluidics for sperm research. Trends Biotechnol. 2015;33:221–9.
81. Muggleton-Harris A, Wittingham DG, Wilson L. Cytoplasmic control of preimplantation development in vitro in the mouse. Nature. 1982;299:460–2.
82. Smith LC, Alcivar AA. Cytoplasmic inheritance and its effects on development and performance. J Reprod Fertil. 1993;48:31–43.
83. Cohen J, Scott R, Schimmel T, Levron J, Willadsen S. Birth of infant after transfer of anucleate donor oocyte cytoplasm into recipient eggs. Lancet. 1997;350:186–7.
84. Barritt JA, Brenner CA, Malter HE, Cohen J. Mitochondria in human offspring derived from ooplasmic transplantation. Hum Reprod. 2001;16:513–6.
85. Cohen J, Scott R, Alikani M, Schimmel T, Munné S, Levron J, et al. Ooplasmic transfer in mature human oocytes. Mol Hum Reprod. 1998;4:269–80.
86. White YA, Woods DC, Takai Y, Ishihara O, Seki H, Tilly JL. Oocyte formation by mitotically active germ cells purified from ovaries of reproductive-age women. Nat Med. 2012;18:413–21.
87. Woods DC, Tilly JL. The next (re)generation of ovarian biology and fertility in women: is current science tomorrow's practice? Fertil Steril. 2012;98:3–10.
88. Demur EL, Herraiz S, De los Santos MJ, Marzal A, Escriba MJ, Buigues A, Pellicer A. Autologous mitochondrial transfer as a complimentary technique to ICSI to improve oocyte and embryo quality in IVF patients. A randomized pilot study. Hum Reprod. 2018;33(Suppl 1):i96.
89. Woods DC, Tilly JL. Autologous germline mitochondrial EnergyTransfer (AUGMENT) in human assisted reproduction. Semin Reprod Med. 2015;33:410–21.
90. Mazur P, Veselovsky V, Masliy Y, Borisov M, Mykytenko D, Zukin V. Three babies born after pronuclear transplantation in young women with unexplained infertility and repeated implantation failure of euploid embryos. Hum Reprod. 2018;33(Suppl 1):i60.
91. Zhang J, Zhuang G, Zeng Y, Grifo J, Acosta C, Shu Y, et al. Pregnancy derived from human zygote pronuclear transfer in a patient who had arrested embryos after IVF. Reprod Biomed Online. 2016;33:529–33.

Sperm Selection Techniques for ICSI

88

Necati Findikli, Ciler Celik-Ozenci,
Munevver Serdarogullari, and Mustafa Bahceci

Although there are species-specific differences regarding the timing of sperm-oocyte fusion during natural fertilization, conception can occur only near the time of ovulation, and only a few sperm cells reach the ampulla or the site of fertilization in humans. Out of many millions of sperm ejaculated, only a few sperm reach the fertilization site. When compared to other species, human sperm seem to have poor quality and a significant degree of heterogeneity in terms of structure and function. However, human sperm can achieve successful fertilization, probably due to less sperm competition when compared to other species [1].

Intracytoplasmic sperm injection (ICSI) has challenged the evolutionary paradigm of "survival of the fittest" [2]. Many of the currently available ICSI-associated techniques (e.g. testicular sperm retrieval) "force" gametes to meet, when this could never occur with natural fertility.

During natural conception, sperm first enter the female reproductive system near the anterior vagina and then rapidly pass through the cervical canal where they have to traverse the cervical mucus. They then enter the uterus and quickly move to the fallopian tubes to fertilize the oocyte. Unique molecules modulate all these events, and their presence and specific function ultimately affect early embryonic development [3, 4]. With ICSI, sperm bypass nearly all biological barriers and filtering steps that would potentially eliminate it from reaching the oocyte.

Current sperm preparation techniques, such as simple wash (SW), swim-up (SU), or density gradient centrifugation (DGC), essentially aim at ameliorating overall quality by eliminating immotile and morphologically abnormal sperm from the initially heterogeneous population found in semen. However, these methods have already been documented as being far away from natural selection that takes place in vivo [5–7].

Besides basic morphologic and viability parameters such as motility, these techniques do not specifically eliminate sperm with DNA fragmentation. Multiple centrifugation steps may also generate oxidative stress themselves, which may inadvertently increase DNA fragmentation levels in vitro [8]. There is a clear need to implement novel sperm selection technologies into our current clinical practice in order to use mature sperm with optimal membrane/organelle structure and healthy genetic/genomic content.

88.1 Success of Current ICSI Applications

Although ICSI is a successful technology, there is major concern when "poorer quality" sperm are selected for microinjection. Defective spermatogenesis may lead to chromosomal, nuclear, membrane, and mitochondrial abnormalities. Sperm may acquire these abnormalities either during production in the testis or during postproduction transport through the testis and storage in the epididymis. Spermatogenesis-related apoptosis, spermiogenesis-related DNA strand breaks due to chromatin remodelling, and post-testicular sperm transport-related DNA fragmentation induced by reactive oxygen species (ROS) can create profound negative effects on sperm health [9].

Currently available robust sperm diagnostic tests are useful to evaluate several morphological or genetic abnormalities, but they cannot yet select functional sperm to use for ICSI. Therefore, indirect markers are mostly taken as the main selection criteria, and this may result in microinjection of poor quality sperm in clinics worldwide [10].

For many years, the success of natural conception has been associated with sperm morphology, and use of morphologically normal sperm is linked to successful pregnancy after ICSI [11]. However, selecting sperm with normal morphology may not necessarily exclude sperm with nuclear

N. Findikli (✉) · M. Bahceci
Bahçeci Fulya IVF Centre, Istanbul, Turkey
e-mail: nfindikli@bahceci.com

C. Celik-Ozenci
Faculty of Medicine, Department of Histology and Embryology, Akdeniz University, Antalya, Turkey

M. Serdarogullari
British Cyprus IVF Centre, Nicosia, Cyprus

G. N. Allahbadia et al. (eds.), *Textbook of Assisted Reproduction*, https://doi.org/10.1007/978-981-15-2377-9_88

defects. The prepared motile sperm fraction may contain a high proportion of sperm with normal morphology, but some of these sperm may still have a high level of DNA fragmentation [12, 13]. One study showed that the absence of normal morphology does not eliminate the chance of getting pregnant, as 29.2% of such cases can achieve pregnancy via natural conception, indicating that morphology per se may not be a strong and effective selection criterion for successful conception in vivo [14].

ICSI has now become the most widely used mode of ART. Establishment of successful pregnancies, even with poor quality sperm, may indicate a corrective role of selecting a single sperm for ICSI from ejaculated, as well as testicular biopsy samples [15–17]. However, whenever a poor sperm with high DNA fragmentation and aneuploidy is microinjected into an oocyte, the risk of potential miscarriage and possible defects in the progeny are increased.

In a recent review by Pereira et al. [18], the long-term safety of ICSI was analyzed, based on data from the past 25 years. Outcomes included congenital malformation rates, cognitive development, and the reproductive health of neonates, children, adolescents, and adults [18]. According to this extensive review, no difference in perinatal outcomes or congenital malformation risks was found when comparing ICSI-conceived and spontaneously conceived (SC) children.

While there are studies reporting adverse side effects of ICSI in perinatal outcomes, the major confounder seems to be the transfer of more than one embryo. Only a few studies report higher malformation rates linked to ICSI children, via national registries [19, 20]. Overall, the growth, development, cognitive function, and general medical and reproductive health (small study populations only) of ICSI children seem to be similar to their SC counterparts. Importantly, however, a possible relationship between increased imprinting defects and autism in ICSI children needs further research.

88.2 Advanced Sperm Selection Techniques

As mentioned previously, currently available diagnostic tests to analyze sperm DNA integrity, aneuploidy, and histone/protamine content involve assessment of the whole semen sample and hence cannot be useful in selecting individual sperm during "live" ICSI. In other words, although these diagnostic tests may be useful in understanding key sperm features in a given sample, these analyzed sperm cannot be later used for ICSI, since analysis requires fixation of the initial material, resulting in loss of viability. In order to overcome this problem, several novel approaches based on antigenic, electric, optic, ultrastructural, and mechanic/dynamic properties of sperm have been developed to help select sperm with the highest genetic integrity as possible.

88.2.1 Electrophoretic/Electrostatic Separation Systems

These systems are mainly based on the fact that mature sperm acquire a negative charge (around −16 to −20 mV) through binding of negatively charged glycoproteins on the sperm surface, as it passes through the epididymis. This is termed the "zeta potential."

Electrophoretic sperm separation was first proposed by Dr. John Aitken, with the first successful pregnancy reported by the same group in 2007 [21]. When utilizing this method in ejaculated, testicular, and frozen sperm samples, the DNA damage was reduced. However, a prospective controlled clinical trial failed to show statistically significant differences in rates of fertilization, embryo cleavage, top quality embryo production, and clinical pregnancy between electrophoretically separated sperm and sperm after DGS [22]. More research is therefore necessary to outline any benefits in selecting sperm based on the zeta potential for contemporary ART applications.

Chan and colleagues have developed a simple "zeta test" for selection of mature sperm [23]. In this method, a sperm sample is washed with serum-free medium and placed into a conical centrifuge tube with positive charge, allowing mature sperm with negative charge to attach on the walls of the tube. The attached sperm cells are then washed with serum-supplemented medium [24, 25]. Two recent studies have showed that this method could be superior in terms of selecting against sperm with DNA fragmentation and improving the fertilization and clinical outcome over conventional DGC [26, 27]. Use of the "zeta test" is easy and appears to be low cost. However, in order to ascertain the beneficial effects, more randomized controlled clinical trials (RCTs) are needed [28].

88.2.2 Magnetic-Activated Cell Sorting

Apoptosis is a programmed cell death which is characterized by specific cellular morphological characteristics and energy-dependent biochemical mechanisms including structural changes in membranes and DNA fragmentation [29]. During apoptosis, loss of membrane integrity leads to phospholipid phosphatidylserine externalization, which has high affinity for annexin V [30].

Annexin V, when combined with magnetic microspheres, can be used as a sperm marker to isolate apoptotic sperm from non-apoptotic ones via a procedure known as magnetic-activated cell sorting (MACS) [31]. Utilization of annexin

V-MACS and DGC has been shown to be effective in separating non-apoptotic sperm with higher motility, viability, and fertilization potential, resulting in an improved clinical pregnancy rate in ICSI cycles [31–33].

However, when utilizing combined DGC and MACS, no statistically difference was found in the live birth rate in ICSI couples using their own or donor gametes with moderate to high sperm DNA fragmentation. Also, use of MACS did not show any reduction in miscarriage rates [34]. Another study confirmed that the MACS-assisted sperm selection approach did not significantly affect the outcome (live birth rate) in couples undergoing ICSI in an oocyte donation program [35].

Besides a technical need to perform several centrifugation steps in order to purify non-apoptotic sperm, the possibility of injecting foreign particles (magnetic microspheres) into the oocytes by microinjecting MACS-sorted sperm has also raised some concerns.

Currently, although reports of successful deliveries are encouraging, this approach also awaits validation by large prospective RCTs in order to find wider clinical application worldwide [36, 37].

88.2.3 Hyaluronic Acid (HA) Binding

Oocytes are surrounded by cumulus cells which contain a high amount of hyaluronic acid (HA) in their extracellular matrix [38]. The sperm plasma membrane contains HA-binding sites that indicate that sperm have achieved a specific development and maturity [25, 39, 40]. Furthermore, sperm that bind to HA have been shown to have more intact or slightly capacitated acrosomes, less DNA deterioration, decreased chromosomal aneuploidy, as well as high motility and viability [39].

Currently, there are two commercially available methods in order to use sperm that binds to HA, namely, "physiological intracytoplasmic sperm injection" (PICSI™) and "Sperm Slow™" (Origio). It is worth noting that both methods require conventional sperm preparation techniques before they are used to select the HA-bound sperm.

In the last decade, several studies have been performed to analyze the efficiency of HA-selected sperm in a clinical setting, although contradictory results have been reported. One study showed that while fertilization rates increased with use of HA-sperm selection, its effect on pregnancy rate was only marginal [40]. Parmegiani and colleagues suggested that HA-sperm selection increases the number of sperm without DNA fragmentation resulting in improvement of embryo quality, while fertilization and pregnancy rates were not affected [41, 42]. However, in 2015, Huang and coworkers found that the sperm DNA integrity ratio did not differ significantly between sperm selected for ICSI from PVP or HA and that a well-trained embryologist can select sperm without DNA abnormality via conventional microscopy [43].

In 2013, a multicenter, double-blinded RCT suggested that the selection of sperm by its binding ability resulted in significant improvements in clinical outcomes and reduced pregnancy loss [44]. In this study, 802 couples were allocated to treatment according to the HA-binding capacity ratio of their sperm, with a low-binding group (<65% bound) and a high-binding group (>65% bound). With regard to implantation rates and clinical pregnancy rates, couples with low HA-binding showed a "promising" but "nonsignificant" increase, whereas the miscarriage rate was significantly lower when HA-bound sperm were used for ICSI.

A meta-analysis of both retrospective and prospective studies showed that when HA-selected sperm was used, while embryo quality and implantation rates improved, fertilization and pregnancy rates did not [45]. In a more recent study, HA-ICSI was demonstrated to improve fertilization rates and the live birth rate, but the difference was not statistically significant since the sample size was small [46].

By contrast, Erberelli and colleagues compared conventional morphology sperm selection and PICSI for male factor couples and found that PICSI achieved a considerably higher chance (almost fivefold) of pregnancy. Moreover, teratozoospermic patients benefited most from PICSI [47].

At this present time, it can be concluded that in order to further evaluate the useful effect of utilizing HA-selected sperm, multicenter RCT studies with a larger sample size in selected patients with male infertility and live birth rate as a primary endpoint are still needed.

88.2.4 Motile Sperm Organelle Morphology Examination

The motile sperm organelle morphology examination (MSOME) technique utilizes high magnification (×6600) of sperm in order to evaluate their nuclear morphology in real time and thus determine sperm with normal chromosomal content, chromatin condensation, and/or DNA integrity [48]. Via this technique, the sperm neck, tail, mitochondria, acrosome, post-acrosomal lamina, and nucleus can be evaluated. Figure 88.1 shows the sperm selected for ICSI under high magnification power.

The MSOME criteria define normal sperm nucleus as smooth, oval, and symmetrical without vacuoles (at most <4% of the nuclear area). However, in different years other MSOME classifications were introduced into the literature:

1. Based on the presence and size of vacuoles: four grades [49].
2. Based on the head shape, vacuoles, and head base: three classes [50].

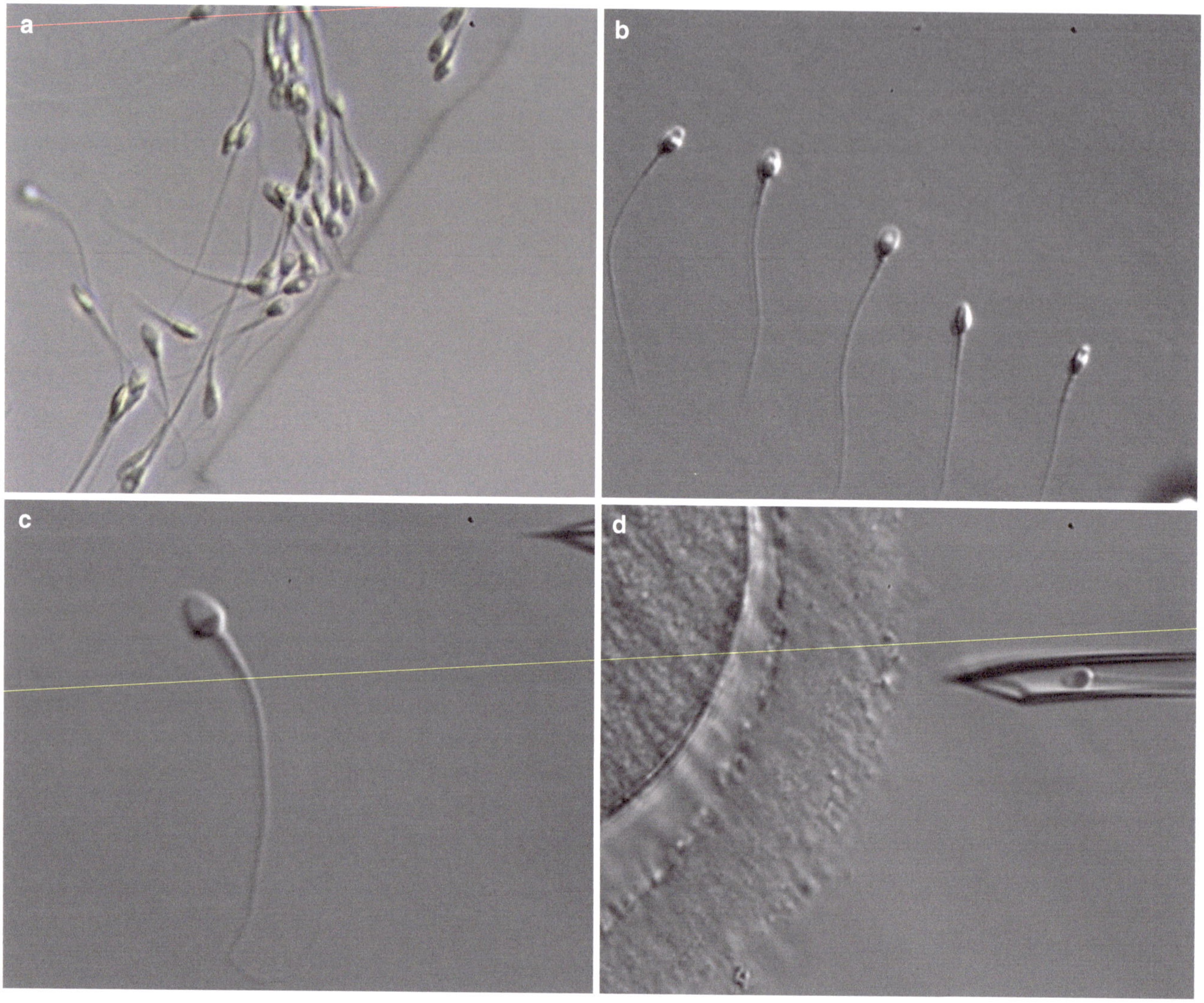

Fig. 88.1 Sperm being selected under high magnification. (**a**) Unselected sperm, (**b**) sperm showing large head-based vacuoles, (**c**) morphologically normal sperm selected for IMSI, (**d**) microinjection of IMSI-selected sperm

3. Five grades [51].
4. Three types [52]. Different classification methods were highly subjective for producing reproducible results.

Only one study has reported the reproducibility of MSOME evaluation which is based on the existence of vacuoles >50% of sperm head [53]. It has been found that small human sperm vacuoles utilizing high magnification technique reflect abnormal chromatin condensation [54]. Sperm defects-associated vacuoles include abnormalities with the acrosome and chromatin compaction [55–57]. However, no increase in DNA fragmentation and in chromosomal aneuploidy has yet to be shown [56, 58].

In patients with at least two previous ICSI failures, Bartoov et al. used MSOME criteria to select motile sperm for ICSI and named the process as "intracytoplasmic morphologically selected sperm injection" (IMSI) [59]. It has been suggested that IMSI technique may eliminate sperm with multiple, small vacuoles which is frequently seen in asthenozoospermic patients, thus allowing the selection of sperm with better chromatin condensation.

According to a systematic literature review, IMSI continues to divide opinion [54]. It may be that only patients with recurrent implantation failure may benefit from this technique, but for now, it can be concluded that routine use of IMSI to increase clinical pregnancy rates and live birth rates and to decrease miscarriage and congenital abnormalities is not supported by current evidence. On the other hand, in patients with high rate of sperm aneuploidy and DNA fragmentation, as well as repeated ICSI failures, IMSI could be beneficial. Prospective RCTs are necessary in order to approve the benefits of utilizing IMSI for other clinical indications.

88.2.5 Birefringency (Double Refraction)

This method utilizes polarized light microscopy and is based on birefringency produced by directing polarized light onto longitudinally oriented protein filaments on the post-acrosomal region of the sperm. By using this technique, sperm concentration, motility, and viability have been shown to correlate with sperm birefringency [60]. Furthermore, the technology can also differentiate acrosome-reacted sperm.

Although the technique still needs further evaluation, sperm selected via a combination of birefringence and MSOME may have reduced DNA fragmentation. In theory, this combination may increase the rate of selecting sperm with intact DNA, by the use of a single microscope [61].

88.2.6 Microfluidics-Based Sperm Selection

Microfluidics-based devices have been gaining importance for sperm selection to mimic the in vivo sperm selection process. Microchannels sort sperm according to density, shape, and motility, thereby eliminating the need for centrifugation steps [62–64].

Microfluidics can be advantageous over conventional sperm preparation methods by offering lower levels of DNA damage and circumventing production of reactive oxygen species (ROS) that can be generated through centrifugation steps during swim-up or density gradient separation [63–65].

However, despite these promising results, current microfluidics-based sperm selection approaches face two important challenges:

1. Although selection efficiency in the proof-of-concept studies is high, quantities are generally too small to be applicable in current clinical practice.
2. Comprehensive validation is still needed for the methods. Further research and extensive RCTs are required to evaluate the safety and usefulness of these approaches.

88.2.7 Selecting Immotile but Viable Sperm for ICSI

For ICSI, viable sperm should be used, with motility being the primary indicator of viability. During ICSI, immotile sperm is a challenge for patients with genetic-based Kartagener's Syndrome and almost all testicular sperm associated with nonobstructive azoospermia.

The World Health Organization (WHO) describes viability testing via eosin-nigrosin staining and the hypoosmotic swelling (HOS) test [66]. With regard to immotile sperm "on the day of ICSI," laser-assisted immotile sperm selection (LAISS) is a possibility [67]. This is an alternative to the HOS test and the sperm tail flexibility test (STFT), but further RCTs are needed to support its application.

Chemical motility enhancers, such as pentoxifylline or theophylline, can also be used, but the long-term effect of potential harm to the gametes requires further research.

88.3 Development of New Technologies for Sperm Selection

This section looks at recent developments in ART using new technologies in addition to conventional and advanced sperm preparation techniques.

88.3.1 Raman Spectroscopy

Raman spectroscopy is based on the principle that every atomic particle produces a unique change or shift in frequency and wavelength (Raman effect) when a photon is directed onto it. It has been recently reported that sperm with intact DNA can be identified by using this innovative noninvasive technology.

Since sperm with normal morphology may have high levels of DNA fragmentation, Raman spectrometry may provide important knowledge about the sperm chromatin and nucleus [24, 68, 69]. Reproducible detection of certain patterns associated with DNA fragmentation have been reported [69]. However, since the analysis has to be performed on fixed sperm samples, the clinical use of such novel sperm selection technique has not yet been reported.

88.3.2 Confocal Light Absorption and Scattering Microscopy

Confocal light absorption and scattering microscope (CLASS) combines confocal microscopy with light-scattering spectroscopy (LSS) [70, 71]. This technology provides an opportunity to examine internal cell structures with highly specific contrast using a physical parameter that differs from other microscopy techniques [24, 71]. Furthermore, the CLASS technique allows individual organelles in living cells to be noninvasively observed [71]. However, CLASS microscopy has not yet been use to analyze sperm ultrastructure [24].

88.3.3 Sperm Chemotaxis

Recent studies show that there are two active sperm guidance mechanisms in mammals. Sperm chemotaxis is known as a cell transport mechanism where sperm is guided towards the egg in natural conception. Sperm thermotaxis, which can be termed as movement of sperm cells along a temperature gradient, may also play an important role [24, 72, 73].

Sperm chemotaxis has been showed in various species including humans, with heat-stable peptides and progesterone as potential attractants [72, 74, 75]. Xie's group has developed a microchannel-based device to monitor sperm motility and chemotaxis which aims to mimic the mammalian female reproductive tract [75]. However, so far there are no reports on the effect of chemotaxis-selected sperm on ART outcomes.

88.4 Conclusion and Future Directions

Our current approaches on selecting the most compatible sperm for ICSI are progressing slowly, from morphology-based approaches to systems involving noninvasive detection of molecular properties that discriminate between healthy and abnormal sperm. Each approach has its own advantages and limitations. While improved clinical outcomes have been reported, nearly all of currently available sperm selection approaches lack properly designed large prospective RCTs to validate their potential in routine clinical use.

Coupled with techniques that mimic natural sperm selection in vivo, there is no doubt that future research will continue to devise and improve novel methods to detect physiologically competent, morphologically normal, and genetically healthy sperm that can be validated for clinical use.

References

1. van der Horst G, Maree L. Sperm form and function in the absence of sperm competition. Mol Reprod Dev. 2014;81(3):204–16. https://doi.org/10.1002/mrd.22277.
2. Palermo G, Joris H, Devroey P, Van Steirteghem AC. Pregnancies after intracytoplasmic injection of single spermatozoon into an oocyte. Lancet. 1992;340(8810):17–8. https://www.ncbi.nlm.nih.gov/pubmed/1351601
3. Krawetz SA. Paternal contribution: new insights and future challenges. Nat Rev Genet. 2005;6(8):633–42. https://doi.org/10.1038/nrg1654.
4. Suarez SS, Pacey AA. Sperm transport in the female reproductive tract. Hum Reprod Update. 2006;12(1):23–37. https://doi.org/10.1093/humupd/dmi047.
5. Beydola T, Sharma RK, Lee W, Agarwal A. Sperm preparation and selection techniques. In: Male infertility practice. 2013. p. 244–51.
6. Mehta A, Sigman M. Identification and preparation of sperm for ART. Urol Clin North Am. 2014;41(1):169–80. https://doi.org/10.1016/j.ucl.2013.08.005.
7. Sakkas D, Ramalingam M, Garrido N, Barratt CL. Sperm selection in natural conception: what can we learn from mother nature to improve assisted reproduction outcomes? Hum Reprod Update. 2015;21(6):711–26. https://doi.org/10.1093/humupd/dmv042.
8. Aitken RJ, Bronson R, Smith TB, De Iuliis GN. The source and significance of DNA damage in human spermatozoa; a commentary on diagnostic strategies and straw man fallacies. Mol Hum Reprod. 2013;19(8):475–85. https://doi.org/10.1093/molehr/gat025.
9. Sakkas D, Alvarez JG. Sperm DNA fragmentation: mechanisms of origin, impact on reproductive outcome, and analysis. Fertil Steril. 2010;93(4):1027–36. https://doi.org/10.1016/j.fertnstert.2009.10.046.
10. Sakkas D. Novel technologies for selecting the best sperm for in vitro fertilization and intracytoplasmic sperm injection. Fertil Steril. 2013;99(4):1023–9. https://doi.org/10.1016/j.fertnstert.2012.12.025.
11. van der Merwe FH, Kruger TF, Oehninger SC, Lombard CJ. The use of semen parameters to identify the subfertile male in the general population. Gynecol Obstet Investig. 2005;59(2):86–91. https://doi.org/10.1159/000082368.
12. Abu Hassan Abu D, Franken DR, Hoffman B, Henkel R. Accurate sperm morphology assessment predicts sperm function. Andrologia. 2012;44(Suppl 1):571–7. https://doi.org/10.1111/j.1439-0272.2011.01229.x.
13. Avendano C, Franchi A, Taylor S, Morshedi M, Bocca S, Oehninger S. Fragmentation of DNA in morphologically normal human spermatozoa. Fertil Steril. 2009;91(4):1077–84. https://doi.org/10.1016/j.fertnstert.2008.01.015.
14. Kovac JR, Smith RP, Cajipe M, Lamb DJ, Lipshultz LI. Men with a complete absence of normal sperm morphology exhibit high rates of success without assisted reproduction. Asian J Androl. 2017;19(1):39–42. https://doi.org/10.4103/1008-682X.189211.
15. Palermo GD, Neri QV, Takeuchi T, Rosenwaks Z. ICSI: where we have been and where we are going. Semin Reprod Med. 2009;27(2):191–201. https://doi.org/10.1055/s-0029-1202309.
16. Virro MR, Larson-Cook KL, Evenson DP. Sperm chromatin structure assay (SCSA) parameters are related to fertilization, blastocyst development, and ongoing pregnancy in in vitro fertilization and intracytoplasmic sperm injection cycles. Fertil Steril. 2004;81(5):1289–95. https://doi.org/10.1016/j.fertnstert.2003.09.063.
17. Vloeberghs V, Verheyen G, Haentjens P, Goossens A, Polyzos NP, Tournaye H. How successful is TESE-ICSI in couples with non-obstructive azoospermia? Hum Reprod. 2015;30(8):1790–6. https://doi.org/10.1093/humrep/dev139.
18. Pereira N, O'Neill C, Lu V, Rosenwaks Z, Palermo GD. The safety of intracytoplasmic sperm injection and long-term outcomes. Reproduction. 2017;154(6):F61–70. https://doi.org/10.1530/REP-17-0344.
19. Belva F, Henriet S, Liebaers I, Van Steirteghem A, Celestin-Westreich S, Bonduelle M. Medical outcome of 8-year-old singleton ICSI children (born >or=32 weeks' gestation) and a spontaneously conceived comparison group. Hum Reprod. 2007;22(2):506–15. https://doi.org/10.1093/humrep/del372.
20. Davies MJ, Moore VM, Willson KJ, Van Essen P, Priest K, Scott H, et al. Reproductive technologies and the risk of birth defects. N Engl J Med. 2012;366(19):1803–13. https://doi.org/10.1056/NEJMoa1008095.
21. Ainsworth C, Nixon B, Jansen RP, Aitken RJ. First recorded pregnancy and normal birth after ICSI using electrophoretically isolated spermatozoa. Hum Reprod. 2007;22(1):197–200. https://doi.org/10.1093/humrep/del351.
22. Fleming SD, Ilad RS, Griffin AM, Wu Y, Ong KJ, Smith HC, et al. Prospective controlled trial of an electrophoretic method of sperm preparation for assisted reproduction: comparison with density gradient centrifugation. Hum Reprod. 2008;23(12):2646–51. https://doi.org/10.1093/humrep/den330.
23. Chan PJ, Jacobson JD, Corselli JU, Patton WC. A simple zeta method for sperm selection based on membrane charge.

Fertil Steril. 2006;85(2):481–6. https://doi.org/10.1016/j.fertnstert.2005.07.1302.
24. Ortega NM, Bosch P. Methods for sperm selection for in vitro fertilization. In vitro fertilization – innovative clinical and laboratory aspects. InTech; 2012.
25. Rappa KL, Rodriguez HF, Hakkarainen GC, Anchan RM, Mutter GL, Asghar W. Sperm processing for advanced reproductive technologies: where are we today? Biotechnol Adv. 2016;34(5):578–87. https://doi.org/10.1016/j.biotechadv.2016.01.007.
26. Kheirollahi-Kouhestani M, Razavi S, Tavalaee M, Deemeh MR, Mardani M, Moshtaghian J, et al. Selection of sperm based on combined density gradient and Zeta method may improve ICSI outcome. Hum Reprod. 2009;24(10):2409–16. https://doi.org/10.1093/humrep/dep088.
27. Nasr Esfahani MH, Deemeh MR, Tavalaee M, Sekhavati MH, Gourabi H. Zeta sperm selection improves pregnancy rate and alters sex ratio in male factor infertility patients: a double-blind, randomized clinical trial. Int J Fertil Steril. 2016;10(2):253–60. https://www.ncbi.nlm.nih.gov/pubmed/27441060
28. Said TM, Land JA. Effects of advanced selection methods on sperm quality and ART outcome: a systematic review. Hum Reprod Update. 2011;17(6):719–33. https://doi.org/10.1093/humupd/dmr032.
29. Elmore S. Apoptosis: a review of programmed cell death. Toxicol Pathol. 2007;35(4):495–516. https://doi.org/10.1080/01926230701320337.
30. Romany L, Garrido N, Motato Y, Aparicio B, Remohi J, Meseguer M. Removal of annexin V-positive sperm cells for intracytoplasmic sperm injection in ovum donation cycles does not improve reproductive outcome: a controlled and randomized trial in unselected males. Fertil Steril. 2014;102(6):1567–75. e1. https://doi.org/10.1016/j.fertnstert.2014.09.001.
31. Gil M, Sar-Shalom V, Melendez Sivira Y, Carreras R, Checa MA. Sperm selection using magnetic activated cell sorting (MACS) in assisted reproduction: a systematic review and meta-analysis. J Assist Reprod Genet. 2013;30(4):479–85. https://doi.org/10.1007/s10815-013-9962-8.
32. Delbes G, Herrero MB, Troeung ET, Chan PT. The use of complimentary assays to evaluate the enrichment of human sperm quality in asthenoteratozoospermic and teratozoospermic samples processed with Annexin-V magnetic activated cell sorting. Andrology. 2013;1(5):698–706. https://doi.org/10.1111/j.2047-2927.2013.00106.x.
33. Lee TH, Liu CH, Shih YT, Tsao HM, Huang CC, Chen HH, et al. Magnetic-activated cell sorting for sperm preparation reduces spermatozoa with apoptotic markers and improves the acrosome reaction in couples with unexplained infertility. Hum Reprod. 2010;25(4):839–46. https://doi.org/10.1093/humrep/deq009.
34. Sanchez-Martin P, Dorado-Silva M, Sanchez-Martin F, Gonzalez Martinez M, Johnston SD, Gosalvez J. Magnetic cell sorting of semen containing spermatozoa with high DNA fragmentation in ICSI cycles decreases miscarriage rate. Reprod Biomed Online. 2017;34(5):506–12. https://doi.org/10.1016/j.rbmo.2017.01.015.
35. Romany L, Garrido N, Cobo A, Aparicio-Ruiz B, Serra V, Meseguer M. Obstetric and perinatal outcome of babies born from sperm selected by MACS from a randomized controlled trial. J Assist Reprod Genet. 2017;34(2):201–7. https://doi.org/10.1007/s10815-016-0838-6.
36. Polak de Fried E, Denaday F. Single and twin ongoing pregnancies in two cases of previous ART failure after ICSI performed with sperm sorted using annexin V microbeads. Fertil Steril. 2010;94(1):351.e15–8. https://doi.org/10.1016/j.fertnstert.2009.12.037.
37. Rawe VY, Boudri HU, Alvarez Sedo C, Carro M, Papier S, Nodar F. Healthy baby born after reduction of sperm DNA fragmentation using cell sorting before ICSI. Reprod Biomed Online. 2010;20(3):320–3. https://doi.org/10.1016/j.rbmo.2009.12.004.
38. Witt KD, Beresford L, Bhattacharya S, Brian K, Coomarasamy A, Cutting R, et al. Hyaluronic acid binding sperm selection for assisted reproduction treatment (HABSelect): study protocol for a multicentre randomised controlled trial. BMJ Open. 2016;6(10):e012609. https://doi.org/10.1136/bmjopen-2016-012609.
39. Mokanszki A, Tothne EV, Bodnar B, Tandor Z, Molnar Z, Jakab A, et al. Is sperm hyaluronic acid binding ability predictive for clinical success of intracytoplasmic sperm injection: PICSI vs. ICSI? Syst Biol Reprod Med. 2014;60(6):348–54. https://doi.org/10.3109/19396368.2014.948102.
40. Nasr-Esfahani MH, Razavi S, Vahdati AA, Fathi F, Tavalaee M. Evaluation of sperm selection procedure based on hyaluronic acid binding ability on ICSI outcome. J Assist Reprod Genet. 2008;25(5):197–203. https://doi.org/10.1007/s10815-008-9223-4.
41. Parmegiani L, Cognigni GE, Bernardi S, Troilo E, Ciampaglia W, Filicori M. "Physiologic ICSI": hyaluronic acid (HA) favors selection of spermatozoa without DNA fragmentation and with normal nucleus, resulting in improvement of embryo quality. Fertil Steril. 2010;93(2):598–604. https://doi.org/10.1016/j.fertnstert.2009.03.033.
42. Parmegiani L, Cognigni GE, Ciampaglia W, Pocognoli P, Marchi F, Filicori M. Efficiency of hyaluronic acid (HA) sperm selection. J Assist Reprod Genet. 2010;27(1):13–6. https://doi.org/10.1007/s10815-009-9380-0.
43. Huang MT, Kuo-Kuang Lee R, Lu CH, Chen YJ, Li SH, Hwu YM. The efficiency of conventional microscopic selection is comparable to the hyaluronic acid binding method in selecting spermatozoa for male infertility patients. Taiwan J Obstet Gynecol. 2015;54(1):48–53. https://doi.org/10.1016/j.tjog.2014.11.006.
44. Worrilow KC, Eid S, Woodhouse D, Perloe M, Smith S, Witmyer J, et al. Use of hyaluronan in the selection of sperm for intracytoplasmic sperm injection (ICSI): significant improvement in clinical outcomes—multicenter, double-blinded and randomized controlled trial. Hum Reprod. 2013;28(2):306–14. https://doi.org/10.1093/humrep/des417.
45. Beck-Fruchter R, Shalev E, Weiss A. Clinical benefit using sperm hyaluronic acid binding technique in ICSI cycles: a systematic review and meta-analysis. Reprod Biomed Online. 2016;32(3):286–98. https://doi.org/10.1016/j.rbmo.2015.12.001.
46. Liu Y, Feenan K, Chapple V, Roberts P, Matson P. Intracytoplasmic sperm injection using hyaluronic acid or polyvinylpyrrolidone: a time-lapse sibling oocyte study. Hum Fertil (Camb). 2017;22:1–8. https://doi.org/10.1080/14647273.2017.1366077.
47. Erberelli RF, Salgado RM, Pereira DH, Wolff P. Hyaluronan-binding system for sperm selection enhances pregnancy rates in ICSI cycles associated with male factor infertility. JBRA Assist Reprod. 2017;21(1):2–6. https://doi.org/10.5935/1518-0557.20170002.
48. Bartoov B, Berkovitz A, Eltes F. Selection of spermatozoa with normal nuclei to improve the pregnancy rate with intracytoplasmic sperm injection. N Engl J Med. 2001;345(14):1067–8. https://doi.org/10.1056/NEJM200110043451416.
49. Vanderzwalmen P, Hiemer A, Rubner P, Bach M, Neyer A, Stecher A, et al. Blastocyst development after sperm selection at high magnification is associated with size and number of nuclear vacuoles. Reprod Biomed Online. 2008;17(5):617–27. https://www.ncbi.nlm.nih.gov/pubmed/18983745.
50. Cassuto NG, Bouret D, Plouchart JM, Jellad S, Vanderzwalmen P, Balet R, et al. A new real-time morphology classification for human spermatozoa: a link for fertilization and improved embryo quality. Fertil Steril. 2009;92(5):1616–25. https://doi.org/10.1016/j.fertnstert.2008.08.088.
51. Mauri AL, Petersen CG, Oliveira JB, Massaro FC, Baruffi RL, Franco JG Jr. Comparison of day 2 embryo quality after conventional ICSI versus intracytoplasmic morphologically selected sperm injection (IMSI) using sibling oocytes. Eur J Obstet

Gynecol Reprod Biol. 2010;150(1):42–6. https://doi.org/10.1016/j.ejogrb.2010.01.004.
52. Perdrix A, Saidi R, Menard JF, Gruel E, Milazzo JP, Mace B, et al. Relationship between conventional sperm parameters and motile sperm organelle morphology examination (MSOME). Int J Androl. 2012;35(4):491–8. https://doi.org/10.1111/j.1365-2605.2012.01249.x.
53. Oliveira JB, Petersen CG, Massaro FC, Baruffi RL, Mauri AL, Silva LF, et al. Motile sperm organelle morphology examination (MSOME): intervariation study of normal sperm and sperm with large nuclear vacuoles. Reprod Biol Endocrinol. 2010;8:56. https://doi.org/10.1186/1477-7827-8-56.
54. Boitrelle F, Guthauser B, Alter L, Bailly M, Bergere M, Wainer R, et al. High-magnification selection of spermatozoa prior to oocyte injection: confirmed and potential indications. Reprod Biomed Online. 2014;28(1):6–13. https://doi.org/10.1016/j.rbmo.2013.09.019.
55. Cassuto NG, Hazout A, Hammoud I, Balet R, Bouret D, Barak Y, et al. Correlation between DNA defect and sperm-head morphology. Reprod Biomed Online. 2012;24(2):211–8. https://doi.org/10.1016/j.rbmo.2011.10.006.
56. Perdrix A, Rives N. Motile sperm organelle morphology examination (MSOME) and sperm head vacuoles: state of the art in 2013. Hum Reprod Update. 2013;19(5):527–41. https://doi.org/10.1093/humupd/dmt021.
57. Perdrix A, Travers A, Chelli MH, Escalier D, Do Rego JL, Milazzo JP, et al. Assessment of acrosome and nuclear abnormalities in human spermatozoa with large vacuoles. Hum Reprod. 2011;26(1):47–58. https://doi.org/10.1093/humrep/deq297.
58. Boitrelle F, Ferfouri F, Petit JM, Segretain D, Tourain C, Bergere M, et al. Large human sperm vacuoles observed in motile spermatozoa under high magnification: nuclear thumbprints linked to failure of chromatin condensation. Hum Reprod. 2011;26(7):1650–8. https://doi.org/10.1093/humrep/der129.
59. Bartoov B, Berkovitz A, Eltes F, Kogosovsky A, Yagoda A, Lederman H, et al. Pregnancy rates are higher with intracytoplasmic morphologically selected sperm injection than with conventional intracytoplasmic injection. Fertil Steril. 2003;80(6):1413–9. https://www.ncbi.nlm.nih.gov/pubmed/14667877
60. Gianaroli L, Magli MC, Collodel G, Moretti E, Ferraretti AP, Baccetti B. Sperm head's birefringence: a new criterion for sperm selection. Fertil Steril. 2008;90(1):104–12. https://doi.org/10.1016/j.fertnstert.2007.05.078.
61. Garolla A, Cosci I, Menegazzo M, De Palo R, Ambrosini G, Sartini B, et al. Sperm selected by both birefringence and motile sperm organelle morphology examination have reduced deoxyribonucleic acid fragmentation. Fertil Steril. 2014;101(3):647–52. https://doi.org/10.1016/j.fertnstert.2013.11.029.
62. Asghar W, Velasco V, Kingsley JL, Shoukat MS, Shafiee H, Anchan RM, et al. Selection of functional human sperm with higher DNA integrity and fewer reactive oxygen species. Adv Healthc Mater. 2014;3(10):1671–9. https://doi.org/10.1002/adhm.201400058.
63. Nosrati R, Graham PJ, Zhang B, Riordon J, Lagunov A, Hannam TG, et al. Microfluidics for sperm analysis and selection. Nat Rev Urol. 2017;14(12):707–30. https://doi.org/10.1038/nrurol.2017.175.
64. Simon L, Emery BR, Carrell DT. Review: diagnosis and impact of sperm DNA alterations in assisted reproduction. Best Pract Res Clin Obstet Gynaecol. 2017;44:38–56. https://doi.org/10.1016/j.bpobgyn.2017.07.003.
65. Shirota K, Yotsumoto F, Itoh H, Obama H, Hidaka N, Nakajima K, et al. Separation efficiency of a microfluidic sperm sorter to minimize sperm DNA damage. Fertil Steril. 2016;105(2):315–21. e1. https://doi.org/10.1016/j.fertnstert.2015.10.023.
66. WHO. WHO laboratory manual for the examination and processing of human semen; 2010.
67. Nordhoff V. How to select immotile but viable spermatozoa on the day of intracytoplasmic sperm injection? An embryologist's view. Andrology. 2015;3(2):156–62. https://doi.org/10.1111/andr.286.
68. Huser T, Orme CA, Hollars CW, Corzett MH, Balhorn R. Raman spectroscopy of DNA packaging in individual human sperm cells distinguishes normal from abnormal cells. J Biophotonics. 2009;2(5):322–32. https://doi.org/10.1002/jbio.200910012.
69. Sanchez V, Redmann K, Wistuba J, Wubbeling F, Burger M, Oldenhof H, et al. Oxidative DNA damage in human sperm can be detected by Raman microspectroscopy. Fertil Steril. 2012;98(5):1124–9e1-3. https://doi.org/10.1016/j.fertnstert.2012.07.1059.
70. Fang H, Qiu L, Vitkin E, Zaman MM, Andersson C, Salahuddin S, et al. Confocal light absorption and scattering spectroscopic microscopy. Appl Opt. 2007;46(10):1760–9. https://www.ncbi.nlm.nih.gov/pubmed/17356619
71. Itzkan I, Qiu L, Fang H, Zaman MM, Vitkin E, Ghiran IC, et al. Confocal light absorption and scattering spectroscopic microscopy monitors organelles in live cells with no exogenous labels. Proc Natl Acad Sci USA. 2007;104(44):17255–60. https://doi.org/10.1073/pnas.0708669104.
72. Eisenbach M, Giojalas LC. Sperm guidance in mammals – an unpaved road to the egg. Nat Rev Mol Cell Biol. 2006;7(4):276–85. https://doi.org/10.1038/nrm1893.
73. Teves ME, Guidobaldi HA, Unates DR, Sanchez R, Miska W, Publicover SJ, et al. Molecular mechanism for human sperm chemotaxis mediated by progesterone. PLoS One. 2009;4(12):e8211. https://doi.org/10.1371/journal.pone.0008211.
74. Teves ME, Barbano F, Guidobaldi HA, Sanchez R, Miska W, Giojalas LC. Progesterone at the picomolar range is a chemoattractant for mammalian spermatozoa. Fertil Steril. 2006;86(3):745–9. https://doi.org/10.1016/j.fertnstert.2006.02.080.
75. Xie L, Ma R, Han C, Su K, Zhang Q, Qiu T, et al. Integration of sperm motility and chemotaxis screening with a microchannel-based device. Clin Chem. 2010;56(8):1270–8. https://doi.org/10.1373/clinchem.2010.146902.

Selecting Sperm with Hyaluronic Acid: Evidence Base for Efficacy and Practical Applications

89

David Miller

Since the first reported successful birth in 1978, assisted reproduction technology (ART) or medically assisted reproduction (MAR) has become a major clinical service for the treatment of infertility, which is estimated to affect 15% of those couples seeking to reproduce. The most recent aggregate figure for the years between and including 2008–2010 indicated that globally, almost 4.7 million treatment cycles were carried out resulting in the birth of over 1.14 million babies [1]. Simple arithmetic shows that the success rate per treatment cycle is approximately 24%, a figure that has remained relatively static in the last 10 years.

Natural cycle success rates among younger women are thought to be similar to those encountered with MAR, and both natural and MAR failures have many common causes (including life-incompatible congenital abnormalities [2]). However, a significant but poorly defined proportion of losses are of unknown cause [3]. If we could better identify and avoid these causes, there is no biological reason preventing improvements in MAR success rates overall. Quality considerations for both sperm and egg are clearly important in this regard, and much research is aimed at understanding how to assess gamete quality and aid the identification and selection of better quality gametes for MAR.

For IVF and IUI, sperm must have the capacity for swimming and fertilizing the egg; hence, good progressive motility is an acceptable quality indicator. Although ICSI removes the need altogether, sperm motility continues to be a good qualitative indicator for most embryologists. While success rates for the two principle interventions (IVF and ICSI) are reasonably well-matched [4], as embryologists have only one chance per egg of choosing the best sperm for injection, alternative, non-destructive methods of quality assessment for ICSI remain desirable. Overall pregnancy rates per treatment cycle estimated at ~35% need to rise if success rates are to increase concomitantly. In addition to this rise, there needs to be a corresponding fall in the rates of pregnancy loss estimated to affect ~8% of all ART cycles [5] and up to 20% of all clinical pregnancies [6].

This chapter focuses on one promising, non-destructive, physiological method for selecting better quality sperm and increasing success rates based on the hypothesis, supported by good evidence, that sperm binding to the naturally occurring polysaccharide, hyaluronic acid (HA) are of better quality than sperm unable to bind to this natural polymer [7–9]. Evidence suggests that a reduction in pregnancy loss appears to be the main clinical improvement arising from sperm captured by this procedure and used for ICSI [8, 10–12]. Although further confirmatory work is needed, in this writer's opinion, the procedure works and, with further optimisation, could bring useful benefits to patients.

89.1 Hyaluronic Acid (HA) and HA-Interacting Proteins

Hyaluronic acid (HA) is a non-sulphated glycosaminoglycan (GAG) composed of repeating disaccharide units of D-glucuronic acid and *N*-acetyl D-glucosamine (Fig. 89.1). In common with the sulphated GAGs, dermatan, keratan and chondroitin sulphates, HA is widely distributed throughout the body and is an important component of extracellular matrix including those of the cervix and the glycocalyx of the cumulus oophorus complex [13, 14].

Sperm express two distinct classes of HA-interacting proteins: hyaluronidases, which as the name signifies are enzymes that digest or degrade HA [15, 16], and HA-binding proteins (HABPs), which can recognise and 'tether' sperm to HA-rich, supporting scaffolds [17, 18]. These two types of proteins have mutually exclusive modus operandi, and while some of the sperm hyaluronidases have been characterised, including PH20/SPAM1 [19], little is known about sperm HABPs.

D. Miller (✉)
Discovery and Translational Science Department, Leeds Institute of Cardiovascular and Metabolic Medicine (LICAMM), University of Leeds, Leeds, UK
e-mail: d.miller@leeds.ac.uk

G. N. Allahbadia et al. (eds.), *Textbook of Assisted Reproduction*, https://doi.org/10.1007/978-981-15-2377-9_89

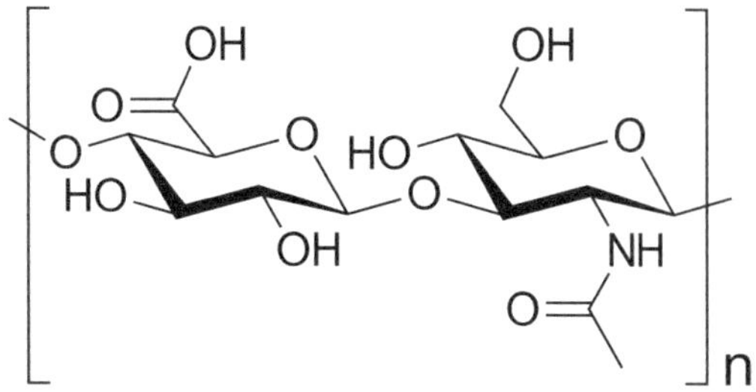

Fig. 89.1 The basic disaccharide repeating subunit of hyaluronic acid. D-glucuronic acid and *N*-acetyl-D-glucosamine are drawn from left to right. The number of repeats (n) varies from hundreds to millions, depending on source and location (courtesy of Wikipedia Commons)

Two such proteins, CD44 [20] and RHAMM [21], have been described in sperm with evidence for additional sperm HABPs reported recently [22]. CD44 is thought to be an important mediator of orchestrated somatic cell migration, which depends on the protein's interaction with HA. While strong, this interaction needs also to be temporary, permitting cell movement to take place and, as importantly, in an organised manner. Disorganised or otherwise abnormal binding (or lack thereof) to HA is thought to confer or promote pathological phenotypes, including malignancy [23]. The precise roles of sperm HABPs, however, remain relatively unclear although their expression in relation to sperm maturity and quality may be physiologically related to the ability of sperm to temporarily 'park' during ascent of the female reproductive tract [24].

Quality indices relating to their HA-binding potential originate from morphological aspects of sperm recovered from the HA-rich endocervix, which correspond most closely with Tygerberg strict criteria [25, 26]. Although the most recent WHO guidelines on semen analysis 'downgraded' the lower reference limit for sperm morphology to ≤5% normal forms [27], sperm shape remains a useful indicator of 'normality' because shape is closely related to density, which is the main physical property responsible for the sedimentation of sperm in a differential density gradient [28].

Early work reported that sperm 'captured' on HA-coated surfaces resemble those enmeshed in and recovered from the endocervical mucus [29]. HA-captured sperm, for example, have less residual cytoplasm, more compact chromatin with fewer aneuploidies and lower levels of DNA fragmentation, all thought to be important indicators of functional fertile sperm [26]. Hence, HA-binding sperm appear to be physically equivalent to, or at least similar to, sperm sedimenting into the 80–90% fraction of a typical discontinuous density gradient [30].

Experimental evidence for this connection has come from several sources. Using a cytogenetic approach, Huszar reported differences in the frequencies of aneuploid sperm recovered from semen and 80% Percoll fractions [31]. He later showed that sperm binding to HA-coated surfaces had lower levels of aneuploidy than sperm in the original unprepared semen samples [32]. Lower levels of DNA fragmentation, more condensed DNA and less residual cytoplasm are encountered among HA-binding sperm [33, 34].

We recently provided further corroborative evidence for these findings by concurrently assaying for DNA fragmentation and DNA compaction levels in density-gradient fractionated and HA-binding/non-binding sperm populations [30]. These experiments showed that the routine differential density gradient preparation of sperm for ART as developed originally in the early 1990s is reasonably good at enrichment of better quality sperm, which are also more motile, presumably because such sperm are more physically mature [28]. Higher motility also confers a greater chance of sperm interacting with and binding to HA, a feature used by the clinically relevant commercial products developed to exploit sperm HA-binding properties for ICSI intervention [35].

89.2 HA-Dependent Products and Processes Developed Specifically for MAR

Being highly hygroscopic, HA-based formulations are in much demand by the cosmetics industry as important additives to moisturising creams and other potions [36]. HA is also widely used to relieve symptoms of mechanically derived inflammation arising from arthritic conditions, often by direct injection to the affected joint [36]. The ability of more mature and motile sperm to recognise and bind HA and the evidence indicating that such sperm are molecularly more competent and therefore more likely to support successful fertilization and subsequent development has spurred efforts leading to its clinical use and commercial exploitation for ART.

At its most basic, this exploitation has led to the development of highly viscous, HA-containing products compositionally similar to EmbryoGlue™. Two such products, 'Sperm Catch' and 'Sperm Slow', are marketed as a more physiological and hence 'safer' alternative to polyvinylpyrrolidone (PVP) commonly used to slow sperm down sufficiently for easier capture prior to ICSI procedures [37]. PVP is a biologically inert compound with no reported toxicity that long before its use in ART practice and procedures was being (and still is) widely used by the food and pharmaceuticals industry [38].

'Sperm Catch' was developed in response to concerns about the potential toxicity of PVP following its unavoidable introduction to eggs and to embryos [37]. In addition to its motility retarding properties, 'Sperm Slow' is also described as a product capable of aiding the embryologist select better quality sperm for potential injection by their dynamic interaction with HA. By adding a droplet of the product to a culture dish and placing it in contact with a droplet of suitably prepared sperm suspended in a typical wash or holding medium, the embryologist can pick from those sperm swimming towards and then contacting the wash buffer/'Sperm Slow' interface (Fig. 89.2). Sperm remaining in contact with the interface are thought to have similar properties to the HA-binding sperm described above. While this may be so, this writer is of the opinion that the sperm/HA interaction observed with 'Sperm Slow' and related products is more of an effect of differential viscosity than physiological HA-binding per se [39].

The 'physiological ICSI' (PICSI) dish is a more engineered product that uses drops or plaques of HA, physically bonded and sitting at one end of a narrow channel cut into the plastic surface of a typical ART-type culture dish (Fig. 89.3). After rehydrating the plaque with a suitable culture medium, a prepared sperm suspension is introduced to the channel, and sperm are given sufficient time to swim towards and interact with the HA plaque. The embryologist can then select tethered sperm for potential injection (see https://fertility.coopersurgical.com/dishes/picsi-dish-for-sperm-selection/).

A related but separate development of the PICSI platform enables estimates of the percentage of HA-binding sperm in a sample to be determined in a manner similar to that used for conventional counting (e.g., using a counting chamber such as a Cell-Vu; Fig. 89.4). A prepared sperm suspension is introduced to the slide chamber, with a micrometre grid etched into its surface and on which HA is bonded. Sperm contacting the substrate either bind to the HA or continue to swim unimpeded. Counting tethered and total sperm allows the proportion of bound sperm to be calculated.

Empirically derived data has shown that most fertile (by the WHO criteria) normozoospermic men have HA-binding scores (HBS) ≥65%. Oligozoospermic and asthenozoospermic men, on the other hand, have lower scores (<65%) with particularly low scores seen in oligoasthenozoospermic men [40–42]. Although, in general, men with lower sperm counts tend to have lower values, being a frequency estimate, HBS has to be considered in the context of the background sperm count and motility measure. Due to the high variation observed in sampled populations, the 65% cut-off for normal/low HBS is somewhat arbitrary. Nevertheless, published data has shown a straightforward positive correlation

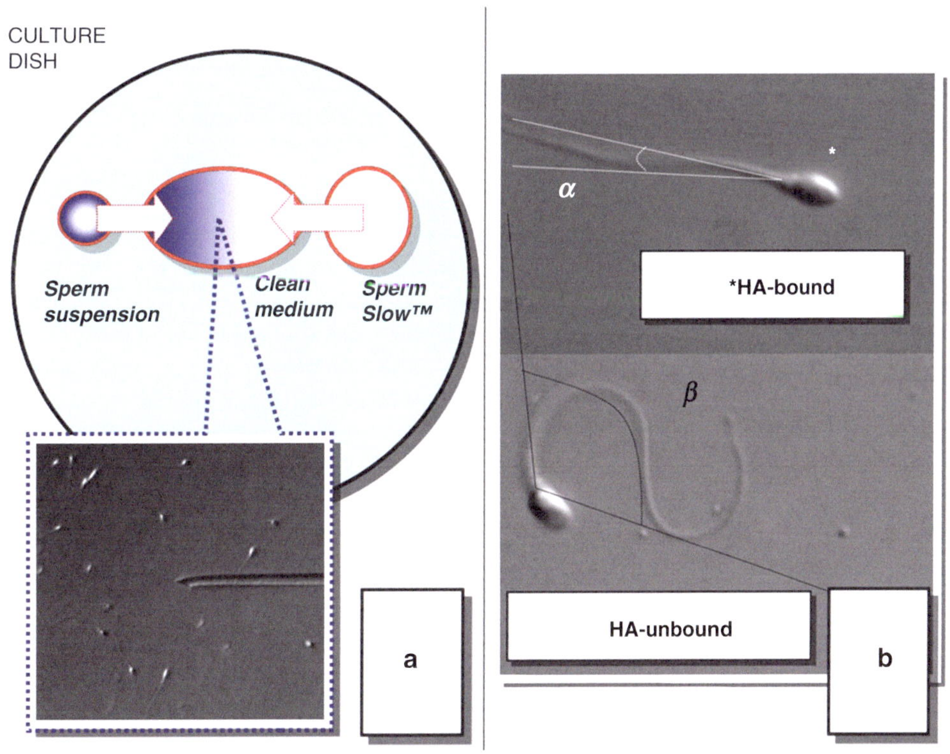

Fig. 89.2 Use of Sperm Slow in clinical practice. (*a*) Droplets of a sperm suspension and Sperm Slow are brought into contact with each other and allowed to interact. Sperm at the interface is selected for injection. (*b*) Close-up view of a sperm interacting with Sperm Slow. Interacting sperm have straightened tails and are relatively immobile (α), while free-swimming sperm have beating tails with a high amplitude (ß) (from Parmegiani L, Cognigni GE, Bernardi S, Troilo E, Taraborrelli S, Arnone A, et al. Comparison of two ready-to-use systems designed for sperm-hyaluronic acid binding selection before intracytoplasmic sperm injection: PICSI vs. Sperm Slow: a prospective, randomized trial. Fertil Steril. 2012 Sep;98(3):632–7, with permission)

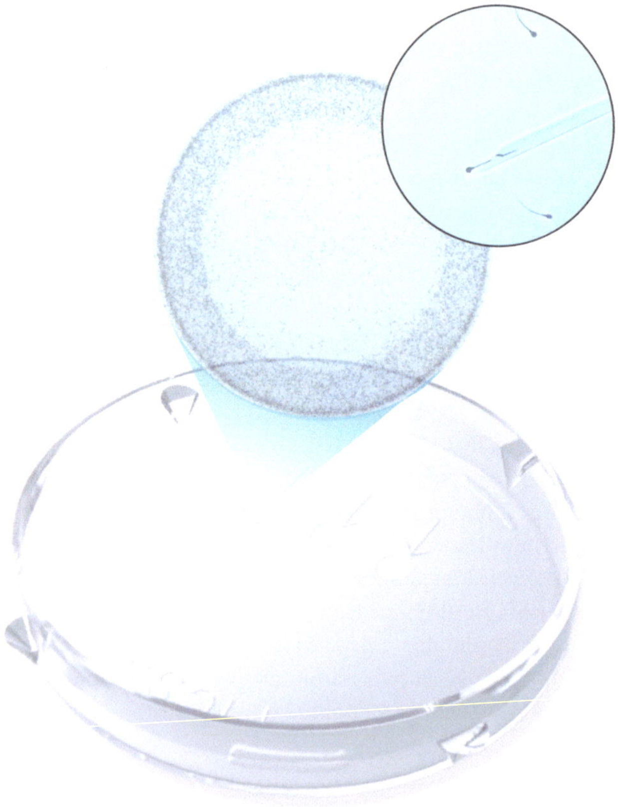

Fig. 89.3 The PICSI platform showing one of the three plaques of HA at one end of the three channels cut into the plastic base. Sperm suspensions placed in the channels swim towards and interact with the HA substrate where they can be selected for injection. (Reproduced with permission of Biocoat Incorporated)

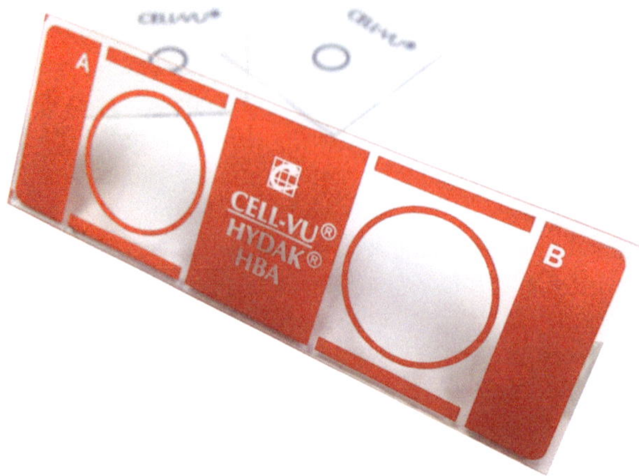

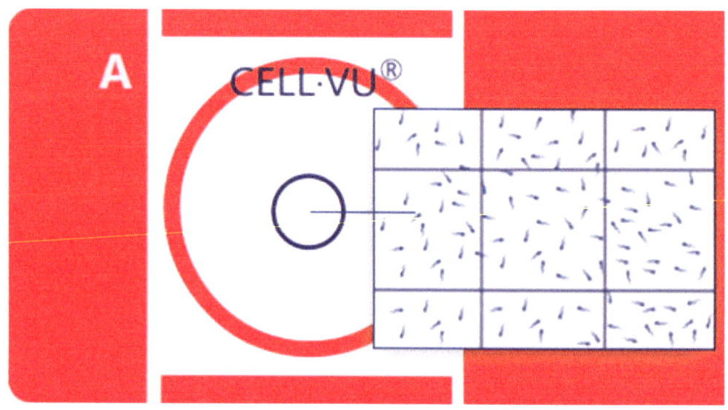

Fig. 89.4 The Hydak HA-binding scoring slide showing the two counting chambers with the grid used to aid sperm counting and assessment of bound versus unbound sperm. (Reproduced with permission of Biocoat Incorporated)

between increasing sperm concentration and motility and increasing HA-binding score [40–42], with studies supporting [11, 41] or not supporting [40, 42, 43] a connection with reported ART outcomes.

89.3 Evidence for Clinical Efficacy of MAR Using HA-Binding Sperm

As ICSI is clearly the target ART for HA-based selection strategies and HA-binding sperm are thought to be of higher overall quality, clinical assessment of HA-binding efficacy in the context of ART is fully justified. Ideally, assessment should be in the form of randomised clinical trials (RCT) of sufficient power. Unfortunately, most reports to date have been insufficiently powered or were not RCTs [7, 11, 12, 35, 44].

Data from four RCTs are available [10, 44–46], one of which [46] was adequately powered from the outset. Parmegiani et al. [45] reported statistically higher numbers of Grade 1 embryos following ICSI using 'Sperm Slow' rather than PVP in the sperm selection process and a significantly improved implantation rate. Parmegiani also reported on the relationship between sperm DNA fragmentation, nuclear morphology and HA-binding capacity [47]. Although sample sizes were small, statistically significant differences in DNA fragmentation and morphology were reported between sperm from the initial sample with swum-up samples, sperm held in PVP or in 'Sperm Slow'. Parmegiani et al. [35] later reported on a small RCT comparing 'Sperm Slow' with PICSI indicating no particular advantage of using either, but this study did not compare with a standard PVP-based procedure.

In a much larger, multicentre RCT of PICSI versus ICSI, Worrilow et al. [10] reported a statistically significant reduction in miscarriage rates in the PICSI arm. The study prospectively stratified and split their cohort into low and normal HBS subgroups prior to the intervention with an equivalent cohort in the normal HBS subgroup not participating in the RCT (to control for seasonality and inter-site variations). The observed lowered miscarriage rate was confined to couples with lower HBS, determined from both the original semen sample and the sperm samples prepared by density gradient centrifugation (the 90% fraction used for ICSI).

There were no differences in other outcomes and live birth was not reported.

Following a retrospective stratification of couples by HBS, Mokanski et al. reported a statistically significant improvement in terms of LBR in their lower (≤60%) HBS subgroup, with a small reduction in LBR reported following PICSI in their >60% HBS subgroup. These data suggested that PICSI could be mildly detrimental to those with a normal semen profile (also indicated by Worrilow's group, who reported a small drop in clinical pregnancy in their PICSI subgroup). Miscarriage rates were also significantly reduced in the PICSI arm but, in this study, confined to the >60% HBS subgroup. Hence, the reported increase in LBR and the reduction in miscarriage may have been mutually exclusive effects of PICSI. The clinical pregnancy rate was significantly higher in Mokanski's PICSI group irrespective of HBS.

In the largest trial of PICSI efficacy undertaken to date, Miller et al. also reported a statistically significant reduction in miscarriage in the PICSI arm (HABSelect [48]). This study's design did not include stratification of couples before or allocation for randomisation by HBS, thus avoiding the potential for patient preselection bias. Taking into account frequently ignored treatment effects and interactions [49], this RCT's primary outcome measure reported a small clinical but statistically insignificant improvement in LBR following PICSI. Of the secondary outcome measures, miscarriage rates were significantly reduced in the PCISI group, and there was no significant difference reported in clinical pregnancy rates. A post-hoc analysis in relation to *clinical pregnancy* pushed the increase in term live birth into statistical significance.

HABSelect obtained HBS from prepared samples, where higher scoring sperm populations might be expected; however, processed sperm samples could still be stratified into normal and subnormal binding groups. Unlike previous studies from the groups led by Mokanski and Worrilow, where benefits of PICSI appeared to lie with couples with a lower HBS, HABSelect reported no clear clinical benefit or statistically significant differences between PICSI and ICSI arms for any of the HBS subcategories. There was also no statistically significant association between HBS and miscarriage rates reported in this study, although a trend for PICSI favouring those with low HBS was apparent, in agreement with the study by Worrilow et al. [41].

The HABSelect study was unusual in reporting beyond the main clinical findings on some mechanistic aspects, associated with patient age and sperm DNA integrity. The mechanistic analysis differed from the clinical analysis by including a hierarchical classification tree interrogation of the trial outcomes [50] and showed (not surprisingly) that older females had generally poorer outcomes and the highest miscarriage rates. The analysis, however, also showed that the protective effects of PICSI manifesting as reduced miscarriage rates fell primarily among those older patients.

Sperm DNA compaction measured by a combination of the sperm chromatin dispersion test [51] and aniline blue staining [52] was also associated with clinical pregnancy, with better compaction statistically more likely to support clinical pregnancy, regardless of PICSI. Sperm DNA fragmentation measured by TUNEL [53], acridine orange [54] and comet [55] assays was only marginally higher in samples associated with miscarriage outcomes, suggesting that PICSI had selected *against* sperm with higher rates of DNA fragmentation and so potentially incompatible with continuing pregnancy.

HABSelect's mechanistic outcomes indicated that if measures of sperm DNA integrity are sought, *original* semen as well as processed samples should be tested. This recommendation harks back to the main objective of processing, which is to enrich for higher quality sperm [30], and indicates the need to be cautious in the choice of sperm sampling for use in DNA integrity tests [56].

A few additional, small studies, mainly using PICSI, have reported either a lowered rate of miscarriage [7, 44] or no differences between interventions and controls [12] leaving a general consensus that sperm selection by HA-binding is most effective at reducing pregnancy loss. The intervention most likely selects for sperm with lower DNA fragmentation although this explanation is tentative and in need of further clarification.

The apparent paradox of HABSelect, where a significant reduction in miscarriage was not translated to a significant increase in live births, can be resolved when considering the relative population sizes and respective frequencies of these clinical outcomes. Miscarriage (~8% of all treatment cycles started [5]) is a relatively infrequent outcome compared with term live births (~25%), so a similar change in their frequencies will have a disproportionately greater and so statistically stronger impact on the smaller population. This effect was reported in the HABSelect study, where reducing the sample population size by *only* considering established clinical pregnancies, pushed the modest difference in term live birth rate favouring PICSI into statistical significance.

89.4 About the Future

In general, recent systematic reviews and data meta-analyses of the relevant literature highlight the deleterious effects of sperm DNA damage on ART outcomes [57–61] but are more equivocal over the beneficial effects of sperm selection aimed at counteracting it [12, 62]. In almost all cases considered by these reports, the highly variable nature of the studies themselves, in terms of design and outcomes, makes their conclusions less robust with the need for further studies.

It is this writer's view that the clinical evidence to date unequivocally supports the efficacy of selecting sperm by HA-binding for reducing miscarriage risk (particularly with older couples). The PICSI platform provided the main evidence for this effect, but there is no reason in principle why alternative HA-binding platforms or processes could not perform similarly if appropriately set up and assessed. The modus operandi appears to be the straightforward selection of sperm for injection with lower levels of DNA fragmentation (perhaps a specific type), and the most likely reason that this has the greatest benefit for older couples is that the capacity for sperm DNA repair by the eggs of older women is weaker [63]. With couples increasingly delaying their attempts to start a family, finding appropriate ways of counteracting their reduced fertility is likely to become more urgent.

The rise of ICSI in the past decade or so has been relentless, and there is justified clinical resistance to its use beyond that for which it was originally intended. On the assumption that conventional IVF offers some protection against fertilization with compromised sperm, there is an argument for restricting the use of ICSI to only those who truly need it [64]. Nevertheless, the trend is clear, and some centres have now abandoned IVF altogether [65].

The relationship between sperm DNA fragmentation and adverse ART outcomes is stronger for failed IVF than for ICSI where the experienced embryologist is relatively competent at avoiding compromised sperm [58] and IVF fails because the oocyte is either not fertilized or implantation of the transferred embryo does not occur. Despite the experience of the embryologist, however, miscarriage associated with higher burdens of sperm DNA fragmentation still occurs following ICSI [60, 61, 66]. Hence, the development of novel, more robust processes for augmenting sperm selection for ICSI is fully justified [12, 67]. Sperm HA-binding for ICSI is the only process that has been rigorously (and realistically) tested to date in a clinical setting and shown to have some efficacy. Compared with the alternatives, HA-based processes like PICSI are relatively inexpensive and unlikely to add much to the cycle cost even taking into account the embryologist's time taken to undertake the additional intervention, although a cost-benefit analysis would be necessary to confirm this prediction.

All gamete selection methods are aimed at overcoming the three major levels of attrition holding back a clinically significant boost in term live birth rates arising from ART. The first level is fertilization, which determines subsequent egg activation and early embryogenesis; the second is implantation and clinical pregnancy which determine the chances of having a live birth or not, and the third is miscarriage which ultimately determines the final birth rate (including stillbirth). Focusing on miscarriage, only HABSelect was a large enough study to show a miscarriage rate matching the generally ART-encountered rates recorded by clinics [5]. Miscarriage is a relatively uncommon outcome of ART. However, unless steps are taken to counteract age-related increases in its risk, the incidence of miscarriage is likely to rise with an increasingly older reproducing population.

Neither of the largest studies on HA-binding reported significant increases in fertilization or clinical pregnancy rates, and we can assume, therefore, that the form of compromised sperm DNA integrity counteracted by HA binding has little influence at these 'lower' levels of progression. HABSelect did provide some evidence that DNA packaging, specifically, better compaction was important for establishing a clinical pregnancy (~35% of all treatment cycles). Taking age-related effects into account and assuming miscarriage rates are reduced as far as possible by interventions like HA selection; increasing the frequency of successful clinical pregnancies is the only route in increasing live birth rates overall.

In its defence, therefore, this writer is of the view that ICSI best ensures that male factors are overcome. Increased ART success rates will then depend on egg quality and a better understanding of the uterine environment into which embryos are ultimately transferred and the culture conditions in which they were maintained.

References

1. Dyer S, Chambers GM, de Mouzon J, Nygren KG, Zegers-Hochschild F, Mansour R, et al. International Committee for Monitoring Assisted Reproductive Technologies world report: assisted reproductive technology 2008, 2009 and 2010. Hum Reprod. 2016;31(7):1588–609.
2. Jenderny J. Chromosome aberrations in a large series of spontaneous miscarriages in the German population and review of the literature. Mol Cytogenet. 2014;7:38.
3. Margalioth EJ, Ben-Chetrit A, Gal M, Eldar-Geva T. Investigation and treatment of repeated implantation failure following IVF-ET. Hum Reprod. 2006;21(12):3036–43.
4. HFEA. A long term analysis of the HFEA Register data, 1991–2006. 2012.
5. Tummers P, De Sutter P, Dhont M. Risk of spontaneous abortion in singleton and twin pregnancies after IVF/ICSI. Hum Reprod. 2003;18(8):1720–3.
6. Garcia-Enguidanos A, Calle ME, Valero J, Luna S, Dominguez-Rojas V. Risk factors in miscarriage: a review. Eur J Obstet Gynecol Reprod Biol. 2002;102(2):111–9.
7. Erberelli RF, Salgado RM, Pereira DH, Wolff P. Hyaluronan-binding system for sperm selection enhances pregnancy rates in ICSI cycles associated with male factor infertility. JBRA Assist Reprod. 2017;21(1):2–6.
8. Nijs M, Creemers E, Cox A, Janssen M, Vanheusden E, Van der Elst J, et al. Relationship between hyaluronic acid binding assay and outcome in ART: a pilot study. Andrologia. 2010;42(5):291–6.
9. Brussow KP, Torner H, Ratky J, Manabe N, Tuchscherer A. Experimental evidence for the influence of cumulus-oocyte-complexes on sperm release from the porcine oviductal sperm reservoir. J Reprod Dev. 2006;52(2):249–57.

10. Worrilow KC, Eid S, Woodhouse D, Perloe M, Smith S, Witmyer J, et al. Use of hyaluronan in the selection of sperm for intracytoplasmic sperm injection (ICSI): significant improvement in clinical outcomes—multicenter, double-blinded and randomized controlled trial. Hum Reprod. 2012;28:306–14.
11. Mokanszki A, Tothne EV, Bodnar B, Tandor Z, Molnar Z, Jakab A, et al. Is sperm hyaluronic acid binding ability predictive for clinical success of intracytoplasmic sperm injection: PICSI vs. ICSI? Syst Biol Reprod Med. 2014;60(6):348–54.
12. McDowell S, Kroon B, Ford E, Hook Y, Glujovsky D, Yazdani A. Advanced sperm selection techniques for assisted reproduction. Cochrane Database Syst Rev. 2014;10:CD010461.
13. Aitken RJ, Bowie H, Buckingham D, Harkiss D, Richardson DW, West KM. Sperm penetration into a hyaluronic acid polymer as a means of monitoring functional competence. J Androl. 1992;13(1):44–54.
14. Cherr GN, Yudin AI, Li MW, Vines CA, Overstreet JW. Hyaluronic acid and the cumulus extracellular matrix induce increases in intracellular calcium in macaque sperm via the plasma membrane protein PH-20. Zygote. 1999;7(3):211–22.
15. Hunnicutt GR, Primakoff P, Myles DG. Sperm surface protein PH-20 is bifunctional: one activity is a hyaluronidase and a second, distinct activity is required in secondary sperm-zona binding. Biol Reprod. 1996;55(1):80–6.
16. Kim E, Yamashita M, Kimura M, Honda A, Kashiwabara S, Baba T. Sperm penetration through cumulus mass and zona pellucida. Int J Dev Biol. 2008;52(5–6):677–82.
17. Ghosh I, Chattopadhaya R, Kumar V, Chakravarty BN, Datta K. Hyaluronan binding protein-1: a modulator of sperm-oocyte interaction. Soc Reprod Fertil Suppl. 2007;63:539–43.
18. Ranganathan S, Ganguly AK, Datta K. Evidence for presence of hyaluronan binding protein on spermatozoa and its possible involvement in sperm function. Mol Reprod Dev. 1994;38(1):69–76.
19. Martin-Deleon PA. Germ-cell hyaluronidases: their roles in sperm function. Int J Androl. 2011;34(5 Pt 2):e306–18.
20. Bains R, Adeghe J, Carson RJ. Human sperm cells express CD44. Fertil Steril. 2002;78(2):307–12.
21. Kornovski BS, McCoshen J, Kredentser J, Turley E. The regulation of sperm motility by a novel hyaluronan receptor. Fertil Steril. 1994;61(5):935–40.
22. Torabi F, Bogle OA, Estanyol JM, Oliva R, Miller D. Zona pellucida-binding protein 2 (ZPBP2) and several proteins containing BX7B motifs in human sperm may have hyaluronic acid binding or recognition properties. Mol Hum Reprod. 2017;23:803–16.
23. Paiva P, Van Damme MP, Tellbach M, Jones RL, Jobling T, Salamonsen LA. Expression patterns of hyaluronan, hyaluronan synthases and hyaluronidases indicate a role for hyaluronan in the progression of endometrial cancer. Gynecol Oncol. 2005;98(2):193–202.
24. Liberda J, Manaskova P, Prelovska L, Ticha M, Jonakova V. Saccharide-mediated interactions of boar sperm surface proteins with components of the porcine oviduct. J Reprod Immunol. 2006;71(2):112–25.
25. Bower L, Serafini P, Wikland M, Moyer D. The use of hyaluronic acid for sperm selection—evaluation of sperm head ultrastructure. Int J Fertil. 1989;34(6):420–4.
26. Prinosilova P, Kruger T, Sati L, Ozkavukcu S, Vigue L, Kovanci E, et al. Selectivity of hyaluronic acid binding for spermatozoa with normal Tygerberg strict morphology. Reprod Biomed Online. 2009;18(2):177–83.
27. WHO. WHO laboratory manual for the examination and processing of human semen. 2010.
28. Mortimer D. Sperm recovery techniques to maximize fertilizing capacity. Reprod Fertil Dev. 1994;6(1):25–31.
29. Fredricsson B, Bjork G. Morphology of postcoital spermatozoa in the cervical secretion and its clinical significance. Fertil Steril. 1977;28(8):841–5.
30. Torabi F, Binduraihem A, Miller D. Sedimentation properties in density gradients correspond with levels of sperm DNA fragmentation, chromatin compaction and binding affinity to hyaluronic acid. Reprod Biomed Online. 2017;34(3):298–311.
31. Kovanci E, Kovacs T, Moretti E, Vigue L, Bray-Ward P, Ward DC, et al. FISH assessment of aneuploidy frequencies in mature and immature human spermatozoa classified by the absence or presence of cytoplasmic retention. Hum Reprod. 2001;16(6):1209–17.
32. Huszar G, Ozkavukcu S, Jakab A, Celik-Ozenci C, Sati GL, Cayli S. Hyaluronic acid binding ability of human sperm reflects cellular maturity and fertilizing potential: selection of sperm for intracytoplasmic sperm injection. Curr Opin Obstet Gynecol. 2006;18(3):260–7.
33. Sati L, Ovari L, Bennett D, Simon SD, Demir R, Huszar G. Double probing of human spermatozoa for persistent histones, surplus cytoplasm, apoptosis and DNA fragmentation. Reprod Biomed Online. 2008;16(4):570–9.
34. Yagci A, Murk W, Stronk J, Huszar G. Spermatozoa bound to solid state hyaluronic acid show chromatin structure with high DNA chain integrity: an acridine orange fluorescence study. J Androl. 2010;31(6):566–72.
35. Parmegiani L, Cognigni GE, Bernardi S, Troilo E, Taraborrelli S, Arnone A, et al. Comparison of two ready-to-use systems designed for sperm-hyaluronic acid binding selection before intracytoplasmic sperm injection: PICSI vs. sperm slow: a prospective, randomized trial. Fertil Steril. 2012;98(3):632–7.
36. Necas J, Bartosikova L, Brauner P, Kolar J. Hyaluronic acid (hyaluronan): a review. Vet Med (Praha). 2008;53(8):397–411.
37. Balaban B, Lundin K, Morrell JM, Tjellstrom H, Urman B, Holmes PV. An alternative to PVP for slowing sperm prior to ICSI. Hum Reprod. 2003;18(9):1887–9.
38. Robinson BV, Sullivan FM, Borzelleca JF, Schwarz SL. PVP: a critical review of the kinetics and toxicology of polyvinylpyrrolidone (povidone). Boca Raton: Lewis; 1990.
39. Vorvolakos K, Coburn JC, Saylor DM. Dynamic interfacial behavior of viscoelastic aqueous hyaluronic acid: effects of molecular weight, concentration and interfacial velocity. Soft Matter. 2014;10(13):2304–12.
40. Tarozzi N, Nadalini M, Bizzaro D, Serrao L, Fava L, Scaravelli G, et al. Sperm-hyaluronan-binding assay: clinical value in conventional IVF under Italian law. Reprod Biomed Online. 2009;19(Suppl 3):35–43.
41. Worrilow KC, Eid S, Woodhouse D, Perloe M, Smith S, Witmyer J, et al. Use of hyaluronan in the selection of sperm for intracytoplasmic sperm injection (ICSI): significant improvement in clinical outcomes—multicenter, double-blinded and randomized controlled trial. Hum Reprod. 2013;28(2):306–14.
42. Ye H, Huang GN, Gao Y, de Liu Y. Relationship between human sperm-hyaluronan binding assay and fertilization rate in conventional in vitro fertilization. Hum Reprod. 2006;21(6):1545–50.
43. Lazarevic J, Wikarczuk M, Somkuti SG, Barmat LI, Schinfeld JS, Smith SE. Hyaluronan binding assay (HBA) vs. sperm penetration assay (SPA): can HBA replace the SPA test in male partner screening before in vitro fertilization? J Exp Clin Assist Reprod. 2010;7:2.
44. Majumdar G, Majumdar A. A prospective randomized study to evaluate the effect of hyaluronic acid sperm selection on the intracytoplasmic sperm injection outcome of patients with unexplained infertility having normal semen parameters. J Assist Reprod Genet. 2013;30(11):1471–5.
45. Parmegiani L, Cognigni GE, Ciampaglia W, Pocognoli P, Marchi F, Filicori M. Efficiency of hyaluronic acid (HA) sperm selection. J Assist Reprod Genet. 2010;27(1):13–6.

46. Witt AM, Burgess K, Hawn TR, Zyzanski S. Role of oral antibiotics in treatment of breastfeeding women with chronic breast pain who fail conservative therapy. Breastfeed Med. 2014;9(2):63–72.
47. Parmegiani L, Cognigni GE, Bernardi S, Troilo E, Ciampaglia W, Filicori M. "Physiologic ICSI": hyaluronic acid (HA) favors selection of spermatozoa without DNA fragmentation and with normal nucleus, resulting in improvement of embryo quality. Fertil Steril. 2010;93(2):598–604.
48. Witt K, Beresford L, Bhattacharya S, Brian K, Coomarasamy A, Hooper R, Kirkam-Brown J, Khalaf Y, Lewis SE, Pavitt S, West R, Miller D. Hyaluronic acid binding sperm selection for assisted reproduction treatment (HABSelect): study protocol for a multicentre randomised controlled trial. BMJ Open. 2016;6:e012609.
49. Harrell FE. Regression modeling strategies: with applications to linear models, logistic regression, and survival analysis. New York: Springer; 2001. xxii, 568 p.
50. Henrard S, Speybroeck N, Hermans C. Classification and regression tree analysis vs. multivariable linear and logistic regression methods as statistical tools for studying haemophilia. Haemophilia. 2015;21(6):715–22.
51. Fernandez JL, Muriel L, Rivero MT, Goyanes V, Vazquez R, Alvarez JG. The sperm chromatin dispersion test: a simple method for the determination of sperm DNA fragmentation. J Androl. 2003;24(1):59–66.
52. Hammadeh ME, Zeginiadov T, Rosenbaum P, Georg T, Schmidt W, Strehler E. Predictive value of sperm chromatin condensation (aniline blue staining) in the assessment of male fertility. Arch Androl. 2001;46(2):99–104.
53. Bach PV, Schlegel PN. Sperm DNA damage and its role in IVF and ICSI. Basic Clin Androl. 2016;26:15.
54. Erenpreiss J, Elzanaty S, Giwercman A. Sperm DNA damage in men from infertile couples. Asian J Androl. 2008;10(5):786–90.
55. Simon L, Proutski I, Stevenson M, Jennings D, McManus J, Lutton D, et al. Sperm DNA damage has a negative association with live-birth rates after IVF. Reprod Biomed Online. 2013;26(1):68–78.
56. Gosalvez J, Caballero P, Lopez-Fernandez C, Ortega L, Guijarro JA, Fernandez JL, et al. Can DNA fragmentation of neat or swim-up spermatozoa be used to predict pregnancy following ICSI of fertile oocyte donors? Asian J Androl. 2013;15(6):812–8.
57. Simon L, Zini A, Dyachenko A, Ciampi A, Carrell DT. A systematic review and meta-analysis to determine the effect of sperm DNA damage on in vitro fertilization and intracytoplasmic sperm injection outcome. Asian J Androl. 2017;19(1):80–90.
58. Cissen M, Wely MV, Scholten I, Mansell S, Bruin JP, Mol BW, et al. Measuring sperm DNA fragmentation and clinical outcomes of medically assisted reproduction: a systematic review and meta-analysis. PLoS One. 2016;11(11):e0165125.
59. Osman A, Alsomait H, Seshadri S, El-Toukhy T, Khalaf Y. The effect of sperm DNA fragmentation on live birth rate after IVF or ICSI: a systematic review and meta-analysis. Reprod Biomed Online. 2015;30(2):120–7.
60. Zhao J, Zhang Q, Wang Y, Li Y. Whether sperm deoxyribonucleic acid fragmentation has an effect on pregnancy and miscarriage after in vitro fertilization/intracytoplasmic sperm injection: a systematic review and meta-analysis. Fertil Steril. 2014;102(4):998–1005.. e8
61. Robinson L, Gallos ID, Conner SJ, Rajkhowa M, Miller D, Lewis S, et al. The effect of sperm DNA fragmentation on miscarriage rates: a systematic review and meta-analysis. Hum Reprod. 2012;27(10):2908–17.
62. Beck-Fruchter R, Shalev E, Weiss A. Clinical benefit using sperm hyaluronic acid binding technique in ICSI cycles: a systematic review and meta-analysis. Reprod Biomed Online. 2015;32:286–98.
63. Menezo Y, Dale B, Cohen M. DNA damage and repair in human oocytes and embryos: a review. Zygote. 2010 Nov;18(4):357–65.
64. Ramsay J. Overuse of ICSI compromises investigation treatment and improvement in male fertility. Predicting the chances of a live birth after one or more complete cycles of in vitro fertilisation: population based study of linked cycle data from 113873 women. Br Med J. 2016.
65. Boulet SL, Mehta A, Kissin DM, Warner L, Kawwass JF, Jamieson DJ. Trends in use of and reproductive outcomes associated with intracytoplasmic sperm injection. JAMA. 2015;313(3):255–63.
66. Zini A. Are sperm chromatin and DNA defects relevant in the clinic? Syst Biol Reprod Med. 2011;57(1–2):78–85.
67. Sakkas D. Novel technologies for selecting the best sperm for in vitro fertilization and intracytoplasmic sperm injection. Fertil Steril. 2013;99(4):1023–9.

Sperm Separation Protocols

90

Rajesh K. Srivastava

Developing an efficient method of sperm separation technique is essential for the successful fertilization using assisted reproductive technologies. Human semen sample is a complex mixture of variable amount of cellular debris, germ cells, and leukocytes and does not have the capacity to fertilize the oocyte instantly after ejaculation. It has to acquire the capacity to be acrosome reacted and fertilize the oocytes in the female genital tract by undergoing a series of complex physiological and biochemical changes termed capacitation [1–2]. It involves the removal of sterols (e.g., cholesterol) and non-covalently bound glycoproteins from sperm cell surfaces. This renders the sperm cell surface receptors to be accessible with an increase in the fluidity of sperm membrane and permeability of Ca^{++}. Due to increased permeability of Ca^{++}, there is an increase in intracellular cAMP which aids sperm to undergo hyperactivation [1–4]. In vivo sperm undergoes the process of capacitation after ejaculation by swimming out from seminal plasma into cervical mucus, but in vitro, to acquire capacitation, sperm has to be removed from seminal plasma by washing it out using different protocols as described in this chapter. It has been shown that prolonged exposure of sperm to seminal plasma (>60 min) is detrimental and hampers the fertilization potential [5] and traces of seminal plasma present in the re-suspended sperm in the media can be harmful [6].

Therefore, when sperm sample has to be used for clinical purposes, like intrauterine insemination (IUI), therapeutic donor insemination (TDI), in vitro fertilization (IVF), or intracytoplasmic sperm injection (ICSI), it is important to remove the semen from the seminal plasma as soon as sample liquefies using different washing protocols with an effort to put least trauma to the sample during preparation. Processed sperm sample has to be re-suspended in a suitable culture medium which is capable of sustaining capacitation.

R. K. Srivastava (✉)
Department of Obstetrics and Gynecology, Andrology Laboratories, Strong Fertility Center, University of Rochester Medical Center, Rochester, NY, USA
e-mail: rajesh_srivastava@urmc.rochester.edu

90.1 Simple Wash Procedure

This is one of the earliest methods to prepare sperm, where semen samples are diluted with Hepes-HTF medium containing 5 mg/ml of human serum albumin (HSA) using centrifugation.

Procedure

1. Mix the semen sample well.
2. Dilute the entire semen sample (1:2) with Hepes-HTF medium with serum to dilute seminal plasma.
3. Transfer diluted sample into more tubes, if total volume is more than 3 ml. There should not be more than 3 ml of sample per tube.
4. Centrifuge at 300–500 × g for 5–10 min.
5. Carefully aspirate and discard the supernatants.
6. Re-suspend the combined sperm pellets if more than one tube was used into one tube in approximately 1 ml of medium by gentle pipetting.
7. Centrifuge again at 300–500 × g for 3–5 min.
8. Carefully aspirate and discard the supernatant.
9. Resulting pellet can be re-suspended in 0.3–0.50 ml of medium depending upon the pellet size.

Although this procedure tends to have a good recovery, other cells, dead spermatozoa, and leucocytes can also accumulate and generate copious amount of reactive oxygen species [7] that can compromise sperm function and DNA integrity. It is therefore not a method of choice. However, where recovery of a few motile sperm is required for achieving fertilization using intracytoplasmic sperm injection (ICSI), it can be useful.

90.2 Direct Swim-Up Method

This method is devised based on the motile sperm's ability to swim out of seminal plasma into the sperm wash buffer, typically Hepes-buffered HTF with 5 mg/ml HSA. Liquefied

G. N. Allahbadia et al. (eds.), *Textbook of Assisted Reproduction*, https://doi.org/10.1007/978-981-15-2377-9_90

sample can be washed once by diluting it with sperm wash buffer, and resultant pellet can be layered under medium in a culture tube or medium can be gently layered over the pellet and left for 30–45 min, so that motile sperm can swim into the medium. However, wash and centrifugation prior to swim-up is not recommended due to the possibility of peroxidative damage to the sperm membranes and due to accumulation of leukocytes and cellular debris in the resultant pellet after centrifugation [8]. Therefore, a direct swim-up method using liquefied semen is recommended [9, 10]. We describe here the direct swim-up technique:

1. Put 2.5 ml of Hepes-HTF medium with 5 mg/ml HSA in three to four 12 × 75 mm 5 ml sterile tubes.
2. Place approx. 0.5 ml aliquots of liquefied semen into the bottom of these tubes. Semen with normal to high counts may require several tubes.
3. Mark the meniscus on the surface of the tube where semen sample meets with the media with a permanent marker.
4. Place caps tightly on the tubes, and incubate for 60 min at 37 °C in an incubator. Tube should be tilted at 45°. This helps in good recovery of motile sperm.
5. Time of incubation should be varied between 30 and 90 min due to the initial count and motility of the specimen, i.e., normal specimens usually only require 30 min to achieve a good concentration in the media layer.
6. Remove the upper layer of media above the meniscus—take care not to aspirate any semen into the pipette. Place the aspirate into a sterile 15 ml conical tube. Repeat for all tubes. Put approximately 4 ml of Hepes-HTF medium with 5 mg/ml HSA.
7. Centrifuge 300–500 × g for 10 min. Remove the supernatant using a sterile Pasteur pipette. Gently dislodge the pellet by tapping. Add 3 ml of medium and centrifuge again for 5 min at 300–500 × g.
8. Re-suspend final pellet to 0.2–0.5 ml with media and assess count and motility.

There is a simple variant of this method where organ culture dish (OCD) can be used successfully and duration of the swim-up can be reduced to 15 min [11]. 0.7 ml of unwashed liquefied semen was transferred under the 2.5 ml of Hepes-HTF medium with HSA in the center well of organ culture dish and incubated at 37 °C for 15 min. Approximately 2 ml of the medium containing motile sperm was removed by a fine tip pipette directed against the edge of the center well. The aspirated medium is centrifuged at 300 × g for 7 min, and the resulting pellet was re-suspended in 1 ml of media and washed again for 5 min at 300 × g, and pellet is reconstituted in 0.5 ml, and then count and motility are assessed. This method works well with good recovery and with frozen sperm as well. It is less time-consuming as compared to multiple tube incubation.

Direct swim-up technique yields good recovery of motile sperm if sperm count and motility are adequate and semen sample is free from cellular contaminants and leukocytes and is successfully used for sperm preparation for IVF and IUI.

90.3 Sperm Preparation Using Discontinuous Density Gradients

This method is most popular and widely used in ART laboratories. It provides best and clean separation of spermatozoa from other cellular debris and contaminants of semen. It is easy to standardize and results are consistent. This method separates spermatozoa based on the density and specific gravity. Mature and morphologically normal spermatozoa have a density of >1.12 g/ml, whereas immature and morphologically abnormal spermatozoa density varies between 1.06 and 1.09 g/ml. Several years ago a commercially available gradient Percoll which was available from Pharmacia Biotech, Uppsala, Sweden, was extensively used for sperm preparation. Percoll is colloidal silica coated with polyvinylpyrrolidone, and 80% (v/v) of it is about 1.10 g/ml. Due to this density, only highly mature spermatozoon could penetrate through the 80% layer which allowed the separation of most mature and morphologically normal spermatozoa. However, Percoll is not recommended anymore for clinical use, and since then various commercial gradients are available now that can be safely and successfully used. Some of the most popular name brands are Isolate from Irvine Scientific (Santa Ana, CA) and PureSperm from Nidacon International, Göteborg, Sweden. These products are tested and found to be as good as Percoll [12]. Here we describe the method of sperm separation using this method [10]:

1. Perform sperm count and motility assessment on the semen sample after 30 min after liquefaction.
2. Transfer 2 ml of 80% PureSperm gradient in a Falcon polystyrene (#2095) 15 ml tube. Do not use polypropylene tube as it may be toxic to sperm.
3. On top of it, layer 2 ml of 40% gradient gently.
4. Pipette same volume of liquefied semen on top of the gradients by touching the semen pipette tip to the top of the 40% gradient. If semen volume is more than 2 ml, make another tube with 80%:40% gradient.
5. Centrifuge at 400 × g for 15 min using a swinging bucket rotor.
6. Aspirate the gradient part without disturbing the pellet. Remove the pellet using a wide bore sterile pipette to a clean tube containing 4 ml of sperm wash buffer, and centrifuge it for 10 min at 200 × g.

7. Remove the supernatant using a fine tip aspiration pipette. Add 2 ml of sperm wash buffer and repeat the centrifugation at 200 × g for 5 min.
8. Re-suspend the washed pellet with 500–1000 μl of sperm wash buffer.

For viscous sample it is difficult to obtain good yield of motile spermatozoa. It is recommended therefore to take few measures to reduce the viscosity before proceeding to sperm preparation. Specimen viscosity can be reduced to some extent by diluting the sample with an equal volume of sperm wash buffer and mixing it using sterile pipette. Let the sample to sit for 5–10 min, and remove the settled debris from the bottom using a sterile Pasteur pipette. Any viscous mass that is still floating in the medium can be carefully removed using a fine bore Pasteur pipette.

In recent years growing attentions are directed to apoptotic markers as indicators of sperm integrity [12–17]. Some studies have compared apoptosis in prepared sperm by swim-up and density gradient centrifugation [18]. Hence, there is a quest to develop sperm preparation protocols that involve minimum trauma because the shearing forces inflicted due to centrifugation stimulate ROS generation in human sperm samples [8, 19].

90.4 Sperm Selection Based on Electrostatic Charges

Some novel methods of sperm selection were developed utilizing the electrokinetic properties of sperm surface membrane. Mature sperm typically exhibit a net negative charge of −16 to −20 mv [20]. This high negative charge on the sperm surface is due to high levels of sialic acid residues which play a role in sperm capacitation and the formation of binding bridges between sperm membrane proteins and oocytes [21]. A procedure of sperm selection based on this property of net negative charge on sperm surface membrane will result in the isolation of more mature, viable, motile, and morphologically normal sperm which are free of DNA damage [22, 23]. Based on these characteristics, two methods have been developed for sperm separation. A simple version is Zeta method [24–26] and a more complex method that separates sperm electrophoretically [27, 28].

90.5 Zeta Method of Sperm Selection

This method is described in detail in [26]. It is recommended that this method should be carried out immediately after semen liquefaction because as more time progresses sperm starts to lose its electrostatic charges. In order to perform this, use polystyrene 15 ml centrifuge tube. It will be better if tubes are checked before to have adequate positive charge and volt meter read 204 kv per square inch. Sperm should be washed using a double density gradient method. Put 0.1 ml of prepared sperm into the tube, and dilute it with 5 ml Hepes-HTF medium without serum. Hold the tube using the cap (never touch anywhere else), and put inside a latex glove with the cap part exposed only. Rotate the tube two to three times gently by holding the cap in clockwise direction, and then let it incubate for a minute which will allow the charged sperm to adhere on the wall of the tube. After the incubation slowly invert the tube to drain off all non-adherent sperm. Centrifuge the tube at 300 × g for 5 min, and then place the tube upside down on a tissue paper to blot off the excess liquid at the mouth of the tube. Put 0.2 ml of Hepes-HTF medium containing 3% or more of serum slowly so that it can trickle down at the bottom detaching the adherent sperm. Pour the medium again on the side wall using a fine tip pipette, and collect the medium at the bottom which has detached sperm. Estimate the count and motility. Sperm selection using zeta methods has increased higher probability in fertilization, implantation, and pregnancy [29, 30].

90.6 Electrophoretic Sperm Separation

Sperm is separated based on the size and charge using electrophoresis [27]. A special device consisting of four chambers is used. There are two inner and two outer chambers. Two polyacrylamide membranes with a pore size of 15 kDA separate the inner and outer chambers. Although free flow of water, small molecules, and ions can occur between the inner and outer chambers, the cell suspension is retained within the inner chamber. A platinum-coated titanium mesh electrode is present in the outer chambers Two 12 v pumps in each electrode chamber circulate the buffer at 1.6 l/min. Each inner chamber has a capacity of 400 μl. One is an inoculation chamber into which semen is deposited, and the other is a collection chamber containing only the buffer. The two inner chambers are separated by a 5 μM polycarbonate membrane. The pore size allows movement of sperm but not the larger leukocyte and precursor germ cells that are commonly present in the semen sample.

Semen sample and buffer are loaded in the two reservoirs and allowed to equilibrate for 5 min before the electric field is applied. The separation and electrode buffer is comprised of 10 mM Hepes, 30 mM Nacl, and 0.2 M sucrose. pH of the buffer was adjusted to 7.4 with an osmolarity of 310 osm/l. The samples were run at the constant applied current of 75 mA and a variable voltage of between 18 and 21 V at room temperature. Purified sample is collected and count, motility, and progression are estimated. Isolated sample collected after this method contained motile, morphologically normal sample and exhibited reduced level of DNA damage. It is also free from contaminating leukocytes and germ cells.

This is a quick method that does not require any centrifugation and recovery which is similar to commonly applied methods like density gradient separation or swim-up.

90.7 Sperm Separation Using Microfluidic Sperm Sorter

In recent years microfluidic sperm sorters (MFSSs) are developed that can be used to separate motile sperm from immotile sperm and from other cellular debris based on fluid dynamics [31–33]. This device has sample inlets, outlets, and sorting channels and a novel passively driven pumping system that provides a steady flow of liquids. These well-designed two parallel laminar flow channels separate motile spermatozoa from immotile spermatozoa. It has been shown that sperm motility and morphology can be increased twofold using this method [32]. It requires no external power or controls. This system does not require any centrifugation and can sort out motile sperm without DNA damage [34].

90.8 Sperm Preparation Using Magnetic-Activated Cell Sorting

The principle behind this method is to bind sperm showing apoptotic marker proteins using Annexin V. Consequently, sperm prepared by this method show reduced level of apoptotic marker proteins, e.g., Fas, phosphatidylserine, Bcl-XL, p53, etc., as compared to routine sperm preparation protocols that require centrifugation [35, 36]. Density gradient-separated sperm is incubated with Annexin V-conjugated microbeads (Miltenyi Biotec, Auburn, CA) for 15 min at room temperature (100 μl microbeads for every ten million sperm) to form a suspension. The suspension is then loaded on a separation column containing a coated-cell matrix containing iron balls which are in turn fitted in a magnet (MiniMACS, Miltenyi Biotec). The spermatozoa with apoptotic markers get retained in the separation column (Annexin-positive fraction), and those with intact membranes are eluted through the column (Annexin-negative). Fluorescence-labeled dye and flow cytometry have confirmed that these sperm have significantly reduced levels of apoptotic markers [37]. It is suggestive therefore that with the use of this method, there is high probability of increase in fertilization potential as revealed in some trials [38, 39].

90.9 Sperm Selection Using Hyaluron Binding

Sperm selection based on its ability to bind hyaluron has shown improved implantation [40] and clinical pregnancy [41]. This technique is based on the concept that spermatozoa bind to hyaluron has completed spermatogenesis. During the process of spermiogenesis, there are alterations in plasma membrane and appearance of hyaluron binding sites. Human sperm that bind to hyaluron appeared to have low DNA fragmentation and normal morphology and exhibit least aneuploidies and are compared to the sperm that bind to zona pellucida which is important for successful fertilization [42]. This sperm selection method can be successfully performed in conjunction with ICSI in specially designed dishes with hyaluron droplets. Sperm head can bind to the hyaluron dots and can be easily picked up for injection in the oocytes.

90.10 Retrograde Ejaculation Sperm Processing

Azoospermia with severely reduced semen volume can be associated with retrograde ejaculation, which is a condition where the sperm are pushed into the bladder (retrograde ejaculation), rather than out through the urethra (antegrade ejaculation). If large numbers of sperm pass into the bladder, then the sperm can be harvested from the urine and used for ART procedures [10]. Patient should abstain from ejaculation for 2–3 days.

1. For 2 days prior, patient should start taking sodium bicarbonate (Alka Seltzer) 650 mg by mouth four times per day and pseudoephedrine (Sudafed) 60 mg by mouth two times per day with an 8 oz of glass before collection of specimen. No alcohol or other drugs (other than those that are necessary) should be taken.
2. On morning of test, patient should urinate, and then take two sodium bicarbonate tablets, and drink one to two glasses of water.
3. The bladder should be emptied approximately 1 h prior to collecting the specimens.

The patient should use masturbation to produce an antegrade semen specimen (if possible). Within 5 min after orgasm, the patient should urinate into another specimen cup(s). Both the antegrade ejaculate (if any) and the post-ejaculatory urine should be presented to the lab. These patients should collect all specimens at the laboratory, so that the sperm can be isolated from the urine quickly.

1. Aliquot all urine into 15 ml sterile conical tubes—approximately 10–15 ml per tube.
2. Record total volume of urine specimen.
3. Centrifuge tubes at 550 × g for 10 min. Discard supernatant.
4. Re-suspend pellets in sperm wash buffer approximately 1–2 ml per tube, depending upon the size of pellet (large pellet, 2–3 ml). Consolidate all aliquots into one 15 ml conical centrifuge tube. If motility is adequate, it can be

processed using density gradient. Remove 10 µl and do a sperm count, and assess the motility and progression following semen analysis method.

If an antegrade specimen is obtained, 10 µl of the semen specimen is assessed for count, motility, and progression as per standard semen analysis protocol.

90.11 Sperm Preparation from Epididymal Aspirates and Testicular Biopsies

Since the advent of ICSI, it is now possible to obtain sperm from men using epididymal sperm aspiration or testicular biopsy, if there is no sperm in the ejaculate due to obstructive or nonobstructive azoospermia. Epididymal aspirates are the suspension of cells usually obtained with fine needles from the epididymis. If epididymal aspirates contain some motile spermatozoa, it can be processed using double density gradient successfully [43]. However, if majority of spermatozoa in the epididymal aspirates are immotile, density gradient separation will be inefficient, and then a simple wash technique will be useful. Often these samples have very poor motility, and incubating sperm with pentoxifylline (2 mg/ml) in sperm wash buffer is quite helpful.

90.12 Sperm Preparation from Testicular Biopsies

Testicular biopsies should be transported to laboratory in a sterile container containing sufficient amount of sperm wash buffer (Hepes-HTF with 5 mg/ml HSA).

1. The biopsy is removed from the container it comes in, using sterile forceps, thoroughly rinsed in sperm wash buffer to remove the blood, placed on the lid of a 60 mm dish in a small drop of sperm wash buffer, and thoroughly minced with a pair of disposable scalpels. Sometimes using a pair of 26 gauge needles bent to an angle of 90° attached with 1 ml disposable syringe is very helpful in finely teasing the seminiferous tubules [10, 44]. Once the tissue is thoroughly minced, use the bottom portion of the 60 mm dish, and place it over the minced tissue, and using fingers inside the lid, press it over at several places to squeeze out the sperm from the tubules. A twisting motion should not be used, as this may break the sperm head from the tail.
2. Once the tissue is well squashed, the lid is rinsed with sperm wash buffer; the sample is collected into a 15 ml centrifuge tube and centrifuged at 800 × g for 5 min.
3. The supernatant is removed and discarded and the sample is suspended in 0.5–1 ml of sperm wash buffer depending on sample size. Vortex the suspension for 20–30 seconds to dislodge spermatozoa from the cells. Take an aliquot (5–10 µl), and put it in 20–30 µl of pentoxifylline solution (2 mg/ml in Hepes-HTF + HSA) in a dish lid covered with oil and kept at 37 °C. Thoroughly examine the droplet under inverted microscope under high power for the presence of a motile sperm. If motile sperm is seen, then sperm preparation can be successfully used. It is always recommended to cryopreserve the sample for future use.

90.13 Conclusions

Routine sperm separation protocols have evolved from simple wash to gradient separation over the years, and the general consensus is that both swim-up and gradient protocols work equally well, although gradient protocol is preferable due to efficient separation of motile sperm even from suboptimal samples [45, 46]; nevertheless, a Cochrane database system review has not found any difference on the clinical outcome by different sperm preparation protocols [47]. There have been several advances made in sperm separation utilizing electrostatic potential and some novel microfluidic procedures with sperm showing significantly reduced apoptotic markers. However, these technologies are still not in routine use. In future, knowledge gleaned from varying DNA methylation patterns of spermatozoa that affect embryo development [48] and sperm RNA analysis [49] may be helpful in devising specific protocols that may help in selecting spermatozoa for better clinical outcome.

References

1. De Jonge C. Biological basis for human capacitation. Hum Reprod Update. 2005;11:205–14.
2. Ikawa M, Inoue N, Benham AM, Okabe M. Fertilization: a sperm's journey to and interaction with the oocyte. J Clin Invest. 2010;120:984–94.
3. Austin CR, Braden AW. Passage of the sperm and the penetration of the egg in mammals. Nature. 1952;170:919–21.
4. Yanagimachi R. Mammalian sperm reaction: where does it begin before fertilization? Biol Reprod. 2011;85:4–5.
5. Rogers BJ, Perrault SD, Bentwood BJ, McCarville C, Hale RW, Soderdahl DW. Variability in the human-hamster in vitro assay for fertility evaluation. Fertil Steril. 1983;39:204–11.
6. Kanwar KC, Yanagimachi R, Lopata A. Effects of human seminal plasma on fertilizing capacity of human spermatozoa. Fertil Steril. 1979;31:321–7.
7. Aitken RJ, Bukingham DW, Bridle J, Gomez E, Baker HW, Irvine DS. Analysis of sperm movement in relation to the oxidative stress created by leukocytes in washed sperm preparation and seminal plasma. Hum Reprod. 1995;10:2061–71.
8. Aitken RJ, Clarkson JS. Significance of reactive oxygen species and antioxidants in defining the efficacy of sperm preparation techniques. J Androl. 1988;9:367–76.

9. Mortimer D. Sperm recovery techniques to maximize fertilizing capacity. Reprod Fertil Dev. 1994;6:25–31.
10. WHO. Laboratory Manual for the examination and processing of human semen. 5th ed. Geneva: World Health Organization, Department of Reproductive Health and Research; 2010.
11. Yin HZ, Srivastava RK, Bar-Ami S, Seibel MM. An unwashed sperm rise method for preparing fresh or frozen sperm using organ culture dishes. Fertil Steril. 1997;68(Suppl 1):S56–7.
12. Centola GM, Herko R, Andolina E, Weisensel S. Comparison of sperm separation methods: effect on recovery, motility, motion parameters, and hyperactivation. Fertil Steril. 1998;70:1173–5.
13. Sakkas D, Mariethoz E, St John JC. Abnormal sperm parameters in humans are indicative of an abortive apoptotic mechanism linked to the fas-mediated pathway. Exp Cell Res. 1999;251:350–5.
14. Ricci G, Perticarari S, Fragonas E, Giolo E, Canova S, Pozzobon C, et al. Apoptosis in human sperm: its correlation with semen quality and the presence of leukocytes. Hum Reprod. 2002;17:2665–72.
15. Sakkas D, Seli E, Bizzaro D, Tarozzi N, Manicardi GC. Abnormal spermatozoa in ejaculate: abortive apoptosis and faulty nuclear remodeling during spermatogenesis. Reprod Biomed Online. 2003;7:428–32.
16. Oehninger S, Morshedi M, Weng SL, Taylor S, Duran H, Beebe S. Presence and significance of somatic cell apoptosis markers in human ejaculated spermatozoa. Reprod Biomed Online. 2003;7:469–76.
17. Agarwal A, Saleh RA, Bedaiwy MA. Role of reactive oxygen species in the pathophysiology of human reproduction. Fertile Steril. 2003;79:829–43.
18. Ricci G, Perticarari S, Boscolo R, Montico M, Guaschino S, Presani G. Semen preparation methods and sperm apoptosis: swim-up versus gradient-density centrifugation technique. Fertil Steril. 2009;91:632–8.
19. Shekarriz M, Thomas AJ Jr, Agarwal A. Effects of time and sperm concentration on reactive oxygen species formation in human semen. Arch Androl. 1995;34:69–75.
20. Isijima SA, Okuno M, Mohri H. Zeta potential of human X- and Y-bearing sperm. Int J Androl. 1991;14:340–7.
21. Calzada L, Salazar EL, Pedron N. Presence and chemical composition of glycoproteic layer on human spermatozoa. Arch Androl. 1994;33:87–92.
22. Aitken RJ, Hanson AR, Kuczera L. Electrophoretic sperm isolation; optimization of electrophoresis conditions and impact on oxidative stress. Hum Reprod. 2011;26:1955–64.
23. Ainsworth C, Nixon B, Aitken RJ. The electrophoretic separation of spermatozoa: an analysis of genotype, surface carbohydrate composition and potential for capacitation. Int J Androl. 2011;34(5 Pt 2):e422–34.
24. Chan PJ, Jacobson JD, Corselli JU, Patton WC. A simple zeta method for sperm selection based on membrane charge. Fertil Steril. 2006;85:481–6.
25. Kam TL, Jacobson JD, Patton WC, Corselli JU, Chan PJ. Retention of membrane charge attributes by cryopreserved-thawed sperm and zeta selection. J Assist Reprod Genet. 2007;24:429–34.
26. Simon L, Ge SQ, Carrell DT. Sperm selection based on electrostatic charge. Methods Mol Biol. 2013;927:269–78.
27. Ainsworth C, Nixon B, Aitken RJ. Development of a novel electrophoretic system for the isolation of human spermatozoa. Hum Reprod. 2005;20:2261–70.
28. Ainsworth C, Nixon B, Jansen RP, Aitken RJ. First recorded pregnancy and normal birth after ICSI using electrophoretically isolated spermatozoa. Hum Reprod. 2007;22:197–200.
29. Kheirollahi-Kouhestani M, Razavi S, Tavaleee M, Deemeh MR, Mardani M, Moshtaghian J, Nasar-Esfahani MH. Selection of sperm based on combined density gradient and zeta method may improve ICSI outcome. Hum Reprod. 2009;24:2409–16.
30. Deemeh MR, et al. The first report of successful pregnancy after ICSI with combined DGC/Zeta sperm selection procedure in a couple with eleven repeated fail IVF/ICSI cycles. Int J Fertil Steril. 2010;4:41–3.
31. Cho BS, Schuster TG, Zhu X, Chang D, Smith GD, Takayama S. Passively driven integrated microfluidic system for separation of spermatozoa. Anal Chem. 2003;75:1671–5.
32. Schuster TG, Cho B, Keller LM, Takayama S, Smith GD. Isolation of motile spermatozoa from semen samples using microfluidics. Reprod Biomed Online. 2003;7:75–81.
33. Wu JM, Chung Y, Belford KJ, Smith GD, Takayama S, Lahann J. A surface modified sperm sorting device with long-term stability. Biomed Microdevices. 2006;8:99–107.
34. Shirota K, Yotsumoto F, Itoh H, Obama H, Hidaka N, Nakajima K, et al. Separation efficiency of a microfluidic sperm sorter to minimize sperm DNA damage. Fertil Steril. 2016;105:315–21.
35. Sakkas D, Moffatt O, Manicardi GC, Mariethoz E, Tarozzi N, Bizzaro D. Nature of DNA damage in ejaculated human spermatozoa and the possible involvement of apoptosis. Biol Reprod. 2002;66:1061–7.
36. Cayli S, Sakkas D, Vigue L, Demir R, Huszar G. Cellular maturity and apoptosis in human sperm: creatine kinase, caspase-3 and Bcl-XL levels in mature and diminished maturity sperm. Mol Hum Reprod. 2004;10:365–72.
37. Lee TH, Liu CH, Shih YT, Tsao HM, Huang CC, Chen HH, et al. Magnetic-activated cell sorting for sperm preparation reduces spermatozoa with apoptotic markers and improves the acrosome reaction in couples with unexplained infertility. Hum Reprod. 2010;25:839–46.
38. de Polak FE, Denaday F. Single and twin ongoing pregnancies in two cases of previous ART failures after ICSI performed with sperm sorted using annexin V microbeads. Fertil Steril. 2010;94:351–8.
39. Rawe VY, Boudri HU, Alvarez SC, Carro M, Papier S, Nodar F. Healthy baby born after reduction of sperm DNA fragmentation using cell sorting before ICSI. Reprod Biomed Online. 2010;20:320–3.
40. Parmegiani L, Cognigni GE, Ciampaglia W, Pocognoli P, Marchi F, Filicori M. Efficiency of hyaluronic acid (HA) sperm selection. J Assist Reprod Genet. 2010;27:13–6.
41. Worrilow KC, Eid S, Woodhouse D, Perloe M, Smith S, Witmyer J, et al. Use of hyaluron in the selection of sperm for intracytoplasmic sperm injection (ICSI): significant improvement in clinical outcomes-multicenter, double-blinded and randomized control trial. Hum Reporod. 2013;28:306–14.
42. Huszar Z, Jakab A, Sakkas D, Ozenci CC, Cayli S, Delpiano E, et al. Fertility testing and ICSI sperm selection by hyaluronic acid binding: clinical and genetic aspects. Reprod Biomed Online. 2007;14:650–63.
43. Ord T, Marcello E, Patrizio P, Balmaceda JP, Silber SJ, Asch RH. The role of the laboratory in the handling of epididymal sperm for assisted reproductive technologies. Fertil Steril. 1992;57:1103–6.
44. Muller CH, Pagel ER. Recovery, isolation, identification, and preparation of spermatozoa from human testis. Methods Mol Biol. 2013;927:227–40.
45. Carrell DT, Kuneck PH, Peterson CM, Hataska HH, Jones KP, Campbell BF. A randomized, prospective analysis of five sperm preparation techniques before intrauterine insemination of husband sperm. Fertil Steril. 1998;69:122–6.
46. Facio CL, Previato LF, Machado-Paula LA, Matheus PC, Araujo EF. Comparison of two sperm processing techniques for low com-

plexity assisted fertilization: sperm washing followed by swim-up and discontinuous density gradient centrifugation. JBRA Assist Reprod. 2016;20:206–11.
47. Boomsma CM, Heineman MJ, Cohlen BJ, Farquhar C. Semen preparation techniques for intrauterine insemination. Cochrane Database Syst Rev. 2007;4:CD004507.
48. Hammoud SS, Nix DA, Zhang H, Purwar J, Carrell DT, Cairns BR. Distinctive chromatin in human sperm package genes for embryo development. Nature. 2009;460:473–8.
49. Ostermeier GC, Goodrich RJ, Diamond MP, Duix DZJ, Krawetz SA. Towards using stable spermatozoal RNAs for prognostic assessment of male factor fertility. Fertil Steril. 2005;83:1687–94.

Embryo Development: From Zygote to Blastocyst

91

Amy Barrie

91.1 Introduction

The purpose of this chapter is to delineate embryo preimplantation development from the zygote stage to the blastocyst stage. This will begin with defining the critical developmental milestones, a discussion regarding novel methods of determining embryo viability (e.g. morphokinetics and metabolomics), and will conclude with a comparison between how embryos develop in vitro and in vivo. During this chapter each pivotal stage in embryo development will be addressed including events such as the activation of the embryonic genome, as well as the concept of cell allocation and polarity. As technology plays a major part in the culture of human embryos in current practice, there will be particular focus throughout on the morphokinetic elements of embryo development made possible by time-lapse imaging (TLI).

91.2 Developmental Milestones

91.2.1 Pronuclear Formation, Breakdown and Scoring

The zygotic stage of preimplantation development is well studied, due to the proliferative work performed in the first few decades of assisted reproductive technologies (ART). A zygote (fertilized oocyte) consists of an oocyte containing two pronuclei (2PN). The presence of 2PN indicates normal fertilization with one pronucleus of paternal origin and one of maternal origin. PN have three main components: a lipid bilayer, a haploid chromosome complement and multiple nucleoli. The nucleoli are small, spherical structures predominantly composed of protein and RNA. They drive the production of ribosomal RNA and participate in the formation of ribosomes. Ribosomes are responsible for translating maternally derived mRNAs into proteins during the G1 and G2 phases of the cell cycle in preparation for DNA replication and mitosis [1].

PN appearance is often asynchronous, whilst their disappearance is usually synchronous. The male PN forms close to the site of sperm entry, whilst the female PN originates at the ooplasmic pole of the meiotic spindle [2]. Once formed, the PN become opposed to one another, usually centrally within the zygote (Fig. 91.1). In mammals, this movement is regulated by the sperm aster, which coordinates a radiating matrix of endoplasmic reticulum bundled with microtubules and separated by clusters of yolk bodies, mitochondria and lipid droplets [3]. This was confirmed by the use of chemicals used to destroy microtubular structures preventing the movement and association of PN [4].

One of the first TLI observations of fertilization used Nomarski differential interference contrast (DIC) optics and a purpose-built switching box allowing an image to be captured every minute [5]. This detailed analysis revealed a defined course of events. Firstly, circular waves of granulation within the cytoplasm were observed (termed a cytoplasmic flare), followed by the extrusion of the second polar body (PB). The formation of the male PN then occurred centrally with the female PN forming at the same time, or shortly afterwards, adjacent to the extrusion site of the second PB. The PN appearance was seen as early as 2 h post-insemination. The PN then became abutted, increased in size, the nucleoli moved within the PN and some amalgamated. The organelles then shrank from the cortex of the ooplasm leaving an obvious cortical zone. Finally, the oocyte decreased in diameter by 6 μm during the course of the observation. The male PN was significantly larger in diameter than the female PN and contained fewer nucleoli.

A. Barrie (✉)
Countess of Chester Hospital, CARE Fertility Chester, Chester, UK
e-mail: amy.barrie@carefertility.com

G. N. Allahbadia et al. (eds.), *Textbook of Assisted Reproduction*, https://doi.org/10.1007/978-981-15-2377-9_91

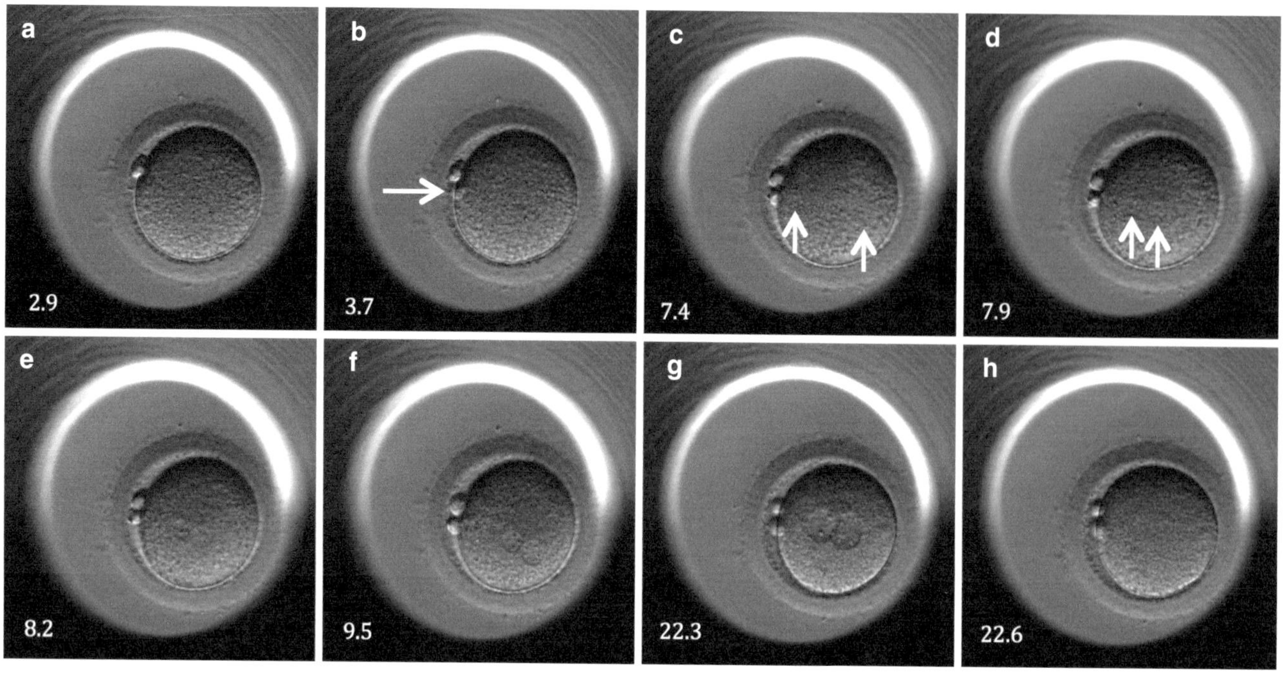

Fig. 91.1 A diagrammatic representation of pronuclei appearance. (**a**) An unfertilized oocyte 2.9 h post injection (hpi). (**b**) The extrusion of the second polar body can be seen (indicated by an arrow) at 3.7 hpi. (**c**) The initial signs of the two pronuclei can be seen at 7.4 hpi. One pronucleus can be seen appearing from the site of polar body extrusion and the other from opposite the polar body extrusion site. (**d**) The abuttal of the two pronuclei begins at 7.9 hpi. (**e**) Pronuclei are abutted at 8.2 hpi. (**f**, **g**) The pronuclei then move within the cytoplasm for over 12 h and by 22.6 hpi the pronuclei have faded (**h**)

Embryo quality has been shown to be related to fertilization events and the periodicity of cytoplasmic waves. For example, good quality embryos arise from oocytes that have more uniform timing and longer cytoplasmic waves. An earlier investigation, not utilising TLI, found that 80% of oocytes had 2PN by 8 h post-ICSI and 99% after 16 h, with some appearing as early as 6 h post-ICSI [6]. This study was repeated with similar results but also found that 100% of IVF-derived embryos had visual PN 14 h post-IVF [7].

Following PN formation, there are approximately 13 h of 'rest' when various stages of the cell cycle are completed. Once complete, the PN membranes disassemble, allowing the maternal and paternal chromosomes to align on the metaphase plate. Timing of PN fading has been linked to embryo quality and viability. This followed a report of 1782 zygotes, where transferred embryos that had undergone early PN fading resulted in a significantly higher cell number and clinical pregnancy rate [8]. However, it should be noted that this study did not utilise TLI and therefore the observations are less precise.

A more recent TLI analysis of fertilization events revealed that, of 1448 embryos, simultaneous PN appearance occurred in 96.4% of zygotes. Optimal ranges for second PB extrusion, PN fading and length of S-phase were also defined. However, there were no significant differences between implanted and non-implanted embryos in the average length of the time taken for the second PB to be extruded or for PN abuttal. A higher implantation rate was observed in zygotes where PN fading took place at 22.2–25.9 h post-ICSI and shorter S-phases were observed (5.7–13.8 h) [9]. Further to this, no embryo with PN fading earlier than 20 h 45 min post-ICSI resulted in a live birth [10].

Before the advent of TLI, and in the early years of IVF treatments, embryologists used the number, size and alignment of nucleoli (also known as nuclear precursor bodies) within the PN to score embryo quality and relate this to the chance of pregnancy. There were two scoring systems developed in conjunction with one another (Table 91.1 and Fig. 91.2).

Observations relating nucleoli distribution, PN size and orientation to embryo morphology, chance of pregnancy and chromosomally normal embryos were then corroborated by others [13]. With the introduction of blastocyst culture media, other embryo morphological features became better able to predict implantation [14–16]. PN scoring was all but forgotten, and when TLI was introduced to clinical practice, it became clear that both the PN and nucleoli are mobile within the zygote and a score given using a static observation could vary on an hourly basis.

In the absence of TLI, a single observation between 16 and 18 h post-insemination/injection is made to identify normal fertilization and PN scoring may be of value, regardless of literature contesting its use. PN are usually scored into three groups: symmetrical, non-symmetrical and abnormal. However, there is now TLI evidence that the morphokinetic timeline of fertilization events in oocytes post-ICSI may vary considerably from those post-IVF [17]. Therefore, a standardisation of timings for embryo observation may not be applicable in a program that utilises both IVF and ICSI as fertilization methods.

Table 91.1 Description of two pronuclear grading schemes

Scott et al. [11]		Tesarik and Greco [12]	
Score	Description	Score	Description
Z1	NPBs (between 3 and 7) Both PNs polarised	P0	NPBs in both PN Polarised if 3 and 7 NPBs Non-polarised if ≥7 NPBs
Z2	NPBs (between 3 and 7) Both PNs non-polarised	P1	>3 NPBs difference between PN
Z3	Alterations in NPB number and/or one polarised PN and one non-polarised PN	P2	<7 NPBs, without polarisation in at least one PN
Z4	PNs asymmetrical and/or PNs separated	P3	>7 NPBs in at least one PN
		P4	<3 NPBs in at least one PN
		P5	One PN polarised and one PN non-polarised

These scoring schemes were used from static observations of human zygotes and embryo, prior to the routine use of clinical time-lapse imaging. Observations were based on the number and distribution of nucleoli (nuclear precursor bodies, NPBs)

91.2.2 Embryo Cleavage and Grading

Following PN fading, the embryo undergoes a series of cleavage events (Fig. 91.3). Arguably, the inaugural method for determining embryo implantation potential is to assess early cleavage. Shoukir et al. [18] first demonstrated that human zygotes cleaving by 25 h post-insemination had a higher viability than those that cleaved later.

More recently, early cleavage has been shown to have less predictive power in terms of implantation [19] likely owing to the advances in embryo selection and the plethora of embryological features that can now be assessed for embryo viability. As far as the link between early cleavage and embryo quality is concerned, there is little literature offering a reason for this. It is reasonable to assume that as early development is under control of the maternal genome [20], it is likely to be an indication of oocyte quality and the ability of maternal RNA to transcribe the necessary tools to allow the embryo to undergo cytokinesis in a timely manner.

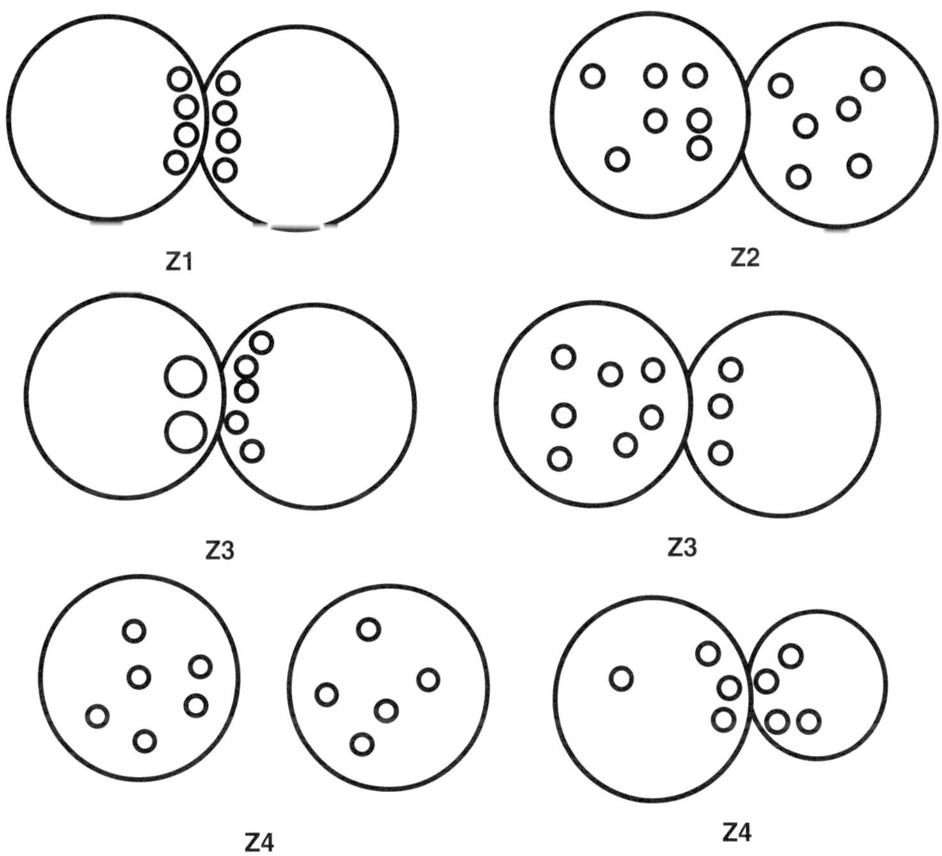

Fig. 91.2 A schematic representation of the pronuclear scoring system (adapted from Scott et al. [11]). Z1 represents 3–7 NPBs with both PN polarised. Z2 is characterised by 3–7 NPBs and both PNs non-polarised. PNs graded as Z3 exhibit alterations in the number of NPBs and/or one polarised and one non-polarised PN. Finally, a Z4 score indicates that the PNs are asymmetrical and/or the PNs are separated

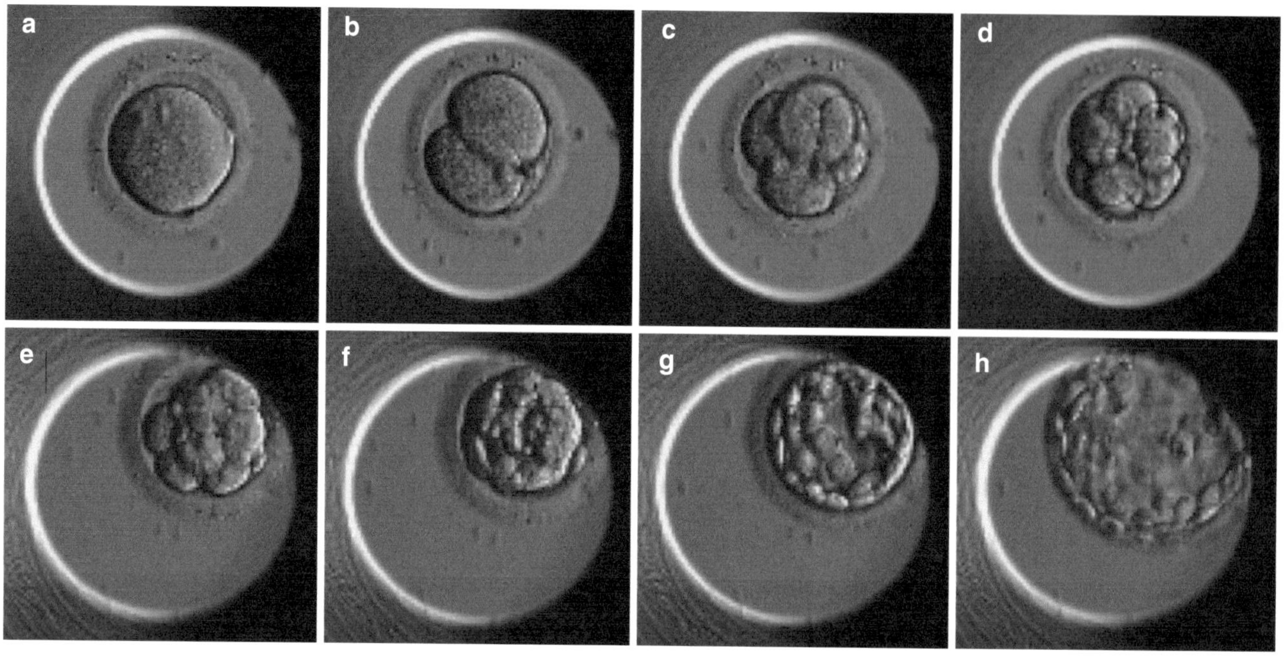

Fig. 91.3 A series of time-lapse images of in vitro embryo development. (**a**) PN formation and abuttal have completed at approximately 24 hpi. (**b**) The embryo should have two distinct, evenly sized blastomeres with less than 10% fragmentation. (**c**) Each blastomere should then cleave to produce four blastomeres on Day 2 of embryo development. (**d**) Each of the four blastomeres should cleave again in close succession to form an eight-cell embryo on Day 3. (**e**) The blastomeres begin compaction where cell membranes begin to breakdown. (**f**) Cavitation should begin at approximately 94 hpi as the embryo begins to form a blastocyst. (**g**) The cavity begins to enlarge and two cell lines are visible; the inner cell mass (ICM) and the trophectoderm. The ICM is indicated by an arrow. (**h**) The embryo should be fully expanded by 118 hpi, the zona thins as the embryo prepares to hatch and implant

Further cleavages then take place during Day 2 and Day 3 of embryo development until the embryo reaches 8–16 cells, where the next phase of embryo development begins. The gold standards for determination of embryo quality and viability should be considered here: fragmentation and cell evenness. These features of embryo development have long been understood to strongly reflect an embryo's ability to create a pregnancy [21, 22]. A variation in blastomere size has also been shown to be linked to increased aneuploidy rates and reduced implantation potential [23, 24]. These critical criteria are described in the UK's national grading scheme [25].

91.2.3 The Cell Cycle

The cell cycle can be broadly split into two phases: interphase and mitotic phase (M-phase). Interphase can then be split into three further stages: the first gap phase (G1), synthesis phase (S-phase) and the second gap phase (G2) (Fig. 91.4).

During the G1-phase the cell physically grows and replicates organelles. The G1-phase takes 5–6 h to complete. A

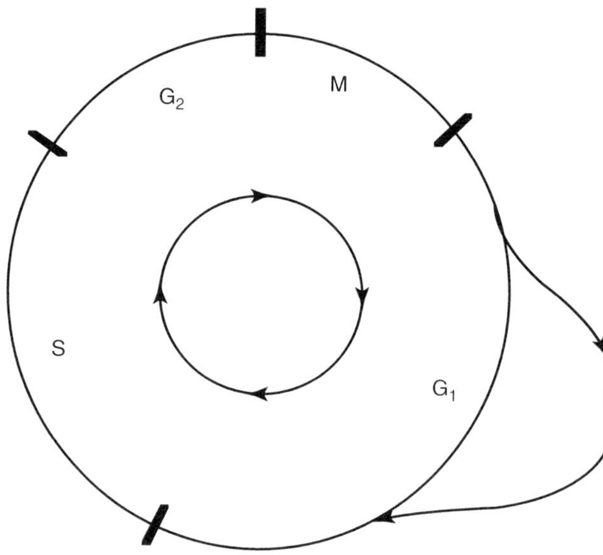

Fig. 91.4 A schematic representation of the mammalian cell cycle (adapted from Collins et al. [26]). In each cell division cycle, chromosomes are replicated during the S-phase and separated to create two genetically identical daughter cells during the M-phase. These events are spaced by intervals of growth and reorganisation (gap phases G1 and G2). Cells cease the cell cycle process following division and can enter a state of quiescence (G0)

complete copy of the DNA in the nucleus is then made in the S-phase, taking 3–5 h. The G2-phase then constitutes the reorganisation of cytoplasmic contents in preparation for the cleavage event and takes 4–6 h to complete. The cell divides its copied DNA and cytoplasm to make two daughter cells during the M-phase and cytokinesis [27, 28]. Cytokinesis involves specification of the cleavage plane, microtubule structure rearrangement and assembly of the contractile ring, followed by ring ingression [29].

Conversely, karyokinesis is well understood occurring in four distinct stages: prophase, metaphase, anaphase and telophase (Fig. 91.5). Broadly, the process of karyokinesis involves the appearance of the spindle apparatus and disintegration of the nuclear membrane (prophase); the movement of the chromosomes towards the centre of the cell arranged on the equatorial plane (metaphase); the splitting of the chromatids to form sister chromosomes (anaphase); and finally, the chromosomes reaching opposite poles, the nuclear membranes reappearing and the spindle disappearing (telophase). The eventual aim of karyokinesis is, following DNA replication, the division into two equal parts each within a daughter cell resulting from cytokinesis.

It should be noted that during oocyte maturation and fertilization, the process of PB formation also involves both karyokinesis and cytokinesis.

91.2.4 Embryonic Genome Activation

The initial stages of embryonic development are dependent on proteins and transcripts that have accumulated in the oocyte during prophase I arrest [30]. Embryonic genome activation (EGA) is necessary for continued development to the blastocyst stage, and three main requirements are needed to be met for this to occur successfully: maternal mRNA degradation, embryonic gene transcription activation and epigenetic changes [31].

Although believed to occur at the four-cell stage for many years [32], interestingly, EGA has been suggested to be independent of cell number, creating speculation that EGA occurs on Day 3 of preimplantation embryo development rather than when a specific cell number is reached [33].

EGA was first brought to light in 1988 [34] following the discovery of distinct aspects of protein synthesis linked to transcriptional activation evident around the four- to eight-cell stage. Others then supported this through the detection of paternal transcripts at the three- and four-cell stages [35].

It is now largely accepted that EGA is a stepwise process [36] with the mouse having at least four periods of major gene transcription [36]. In humans, there is also evidence of a multilevel gene induction process [35, 37, 38].

There have been a number of investigations scrutinising the differential expression of various genes at the early embryonic development stage compared to the blastocyst stage. One of the more recent of these confirmed that human oocytes are well-equipped with transcripts and proteins to support preimplantation development [39]. Further to this, and in corroboration with other investigations, it has been demonstrated that during EGA, the maternal gene downregulation far outweighs the embryonic gene upregulation where 147 maternal genes were depleted and just 6 genes of embryonic origin were upregulated [31, 33]. Using TLI, some researchers believe that development to the blastocyst stage can be predicted from morphokinetics observed up to the four-cell stage [40] suggesting that successful implantation is highly influenced by maternal factors [41].

91.2.5 Compaction, Cell Allocation and Polarity

The process of compaction is the first evidence of embryo differentiation. Little is known about the details of compaction in humans including the underlying mechanisms and processes controlling it.

Much of the insight into the process of compaction in humans has been extrapolated from the well-studied mouse model. Compaction commences with flattening of the blastomeres and redistribution of microvilli [42, 43]. Cell adhesions, gap and tight junctions appear, with cytoplasmic polarisation. As a consequence, the blastomeres resulting from the next cleavage round segregate to inside (apolar) and outside (polar) cells [44–46] to form the inner cell mass and trophectoderm, respectively [47].

Using scanning electron microscopy (SEM), it was found that noncompacted cells on Day 4 had considerably fewer microvilli compared to compacted counterparts. Polarisation was also seen as a flattened microvilli-free area with distinct borders at the sites of contact between cells, which frequently contained small, cytoplasmic blebs. The free surfaces of the blastomeres were covered by microvilli of an increased density compared to that of cleavage-stage embryos. In addition, it was shown that compaction was related both to total blastomere number and embryonic age; Day 3 embryos with 10–12 blastomeres demonstrated some polarisation, but none of them were classified as compact. However, in contrast, most Day 4 embryos were compact, including some with only ten blastomeres [48].

SEM has since demonstrated that the human embryo does not develop surface polarity before the eight-cell stage [49], confirmed by others [50].

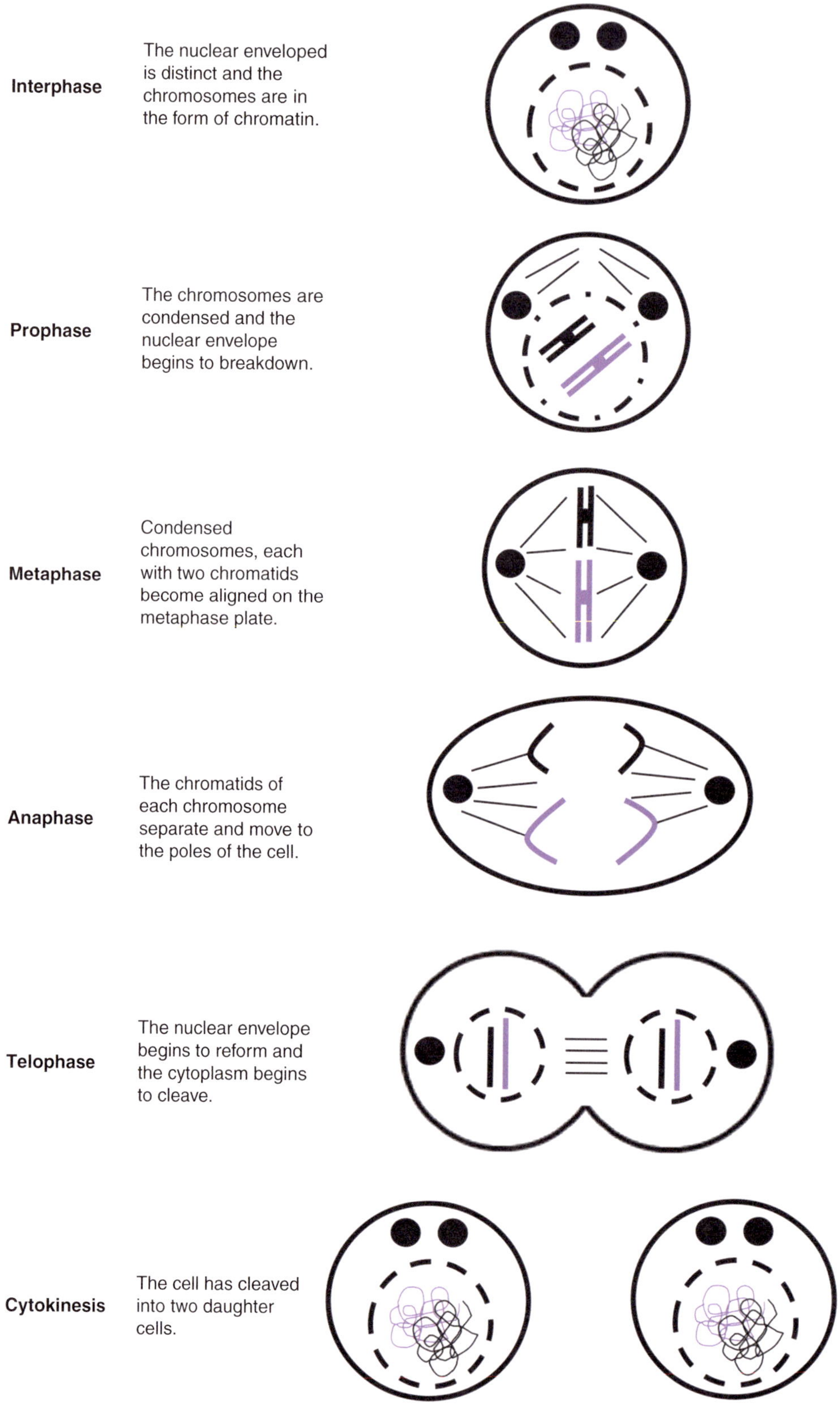

Fig. 91.5 A schematic representation of karyokinesis. The cell progresses through the stages from interphase to cytokinesis with the resultant cells carrying a diploid chromosome complement. For illustration purposes, the images are shown with two chromosomes only

In the human, embryos that have not yet compacted by Day 4 have been shown to have reduced developmental capacity [51–53]. Embryos that compact earlier than expected (eight-cell stage) have also been shown to have a higher implantation potential [54, 55], and early compaction could be a positive indicator of embryonic potential where 20% embryos are considered good quality compacted earlier compared to 12.5% considered to be poor quality [56].

TLI has revealed that 22.6% embryos commenced compaction at the eight-cell stage, 13.9% initiated compaction before the eight-cell stage and 86.1% initiated compaction at the eight-cell stage or later [54, 55]. Of these, 49.5% developed into good quality blastocysts, whereas, and conversely to reports from Desai et al. [54] and Skiadas et al. [55], just 18.8% embryos initiating compaction before the eight-cell stage developed into good quality blastocysts [57]. In addition, 93.8% embryos initiating compaction before the eight-cell stage had a significantly higher proportion of multinucleated blastomeres.

The fate of cells within the preimplantation embryo has been largely investigated in the mouse model. As a result, the following two hypotheses exist for cell fate:

1. Polarity predetermination takes place prior to the two-cell stage, where cells adopt positions depending on the cell division orientation along the animal-vegetal axis [58].
2. The embryo is entirely symmetrical and has no animal-vegetal axis and no predisposition to a pattern [59].

A gene profiling investigation has shown a common transcript pattern in blastomeres analysed in five-, six- and eight-cell stage embryos [31], supporting the latter of these hypotheses. However, TLI allows for subtle morphological features of embryos undergoing compaction to be investigated, and it could also be possible to build on the hypothesis presented by Edwards and Hansis through observations of cleavage planes.

91.2.6 Blastocoel Formation and Expansion

Following completion of compaction, the formation of the blastoceol cavity is initiated (Fig. 91.6).

There is a significant increase in ATP production as the embryo develops into blastocyst stage [60]. This is reflected by the increase in oxygen consumption between the morula and blastocyst stages [61, 62]. One of the two major consumers of ATP is the Na+/K+ ATPase pump [63] which allows, through the transport of Na+ and K+ through the cell

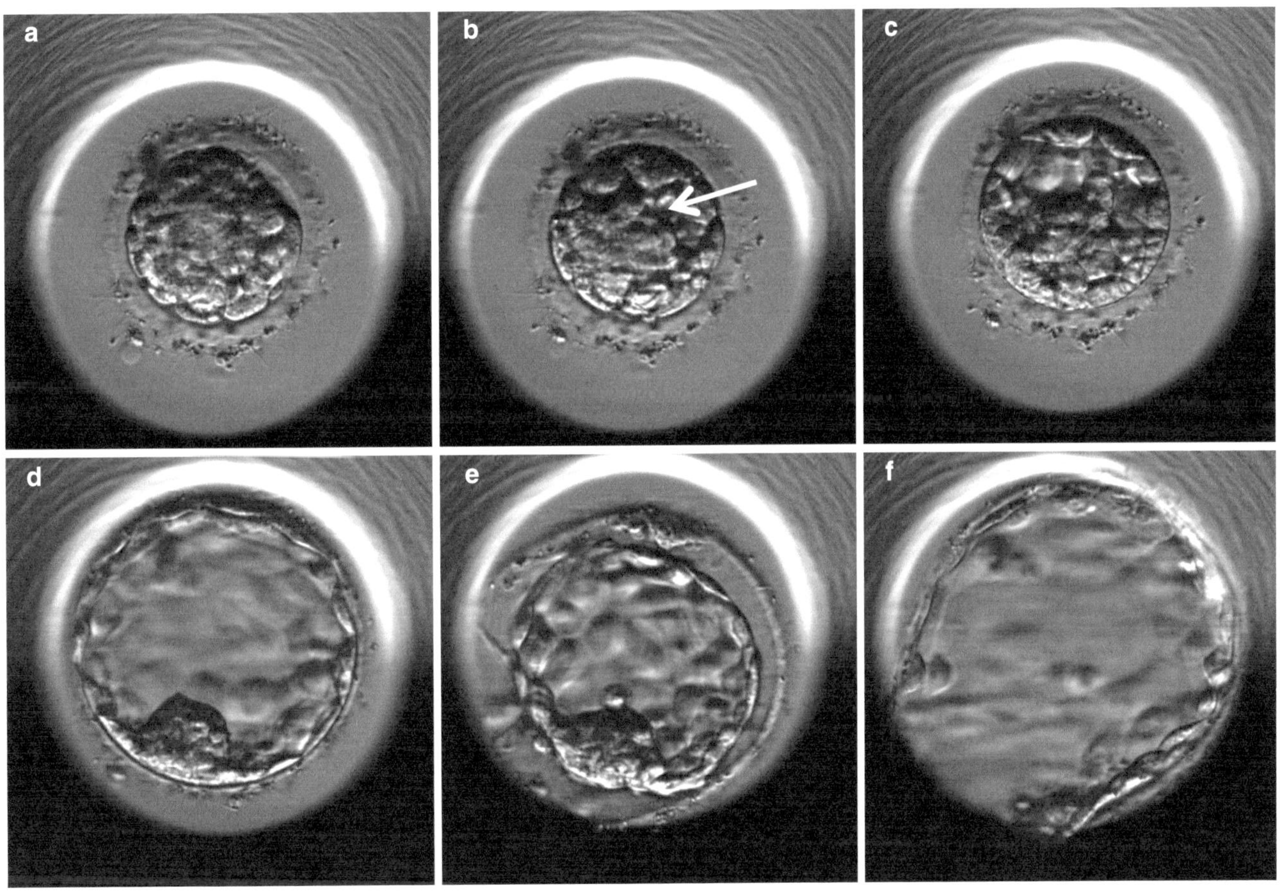

Fig. 91.6 Time-lapse images detailing blastocyst formation. (**a**) The embryo becomes a morula on Day 4 where cell membranes are lost. (**b**) Cavitation begins, indicated by an arrow, through the influx of water via the Na+/K+ ATPase. (**c**) The zona pellucida (ZP) begins to thin as the cavity increases in size and the two cell lines are formed. (**d**) The embryo is fully expanded, the ZP is barely visible, and the inner cell mass and the trophectoderm are well formed. (**e**) In vitro, some embryos are seen to undergo a collapsing process; in this image, the embryo undergoes a rapid collapse and re-expansion. (**f**) After a series of collapses, the embryo breaches the ZP to begin hatching

membrane, the transport of water into the cell and blastocoel cavity formation [64] (Fig. 91.7).

The contribution of the Na+/K+ ATPase pump to the production of the blastocoel cavity in human embryos was demonstrated via the relationship between pump activity and the expansion stages. Pump activity was similar at the morula and early blastocyst stages (27.7 pmol/embryo/h to 24.5 pmol/embryo/h, respectively) and then increased to

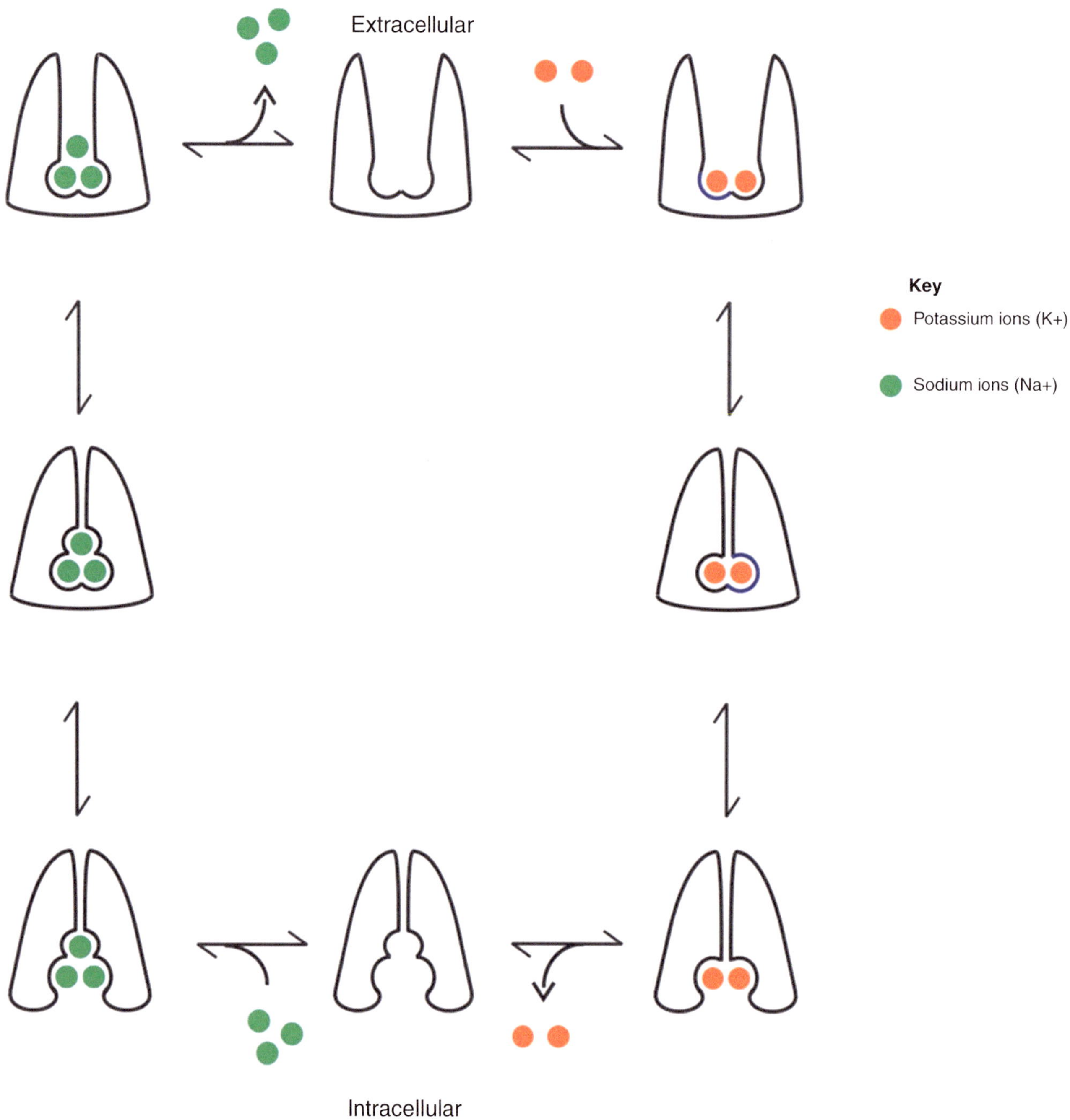

Fig. 91.7 A schematic representation of the sodium-potassium (Na+/K+) ATPase pump (adapted from Castillo et al. [65]). By using ATP, this protein-bound transporter is able to move sodium and potassium ions across the membrane against their concentration gradients. This activity causes the movement of water through osmosis dictated by the concentrations of sodium and potassium ions in the intra- and extracellular compartments

94.5 pmol/embryo/h at the expanding blastocyst stage before decreasing to 33.5 pmol/embryo/h at the expanded blastocyst stage [66].

During expansion, some embryos pass through a series of 'collapses', the purpose of which are largely unknown. It has been suggested that these collapses, and subsequent expansions, are to aid in hatching [67]. There is a paucity of research regarding the importance of this phenomenon; however, a TLI investigation of 277 embryos found that 54% embryos underwent no collapse, 22% underwent a single collapse and 24% underwent multiple collapses (average 2.9, range 2–9 contractions). In terms of the significance of these contractions, the live birth rate decreased progressively from no, single and multiple contractions (36%, 31%, 14%) indicating that the presence of multiple collapses is correlated with a reduction in live birth rate [68].

91.2.7 Blastocyst Hatching

Blastocyst hatching is a crucial event in preimplantation embryo development necessary to achieve implantation. However, the exact molecular processes underpinning the hatching mechanism remain unclear [69].

Hatching is primarily initiated by the exertion of hydrostatic pressure caused by blastocoel cavity growth, aided by the secretion of proteases to digest the zona pellucida (ZP) [70–72]. Human blastocysts hatch in a fully distended state, and the ZP remains largely intact and undigested [69]. In other species, such as the hamster, the ZP completely dissolves, and the blastocyst hatches in a collapsed state [73]. Common factors for mammalian blastocyst hatching are that the process involves dynamic actin-based trophectodermal projections together with a variety of autocrine and paracrine molecules [71].

The process of mammalian hatching remains a topic of keen interest. A recent review highlighted that both pro- and anti-inflammatory cytokines are potentially required to maintain normal embryo development and blastocyst hatching [69]. There may be functionally critical and indispensable cytokines, such as LIF [74], and cytokine receptors, such as IL-11R [75, 76] that orchestrate hatching and could be important indicators of embryo viability.

With TLI, hatching can be visualised with a greater degree of interest. There have been numerous reports in the literature of monozygotic twinning due to potential atypical hatching [77–79]. TLI can highlight embryos with atypical hatching patterns, and this could then be related to embryo quality or viability and potentially lead to the deselection of these embryos for transfer [80].

91.3 Morphokinetics

The first application of TLI in embryology was recorded in 1968, when chick embryos exposed to teratogenic doses of hypoxia were analysed [81]. Following this, studies relating to preimplantation embryonic development were published [82–84].

One of the earliest clinical applications of TLI was reported in 1997 regarding PB extrusion and PN formation [5]. Subsequently, two further TLI studies reported fragment internalisation in human embryos [85] and blastocoel collapse in mouse embryos [86].

From 2008 onwards, there have been numerous TLI studies of human preimplantation embryonic development to help determine embryo viability [17, 87, 88]. Whilst TLI for clinical application is now used worldwide, a Cochrane review showed there was no conclusive evidence of a difference in clinical pregnancy, miscarriage, live birth and stillbirth rates per couple randomised using TLI compared to standard incubation without TLI [89].

Basic embryo grading (blastomere number/size/evenness and proportion of fragmentation) remains the gold standard for embryo selection. However, static observations inevitably expose the embryo to suboptimal temperatures and gas concentrations when observations take place (out of the incubator) and restrict the overview of embryo development.

91.3.1 Identification of Useful Morphokinetic Parameters

TLI observations of embryo development have been termed morphokinetics and relate to the time an embryo reaches certain cell stages. For example, the time an embryo reaches two cells would be termed t2, and the time to reach three cells would be termed t3, four cells t4 and so on. Many morphokinetic parameters have been correlated with the embryo's ability to create a pregnancy both in humans (reviewed by [90]) and animals. These include the following:

- Appearance and disappearance of PN and nuclei at each cell stage [5, 10, 17, 91]
- Length of time between early cytokineses [92–94]
- Initiation of blastulation [95]

91.3.2 The Development of Embryo Scoring Algorithms

Following the identification of various morphokinetic parameters that could predict an embryo's ability to implant, these parameters were used to develop embryo scoring algorithms

(ESAs). ESAs incorporate a set of instructions for the user where, depending on the answers to the questions asked, a result is given that will aid in the selection of the best embryo for transfer.

Many ESAs have been published, each incorporating different morphokinetic parameters and optimum timings of morphokinetic parameters [40, 94, 95]. Since many clinics record morphokinetics differently, it became clear that a consensus was required—this was published in 2014 [96]. However, it has been suggested that the use of these ESAs in laboratories other than those in which they were developed may cause them to lose their diagnostic capabilities. Furthermore, this may be due to subtle environmental, treatment and patient-specific parameters such as differing stimulation regimes and varying treatment types (IVF or ICSI), a patient's endogenous hormone levels and also their age. This is now the direction many are taking in terms of research where it is becoming clear that ESAs to be used for all patients are ineffective.

91.3.3 Identification of Abnormal Embryo Development Using TLI

Further embryological phenomena have been observed using TLI, including direct cleavage from one to three cells ([97], see Fig. 91.8) and reverse cleavage ([98], see Fig. 91.9). The ability of such embryos to create a pregnancy

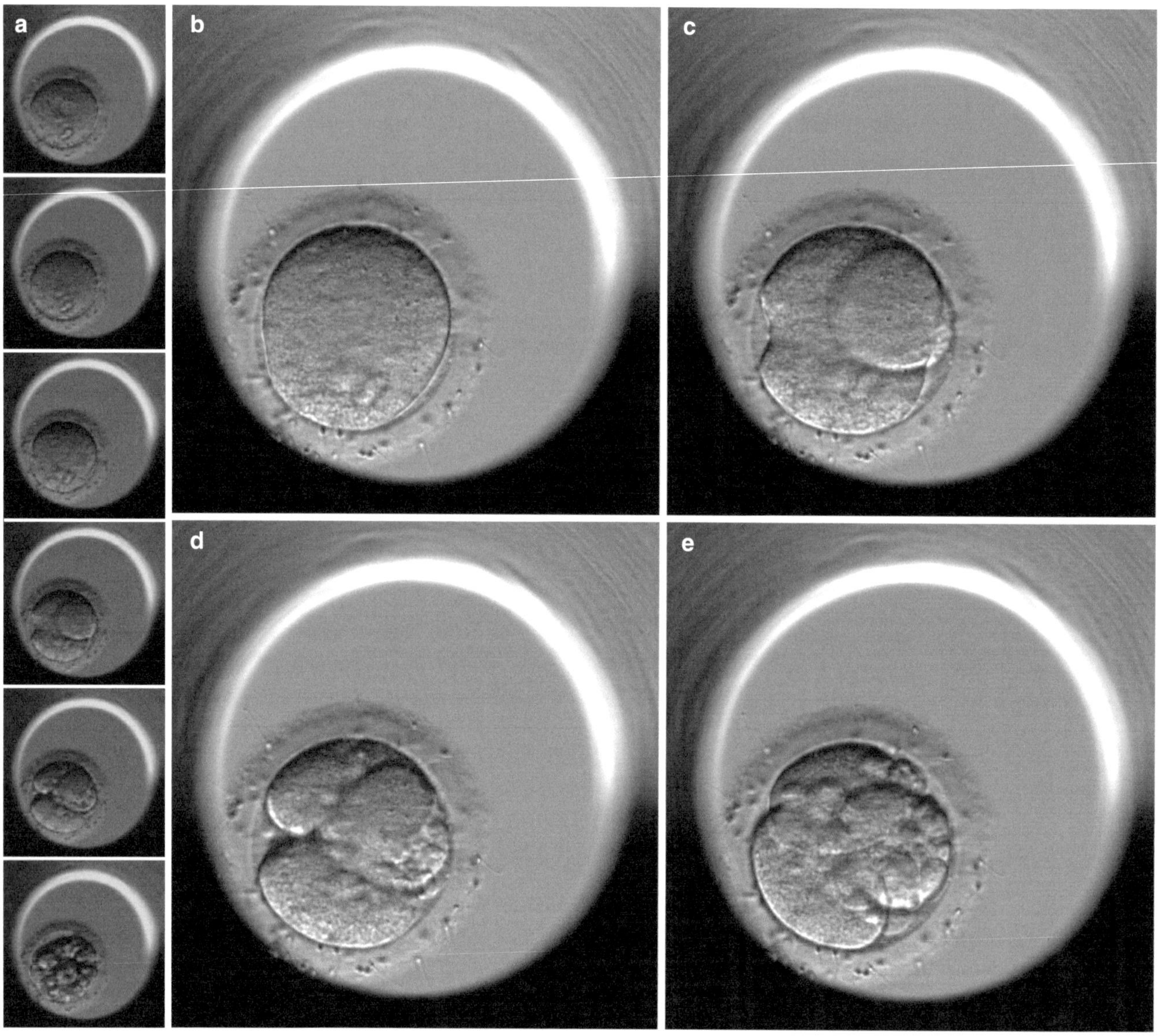

Fig. 91.8 Time-lapse images of an embryo undergoing direct cleavage. (**a**) A timeline of the embryo from 22.9 to 112 hpi. The final image indicates the stage that the embryo reaches after 5 days of culture. (**b**) Enlarged image of 28.9 hpi. (**c**) Enlarged image of 0.2 h later (29.1 hpi) where the cleavage furrow of the division into three cells can be seen. (**d**) Enlarged image of 29.4 hpi where three clear cells can be seen. (**e**) Enlarged image of 33.1 hpi where the division event has completed and three cells can be seen clearly

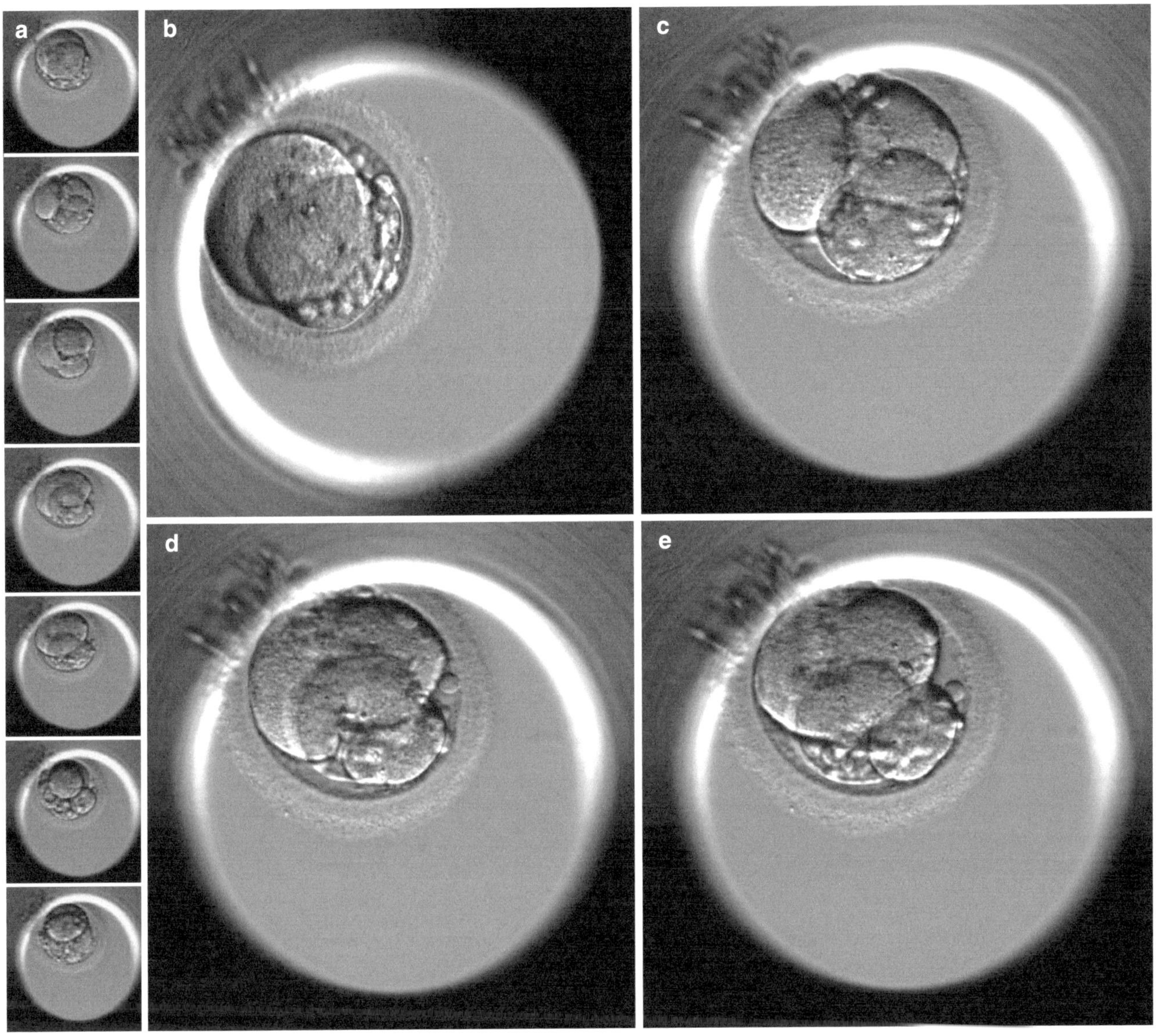

Fig. 91.9 Time-lapse images of an embryo undergoing reverse cleavage. (**a**) Timeline from 43.3 to 121.8 hpi. The final image indicates the stage that the embryo reaches after 121.8 hpi of culture. (**b**) Enlarged image of 43.3 hpi where the embryo has two blastomeres. (**c**) Enlarged image of 49.4 hpi where one blastomere has cleaved to produce a three-cell embryo. (**d**) Enlarged image of 51.6 hpi, 2.2 h after image (**c**), two blastomeres can be seen reverse cleaving. (**e**) Enlarged image of 60.3 hpi, 8.7 h after image (**d**), the two blastomeres have now completely fused and the embryo has two blastomeres

has been shown to be significantly reduced [99]. Strangely, embryos exhibiting cleavage anomalies, such as reverse cleavage, have been reported to have a 40% utilisation rate [100].

Other morphokinetic phenomena that might gain more attention due to TLI include the following:

- Absent cleavage (the process by which a blastomere undergoes a pseudo division (seen as a 'roll') that does not produce two discernable blastomeres but a single blastomere containing multiple nuclei) (Fig. 91.10)
- Chaotic cleavage (apparent cleavage not creating distinctive blastomeres but what appears to be many fragments) (Fig. 91.11)
- Cell lysis

All of these could give the embryologist more information regarding the most viable embryo in a patients' cohort.

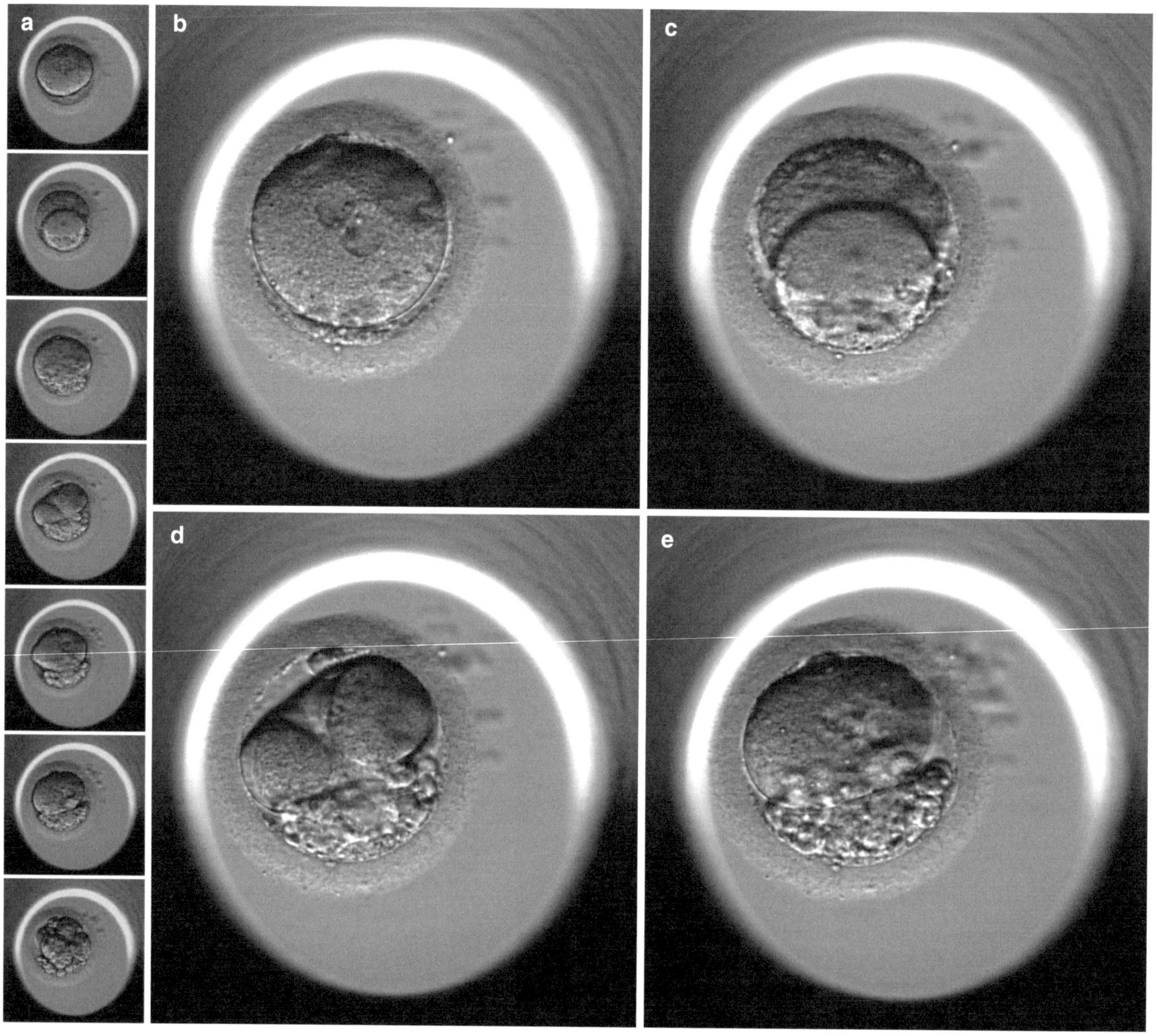

Fig. 91.10 Time-lapse images of an embryo undergoing an abnormal division event termed absent cleavage. (**a**) Timeline from 26.6 hpi to 139.1 hpi. The final image indicates the stage the embryo reaches after 139.1 hpi of culture. (**b**) Enlarged image of 26.6 hpi where two pronuclei can be seen indicating normal fertilization. (**c**) Enlarged image of 29.9 hpi where it appears that two blastomeres have been formed; however, just 1 h later in image (**d**) these two blastomeres are no longer evident. (**e**) Enlarged image at 39.9 hpi where only one clear blastomere can be seen with multiple nuclei indicating that effective cleavage has not occurred

91.4 Embryo Metabolism

Metabolism is arguably one of the most studied areas of preimplantation embryo development getting substantial and continued attention since the early 1970s. It has long been known that metabolism changes from anaerobic to aerobic in line with the EGA [101] and that the substrate requirements change accordingly [60, 102]. Pyruvate uptake exceeds that of glucose in early developmental stages, with glucose becoming a dominant substrate in the blastocyst [103] most likely due to the energy demands of the Na+/K+ ATPase pump required to form the blastocoel cavity [104]. Amino acids are also important for embryo metabolism not only as precursors for protein synthesis but as cell membrane transporters, among others [105, 106].

The 'quiet' embryo hypothesis, proposed in 2002, denotes that embryos with a relatively low metabolism have a higher embryo viability [107]. This hypothesis was then developed to give the idea of a 'quiet range' [108] where categories of quietness were considered owing to the fact that a metabolism that is too quiet may represent an embryo about to arrest. This was further developed into the 'Goldilocks principle'. This states that, rather than a quiet metabolism, embryo metabolism must fall within certain margins, as opposed to

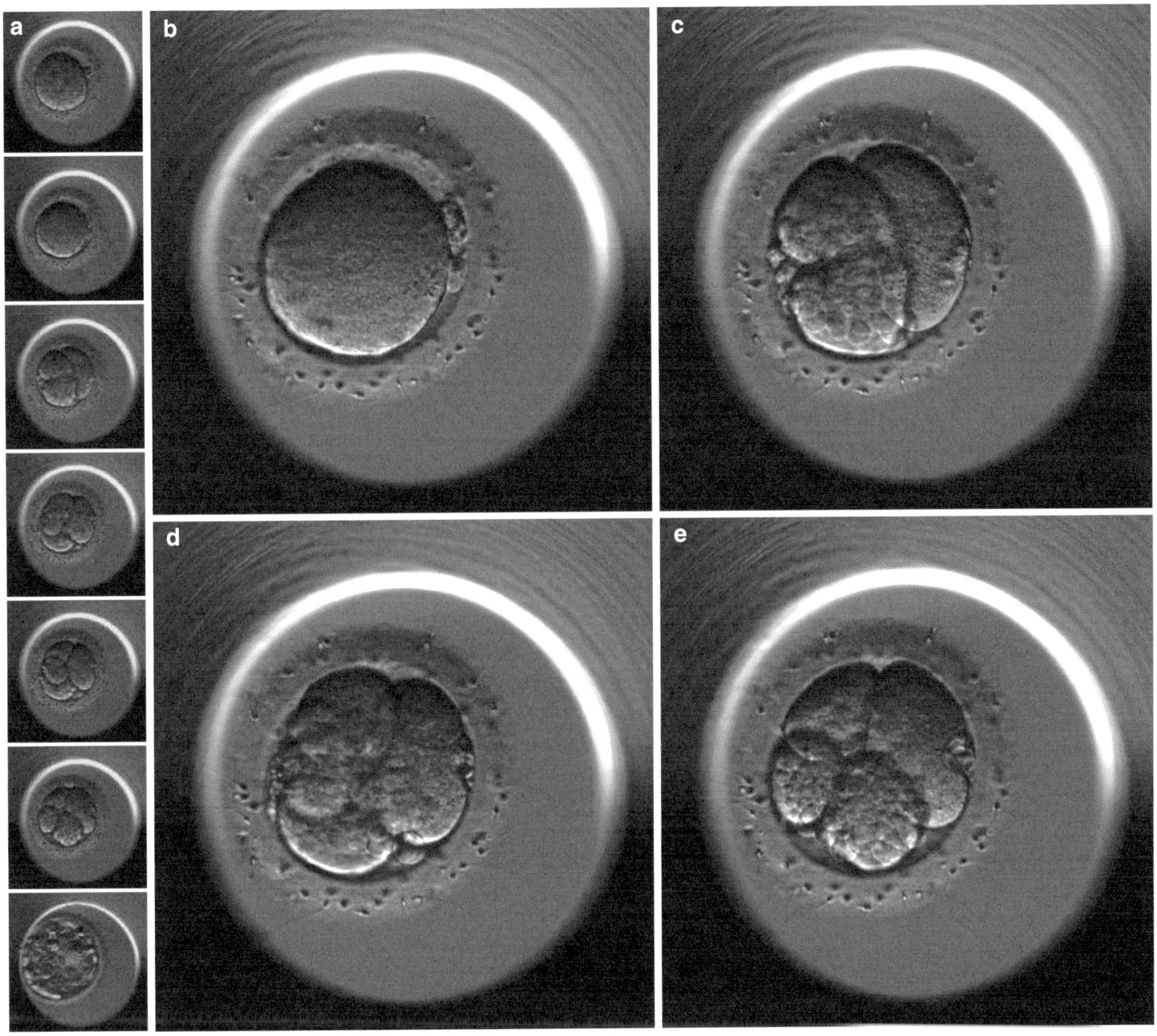

Fig. 91.11 Time-lapse images of an embryo undergoing an abnormal division event termed chaotic cleavage. (**a**) Timeline of embryo development from 21.9 hpi to 138.6 hpi where the final image indicates the stage that the embryo reaches at the end of its culture period. (**b**) Enlarged image of 27.4 hpi showing the frame immediately prior to the cleavage event. (**c**) Enlarged image of 29.1 hpi where three blastomeres are observed. (**d**) Enlarged image of 30.9 hpi where up to five blastomeres can be seen. (**e**) Enlarged image of 35.0 hpi, where the embryo has completed its division event and settled with four blastomeres of uneven size

reaching extremes, much like the Goldilocks fairy tale. The existence of a 'Goldilocks zone' has been proposed (insinuating 'just the right amount') within which embryos with maximum developmental potential can be categorised [104].

91.4.1 Using Metabolomics to Determine Embryo Viability

It is an attractive principle to be able to quantify an embryo's substrate use and waste production and relate this to likelihood of implantation. As such, there have been a number of studies of the embryo metabolome, using spent culture media samples, each finding a significant correlation between implantation potential and the embryo's metabolomic profile or 'viability score' (VS) [109, 110].

More specifically, nuclear magnetic resonance spectroscopy (NMRS) has been used to deduce relationships between specific metabolites, such as amino acid turnover, and an embryo's implantation potential. It has been concluded that:

- An increase in asparagine and decreased glycine and leucine in spent embryo culture media correlated with viable pregnancies [111].

- The ratio between glutamate and alanine/lactate was higher for implanted embryos [112].

A significant correlation between five oxidative metabolism biomarkers and implantation potential has also been proposed [113, 114]. However, it transpired that morphology scores did not correlate with the embryonic metabolic activity, in terms of oxidative metabolism, and pregnancy outcome, with >85% of transferred embryos classed as top morphological grade but only 27% resulting in pregnancy [114].

Whilst metabolomic profiling as a method of embryo selection continues to be a hive of research activity, there have not yet been any significant developments for the clinical implementation of this embryo selection method.

91.5 The In Vitro Versus In Vivo Environment

It is logical that for successful embryo development, the in vitro environment should mimic that of the in vivo situation as closely as possible. However, in practice it is not always possible to, firstly, know specific in vivo environmental factors and, secondly, to implement them. Osmolality is a classic example of this disparity.

Commercially available culture media have a range of osmolality from 255 to 298 mOsm/kg, yet the in vivo environment may have an osmolality as high as 360 mOsm/kg [115]. Interestingly, an in vitro osmolality >300 mOsm/kg has been shown to cause severe developmental retardation in the resulting offspring [116, 117].

Oxygen concentration is a further example of the difference between the in vitro and in vivo environment. Historically, embryos were cultured at atmospheric oxygen concentrations (20%). However, it has been shown that the oxygen concentration in vivo is considerably lower (5%) than the atmospheric level [118]. There is a wealth of evidence, including a Cochrane review, showing that culturing embryos at low oxygen concentration (using a trigas system) provide a clinical benefit [119].

91.6 Conclusion

The purpose of this chapter was to delineate embryo development from the zygote to the blastocyst. It is clear that there remains much to learn regarding preimplantation embryo development and not only is there a lack of basic scientific knowledge in some areas but the significance of various embryonic processes is yet to be elucidated. With the introduction of new technologies such as TLI and noninvasive metabolics, some of the less clear phenomenon can be addressed, such as the processes underpinning compaction, hatching and blastocyst collapse. A large part of the success of reproductive technologies lies with the preimplantation embryo, and the more information that can be gathered about these first few crucial days of development, the more likely it is that successful treatment will follow.

References

1. Cooper GM, Sunderland MA. The cell: a molecular approach. 2nd ed. Sunderland: Sinauer Associates; 2000.
2. Wright G, Wiker S, Elsner C, Kort H, Massey J, Mitchell D, et al. Observations on the morphology of pronuclei and nucleoli in human zygotes and implications for cryopreservation. Hum Reprod. 1990;5(1):109–15.
3. Longo FJ. Sperm aster in rabbit zygote: its structure and function. J Cell Biol. 1976;69(3):539–47.
4. Schatten G. The supramolecular organization of the cytoskeleton during fertilization. Subcell Biochem. 1984;10:359–453.
5. Payne D, Flaherty SP, Barry MF, Matthews CD. Preliminary observations on polar body extrusion and pronuclear formation in human oocytes using time-lapse video cinematography. Hum Reprod. 1997;12:532–41.
6. Nagy ZP, Liu J, Joris H, Devroey P, Van Steirteghem A. Time-course of oocyte activation, pronucleus formation and cleavage in human oocytes fertilized by intracytoplasmic sperm injection. Hum Reprod. 1994;9(9):1743–8.
7. Nagy ZP, Janssenswillen C, Janssens R, De Vos A, Staessen C, Van de Velde H, et al. Timing of oocyte activation, pronucleus formation and cleavage in humans after intracytoplasmic sperm injection (ICSI) with testicular spermatozoa and after ICSI or in-vitro fertilization on sibling oocytes with ejaculated spermatozoa. Hum Reprod. 1998;13(6):1606–12.
8. Fancsovits P, Toth L, Takacs ZF, Murber A, Papp Z, Urbancsek J. Early pronuclear breakdown is a good indicator of embryo quality and viability. Fertil Steril. 2005;84(4):881–7.
9. Aguilar J, Motato Y, Escriba MJ, Ojeda M, Munoz E, Meseguer M. The human first cell cycle: impact on implantation. Reprod Biomed Online. 2014;28(4):475–84.
10. Azzarello A, Hoest T, Mikkelsen AL. The impact of pronuclei morphology and dynamicity on live birth outcome after time-lapse culture. Hum Reprod. 2012;27:2649–57.
11. Scott L, Alvero R, Leondires M, Miller B. The morphology of human pronuclear embryos is positively related to blastocyst development and implantation. Hum Reprod. 2000;15(11):2394–403.
12. Tesarik J, Greco E. The probability of abnormal preimplantation development can be predicted by a single static observation on pronuclear stage morphology. Hum Reprod. 1999;14:1318–23.
13. Nagy ZP, Dozortsev D, Diamond M, Rienzi L, Ubaldi F. Pronuclear morphology evaluation with subsequent evaluation of embryo morphology significantly increases implantation rates. Fertil Steril. 2003;80(1):67–74.
14. James AN, Hennessy S, Reggio B, Wiemer K, Larsen F, Cohen J. The limited importance of pronuclear scoring of human zygotes. Hum Reprod. 2006;21(6):1599–604.
15. Salumets A, Hyden-Granskog C, Suikkari AM, Tiitinen A, Tuuri T. The predictive value of pronuclear morphology of zygotes in the assessment of human embryo quality. Hum Reprod. 2001;16(10):2177–81.
16. Weitzman VN, Schnee-Riesz J, Benadiva C, Nulsen J, Siano L, Maier D. Predictive value of embryo grading for embryos with known outcomes. Fertil Steril. 2010;93(2):658–62.

17. Lemmen JG, Agerholm I, Ziebe S. Kinetic markers of human embryo quality using time-lapse recordings of IVF/ICSI-ferilized oocytes. Reprod Biomed Online. 2008;17:385–91.
18. Shoukir Y, Campana A, Farley T, Sakkas D. Early cleavage of in-vitro fertilized human embryos to the 2-cell stage: a novel indicator of embryo quality and viability. Hum Reprod. 1997;12(7):1531–6.
19. de los Santos MJ, Arroyo G, Busquet A, Calderon G, Cuadros J, Hurtado de Mendoza MV, Moragas M, Herrer R, Oritz A, Pons C, Ten J, Vilches MA, Figueroa MJ. ASEBIR Interest Group in Embryology. Fertil Steril. 2014;101(4):981–7.
20. Jeanblanc M, Salvaing J, Mason K, Debey P, Beaujean N. Embryonic genome activation. Gynecol Obstet Fertil. 2008;36(11):1126–32.
21. Van Royen E, Mangelschots K, De Neubourg D, Valkenburg M, Van de Meerssche M, Ryckaert G, et al. Characterization of a top quality embryo, a step towards single embryo transfer. Hum Reprod. 1999;14(9):2345–9.
22. Ziebe S, Petersen K, Lindenbery S, Andersen AG, Gabrielsen A, Andersen AN. Embryo morphology or cleavage stage: how to select the best embryos for transfer after in-vitro fertilization. Hum Reprod. 1997;12(7):1545–9.
23. Hardarson T, Hanson C, Sjogren A, Lundin K. Human embryos with unevenly sized blastomeres have lower pregnancy and implantation rates: indications for aneuploidy and multinucleation. Hum Reprod. 2001;16:313–8.
24. Van Royen E, Mangelschots K, Vercruyssen M, De Neubourg D, Valkenburg M, Ryckaert G, et al. Multinucleation in cleavage stage embryos. Hum Reprod. 2003;18(5):1062–9.
25. Cutting R, Morrol D, Roberts SA, Pickering S, Rutherford A. BFS and ACE. Elective single embryo transfer: guidelines for practice British Fertility Society and Association of Clinical Embryologists. Hum Fertil. 2008;11(3):131–46.
26. Collins K, Jacks T, Pavletich NP. Cancer and the cell cycle. PNAS. 1997;94(7):2776–8.
27. Alberts B, Johnson A, Lewis J, Raff M, Roberts K, Walter P. Molecular biology of the cell. 5th ed. New York: Garland Science; 2007.
28. Imoto Y, Yoshida Y, Yagisawa F, Kuroiwa H, Kuroiwa T. The cell cycle, including the mitotic cycle and organelle division cycles, as revealed by cytological observations. J Electron Microsc. 2011;60:117–36.
29. Eggert US, Mitchison TJ, Field CM. Animal cytokinesis: from parts list to mechanisms. Annu Rev Biochem. 2006;75:543–66.
30. Assou S, Anahory T, Pantesco V, Le Carrour T, Pellestor F, Klein B, et al. The human cumulus-oocyte complex gene-expression profile. Hum Reprod. 2006;21(7):1705–19.
31. Galán A, Montaner D, Póo ME, Valbuena D, Ruiz V, Aguilar C, et al. Functional genomics of 5- to 8-cell stage human embryos by blastomere single-cell cDNA analysis. PLoS One. 2010;26:e13615.
32. Nothias JY, Majumder S, Kaneko KJ, DePamphilis ML. Regulation of gene expression at the beginning of mammalian development. J Biol Chem. 1995;270(38):22077–80.
33. Dobson AT, Raja R, Abeyta MJ, Taylor T, Shen S, Haqq C, et al. The unique transcriptome through day 3 of human preimplantation development. Hum Mol Genet. 2004;13:1461–70.
34. Braude P, Bolton V, Moore S. Human gene expression first occurs between the four- and eight-cell stages of preimplantation development. Nature. 1988;332:459–61.
35. Taylor DM, Ray PF, Ao A, Winston RM, Handyside AH. Paternal transcripts for glucose-6-phosphate dehydrogenase and adenosine deaminase are first detectable in the human preimplantation embryo at the three- to four-cell stage. Mol Repr Dev. 1997;48:442–8.
36. Latham KE, Schultz RM. Embryonic genome activation. Front Biosci. 2001;6:748–59.
37. Ao A, Erickson RP, Winston RM, Handyside AH. Transcription of paternal Y-linked genes in the human zygote as early as the pronucleate stage. Zygote. 1994;2:281–7.
38. Artley JK, Braude PR, Johnson MH. Gene activity and cleavage arrest in human pre-embryos. Hum Reprod. 1992;7:1014–21.
39. Kakourou G, Jaroud S, Tulay P, Heath C, Serhal P, Harper JC, et al. Investigation of gene expression profiles before and after embryonic genome activation and assessment of functional pathways at the human metaphase II oocyte and blastocyst stage. Fertil Steril. 2013;99:803–14.
40. Wong CC, Loewke KE, Bossert NL, Behr B, De Jonge CJ, Baer TM, et al. Non-invasive imaging of human embryos before embryonic genome activation predicts development to the blastocyst stage. Nat Biotechnol. 2011;28:1115–21.
41. Niakan KK, Han J, Pedersen RA, Simon C, Reijo Pera RA. Human pre-implantation embryo development. Development. 2012;139:829–41.
42. Handyside AH. Distribution of antibody- and lectin-binding sites on dissociated blastomeres from mouse morulae: evidence for polarization at compaction. J Embryol Exp Morphol. 1980;60:99–116.
43. Reeve W, Ziomek C. Distribution of microvilli on dissociated blastomeres from mouse embryos: evidence for surface polarization at compaction. J Embryol Exp Morphol. 1981;62:339–50.
44. Biggers JD, Bell JE, Benos DJ. Mammalian blastocyst: transport functions in a developing epithelium. Am J Phys. 1988;255(4 Pt 1):C419–32.
45. Johnson MH, Chisholm JC, Fleming TP, Houliston E. A role for cytoplasmic determinants in the development of the mouse early embryo? J Embryol Exp Morphol. 1986;97(Suppl):97–121.
46. Lee S, Gilula NB, Warner AE. Gap junctional communication and compaction during preimplantation stages of mouse development. Cell. 1987;51(5):851–60.
47. Saini D, Yamanaka Y. Cell polarity-dependent regulation of cell allocation and the first lineage specification in the preimplantation mouse embryo. Curr Top Dev Biol. 2018;128:11–35.
48. Nikas G, Ao A, Winston RM, Handyside AH. Compaction and surface polarity in the human embryo in vitro. Biol Reprod. 1996;55(1):32–7.
49. Dale B, Tosti E, Laccarino M. Is the plasma membrane of the human oocyte reorganized following fertilization and early cleavage? Zygote. 1995;3:31–6.
50. Mottla GL, Adelman MR, Hall JL, Gindoff PR, Stillman RJ, Johnson KE. Lineage tracing demonstrates that the blastomeres of early cleavage stage human pre-embryos contribute to both trophectoderm and inner cell mass. Hum Reprod. 1995;10:384–91.
51. Ebner T, Moser M, Shebl O, Sommergruber M, Gaiswinkler U, Tews G. Morphological analysis at compacting stage is a valuable prognostic tool for ICSI patients. Reprod Biomed Online. 2009;18:61–6.
52. Pantos K, Makrakis E, Chronopoulou M, Biba M, Perdikaris A, Dafereras A. Day 4 versus day 3 embryo transfer: a prospective study of clinical outcomes. Fertil Steril. 2008;89:573–7.
53. Tao J, Tamis R, Fink K, Williams B, Nelson-White T, Craig R. The neglected morula/compact stage embryo transfer. Hum Reprod. 2002;17:1513–8.
54. Desai NN, Goldstein J, Rowland DY, Goldfarb JM. Morphological evaluation of human embryos and derivation of an embryo quality scoring system specific for day 3 embryos: a preliminary study. Hum Reprod. 2000;15:2190–6.
55. Skiadas CC, Jackson KV, Racowsky C. Early compaction on day 3 may be associated with increased implantation potential. Fertil Steril. 2006;86:1386–91.
56. Le Cruguel S, Ferre-L'Hotellier V, Moriniere C, Lemerie S, Reynier P, Descamps P, et al. Early compaction at day 3 may be

a useful additional criterion for embryo transfer. J Assist Reprod Genet. 2013;30:683–90.
57. Iwata K, Yumoto K, Sugishima M, Mizoguchi C, Kai Y, Iba Y, et al. Analysis of compaction initiation in human embryos by using time-lapse cinematography. J Assist Reprod Genet. 2014;31(4):421–6.
58. Edwards RG, Hansis C. Initial differentiation of blastomeres in 4-cell human embryos and its significance for early embryogenesis and implantation. Reprod Biomed Online. 2005;11:206–18.
59. Cauffman G, De Rycke M, Sermon K, Liebaers I, Van de Velde H. Markers that define stemness in ESC are unable to identify the totipotent cells in human preimplantation embryos. Hum Reprod. 2009;24(1):63–70.
60. Leese HJ. Metabolic control during preimplantation mammalian development. Hum Reprod Update. 1995;1:63–72.
61. Houghton FD, Thompson JG, Kennedy CJ, Leese HJ. Oxygen consumption and energy metabolism of the early mouse embryo. Mol Reprod Dev. 1996;44(4):476–85.
62. Thompson JG, Partridge RJ, Houghton FD, Cox CI, Leese HJ. Oxygen uptake and carbohydrate metabolism by in vitro derived bovine embryos. J Reprod Fertil. 1996;106(2):299–306.
63. McBride BW, Kelly JM. Energy cost of absorption and metabolism in the ruminant gastrointestinal tract and liver: a review. J Anim Sci. 1990;68(9):2997–3010.
64. Watson AJ, Barcroft LC. Regulation of blastocyst formation. Front Biosci. 2001;1(6):D708–30.
65. Castillo JP, Rui H, Basilio D, Das A, Roux B, Latorre R, et al. Mechanism of potassium ion uptake by the Na+/K+ ATPase. Nat Commun. 2015;6:7622. https://doi.org/10.1038/ncomms8622.
66. Houghton FD, Humpherson PG, Hawkhead JA, Hall CJ, Leese HJ. Na+, K+, ATPase activity in the human and bovine preimplantation embryo. Dev Biol. 2003;263(2):360–6.
67. Yumoto K, Iwata K, Sargent CH, Kai Y, Imajyo A, Iba Y, et al. Dynamic analysis of the relationship between the collapse of blastulation and hatching in human blastocysts using time-lapse cinematography. Fertil Steril. 2012;97:S30.
68. Bodri D, Sugimoto T, Yao Serna J, Kawachiya S, Kato R, Matsumoto T. Blastocyst collapse is not an independent predictor of reduced live birth: a time-lapse study. Fertil Steril. 2016;105:1476–83.
69. Seshagiri PB, Vani V, Madhulika P. Cytokines and blastocyst hatching. Am J Reprod Immunol. 2016;75(3):208–17.
70. Mishra A, Seshagiri PB. Evidence for the involvement of a species-specific embryonic protease in zona escape of hamster blastocysts. Mol Hum Reprod. 2000;6:1005–12.
71. Seshagiri PB, Sen Roy S, Sireesha G, Rao RP. Cellular and molecular regulation of mammalian blastocyst hatching. Rev J Reprod Immunol. 2009;83:79–84.
72. Sireesha GV, Mason RW, Hassanein M, Tonack S, Navarrete Santos A, Fischer B, et al. Role of cathepsins in blastocyst hatching in the golden hamster. Mol Hum Reprod. 2008;14:337–46.
73. Mishra A, Seshagiri PB. Successful development in vitro of hamster 8-cell embryos to 'zona-escaped' and attached blastocysts: assessment of quality and trophoblast outgrowth. Reprod Fertil Dev. 1998;10:413–20.
74. Stewart CL, Kasper P, Brunet LJ, Bhatt H, Gadi I, Kontegen F, et al. Blastocyst implantation depends on maternal expression of leukemia inhibitory factor. Nature. 1992;352:76–9.
75. Bilinski P, Roopenian D, Gossler A. Maternal IL-11Ra function is required for normal decidua and fetoplacental development in mice. Genes Dev. 1998;12:2234–43.
76. Robb L, Li R, Hartley L, Nandurkar HH, Koentgen F, Begley CG. Infertility in female mice lacking the receptor for interleukin-11 is due to a defective uterine response to implantation. Natl Med. 1998;4:303–8.
77. Behr B, Milki AA. Visualization of atypical hatching of a human blastocyst in vitro forming two identical embryos. Fertil Steril. 2003;80:1502–3.
78. Sheiner E, Kivilevitch Z, Levitas E, Sonin Y, Albotiano S, Har-Vardi I. Monozygotic twins following blastocyst transfer: a report of two cases. Eur J Obstet Gynecol Reprod Biol. 2001;98:135–8.
79. Van Langendonckt A, Wyns C, Godin PA, Toussaint-Demylle D, Donnez J. Atypical hatching of a human blastocyst leading to monozygotic twinning: a case report. Fertil Steril. 2000;74:1047–50.
80. Sutherland K, Leitch J, Lyall H, Woodward B. Time-lapse imaging of inner cell mass splitting with monochorionic triamniotic triplets after elective single embryo transfer: a case report. Reprod Biomed Online. 2018;
81. Grabowski CT, Schroeder RE. A time-lapse photographic study of chick embryos exposed to teratogenic doses of hypoxia. Exp Hematol. 1968;19(3):347–62.
82. Alexandre H, Mulnard J. Time-lapse cinematography study of the germinal vesicle behaviour in mouse primary oocytes treated with activators of protein kinases A and C. Gamete Res. 1988;21(4):359–65.
83. Milligan MP, Harris S, Dennis KJ. Comparison of sperm velocity in fertile and infertile groups as measured by time-lapse photography. Fertil Steril. 1980;34:509–11.
84. Schatten H, Schatten G. Surface activity at the egg plasma membrane during sperm incorporation and its cytochalasin B sensitivity. Scanning electron microscopy and time-lapse video microscopy during fertilization of the sea urchin *Lytechinus variegatus*. Dev Biol. 1980;78(2):435–49.
85. Hardarson T, Lofman C, Coull G, Sjogren A, Hamberger L, Edwards RG. Internalization of cellular fragments in a human embryo: time-lapse recordings. Reprod Biomed Online. 2002;5:36–8.
86. Niimura S. Time-lapse videomicrographic analyses of contractions in mouse blastocysts. J Reprod Dev. 2003;49(6):413–23.
87. Arav A, Aroyo A, Yavin S, Roth Z. Prediction of embryonic developmental competence by time-lapse observation and 'shortest-half' analysis. Reprod Biomed Online. 2008;17(5):669–75.
88. Mio Y, Maeda K. Time-lapse cinematography of dynamic changes occurring during in vitro development of human embryos. Am J Obstet Gynecol. 2008;199:660.e1–5.
89. Armstrong S, Bhide P, Jordan V, Pacey A, Farquhar C. Time-lapse systems for embryo incubation and assessment in assisted reproduction. Cochrane Database Syst Rev. 2018;25(5):CD011320. https://doi.org/10.1002/14651858.
90. Kirkegaard K, Agerholm IE, Ingerslev HJ. Time-lapse monitoring as a tool for clinical embryo assessment. Hum Reprod. 2012;27(5):1277–85.
91. Scott L. The origin and consequences of day 2 multinucleation of human embryos. Abstracts of the 26th annual meeting of ESHRE. Rome; 2010, vol. 25. p. 204.
92. Cruz M, Garrido N, Herrero J, Perez-Cano I, Munoz M, Meseguer M. Timing of cell division in human cleavage stage embryos is linked with blastocyst formation and quality. Reprod Biomed Online. 2012;25:371–81.
93. Herrero J, Tejera A, Ramsing N, Romero JL, Rubio I. Establishing the optimal time ranges of key events during development using time lapse video cinematography. Fertil Steril. 2011;96(Suppl):S102.
94. Meseguer M, Rubio I, Cruz M, Basile N, Marcos J, Requena A. Embryo incubation and selection in a time-lapse monitoring system improves pregnancy outcome compared with a standard incubator: a retrospective cohort study. Fertil Steril. 2012;98:1481–9.
95. Campbell A, Fishel S, Bowman N, Duffy S, Sedler M, Hickman CF. Modelling a risk classification of aneuploidy in human

embryos using non invasive morphokinetics. Reprod Biomed Online. 2013;26:477–85.

96. Ciray HN, Campbell A, Agerholm IE, Aguilar J, Chamayou S, Esbert M, et al. Proposed guidelines on the nomenclature and annotation of dynamic human embryo monitoring by a time lapse user group. Hum Reprod. 2014;29:2650–60.
97. Rubio I, Kuhlmann R, Agerholm I, Kirk J, Herrero J, Escriba MJ, et al. Limited implantation success of direct cleave human zygotes: a time lapse study. Fertil Steril. 2012;98:1458–63.
98. Hickman CFL, Campbell A, Duffy S, Fishel S. Reverse cleavage: its significance with regards to human embryo morphokinetics, ploidy and stimulation protocol. Hum Reprod. 2012;27(Suppl. 2).
99. Barrie A, Homburg R, McDowell G, Brown J, Kingsland C, Troup S. Preliminary investigation of the prevalence and implantation potential of abnormal embryonic phenotypes assessed using time-lapse imaging. Reprod Biomed Online. 2017;34(5):455–62.
100. Desai NN, Ploskonka S, Goodman LR, Austin C, Goldberg J, Falcone T. Analysis of embryo morphokinetics, multinucleation and cleavage anomalies using continuous time lapse monitoring in blastocyst transfer cycles. Reprod Biol Endocrinol. 2014;12:54.
101. Martin KL. Nutritional and metabolic requirements of early cleavage stage embryos and blastocysts. Hum Fertil. 2000;3:247–54.
102. Lane M, Gardner DK. Amino acids and vitamins prevent culture-induced metabolic perturbations and associated loss of viability of mouse blastocysts. Hum Reprod. 1998;13:991–7.
103. Gott AL, Hardy K, Winston RM, Leese HJ. Non-invasive measurement of pyruvate and glucose uptake and lactate production by single human preimplantation embryos. Hum Reprod. 1990;5:104–8.
104. Leese HJ, Guerif F, Allgar V, Brison D, Lundin K, Sturmey RG. Biological optimisation, the Goldilocks principle, and how much is lagom in the preimplantation embryo. Mol Reprod Dev. 2016;83:748.
105. Bavister BD, Leibfried ML, Lieberman G. Development of preimplantation embryos of the golden hamster in a defined culture medium. Biol Reprod. 1983;28:235–47.
106. Devreker F, Hardy K, Van den Bergh M, Vannin AS, Emiliani S, Englert Y. Amino acids promote human blastocyst development in vitro. Hum Reprod. 2001;16:749–56.
107. Leese HJ. Quiet please, do not disturb: a hypothesis of embryo metabolism and viability. BioEssays. 2002;24:845–9.
108. Leese HJ, Baumann CG, Brison DR, McEvoy TG, Sturmey RG. Metabolism of viable mammalian embryo: quietness revisited. Mol Hum Reprod. 2008;14:667–72.
109. Scott R, Seli E, Miller K, Sakkas D, Scott K, Burns DH. Non invasive metabolomic profiling of human embryo culture media using Raman spectroscopy predicts embryonic reproductive potential: a prospective blinded pilot study. Fertil Steril. 2008;90:77–83.
110. Seli E, Sakkas D, Scott R, Kwok SC, Rosendahl SM, Burns DH. Noninvasive metabolomic profiling of embryo culture media using Raman and near-infrared spectroscopy correlates with reproductive potential of embryos in women undergoing in-vitro fertilisation. Fertil Steril. 2007;88:1350–8.
111. Brison DR, Houghton FD, Falconer D, Roberts SA, Hawkhead J, Humpherson PG, et al. Identification of viable embryos in IVF by non-invasive measurement of amino acid turnover. Hum Reprod. 2004;19:2319–24.
112. Seli E, Botros L, Sakkas D, Burns DH. Non-invasive metabolomic profiling of embryo culture media using proton nuclear magnetic resonance correlates with reproductive potential of embryos in women undergoing in-vitro fertilisation. Fertil Steril. 2008;90:2183–94.
113. Hardarson T, Rogberg L, Ahlstrom A, Wikland M, Rose P, Burns D. Non-invasive assessment of embryo reproductive potential: metabolomic profiling of biomarkers of oxidative metabolism (OM) during embryo development. Fertil Steril. 2007;88:S307–8.
114. Vergouw CG, Botros LL, Roos P, Lens JW, Schats R, Hompes PG, et al. Near infrared spectroscopy as a tool to predict embryo viability: a novel, non invasive method for embryo selection. Hum Reprod. 2007;23:1499–504.
115. Quinn P. Media and embryo interactions – antibiotics in culture media, solutions, and Systems in Human ART. Cambridge: Cambridge University Press; 2014.
116. Richards T, Wang F, Liu L, Baltz JM. Rescue of postcompaction-stage mouse embryo development from hyper-tonicity by amino acid transporter substrates that may function as organic osmolytes. Biol Reprod. 2010;82:769–77.
117. Swain JE, Cabrera L, Xu X, Smith GD. Microdrop preparation factors influence culture-media osmolality which can impair mouse embryo preimplantation development. Reprod Biomed Online. 2012;24:142–7.
118. Catt JW, Henman M. Toxic effects of oxygen on human embryo development. Hum Reprod. 2000;15:199–206.
119. Bontekoe S, Mantikou E, van Wely M, Seshadri S, Repping S, Mastenbroek S. Low oxygen concentrations for embryo culture in assisted reproductive technologies. Cochrane Database Syst Rev. 2012;11:CD008950.

92 Time-Lapse Monitoring

Csaba Pribenszky and Peter Kovacs

92.1 Background

Almost 40 years have passed since the first successful in vitro fertilization (IVF) treatment [1]. Since then many aspects of IVF have continued to evolve and undergone significant changes. These have included controlled ovarian hyperstimulation (COH) protocols to augment oocyte and embryo yield. Culture conditions have improved to allow extended culture to the blastocyst stage, and cryopreservation of supernumerary embryos has enabled patients to have multiple embryo transfers while undergoing one cycle of COH and oocyte retrieval.

Unfortunately, IVF outcomes still remain relatively low with live birth rates ranging from 54.4% per retrieval under 35 years to 3.9% among those over 42 years according to the Society of Assisted Reproductive Technology (SART) 2014 report and a 23.7% delivery rate per retrieval in women all ages combined based on the European Society of Human Reproduction 2012 report. Clearly, the desire to increase the number of cycles that result in successful outcomes is of paramount. Success can be measured in many ways, but most consider the birth of a healthy, full-term singleton as the ultimate measure [2]. However, to further optimize outcomes, the transfer of multiple embryos is often entertained resulting in a multiple gestations. Furthermore, pregnancy-related maternal, fetal, and neonatal complications are more frequent with multiple gestations [3, 4]. Neonatal outcome can be expected to be ideal following a singleton pregnancy. Thus, the transfer of a single embryo (SET) at a time provides the highest chance for a singleton gestation.

SET, however, is still not uniformly accepted. According to the 2014 SART data report, the mean number of embryos transferred was 1.6 under the age of 35 and 2.6 over 42, while only 1/3 of cycles under the age of 35 involved elective SET [5]. According to 2012 ESHRE data, only approximately 30% of cycles involved SET [6].

There are several potential explanations for this trend in practice. Many couples feel that they can improve their chances if multiple embryos are replaced, while some can only afford one treatment and wish to maximize their chances. Furthermore, IVF clinics compete with each other and usually report intermediate outcome parameters such as pregnancy rate (PR) but not perinatal outcomes to attract potential patients [7]. Finally, the current embryo evaluation methods that rely on once-a-day evaluation of cleavage rate and morphology are ineffective in identifying the embryo with the highest implantation potential [8].

The call for identifying a better assessment tool for embryo quality has the potential to mitigate the transfer of multiple embryos. Time-lapse monitoring (TL) is a laboratory tool that has attempted to respond to the need for improved embryo evaluation. Its use provides significantly more data on embryo development kinetics and morphology without the need to remove embryos from their optimal culture conditions. This additional information has the potential to be used for optimal embryo selection. This chapter will review our current knowledge on the clinical application to TL monitoring and discuss future directions with the use of this technology.

92.2 Time-Lapse Technology

In order to achieve optimal fertilization and embryo development, embryos are cultured under tightly controlled conditions (temperature, pH, culture medium composition, gas concentration, etc.) [9–12]. Whenever they are removed from the incubator, the optimal environment is compromised. According to current standards, embryos are assessed daily or every other day for cell cleavage and morphology under light microscopy [8]. This allows the embryos to spend as much time as possible undisturbed in

C. Pribenszky
University of Veterinary Medicine, Budapest, Hungary

P. Kovacs (✉)
IVF Center, Kaali Institute, Budapest, Hungary

G. N. Allahbadia et al. (eds.), *Textbook of Assisted Reproduction*, https://doi.org/10.1007/978-981-15-2377-9_92

the incubators but, on the other hand, limits the information that can be ascertained.

The past two decades have seen various technologic innovations aimed to learn more about early in vitro embryo development including metabolomics, proteomics, preimplantation genetic screening (PGS), and now most recently TL monitoring [13]. TL monitoring relies on the analysis of digital images taken by a camera that is either part of the incubator or is placed into a standard incubator. Images are taken at preset 5–20 min intervals. Time-lapse units now come with custom-made software that creates a short film based on the images and allows analysis by fast-forwarding, rewinding, blow-up images as well as the analysis of embryos in multifocal planes. Some programs provide algorithms that help the embryologist with optimal embryo selection for transfer. Computer-aided analysis of the images enables one to measure the precise timing of kinetic events and to observe transient morphologic changes and their dynamics. This is all achieved without the need to remove the embryo from incubators, potentially even during the entire duration of embryo culture [14].

92.3 Time-Lapse Parameters

As a starting point, time of fertilization is typically defined as the midpoint of the time interval of the injection of the oocyte cohort with intracytoplasmic sperm injection (ICSI) or the time when the semen droplet is added to the oocyte cohort during IVF. Then various parameters can be evaluated and annotated during analysis. These include time to pronuclear fading/breakdown and appearance of the 2, 3, 4, 5, … 8 cell stages (tpnf, t_2, t_3, t_4, t_5, … t_8) from the time of fertilization. Duration of the cell cycles (CC; CC1: 2PN → 2 cell; CC2: 2 → 3 cell, CC3: 4 → 5 cell cleavage), as well as the synchronicity of the divisions (S_1: cleavage furrow → 2 cells, S_2: t_4–t_3; S_3: t_8–t_5), can be calculated. Furthermore, timing of the morula stage, start of blastulation, and time to reach the expanded blastocyst stage can be measured. These kinetic events as well as any mathematical formula based on them can be used to build algorithms for embryo selection [15–19]. Beyond the precise timing of kinetic parameters, transient or permanent morphologic changes (fragmentation, vacuolization, blastocyst pulsation) can also be followed by TL monitoring. This includes abnormal early embryonic events including multinucleation, direct cleavage, or uneven blastomere size that could be missed by the traditional daily-once observation (Fig. 92.1a, b) [16, 20].

92.4 Time-Lapse Equipment

There are various commercially available TL units. While they utilize the same concept of embryo observation, there are important differences as well. Some units are incubators with a built-in camera (e.g., Embyoscope, Geri, ESCO Miri), while others have to be placed into larger incubators (Primo Vision). Some units require single embryo culture, while others allow group culture in special dishes ("well-of-the-well") that still allows individual embryo observation with the added benefit of communication between embryos (Fig. 92.2a–c) [21]. Some equipment utilizes dark field technology, while others use bright field illumination. The number of embryos that can be monitored simultaneously differs as well. The technical differences of the currently available TL units are compared in Table 92.1.

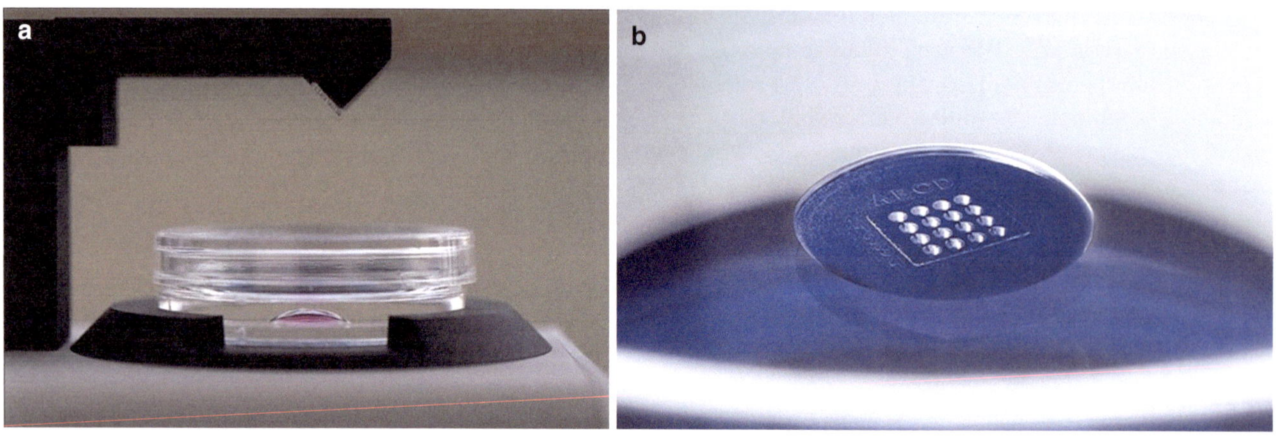

Fig. 92.1 (**a** and **b**) Beyond the precise timing of kinetic parameters, transient or permanent morphologic changes (fragmentation, vacuolization, blastocyst pulsation) can also be followed by TL monitoring, including abnormal early embryonic events including multinucleation, direct cleavage, or uneven blastomere size that could be missed by the traditional daily-once observation

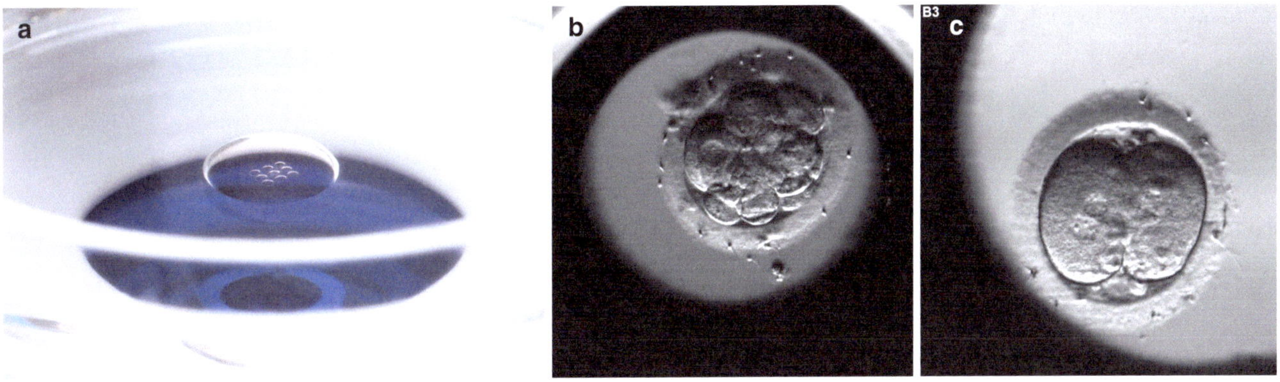

Fig. 92.2 (**a–c**) Some units require single embryo culture, while others allow group culture in special dishes ("well-of-the-well") that still allows individual embryo observation with the added benefit of communication between embryos

Table 92.1 Comparison of the technical parameters of the commercially available time-lapse systems

	Illumination	Microscope incubator	Culture dish	Embryo culture	Software
Primo Vision Evo http://www.vitrolife.com/en/Products/Primo-Vision-Time-Lapse-System/	Bright field	Microscope placed in standard incubator	9–16 well Primo Vision embryo culture dishes	Group culture, evaluation in 11 focal planes, up to 96 embryos	Comes with software, universal embryo evaluating algorithm
Embryoscope/Embryoscope+ http://www.vitrolife.com/en/Products/EmbryoScope-Time-Lapse-System/	Bright field	Incubator with integrated time-lapse system	Embryoslide (12–16 embryo/slide); simultaneous evaluation of up to 15 patients	Single culture, seven focal planes, 6 × 12 or 15 × 16 embryos	Comes with software, universal embryo evaluating algorithm
GERI Genea	Bright field	Incubator with integrated time-lapse system, six chambers each equipped with a camera	Multi-well Geri dish	Single culture	Comes with software
ESCO Miri http://www.escoglobal.com/product/art-equipment/time-lapse-incubator/MRI-TL/	Bright field	Incubator with integrated time-lapse system; 6 individual chambers, up to 84 embryos	Culture coin dish	Culture coin dish 14 embryos in individual wells (single culture)	Comes with software
EEVA	Dark field	Microscope placed in standard incubator	EEVA dish	Group culture, single focal plane evaluation	Automated, software scores blastocyst formation potential

92.5 Safety

It is important to establish the safety of any new technology. One concern raised is the periodic light exposure when images are taken. With that said, light exposure is significantly lower with all available units when compared to standard out-of-incubator evaluation, and the use of detrimental short wavelength is also avoided [16, 22]. Other issues include possible electromagnetic effects, fumes from lubricants, and heat accumulation from the moving parts of the equipment. Various equipment on the market likely differ regarding these aspects due to technical differences.

To date, studies have not found any detrimental effects of TL technology on fertilization rates, cleavage or blastocyst stage morphology, and implantation or pregnancy rates [16, 22–26]. The following is a review of the existing literature.

92.6 Prospective and Retrospective Observational Data

Early work using TL technology was purely descriptive [23, 27]. More recent studies have collected information on morphologic changes and measured timing of certain cleavage events. Data collected from multiple cycles has led to the accumulation of large databases where laboratory and clinical outcomes have been correlated with TL parameters. In order to best assess these data sets, only the correlation with specific markers and embryos with known implantation data (KID) should only be considered.

With that said, various groups have tested different endpoints in their studies (Tables 92.2 and 92.3). Wong et al. tested the embryos' ability to turn into a good quality blastocyst. Frozen pronuclear stage embryos were observed using the EEVA system, but embryos that reached the blas-

Table 92.2 Prospective and retrospective cohort studies evaluating time-lapse technology

	Type of study	Outcome studied	Parameter studied	Outcome	TL system
Wong et al. [15]	Cohort study of frozen-thawed embryos (cryopreservation at zygote stage)	BC development (embryos not transferred)	S_1, CC_2, S_2	Studied parameters when in optimal range predictive of BC development	EEVA
Meseguer et al. [16]	Retrospective analysis, normal responder patients using own oocytes and donor oocyte cycles; 247 embryos with known implantation	Implantation rate	$CC_2 < 5$ h, multinucleation and uneven blastomere size excluded, t_5, CC_2, S_2 (Meseguer decision tree based on in and out of range kinetic parameters)	Studied parameters when in optimal range predictive of implantation	Embryoscope, 21% O_2
Rubio et al. [28]	Retrospective study, donor oocytes and own oocytes ($N = 1659$ transferred embryos)	Implantation rate	Direct cleavage: $CC_2 < 5$ h	Embryos with CC_2 <5 h min chance (1.2%) to implant	Embryoscope, 21% O_2
Cruz et al. [29]	Retrospective analysis, donor oocyte treatments, ET on D5	BC development Implantation rate (embryos with known implantation)	t_5, S_2 (four categories based on in and out of range values); uneven blastomeres at two-cell stage, direct cleavage one to three cells	Symmetric blastomeres and no direct cleavage predictive of BC development, t_5/S_2 categories not predictive of implantation	Embryoscope, 21% O_2
Conaghan et al. [30]	Prospective study to predict usable blastocyst formation by D3	Blastocyst development rate	S_1, CC_2, S_2	CC_2 and S_2 when in optimal range predictive of usable blastocyst development	EEVA, O_2 conc. not specified
Meseguer et al. [24]	Retrospective study, own and donated oocytes, TL incubation vs. standard incubation	Clinical pregnancy rate	Standard morphology vs. t_5, CC_2, S_2 (Meseguer decision tree) in TL cycles	20.1% average improvement in CPR	Embryoscope, 21% O_2
Azzarello et al. [31]	Prospective cohort study of 159 zygotes from women under 39 years	Live birth (embryos with known implantation data)	Pronuclear fading, pronuclear breakdown (PNB)	PNB is higher when transfer results in live birth; no live birth when PNB < 20 h:45 min	Embryoscope, 5% O_2
Chamayou et al. [32]	Retrospective analysis, patients <40 years	Implantation, clinical pregnancy	Various kinetic parameters	Predictive of BC development: t_1, t_2, t_4, t_7, t_8, time to visible pronuclei, S_3 parameter predictive of implantation: CC_3	Embryoscope, 5% O_2 Different parameters predict BC development and implantation
Dal Canto et al. [33]	Retrospective analysis of TL data, women 27–42 years, D3 and D5 ET ($n = 71$ cycles)	Cleavage times	BC development	Up to six cells no difference; t_7 and t_8 are shorter in embryos that reached BC stage; $t_8 - t_4$ and $t_8 - t_5$ are shorter in embryos that reached BC stage; t_8 shorter in embryos that implanted but t_5 did not differ	Embryoscope, 5% O_2
Basile et al. [34]	Two-phase study (I: algorithm building $N = 765$ cycles), II: algorithm testing ($N = 885$ cycles); donor oocytes, own oocytes; D3 ET	Direct cleavage, multinucleation, uneven blastomeres; t_2, t_3, t_4, t_5, CC_2, S_2, only embryos with known implantation data	Implantation	Phase I: t_3, CC_2, and t_5 most relevant (based on in and out of range eight categories created) Phase II: sig. decline in implantation as moving from all three parameters in range to none in range	Embryo scope, 21% O_2

Table 92.2 (continued)

	Type of study	Outcome studied	Parameter studied	Outcome	TL system
Siristatidis et al. [35]	Prospective cohort study of 239 ICSI cycles (169 standard culture and morphology based selection vs. 70 cycles using TL culture and selection based on kinetic markers	Clinical and ongoing PR; live birth rate	t_2, CC_2, t_3, S_2, t_4, CC_3, t_5, S_3, t_8 (in TL group the embryo(s) with the most in range parameters was selected for transfer)	Clinical pregnancy rate TL vs. control: 65.7% vs. 39.0% ($p < 0.001$) Ongoing pregnancy TL vs. control: 55.7% vs. 31.3% ($p < 0.001$) Live birth TL vs. control: 45.7% vs. 28.4% ($p = 0.01$)	Primo Vision, atmospheric O_2
Motato et al. [36]	Retrospective analysis, three phases: 1 algorithm building to predict BC, 2 algorithm building to predict implantation, 3 validation of implantation algorithm Own and donated oocytes	BC development	t_2, t_3, t_4, t_5, t_6, t_7, t_8, t_9, tM, tBC, t expand BC, t hatching BC, $t_3 - t_2$, $t_5 - t_3$, $t_5 - t_2$, $t_8 - t_5$	For BC development best model is based on tM and $t_8 - t_5$ (four categories based on in and out of range) *but* little utility to predict BC For IR best model is based on tEB and $t_8 - t_5$ (four categories based on in and out of range) poor performance	Embryoscope O_2 not specified
VerMilyea et al. [37]	Retrospective analysis based on data from 6 clinics, 331 embryos with known implantation data; fresh IVF, ICSI cycles	Clinical pregnancy, implantation	CC_2, S_2 CC_2 9.33≤ and ≤11.45 h and S_2 ≤1.73 h Two category results: EEVA high when both in range and EEVA low when one or both out of range Three category outputs: high, CC_2 and S_2 in range; EEVA medium, CC_2 9.33≤ and ≤12.65 h and S_2 ≤4 h; EEVA low, out of the above ranges	Two category results: EEVA high vs. low IR: 37% vs. 23% ($p = 0.003$) Three category results: high vs. medium vs. low IR: 37% vs. 35% vs. 15% (p: sig. between high vs. low and medium vs. low)	EEVA system Different clinic specific protocols, culture medium, O_2 concentration
Milewski et al. [38]	Retrospective analysis of embryos that developed to BC stage ($n = 156$) vs. those that did not ($n = 276$)	BC development	t_2, t_3, t_4, t_5; CC_2; S_2	A score created based on t_2, t_5, and CC_2 is predictive of BC development	Embryoscope, 5% O_2
Petersen et al. [17]	Retrospective analysis; data from 24 clinics	Implantation	t_3 − tPNf; t_3; $(t_5 - t_3)/(t_5 - t_2)$; cell count at 66 h	Five scores assigned based on time-lapse parameters and cell count at 66 h; sevenfold increase in implantation rates from score 1 to score 5; model is predictive regardless of IVF vs. ICSI or low O_2 vs. atmospheric O_2	TL system not specified; both 5% and atmospheric O_2 concentration

From Kovacs P. Time-lapse embryoscopy: do we have an efficacious algorithm for embryo selection? Journal of Reproductive Biotechnology and Fertility. 2016;5:1–12. Reprinted with permission from SAGE Ltd.
BC blastocyst, *ET* embryo transfer, *D5* day 5, *D3* day 3, *CPR* clinical pregnancy rate

tocyst stage were not transferred [15]. The IVI group lead by Marcos Meseguer tested early kinetic and morphologic markers to various clinical outcomes (implantation rate, pregnancy rate, live birth rate) in a number of clinical trials [16, 28, 29, 39]. Others relied more on the analysis of late, blastocyst stage markers and correlated kinetic events with aneuploidy [18, 19]. A combined analysis of available data is further complicated by the different patient populations (own vs. donor oocytes, fresh vs. frozen oocytes), the day of transfer (day 2 vs. day 3 vs. day 5 transfers), the type of equipment used (dark field vs. bright field evaluation, incubators with built-in cameras vs. TL unit placed into incubators), and different culture conditions (atmospheric vs. low oxygen concentration, culture media used). Thus, it is not surprising that various studies have identified different kinetic and morphologic markers to be associated with various degrees of predictive ability for the selected outcome.

Table 92.3 Results of studies evaluation aneuploidy and time-lapse technology

	Type of study	Outcome studied	Parameter studied	Outcome	TL system
Campbell et al. [18]	Retrospective analysis, patients undergoing ICSI-PGS	Aneuploidy	tSC (initiation of compaction), tSB (start of blastulation), tB (full blastocyst development)	All parameters delayed in aneuploidy embryos	Embryoscope, 5% O_2
Campbell et al. [19]	Retrospective analysis using aneuploidy risk model based on tSB and tB	Implantation (embryos with known implantation)	Low risk: tSB < 96.2 h, tB <122.9 h Medium risk: tSB ≥ 96.2 h, tB <122.9 h High risk: tB ≥122.9 h	High risk: none implanted Low risk: 74% increase in implantation rate when compared to all three risk categories	Embryoscope 5% O_2
Basile et al. [39]	Retrospective analysis of patients undergoing PGS	Euploidy–aneuploidy risk based in TL parameters	$t_5 - t_2$ and CC_3; four categories established based on in and out of range values	The proportion of euploid embryos decreases across the categories (highest when $t_5 - t_2$ and CC_3 are in range and lowest when both out of range)	Embryoscope
Chavez et al. [40]	Cohort of frozen-thawed zygotes cultured to D2	Aneuploidy	S_1, CC_2, S_2	Majority of aneuploidy embryos display time intervals outside the normal range; aneuploid embryos more likely to be fragmented	EEVA, 5% O_2

From Kovacs P. Time-lapse embryoscopy: do we have an efficacious algorithm for embryo selection? Journal of Reproductive Biotechnology and Fertility. 2016;5:1–12. Reprinted with permission from SAGE Ltd.

Thus, the predictive ability of the markers can be increased if multiple markers are analyzed creating algorithms for embryo selection. Research groups have proposed different algorithms based on their own data sets, obtained from their patient population using clinic specific embryology and transfer protocols. The three best-known models are the Wong model, Meseguer hierarchical model, and Petersen KID score (for details see Table 92.2). The Wong model relies on three early markers (S_1, S_2, CC_2) that are predictive of blastocyst formation using dark field TL technology [15]; the Meseguer model is based on in and out of range (t_5, CC_2, and S_2 time ranges), and in addition abnormal early morphologic parameters are used as exclusion criteria [16], while the Petersen model (KID score) is based on five kinetic and one morphological event [17]. The data for the Petersen model was collected from several clinics with local laboratory protocols in a heterogeneous patient population and therefore is considered universally applicable. The other models are clinic specific, and prior to introduction into daily practice, local evaluation and/or adjustments are recommended. This however requires the collection of data on hundreds of KID embryo observations, and this is not practical for smaller clinics.

External validation of these models (different clinics, different patient populations, different culture conditions) is imperative prior to implementing such algorithms. Unfortunately, none of the external validation attempts have been successful to date [41, 42]. To date, there are many reviews and observational studies discussing the value of time-lapse monitoring in routine laboratory practice [22, 41, 43–45]. Some suggest that investing in time-lapse and changing the daily routine would not lead to clinical benefits [25, 46].

Table 92.4 The number of randomized patients and those who have completed the protocols in the seven RCTs potentially eligible for the meta-analysis

Randomized controlled trials	No. of randomized patients	No. of patients completed the protocol	Included in the analysis[a]
Kahraman et al. [49]	76	64	Yes
Rubio et al. [28]	856	843	Yes
Park et al. [53]	364	361	No
Siristatidis et al. [35]	244	239	Yes
Goodman et al. [51]	300	235	Yes
Wu et al. [52]	49	31	No
Kovacs et al. 2017	161	139	Yes

[a]Undisturbed culture and TL imaging information is used for evaluation

92.7 Prospective Randomized Studies, Meta-analysis

It has been suggested that any new technology should be verified and tested by randomized controlled trials (RCT) before general implementation into routine clinical use [47]. A 2015 Cochrane review based on three randomized trials [28, 48, 49] with 994 patients concluded that there was insufficient evidence for the benefit of time-lapse imaging [50]. Since its publication, another four RCTs have been published examining the effect of TL intervention on clinical outcomes suggesting as best evidence to support changes in clinical practice. The conclusions were that TL embryo monitoring offers undisturbed culture conditions and provides significantly more morphokinetic data compared to the standard, daily-once out-of-incubator evaluation and needs to be considered [35, 51–54] (Table 92.4). A review of these studies considering the utilization of the full benefits is as follows.

Table 92.5 Clinical outcome achieved in the individual studies and the cumulative results (OR) with respect to ongoing pregnancy rate and live birth

Ongoing pregnancy rate					
Study	Intervention (event/total)	Controls (event/total)	Odds ratio	95% CI	Weight (%)
Kahraman et al. [49]	20/33	19/31	0.97	0.36–2.65	6.82
Rubio et al. [28]	226/438	169/405	1.49	1.13–1.96	42.80
Siristatidis et al. [35]	39/70	53/169	2.75	1.55–4.88	17.60
Goodman et al. [51]	81/119	73/116	1.26	0.73–2.15	19.28
Matyas et al. [54]	34/68	26/71	1.73	0.88–3.41	13.50
Total	400/728	340/792	1.59	1.21–2.10	100.00
Live birth					
Study	Intervention (event/total)	Controls (event/total)	Odds ratio	95% CI	Weight (%) Random
Kahraman et al. [49]	18/33	17/31	1.00	0.64–1.55	27.41
Siristatidis et al. [35]	32/70	48/169	1.61	1.13–2.28	38.84
Matyas et al. [54]	34/68	26/71	1.37	0.93–2.01	33.75
Total	84/171	91/271	1.33	1.02–1.74	100.00

Kahraman et al. performed a single-center RCT with a 1:1 randomization at oocyte retrieval. Embryoscope TL unit was used with 5% O_2, and fresh elective SET was performed on day 5 (D5). Good responder patients under the age of 35 were recruited. Embryo selection in the TL group was according to D5 morphology and the Meseguer hierarchical model vs. D5 morphology in controls (ongoing PR: 60.6% TL vs. 61.3% control) [49] (results shown in Table 92.5).

Rubio et al. performed a multicenter RCT with a 1:1 randomization on the day before oocyte collection. They also used the Embryoscope but with atmospheric 21% O_2 concentration. These transfers involved fresh and frozen eSET or double embryo transfer (DET) on day 3 (D3) or D5. Patients under the age of 38 years using own oocytes or undergoing donor oocyte treatment were included. Selection in the TL group was according to the Meseguer hierarchical model vs. D3 or D5 morphology in the control group (ongoing pregnancy rate: 51.4% in TL vs. 41.7% in control groups). However, culture conditions differed between the TL and control groups not just based on different, undefined standard incubators used in the control group but also because of different volumes of culture media used between the groups. One might also criticize the study as the embryos in the control group were removed from the incubator for morphology checkups at least twice, while in the time-lapse group, out-of-incubator evaluation did not occur, but this feature is an inherent benefit with TL systems that minimize embryo handling [28] (results shown in Table 92.5).

Park et al. reported in a single-center RCT with a 2:1 randomization ratio after retrieval. In this study, the Embryoscope was used for incubation in the "time-lapse" group at 21% O_2, and eSET or DET were performed on day 2 (D2). Patients under the age of 40 were eligible. Out of 364 randomized participants, 361 completed the protocol. Embryo selection was based on morphology in both groups, so visual information provided by TL was not used for embryo evaluation [53]. Results favored conventional culture over TL. However, there are several weaknesses in this study that have to be considered carefully including the transfer of embryos on D2. A short, 2-day culture period is inadequate to show benefit of an undisturbed culture concept. Furthermore, there was an unexplained, exceptionally high early pregnancy loss rate reported (33.3% vs. 10.2%) in the TL group. Finally, embryo evaluation was based on morphology alone, and no advantage of any morphokinetic algorithm was taken for embryo selection. Since this study did not take advantage of the full benefits of the TL system, it was excluded from the most updated meta-analysis detailed later.

Siristatidis et al. published a single-center RCT, with a randomization after oocyte retrieval in a 3:7 allocation ratio. Primo Vision time-lapse monitoring system was used for the study, at 21% O_2. Fresh eSET, DET, or triple embryo transfer (TET) was performed on D2 or D3. Patients under the age of 42 years were eligible for the study. Embryo selection in the TL group was based on in and out of range kinetic markers (t_2, CC_2, t_3, S_2, t_4, CC_3, t_5, S_3, t_8), whereas D2 or D3 morphology was used in the control group (ongoing PR: 55.7% TL vs. 31.3% control) [35] (results shown Table 92.5).

Goodman et al. performed a single-center RCT, with a 1:1 randomization at retrieval. Embryoscope was used at 5.5% O_2, and eSET or DET was performed on D3 or D5. Patients under the age of 43 were eligible for the study. Embryos in the TL group were primarily evaluated using standard morphologic assessment, and then further ranking was applied based on TL markers (CC_2, t_5, and S_2, S_3, tSB) plus cleavage abnormalities, while standard morphology was assessed in the control group (ongoing PR: 68% TL vs. 62.9% control) [51] (results shown in Table 92.5).

Wu et al. randomized (1:1) patients at retrieval to embryo culture in Embryoscope at 5% O_2 and ET on D3 versus con-

Table 92.6 Analysis of cumulative results by Chi-square test

	Absolute numbers (event/total)	Mean	Absolute numbers (event/total)	Mean (%)	*p*-value
Ongoing pregnancy	400/728	54.9	340/792	42.9	<0.001
Early pregnancy loss	72/472	15.3	92/432	21.3	0.02
Stillbirth	9/171	5.3	7/271	2.6	0.14
Live birth	84/171	49.1	91/271	33.6	<0.00

trols using standard incubators for embryo culture. Embryo selection for transfer was based on morphology in both TL and control groups [52]. The study was considered a RCT; however, it was a pilot study, ultimately underpowered, and it did not take TL information into consideration at embryo evaluation and selection and thus was not considered for the updated meta-analysis evaluating the full benefits of TL systems.

Kovacs et al. reported a multicenter RCT with randomization in 1:1 ratio prior to the start of COH for IVF. Primo Vision time-lapse system was used at 5% O_2, and eSET was performed on D5. Good prognosis patients under the age of 36 were eligible for the study. Embryo selection was performed based on a composed score consisting of kinetic parameters (CC_1, CC_2, S_1, S_2, t_5) and scores for blastocyst morphology in the TL arm vs. D5 morphology in the control group (ongoing PR: 50% TL vs. 36.6% control) (results shown in Table 92.5).

92.7.1 Analysis of the Cumulative Outcome and Synthesis of Results

In an up-to-date meta-analysis, which excluded 2 of the 7 identified RCTs, data from 1637 randomized patients who completed the protocol (in total 1528 cycles) were included. Outcome measures were pregnancy rate (PR) defined as a rise in β-human chorionic gonadotropin (βhCG) and ongoing pregnancy rate (OPR) as presence of gestational sac or fetal heartbeat detected by ultrasound observed between weeks 5 and 16. Early pregnancy loss was defined as positive βhCG that did not continue into a clinical pregnancy. Live birth data were evaluated where available. A random effect model was applied when appropriate, and pooled results were presented as odds ratio (OR). Categorical variables were presented as percentages. Results of the cumulative analysis are shown in Tables 92.5 and 92.6.

The results which utilized both TL culture- and TL algorithm-based embryo evaluation in the intervention arms showed an increase of the OPR from 42.9% to 54.9% by using TL for continuous embryo assessment compared to conventional daily embryo evaluation at fixed time points (OR: 1.59; CI: 1.208–2.096; $p < 0.001$). In addition, early pregnancy loss was significantly reduced from 21.3% to 15.3% (OR: 0.66; CI: 0.469–0.935; $p = 0.019$). In the three studies that reported pregnancy outcome, stillbirth rates did not differ between the groups (2.6% vs. 5.3%; OR: 2.388; CI: 0.694–8.215; $p = 0.167$); however there was a significant difference in live birth rates in favor of the use of TL systems: 33.6% vs. 49.1% (OR: 1.741; CI: 1.165–2.600; $p = 0.007$).

92.8 Concluding Remarks and Future Directions

There appears to be growing evidence for the clinical benefit of using imaging systems in human IVF. The combined effect of higher chance of ongoing pregnancy, reduced risk of early pregnancy loss, and higher live birth rate after embryo assessment by TL suggests a benefit on clinical outcomes and may warrant a change of routine practice of embryo assessment. External validation of any new algorithm for day 3 or 5 transfer is needed. Furthermore, other needs include the automatization of the annotations making time-lapse a robust and universal tool for undisturbed culture and embryo evaluation in human IVF treatments. Beyond these clinical benefits, TL also simplifies and makes the daily workload in an embryology lab more flexible and can be used for quality control, training, and patient education.

References

1. Steptoe PCV, Edwards RG. Birth after the reimplantation of human embryo. Lancet. 1978;2:366.
2. Heijnen EM, Macklon NS, Fauser BC. What is the most relevant standard of success in assisted reproduction? The next step to improving outcomes of IVF: consider the whole treatment. Hum Reprod. 2004;19:1936–8.
3. Kovacs P. Multiple pregnancies after ART and how to minimize their occurrence. Curr Women's Health Rev. 2012;8(4):289–96.
4. Conde-Agudelo A, Belizán JM, Lindmark G. Maternal morbidity and mortality associated with multiple gestations. Obstet Gynecol. 2000;95:899–904.
5. https://www.sartcorsonline.com/rptCSR_PublicMultYear.aspx?reportingYear=2014
6. European IVF-Monitoring Consortium (EIM); European Society of Human Reproduction and Embryology (ESHRE), Kupka MS, D'Hooghe T, Ferraretti AP, et al. Assisted reproductive technology in Europe, 2011: results generated from European registers by ESHRE. Hum Reprod. 2016;31:233–48.
7. Kulkarni AD, Jamieson DJ, Jones HW Jr, Kissin DM, Gallo MF, Macaluso M, et al. Fertility treatments and multiple births in the United States. N Engl J Med. 2013;369:2218–25.
8. Alpha scientists in reproductive medicine and ESHRE special interest group of embryology. The Istanbul consensus workshop

on embryo assessments: proceedings of an expert meeting. Hum Reprod. 2011;26:1270–83.
9. Swain JE. Optimal human embryo culture. Semin Reprod Med. 2015;33:103–17.
10. Swain JE. Decisions for the IVF laboratory: comparative analysis of embryo culture incubators. Reprod Biomed Online. 2014;28:535–47.
11. Bontekoe S, Mantikou E, van Wely M, Seshadri S, Repping S, Mastenbroek S. Low oxygen concentrations for embryo culture in assisted reproductive technologies. Cochrane Database Syst Rev. 2012;7:CD008950.
12. Marianowski P, Dąbrowski FA, Zyguła A, Wielgoś M, Szymusik I. Do we pay enough attention to culture conditions in context of perinatal outcome after in vitro fertilization? Up-to-date literature review. Biomed Res Int. 2016;2016:3285179.
13. Montag M, Toth B, Strowitzki T. New approaches to embryo selection. Reprod Biomed Online. 2013;27:539–46.
14. Kovacs P. Embryo selection: the role of time lapse monitoring. Reprod Biol Endocrinol. 2014;15:124.
15. Wong CC, Loewke KE, Bossert NI, Behr B, De Jonge CJ, Baer TM, et al. Non-invasive imaging of human embryos before embryonic genome activation predicts development to the blastocyst stage. Nat Biotechnol. 2010;28:1115–24.
16. Meseguer M, Herrero J, Tejera A, Hilligsoe KM, Ramsing N, Remohi J. The use of morphokinetics as a predictor of embryo implantation. Hum Reprod. 2011;26:2658–71.
17. Petersen BM, Boel M, Montag M, Gardner DK. Development of a generally applicable morphokinetic algorithm capable of predicting the implantation potential of embryos transferred on Day 3. Hum Reprod. 2016;31:2231–44.
18. Campbell A, Fishel S, Bowman N, Duffy S, Sedler M, Fontes Lindeman Hickman C. Modelling a risk classification of aneuploidy in human embryos using non-invasive morphokinetics. Reprod Biomed Online. 2013;26:477–85.
19. Campbell A, Fishel S, Bowman N, Duffy S, Sedler M, Thornton S. Retrospective analysis of outcomes after IVF using an aneuploidy risk model derived from time-lapse imaging without PGS. Reprod Biomed Online. 2013;27:140–6.
20. Rubio I, Kuhlmann R, Agerholm I, Kirk J, Herrero J, Escriba M-J, et al. Limited implantation success of direct-cleaved human zygotes: a time-lapse study. Fertil Steril. 2012;98:1458–63.
21. Vajta G, Korosi T, Du Y, Nakata K, Ieda S, Kuwayama M, et al. The well-of the-well system: an efficient approach to improve embryo development. Reprod Biomed Online. 2008;17:73–81.
22. Kirkegaard K, Agerholm IE, Ingerslev HJ. Time-lapse monitoring as a tool for clinical embryo assessment. Hum Reprod. 2012;27:1277–85.
23. Mio Y, Maeda K. Time-lapse cinematography of dynamic changes occurring during in vitro development of human embryos. Am J Obstet Gynecol. 2008;199:660.e1–5.
24. Meseguer M, Rubio I, Cruz M, Basile N, Marcos J, Requena A. Embryo incubation and selection in a time-lapse system improves pregnancy outcome compared with standard incubator: a retrospective cohort study. Fertil Steril. 2012;98:1481–91.
25. Wong C, Chen AA, Behr B, Shen S. Time-lapse microscopy and image analysis in basic and clinical embryo development research. Reprod Biomed Online. 2013;26:120–9.
26. Cs P, Mátyás S, Kovács P, Losonczi E, Zádori J, Vajta G. Case report: pregnancy achieved by transfer of a single blastocyst selected by time-lapse monitoring. Reprod Biomed Online. 2010;21:533–6.
27. Payne D, Flaherty SP, Barry MF, Matthews CD. Preliminary observations on polar body extrusion and pronuclear formation in human oocytes using time-lapse video cinematography. Hum Reprod. 1997;12:532–41.
28. Rubio I, Galán A, Larreategui Z, Ayerdi F, Bellver J, Herrero J, et al. Clinical validation of embryo culture and selection by morphokinetic analysis: a randomized, controlled trial of the EmbryoScope. Fertil Steril. 2014;102:1287–94.e5.
29. Cruz M, Garrido N, Herrero J, Perez-Cano I, Munoz M, Meseguer M. Timing of cell division in human cleavage-stage embryos is linked with blastocyst formation and quality. Reprod Biomed Online. 2012;25:371–81.
30. Conaghan J, Cjhen AA, Willman SP, Ivani K, Chenette PE, Boostanfar R, et al. Improving embryo selection using a computer-automated time-lapse image analysis test plus day 3 morphology: results from a prospective multicenter trial. Fertil Steril. 2013;100:412–9.
31. Azzarello A, Hoest T, Mikkelsen AL. The impact of pronuclei morphology and dynamicity on live birth outcome after time-lapse culture. Hum Reprod. 2012;27:2649–57.
32. Chamayou S, Patrizio P, Storaci G, Tomaselli V, Alecci C, Ragolia C, et al. The use of morphokinetic parameters to select all embryos with full capacity to implant. J Assist Reprod Genet. 2013;30:703–10.
33. Dal Canto M, Coticchio G, Mignini Renzini M, De Ponti E, Novara PV, Brambillasca F, et al. Cleavage kinetics analysis of human embryos predicts development to blastocyst and implantation. Reprod Biomed Online. 2012;25:474–80.
34. Basile N, Vime P, Florensa M, Aparicio Ruiz B, García Velasco JA, Remohí J, et al. The use of morphokinetics as a predictor of implantation: a multicentric study to define and validate an algorithm for embryo selection. Hum Reprod. 2015;30:276–83.
35. Siristatidis C, Komitopoulou MA, Makris A, Sialakouma A, Botzaki M, Mastorakos G, et al. Morphokinetic parameters of early embryo development via time lapse monitoring and their effect on embryo selection and ICSI outcomes: a prospective cohort study. J Assist Reprod Genet. 2015;32:563–70.
36. Motato Y, de los Santos MJ, Escribe MJ, Ruiz BA, Remohí J, Meseguer M. Morphokinetic analysis and embryonic prediction for blastocyst formation through an integrated time-lapse system. Fertil Steril. 2016;105:376–84.
37. VerMilyea MD, Tan L, Anthony JT, Conaghan J, Ivani K, Gvakharia M, et al. Computer-automated time-lapse analysis results correlate with embryo implantation and clinical pregnancy: a blinded, multi-Centre study. Reprod Biomed Online. 2014;29:729–36.
38. Milewski R, Kuc P, Kuczynska A, Stankiewicz B, Łukaszuk K, Kuczyński W. A predictive model for blastocyst formation based on morphokinetic parameters in time-lapse monitoring of embryo development. J Assist Reprod Genet. 2015;32:571–9.
39. Basile N, del Carmen Nogales M, Bronet F, Florensa M, Riqueros M, Rodrigo L, et al. Increasing the probability of selecting chromosomally normal embryos by time-lapse morphokinetics analysis. Fertil Steril. 2014;101:699–704.
40. Chavez SL, Loewke KE, Han J, Moussavi F, Colls P, Munne S, et al. Dynamic blastomere behavior reflect human embryo ploidy by the four-cell stage. Nat Commun. 2012;3:1251. https://doi.org/10.1038/ncomms2249.
41. Freour T, Le Fleuter N, Lammers J, Splingart C, Reignier A, Barrière P. External validation of a time-lapse prediction model. Fertil Steril. 2015;103:917–22.
42. Kirkegaard K, Campbell A, Agerholm I, Bentin-Ley U, Gabrielsen A, Kirk J, et al. Limitations of a time-lapse blastocyst prediction model: a large multicentre outcome analysis. Reprod Biomed Online. 2014;29:156–8.
43. Kaser DJ, Racowsky C. Clinical outcomes following selection of human preimplantation embryos with time-lapse monitoring: a systematic review. Hum Reprod Update. 2014;20:617–31.
44. Rakowsky C, Kovacs P, Martins WP. A critical appraisal of time-lapse imaging for embryo selection: where are we and where we need to go? J Assist Reprod Genet. 2015;32:1025–30.

45. Montag M, Liebenthron J, Köster M. Which morphological scoring system is relevant in human embryo development? Placenta. 2011;32(Suppl 3):S252–6.
46. Armstrong S, Vail A, Mastenbroek S, Jordan V, Farquhar C. Time-lapse in the IVF-lab: how should we assess potential benefit? Hum Reprod. 2015;30:3–8.
47. Harper J, Magli MC, Lundin K, Barratt CL, Brison D. When and how should new technology be introduced into the IVF laboratory? Hum Reprod. 2012;27:303–13.
48. Kovacs P, Matyas SZ, Forgacs V, Sajgo A, Rarosi F, Pribenszky CS. Time-lapse embryo selection for single blastocyst transfer – results of a multicenter, prospective, randomized clinical trial (O-295). Fertil Steril. 2013;100(Suppl 3):S90.
49. Kahraman S, Cetinkaya M, Pirkevi C, Yelke H, Kumtepe Y. Comparison of blastocyst development and cycle outcome in patients with eSET using either conventional or time lapse incubators. A prospective study of good prognosis patients. J Reprod Stem Cell Biotechnol. 2012;3:55–61.
50. Armstrong S, Arroll N, Cree LM, Jordan V, Farquhar C. Time-lapse systems for embryo incubation and assessment in assisted reproduction. Cochrane Database Syst Rev. 2015;2:CD011320.
51. Goodman LR, Goldberg J, Falcone T, Austin C, Desai N. Does the addition of time-lapse morphokinetics in the selection of embryos for transfer improve pregnancy rates? A randomized controlled trial. Fertil Steril. 2016;105:275–85.
52. Wu Y-G, Lazzaroni-Tealdi E, Wang Q, Zhang L, Barad DH, Kushnir VA, et al. Different effectiveness of closed embryo culture system with time-lapse imaging (EmbryoScopeTM) in comparison to standard manual embryology in good and poor prognosis patients: a prospectively randomized pilot study. Reprod Biol Endocrinol. 2016;14:49.
53. Park H, Bergh C, Selleskog U, Thurin-Kjellberg A, Lundin K. No benefit of culturing embryos in a closed system compared with a conventional incubator in terms of number of good quality embryos: results from an RCT. Hum Reprod. 2015;30:268–75.
54. Matyas SZ, Kovacs P, Forgacs V, Sajgo A, Pribenszky CS. Selection of single blastocyst for transfer using time-lapse monitoring during in vitro fertilization in good prognosis patients: a randomized controlled trial. Hum Reprod. 2015;30(Suppl 1):i119.

Correction to: Textbook of Assisted Reproduction

Gautam Nand Allahbadia, Baris Ata, Steven R. Lindheim, Bryan J. Woodward, and Bala Bhagavath

Correction to:
G. N. Allahbadia et al. (eds.), *Textbook of Assisted Reproduction*, https://doi.org/10.1007/978-981-15-2377-9

The original version of the book has been revised with the following corrections in the book's front matter.

1. Affiliation of Dr. Baris Ata in the FM has been updated as
   Division of Reproductive Endocrinology and Infertility,
   Department of Obstetrics and Gynecology,
   Koç University School of Medicine,
   Istanbul, Turkey.
2. The below corrections are made in the list of contributors section in the front matter of the book.
   - Name of Dr. Alteri has been revised to Alessandra Alteri
   - Degree of Dr. Amy Barrie has been updated as PhD
   - Degree of Christophe Blockeels has been updated as PhD, MD
   - Degree of Ivor Cullen has been updated as Ivor Cullen, MD
   - Name and degree of Dr. Racheal Cutting, MB, has been changed as Rachel Cutting, MBE
   - Dr. Petra De Sutter, Department of Reproductive Medicine, Gent University Hospital, Gent, Belgium should read as Dr. Petra De Sutter, Department of Reproductive Medicine, Ghent University Hospital, Ghent, Belgium.
   - Dr. Chloë De Roo, MD, Department of Reproductive Medicine, Gent University Hospital, Ghent, Belgium should read as Dr. Chloë De Roo, MD, Department of Reproductive Medicine, Ghent University Hospital, Ghent, Belgium.
   - Dr. Sylvie Lierman, BSc, Department of Reproductive Medicine, Gent University Hospital, Ghent, Belgium should read as Dr. Sylvie Lierman, BSc, Department of Reproductive Medicine, Ghent University Hospital, Ghent, Belgium.
   - Dr. Kelly Tilleman, PhD, Department of Reproductive Medicine, Gent University Hospital, Gent, Belgium should read as Dr. Kelly Tilleman, PhD, Department of Reproductive Medicine, Ghent University Hospital, Gent, Belgium.
   - Degree of Dr. Sheryl Homa, MD, has been changed as Sheryl Homa, PhD
   - Name and degree of Dr. Eleanor Taylor T has been changed as Eleanor Taylor, PhD
3. In Chapter 42, the coauthor Racheal Cutting's name has been changed as Rachel Cutting.

The updated online version of this book can be found at
https://doi.org/10.1007/978-981-15-2377-9
https://doi.org/10.1007/978-981-15-2377-9_42

G. Allahbadia et al. (eds.), *Textbook of Assisted Reproduction*, https://doi.org/10.1007/978-981-15-2377-9_93

MIX
Papier aus verantwortungsvollen Quellen
Paper from responsible sources
FSC® C105338

If you have any concerns about our products,
you can contact us on
ProductSafety@springernature.com

In case Publisher is established outside the EU,
the EU authorized representative is:
Springer Nature Customer Service Center GmbH
Europaplatz 3, 69115 Heidelberg, Germany

Printed by Libri Plureos GmbH
in Hamburg, Germany